Obstetrics
and
Gynecology

Obstetrics and Gynecology

8th Edition

With 562 illustrations

ASSOCIATE EDITORS

William J. Ledger, M.D.

Given Foundation Professor of Obstetrics and
  Gynecology
Cornell University Medical College;
Obstetrician and Gynecologist in Chief
The New York Hospital
New York, New York

Russell K. Laros, Jr., M.D.

Professor and Vice-Chairman
Department of Obstetrics and Gynecology
University of California School of Medicine
San Francisco, California

John H. Mattox, M.D.

Chairman
Department of Obstetrics and Gynecology
Sisters of Charity Hospital;
Associate Clinical Professor
State University of New York at Buffalo
Buffalo, New York

J. Robert Willson, M.D.

Adjunct Professor
Department of Obstetrics and Gynecology
University of New Mexico School of
  Medicine
Albuquerque, New Mexico

Elsie Reid Carrington, M.D.

Adjunct Professor
Department of Obstetrics and Gynecology
University of New Mexico School of
  Medicine
Albuquerque, New Mexico

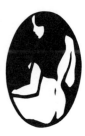

The C.V. Mosby Company

ST. LOUIS • WASHINGTON, D.C. • TORONTO   1987

MOSBY

A TRADITION OF PUBLISHING EXCELLENCE

Editor: Stephanie Bircher
Assistant Editor: Anne Gunter
Project Editor: Patricia Gayle May
Production Editor: Mary E. Drone
Book Design: Elizabeth K. Fett

8th Edition

The C.V. Mosby Company
11830 Westline Industrial Drive, St. Louis, Missouri 63146

Library of Congress Cataloging-in-Publication Data

Willson, J. Robert (James Robert), 1912-
    Obstetrics and gynecology.

    Includes bibliographies and index.
    1. Gynecology. 2. Obstetrics. I. Carrington,
Elsie Reid, 1912-   . II. Laros, Russell K.,
1936-   . III. Ledger, William J., 1932-   .
IV. Mattox, John H. V. Title. [DNLM: 1. Genital
Diseases, Female. 2. Obstetrics. WP 100 W742o]
RG101.W75 1987   618   87-1605
ISBN 0-8016-5650-9

GW/VH/VH 9 8 7 6 5 4 3 2 1   01/C/012

Contributors

ELSIE REID CARRINGTON, M.D.

Adjunct Professor
Department of Obstetrics and Gynecology
University of New Mexico School of Medicine
Albuquerque, New Mexico

MICHAEL J. DALY, M.D.

Professor and Chairman
Department of Obstetrics and Gynecology
Temple University School of Medicine
Philadelphia, Pennsylvania

KATHY HOTELLING, Ph.D.

Assistant Professor
Department of Psychiatry
Temple University School of Medicine
Philadelphia, Pennsylvania

REBECCA JACKSON, M.D.

Assistant Professor
Family, Community and Emergency Medicine
University of New Mexico School of Medicine
Albuquerque, New Mexico

RUSSELL K. LAROS, Jr., M.D.

Professor and Vice-Chairman
Department of Obstetrics and Gynecology
University of California, San Francisco
San Francisco, California

WILLIAM J. LEDGER, M.D.

Given Foundation Professor of Obstetrics and
 Gynecology
Cornell University Medical College;
Obstetrician and Gynecologist in Chief
The New York Hospital
New York, New York

JOHN H. MATTOX, M.D.

Chairman
Department of Obstetrics and Gynecology
Sisters of Charity Hospital;
Associate Clinical Professor
State University of New York at Buffalo
Buffalo, New York

KATE MOFFIT MUSELLO, M.D.

Attending Obstetrician/Gynecologist
Lower Shore Obstetrics and Gynecologic Center
Princess Anne, Maryland

J. ROBERT WILLSON, M.D.

Adjunct Professor
Department of Obstetrics and Gynecology
University of New Mexico School of Medicine
Albuquerque, New Mexico

Preface

The eighth edition of *Obstetrics and Gynecology,* as were those preceding it, was prepared specifically for students rather than for practicing obstetrician-gynecologists. The term "student" has a broad connotation. It encompasses medical students, house officers, and practicing physicians, as well as nurse-midwives, nurse-practitioners, and others who provide health care for women. Our concentration on normal reproductive physiology and on the anatomic, pathologic, and functional changes that may disrupt the reproductive processes makes *Obstetrics and Gynecology* an appropriate text for medical students, obstetric-gynecologic residents, and others who are learning the basic principles of the specialty. It should also be helpful to those in other disciplines, particularly internists and family physicians. The diagnostic and therapeutic methods that are discussed can be carried out in ambulatory settings or in the hospital, and extensive experience in the field of obstetrics-gynecology is not necessary for most of them.

We have deliberately omitted descriptions of operative technics, except those such as episiotomy and low forceps delivery that are performed by physicians who are not necessarily experienced obstetrician-gynecologists. We have not included complicated therapeutic regimens such as chemotherapy for ovarian cancer. These require experience and expertise beyond those of the average obstetrician-gynecologist and are more appropriately considered in specialized publications. However, we have retained the concept of dividing the material into that which we consider to be basic information with which every physician who treats women should be familiar and that which is more advanced. The latter, set in small type, together with comprehensive references, are readily available to those who want to acquire more than a basic understanding of female reproductive disorders. Whenever possible we have included review articles that not only cover individual subjects thoroughly but contain extensive references.

Each chapter has been revised extensively, and several have been almost completely rewritten. Outmoded diagnostic and therapeutic procedures have been replaced with those that are more accurate and effective. The material has also been rearranged, and chapters have been combined to present the information in more logical sequence. For example, Sexual Responses of Women is now a chapter in its own right; Dysmenorrhea and the Premenstrual Syndrome are also presented separately. The chapters on benign and malignant cervical diseases have been combined, as have those on benign and malignant uterine diseases. A new chapter, Sexual Assault, prepared by Doctors Kate Moffit Musello and Rebecca Jackson, has been added.

Several new contributers, each selected because of special interest and expertise in specific areas, have been added. Dr. John H. Mattox is now responsible for the chapters on normal and abnormal menstruation, endometriosis, abortion, and infertility. Dr. Russell K. Laros, Jr. has revised the chapters on fertilization, placental and fetal development, the physiology and some of the disorders of pregnancy, and the care of the infant. Dr. Kathy Hotelling has joined Dr. M.J. Daly in revising the chapters on psychology, sexual responses, dysmenorrhea, and the premenstrual syndrome. Dr. William J. Ledger's contributions have been expanded to include infectious diseases and genital tract disorders during pregnancy and vaginal diseases, in addition to obstetric-gynecologic infections and normal and abnormal labor.

We hope that the improvements and additions to this edition of *Obstetrics and Gynecology* will enhance its value both as a textbook and as a reference for those who are responsible for providing obstetric and gynecologic care.

J. Robert Willson
Elsie Reid Carrington

Contents

1 Introduction, 1
J. ROBERT WILLSON

2 Diagnostic methods in obstetrics and gynecology, 13
J. ROBERT WILLSON

3 Pediatric gynecology, 36
ELSIE REID CARRINGTON

4 Psychology and life stages of women, 52
MICHAEL J. DALY AND KATHY HOTELLING

5 Sexual responses of women, 61
MICHAEL J. DALY AND KATHY HOTELLING

6 Sexual assault, 70
KATE MOFFIT MUSELLO AND REBECCA JACKSON

7 Normal menstruation, 76
JOHN H. MATTOX

8 Abnormal uterine bleeding, 88
JOHN H. MATTOX

9 Amenorrhea, 97
JOHN H. MATTOX

10 Dysmenorrhea and the premenstrual syndrome, 115
MICHAEL J. DALY AND KATHY HOTELLING

11 Endometriosis, 122
JOHN H. MATTOX

12 The breast, 133
ELSIE REID CARRINGTON

13 Fertilization; development, physiology, and disorders of the placenta; fetal development, 142

RUSSELL K. LAROS, Jr.

14 Infertility, 177

JOHN H. MATTOX

15 Family planning, 192

J. ROBERT WILLSON

16 Abortion, 210

JOHN H. MATTOX

17 Ectopic pregnancy, 225

J. ROBERT WILLSON

18 Gestational trophoblastic neoplasms, 239

J. ROBERT WILLSON

19 Physiology of normal pregnancy, 251

RUSSELL K. LAROS, Jr.

20 Diagnosis and duration of pregnancy and prenatal care, 273

J. ROBERT WILLSON

21 Infectious diseases during pregnancy, 293

WILLIAM J. LEDGER

22 Endocrine disorders during pregnancy, 298

RUSSELL K. LAROS, Jr.

23 Diseases of the respiratory system, the circulatory system, and the blood during pregnancy, 313

RUSSELL K. LAROS, Jr.

24 Digestive tract disorders during pregnancy, 326

J. ROBERT WILLSON

25 Urinary tract disorders during pregnancy, 335

J. ROBERT WILLSON

26 Genital tract disorders during pregnancy, 343

WILLIAM J. LEDGER

27 Disorders of the nervous system, the skin, and the bones and joints during pregnancy, 356

ELSIE REID CARRINGTON

28 Hypertensive disorders during pregnancy, 364
RUSSELL K. LAROS, Jr.

29 Bleeding during late pregnancy, 380
J. ROBERT WILLSON

30 Determination of position and lie, 393
J. ROBERT WILLSON

31 Labor and delivery, 400
WILLIAM J. LEDGER

32 Obstetric analgesia and anesthesia, 434
J. ROBERT WILLSON

33 Third stage of labor and postpartum hemorrhage, 444
J. ROBERT WILLSON

34 Care of the infant during pregnancy and labor and after delivery, 456
RUSSELL K. LAROS, Jr.

35 Dystocia and prolonged labor, 474
WILLIAM J. LEDGER

36 Pelvimetry; dystocia from contracted pelvis, 494
WILLIAM J. LEDGER

37 Multifetal pregnancy, 507
J. ROBERT WILLSON

38 Breech delivery, 517
J. ROBERT WILLSON

39 Forceps delivery, 533
J. ROBERT WILLSON

40 Cesarean section, 541
J. ROBERT WILLSON

41 Immediate and remote effects of childbirth injury; uterine retroplacement, 548
J. ROBERT WILLSON

42 Obstetric and gynecologic infections, 577
WILLIAM J. LEDGER

43 The puerperium, 598
J. ROBERT WILLSON

44 Diseases of the vulva, 608
J. ROBERT WILLSON

45 Diseases of the vagina, 621
WILLIAM J. LEDGER

46 Benign and malignant diseases of the cervix, 627
J. ROBERT WILLSON

47 Benign and malignant diseases of the uterus, 649
J. ROBERT WILLSON

48 Ovarian neoplasms, 666
J. ROBERT WILLSON

49 Aging, 680
J. ROBERT WILLSON

Obstetrics
and
Gynecology

1

J. Robert Willson

Introduction

It might appear that physicians who confine their professional activities to the treatment of pregnant women (obstetrics) and patients with dysfunctioning genital organs (gynecology) are limiting their practice rather severely. On the contrary, obstetricians and gynecologists must be familiar with many fields of medicine because their patients vary in age from those newly born to senescent women. It is possible for women with medical conditions such as hypertension, tuberculosis, rheumatic heart disease, diabetes, multiple sclerosis, and a host of others to conceive; and all manner of acute medical and surgical conditions may develop during pregnancy.

Gynecologists must be pediatricians, internists, endocrinologists, and surgeons, since they treat females of all ages and often are the first persons consulted because of symptoms that arise in structures other than the genital organs. They must also be familiar with the basic principles of psychiatry and be able to recognize the emotional problems that so frequently manifest themselves in sexual disorders.

The American Board of Obstetrics and Gynecology was organized in 1930, training facilities for obstetrician-gynecologists were expanded, and women began to consult specialists rather than family physicians who had previously provided most obstetric care. At present about 80% of deliveries in the United States are performed by obstetrician-gynecologists in practice or in training.

In the past, family physicians treated women with gynecologic problems, and general surgeons performed most gynecologic operations. The obstetrician-gynecologist has gradually assumed responsibility for much gynecologic care. Obstetrician-gynecologists introduced the concept of periodic health examinations on a large scale. These examinations were directed toward the discovery of asymptomatic pelvic disease. More and more women are coming to obstetrician-gynecologists at regular intervals for such examinations.

Obstetrician-gynecologists often provide considerable amounts of general medical care for their own patients. A survey of Fellows of the American College of Obstetricians and Gynecologists indicates that 57% of those responding serve as principal providers of medical care for at least half of their patients, and 36% serve as providers for more than half. This is not surprising, since an obstetrician-gynecologist often has provided care for an individual patient before her marriage, during pregnancies, and at regular periodic examinations after childbearing is completed.

Unfortunately, physicians cannot respond adequately to the steadily increasing demands for obstetric-gynecologic care. In fact, they cannot even cope with all serious problems. For example, in

1986 about 6800 women died with cancer of the cervix, a disease that can be diagnosed so early that it can be eradicated almost without exception. The deaths occurred because these women were not screened for early cellular changes. An additional 2900 died of other malignant uterine tumors; most of them might have been treated successfully had they consulted their doctors early. In the same year, 39,900 women died of breast cancer, another malignancy that can be diagnosed in its earliest stages by effective techniques that are not yet readily available to all women.

Unfortunately, lung cancer, a preventable disease, is increasing in women. In 1986 about 41,000 women died of this disease, an increase from about 36,000 in 1984. Lung cancer has surpassed breast cancer as a cause of death in women.

In 1981 there were 336 maternal deaths, most of them preventable; 30,618 neonatal deaths; and 21,012 fetal deaths, many of these also preventable. There are vast unmet needs in general nutrition and health care and in health education, notably in sex and family living.

In most countries throughout the world the management of normal pregnancy, labor, and delivery is the responsibility of midwives. The traditional midwife in more primitive societies rarely has training other than that as an apprentice to an untrained mentor, and her practice is uncontrolled. In more advanced countries, midwives must meet stringent educational requirements, and the limitations of their practice are established in specific government regulations.

The outcome of obstetric care provided by midwives is determined by their training and skill, by the availability of physician consultants and of facilities to which women with complications can be referred, and by the regulations governing practice and consultation. Both maternal and perinatal mortalities are high in underdeveloped countries where untrained midwives have no supporting facilities and the general level of health is low. In contrast, maternal and perinatal mortalities are among the lowest in the world in countries such as the Netherlands and the United Kingdom where midwives,

who are responsible for much of the obstetric care in normal cases, are well trained and work closely with obstetrician-gynecologist consultants.

Obstetric-gynecologic care can be improved and made more acceptable to women of any economic or social class through the development of *health care teams* composed of obstetrician-gynecologists, nurse-midwives, obstetric-gynecologic nurse practitioners, and specially trained aides. Each can be made responsible for the area of care that is appropriate on the basis of training and ability. For example, the nurse-midwife can provide much of the prenatal care and education for *all* pregnant women and delivery and care after delivery for those in whom normal deliveries are anticipated. Nurse-midwives or trained obstetric-gynecologic nurses can provide contraceptive counseling, perform periodic health examinations on well women, diagnose and treat minor gynecologic conditions such as vaginitis, and be responsible for a comprehensive health education program. With such capable associates, physicians could concentrate on women with high-risk pregnancies and with gynecologic problems that require their special skills; they would serve as immediately available consultants to associates working in their offices and be responsible for women who require special care during labor and delivery and for gynecologic operations.

Such teams can extend care into areas where there are no physicians, with nonphysician workers serving as screening and triage agents who refer women needing special care to an appropriate physician. It is essential that such a system be organized to deliver medical care to women of all socioeconomic classes. The model is not one that is appropriate only for poor women.

FACILITIES FOR OBSTETRIC CARE

Most births occur in hospitals, but more and more women are requesting out-of-hospital confinement. In 1981 approximately 99% of all births occurred in hospitals, 96.5% of deliveries were by physicians, 1.5% by midwives, and 1.2% by others. The remaining births occurred out of hospitals; 0.3% by physicians, 0.4% by midwives, and 0.4% by others.

HOSPITAL OBSTETRIC SERVICES

The remarkable decreases in maternal and perinatal mortality and morbidity were achieved not only by increasing the number of skilled obstetrician-gynecologists but by simultaneously improving hospital obstetric services that in the past had been unorganized and in which obstetric practice was unregulated. In most hospitals any physician with staff privileges was allowed to perform deliveries and even to perform obstetric operations without regard to training and ability. Most hospital obstetric services are now organized; staff privileges are awarded on the basis of competence, and hospitals make available essential services and equipment designed to make labor and delivery safe.

A national survey of maternity care by the American College of Obstetricians and Gynecologists pointed out several important inadequacies in hospitals in which women are delivered. As a general rule the facilities provided by hospitals in which fewer than 2000 women are delivered yearly are less adequate than those with larger services. Constant 24-hour coverage of the labor-delivery area was provided by registered nurses in almost all large services but in only 40% of hospitals with less than 250 deliveries each year. In 93% of hospitals with large services, emergency cesarean section could be performed in less than 40 minutes; this was possible in only 63% of hospitals with small services. In addition, intensive newborn care by experienced pediatricians was more readily available in larger hospitals.

Hospital-related maternal deaths in Michigan indicate the importance of these findings.* From 1966 to 1971 there were 973,252 live births after 20 or more completed weeks of gestation in hospitals and 154 maternal deaths, a rate of 1.58/ 10,000 live births. The maternal death rate varied

*From Rice, Gerald, Chief Bureau of Maternal and Child Health, Michigan Health Department: Personal communication.

according to the size of the hospital obstetric service as follows:

Annual live births in hospital	Maternal mortality
1-100	4.24
101-500	1.86
501-1000	1.52
1001-2000	1.70
2001 plus	1.35

Each maternal death was studied, responsibility was assigned, and avoidable factors were indicated by the members of the Michigan Maternal Mortality Subcommittee of the Committee on Maternal and Perinatal Health. The maternal death rates associated with avoidable factors were higher in small hospitals than in larger ones as follows:

Annual live births in hospital	Maternal mortality with avoidable factors
1-100	2.83
101-500	1.72
501-1000	1.14
1001-2000	1.29
2001 plus	0.96

In recent years these figures have changed. Perinatal centers, which have the facilities and personnel to manage the most complicated pregnancies, have been developed. More and more physicians, both family practitioners and obstetrician-gynecologists, are using such centers, and the end result is an improved outcome for both mothers and their infants.

An example of the change is indicated in a report of the outcome of obstetric care in Iowa hospitals of several levels of sophistication. Level Ia maternity units, in which fewer than 500 deliveries are conducted each year, are staffed by family physicians. Obstetrician(s) and pediatrician(s) staff level Ib institutions. All level I hospitals are designed to serve only low-risk obstetric patients and healthy newborn infants. Level II maternity units serve patients at moderate risk, and intensive obstetric and perinatal care is available in level III hospitals. Although 37% of deliveries are now conducted in level I units, the percentage of neonatal deaths in these hospitals has declined substantially. Neonatal mortality rates were 2.7/1000 live births in level Ia hospitals, 4.6 in level Ib hospitals, 5.5 in level II hospitals, and 17.6 in level III hospitals. More and more mothers with complications are being transferred to hospitals that are better equipped to manage the problems. Transfers can be made during pregnancy when a condition such as diabetes or hypertension is recognized or during labor when the need for a higher level of care becomes necessary.

ALTERNATIVE BIRTH CENTERS

The increasing use of technologic innovations during normal labor has led many women to seek less complicated alternative methods of obstetric care. They reason that a completely normal pregnancy and delivery can be managed successfully by a qualified nurse-midwife, without interference and without mechanical monitoring equipment. Some even contend that delivery at home is safer than delivery in a hospital. The former concept is correct; the latter is not.

Alternative birth centers have been developed in an attempt to avoid the use of scientifically oriented hospital labor-delivery areas, while providing many safeguards that cannot be made available during delivery at home. Such centers are specifically designed for women whose pregnancies have been uncomplicated and for whom normal labor and delivery is anticipated. Most centers are located in or near hospital labor-delivery areas, but some have no direct physical connection with a hospital. The centers are alike in that the atmosphere is more like that of a home than a hospital. The patients labor and deliver in a comfortable bed where they remain with the newborn infant until they are discharged, usually within a few hours. Their families can be with them. The centers are staffed by personnel who are both well trained and experienced in providing care during labor and who support the concept of helping the perfectly normal pregnant woman have her baby as naturally as possible. The labor can be managed by nurse-midwives or physicians, and either can conduct the delivery.

Hospital-based centers are usually located near or within the regular labor-delivery area, which permits prompt consultation with a physician whenever it is necessary and immediate transfer when a complication arises. Freestanding centers have agreements with nearby hospitals that permit the immediate transfer of patients when a complication develops. They also are prepared to provide emergency care during transfer. Such precautions are essential because from 15% to 25% of carefully screened patients develop complications during labor or after delivery that require more sophisticated care than can be provided in an alternative birth center.

Many of the problems that arise during labor can be anticipated and prevented by careful patient selection. Only women in whom a completely normal pregnancy, labor, and delivery is anticipated should be selected for care at a center. Some of these will be transferred during pregnancy, for example, when the membranes rupture prematurely, if an abnormal position is diagnosed, if hypertension is recognized, if bleeding occurs, or if labor begins prematurely. The most common reasons for transfer during labor are failure to progress, abnormal fetal position, and fetal distress.

The progress of labor is followed by physical assessment of the quality of the contractions, cervical dilatation, and descent of the presenting part. The fetal heart is monitored by frequent auscultation. Spontaneous delivery is supervised by the nurse-midwife or physician.

The results of delivery in alternative birth centers in which patients are properly screened, in which meticulous care is provided during labor and delivery, and from which patients with complications are transferred to hospitals promptly are excellent.

A comparison of 250 patients who delivered in the Birth Center of Jackson and who were carefully matched with 250 who were delivered in the Jackson Memorial Hospital, a level III unit, indicates significant differences. Of Birth Center patients, 21% were transferred during labor because they required hospital care, but the outcomes were analyzed with the other Birth Center patients. Intravenous fluids were administered to all hospital patients, but to only 28% of Birth Center patients; 14% of hospital patients and 6% of Birth Center patients were delivered by cesarean section, and labor was augmented twice as often in hospital patients. Birth Center babies weighed more, and there was one instance of shoulder dystocia; but Apgar scores were similar.

Since the cost of obstetric care for women with normal pregnancies in birth centers is about half that for hospital delivery, it seems likely that more women will seek care in low-risk units.

HOME DELIVERY

Conversely, home delivery is far from safe. Neither the necessary safety support nor an adequate number of competent attendants is available, and transfer to a hospital when a complication arises is usually delayed. Few trained midwives or physicians will agree to perform deliveries in the home. This has led to the appearance of untrained birth attendants who are willing to do so. In many instances their only qualifications are that they have had children themselves or that they have assisted others in having babies. As might be anticipated, the results can be disastrous. In the states that maintain statistics concerning outcome of delivery, perinatal mortality is from two to five times higher in home than in hospital delivery.

The outcome, however, is influenced by prenatal selection of patients and by the experience of the attendant. Burnett and associates reported the following perinatal mortalities for home deliveries in North Carolina: (1) planned home delivery, patients screened in a health department clinic and delivered by a physician or an approved lay-midwife: 4/1000 live births; (2) planned home deliveries if the attendant was neither a physician nor an approved lay-midwife: 30/1000 live births, and (3) unplanned home delivery (usually precipitous): 120/1000 live births.

If one compares the result of delivery at home and in an alternative birth center, the only logical conclusion is that the risks of home delivery are usually too great to assume.

BIRTHRATES

The *birthrate,* the number of live births per 1000 population, varies from year to year, depending on a multitude of factors. The rate fell progressively from 30 in 1910 to 18.4 in 1933. It is interesting that this low rate was attained before the present sophisticated contraceptive methods were available and undoubtedly represents a calculated mass decision to prevent pregnancy because of the severe financial depression.

Most couples were forced to delay starting their families because of World II, but the birthrate started upward in 1940 and rose steeply after 1945, reaching a peak of 26.6 in 1947. It was 25 with 4,254,784 births in 1957 and 23.3 with 4,268,326 births in 1961. The birthrate continued to fall, reaching 17.8 with 3,520,959 births in 1967.

An increase in the number of births was anticipated in 1969 because of the large number of young people who were born during the "baby boom" of the 1940s. The number of women between the ages of 15 and 45 years increased from 42,336,000 in 1970 to about 56,000,000 in 1985. However, the anticipated increase in births did not occur. By 1975 the birthrate had decreased to 14.8 with 3,144,198 births. In recent years both total births and birthrates have increased slightly, but the birthrate appears to have stabilized. In 1979 the birthrate was 15.9, and 3,494,398 live births were registered. Comparable figures for 1981 were 15.8 and 3,629,238.

The predicted vast increase in the number of births was based on continuing high birthrates rather than on the present low ones, which were not expected. Once again the young people of the country have made considered decisions to limit family size. In contrast to the 1930s, however, reliable methods for preventing pregnancy are readily available, and abortions can be obtained legally if contraception fails. There is no certain way of predicting the reproductive rates for the future, but some increase in the *number* of births is inevitable. Even though birthrates remain low, an increasing number of women will enter the childbearing years. In addition, the birthrate may rise because women who have postponed pregnancy and are now in their late twenties and early thirties will become pregnant and because a slight increase in family size may again become popular.

The *fertility rate,* the births per 1000 women between the ages of 15 and 45 years, is a better indication of reproductive patterns than the birthrate. The fertility rate in the United States rose from 75.8 in 1936 to 122.9 in 1957. It fell to 87.2 in 1967 and to 67.8 in 1977. In 1981 the fertility rate was 67.4.

Even the fertility rate does not provide complete information concerning pregnancy because it does not include spontaneous and induced abortions. In 1979, 1,238,987 legal abortions, 358/1000 live births, were reported in the United States.

OUT-OF-WEDLOCK PREGNANCIES

Both the number and ratio (number of births per 1000 unmarried women) of births to unmarried women are increasing. In 1950 there were 141,600 (ratio 39.8); in 1960, 224,300 (ratio 52.7); in 1970, 398,700 (ratio 106.9); and in 1977, 515,700 (ratio 155). The numbers continue to increase. In 1981 686,605 unmarried women bore children (ratio 189.2). Of these, 377,050 were white (ratio 115.9), and 328,879 were black (ratio 559.5). Following are the number and ratios of illegitimate births in 1981 by age of the mother:

Age	Number	Ratio	
		White	Black
<15	8,589	763.2	988.2
15-19	259,239	348.6	861.8
20-24	246,919	124.0	574.2
25-29	109,174	55.6	379.0
30-34	43,300	47.5	303.9
35-39	14,281	66.5	295.1
40 plus	3,103	89.8	306.4

The reported births represent only a small fraction of total out-of-wedlock conceptions. Estimates based on correlating the wedding date with the date the first child is born indicate that more than 50% of women of all ages are already pregnant at the time of their marriage. In addition, many births to unmarried women are not reported as such.

TEENAGE PREGNANCY

An out-of-wedlock pregnancy is a problem at any age, but it may be disastrous to a teenager.

Before legal abortion became available, the alternatives were to marry or to remain pregnant, usually giving the baby up for adoption. Neither alternative was a satisfactory solution in most instances. Teenage marriages, particularly those forced by pregnancies, are notoriously unsuccessful, and the alternative of remaining pregnant is inadequate for most girls. Whatever the choice, the result was disrupted education, which too often was not resumed; broken marriages; and often repeated out-of-wedlock pregnancies.

Unfortunately, the availability of effective contraceptive methods has made no remarkable change in the number of teenagers who conceive. The principal difference has been in the number of births. The conception rate of women ages 12 to 19 was 53.8 in 1976; in 1978 it increased to 56.9. In 1976, 570,672 teenagers were delivered, whereas the pregnancies of 314,217 were terminated by abortion. Comparable figures for 1978 were 554,179 deliveries and 357,028 abortions.

Fetal, neonatal, and postneonatal death rates are higher in teenage pregnancies than in those of mature married women. The fetal death ratios for various age groups of pregnancies in married and unmarried women are listed in Table 1-1. The curves for neonatal and postneonatal deaths demonstrate a similar disadvantage for young girls. The highest mortalities occur in girls of the lowest socioeconomic groups, those who have had the least education, and those who have had more than one baby before they reach the age of 20 years.

The solution is far more complex than a simplistic approach of making contraceptives available to all girls entering their teens. Most young girls have little accurate and useful information concerning reproduction and, in many communities, no way of learning more. Parents are likely to avoid sexual discussions; and either there are no effective sex education courses in schools, or they do not include instruction in contraception. Some girls may be forced into premature sexual activity by the pressure of their peers; others are seeking love and attention, which they think they can get in no other way. Some have unprotected coitus because they know little about contraception and counseling

TABLE 1-1 Fetal death ratios (1980)

Age	Total deaths	Legitimate White	Legitimate Black	Illegitimate White	Illegitimate Black
<15	147	33.6	20	17.8	20
15-19	3784	9.2	14.8	10.4	13.9
20-24	6721	7.5	12.6	11	13.7
25-29	5549	7.1	12.8	12.9	15.9
30-34	3160	8.4	14.5	17.8	19.6
35-39	1249	13.6	20.5	22	27.9
40 plus	402	25.9	36.6	29.8	44.3

TABLE 1-2 Percentages of live births by months since last birth (1981)

Months	<15 White	<15 Black	15-19 White	15-19 Black	20-24 White	20-24 Black	25-29 White	25-29 Black
1-11	1.47	17.1	6.1	6.4	2.1	2.4	0.8	1.0
12-17	44.1	46.9	31.7	31.5	16.2	16.5	8.4	8.9
18-23	20.6	16.6	24.9	24.2	19.4	18.6	14.3	13.8
24-35	—	—	24.4	24.2	28.3	27.0	26.9	25.2
36-47	—	—	7.6	8.1	15.7	15.5	17.3	16.5

is not available to them. Others fail to use contraceptives because of an unconscious wish to become pregnant to fill an emotional need. Pregnancy in more mature unmarried women often is a result of carelessness in the use of contraception.

The obvious solution, and it will not come soon, is basic and effective sex education at home and in schools, opportunities to discuss personal problems of sex and reproduction with understanding parents and counselors, and readily available contraception for those who are sexually active.

Counseling also is important for teenage girls who already have conceived. The initial decision is between abortion and remaining pregnant. Those who choose the latter must be permitted to continue their education. They, as well as those who select abortion, need continuing counseling and the best medical care.

An important objective in counseling is to provide the patient with an understanding of why she became pregnant and to help her develop the motivation to prevent a recurrence. Without such motivation, as many as 50% of teenagers will be pregnant within a year after delivery. Comparative figures of months between births are displayed in Table 1-2. It is obvious that teenagers are more likely to conceive soon after a pregnancy than are more mature women.

MATERNAL MORTALITY

A *maternal death* is the death of any woman from any cause during pregnancy or within 42 days of the termination of pregnancy, irrespective of the duration of pregnancy or its site. A *direct obstetric death* is one resulting from a complication of pregnancy itself—from intervention, from omissions of or incorrect treatment, or from a chain of events resulting from any of the preceding. An example is a death from postpartum hemorrhage. An *indirect obstetric death* is one resulting from a disease that had existed previously or that developed during pregnancy, but the course of which was aggravated by the physiologic effects of pregnancy. An example is serious rheumatic heart disease with decompensation during the period of maximum cardiac stress. A *nonobstetric death* is one resulting from an incidental cause unrelated to pregnancy. An example of a nonobstetric death is one resulting from injuries sustained in an automobile accident or death from a brain tumor.

The *maternal mortality* is the number of maternal deaths from direct causes per 100,000 live births as indicated in the following equation:

$$\frac{\text{Number of direct maternal deaths}}{\text{Total live births}} \times 100{,}000 = \text{Maternal mortality}$$

Maternal death rates vary considerably in different parts of the country and with different classes of patients. The mortality is higher in nonwhite patients than in either white nonprivate or white private patients. This undoubtedly occurs because the nonwhite patients include the most impoverished and least well-educated people in the United States. There is a higher incidence of medical complications such as essential hypertension, anemia, malnutrition, and preeclampsia-eclampsia among this group of patients, and these conditions often remain untreated. The patients frequently do not seek prenatal care, entering the hospital only after labor has begun; if they do register in clinics, they often appear late in pregnancy, attend irregularly, and cannot afford adequate diets and medications. The death rate is highest in urban communities and in the southeastern states, where the concentration of nonwhite patients and those of low economic status is greatest. Maternal mortality is lowest in the Northwest, parts of New England, and the upper Midwest, where the population is more homogeneous with fewer blacks and less poverty and malnutrition. Reduction in maternal mortality therefore must be a concern of educators, sociologists, and economists, as well as physicians.

The maternal mortality in 1930 was more than 600/100,000 live births. The rate has fallen steadily to a level of 9.2 in 1981. The causes of the 336 maternal deaths in 1981 are listed in Table 1-3.

Tabulations of causes of maternal mortality do not reflect the overlap of all responsible contributing factors, since they include only the primary cause listed on the death certificate. For example, most deaths listed as "abortion" are caused by infection; and many women who die of puerperal sepsis also had hemorrhage following delivery, which may represent a major factor in their deaths. In addition, indirect and nonobstetric deaths may be listed under specific causes such as heart disease and do not appear as deaths of pregnant or recently delivered women.

The reduced maternal death rate is a result of many factors, which include an increase in hospital deliveries, the development of perinatal centers, the availability of blood, and the ability to treat infection effectively. In addition, there are many more highly trained and skillful obstetricians in all parts of the United States with whom general practitioners can consult when a complication develops. Most hospital staffs are organized and have estab-

TABLE 1-3 Causes of maternal deaths (1982)

Cause	Total number
Puerperal complications	93
Toxemia	60
Ectopic pregnancy	48
Hemorrhage	44
Abortion	16
Other direct causes	64
Indirect causes	11

lished rules by which obstetric practice in the institution is governed. Those without special training and experience are required to seek consultation for serious complications and for abnormalities of labor. This is in contrast to the previous situation, when any staff member, regardless of ability, was permitted to perform any type of operative procedure or manage any complication without seeking help.

An important factor in the reduction of maternal mortality was the development of state and local Maternal Mortality Review Committees in the early 1930s. The complete care of each pregnant woman who dies is reviewed by a committee of obstetrician-gynecologists who determine the cause and assign responsibility for the death to the primary physician, the consultant, the patient, the institution, or the community. The principal reason for these committees is physician education, and the result has been a dramatic reduction in maternal mortality. Maternal Mortality Review Committees represent the first organized peer review system to be developed in the United States.

Maternal mortality can be reduced even further. It should be possible at least to eliminate deaths from hemorrhage and infection, both of which can be prevented or treated if they occur. Deaths from abortion can be eliminated or reduced to a minimum by making reliable contraceptive methods and legal abortion available to everyone who wants them. There may be an irreducible minimum of obstetric deaths, but it can only be reached if every physician concentrates on preventing or detecting and correcting potentially lethal abnormalities and if the facilities in which pregnant women are treated are optimal.

PERINATAL MORTALITY (Fig. 1-1)

A *fetal death* is the death before or during birth of a fetus weighing 500 g or more. No heartbeat, cord pulsation, respiratory activity, or movement of voluntary muscle can be detected after birth. If the weight is unknown, fetal death is diagnosed if the pregnancy duration is of 20 completed weeks or more as measured from the first day of the last normal menstrual period.

A *liveborn infant* is one in which signs of life, including breathing, cord pulsation, heartbeat, or voluntary muscle movement, can be detected after its complete expulsion from the vagina. A *neonatal death* is the death within the first 28 days of life of a liveborn infant weighing at least 500 g or after 20 completed weeks of pregnancy. A *hebdomadal death* is the death within the first 7 days of life of a liveborn infant weighing 500 g or more.

The term *perinatal death* is an inclusive one, indicating the death of a fetus weighing 500 g or more before or during labor and of a liveborn infant within the first 28 days of life.

The *fetal mortality* is the number of fetal deaths per 1000 births of liveborn *and* dead-born infants. The *neonatal mortality* is the number of deaths per

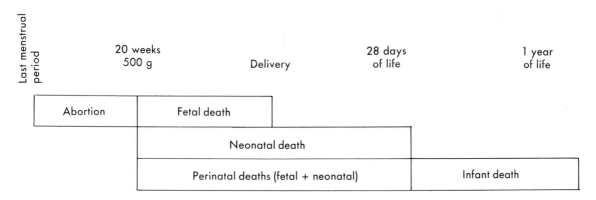

Fig. 1-1. Abortion, perinatal, and infant mortality.

1000 births of *liveborn* infants. The *perinatal mortality* is the number of fetal plus the number of neonatal deaths per 1000 births of live and dead infants. *Infant mortality* includes deaths that occur between the twenty-eighth day and the end of the first year of life.

Most states require that the deaths of all infants born after 20 or more weeks of pregnancy be reported; in some states it is necessary to report deaths from pregnancies of less than 20 weeks' duration.

Perinatal mortalities based on births of all infants weighing more than 500 g include many who are too immature to survive, even under the most advantageous conditions. A more realistic method is to base the calculation on births of infants who are likely to live if they are born in good condition and if facilities for intensive neonatal care are available. These are infants who weigh more than 800 g or those with gestation periods of at least 27 weeks. This does not mean, of course, that the large number of deaths of smaller infants can be ignored, because spontaneous abortions and immature births constitute one of the most important causes of infant loss.

There are many reasons for perinatal deaths; some deaths, such as those associated with hypertension and other acute and chronic diseases in the mother, complications of labor, infections, and birth injuries, can often be prevented. Those caused by congenital malformation, cord entanglement, and certain disorders of placental function cannot yet be controlled. The latter, however, are in the minority.

If a postmortem examination is performed on every infant who dies and if attending obstetricians will review the management of the pregnancy and delivery, they may find an obvious cause for the death of the baby. The application of this information to similar situations in the future may help prevent other deaths. Most hospitals hold regular mortality conferences in which obstetricians, pediatricians, and pathologists participate; interested individual physicians can accomplish the same things by reviewing the deaths of their own patients.

Fetal deaths. The World Health Organization has recommended the term *fetal death* to replace the older terms, *stillbirth* and *abortion*. Fetal deaths are classified as follows:

Group I: Early fetal deaths—less than 20 completed weeks of pregnancy
Group II: Intermediate fetal deaths—20 through 27 completed weeks of pregnancy
Group III: Late fetal deaths—28 or more completed weeks of pregnancy
Group IV: Unclassified

In 1980 there were 33,353 fetal deaths of 20 weeks or more. The *fetal mortality ratio* was 9.2/1000 births.

The total number of fetal deaths cannot be determined accurately because most states do not require the reporting of deaths from pregnancies of less than 20 weeks' duration; 10% to 15% or more of all pregnancies terminate in spontaneous abortion.

The most common causes of fetal deaths are *anoxia* (many of these deaths are associated with abruptio placentae, placenta previa, hypertension, maternal diabetes, prolapsed cord, and abnormal labor), *congenital anomalies,* and *infection.* In one third to one half of fetal deaths no cause can be determined, even though an autopsy is performed.

Neonatal deaths. In 1980, 30,618 liveborn infants died during the first 28 days after birth. The *neonatal mortality rate* was 8.5.

The reduction in the number of neonatal deaths has been less spectacular than that of maternal deaths. The neonatal mortality fell from 39.7 between 1920 and 1924 to 28.8 in 1940, to 20 in 1951, and to 10.9 in 1976.

Since most perinatal deaths occur in low-birth-weight infants, there are two possible causes for the relatively rapid improvement in recent years: a lower incidence of prematurity and improved care for small infants. The latter is the more likely cause. The delivery of infants weighing between 1000 and 1500 g decreased at a rate of about 1.7%/yr in white women and about 9.0%/yr in black women during the 1970s. Births of infants weighing less than 1000 g changed even less: a decrease of about 0.6%/yr occurred in white women, but the number delivered in black women actually increased at a rate of about 0.4%/yr.

Clearly, the principal reason for the improvement is that more women with pregnancy complications are now being treated in perinatal centers where specially trained teams provide intensive care both for mothers during pregnancy and labor and for their newborn infants.

Neonatal deaths in 1980 resulted primarily from the causes listed in Table 1-4.

Prevention of neonatal mortality. Approximately half of all neonatal deaths occur in premature infants who are unable to cope with the hazards of an independent existence. The most obvious way to reduce neonatal mortality therefore is to reduce the premature delivery rate. Although it is possible to accomplish this in certain patients, our understanding of many of the causes of premature labor is as yet incomplete, and we cannot always prevent it.

Most neonatal deaths occur with *high-risk pregnancies;* therefore it is essential that women with conditions associated with increased perinatal mortality be given special attention during pregnancy and labor. The principal problems of delivery are breech and other malpresentations, prolapsed cord, placenta previa, and abruptio placentae. *High-risk pregnancies are best managed in perinatal centers.*

Illegitimate pregnancies and pregnancies at the extremes of the reproductive years are accompanied by increased prematurity and fetal and neonatal death rates. It is essential therefore that sexually active teenagers and women who want no more children be provided with reliable contraceptive methods.

Socioeconomic factors in perinatal mortality. Perinatal mortality from all causes is higher in poor women than in middle- and upper-class women. The general health of more affluent women is better, they are better nourished, they have relatively easy access to physicians, and they know how to use medical care facilities. Poor women are likely to be congenitally malnourished and anemic, and they live in unfavorable environments. They are more likely to have more pregnancies at short intervals than are upper-class women. Medical care facilities available to poor women may be limited and inappropriate, and access to these facilities may be difficult. As a consequence, they use the facilities principally for serious acute illnesses rather than for health maintenance.

Adequate prenatal care alone, although obviously important in determining the outcome of high-risk pregnancies, is only a partial solution for the reproductive problems associated with poverty. Poor women must first be adequately fed and housed so they will no longer need to think only in terms of day-to-day existence. Physicians have little control over these aspects of the total problem,

TABLE 1-4 Neonatal mortality (1980)

Cause	Number	Percent of total
Congenital anomalies	6701	21.9
Respiratory distress syndrome	4721	15.4
Immaturity alone	3615	11.8
Major complications of pregnancy, labor, and delivery	1696	5.5
Asphyxia	1438	4.7
Infections	1053	3.4
Birth trauma	1033	3.4
Neonatal hemorrhage	960	3.1
Complications of cord and placenta	981	3.2
Pneumonia	241	0.8

but they do have the responsibility of making certain that appropriate medical care facilities are made available and that acceptable educational programs, designed to help women learn to use these facilities, are instituted. Better general health alone will improve the outcome of pregnancy, but even this cannot be accomplished without concomitant social and economic advances.

NONLETHAL EFFECTS OF THE BIRTH PROCESS

Not all infants who are born alive are normal. Approximately 7% of all liveborn infants have structural or functional defects. Less than half of these defects are diagnosed during the early postnatal period; the rest appear weeks or even years later.

It is difficult to determine how many of these conditions could have been prevented by better obstetric care, because many are caused by unrecognized chromosomal conditions or teratogenic stimuli during pregnancy. Many individuals, however, particularly those who are mentally defective, might have been normal had they not been born prematurely, been injured during labor and delivery, or suffered hypoxia. Improvements in these figures must await more information concerning the prevention of premature labor, sensitive instruments that will detect early intrauterine hypoxia, precise methods for determining the need for delivery, and improvements in the treatment of respiratory distress following delivery.

REFERENCES

American College of Obstetricians and Gynecologists: Guidelines for vaginal delivery after previous cesarean birth, ACOG Newsletter **29**(1):8, 1985.

Apgar, V.: Birth defects: their significance as a public health problem, J.A.M.A. **204**:79, 1968.

Barton, J.J., Rovner, S., Puls, K., and Read, P.A.: Alternative birthing center: experience in a teaching obstetric service, Am. J. Obstet. Gynecol. **137**:377, 1980.

Burnett, C.A., III, Jones, J.A., Rooks, J., Chen, C.H., Tyler, C.W., Jr., and Miller, C.A.:; Home delivery and neonatal mortality in North Carolina, J.A.M.A. **244**:2741, 1980.

Fox, L.P.: A return to maternal mortality studies: a necessary effort, Am. J. Obstet. Gynecol. **152**:379, 1985.

Fuchs, V.R.: Expenditures for reproduction-related health care, J.A.M.A. **255**:76, 1986.

Hein, H.A.: The status and future of small maternity services in Iowa, J.A.M.A. **255**:1899, 1986.

Kiely, J.L., Paneth, N., and Susser, M.: Fetal death during labor: an epidemiologic indicator of level of obstetric care, Am. J. Obstet. Gynecol. **153**:721, 1985.

Potter, E.L.: Pathology of the fetus and newborn, Chicago, 1952, Year Book Medical Publishers, Inc.

Scupholme, A., McLeod, A., and Robertson, E.: A birth center affiliated with the tertiary care center: comparison of outcome, Obstet. Gynecol. **67**:598, 1986.

Wegman, M.E.: Annual summary of vital statistics-1984, Pediatrics **76**:861, 1985.

2

J. Robert Willson

Diagnostic methods in obstetrics and gynecology

An accurate medical history and a complete physical examination are at least as important for pregnant women and those with gynecologic disorders as for medical and surgical patients. Chronic diseases may influence the course of pregnancy adversely, and many gynecologic patients who are likely to be in the older age groups have medical conditions of which they may be unaware. The principles of history taking and examination do not differ from those for other patients.

HISTORY

The patient should be encouraged to tell her story in her own words, even though this may be a prolonged process. Details can be filled in by questions that will provide the additional information necessary to complete the recital. Questions should be phrased simply in words the patient can understand easily; too many patients will answer "no" to questions they cannot understand rather than display what they presume to be ignorance.

Family history. Particular reference should be made to medical conditions such as cancer, diabetes, and vascular disease; to emotional problems; and to the patient's relationships with her parents and siblings.

Past medical history. Serious illnesses and the details of operative procedures should be noted. In the systemic review, particular interest should be directed toward endocrine disorders, cardiovascular diseases, diseases and dysfunctions of the urinary tract (infection, urinary control), and symptoms of pelvic relaxation.

Menstrual history. Many women find it difficult to discuss the details of menstrual function candidly with an unfamiliar person, particularly a man. Nevertheless, those who have made up their minds to consult a physician because of a pelvic complaint usually are willing to discuss reproductive function in considerable detail. If they are not, the possibility of a psychosexual problem should be considered.

The menstrual history should include the age at which periods began and the type of flow at onset (regular, irregular, interval), preparation for menstruation and reaction to its onset, frequency and duration of periods and amount of bleeding (number of well-saturated or stained pads, clots, color), pain (type, when it began, how long it lasts, how much interference with activity, what medications required for relief), date of onset of the last *normal* menstrual period and of the previous *normal* period, intermenstrual bleeding (duration, amount, relationship to menses, pain, relation to trauma), and relationship of other symptoms to menstruation.

Vaginal discharge. Information concerning vaginal discharge should include how long it has been present; its relation to menses, coitus, or other stimuli; bleeding; irritation; and previous treatment.

Obstetric history. Each pregnancy should be listed chronologically with information concerning prenatal complications, duration, type of termination, complications of labor, and puerperium; sex and weight of infants and their subsequent development; and patient's reactions to pregnancy and her evaluation of labors.

Sexual and marital history. Many physicians are reluctant to inquire into sexual functions and relationships, but the answers may provide clues as to the basis of symptoms or they may indicate serious emotional disturbances. Physicians may deliberately avoid asking these questions because they are embarrassed, because they feel inadequate to cope with the problems that may surface, or because they may precipitate long, tearful sessions that will interrupt their already busy schedules.

An important area to explore, because it may help to explain sexual dysfunction, is what preparation the patient had for marriage or before initiating sexual activity and who provided the information (for example, mother? friends? sex education classes in school?). One should next inquire about age at first coitus, the reaction to it, and the number of sexual partners the patient has had. This information is important, because it may indicate the risk of developing cervical cancer (Chapter 46) and suggest possible psychologic problems. Other questions concern the frequency of sexual relations and reaction to coitus, with particular reference to whether it is an enjoyable experience, whether it is painful, and whether and how often the patient experiences orgasm. The number of marriages, the duration of each, the reason for termination, and the stability of the present relationship should be determined. Patients should also be asked about the contraceptive method they are using.

Present illness. The chronologic account of the problem should be obtained, including the applicable details of menstrual disturbance and symptoms referable to pelvic structures.

PHYSICAL EXAMINATION

A complete general physical examination should be performed on new patients with the exception of those referred from other physicians only for gynecologic evaluation. The *basic gynecologic examination* includes recording the weight and blood pressure, palpation of the breasts, and abdominal, vaginal, and rectal examinations.

Abdominal examination. In most instances abdominal tenderness caused by painful lesions of the pelvic structures is located low in the abdomen. Tenderness in the upper abdomen, near the umbilicus, in the region of the cecum, and along the course of the descending colon is less characteristic of disease in the pelvic organs.

Pelvic examination. The pelvic examination is performed with the patient in lithotomy position, suitably draped with a sheet, her feet in stirrups, and her buttocks hanging just over the lower end of the table. Unless the physician wishes to obtain a specimen of urine by catheter or to check for urinary control, the patient should void immediately before the examination.

The external genitals are inspected in a good light. A note should be made of developmental anomalies, hair distribution, clitoral size, skin changes, discharge, irritation, new growths, and enlargements of Bartholin's glands.

A *warmed speculum* moistened with water is gently inserted into the vagina to expose the cervix. Lubricating jelly may interfere with accurate evaluation of vaginal and cervical secretions. The labia minora and majora are separated with thumb and index finger to expose the introitus. As the tip of the speculum is inserted into the vaginal opening, downward pressure is exerted posteriorly to expand the size of the introitus enough to admit the speculum with a minimum of discomfort. The urethral meatus is the most sensitive structure in the area; hence every precaution must be made to protect it. Pain produced by the speculum may make the rest of the examination much more difficult. Material is collected from the cervix for cytologic examination, and, when indicated, a sample of the fluid from the vaginal canal is obtained for culture or for microscopic study.

After the exposed cervix has been wiped clean with dry cotton, a note is made of its color, size, and configuration; and any obvious lesions are described minutely. The canal is probed in an attempt to provoke bleeding, and a biopsy of the cervix is performed when indicated. As the speculum is slowly withdrawn, the vaginal walls are inspected.

One or two fingers are then inserted into the vagina to depress the posterior wall as the patient holds her breath and ''bears down.'' If the muscular supports of the bladder and rectum have been damaged, these structures will bulge through the open introitus as intraabdominal pressure is increased. The uterus also may be forced downward if its supports have been weakened.

Although it is not possible to visualize the body of the uterus and the adnexal structures, their size, shape, position, mobility, and sensitivity can usually be determined by *bimanual examination* (Figs. 2-1 to 2-4), in which the index fingers alone or the index and second fingers of one hand are inserted into the vagina while those of the other hand palpate through the abdominal wall. The accuracy with which bimanual examination can be performed is determined by the thickness of the abdominal wall,

the patient's ability to relax her voluntary muscles, and whether a painful lesion is present. Nothing can be done about obesity, but it is possible to perform pelvic examinations on most women, even virgins, without causing undue pain. Two fingers can usually be inserted into the vagina of most multiparous women, but this is not often possible when the hymen is intact. If one learns to perform pelvic examination using only the index finger, one can examine almost anyone without causing pain.

The consistency of the cervix and the direction in which it points are determined, and the cervix and uterus are pushed upward and from side to side to determine whether it is mobile or fixed and to detect pain produced by motion. The body of the uterus is located; and its size, shape, and consistency are determined by palpating it between the finger in the vagina and the fingers pushing the abdominal wall structures inward.

An attempt is then made to feel each tube and ovary between the fingertips of the vaginal and abdominal hands. The right adnexum can be outlined most accurately with the fingers of the right hand in the vagina and those of the left hand palpating abdominally. The left adnexum can be felt best with the fingers of the left hand in the vagina. Normal tubes cannot be felt as distinct structures, and it may be difficult to feel normal ovaries unless

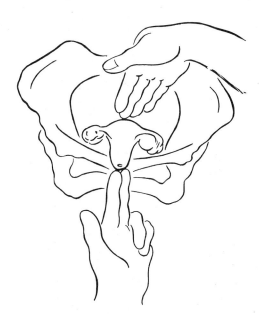

Fig. 2-1. Bimanual palpation of uterus.

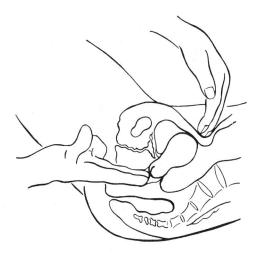

Fig. 2-2. Bimanual palpation of uterus.

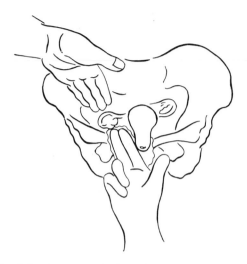

Fig. 2-3. Bimanual palpation of normal adnexal structures.

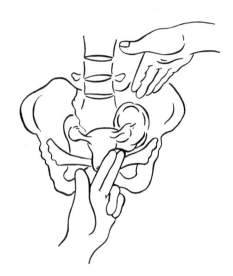

Fig. 2-4. Bimanual palpation of adnexal mass.

the patient is very thin or the abdominal wall is relaxed; but she may experience momentary discomfort as the ovary is squeezed between the tips of palpating fingers. Adnexal masses can usually be felt if the patient can relax her abdominal muscles and if she is not too obese.

The posterior surfaces of the uterus and broad ligaments, the uterosacral ligaments, the posterior cul-de-sac, and the structures on the lateral pelvic walls can be felt more accurately by rectal than by vaginal palpation. Rectocele and other lower bowel lesions such as polyps and carcinoma can also be felt. *A rectal or rectovaginal examination should be performed as a part of every pelvic examination.*

DIAGNOSTIC TESTS

In many women the information obtained from the history and the physical examination is enough to indicate what treatment, if any, is required. In others, further study is necessary before a treatment plan can be developed. Most organic gynecologic disorders are caused by infection, endocrine dysfunction, tumor growth, and the late effects of childbirth injury; of these the last can usually be diagnosed without difficulty by physical examination alone, but it is necessary to perform certain laboratory studies to identify the type of tumor, the

infecting organism, or the hormone disorder. Many diagnostic tests are simple and can be performed in the physician's office, requiring little equipment other than a microscope and stains for bacteria. Some can be done only in elaborate and specialized laboratories.

Urine examination. The microscopic examination of a catheterized or clean voided specimen of urine often is helpful, because infections occur so frequently in women. Urine tests are best performed in the office, because the examination of the sediment of freshly collected urine is far more revealing than that which has stood for several hours awaiting transportation to the laboratory. Unless the specimen is refrigerated, any bacteria present may multiply many times. There is little point in performing a microscopic examination on voided urine in women unless special precautions are taken to prevent contamination by vulvar debris (clean voided specimen).

Blood examination. Hemoglobin and hematocrit determination may aid in the diagnosis of certain gynecologic conditions, particularly those associated with intraperitoneal bleeding or when one suspects that blood loss with menstruation is excessive. White blood cell counts are important when infection is suspected; for example, whenever it is

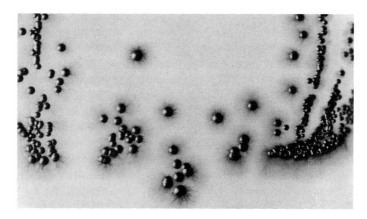

Fig. 2-5. Colonies of yeastlike organisms on Nickerson's medium.

necessary to differentiate between a minor pelvic disorder and appendicitis or between tubal pregnancy and acute salpingo-oophoritis.

Cultures, smears, and suspensions of vaginal secretions. One should try to identify the organisms responsible for the various types of pelvic infection. In some instances this can be accomplished in the physician's office, but in others it is necessary to send the specimens to a laboratory. Crusts or exudates should be removed so that material for bacterial culture can be obtained directly from the infected area with a sterile swab, by scraping the lesion, or by removing small bits of tissue. The cotton swab, scrapings, or tissue should be placed in nutrient broth at once to prevent drying and should be transported to the laboratory as soon as possible. Special precautions are necessary when anaerobic organisms are suspected.

CULTURES. Bacterial cultures are most informative for the study of localized infections, such as gonorrhea or ulcerated lesions; they are least helpful in evaluating chronic cervicitis or chronic vaginitis.

Gonorrhea can be diagnosed more accurately by culture of cervical and urethral secretions than by clinical examination or by stained smear (Chapter 42). The material for culture is best obtained from the cervical crypts rather than purulent exudate in the vaginal canal.

The cervix is exposed and wiped clean, and a dry swab is inserted into the canal and rotated.

Infected material can be expressed from the crypts by closing the blades of the speculum and squeezing the cervix. The applicator should be left in the cervical canal for at least 30 seconds.

Thayer-Martin culture medium, which inhibits growth of organisms other than gonococci, is inoculated with the cervical secretions and maintained under anaerobic conditions until it reaches the laboratory.

Cultures are also helpful in the diagnosis of *vaginal candidiasis* if the characteristic mycelia cannot be identified in saline suspension of the vaginal secretions. The material is obtained with a dry swab from the inflamed vaginal wall and streaked on the culture medium. *Candida* organisms can be grown in the physician's office on Nickerson's medium or Pagano-Levin medium without special equipment. The surface of the commercially prepared slant is streaked with the discharge, and within 48 hours characteristic colonies will appear (Fig. 2-5). Bacteria do not grow on these media, and the tubes can be kept at room temperature.

STAINED SMEARS. A Gram stain of cervical or vaginal secretions may provide information necessary to initiate appropriate treatment while awaiting the reports of bacterial cultures. This is particularly important in the treatment of septic abortions and suspected gonococcal, clostridial, and other serious acute infections.

SUSPENSIONS. If a small amount of vaginal discharge is examined under the microscope without staining, trichomonads and yeastlike organisms can be detected if they are present. An unlubricated speculum is inserted into the vagina, and a specimen of the secretion is collected with a dry cotton swab, which is immediately placed in a small test tube containing about 1.25 cm of warm physiologic saline solution and agitated. A drop of the suspension is placed on a clean glass slide, covered with a coverslip, and examined under the microscope without staining. The trichomonads are actively motile and slightly larger than a leukocyte.

Yeastlike organisms can be identified if several drops of 10% aqueous potassium hydroxide solution are added to the suspension. This dissolves epithelial cells and red and white blood cells, leaving the mycelia and spores.

Whenever there is an acute *Trichomonas* or *Candida* vaginitis, one sees a predominance of white blood cells and few vaginal epithelial cells in the suspended material. This is in contrast to the normal vaginal secretions in which there are relatively few leukocytes as compared with epithelial cells, even during the postovulatory phase of the cycle or after the menopause when one expects to see them.

HORMONE ASSAY

It is not often necessary to concern oneself with the exact endocrine status of women with gynecologic conditions resulting from infections, injury, or congenital anatomic anomalies, but disturbances in production and metabolism of reproductive hormones may be important as causes of menstrual abnormalities and infertility.

One can determine *if* the ovary is producing estrogen or *if* a woman is ovulating by simple inexpensive tests that can be done in the office; these may provide enough information on which to base treatment.

Laboratory assay is required when more precise information concerning hormone production is necessary. Examples of conditions for which accurate assay is essential are the follow-up of patients who have been treated for hydatidiform mole; the evaluation of women suspected of having anterior pituitary dysfunction; the diagnosis of hormone-secreting ovarian neoplasms; and the evaluation of

women with amenorrhea, infertility, or hirsutism and those suspected of having adrenal hyperplasia.

The first consideration is the information needed. For example, must one know *only* whether a woman is producing estrogen? This question can be answered by simple office procedures. Such tests are not quantitative, and a more precise laboratory assay is necessary to determine how much estrogen is being produced.

Measuring reproductive hormone function is different from measuring activity of other endocrine organs. Thyroid function, for example, varies little from day to day, and one can usually assess thyroid activity reasonably accurately with a set of tests performed on one occasion. This is not true of ovarian function, which changes from day to day throughout the menstrual cycle. It is easy to get a false impression of reproductive endocrine function if one fails to relate the results of the test to the day of the cycle or if one accepts a single study as representative of a constantly changing production of hormones.

In short, endocrine assays are expensive, and they provide little useful information if they are ordered indiscriminately and unless they are performed in a laboratory in which the techniques are well designed and carefully controlled. Before an assay is ordered, one should have decided whether it will provide the information needed and also whether equally satisfactory information can be obtained by a simpler and less expensive method.

Tests for estrogenic activity

Examination of vaginal smears. Estrogen stimulates the growth of vaginal epithelial cells. The basal and parabasal cells respond to this hormone by proliferating and becoming cornified. During periods of physiologic low estrogen production, before puberty, and after the menopause, the vaginal epithelium is thin and made up almost entirely of basal and parabasal cells. The cells contain little or no glycogen. Estrogen produced by the active ovaries of mature women stimulates epithelial cell growth. Basal and parabasal cells proliferate, and the epithelium becomes thicker as the cells grow and cornify. The glycogen content of the stimulated epithelial cells increases as cornification progresses. These changes can be demonstrated by examining stained spreads of exfoliated cells in vaginal secretions. Glycogen can be identified by inverting a dried smear of vaginal secretions over a dish containing Lugol's solution. The iodine vapor stains glycogen-containing cells brown.

The presence of systemic estrogen activity may be assumed when a smear of cellular material collected from the upper vagina and stained by the Papanicolaou technique or simply with methylene blue reveals cornified or precornified cells (Fig. 2-6). Estrogenic effect can be considered absent when cells are predominantly from the basal and parabasal layers.

A rough measure of estrogenic effect is the *maturation index;* that is the proportions of parabasal, precornified (intermediate), and cornified (superficial) cells in each 100 vaginal mucosal cells counted. Absence of estrogen is indicated by a predominance of parabasal cells (100:0:0). With a small amount of estrogen there is cellular stimulation and more precornified cells

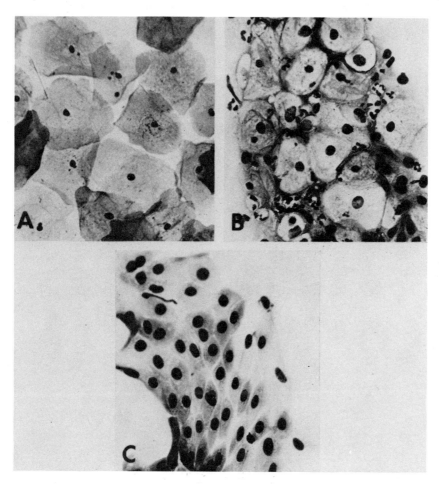

Fig. 2-6. Estrogen-induced changes in vaginal epithelial cells. **A,** Cornified (superficial) cells, a strong estrogen effect. **B,** Intermediate cells and parabasal cells, smaller rounder cells with large nuclei. **C,** Clump of basal cells, vaguely outlined with large nuclei, indicating lack of estrogen. (From Riley, G.: Clin Obstet. Gynecol. 7:432, 1964.)

(10:80:10). At ovulation the numbers of precornified and cornified cells are about equal (0:40:60), and with increasing estrogen stimulation the percentage of cornified cells increases even more.

Examination of cervical mucus. Papanicolaou (1946) described an interesting pattern of arborization, or ferning, in cervical mucus spread on a clean glass slide and allowed to dry. The intensity of ferning is determined by the concentration of sodium chloride and other electrolytes in the cervical secretion; the greater the amount, the more pronounced the ferning. Electrolyte concentration is controlled by estrogen; the higher the concentration of estrogen the more complete the arborization.

Ferning is absent immediately after menstruation when estrogen is low (Fig. 2-7). It increases progressively to the maximum at the time of ovulation when the estrogen concentration peaks (Figs. 2-8 and 2-9). Arborization does not occur in cervical mucus from untreated castrated women and from women after the menopause, but it can be induced in such women by the administration of small amounts of estrogen.

Ferning is inhibited by progesterone; hence the pattern is not present during the postovulatory phase of the normal menstrual cycle and during pregnancy.

A negative test (no ferning) indicates either the absence of estrogen or the presence of fern-inhibiting progesterone.

To obtain mucus, an unlubricated speculum is inserted into the vagina, exposing the cervix from which the visible discharge is wiped. A cotton-tipped applicator is gently inserted into the cervical canal and rotated. The mucus that adheres to the cotton swab is spread on a clean slide and allowed to dry at room temperature. The dried, unstained spread is scanned under the low power of the microscope.

If the cervical mucus is so scant and tenacious that it is difficult to obtain an adequate quantity by means of the cotton-tipped applicator, a sample can

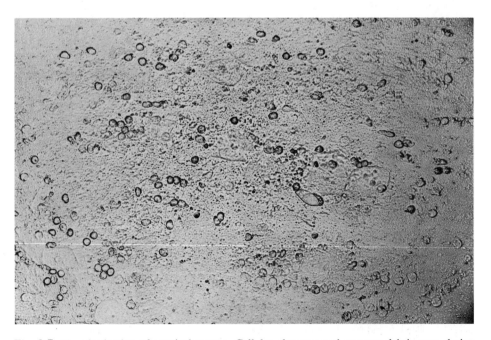

Fig. 2-7. No arborization of cervical mucus. Cellular elements and mucous debris seen during premenstrual and immediate postmenstrual phases of cycle, after the menopause, and during pregnancy. ($\times$153.)

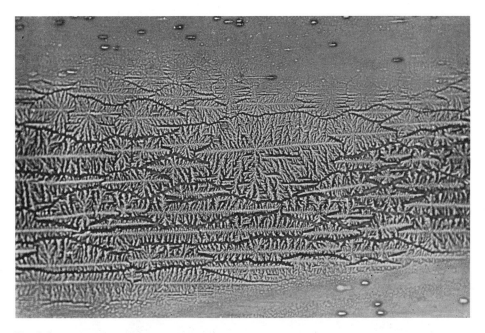

Fig. 2-8. Moderate arborization of cervical mucus: a layer of arborization between two cellular areas. This type of smear indicates moderate estrogen activity.

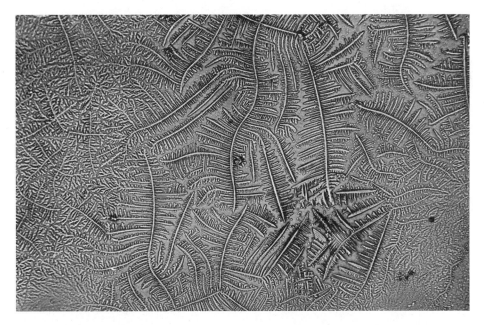

Fig. 2-9. Complete arborization of cervical mucus seen in midcycle at peak of unopposed estrogen activity. ($\times 164$.)

be obtained with a uterine dressing forceps (Fig. 2-10).

The slides used for examination of cervical mucus should be washed, and the instruments sterilized in distilled water when the local water supply has a high salt content; the electrolytes in tap water may produce a false arborization. Also, in obtaining cervical mucus, the physician should be careful not to injure the cervix because blood mixed with the mucus may inhibit arborization.

Endometrial biopsy. Since estrogen produces characteristic endometrial proliferation, one can detect estrogenic activity by studying the histologic pattern of endometrium obtained with a biopsy curet (Fig. 2-11). An unstimulated or atrophic pattern indicates an estrogen deficiency. A more com-

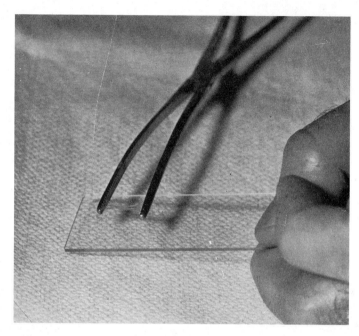

Fig. 2-10. Fern test. Mucus obtained from cervical canal with forceps is spread on glass slide and allowed to dry.

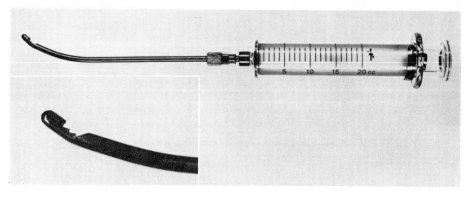

Fig. 2-11. Endometrial biopsy suction curet (Novak). Inset shows detail of serrated fenestration.

plete endometrial sample can be obtained by *suction curettage* (vabra aspiration) similar to that used to terminate early pregnancies.

Immunologic estrogen assays. Estrogens can be extracted from plasma and urine and may be separated from other lipids and steroid hormones. The isolated estrogens may then be quantitated.

Radioimmunoassay techniques for the measurement of plasma estrone, estradiol, and estriol enable one to quantitate picogram quantities of these compounds in serum. The plasma concentrations of estradiol during the early follicular phase of the normal menstrual cycle are in the range of 25 to 75 pg/ml and during the midcycle peak 200 to 600 pg/ml, respectively. During the luteal phase the concentrations fall to a level of 100 to 300 pg/ml for estradiol. In postmenopausal women the concentrations of hormones are as low as 5 to 25 pg/ml for estradiol (Fig. 2-12).

Tests for progesterone

Progesterone activity can be detected by simple tests, but precise measurements require complicated assay.

Basal body temperature charts. Since progesterone has a thermogenic property, a sustained rise in the basal body temperature during the latter half of the menstrual cycle is presumptive evidence of progesterone activity. A monophasic curve is suggestive of absent or deficient progesterone secretion (see tests for ovulation).

Premenstrual endometrial biopsy. Histologic examination of tissue removed by curettage or by endometrial biopsy several days before the onset of the flow is the most accurate method for the determination of progesterone activity. A late secretory endometrium is indicative of an adequate progesterone effect, whereas an endometrium in the proliferative phase or with a scant progesterone effect during the premenstruum indicates absent or inadequate progesterone secretion.

Examination of cervical mucus. Examination of cervical mucus may be of value in determining progesterone activity. If arborization is complete at midcycle and has disappeared a few days later, it can be assumed that the change was brought about by the fern-inhibiting effect of progesterone. An adequate evaluation requires at least two tests, one at midcycle showing advanced arborization and a second 5 to 7 days after showing absence of ferning.

Assays for progesterone. Competitive protein-binding and radioimmunoassay procedures are used for the determination of plasma progesterone levels, which increase from low follicular phase levels (0.4 to 1 ng/ml) to significantly elevated concentrations (5 to 20 ng/ml) during the luteal phase (Fig. 2-12). These luteal phase progesterone levels drop before the onset of the next menstruation or rise sharply in early pregnancy under the stimulus of chorionic gonadotropin. Plasma progesterone concentration increases throughout the course of pregnancy.

Tests for gonadotropins

Concentrations of anterior pituitary gonadotropins in peripheral blood can be determined by radioimmunoassay, which not only distinguishes between follicle-stimulating hormone (FSH) and luteinizing hormone (LH) but also measures minute amounts of the hormones in small volumes of serum.

The pattern of FSH and LH secretion during a normal menstrual cycle is depicted in Fig. 2-12. The details of the changes are described in Chapter 7.

Tests for androgens

Radioimmunoassay procedures are used for the measurement of *testosterone* in serum. During the normal menstrual cycle, the plasma testosterone level is 0.2 to 0.8 ng/ml. In normal males the concentration of testosterone is 5.96 ± 2.02 ng/ml of serum.

Radioimmunoassay procedures are also available for measuring androstenedione and dehydroepiandrosterone in plasma.

Tests for ovulation

Without ovulation, reproduction is impossible. This makes it important not only to be able to detect ovulation but also to time its occurrence with some degree of accuracy. The only certain method to document ovulation is to recover an ovum, which is impractical, or by the initiation of pregnancy. However, a number of fairly reliable indirect evidences that ovulation has occurred may be used to determine and to time this event.

The cervix and cervical mucus. About 2 days before ovulation the cervix is soft, the external os is dilated, and mucus production is at a peak. The mucus is clear, abundant, watery in consistency, exhibits maximum *spinnbarkheit* (ability to stretch under tension) and maximum arborization. This is a response to rising concentrations of estrogens, which peak about 1 day before the LH surge.

If cervical mucus demonstrates complete ferning at about midcycle and, when examined again 7

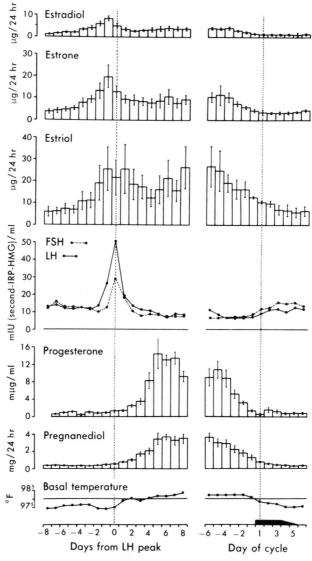

Fig. 2-12. Means of serum LH and FSH levels; serum progesterone concentration; 24-hour urinary estrone, estradiol, estriol, and pregnanediol excretions; and basal body temperatures in five normal women. Data are plotted both in terms of days from midcycle LH and FSH peak, from approximate time of ovulation, and from onset of menstruation. Vertical bars indicate standard errors. (From Goebelsmann, U., Snyder, D.L., and Jaffe, R.B.: Unpublished data.)

days later, is thick, scanty, and no longer ferns, ovulation probably has occurred. Progesterone inhibits the estrogen-produced arborization.

With an anovulatory cycle, ferning gradually increases to a maximum and then gradually decreases as the follicle regresses and estrogen secretion decreases. The gradual loss of arborization is a result of declining levels of unopposed estrogen.

Basal body temperature charts. The occurrence and timing of ovulation can be determined by recording the basal body temperature daily throughout a cycle. During the preovulatory estrogen phase the basal temperatures remain at a relatively low level. A slight drop, as compared with the waking temperature of the preceding day, and a sharp rise of at least 0.3 C (0.6 F) on the following day are typical of ovulation. The rise is maintained with minor fluctuations until a day or two before the onset of menstruation, at which time it drops. When these daily fluctuations are charted, they produce a typical *biphasic curve,* which is indicative of progesterone production and, presumably, of

ovulation (Fig. 2-13). Since the rise in temperature is caused by the thermogenic effect of progesterone, ovulation probably occurs about a day or two before the thermal shift.

A *monophasic curve,* which indicates complete failure of ovulation, is one in which the temperature level remains low throughout the cycle (Fig. 2-14).

In cycles in which ovulation and fertilization have occurred, the rise is maintained past the date of the expected menstrual period (Fig. 2-15).

The patient is provided with a chart similar to the one illustrated in Fig. 2-13 and with a thermometer, which she is taught to read (Fig. 2-16). The thermometer is kept at the bedside, and the temperature is taken immediately on awakening and before arising at approximately the same time each morning. The thermometer is allowed to remain in the mouth for 5 minutes, is read, and is shaken down after the reading is recorded on the chart. For proper evaluation, accurate temperature recordings should be kept over a period of at least three menstrual cycles.

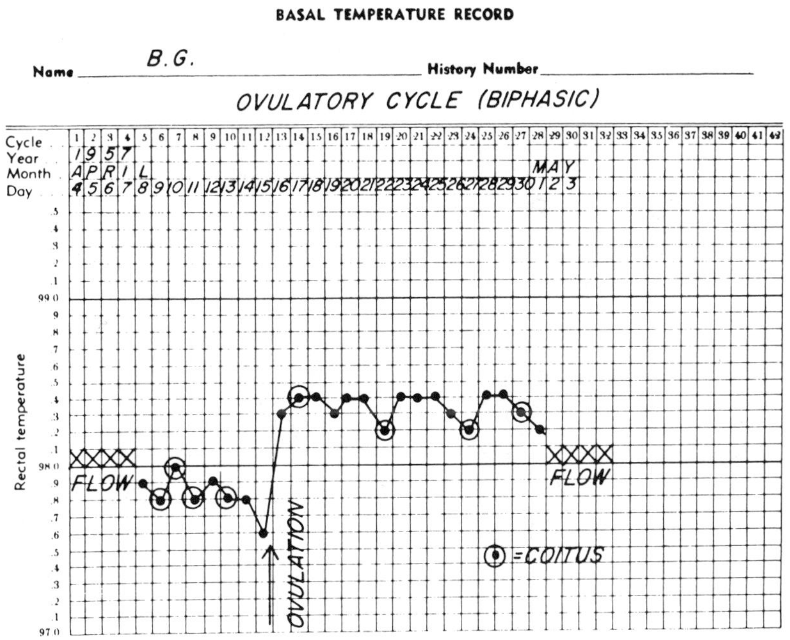

Fig. 2-13. Basal body temperature chart showing biphasic curve indicative of ovulatory cycle. Note drop and sharp rise at time of ovulation.

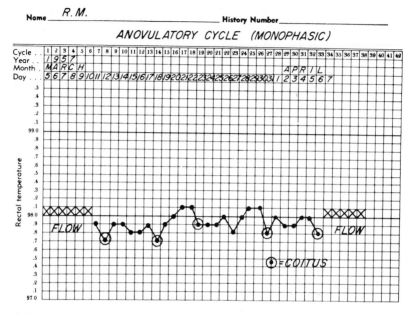

Fig. 2-14. Basal body temperature chart (anovulatory cycle). Note flat monophasic curve.

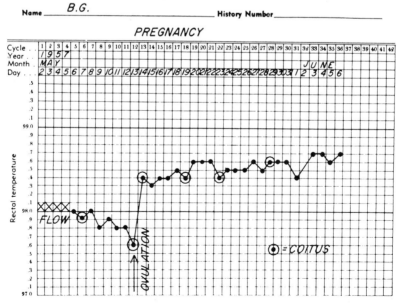

Fig. 2-15. Basal body temperature chart. Persistent elevation and absence of menstruation are suggestive of pregnancy.

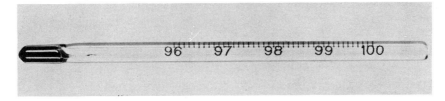

Fig. 2-16. Special thermometer for recording basal body temperature.

Zuspan and Zuspan reported that an almost identical temperature curve can be obtained by taking temperatures at 5 PM or at bedtime rather than on awakening. Although the 5 PM temperatures are slightly higher than those in early morning, the late afternoon schedule may be quite appropriate for women whose schedules of arising and retiring are irregular or for those who cannot adjust to the basal temperature regimen.

The basal body temperature curve is an inexpensive method for determining ovulation. It has the advantage of simplicity and the feasibility of repeated observations over a period of several months. In addition, it is a fairly accurate guide to the timing of ovulation. However, despite these advantages, this method should not be used for unduly long periods, since it may become a source of irritation and anxiety to the patient and her partner.

Endometrial biopsy. Histologic examination of a piece of endometrium removed either by curettage or by biopsy 3 to 5 days before the onset of a normal menstrual period should demonstrate a late secretory endometrium. The limitations of this method are that it indicates only what has happened in one isolated cycle and that the expense and discomfort involved make it impractical to repeat the test during several cycles. To obviate the possibility of interfering with an early pregnancy in women who are trying to conceive, some authors have suggested that the endometrial biopsy be obtained during the first few hours of the menstrual flow. This is not always practicable, and, furthermore, the histologic picture of the endometrium during the bleeding phase when it is disintegrating is not nearly so well defined as it is during the premenstruum.

That the risk of interrupting pregnancy is not great is suggested by the experience of Rosenfeld and Garcia. They obtained endometrial biopsies during the cycles in which 18 infertile patients conceived; 14 delivered normal infants at term, one delivered prematurely, one aborted, and two were lost to follow-up.

The tissue can be obtained in the physician's office without anesthesia. The patient is placed in lithotomy position, and a bimanual examination is performed to determine the status of the pelvic viscera and, particularly, the position of the uterus. The cervix is exposed and cleansed, its anterior lip is grasped with a tenaculum forceps, and a sound is passed into the uterine cavity. A narrow suction tube–curet is inserted to the fundus of the uterus and pressed firmly against the anterior wall, and suction is applied as the instrument is slowly withdrawn. Strips of endometrium can also be removed with a small biopsy curet without suction. An attempt is then made to obtain specimens from the posterior and lateral walls. The strips of tissue are placed in 10% formalin solution and are submitted to the pathologist for histologic examination.

Hormone assay. Serum progesterone levels are significantly increased after ovulation. No comparable change occurs during anovulatory cycles.

Examination of cervical mucus, temperature curves, endometrial biopsy, and progesterone assay will usually indicate that ovulation has occurred or at least that progesterone is being secreted. None of these tests, however, is of value in determining the exact time of ovulation. It may be possible to anticipate ovulation by the use of *rapid estradiol assay* to detect maximum estrogen concentrations that occur about 24 to 36 hours before ovulation, by *rapid LH assay* to detect the LH surge that occurs about 12 hours before follicle rupture, and by monitoring follicle growth by daily ultrasound studies.

TESTS FOR PREGNANCY

Soon after the ovum is fertilized, the trophoblast begins to secrete human chorionic gonadotropin (hCG). The detection of this hormone is the basis of all pregnancy tests.

hCG can be detected as early as 7 to 9 days after fertilization by the highly sensitive techniques of beta-subunit radioimmunoassay and radioreceptor assay. The production of hCG increases rapidly; the serum concentrations double about every 48 hours during the early weeks of pregnancy. Serum levels and urinary excretion of hCG rise to a peak at about the sixtieth or seventieth day after conception and then decline toward a lower plateau, which is maintained throughout the second and third trimesters. Pregnancy tests generally remain positive throughout gestation or as long as viable trophoblastic tissue is in contact with the maternal circulation.

Immunologic tests. Immunologic pregnancy tests are based on the reaction of urinary hCG with antiserum to chorionic gonadotropin (rabbit anti-hCG). Most pregnancy tests use the agglutination inhibition principle as an indicator. Either latex particles (slide tests) or sheep erythrocytes (test tube assay) are used.

In the former tests, 1 drop of urine to be tested and 1 drop of antiserum against chorionic gonadotropin are stirred together for 30 seconds on a glass slide. Two drops of a suspension of latex particles that have been coated with hCG are added and mixed. The slide is then rocked gently for 2 minutes to ensure complete exposure of the latex particles to the fluid. Urine from a nonpregnant woman contains no chorionic gonadotropin; therefore the antiserum is free to react with the latex particles coated with hCG, causing them to agglutinate (negative test). This agglutination appears as a fine flocculation. If the woman is pregnant, the hCG in the urine will neutralize the antiserum, thus preventing agglutination of the latex particles (positive pregnancy test).

In the hemagglutination inhibition test (test tube assay) a small volume of urine is mixed with the antiserum, and a supension of sheep erythrocytes coated with hCG is added. Within 2 hours, either a mat of agglutinated red cells has settled to the bottom of the test tube (negative test), or a ring of nonagglutinated red cells has formed (positive test).

Although the hemagglutination inhibition test is a 2-hour test as compared with the 2-minute slide tests, it is more accurate and sensitive than currently available slide tests. The hemagglutinin inhibition tests are sensitive enough to detect 500 to 1000 international milliunits (ImU) hCG per milliliter of urine and will usually be positive by about 6 weeks after the first day of the last menstrual period. The slide tests are even less sensitive, detecting no less than 1500/ml of urine; they may not be positive until 7 or more weeks after the last period began.

The false-negative rate for these tests is high if they are performed too early. If pregnancy is suspected, a negative test should be repeated in 7 to 10 days. These tests also may react positively to the urine of women who are not pregnant. The alpha subunits of hCG and LH are so much alike that they may stimulate identical immunologic responses. Thus a high concentration of LH, for example, in postmenopausal women, may occasionally produce a positive reaction for pregnancy.

A new, highly sensitive immunoassay technic designed to detect concentrations of hCG as low as 40 ImU/ml in urine are available. These *monoclonal antibody tests* use two types of antibodies that react to different areas of the hCG molecule. The first immobilize hCG molecules on a membrane; the second, combined with an enzyme that produces a color change, attach to the captured hCG molecules. If hCG is present, a characteristic color appears on the membrane. If there is no hCG, the color of the membrane is unchanged. The necessary materials are supplied in kit form, and tests can be run in 10 to 20 minutes. Monoclonal antibody tests are far more sensitive than the ordinary immunologic tests and can be used to detect hCG soon after implantation and in women suspected of having ectopic pregnancies.

Radioimmunoassay and radioreceptor assay. Although the alpha subunits of hCG and LH are identical chemically, the beta subunits are different. Thus one can prepare a specific antibody against the beta subunit of hCG that will not react with LH. *Beta-subunit radioimmunoassay* on serum is highly sensitive but is not practical for routine use as a pregnancy test. The assay is expensive and takes at least 48 hours for completion.

Radioreceptor assay for serum hCG can be run in 2 hours or less, is specific, and is highly sensitive, detecting levels of hCG of less than 10 ImU/ml. With this test one can detect a pregnancy a day or two after implantation. The test can also measure the minute amounts of hCG secreted with ectopic pregnancy, whereas standard pregnancy tests are negative in at least 50%. It also is helpful in evaluating patients who may be aborting; hCG production is either decreased or does not increase at the expected rate if the pregnancy is disturbed. This is not likely to be evident with standard pregnancy tests. Assays for the beta subunit of hCG are also important in following regression of hormone production after treatment for gestational trophoblastic neoplasms.

Basal body temperature charts. A persistent elevation of the basal body temperature for 7 to 10 days after a missed menstrual period is suggestive of early pregnancy. Therefore, when basal temperatures are being kept, as in cases of infertility, a sustained high level for a period of 3 weeks may be considered as a presumptive positive test for pregnancy. The rise is caused by the thermogenic effect of progesterone.

Evaluation of pregnancy tests. Ordinarily, the diagnosis of pregnancy can be made without the laboratory procedures described. However, there are situations in which the history and physical findings are inconclusive or in which a complication such as threatened abortion or ectopic pregnancy is suspected but cannot be confirmed. Under these circumstances, tests for the beta subunit of hCG may prove to be an invaluable aid in diagnosis.

The standard hormone tests for pregnancy are about 98% accurate when carried out by hemagglutination inhibition procedures, when done properly, and when 4 to 6 weeks have elapsed since fertilization. Slide tests are less accurate in early pregnancy.

False-negative tests are encountered more frequently than false positive. The most common reasons for a false-negative test are performing the test too early in pregnancy before there is sufficient circulating hormone or technical errors either in handling or storing of the test urine. Negative standard pregnancy tests are encountered in intrauterine fetal death unless a considerable amount of viable trophoblast tissue is present. A negative standard pregnancy test, which occurs in about half of ectopic pregnancies, never excludes the diagnosis.

False-positive tests may be obtained early in the menopause or in other gonadal deficiencies in which there is an overproduction of pituitary LH and because of errors in technique. False-positive tests may be encountered in patients who have been taking tranquilizing drugs, notably promazine or one of its derivatives.

It must be emphasized that all of these tests demonstrate the production of chorionic gonadotropin and do not necessarily indicate the presence of a normal pregnancy. The only thing we can conclude from a positive pregnancy test is that there is a source of gonadotropin, which may be a normal pregnancy.

TESTS FOR CANCER

Some of the common benign cervical lesions look much like cancer grossly and can only be differentiated by special tests, all of which require highly trained personnel for their interpretation. The specimens must be properly collected and carefully handled so that they will provide the maximum amount of information. These tests are discussed in detail in Chapter 46.

Schiller's test. Normal cervical squamous epithelial cells contain glycogen and are immediately stained dark brown when painted with Lugol's iodine solution (positive Schiller test). Abnormal epithelial cells and columnar cells are devoid of glycogen and therefore do not stain. The Schiller test is not diagnostic of cancer of the cervix, but it does indicate areas of abnormal epithelium from which tissue for microscopic study can be obtained. The test will also be negative in premenarchal girls, postmenopausal women, and other estrogen-deficient states.

Cytologic examination. A cytologist can detect abnormal cervical cells in specially prepared and stained spreads from the cervix. The most accurate results are obtained when the material is collected from the cervical canal (endometrial and endocervical secretions) and from the junction of the squamous and columnar epithelium (Fig. 2-17). This is the area at which squamous cell cancer usually originates. The former specimen is obtained by rotating a saline-moistened cotton swab within the cervical canal (Fig. 2-18) or by aspirating the secretion with a pipette. Material from the squamocolumnar junction is collected by scraping and abrading the area with a special spatula and transferring the material to a clean glass slide, which is then stained and read by the cytologist.

Cytologic examination is a screening procedure that indicates patients in whom further study is necessary. Whenever abnormal cells are found on a cytologic spread, more precise investigation, usually by colposcopy, biopsy, and endocervical curettage, is necessary. Cytologic studies should be obtained as a part of the periodic examination, even though the cervix appears normal because the earliest carcinomas are not obvious clinically.

Cytologic examination is of little help in screening for endometrial cancer. Abnormal endometrial cells can be detected in only a small percentage of women with invasive endometrial lesions.

Cervical biopsy. Histologic examination of tissue removed from the cervix is an important part of the study of cervical lesions because it permits more precise diagnosis than that by either gross inspection or cytologic examination. Small bits of

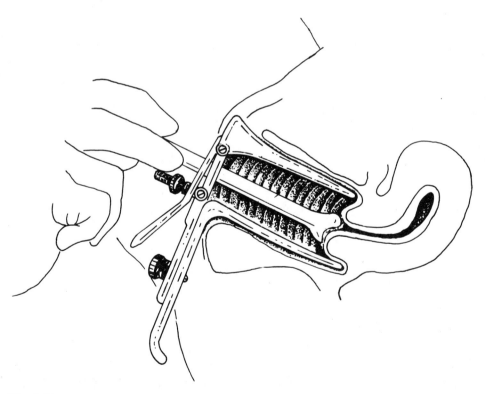

Fig. 2-17. Cytologic examination. Material obtained by rotational scrape of the squamocolumnar junction.

tissue can be removed with a *punch biopsy instrument* in the physician's office without causing undue pain or alarming bleeding. This procedure is most valuable when a small lesion such as a polyp can be removed completely, but it also is helpful in the study of larger lesions, particularly those having the gross appearance of cancer. If several bits of tissue are taken from such a lesion and invasive carcinoma is diagnosed, the physician may proceed directly to treatment. If carcinoma in situ, cervicitis, or some similar condition is diagnosed, further study is indicated.

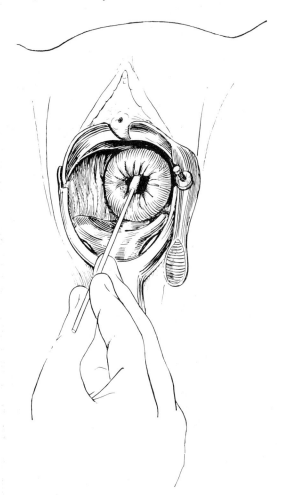

Fig. 2-18. Cytologic examination. Secretions are obtained by rotating a saline-moistened cotton swab in cervical canal.

Cone biopsy, with which the visible cervical lesion, the squamocolumnar junction, and most of the cervical canal are removed, must be performed under anesthesia. This procedure is indicated in women with dysplasia or carcinoma in situ diagnosed by cytologic examination or random punch biopsy, if colposcopic examination is not available or if the entire endocervical canal cannot be seen through the colposcope. If multiple sections are cut from the removed cone of tissue, the pathologist can make a more exact diagnosis than can be made from the small bites obtained by punch biopsy.

Colposcopy. The colposcope is a binocular magnifying instrument through which one can detect epithelial changes that are not visible by gross inspection. Expert colposcopists can identify the early changes in cervical and vaginal epithelium that precede the development of invasive cancer.

Under certain conditions colposcopy can replace cone biopsy in evaluating the cause of abnormal cervical cytologic studies. Tiny areas of dysplasia, carcinoma in situ, and invasive cancer can be seen and biopsied (colposcopic-directed biopsy). This is far more accurate than are random punch biopsies.

The requirement for accurate colposcopy is a skillful colposcopist who is able to inspect the portio vaginalis, the transformation zone, the squamocolumnar junction, and the entire cervical canal. If this is impossible, the examination is inadequate, and additional studies such as cone biopsy are imperative in evaluating the cervix when cytologic analysis suggests the possibility of an abnormality.

Endometrial biopsy. Enough endometrium can be obtained by office biopsy to determine its histologic pattern, but it is impossible with usual techniques to remove as much tissue as with dilatation and curettage. The principal role of endometrial biopsy therefore is the study of menstrual abnormalities presumed to be caused by disordered ovarian function.

It may be possible to diagnose carcinoma of the endometrium by office biopsy if much of the tissue has undergone neoplastic change, but scattered foci may be missed when only several small pieces of tissue are removed. Endometrium can also be obtained by *suction curettage,* like that used to terminate early pregnancy. More tissue can be removed by this technique than with a small biopsy curet. Endometrial biopsy alone cannot be considered an adequate procedure to eliminate suspected endometrial cancer.

Attempts have been made to improve the accuracy of office biopsy. With *endometrial wash techniques,* saline solution is injected under pressure, collected, and spun down; the tissue to be examined represents cells washed off the surface epithelium, small bits of tissue, and the exfoliated cells in the uterine cavity. Although the procedure provides more tissue from a larger surface area, it too is less accurate than dilatation and curettage.

As is true with cervical biopsy, one can proceed directly to treatment if invasive cancer is diagnosed on tissue removed by office endometrial biopsy. A report of hyperplasia, particularly if it is atypical, is usually an indication for more complete curettage.

Vulvar disease. Early carcinoma of the vulva may be multicentric and in its earliest phase presents no characteristic gross appearance. Areas of abnormal tissue can be detected by applying 1% aqueous toluidine blue solution to the vulva, permitting it to dry, and then sponging the vulva with 1% acetic acid. Ulcerated, excoriated, or abraded areas retain a dark blue stain. Although this test is not specific for malignancy, it does indicate areas of abnormal tissue that should be biopsied.

Adequate biopsies can be obtained with a Keyes dermatologic punch. Several specimens can be obtained from various areas of the vulva. If there is a distinct proliferative or ulcerated lesion, the biopsy can be performed with a punch biopsy instrument or by excising a wedge of tissue. These are all outpatient procedures that can be performed with local anesthesia.

X-RAY FILM EXAMINATION

The most important use of x-ray film examination in gynecology is for hysterosalpingography, by which small intracavitary uterine lesions as well as abnormalities in the tubes can be detected (Chapter 14). Special x-ray film studies are also useful in differentiating bowel or urinary tract abnormalities from disorders of the reproductive organs.

X-ray film examinations are used infrequently during pregnancy. The number of fetuses and their age, size, growth pattern, and position can be determined as accurately by ultrasound, which has no deleterious effect on fetal and gonadal tissues. Although x-ray film study is more accurate than ultrasonography for determining the size and shape of the maternal pelvic cavity, such examinations are seldom necessary.

X-ray film studies during the first few weeks of pregnancy are more likely to disturb fetal growth than are those during the second and third trimesters, when the organs are reasonably well formed. The tissues are particularly susceptible from the second to the sixth week after conception, when it may be difficult to diagnose pregnancy. After the primary organ systems have developed and the embryonic cells are transformed into those with adult characteristics, it is less likely that ordinary diagnostic procedures will influence fetal development.

X-ray film studies, except those of an emergency nature, should not be performed during the first trimester and, in fact, are best avoided throughout the entire pregnancy. X-ray film studies that are required for the diagnosis of serious medical and surgical conditions (for example, when intestinal obstruction is suspected) must be performed regardless of the stage of pregnancy. The radiologist should know that the patient is pregnant so that techniques designed to reduce radiation to a minimum can be used.

One should seldom have to consider the need for therapeutic abortion because of radiation during pregnancy if adequate protective measures are observed consistently. Most of the questions concerning possible fetal damage arise because pregnancy is not eliminated by history, physical examination, and pregnancy tests before the studies are ordered.

The American College of Obstetricians and Gynecologists and the American College of Radiology have developed the following guidelines for the use of diagnostic x-ray film studies in fertile women*:

1. The use of x-ray examinations should be considered on an individual basis. Concern over harmful effects should not prevent the proper use of radiation exposure when significant diagnostic information can be obtained. Preexamination consultation with a radiologist may be useful in obtaining optimal information from the x-ray exposure.

2. There is no measurable advantage to scheduling diagnostic x-ray examinations at any particular time during the menstrual cycle.

3. The degree of risk involved in an x-ray examination if the person is pregnant, or should become pregnant, should be explained to the patient and documented in her record.

They also state*:

The problem of defining . . . risks is complicated because the effects attributed to x-ray exposures also occur in the absence of such exposures. From radiobiological literature, using linear extrapolation, it may be concluded that the hypothetical risk of an observable anomaly in a fetus from diagnostic radiation does not exceed 1 to 5/1000/rad. This is substantially less than the natural incidence of 40/1000 of observed birth anomalies.

Ninety-five percent of women scheduled for x-ray examination will not be pregnant. If a pregnancy should occur, it is better that x-ray exposure be during the first and second weeks following conception than later, since the next four weeks are probably the most critical with respect to reproduction of observable anomalies in the unborn child.

One can infer from the preceding statement that abortion is not often necessary unless the woman has had multiple studies during the third to sixth weeks after conception.

ULTRASOUND

High-frequency sound waves send back echoes whenever there is a change in density of the tissues

---

*From Executive Board, American College of Obstetricians and Gynecologists: Guidelines for diagnostic x-ray examination of fertile women: statement of policy, Chicago, 1977, The College.

through which they are passing. This technique is useful in diagnosing both normal and abnormal pregnancy during the early weeks, in identifying multifetal pregnancy and fetal anomalies, in differentiating hydatidiform moles from normal pregnancy, in diagnosing missed abortion and intrauterine fetal death, as an aid in diagnosing ectopic pregnancy, in identifying abnormalities in amniotic fluid volume, in measuring the biparietal diameter of the fetal skull, in assessing fetal size and the rate of fetal growth, for placental localization, and in the differential diagnosis of various uterine and ovarian enlargements. These are discussed in detail in appropriate sections of the book. Diagnostic sound waves appear to have no deleterious effect on maternal or fetal tissues.

MAGNETIC RESONANCE IMAGING

Magnetic resonance imaging is based on the principle that nuclei of certain atoms possess the property of angular momentum, or spin, which makes them function as magnets. In a magnetic field the atoms assume positions either parallel to or opposite from the direction of the field. The tissue images provided by this technique are far superior to those of ultrasound and eliminate the potential dangers from radiation associated with CT scans. Since there are no known ill effects on tissue, magnetic resonance imaging has an important potential for use in obstetrics and gynecology, but it is too early to evaluate its contribution.

LAPAROSCOPY

The development of high-intensity, fiberoptic light sources has led to a reevaluation of an old method of examining the peritoneal cavity. With the laparoscope, which is inserted through a subumbilical incision after pneumoperitoneum has been established, it is possible to inspect the contents of both the pelvis and the upper abdomen. The view of the pelvic organs is usually excellent; one looks down from above and can see the bladder, the anterior surface of the uterus, the adnexa, and the posterior cul-de-sac.

The principal *indications* for laparoscopy are the evaluation of pelvic pain, for inspection of small uterine or ovarian masses, infertility, endocrinopathies, amenorrhea, congenital anomalies and ascites. The main *complications* are hemorrhage from punctured blood vessels and perforation of a hollow viscus.

HYSTEROSCOPY

The advantages of diagnosing intrauterine disease by direct inspection rather than indirectly by palpating the cavity with a curet and by histologic examination of the endometrium are obvious. Hysteroscopy was first described in 1869, but is has been used little. Improved instruments and lighting sources have been designed, and hysteroscopy may become an important diagnostic aid.

AMNIOCENTESIS

A variety of examinations can be performed on amniotic fluid. Almost all tests performed during early pregnancy are to diagnose genetic defects (Chapter 34). The majority performed during the third trimester are to obtain fluid for examination in Rh disease (Chapter 34) and to assess fetal maturity (Chapter 20).

The aim of *genetic amniocentesis* is to detect fetal chromosomal and biochemical abnormalities during early pregnancy so that parents may either obtain an abortion or plan for the care of the child if a defect is present. Fetal cells in amniotic fluid are cultured for karyotyping, identification of certain enzymatic deficiencies, and determination of fetal sex. The fluid can also be assayed for its alpha-fetoprotein content, which may indicate neural tube defects.

The majority of amniocenteses are performed to detect chromosomal abnormalities, which increase with maternal aging. Tsuji and Nakano karyotyped 256 specimens of fetal tissue that were removed during elective abortions of presumably normal pregnancies. Trisomies were identified in 1.6% of specimens from mothers 35 to 39 years of age, in 6.0% from those between 40 and 44, and in 25% from those between 45 and 49. Others have reported a similar pattern of increase with aging. Some abnormalities of carbohydrate, lipid, and protein metabolism can be diagnosed by studying cultured or uncultured cells. The determination of

fetal sex is important in considering the possible outcome of sex-linked genetic disorders.

Genetic amniocentesis is usually performed at about 16 weeks. Before this there may be too little amniotic fluid and too few shed cells to ensure a successful result. If done much later, the pregnancy may be so far advanced when the results are available that the possibility of abortion is eliminated. Genetic amniocentesis is an outpatient procedure performed with local infiltration anesthesia and ultrasound guidance.

The *principal indications* for genetic amniocentesis are:

1. Maternal age of 35 years or more
2. Chromosomal abnormality in a previous child
3. Known chromosomal abnormality in either parent
4. Metabolic disorder in a previous child
5. History of a sex-linked genetic disorder
6. Family history of chromosomal or enzymatic abnormality or of neural tube defects

The *potential complications* are infection of either mother or fetus, injury to the fetus, fetomaternal transfusion with possible Rh alloimmunization if a placental blood vessel is punctured, and abortion. Infection can be kept at a minimum by using meticulous sterile technique. One can usually avoid injuring the placenta by identifying its position with ultrasound and selecting a puncture site beyond its edge. Crandall and co-workers found that genetic amniocentesis did not increase the rates of abortion, preterm delivery, fetal or neonatal death, or neonatal complications in 2000 cases. Leschot, Verjaal, and Treffers suggested that fetal death within 3 weeks of midtrimester amniocentesis occurs in about 0.5% of cases when experienced operators perform the procedures.

The accuracy of genetic amniocentesis is limited. Occasionally, fetal cells will not grow in the culture, minor chromosomal abnormalities may not be detected, and the techniques for diagnosing many of the metabolic disorders are still in the experimental stages or not even available. There is no way to detect anomalies such as cleft palate, club foot, and other similar defects by studing amniotic fluid.

Because of the importance of accurate diagnosis and the potential complications, amniocentesis should be performed in a perinatal center where the procedures are done regularly and where facilities are available for prompt and accurate evaluation of the cells and fluid.

Amniocentesis during late pregnancy, although easier, is not without danger. Several cases of fetal death from hemorrhage after the puncture of an umbilical vessel have been recorded.

CHORIONIC VILLUS SAMPLING

A major disadvantage of amniocentesis is that it cannot be performed much before the sixteenth gestational week. It is possible to obtain the same information during the first trimester by examining cells obtained from the chorion frondosum. A sampling catheter is inserted through the internal cervical os with ultrasound monitoring, and villous material is aspirated and examined by the same methods used for fetal cells obtained from amniotic fluid. The technique has not yet been completely evaluated; but when its safety and diagnostic accuracy are proved, it should become a valuable adjunct to early assessment of the fetus.

FETOSCOPY

Fetoscopy, or amnioscopy, is a technique that permits direct inspection of the fetus and placenta through an endoscope, which is introduced through the maternal abdominal and uterine walls. The available instruments have a limited field of vision, and it is not yet possible to inspect the entire fetus and amnionic cavity. Fetal blood samples can be obtained from a placental vein, and the skin can be biopsied.

REFERENCES

Batzer, F.R.: Guidelines for choosing a pregnancy test, Contemp. Obstet. Gynecol.: **23**:42, 1986.

Crandall, B.F., Howard, J., Lebherz, T.B., Rubinstein, L., Sample, W.F., and Sarti, D.: Follow-up of 2000 second-rimester amniocenteses, Obstet. Gynecol. **56**:625, 1980.

Diagnostic ultrasound imaging in pregnancy. Report of a consensus development conference. NIH Publication No. 84-667, Bethesda, Md., 1984, National Institutes of Health.

Elias, S., Simpson, J.L., Martin, A.O., Sabbagha, R.E., Gerbie, A.B., and Keith, L.G.: Chorionic villus sampling for first-trimester prenatal diagnosis: Northwestern University Program, Am., J. Obstet, Gynecol. **152**:204, 1985.

Goebelsmann, U., Midgley, A.R., Jr., and Jaffe, R.B.: Regulation of human gonadotropins. VII. Daily individual urinary estrogens, pregnanediol, and serum-luteinizing and follicle-stimulating hormones during the menstrual cycle, J. Clin. Endocrinol. Metab. **29**:1222, 1969.

Golbus, M.S. et al.: Prenatal genetic diagosis in 3000 amniocenteses, N. Engl. J. Med. **300**:157, 1979.

Landesman, R., and Saxena, B.B.: Results of the first 1000 radioreceptorassays for the determination of human chorionic gonadotropin: a new, rapid, reliable, and sensitive pregnancy test, Fertil. Steril. **27**:357, 1976.

Leschot, N.J., Verjaal, M., and Treffers, P.E.: Risks of midtrimester amniocentesis: assessment in 3000 pregnancies, Br. J. Obstet. Gynaecol. **92**:804, 1985.

Lindemann, H.: Historical aspects of hysteroscopy, Fertil. Steril. **24**:230, 1973.

Mikhail, G.: Hormone assays and the gynecologist, Fertil. Steril. **27**:229, 1976.

Papanicolaou, G.: General survey of vaginal smear and its use in research and diagnosis, Am. J. Obstet. Gynecol. **51**:316, 1946.

Roberts, N.S., Dunn, L.K., Weener, S., Godmilow, L., and Miller, R.: Midtrimester amniocentesis—indications, technics, risks, and potential for prenatal diagnosis, J. Reproduc. Med. **28**:167, 1983.

Rosenfeld, D.L., and Garcia, C.R.: Endometrial biopsy in the cycle of conception. Fertil. Steril. **26**:1088, 1975.

Roy, S., Klein, T.A., Scott, J.Z., Kletzky, O.A., and Mishell, D.R., Jr.: Diagnosis of pregnancy with a radioreceptor assay for hCG. Obstet. Gynecol. **50**:401, 1977.

Sabbagha, R.E.: Diagnostic ultrasound applied to obstetrics and gynecology, New York, 1980, Harper & Row, Publishers.

Tompkins, P.: The use of basal temperature graphs in determining the date of ovulation, J.A.M.A. **124**:698, 1944.

Tsuji, K., and Nakano, R.: Chromosome studies of embryos from induced abortions in pregnant women age 35 and over, Obstet. Gynecol. **52**:542, 1978.

Zondek, B., and Rozin, S.: Cervical mucus arborization: its use in the determination of corpus luteum function. Obstet. Gynecol. **3**:463, 1954.

Zuspan, K.J. and Zuspan, F.P.: Thermogenic alterations in women. II. Basal body, afternoon, and bedtime temperatures, Am. J. Obstet. Gynecol. **120**:441, 1974.

3

Elsie Reid Carrington

Pediatric gynecology

Genital disorders most often encountered in girls from infancy to adolescence include various local infections, injuries, congenital anomalies, and abnormal sexual development. The disorders during the adolescent years are primarily those related to menstrual function. The differences in adult and adolescent anatomy and physiology alter the method of examination and the interpretation of findings.

Pelvic examination can be performed at any age from birth on, usually without anesthesia and without psychologic trauma.

Normal variations from adult genitals include a more anterior location of the introitus and a relative prominence of the clitoris, which may measure 1 to 1.5 cm. During the first few days after birth, the breasts and genitals are swollen, and the latter are moistened by clear secretions from the estrogen-stimulated vagina. The endometrium also is stimulated, and estrogen-withdrawal bleeding may occur within 3 to 5 days of delivery because the placental source of estrogen is no longer present.

All estrogen effects disappear after 2 to 3 weeks and do not return until puberty when ovarian function is initiated. During this intermediate period, the vaginal epithelium is thin, uncornified, and red. The vaginal smear is made up of basal and parabasal cells, and the vaginal pH is alkaline.

Fine, short pubic hairs may be noted in young girls as a response to normal levels of androgens. The hymen is redundant and with strain may protrude beyond the surrounding parts. The hymenal opening changes little in size throughout the prepubertal period and is as adequate for passage of the same instruments in the infant as in the girl of 10 years of age. Bartholin's, paraurethral, and cervical glands are rudimentary and virtually functionless.

The vaginal portion of the cervix is flat, and the endocervical epithelium extends for a short distance over the surface. This should not be interpreted or treated as an erosion or cervicitis (Fig. 3-1).

Since the posterior fornix is short and the cul-de-sac almost nonexistent, it is difficult to advance the examining finger high enough vaginally to outline pelvic structures. Rectal palpation is more informative. The long axis of the uterus is parallel to the long axis of the body in contrast to the anteverted position in the adult (Fig. 3-2). The total length is 2.5 to 3 cm with reversal of the adult cervix-corpus ratio, the cervix in the immature female comprising two thirds of the entire organ. Complete reversal of the ratio does not occur until full maturation, which can be within a few months or as long as several years after the menarche.

The vaginal vault and cervix can be seen through a small, well-lubricated vaginoscope or urethro-

36

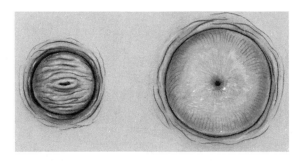

Fig. 3-1. Appearance of immature cervix compared with mature nulliparous cervix.

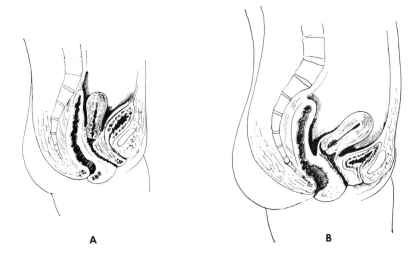

Fig. 3-2. Comparison of immature, **A,** and mature, **B,** pelvic organs. In immature organs the uterus is horizontal, the cervix comprises two thirds of the organ, and the vaginal fornices are short.

scope. Makeshift instruments such as a nasal speculum or an otoscope are inadequate because they are too short to expose the upper vagina and cervix. If vaginal smears or cultures are to be obtained, a combined rectovaginal examination is better tolerated than instrumentation of the vagina alone. While the patient's attention is diverted by rectal examination, a cotton-tipped applicator moistened in sterile saline solution is rolled through the hymenal opening. The thin rectovaginal septum makes possible a clear outline of the vaginal tract between the examining finger and the applicator (Fig. 3-3).

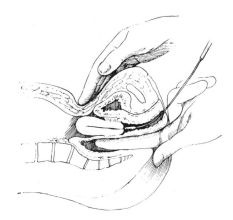

Fig. 3-3. "Combined examination" in child with rectal palpation and vaginal sound or applicator.

GYNECOLOGIC PROBLEMS IN PREADOLESCENTS

Vulvovaginitis. Investigation of infections involving the external genitals should include pelvic examination; culture of the discharge; perianal examination, particularly for pinworm ova; and urinalysis to exclude urinary tract infection and diabetes.

Any sexually transmitted disease in a child should suggest the possibility of sexual abuse.

ACUTE GONORRHEAL VULVOVAGINITIS. Acute gonorrheal vulvovaginitis produces an intense inflammatory reaction, edema of the vulva, and a profuse purulent vaginal discharge. Cervical, paraurethral, and Bartholin's glands are poorly developed and are rarely involved, but an associated specific proctitis is not uncommon. Upper genital tract infections are extremely rare. Systemic reactions are minimal.

Parenteral penicillin is the drug of choice. Tetracycline can be used in penicillin-sensitive patients.

CHLAMYDIAL TRACHOMATIS INFECTIONS. *Chlamydia trachomatis* is now considered the most common cause of sexually transmitted diseases in women and of ophthalmia neonatorum in the infant. Golden and associates recently focused attention on young females and found that chlamydial cervicitis was at least as common (10.2%) as gonorrheal infections (9.7%) in 186 adolescent girls aged 12 to 17 years. One third of the teenagers were pregnant. Cervical erosion and a mucopurulent discharge are usually noted. Smears show characteristic evidence of infection, although both chlamydial and gonorrheal cervicitis are frequently asymptomatic. Mixed infections are common. Culture or an immunofluorescent staining technique is necessary for diagnosis. *C. trachomatis* has been found in pure culture from samples obtained by laparoscopy in patients with salpingitis and perihepatitis.

Chlamydial vaginitis found in a young child can occur by eye-to-vagina transmission but should also raise suspicion of sexual abuse. Therapy with erythromycin or sulfonamides is effective. The risk of subsequent infertility in untreated adolescents is unknown, but for their neonates the risk of eye or respiratory infections, including pneumonia, is 20% to 30%.

HEMOLYTIC STREPTOCOCCAL VAGINITIS. Hemolytic streptococcal vaginitis is more often the cause of bloody or serosanguineous discharge than is a foreign body, although the possible presence of the latter should not be overlooked. Evidence of genital infection generally appears 2 to 4 weeks after a streptococcal infection elsewhere, particularly in the throat or skin, or after scarlet fever. Diagnosis is made by culture. Antibiotic therapy is indicated for 5 to 7 days.

NONSPECIFIC VAGINITIS. Nonspecific vaginitis is characterized by a relatively low-grade, often persistent mixed infection. Local irritation by scratching or manipulation is a common cause. Intestinal *pinworm infestations* should be suspected in any persistent or recurrent nonspecific vaginitis, and examination should be made for ova and parasites.

Treatment consists of good local hygiene and removal of irritation. Antibiotics usually are unnecessary. Pinworm infestations, when present, must be eradicated. Sitz baths two or three times a day, the application of a protective ointment (plain Lassar's paste, half strength) to the vulva, then good local cleansing once a day is usually sufficient. When inflammation of vulvovaginal tissues is intense, the oral administration of appropriate antibiotics gives more prompt relief than do local measures alone.

Estrogen therapy is indicated for persistent or recurrent vaginitis because cornification of the epithelium and reduction of the vaginal pH increases local tissue resistance. Steroidal estrogen such as Premarin, with dosage adjusted to size of the patient, is usually given daily for 21 days. Oral preparations are as effective as suppositories and far more readily accepted. Breast stimulation may occur but is reversed when the hormone is discontinued.

MONILIAL VAGINITIS. Candidiasis is uncommon except in diabetic children and in children following antibiotic administration. A urine or blood glucose determination is indicated in every case.

TRICHOMONAS. *Trichomonas* infections are rare, but, when present, trichomonads are usually found in the urine as well as in the vaginal discharge. Treatment with metronidazole is effective.

VAGINAL FOREIGN BODY. The presence of a persistent vaginal discharge accompanied by pain suggests a foreign body. Endoscopic inspection of the vaginal canal and combined rectovaginal palpation offer the best means of localization. X-ray film or ultrasound examination is necessary if the foreign body has migrated into adjacent tissues. A nonspecific vaginitis occurs secondarily and requires treatment.

LICHEN SCLEROSUS. Lichen sclerosus usually is diagnosed in older women, but it sometimes occurs in children. It is discussed in detail in Chapter 44. Surgery, other than biopsy for diagnosis, is contraindicated.

LABIAL AGGLUTINATION. Labial agglutination may occur congenitally or as the result of infection or irritation, which denudes the thin membrane and leads to adhesion of the labia minora in the midline. A characteristic livid line, extending vertically down the center of the membrane, distinguishes agglutination from the less commonly encountered imperforate hymen or vaginal atresia.

This condition is self-limiting and disappears as puberty approaches and estrogen levels rise, but it usually should be treated before that because the agglutination encourages pocketing of urine, irritation, and infection.

Application of an estrogen cream twice daily induces cornification of the epithelium, and spontaneous separation will usually occur within 2 weeks. Reagglutination can be prevented by regular perineal cleansing.

On rare occasions the agglutination does not respond to estrogen. The labia can be separated by quick, firm pressure on the adherent area with a small probe (Fig. 3-4). Reagglutination can be prevented by local estrogen ointment until the raw areas heal and by regular perineal cleansing.

PROLAPSED URETHRA. Bleeding, the appearance of a mass at the vaginal orifice, and pain, particularly with micturition, suggest prolapse of the urethral mucosa (Fig. 3-5). The congested edematous mass may occlude the vaginal orifice and is likely to be misinterpreted as vaginal prolapse or genital tumor. Although no lumen is visible, a lubricated

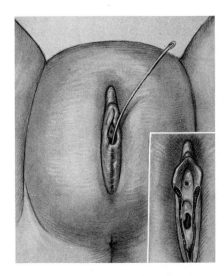

Fig. 3-4. Labial agglutination. Separation by pressure on probe is rarely necessary.

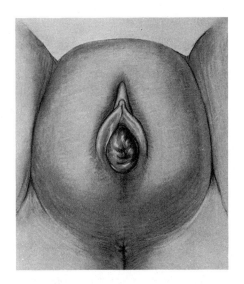

Fig. 3-5. Prolapsed urethra.

catheter inserted in the center of the mass will seek the bladder and confirm the diagnosis.

Reduction of the prolapse can be accomplished occasionally; but necrosis often is present, and excision of the redundant tissue at the meatal line of demarcation is necessary. An indwelling catheter should be left in place overnight. Recurrences or late sequelae are unusual.

TRAUMA. Most injuries to the female genitals produce no permanent damage. Bleeding can usually be controlled by pressure. Deep lacerations requiring suturing heal with little scarring. The location of the urethra provides protection against actual injury, but urinary retention as a result of edema and spasm is not uncommon. Reassuring the parents that local genital injuries will not interfere with future functions is one of the most important aspects of treatment.

Trauma caused by *rape* can be a devastating experience for a young child. Team approach, including physician, nurse, psychiatrist, and security officer, is vital to management of the overall problem in order to begin dealing promptly with potentially long-term psychosocial effects of rape. If trauma is marked or if bleeding persists, examination under anesthesia is necessary to rule out upper genital tears or penetration of the peritoneal cavity.

In the usual case, rape results in circumferential tears, abrasions, and ecchymosis. These evidences or the demonstration of sperm about the genitals are indications for prophylactic penicillin therapy. A single 2 ml injection of long-acting penicillin containing 600,000 U/ml should provide protection against either gonorrhea or syphilis. Since normal variations in patency of the hymenal ring can be misleading to the most experienced examiner, the diagnosis of sexual assault should not be made in the absence of characteristic signs (Chapter 6).

CONGENITAL ANOMALIES

Because of the close embryologic relationship of the genital and urinary tracts, developmental anomalies observed in one system warrant thorough examination of both.

Imperforate hymen. Imperforate hymen is an exception in that it usually occurs as an isolated anomaly. Surgical correction is desirable when the diagnosis is made but is imperative at puberty. Simple puncture of the membrane will heal over and is inadequate. Cruciate incisions across the membrane will maintain patency.

Vaginal agenesis. Complete vaginal agenesis is gener-

ally associated with absent or rudimentary development of the uterus and tubes. Ovarian development usually is normal. It is unlikely that a rudimentary uterus will respond to stimulation, and the need for providing a menstrual outlet arises only on the rare occasion when the uterus is normal. Although the karyotype is usually that of normal 46 XX women, a mosaicism has been reported occasionally. Extragenital anomalies involving the urinary tract, the skeletal system, and the ear are found in approximately one third of cases. Periodic examinations during adolescence will clarify the status of the uterus and at the same time offer opportunities to assist the young girl's social adjustment when necessary and to make psychologic preparation for future treatment. There are several operative and nonoperative methods for correcting this defect. With gradual dilatation method in 21 patients, Rock and co-workers achieved functional success in nine cases (43%), whereas all 79 cases treated surgically with the authors' modifications of the McIndoe technique were functionally successful. The procedure selected should be performed soon after puberty.

Ectopic ureter with vaginal terminus. Ectopic ureter in the female most often terminates in the vaginal vault or the vestibule; hence there usually is constant loss of urine from the vagina. If the terminus is closed, the *ureterocele* thus formed appears as a cystic mass that protrudes from

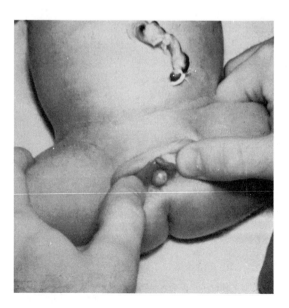

Fig. 3-6. Ectopic ureter with ureterocele.

the vagina (Fig. 3-6). This is the most common "vaginal cyst" in infants. If the ectopic ureter is patent, constant irritation from urine promotes infection, and a vaginitis may be the first sign.

Direct visualization of a vaginal ureteral orifice is frequently impossible, even with anesthesia. Instillation of methylene blue into the bladder will rule out a vesicovaginal communication. X-ray film examination after the instillation of radiopaque media into the vagina and into the ectopic channel, if possible, and intravenous pyelography will outline both tracts most effectively. It is imperative that the entire urinary system be visualized before surgery. Removal of the ectopic ureter and the associated portion of the kidney is the treatment of choice.

Vaginal ectopic anus. Imperforate anus associated with a rectovaginal communication in the female infant represents erratic migration of the hindgut, occurring by 6 to 8 weeks of embryonic life (Fig. 3-7).

A skin dimple is visible at the normal anal site, surrounded by an intact external sphincter muscle. The rectum ends blindly above this area, and a fistulous tract passes forward to the genital region at various levels from the posterior fornix to the perineum. A few muscle fibers usually surround the opening and prevent gross incontinence.

If the fistulous tract and its orifice provide an adequate lumen, correction should be deferred until definitive measures are feasible. Mobilization of the rectum downward and backward through the external sphincter can then be performed.

NEOPLASMS

Tumors of the genital tract are important not because of their frequency but because of their highly malignant potential. An exception is the high frequency of benign vaginal and cervical lesions found in young women exposed to diethylstilbestrol (DES) during the first 18 weeks of intrauterine life and the unusual but significant occurrence of clear cell adenocarcinoma of the vagina or cervix in DES-exposed women. Herbst and coworkers, who first perceived an association between DES and this rare vaginal malignancy, expeditiously established a Registry of Clear Cell Adenocarcinoma of the Genital Tract in Young Females in 1971. Data from this source and from numerous screening clinics throughout the country provide the rationale for examination and management of young women at risk.

VAGINAL ADENOSIS AND CERVICAL ECTOPY

Characteristic benign lesions found in at least 80% of women with a history of *fetal exposure to DES* or related synthetic nonsteroidal estrogens, and anatomic deformities found in about 20%, give clear evidence of the teratogenic potential of this group of drugs. Remnants of müllerian anlage persist beneath the vaginal plate of squamous epithelium where glandular elements are not normally found. Most of the glands are lined by mucin-

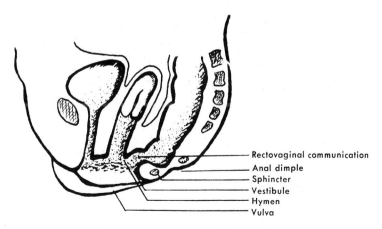

Rectovaginal communication
Anal dimple
Sphincter
Vestibule
Hymen
Vulva

Fig. 3-7. Vaginal ectopic anus.

secreting columnar cells resembling those of the endocervix. In some the lining cells are smaller and resemble tubal or endometrial cells. They may be completely buried beneath the vaginal epithelium, but often ostia of the glands and their secretions are visible on the surface.

Eversion, or ectropion, of the cervix is common. Deformities of the vagina or cervix occur mainly in the form of transverse ridges. The terms, "ridges," "vaginal hood," "cervical collar," and "cockscomb cervix" are used, depending on the appearance and extent of the deformity (Fig. 3-8).

Upper genital tract abnormalities also occur more frequently in exposed females. These include reduced size and shape of the uterus, synechiae, and constricting bands. The incidence of premature labors and pregnancy failures caused by uterine abnormalities and by incompetence of an anomalous cervical os is increased.

Effects on intrauterine-exposed males are controversial. McGill, Schumacher, and Bibbo and

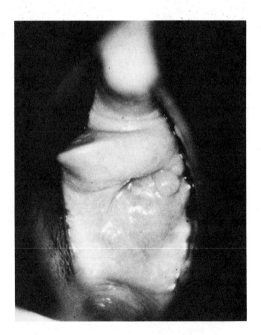

Fig. 3-8. Colposcopic appearance of cervix and upper vagina in 19-year-old woman exposed to DES in utero. Note anterior cervical abnormality (cockscomb) and adenosis of posterior cervix and upper vagina.

other investigators have reported an increased occurrence of morphologic and functional abnormalities in DES-exposed males. Epididymal cysts, hypoplastic testes, and capsular induration of the testes were found in 25.8% of the study group as compared with 6.8% of controls. Low sperm counts were observed in 29% of the study patients and in none of the controls. Neoplasms have not been reported. Leary and associates could not confirm these findings. Their study of 828 DES-exposed males failed to show an increased risk of genitourinary abnormalities or sterility as compared with 677 matched controls. They also concluded that the risk of neoplastic growths was not increased.

CLEAR CELL ADENOCARCINOMA

More than 90% of the young women exposed to DES in utero who subsequently develop this rare type of lower genital tract malignancy have reached puberty or beyond. Ages at the time of diagnosis range from 7 to 29 years. It is therefore likely that stimulation of the anomalous glandular epithelium plays a key role in their growth. The risk of adenocarcinoma in DES-exposed women was estimated by Herbst and associates to be between 1.4/1000 to 1.4/10,000 exposed females. By 1984 the National Collaborative DES Adenosis Project had accumulated large numbers of DES-exposed and matched control cases who were examined annually over a 7-year period. These studies indicate that the incidence of cervical dysplasia and carcinoma in situ, calculated as the number of cases per 1000 person years of follow-up, was 15.7 in those who had been exposed to DES and 7.9 in controls.

Neoplastic lesions arise most commonly in the upper half of the vagina or in the cervix. They may be polypoid or nodular, friable, and hemorrhagic (Fig. 3-9). Clear, hobnail-shaped cells are most characteristic, although some lesions appear highly undifferentiated with solid, papillary, or cystic areas. Vaginal adenosis occurs in proximity to the tumor in almost all instances, but transition of the benign to a malignant lesion has not been demonstrated. Metastasis occurs locally at first and then in the regional or paraaortic nodes. Pulmonary and supraclavicular node metastases occur frequently in recurrent disease.

Examination and management of DES-exposed women. Every young woman whose mother received DES during pregnancy should be considered at risk of adenosis or adenocarcinoma of the lower genital tract. All should be examined regardless of age if symptoms appear, otherwise beginning about age 12 to 14, before the risk of malignancy becomes significant. Symptoms are vaginal bleeding, discharge, or pain, although about 20% of malignant and most benign lesions are asymptomatic.

The screening pelvic examination includes direct visual inspection, which may reveal patchy red areas of adenosis, cervical ectropion or eversion, or marked mucus secretion. Because adenosis may be entirely submucosal, palpation of the entire vagina is necessary to detect small nodular structures.

Cytologic examination is not wholly reliable for diagnosis of this malignancy. False-negative results have been found in approximately 20% of cases.

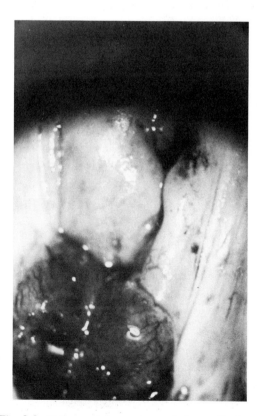

Fig. 3-9. Colposcopic appearance of clear cell adenocarcinoma of vagina in 16-year-old girl exposed to DES in utero. Vascularity is prominent.

This can be minimized if material for smears is obtained by direct scraping of visible lesions, the upper vagina, and the cervix rather than by swabbing. Application of Schiller's solution or half-strength Lugol's solution to the cervix and vagina will delineate abnormal nonglycogenated areas. Biopsies should be obtained from areas that appear suspicious or that fail to take the iodine stain. *Colposcopic examination* has proved to be of particular value in diagnosis of adenosis, interpretation of findings in the surrounding transformation zone of squamous metaplasia or dysplasia, and in selection of suspicious areas for biopsy.

Treatment of adenosis is conservative, with follow-up examinations at 6- to 12-month intervals. Improvement with time or after pregnancy is not uncommon. This is observed particularly in cases with extensive cervical ectopy and apparent deformity of the cervix. Replacement of columnar epithelium by squamous metaplasia and a smoothing of cervical ridges have been observed within a 3- to 5-year period.

If adenocarcinoma is diagnosed early, cures have been effected in a high percentage of cases primarily by surgical therapy. Because metastasis in recurrent disease is so frequently to the lung and supraclavicular nodes, clinical and x-ray film examinations of these areas should be included in the follow-up. Fortunately, a high proportion of patients seek a physician at an early stage of the disease. In the analysis by Herbst and co-workers of 346 cases, 54% were stage I. The 5-year survival rate for all 346 patients was 78%.

MIXED MESODERMAL TUMORS

Sarcoma botryoides arises from mesenchymal tissue of the cervix or vagina and appears as an edematous grapelike mass of tissue that bleeds readily on touch (Fig. 3-10). Extension proceeds locally, involving all pelvic structures. Distant metastasis is not characteristic. The neoplasm is resistant to x-ray or radium therapy and curable only by early radical extirpation.

Ovarian neoplasms are occasionally encountered in preadolescents. Dermoid cyst is the most common type

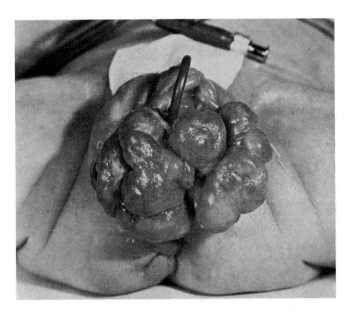

Fig. 3-10. Sarcoma botryoides.

and is more likely to cause symptoms as a result of torsion rather than size. Karrer and Swenson reported a case of twisted ovarian cyst in a newborn infant and reviewed 25 cases of ovarian cysts in infants under 1 year of age. Feminizing tumors must be considered in connection with precocious puberty in the young girl. Masculinizing tumors are discussed later in this chapter.

Abell and Holtz studied 188 primary ovarian neoplasms from patients under the age of 20 years. Forty percent of these were of nongerm cell origin, the majority arising from coelomic epithelium or its derivatives. The behavior of these and 113 germ cell neoplasms found in young girls is discussed in detail by the authors.

ABNORMAL SEXUAL DEVELOPMENT

Classification of intersexual states is based on morphologic criteria, including (1) sex chromatin, (2) sex chromosomal constitution, (3) structure of the gonads, (4) structure of internal genital organs, and (5) structure of external genital organs. Management of intersexual problems, however, is influenced by the hormonal status evoked by the disorder and by psychologic factors, the sex of rearing, and the gender role. *The types of sexual abnormalities encountered can be characterized in terms of the three distinctive stages of sexual development: (1) gonadal, (2) differentiation of the internal genitals,* and *(3) differentiation of the external genitals.*

Genetic sex is determined at the time of fertilization. The sequence of events leading to gonadal differentiation begins with the appearance of the undifferentiated gonad at the fourth week of embryonic life: the germ cells then migrate from the entoderm to the yolk sac along the hindgut and beyond to enter the primitive gonad; finally, gonadal sex is determined by the sex-controlling genes in the X and Y chromosomes. The Y chromosome, or a specific portion (pericentric), must be present to induce development of the testis. An H-Y histocompatibility antigen, the location of which has been recently identified near the testis-determining gene on the Y chromosome, appears to play a determinant role in gonadal differentiation. At about 7 to 8 weeks after conception, the seminiferous tubules and then Leydig cells appear, and the latter begin to produce testosterone, which is essential for any further male development.

Both wolffian (mesonephric) and müllerian (paramesonephric) ducts are present in the early embryo. Differentiation of the internal genitals is controlled by hormones, but female development can proceed autonomously. Early in embryonic life the testis produces *müllerian-inhibiting substance,* which causes regression of the müllerian ducts. The early testis also produces testosterone, the essential factor in differentiation of the wolffian ducts into vas deferens, epididymis, and seminal vesicles. If an ovary is present or even in its absence, as in ovarian agenesis XO, the wolffian system, lacking testosterone stimulation, regresses; and the müllerian duct differentiates into uterus, fallopian tubes, and upper vagina.

The last stage, or differentiation of the external genitals, involves common primordial structures in both sexes. Androgen stimulation of the genital tubercle, folds, and swellings is essential for differentiation into male external genitals; otherwise, female phenotypia prevails. During intrauterine life, masculinization of the female external genitals is caused by androgen excess (congenital adrenal hyperplasia) or by the effects of maternal androgenic drugs or masculinizing tumors. The internal genitals are unaffected and remain distinctly female in the absence of a testis and testicular production of müllerian-inhibiting substance.

Certain intersexual states are not evident until puberty, when hormonal effects on secondary sex characteristics are inappropriate or lacking. These include gonadal dysgenesis without other physical stigmata, testicular feminization, Klinefelter's syndrome, and mild forms of congenital adrenal hyperplasia with postpubertal virilization.

Sexual ambiguity of the newborn

The proper *assignment of sex of the newborn infant* is one of the first obligations of the obstetrician. Cases of doubtful sex noted at birth involve abnormalities in development of the external genitals, and these fall into four main groups: (1) *congenital adrenal hyperplasia,* (2) *nonadrenal masculinization caused by maternal environmental factors,* (3) *male pseudohermaphroditism with incomplete development of the external genitals,* and (4) *true hermaphroditism.*

Congenital adrenal hyperplasia is the most frequent cause of distinct virilization of the newborn infant. The

disorder is an inborn error in metabolism and may be hereditary. There is impairment or block of the synthesis of cortisol caused by specific defects in steroid hydroxylating enzyme.

In order of frequency, deficits occur in C-21 hydroxylase, C-11 hydroxylase, and 3-beta-ol dehydrogenase. Impairment of C-21 hydroxylation of the 17-alpha-hydroxyprogesterone is followed by diminution in the biosynthesis of deoxycortisol (compound S) and in turn by reduction in cortisol. Since the rate of adrenocorticotropic hormone (ACTH) secretion by the pituitary is regulated by cortisol feedback, diminution of this hormone results in excessive ACTH secretion and overstimulation of the adrenal glands, with resultant hyperplasia of the zona reticularis. Overproduction of androgenic hormones ensues in response to ACTH stimulation, since the metabolic pathway for these end products remains unimpaired.

When deficit of C-21 hydroxylase is incomplete, the condition is known as *compensated congenital adrenal hyperplasia,* and the clinical characteristics are limited to virilization. In approximately a third of cases the deficit is so great that virilization is accompanied by the *salt-losing syndrome* resulting from critical reduction of cortisol. This aspect of congenital adrenal hyperplasia may be temporary or permanent in nature in contrast to the virilization that is always progressive if untreated.

The clinical characteristics in the newborn are shown in Fig. 3-11. These include relative persistence of the urogenital sinus, accentuation of the labial folds, and enlargement of the clitoris. A small vagina usually communicates with the urethra. The single opening is located at the base of the enlarged clitoris and suggests hypospadias. The appearance can be so perplexing that determination of sex on the basis of external examination alone is impossible. Chromosome studies for determination of sex, rectal palpation of the uterus, and visualization of the cervix by endoscopy or the urinary and genital tracts by x-ray film examination after radiopaque instillation aid in diagnosis (Fig. 3-12). Elevated 17-ketosteroid and pregnanetriol levels are diagnostic. Amounts of pregnanetriol normally excreted by the female are insignificant up to the the age of 10 years.

Treatment. Cortisone will reverse the symptoms. Early diagnosis of sex and the establishment of a plan for the child's future are of the utmost importance. Surgical correction includes excision of the clitoris, which should be done before the age of 3 years, and reconstruction of the vagina when the need arises. Cortisone therapy must be continued, and at puberty oral estrogens can be added

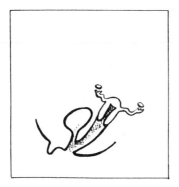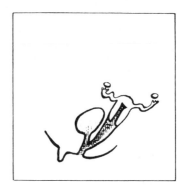

Fig. 3-11. Persistence of urogenital sinus in females with congenital adrenal hyperplasia; these are usual sites of communication between urethra and vagina.

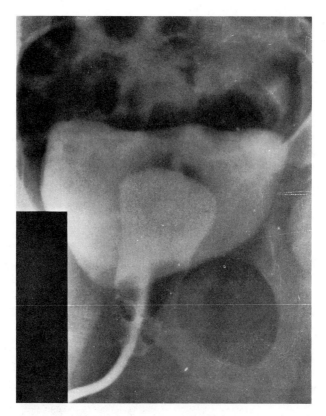

Fig. 3-12. Female pseudohermaphrodite. Retrograde instillation of dye through persistent urogenital sinus. Vagina and lower urinary tracts are visualized separately above common perineal opening.

to the therapeutic regimen to improve development of the secondary sex characteristics.

Adrenal tumors. Virilizing symptoms appearing in young children are far less likely to be caused by adrenocortical tumor than by hyperplasia. Administration of cortisone helps in the differential diagnosis, since the marked reduction in 17-ketosteroid levels that characteristically occurs in patients with hyperplasia has little or no effect on high levels when a tumor is present. Of eight cases of these tumors found by Lee, Winter, and Green in children aged 15 months to 5 years, five were females. Virilization was present in all instances; and in most cases a cushingoid appearance, rarely seen in childhood, was apparent. Excessive linear growth is also common despite hypercortisolism. Serum cortisol and androgen levels were elevated in all cases. None of the tumors was suppressible in response to cortisone. Unless the tumor is small, ultrasound or computed tomography is a useful aid in diagnosis. Small tumors may be identified by arteriography.

Treatment requires surgical removal with preoperative administration of stress dosages of cortisone that are tapered off during the postoperative period. Of the eight cases, six tumors were adrenal adenomas, two showing pleomorphism; and two were adenocarcinomas.

Nonadrenal virilization. Masculinization of the female fetus can occur when certain progestins are administered to the expectant mother during early pregnancy. Except for the importance of accurate diagnosis, this type of masculinization does not pose a serious problem, since effects are limited to the external genitals.

The clitoris is enlarged, and the labial folds may be firmly fused in the midline, giving an ambiguous impression of the sex (Fig. 3-13). There is no interference with differentiation of the müllerian and wolffian ducts; and therefore the vagina, uterus, and tubes are normal. The fetal ovary is unaffected.

In contrast to adrenal female pseudohermaphroditism, progressive virilization does not occur. Instead, growth and development are normal; secondary sex changes and menstrual and reproductive functions are not affected, although the latter aspect deserves further exploration as most of these individuals reach maturity.

Diagnosis is made by (1) buccal smear, which should show chromatin-positive nuclei characteristic of normal females; (2) normal 17-ketosteroids and pregnanetriol excretion; and (3) a history of oral or intramuscular administration of progestins to the expectant mother before the twelfth and through the fifteenth or sixteenth week of gestation, usually for threatened or habitual abortion.

Treatment begins with reassurance of the parents. Removal of the clitoris if significantly enlarged and surgical correction of the fused labia are not difficult and should

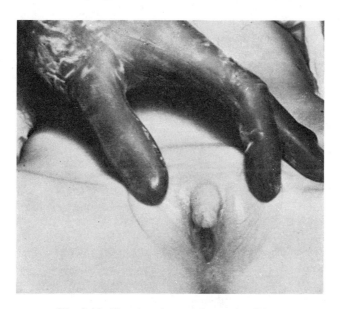

Fig. 3-13. Nonadrenal pseudohermaphroditism.

be done before the age of 3 years. Hormone therapy is not needed.

Male pseudohermaphroditism. Physical characteristics of individuals with male pseudohermaphroditism show gradations of abnormality. The external genitals may appear feminine, doubtful, or masculine. The feminine type, *testicular feminizing syndrome,* is most common.

For the types in which feminization is incomplete, extreme caution in the assignment of sex is particularly urgent in this condition.

A buccal smear for sex chromatin analysis is negative, since the chromosomal complement is usually 46 XY and one is tempted to make an assignment of male sex on this cursory examination; yet subsequent development tends to proceed along female lines. This problem is discussed in Chapter 9.

The assignment of a contradictory sex at birth is a difficult commitment for both the physician and the family. In difficult problems such as this the final solution should not be reached without recourse to the many sources of information now available in the fields of cytogenetics, endocrinology, and psychosexual development.

True hermaphroditism, in which both male and female gonads are present, is rare. In the newborn infant there are no distinguishing physical chromosomal or hormonal changes that can be considered diagnostic of true hermaphroditism. Since the testicular androgens are responsible for masculinization of the external genitals, and since testicular tissue is present in true hermaphroditism, it is not surprising that male external genital configuration predominates in a ratio of approximately 3:1. Yet it is of the utmost importance to establish the dominant sex as soon after birth as possible so that the optimal choice of gender may be made. Both the confirmation of diagnosis and the treatment require laparoscopy or laparotomy.

Treatment consists of removal of the contradictory gonad. Hormone therapy may be necessary at puberty if the appearance of appropriate secondary sex characteristics is delayed.

Sexual precocity

Manifestations of precocious puberty are either isosexual or heterosexual. *Isosexual types* in the female child are dependent on early or abnormal estrogen stimulation that may be pituitary (constitutional), neurogenic, or ovarian in origin. Effects are entirely feminizing. *Heterosexual types,* resulting in virilization, are usually caused by increased adrenocortical activity.

True and pseudoisosexual precocity. The onset of puberty has a wide normal range. Early appearance of secondary sex characteristics usually represents *sensitive end-organ response* to minimal hormone stimulation, but the occurrence of the menarche before the age of 10 years is unusual and deserves investigation.

The most common type of isosexual precocious puberty is "constitutional," in which *idiopathic hypothalamic-pituitary-ovarian activation* occurs. No abnormalities other than early maturity are associated. Hypothalamic, pituitary, ovarian, and adrenal hormones reach normal adult levels; menstruation is ovulatory; and pregnancy is possible. Rarely, *central nervous system lesions* may produce true isosexual precocity and result in full maturation with normal hormonal relationships.

Social adjustment poses the most serious problem for these children. Sexual awakening and receptivity are far in advance of mental and emotional maturity. Children with idiopathic precocious puberty can be treated with medroxyprogesterone acetate (Depo-Provera), 400 mg, intramuscularly every 2 to 4 months. This will inhibit gonadotropin secretion, menstruation, and breast development. The medication should be continued until bone age and chronologic age are compatible. Another type of treatment is the administration of long-acting gonadotropin-releasing hormone (GnRH) agonists, which reverse all the precocious changes.

Precocious sexual development and uterine bleeding resulting from *feminizing tumors of the ovary* are estrogen induced and anovulatory. Hence pregnancy does not occur, but in other respects clinical features of this type of precocity do not differ from other isosexual varieties.

Examination under anesthesia may reveal an ovarian mass, but in some instances actively functioning feminizing tumors are too small to be outlined. Under these circumstances it may be difficult to differentiate ovarian and constitutional types. In ovarian types the vaginal smear shows a more pronounced unopposed estrogen effect with consistent cornification throughout the cycle, and gonadotropin excretion is low or absent. In association with constitutional precocious puberty the vaginal smear usually shows less pronounced cornification, and there are cyclic changes; gonadotropin excretion attains mature levels. When the diagnosis cannot be otherwise made, laparotomy is indicated. Removal of the involved ovary results in cessation of bleeding, but regression of secondary sex characteristics may be incomplete.

Rarer causes for pseudoprecocity include advanced *hypothyroidism, estrogen-producing adrenal tumors,* and *Albright's syndrome.*

Heterosexual precocity. Virilization is the striking manifestation of heterosexual precocity and is usually caused by an adrenal lesion. When evident at birth, congenital adrenal hyperplasia is most likely, whereas after the first year of life the onset of an adrenogenital syndrome is usually caused by an adrenal tumor or a mild delayed type of adrenal hyperplasia. Virilization appearing in puberty and in early adulthood is associated with adrenal or ovarian tumors, the incomplete form of male pseudohermaphroditism, and delayed or acquired adrenal hyperplasia. These disorders and their management are discussed earlier in this chapter and in Chapters 9 and 48.

GYNECOLOGIC PROBLEMS IN ADOLESCENT GIRLS

Menarche. The sequence of events leading to the menarche, or first menstrual period, is illustrated in Fig. 3-14. Characteristic body changes precede the menarche by several years. Various factors—genetic, socioeconomic, and general health of the individual—influence the age of onset of menstruation.

There is increasing evidence that the primary stimulus for initiation of these changes originates in the hypothalamus and is mediated through the pituitary gland. Harris transplanted the pituitary from prepubertal rats into adult female hypophysectomized hosts and found that estrus cycles were resumed and pregnancies achieved. In the human, pituitary hormones that are low during childhood show a sharp rise 1 to 4 years before the menarche. Increasing amounts of estrogenic and androgenic hormones are secreted, and secondary sex changes become apparent.

Growth spurt is greatest during this time, the protein requirement being three times that of the adult. Growth continues for another 3 years or so

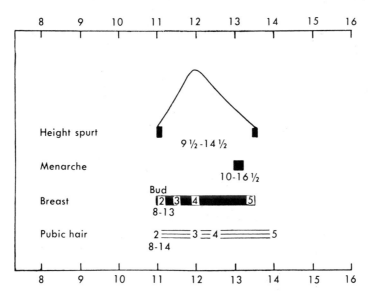

Fig. 3-14. Diagram of sequence of events of adolescence in girls. An average girl is represented; range of ages within which some events may occur is given by figures placed below them. (From Tanner, J.M.: Growth at adolescence, ed. 2, Oxford, England, 1962, Blackwell Scientific Publications, Ltd.)

after the onset of menstruation, but the rate is slower and rarely exceeds 5 cm (2 inches). Ossification centers gradually disappear, and growth is complete. Thus girls in whom the menarche occurs at an early age are likely to be shorter as adults than those in whom its appearance is late.

Apparently, there is considerable variation in the sensitivity of breast tissue and the pubic hair follicles to stimulation by estrogen and androgen, respectively. This phenomenon explains the early appearance of breast development and pubic hair growth in many girls in whom endocrine function and onset of menstruation are normal.

EARLY MENARCHE. The onset of menstruation before the age of 10 years is precocious and should be investigated. This problem is discussed under abnormal sexual development in this chapter.

LATE MENARCHE. Absence of menstruation beyond the sixteenth year, *primary amenorrhea,* should be considered abnormal, and the possibility of a disorder of genetic origin should be given careful consideration in all such cases. Chromosomal abnormalities are found in approximately 40% of phenotypic females in whom menarche is delayed beyond the sixteenth year. Instances in which the menarche has occurred as late as the twenties are rare.

Primary amenorrhea is discussed in detail in Chapter 9.

Adolescent dysfunctional uterine bleeding. Menstrual irregularities, so common at this time of life, are usually the result of fluctuating, unopposed estrogen production by the immature, nonovulating ovary; but even in young girls the possibility of systemic or pelvic lesions must be eliminated before the diagnosis of dysfunctional uterine bleeding is made.

Although a reasonable time must be allowed for the establishment of a full ovulatory cycle, adolescent dysfunctional uterine bleeding is not necessarily self-limiting. In a long-range study of 538 adolescents with menstrual disorders conducted by Southam and Richart, 291 cases were diagnosed as dysfunctional uterine bleeding. The follow-up period was as long as 25 years. These authors showed that, if symptoms persist for a period of 4 years or more, there is a fifty-fifty chance for future irregularities, a diminution in reproductive potential, and an increased risk of uterine neoplasm.

Abnormal bleeding is discussed in detail in Chapter 8.

Dysmenorrhea. Primary dysmenorrhea, the most common menstrual disorder in adolescent girls, is discussed in detail in Chapter 10.

REFERENCES

Abell, M.R., and Holtz, F.: Ovarian neoplasms in childhood and adolelscence. II. Tumors of non-germ cell origin, Am. J. Obstet. Gynecol. **93:**850, 1965.

Bongiovanni, A.M., and Eberlein, W.R.: Symposium: adrenal steroids; defects in steroidal metabolism of subjects with adrenogenital syndrome, Metabolism **10:**917, 1961.

Capraro, V.J., editor: Pediatric and adolescent gynecology, Clin. Obstet. Gynecol. **20:**531-663, 1977.

Carrington, E.R.: Laboratory examination of the pediatric gynecologic patient, Symposium on Pediatric and Adolescent Gynecology, Ann. N.Y. Acad. Sci. **142:**623, 1967.

Golden, N., Hammerslag, M., Neuhoff, S., and Gleyzer, A.: Prevalence of *Chlamydia trachomatis* cervical infection in female adolescents, Am. J. Dis. Child. **138:**562, 1984.

Hanssen, W.P., Westrom, L., and Mardh, P.-A.: Perihepatic and chlamydial salpingitis, Lancet **1:**901, 1980.

Harris, G.W.: Neural control of the pituitary gland, London, 1955, E. Arnold, Ltd.

Herbst, A.L., Cole, P., Colton, T., Robboy, S.J., and Scully, R.E.: Age-incidence and risk of DES-related clear cell adenocarcinoma of the vagina and cervix, Am. J. Obstet. Gynecol. **128:**43, 1977.

Herbst, A.L., Kurman, R.J., Scully, R.E., and Poskanzer, D.C.: Clear-cell adenocarcinoma of the genital tract in young females; registry report, N. Engl. J. Med. **287:**1259, 1972.

Herbst, A.L., Norusis, M.J., Rosenow, P.J., Welcj, W.R., and Scully, R.E.: An analysis of 346 cases of clear cell adenocarcinoma of the vagina and cervix with emphasis on recurrence and survival, Gynecol. Oncol. **7:**111, 1979.

Jones, G.S.: Diagnostic evaluation of patients with intersexuality, Symposium on Pediatric and Adolescent Gynecology, Ann. N.Y. Acad. Sci. **142:**729, 1967.

Jones, H.W., and Heller, R.H.: Pediatric and adolescent gynecology, Baltimore, 1966, The Williams & Wilkins Co.

Kaufman, R.H., Binder, G.H., Gray, P.M., and Adam, E.: Upper genital tract changes associated with exposure in utero to DES, Am. J. Obstet. Gynecol. **128:**51, 1977.

Karrer, F.W., and Swenson, S.A.: Twisted ovarian cyst in a newborn infant, Arch. Surg. **83:**143, 1961.

Koo, G.C., Wachtel, S.S., Krupen-Brown, K., Mittl, L.R., Breg, W.R., Genel, M., Rosenthal, I.M., Borgaonkar, D.S.,

Miller, A.D., Tantravahi, R., Schreck, R.R., Erlanger, B.F., and Miller, O.J.: Mapping the locus of the H-Y gene on the human Y chromosome, Science **198:**940, 1977.

Leary, F.J., Ressengule, L.J., Kurland, L.T., O'Brien, P.C., Emslander, R.F., and Noller, K.L.: Males exposed in utero to diethylstilbestrol, J.A.M.A. **252:**2984, 1984.

Lee, P.D.K., Winter, R.J., and Green, O.C.: Virilizing adrenocortical tumors in childhood: eight cases and a review of the literature, Pediatrics **76:**437, 1985.

McGill, W.B., Schumacher, G.F.B., and Bibbo, M.: Pathological semen and anatomical abnormalities in the genital tract in human male subjects exposed to DES in utero, J. Urol. **117:**477, 1977.

Mishell, Jr., D.R.: Disorders of sexual differentiation. In Mishell, D.R., Jr., and Davajan, V.: Reproductive endocrinology, infertility and contraception, Philadelphia, 1979, F.A. Davis Co.

Paradise, J.E., and Campos, J.M., Friedman, H.M., and Frishmuth, G.: Vulvovaginitis in premenarchal girls: clinical features and diagnostic evaluation, Pediatrics **70:**193, 1982.

Robboy, S.J., Noller, K.L., O'Brien, P., Kaufman, R.H., Townsend, D., Gundersen, J., Lawrence, W.D., Bergstral, E., McGorray, S., Tilley, B., Anton, J., and Chazen, G.: Increased risk of cervical and vaginal dysplasia in 3980 diethylstilbestrol-exposed young women: experience of the National Collaborative Diethylstilbestrol Adenosis Project, J.A.M.A. **252:**2979, 1984.

Rock, J.A., Reeves, L.A., Retto, H., Baremki, T.A., Zacur, H.A., and Jones, H.W., Jr.: Success following vaginal creation for müllerian agenesis, Fertil. Steril. **39:**809, 1983.

Southam, A.L., and Richart, R.M.: Prognosis for adolescents with menstrual abnormalities, Am. J. Obstet. Gynecol. **94:**637, 1966.

Tanner, J.M.: Growth at adolescence, ed. 2, Oxford, England, 1955, Blackwell Scientific Publications, Ltd.

Varner, R.E., Younger, J.B., and Blackwell, R.E.: Müllerian dysgenesis, J. Reprod. Med. **30:**443, 1985.

4

Michael J. Daly and Kathy Hotelling

Psychology and life stages of women

The physician who manages obstetric and gynecologic health problems appropriately must have a knowledge of psychology, as well as anatomy, physiology, and pathology. As the understanding of physiologic functions has expanded, physicians have learned that a complex feedback system, influenced by psychologic, physical, and sociocultural factors, exists. These factors can act independently and in combination to produce physical illness. Since sexuality and pregnancy, which are integral aspects of obstetrics and gynecology, are affected by this feedback system, an understanding of the psychology of women allows obstetrician-gynecologists to make more accurate diagnoses and to direct their therapeutic efforts in a more effective way than is otherwise possible. Special consideration must be directed toward life events and stages of individual and socially transmitted attitudes toward sexuality. Although this chapter cannot be exhaustive in exploring the components of women's psychology (numerous books have been written on this subject), the material covered here provides an introduction to and raises issues of particular relevance to obstetric and gynecologic care.

Traditionally, several assumptions about women and their physical and mental health have been made. These assumptions often operate to deny an individual's experience and thus influence treatment of health problems negatively. Women who are aware of these assumptions are hesitant to seek medical treatment because they fear that their individuality will not be taken into account and that the assumptions will bias their treatment. They may feel neither safe nor comfortable in seeking treatment unless an emergency arises. It is important for physicians to be aware of these societal assumptions and actively work to keep them from influencing their interactions with their female patients.

The first such assumption is that women's health concerns are often "all in their minds." Although physical health can be affected by mental health, this does not mean that psychologic processes automatically account for symptoms. Symptoms may be primarily from organic causes or from psychologic stress situations, but usually there is an interplay between psychologic and physical factors.

A second assumption is that all women are heterosexual. This is demonstrated when questions about sexuality, "intercourse," and birth control are asked. It is estimated that 10% of women are lesbians. Thus how one approaches questions related to sexuality is important, so that an atmosphere is created in which lesbians are comfortable in sharing their health concerns. For example, using a term such as "sexual partner" connotes the possibility of that person being male or female.

The question "Is birth control a concern to you?" is a better question to ask than "What kind of birth control do you use?" because it recognizes that not all women are sexually active with men. With an open mind concerning the sexual experiences of patients, gynecologists can provide the best possible treatment for them. A knowledge of the types of sexually transmitted diseases that lesbians are likely to acquire is essential.

A related assumption is that lesbians are promiscuous. As with heterosexual persons, lesbian life-styles include both monogamous and nonmonogamous ways of being.

Another unjustified assumption is that all women desire to have children. As more options become available to women, many are choosing to remain childless. On the other hand, lesbians may choose to have children, contrary to the belief that they do not have this interest.

THE WOMAN AND HER PHYSICIAN

The proper treatment of any obstetric or gynecologic patient is based on an understanding of the complex interplay of events and attitudes that affect her personality. The patient consults the phsician because she is concerned about her health. The cause of an illness, which is the primary concern of the physician, is less significant for the patient. She seeks reassurance and relief of symptoms. It is therefore important for the physician to recognize what motivates the patient to seek medical attention.

Almost every successful therapeutic outcome depends on the understanding and cooperation of the patient. She must follow instructions relating to medications and other therapy. To establish the best plan of management, the physician must try to understand the patient's emotional state. Frequently, this is done by intuition, but there should also be a more objective approach. Many physicians hesitate to explore a patient's emotional state because they do not know how to respond to the information that surfaces. They may also fear a negative reaction from the patient or fear that they may cause her additional discomfort. If the interview is conducted skillfully, the patient will usually realize

that the physician is seeking a more complete understanding of the factors contributing to her condition and is acting in her best interest. Some women, however, will not be open about their emotions. Their reluctance should be honored by the physician.

The evaluation of a patient's personality need not entail a lengthy study. The patient's verbal and nonverbal behavior often expresses how comfortable she is with herself and her physician. An observant physician will note her personal hygiene, her speech patterns (including speed, tone, hesitancy, and directness), and her body carriage, all of which serve as indicators of her emotional state. The initial impressions can be confirmed or refuted by later observations and by questions asked during the interview.

When the physician obtains a patient's history, he or she must realize that the patient brings with her a unique set of experiences and certain ingrained cultural attitudes about her body and her sexuality. Incidents of incest, rape, abortion, physical and emotional abuse, and other life experiences interact with cultural myths and attitudes about sex to produce her response to the physician and to the physical examination. Although her experiences and attitudes may not be pleasant or even socially acceptable, they involve important facets of her personality. They will also have a bearing on how she gives her medical history, responds to her physical examination, and participates in her treatment.

Important information to be obtained from the history includes the age when menstruation first began, how she felt about the first period, from whom she received her information about menstruation, and what the attitudes toward menstruation were among her parents, siblings, and friends.

Some patients may experience difficulty in discussing menstruation, especially with male physicians, because of the personal nature of this normal function and of various societal views toward it. Prejudice against the menstruating woman is evident in many cultures, even in the United States. She is often viewed as unclean or dangerous, and menstruation may be considered a reason for isolation. The physician should be aware that these societal attitudes may play a part in a woman's negative attitude toward herself and her body.

Important aspects of the patient's sexual life should also be discussed. These include the degree of sexual satisfaction and her response to it, any occurrences of rape or incest, sexual preference, pregnancies, and attitudes toward sexual relations. The degree of openness about sexual issues in the patient's family, culture, and religion will affect how she responds to the taking of this sexual history. Although it is now more acceptable to discuss sexual issues than it used to be, such discussions may remain taboo for some women, and questions may produce much anxiety. The timing and manner in which she first received information about sex will influence the patient's response. A young girl usually learns about sex and sexual attitudes from her mother, but she may have obtained additional information from siblings, friends, her father, and written materials.

A patient who is experiencing her first gynecologic examination is usually anxious and fearful. A thorough and frank explanation of the procedure before it commences and as it goes along will usually lessen her fear. For other patients, discussion of previous experiences with gynecologic examinations will help the physician understand the patient's response to the situation. The physician might even recommend several books that can help girls and women understand their bodies.

The patient's reactions during the physical examination should be observed closely. A pelvic examination can be difficult for women and physicians alike because of the sexual implications inherent in the situation. However, by approaching the examination in a professional and confident manner, the physician can reduce the patient's anxiety. He should tell her that her anxiety and concern about modesty are natural and will receive consideration. If she is unduly anxious or tense, the physician should stop the examination and discuss the source of tension. Occasionally, the physician is confronted with a woman who refuses a pelvic examination. No physician can assume responsibility for treating a patient who will not permit the examination necessary to make a diagnosis.

FEMININITY AND MASCULINITY

Society exerts a considerable influence on the expectations and therefore the personality characteristics and behavior of its members; this is reflected by the roles that it assigns to individuals. Until recently, women in our society have been expected to pursue the roles of wife and mother, whereas men were assigned the roles of worker and leader. As a result, femininity and masculinity have traditionally been viewed as mutually exclusive concepts with attendant expectations, behaviors, and personality characteristics being socially transmitted and attributed to females and males, respectively. *Femininity* refers to an expressive concern for others and includes such qualities as nurturance, passivity, gentleness, and dependence. *Masculinity* connotes an instrumental orientation (focus on meeting goals) and includes such qualities as ambition, independence, self-reliance, and leadership.

However, since the early 1960s, the women's movement, an increased number of households headed by females, and effective birth control have expanded the roles of women. With this expansion has come the concept of androgyny, which asserts that "feminity" and "masculinity" are not mutually exclusive categories and that both females and males can develop personality characteristics from each traditional arena. For example, careers for women have become commonplace; this has emphasized the need for assertive behavior and independence in women who choose this life-style.

Although the possibilities available to women are exciting, they also may be anxiety producing and frightening. No longer is a woman sure she will be, or wants to be, a mother; this in turn may affect her view of birth control, sterilization, and sexuality in general.

Even though more opportunities are available to women, parental expectations still influence the female child and may run counter to her internal needs and desires. This adds to the difficulty in carving out her life among the many possibilities and may cause emotional strain and ambivalence about her choices, including motherhood and sexuality.

Although societal and parental attitudes toward behavior are impactful, inherited anatomy and physiology cannot be discounted in their influence on the development of certain traits. Animal research indicates that there is a female brain and a male brain. These formations take place in the developing fetus under the influence of the sex hormones. Fetal androgens are necessary in rats and other animals for the development of the male brain and subsequent adult sex behavior. Studies of disorders of human sexual differentiation indicate that in humans, as well as in lower animals, there is a fetal organization of neural structures in the hypothalamus and that these portions of the brain are organized along male or female lines. These areas not only mediate hormonal and reproductive function but also influence behavior.

The reciprocal influence of body on mind should also be considered. A male has an observable organ, the penis, whereas a female's sexual organs for the most part are not observable. Sexual feelings of the male are easily identified with erection, whereas for the female sexual feelings are more difficult to identify with a particular bodily change. These differences may at times influence behavior. In addition, a woman is well aware that one of the possibilities of her body is to have children. As a result of this possibility, women have been encouraged to develop nurturance and other personality characteristics that promote caretaking of children.

In summary, personality characteristics of both females and males are strongly influenced by societal expectations and roles, as well as by anatomy. It must be recognized that there is a continuum of personality attributes that are available to both female and males and that preclude preconceived notions of how an individual "should" be.

LIFE STAGES OF THE FEMALE

The function of the genital system is reproduction—a function that is intimately interrelated with the psychology of women. Although the reproductive system is present at birth, it does not become operative until some years later. It is relatively dormant in childhood, is activated during puberty,

continues its activity during the reproductive years, and becomes relatively dormant again after menopause. Thus the sexual life cycle of the human female is divided into the following phases: (1) childhood, (2) puberty-adolescence, (3) maturity, (4) climacteric-menopause, and (5) postmenopause (senescence).

Childhood. During childhood, which is a period of general physical growth but of little genital development, the basic personality of the individual is established. The child's psychologic development is divided into oral, anal, phallic, and latency phases.

During the first 3 years of life the gender identity of the female is established. This gender identify is different from an awareness of sexual organs. Rather, it is an awareness derived from attitudes of the parents toward the child and from the identification models they appear to value.

In the earliest phase the infant forms an identification with the mother that prevents the child from distinguishing between itself and its mother. As the child matures, a gradual process of individualization takes place. This maturation process is different for girls and boys. To develop a masculine identity, boys must separate and differentiate themselves as separate individuals. Thus, whereas the daughter and mother must separate to some degree to allow the daughter to become a person in her own right, they also remain connected so that the daughter can have a role model. As a result, a girl's identity may be more difficult to achieve than that of a boy, since the psychologic developments are distinctly different. In a society in which separation and individuation are hallmarks of adulthood, a girl's connection to her mother can appear to some people to be a developmental failure. Also, although this connection will affect a female throughout the years, it may run counter to what she needs or wants for her own development.

During the *oral phase,* which lasts from birth to about 1½ years of age, the infant's primary concern is the satisfaction or dissatisfaction of the gastrointestinal system. The child also begins to learn to differentiate herself from the world around her.

During the *anal phase,* which lasts from 1½ to

3 years of age, the main concern is mastery of the musculature. This phase centers around the anal-urethral functions, since this is the first major area that parents expect the child to learn to control. Many of the woman's attitudes toward her genitals and sexuality have their roots in this phase because of the physical closeness of the anus, urethra, and vagina.

During the *phallic phase,* which lasts from 3 to 6 years of age, the child becomes interested in the genital organs and the differences between the sexes. Freud hypothesized that girls in this phase developed "penis envy," to which he ascribed great significance. Today, penis envy is seen less as a physical symbol connoting a woman's negative view of her body and sexuality than as a symbol of the powerlessness that women so often feel in the social realm.

During this phallic phase the young girl is attempting to solve oedipal conflicts revolving around her desire for her father. Masturbation occurs during this phase in both sexes, and parents may need help in understanding that this is a natural phenomenon.

During the *latency phase,* which lasts from 6 years of age to puberty, the young girl begins to apply her mastery of her body. She also changes focus from interpersonal relationships within the family to those in the outside world. She develops an interest in school and friends. Sexual interests, however, are sublimated by games, studies, and other social activities.

Adolescence. Adolescence is marked by the beginnings of sexual development. The sexual endocrine system matures and brings about many anatomic and psychologic changes. The most significant physical changes are growth of pubic and axillary hair, development of the breasts, and the onset of menstruation. These physical changes are accompanied by an upsurge in sexual feelings.

Adolescence is also a time when both girls and boys seek independence from their parents and turn to peer groups for support and role models. Peer groups exert a powerful influence and establish standards of behavior by which the adolescent practices being an adult. Adolescent girls continue to define their identity in the context of relationships, but the critical task is to separate themselves from the needs and expectations of parents and others. During this transition to adulthood, the adolescent girl is faced with a conflict between her own needs and those of others. This conflict is best exemplified by the girl who "lets" her boyfriend have intercourse with her even though she may not want to engage in it. Similar dilemmas often occur throughout a woman's life and can be the cause of great anxiety.

A young girl's *reactions to the first menstrual period* are determined by her preparation for the event and by her feelings about her own body. If she has not been told what to expect, she may believe that she has some kind of internal injury. Some girls have difficulty accepting menstruation because they cannot confront their impending adulthood and its attendant responsibilities, sexual and otherwise. Others may be disappointed because the miraculous changes they expected with this first sign of adulthood do not appear.

Ambivalent feelings about menstruation are reflected in its many nicknames such as "the curse," "being unwell," or "falling off the roof." None of these terms denotes a positive experience. In most primitive societies, actual taboos are connected with the menstrual period.

Many menstrual disorders arise from emotional factors rather than from pituitary or ovarian failures. Excessive tension such as that engendered by going away to school can cause a young girl to miss a period. Conversely, a postmenopausal woman who has been separated from important people in her life may experience vaginal bleeding. A woman with strong conflicts about becoming pregnant may even develop amenorrhea, as in pseudocyesis. The weight loss and nutritional imbalances of anorexia nervosa and bulimia, which are psychologic disorders primarily found in women, may be associated with amenorrhea and dysmenorrhea.

Physicians should help parents communicate to their daughters the fact that menstruation is not a sickness but a normal function. There need be no restrictions on physical activity during the menstrual period.

Adolescence is the time when young girls are in

need of sexual education. A parent's acceptance, warmth, and understanding are as important as factual data. Many parents do not know how to provide this education and will bring the adolescent girl to the physician for instruction. The physician's best approach is to find out first what the young girl knows and believes about sex. Misconceptions and unpleasant emotional reactions can then be addressed and dispelled.

Maturity. Maturity is the phase in which regular menstruation and reproduction are the chief functions of the genital system. This phase lasts about 35 years and is often spoken of as the childbearing years. Information about marriage and childbirth, contraception, and general health care should be made available to all women in this phase of life.

PREGNANCY. The ability to have children is important for many reasons. Many societies place great value on women who are fertile and consider infertility to be a reason for discarding a wife. In almost every culture, a woman's status is enhanced by her ability to have children. Many women have a sense of incompleteness if they cannot have children. It is an experience unique to their sex and a clear-cut sign of maturation. They may also have a deep emotional drive to reproduce something of themselves and to thus attain some assurance of immortality.

Like other developmental steps, pregnancy induces new conflicts and may precipitate the re-emergence of older, unresolved conflicts. Even though it is desired, it may also produce ambivalent feelings. This is because pregnant women may be concerned about future responsibilities, the effect of children on their careers, and the anticipated changes in her relationships with others. Children present a challenge to any woman's ability to give of herself. They also force her to fall back on her own life experiences. She may view her mother as a model to be copied or rejected. Pregnancy may conjure up fears of physical discomfort, pain, or injury that she may not want to accept because of difficulty during previous pregnancies or the feeling that a child is "not worth" the pain. These fears can be diminished by familiarizing her with the childbearing. Pregnancy may also arouse a woman's feelings of inadequacy. It is necessary for the

physician to observe the pregnant patient closely because of all the conflicting emotions that can arise. Positive feelings toward the pregnancy are appropriate, but negative reactions that the patient may be afraid or ashamed to express can cause physical symptoms.

Physicians should be aware of these influences and should not let personal beliefs and feelings about pregnancy determine his advice. An example is a sterilization request from a young woman who has had only one or two children or none at all. Many physicians consider this to be an indication for a psychiatric referral, but they should realize that this can be a healthy decision for many valid reasons.

In the *first trimester,* the child-to-be is not yet a reality for the expectant mother. The fetus is, in a sense, a part of her body rather than a separate individual. Her conflicting feelings about the pregnancy may cause the expectant mother to lose interest in her sexual partner, her family, and the world around her.

During the *middle trimester,* fetal movements, her increasing size, and other changes make the expectant mother aware that the child is a separate entity. She also begins to fantasize about the child. Physicians can help a woman make the emotional transition to motherhood by allowing her to hear the fetal heart sounds and by exhibiting an understanding attitude. Women may report either increased feelings of dependency or a desire to be alone at this time.

In the *last trimester,* the patient feels a mounting tension and increasing physical discomfort. She is usually eager for labor to begin. During this stage she may also develop fears of death during childbirth. These fears in turn may cause insomnia and depression.

During the patient's early visits, the physician must gradually get to know her and attempt to develop a feeling of trust. He should exhibit concern for the patient's well-being; for her diet, weight, and vitamin and iron intake; and for any medical complications she may exhibit.

During the second trimester, the physician or an obstetric nurse should begin to discuss breast-feeding, and the patient should be encouraged to express her feelings about it. An overly anxious mother will be unable to breast-feed because of inadequate milk production and because the infant will sense her anxiety. Also, it is during the second trimester that the mother-to-be will start to plan for the baby by making clothes and decorating a room. This is an excellent time for the patient and her partner to consider a course in childbirth education. It is perfectly acceptable for them to decide against childbirth classes as long as the decision does not compromise the outcome.

During the third trimester, the patient often develops a wish "to get it over with." Most women ask, "Do you think the baby will come early, Doctor?" Often she will experience insomnia. Her physical condition may be the most obvious cause, but the physician may also find that the insomnia is caused by dreams of death. Since the darkness of night is so often associated with loneliness and death, the same patient may be able to sleep easily during the day, and the physician should recommend that she try this.

During labor the patient faces the reality of having a baby and the accompanying fear of injury and death. On entering the hospital, the patient's contractions may stop because of Selye's fear and fight reaction. In most cases labor can be reestablished by the judicious use of medication and by reassuring the patient about her fears. The physician or labor coordinator is usually the only familiar person in the strange environment of the hospital and therefore the only person with whom the patient feels secure.

As labor progresses, the patient may worry about how much she should let herself go or move about or when to ask for assistance. She may also worry about getting messy and feel that she is losing dignity and respect. Unfortunately, delivery room personnel can often reinforce these feelings by crude, impersonal, or unsympathetic behavior. By the time full dilatation approaches, she may feel that she cannot go on.

During labor and delivery, anything the physician can do to help the patient participate in the process will add to her sense of well-being and accomplishment afterward. A calm, confident, and reassuring attitude on the part of the physician will allow the labor to progress in a comfortable manner. The physician need actively intervene only when complications arise.

After the delivery and for varying lengths of time, the mother may feel somewhat estranged from the infant. She may not be sure this is really her baby, especially if she was asleep during the delivery or did not see the baby immediately after birth. For 9 months she has envisioned the baby only in her imagination, and she may have difficulty adjusting her fantasied image of the baby to the real infant. Most women become more comfortable with their child as they begin to care for it. This process is called *bonding,* and it generally takes place naturally as time goes on. Bonding is a natural process that will take place if the mother and infant are together.

The new mother may have many preconceived feelings and ideas about her infant. If her relationship with her own mother has been good, she will have little conflict in her new role. However, many problems can arise if she feels anger or hate toward her mother. This is because so many seemingly instinctive things she does for her child have been modeled on the actions of her mother. If she finds fault with the way her mother raised her, she will experience many self-doubts in raising her own child.

About the third day after delivery, many patients experience a short period of depression or the "postpartum blues." This may be because of a drop in estrogen levels, causing an increase in the brain monamine oxydase. Depression may also deepen because the reality of having a baby rarely lives up to the expectations that were built up before delivery. The new mother may feel a lack of support from her partner or other significant figures at this time. She may also find that becoming a mother has revived memories of her own unpleasant childhood experiences. "Postpartum blues" are self-limiting and should not be confused with postpartum psychosis.

Postpartum psychosis, which occurs once or twice per every 1000 deliveries, is not a discrete nosologic entity. All types of reactions such as schizophrenia, affective disorders, psychoneurotic disorders, and deliriums have been reported. The symptoms are produced by the combined effect of biologic, social, and psychologic factors on a sensitized ego. The illness may start at any time during pregnancy, labor, or the period following delivery.

The treatment and prognosis of the condition will depend on the underlying problems brought out by the stress of pregnancy and delivery.

GYNECOLOGIC. The studies of Selye on the general adaptation syndrome and the response of endocrine glands to stress have led many investigators to appreciate the function of *stress in altering physiologic functions*. The effects or stress can be transmitted in many ways to the female organs and the endocrine system. There is a direct pathway from the hypothalamus to the autonomic nervous system. There can also be an indirect neurologic influence on the entire endocrine system through the cerebral cortex, the hypothalamus, and the pituitary gland. The manner in which emotions influence the female endocrine system was demonstrated in a study by Benedek (a psychoanalyst) and Rubenstein (an endocrinologist). Benedek was able to predict ovarian function on the basis of unconscious processes and dreams.

When an emotional conflict is manifested through the mechanisms just related, physical symptoms may arise. For example, a patient may consult a physician because of irritating vaginal discharge. If saline suspension reveals the presence of trichomanads, a diagnosis can be made. However, the physician must wonder if the diagnosis is a complete one. Prescribing treatment is usually insufficient. Such parasites are found in many women who have no symptoms, and symptoms often arise only during periods of stress and sexual tension. A sympathetic physician who shows a genuine interest in any emotional problems the patient may have can be a great assistance at this time.

Gynecologic patients often wish to discuss *problems concerning sexual relations*. They often bring up a sexual problem as an apparent afterthought. Regardless of when or how a patient presents a problem about lack of sexual enjoyment, dyspareunia, or frigidity, the problem is significant to her. Although the cause of these symptoms may also be relatively minor, it can be a serious emotional disturbance. A physician who is interested may be able to solve the minor problems. However, if the patient seems unduly disturbed about the discussion, consultation with a psychiatrist is indicated.

The *infertile couple* can present a difficult problem for the physician. Their inability to conceive can have many organic causes, but, not infrequently, emotional problems may be a factor. An example of such a phenomenon is the previously infertile woman who becomes pregnant after a dilatation and curettage that has been done strictly for diagnostic purposes. Perhaps she is able to conceive because the physician has reassured her and helped her with some emotional conflict. One should be aware of the fact that she may also experience emotional problems during her pregnancy.

Any *operation,* particularly one on the reproductive organs, can have a symbolic meaning for the patient. The psychologic impact of a hysterectomy, for example, is complex. A woman who has undergone a hysterectomy must confront the fact that she can no longer menstruate or reproduce. She must also deal with negative responses to the procedure from others and with any unconscious feelings she may have about her uterus. Although most women know rationally that a hysterectomy will not affect their day-to-day functioning or sexuality, they may still be anxious about this until they are reassured by the physician. If he does not handle the problem well, the patient may develop postoperative orgasmic dysfunction, other psychophysiologic complaints, or pain. This type of surgery may also affect the woman's partner psychologically. A patient who has had a hysterectomy may also experience depression caused by the loss of a bodily organ. It is important that the physician prepare a woman facing a hysterectomy for the grieving process and to support her during it.

Climacteric. The climacteric, like adolescence, is a transitional stage. Its primary manifestation, the cessation of menstruation, usually is preceded by several months of irregular ovulation and the appearance of symptoms. These are indications of the waning of ovarian function. The menopause usually occurs at about 50 years of age.

There is also a *psychologic "menopause"* that arises whenever a woman begins to realize that she is approaching the end of her childbearing years. This is a significant milestone for most women, indicating that they are getting old, approaching death, and perhaps losing their position of value in the world. Many women develop depressions during this period that may be difficult to diagnose. They may seek treatment for symptoms such as fatigue, anorexia, insomnia, irritability, and constipation, which they may attribute to menopause rather than to emotional difficulty in adjusting to aging. The physician may help such a patient by reminding her that she is a useful member of society and by encouraging her to participate in her usual activities or to develop new ones. The woman who has dedicated her life to bearing and caring for children may have the most difficulty adjusting to menopause. She must be helped to channel her energies into new areas—work, hobbies, organizations, or grandchildren. She needs to regain the old feeling of being needed and valued.

Senescence. Senescence begins with the complete cessation of menstruation and continues until the end of life. It is marked by the progressive atrophy of the genital and other bodily organs. A woman in this phase may be disturbed by the loss of physical beauty, especially if she has previously put great emphasis on her attractiveness. Pelvic relaxations that once produced little discomfort now tend to produce symptoms and often require surgical correction because of the loss of estrogenic stimulation of the supporting structures. Cancer of the uterus and the vulva and other general medical conditions often develop during this period.

Psychologically, this is also a period of great adjustment. The woman often has to give up many things that are of great importance to her such as her home, her grown children, a job, and social prestige. She may also experience a decrease in her economic status. All these things lead to great insecurity. The woman who has been dependent on a rigidly scheduled existence throughout most of her life will find it difficult to adjust to these changes and may develop psychologic or psychophysiologic symptoms.

SUMMARY

The obstetric or gynecologic patient should be evaluated as a total person. Her personality should not be ignored just because the physician believes it will be too time-consuming to deal with that aspect of her care. The physician can make a quick evaluation of the patient's psychologic makeup by paying attention to her attitudes and behavior and by asking a few key questions. All this can be accomplished during the history-taking and physical examination. Emotional and organic problems cannot be totally separated, and a diagnosis should not be made by an exclusionary process, but on the basis of a total evaluation and a positive finding. Therapy will then be more effective, and most emotional and physiologic problems can be managed competently.

REFERENCES

Benedek, T., and Rubenstein, B.B.: The sexual cycle in women, Psychosom. Med. **3**(1, 2), 1942.

Boston Women's Health Collective: the new our bodies, ourselves, New York, 1984, Simon and Schuster.

Chickering, A.W.: Education and identity, San Francisco, 1969, Jossey-Bass, Inc., Publishers.

Chodorow, N.: The reproduction of mothering, Berkeley, 1978, University of California Press.

Cooke, C.W., and Dworkin, S.: The ms. guide to a woman's health, New York, 1981, Berkeley Publishing Corp.

Freud, S.: Female sexuality (collected papers), vol. 5, London, 1950, The Hogarth Press, Ltd.

Gilligan, C.: In a different voice, Cambridge, 1982, Harvard University Press.

Gove, W., and Tudor, J.: Adult sex roles and mental illness, Am. J. Sociol. **78**:812, 1973.

Kaplan, A.G., and Bean, J.P.: Beyond sex-role stereotypes, Boston, 1976, Little, Brown & Co.

Paffenberger, R., Steinmetz, C.H., Pobler, B.G., and Hyde, R.T.: The picture puzzle of the postpartum psychosis, J. Chronic Dis. **13**:161, 1961.

Selye, H.: The general adaptation syndrome and the diseases of adaptation, J. Clin. Endocrinol. **6**:117, 1946.

Shephard, B., and Shephard, C.: The complete guide to women's health, Tampa, Fla., 1982, Mariner Publishing Co., Inc.

5

Michael J. Daly and Kathy Hotelling

Sexual responses of women

The human female responds to sexual feelings or sexual stimulation in varying degrees from infancy to death. Some women are unable to find sexual gratification because of somatic, endocrine, or psychosocial problems. The physicians from whom these women seek help need to be knowledgeable in human sexuality.

NORMAL SEXUAL RESPONSE

Sexual response may result in an orgasm, which physically is the fine, involuntary contraction of the vagina and pelvic muscles. This climax may be triggered as an autoerotic response or through heterosexual or homosexual stimulation. An orgasm is dependent on the close integration of several systems: the endocrinologic, the psychologic, and the somatesthetic. A woman's sexual satisfaction is not as dependent on the climax as is a man's. However, inhibition of sexual fulfillment may cause a variety of symptoms such as depression, pruritus vulvae, pelvic pain, or fatigue.

Endocrinologic role

All mammals have subcortical centers responsible for sexual activity in the hypothalamus and upper midbrain. In lower orders of mammals these areas are primarily activated by gonadal hormones. This is why the female dog will accept the male only when she is in heat. In human beings the higher cortical centers inhibit this hormonal influence so that the sexual response in women is independent of their ability to conceive. The libido of most women, however, is affected by the menstrual cycle. Many women are more sexually active before ovulation and before menstruation than at other times during their cycles. However, under the proper circumstances, a woman is able to respond sexually at any time.

Estrogen exerts a minimal effect on the sexual desire of women. Progesterone has a tranquilizing effect. The sexually unresponsive female is not affected by massive doses of estrogen or progesterone. The libido of a responsive female may be increased with the administration of testosterone. This is probably brought about by the increase in clitoral size and sensitivity without direct influence on the psyche. Hormonal therapy will not alleviate orgasmic dysfunction or dyspareunia, except that caused by atrophic vaginitis.

The effect of testosterone on the development of the fetus is important. In experimental animals, if androgen stimulation is blocked in genetic males, the fetus will develop into a female anatomically, physiologically, and behaviorally. Conversely, androgen stimulation in appropriate amounts will produce masculinization of the external genitals of a genetic female. Money studied a group of women who had androgen stimulation as fetuses. Although their subsequent development was en-

61

tirely as women, he was able to demonstrate a difference in personality in the direction of more male traits.

Psychosocial role

The psychosocial factors that are essential to the physiologic response of a climax in the female include (1) her comfort with her body and particularly her genitals, (2) acceptance of herself as a sexual person, (3) ability to relate with another, and (4) integration of her role into the whole personality. These factors are determined by a complex interrelationship of social, cultural, familial, developmental, physiologic, and interpersonal influences. The imprinting from these psychosocial experiences leaves both positive and negative impressions in the psyche of the mature woman. The balance of these forces determines the sexual fulfillment of any given woman.

Somatesthetic role

A woman's whole body responds to a greater degree to emotional stimulation than does that of the male. Erotic responses may be stimulated by being looked at, words of love, and particularly touch. Specific areas of response are the skin, lips, mouth, breasts, abdomen, thighs, and genital region. The response of the pelvis is vascular dilatation and pelvic congestion, resulting in vaginal lubrication from transudation of a mucoid material from the engorged vessels around the vagina. In addition, a woman's body responds with the development of myotonia.

The gross anatomic reaction of the female has been divided into four phases by Masters and Johnson: (1) excitement, (2) plateau, (3) orgasm, and (4) resolution. The skin, breasts, clitoris, vagina, and uterus change during these phases.

The normal woman's sexual response is the sum total of psychologic response to physical stimulation, which reaches a climax in an autonomic reflex arc, producing multiple somatic responses. There is no difference in the anatomic response of the pelvis to orgasm whether it be stimulated by manipulation of the breasts, clitoris, or vagina or even by fantasy. In addition to the physiologic responses listed in Table 5-1, the uterus elevates and contracts. The human female differs from the male in that she may go from one orgasm to another without going through the resolution phase.

Sexual attitudes and behavior

We are in a period of changing attitudes and practices regarding sex. The concepts of modesty, chastity, and sexual inhibition have been under attack. A woman's position is now equal to that of the man. An important causative factor in this change is the development of safe, reliable contraceptives, which removes a principal block to a freer sexual life for women, the fear of pregnancy. Just as important a block has been the use of sex for power and control over women, which existed in the past. Sexism and male chauvinism have been challenged, and increasing numbers of women are demanding the right to control their bodies and to

TABLE 5-1 Anatomic sexual responses of the female

Phases	Skin	Breasts	Clitoris	Vagina
Excitement	Increased sensitivity	Nipple erection	Vasocongestion tumescence	Lubrication
Plateau	Maculopapular flush	Increased breast size	Gland retraction	Expansion of inner two thirds and vasocongestion in outer one third
Orgasm	No change	No change	No specific change	Involuntary contractions
Resolution	Perspiration	Loss of nipple erection	Loss of congestion and retraction	Loss of vasocongestion

express themselves sexually in a more active way. Fifty percent of adolescents are now sexually active.

The physician often is thrown into the middle of this conflict of value systems. This is particularly true when one is consulted by an adolescent girl desiring contraception. Questions that are important include the following. Has the patient developed a sexual value system for herself? What is the physician's responsibility to the patient, the parents, and society? Why is the girl becoming sexually active? The pleasure in sex is obvious. Since the main practical danger, pregnancy, can be removed, why not indulge? There can be an examination of the girl's moral and religious ideals in a nonjudgmental way. Sex can be discussed as a reflection of the girl's self-esteem. Is there a deep commitment to a partner, a temporary liaison, or a bartering transaction? The physician can thus help the young woman discover how she wishes to relate to her sexual partner.

Sexual expression and love

Probably no other word is more difficult to define than love, although poets, novelists, and philosophers throughout history have written about it. Usually there is a component of love in sexual relationships; however, humans may participate in sexual activities for pleasure alone, through masturbation or heterosexual or homosexual relationships. Some humans as part of their concept of love choose freely the option of exclusivity of their sexual partners, giving up variety, whereas others choose variety as their life-style. Although homosexuality and heterosexuality need not be entirely separate paths, bisexuality is practiced by a minority of women and men in our society.

Some individuals are sexually excited by transvestism, sadomasochism, exhibitionism, voyeurism, and sexual experiences with animals. There has recently been an increased demand for operative and endocrine treatment by unhappy transsexuals requesting a change in their gender. Before any significant operative intervention is attempted, these patients must be well evaluated and must live a year in their desired sexual role. Endocrine therapy may be used during this trial period. Many practices that a number of people consider perverse because they are connected with aberrant sexuality are a part of normal heterosexual intercourse. At times, physicians will be called on to reassure the patient in this area.

Sexual history

The sexual history should be an integral part of every medical history because pertinent sexual and psychosocial data are essential to evaluate the patient as a whole person. It should reflect the chronologic framework of the patient's life, including sexual attitudes, feelings, expectations, experiences, and environmental changes and practices.

The comfort of both the historian and the patient in obtaining this emotionally charged information is essential. The sexual value system of the patient and how these values affect her psychosocial relationships should be considered. In addition, the history should provide information to determine the onset, severity, and duration of sexual dysfunction, if such a problem exists.

Obtaining the sexual history. A good method of starting to gather sexual information is to ask the patient about her sexual satisfaction. One should pay close attention to both verbal responses and nonverbal communication. If the patient reacts with a great deal of anxiety and tension, no further probing in this area should be attempted at this time. The reaction, however, suggests that this is an area of tension for the patient that might well be explored later. If the patient responds without a great deal of anxiety, an open-ended history should be obtained. The physician is primarily a listener and does not lead the patient, but if she strays from the subject, the physician should point this out.

During the questioning, one should (1) convey an aura of comfort and trust, (2) provide factual knowledge when it is appropriate, and (3) create an atmosphere free of discernible prejudice toward the sexual values, ideals, or practices discussed by patients. This in no way means that physicians need change their own behavior patterns but rather that they should relate to patients in a nonjudgmental way. They can logically point out to their patients self-destructive behavior.

Format of history. The history should include the following information:

1. Baseline sexual data, including early sexual experiences and, if appropriate, early fantasies, as well as sexual knowledge
2. Sexual preference
3. Each stage of the life cycle and significant events (such as early childhood, adolescence, premarital experiences, marriage, middle age, menopause, and old age) as they relate to sexual influences

SEXUAL PROBLEMS OF FEMALES

The sexual problems for which women seek help are *inhibitions of sexual desire, excitement, and orgasm.* There are also separate or associated complaints of *dyspareunia* and *vaginismus.* These complaints, when functional, have their origin in anxiety, guilt, identity problems, and difficulties of interpersonal relations. Prohibitions and guilts learned early in life are of particular significance. If they are strong they can produce a *primary sexual dysfunction,* which is a situation in which lack of desire, excitement, and orgasm have been present the whole life. It has a poor prognosis, although it is not hopeless. *Secondary sexual dysfunction* occurs when there has been a period of enjoying sex followed by a regression in the ability to find satisfaction. If this secondary sexual dysfunction is caused by physical changes or has been of a short duration, the prognosis for return to satisfying sexual experiences is good. In those patients in whom secondary dysfunction is long-standing, successful therapy may be difficult, since strong inhibiting reactions such as anxiety, guilt, anger, or even hostility have been built up. The most frequent problem of secondary sexual dysfunction in women of reproductive age is the loss of sexual desire. In older women dyspareunia from atrophic vaginal changes is more common.

Sexual dysfunction is marked by specific levels of sensory deprivation that have their origin in the fear of sexual situations, the denial of personal sexual identity, rejection of the partner, the circumstances of the particular sexual encounter, or poor communication both verbally and nonverbally. Since most patients find sexual problems difficult to discuss, the physician should realize that no matter how the subject is presented, it is of great importance to the patient. O'Connor and Stern have noted that women with sexual problems have other types of complaints more often than do men.

Dyspareunia

Dyspareunia means painful intercourse. The symptom may indicate local organic disease in the pelvis or result from psychologic conflicts.

Local causes. *Any condition that obstructs the entrance of the vagina or narrows the vaginal tube* may interfere with intercourse. This obstruction may be congenital, the result of scarring from birth injury or an operation, or the result of atrophy. *Vaginal and vulvar infections* may render the tissue so sensitive that coitus becomes either painful or impossible. Less often, pelvic lesions such as *salpingo-oophoritis, endometriosis, prolapsed ovaries,* and *retroversion of the uterus* may be responsible for dyspareunia. *Atrophic vaginitis* caused by estrogen lack may cause dyspareunia in postmenopausal women.

A less common cause of organic dyspareunia is a *rigid hymen* that interferes with intromission. Each coital attempt is thwarted by the narrow orifice and by the pain that the young woman experiences as a result of this. Usually the couple will seek medical advice soon after marriage, but some couples allow this situation to continue for months or even years, suggesting an emotional difficulty.

We have encountered several instances of rigid, intact hymens in women who consulted us because of infertility of several years' duration and in a few women who came for prenatal care. None of these patients complained of dyspareunia. Actually, they had never had normal intercourse. After the first few unsuccessful attempts to penetrate the obstructing membrane, their husbands became discouraged and contented themselves with ejaculation outside the vagina.

The pain experienced in early attempts at intercourse is tolerated without much concern by most women. The fearful, anxious woman may react by tensing the muscles that surround the introitus of the vagina; and, if this persists, a condition known as *vaginismus* develops. This spasmodic reaction almost completely closes the entrance of the vagina, thus making intercourse virtually impossible. When examining a woman with this problem, the physician usually will find tightening of the thigh muscles and spasm of the levator ani muscles.

The psychologic mechanism that is usually responsible for vaginismus is an inordinate fear of injury to the genitals, which may have been conditioned by experiences in childhood. Some of these experiences are related to sex only through the fantasy life of the child. Many guilt feelings about sexuality find expression in a tendency to overemphasize the pain. This condition may be a reflection of the overall relationship to the partner. Therefore the symptom can be an unconscious expression of anger, revenge, control, rejection, and fear directed toward the man. For some women these feelings may have been a result of rape.

Treatment. Dyspareunia caused by local inflammatory lesions, painful scars, or pelvic disorders is usually amenable to either medical or surgical correction. When the cause of difficulty is a thick, rigid hymen, gentle but forceful dilatation with graduated dilators, which is repeated at regular intervals by the physician, sexual partner, or patient, is preferable to the often-recommended incision or divulsion of the hymen under anesthesia. The dilatation causes a mild discomfort. It also demonstrates to the patient that she is capable of withstanding the discomfort of admitting her partner's penis.

Cooperation with her partner should be sought and encouraged. Discussion with the partner regarding the technique of the sexual act should take place during treatment. Suggestions relating to sex play and the use of lubricating jelly may be helpful. A need for a gentle but firm approach on the part of the sexual partner should be stressed. Communication between the couple is the key to solving many of these problems. There is usually a breakdown in this area because the mutual frustration has led to unexpressed anger. The couple may also have guilt about discussing sex or wanting to enjoy it. They may be helped by reading and discussing material relating to the subject together.

These measures often succeed in correcting the sexual difficulty by establishing better communication and relieving anxiety, fear, or guilt. In more refractory patients, behavior therapy or psychotherapy may be indicated. Psychotherapy is directed toward helping the patient gain awareness of her sexual self and uncovering unconscious fears or hostility relating to men, the sex act, or the sexual organs. The techniques of behavior therapy are directed toward retraining the woman to experience sex without unpleasant emotions.

Psychosexual dysfunction

Because of the unpleasant connotations and the lack of specificity in diagnosis, the terms frigidity and impotence should be eliminated from medical nomenclature. Preferable diagnostic labels are *inhibited sexual desire, inhibited sexual excitement,* and *inhibited female orgasm.* They more clearly define the problematic area as sexual feelings progress from mental representations to complete sexual satisfaction. A detailed history examining these three areas is most important in establishing a diagnosis. It is important to realize that many psychoses and neuroses can present as sexual problems. In most cases, the more generalized emotional state should be treated first. Sexual problems can also present when the difficulty is primarily in the area of interpersonal relationships. Under these circumstances, the relationship with the partner should be treated first.

Inhibited sexual desire. This is a persistent and pervasive inhibition of sexual desire. The judgment that this is the appropriate diagnosis is made by the clinician taking into account factors that influence sexual desires such as age, health, and individual circumstances. It cannot be separated from the context of the whole life. It is particularly important to examine the occurrence and frequency of sexual thoughts and fantasies. In many cases the woman will not be distressed by this symptom. A study by Frank, Anderson, and Rubinstein in 1978 of middle to high socioeconomic class women with "successful marriages" discovered 48% with this complaint. Two percent reported no intercourse, and 8% had less than one sexual encounter per month.

Inhibited sexual excitement. This diagnosis can be made when there is a partial or complete failure to attain or maintain the lubrication; that is, to maintain the swelling response of sexual excitement until completion of the sexual act. In Frank, Anderson, and Rubinstein's study, 33% of women complained of this difficulty. Usually the amount of sexual activity is adequate.

Inhibited female orgasm. Orgasm is delayed or absent after an excitement phase that is judged by the clinician to be adequate in focus, intensity, and duration. If the woman achieves orgasm by non-coital manual clitoral stimulation or if she requires manual stimulation of the clitoris during intercourse, diagnosis can be difficult. In some cases, these are considered to be normal variations.

Most women do not reach a climax during every sexual exposure. This by no means classifies them as being nonresponsive sexually. It is important to discover what type of mental activity and physical stimulation produces sexual feelings. If the woman can have sexual feeling, it is informative to discover the mental and physical acts surrounding the moments when a block to the natural progress toward orgasm appears.

Etiologic factors. The cause of sexual dysfunction may be somatic, environmental, coital, or psychogenic. These etiologic factors are closely interrelated, and each factor has some effect on the others.

SOMATIC FACTORS. Patients who experience pain at intercourse because of a genital lesion or abnormality can hardly be expected to look forward to the act with pleasurable anticipation. The obvious solution is to correct the lesion, whether it be an abnormal hymen, vaginitis, or a severely retroverted uterus.

ENVIRONMENTAL FACTORS. Some of the problems of everyday living can affect the libido adversely. A woman who is overworked, is plagued by financial problems, or suffers from poor health is often uninterested in sex. The increase in desire for sex on vacations occurs because of an ability to put these deterrents aside.

A common unhappy environmental situation is fear on the part of the couple of being overheard in the act of coitus. Young couples living with parents often are inhibited in their lovemaking by this possibility; a similar situation is the presence of children in or near the parents' bedroom. The daily fluctuations of love and anger between the couple are also influential.

COITAL FACTORS. Many women who have per-

fectly normal sexual desires and inclinations remain relatively unresponsive because of inappropriate coital techniques. The failure to recognize the woman's desire for preliminary caresses and sex play accompanied by endearing expressions of love frequently accounts for lack of interest or actual distaste for coitus. At times, however, sex without love can be very satisfying.

Obviously, serious sexual difficulties in the man such as impotence or premature ejaculation will alter the response of the woman. They are especially difficult to manage if the couple cannot communicate about them.

It is important to realize that a woman must take pleasure in coitus—a mate alone cannot make her respond.

PSYCHOGENIC FACTORS (CONSCIOUS AND UNCONSCIOUS). Conscious thoughts, feelings, and attitudes play a major role in some cases of orgasmic dysfunction. These interfere with the necessary excitement of anticipation that heightens a woman's sexual desire. A woman who resents her partner's preoccupation with work or recreational activities and interprets them as indifference to her may retaliate by sexual coolness, since she may consider intercourse to be a means for her partner to use her. Some women consciously remain passive during coitus because of a mistaken notion that conception is more likely to occur if they participate actively and derive pleasure from the act. A few consider it unladylike to seem to enjoy intercourse or to assume an aggressive or active role. Some men think the same, and the woman may respond to this. Sexual intercourse is an interaction between two people, and it is almost impossible for one partner to have a problem that isn't related to difficulties in the other.

Most women who are unable to enjoy intercourse and certainly those who have an aversion to it harbor some unconscious childhood sexual fantasy that they have inappropriately carried into adulthood. It may be fear of injury, feelings of guilt, a continued attachment to the father, a disappointing relationship with a significant male figure, or hostility toward men. Other realistic experiences such as molestation during childhood, rape, or incest may be responsible for their fears.

Many *medications,* especially those that are psychoactive or that affect the autonomic nervous system such as antihypertensive drugs decrease libido. Physicians who are cognizant of this effect can help simply by informing the patient of the source of the decreased sexual drive. This knowledge will help the patient rid herself of the anxiety and guilt that accompanies the unexplained lack of responsiveness that in turn can cause more problems.

The woman may wish to express her hostility by defeating the man in his attempts to please her. She may be so afraid to lose control that she cannot contemplate the strong emotions felt during orgasm. Occasionally, a woman will equate orgasm with loss of bowel control. Other women have a maternal attitude toward men and approach intercourse with the idea of only satisfying and pleasing the man. These women may never have an orgasm but will rarely complain. Extremely narcissistic people have difficulty experiencing an orgasm because they cannot identify with the pleasure of their partner. Many women who do not enjoy sex with men see their role as one of being used. If the woman's role is complete surrender, the enjoyment of sex can be interpreted by the woman as a link in the chains of slavery. Homosexual women may also have dysfunctional problems.

Prophylaxis. A great deal may be accomplished by the enlightened physician in the prevention of this all too common disability, but the first and most important prerequisite for sexual adequacy in the woman is a childhood atmosphere characterized by affection, understanding, and a sane and sensible attitude on the part of parents toward the little girl's sexual curiosity and activity. Intimidation or punishment for childhood sexual activity such as masturbation and exposure of the genitals does much more harm than the acts themselves. The experience of affectionate and loving parents is important in developing the proper attitudes concerning sex.

Adequate education at puberty that enlightens the girl in matters of menstruation, sexuality, emotional interactions of the sexes, and pregnancy without engendering fear of injury or disease is of considerable value. The calm, accepting manner of the presenter is more important than the educational material. Unembarrassed explanations and preparation for the menarche should be made by the girl's mother. Careful premarital examination and a frank discussion between the couple and the physician regarding the techniques of coitus and family planning are most helpful in clearing up misunderstandings and in preventing sexual disharmony.

Treatment. Treatment of women with sexual dysfunction may range from rather simple to most complicated types of therapy, depending on the cause and the degree of the pathologic condition. Sexual disorders are symptomatic, and only an intense study can reveal the real difficulty.

The first step is the taking of a history of the patient's sexual experiences. A physician who displays a sincere interest in the woman's problem and gains her confidence can obtain information concerning relevant childhood experiences, parental attitudes toward her and her siblings, and data evaluating the adequacy of her mate. One should keep in mind that problems in the patient's personality and interpersonal relations are reflected in the couple's sexual adjustment. If the sexual problem seems to result from some environmental, somatic, or coital factor, it is usually amenable to physical treatment or supportive therapy, often in the form of reeducation, reorientation, and manipulation of the environment.

Additional frank discussion with the sexual partner separately and with the couple together often can help the man recognize the woman's needs and thus pave the way for a more satisfactory sexual adjustment through increased communication. On the other hand, prudishness on the part of the woman, as indicated by aversion to so-called abnormal positions during intercourse or to certain types of sex play, can sometimes be overcome by the physician's tactful suggestion that there is nothing wrong in this type of experimentation if it culminates in mutual satisfaction. If the patient does not respond to reassurance and reeducation, the couple should be evaluated for referral.

It is important to keep in mind that couples who have lived for many years with a sexual dysfunction have made many adjustments. This delicate balance can be threatened by the suggestion that the sexual problem can be corrected; the couple can react with fear and resistance to such a suggestion. An example is that of a woman who has made an adjustment to an unhappy marriage by withholding from her husband the knowledge that she enjoys sex. The removal of her symptom becomes a threat because she has to recognize the depth of her anger and may be forced to act on it, perhaps by fighting, obtaining a divorce, or having an affair.

In the past many types of treatment have been used. Behavior therapy, psychotherapy, and psychoanalysis have received the most recognition, and each is effective when the proper patient choice is made. O'Connor and Stern found a 77% improvement rate from psychoanalytic treatment in 96 cases of functional sexual disorders (61 females, 35 males). Behavior therapists have reported higher cure rates with relaxation and desensitization techniques.

The methods of behavior therapy, psychotherapy, and psychoanalysis can be used flexibly in the same case. Many techniques have been combined in the development of a new sex therapy.

COMBINED SEX THERAPY. The concept of treating dysfunctional problems in humans by focusing on altering behavior is not new. For many years this form of therapy has been viewed with some skepticism. The interest in using these techniques to treat sexual problems of men and women was initiated by Masters and Johnson and confirmed by others. Their therapy is a combination of behavior therapy, psychotherapy, conjoint therapy, and marriage counseling.

Following are the principles of combined sex therapy:

1. *Co-therapists.* A woman therapist and a man therapist are used. Although there are insufficient data at this time to prove that the co-therapy team is more effective than a single therapist, it would seem that this form of approach might allow for identification, support, and understanding to a degree that is not possible with a single therapist. Kaplan found that the co-therapist is unnecessary and that the most important factor in cure is quick intensive intervention of the therapist.

2. *Sexual unit.* Both partners are involved in the therapy sessions and responsible for the outcome, although the sexual problem may be present in only one partner.

3. *Sensate focus.* Awareness of one's self as a sexual person is developed. The couple is placed in a nondemanding situation in which they learn to perceive the pleasure of the sensations of touch, vision, smell, and sound. They learn to communicate what pleases and displeases them. Intercourse is prohibited at this time to help focus attention and to remove pressure for performance.

4. *Communication.* The couple communicates both verbally and nonverbally as each partner develops a realization of the erotic body areas, including skin, mouth, ears, breasts, and, finally, genitals. At different times one partner may be the recipient and the other the giver, with roles being reversed when appropriate.

5. *Removal of stress.* It is important that neither partner be placed in a stressful position. The couple is reassured that their anatomy and physiology are functioning properly and that orgasm is a natural process that can be blocked by the processes of the mind. Too much thought about performance and the injury to self-esteem, which occurs when there is failure, is presented as a major problem. Partners are alerted to be aware of anxiety and worry as the blocking agents to the pleasures of sex. These feelings must be dispelled before the problem can be solved.

6. *Masturbation.* Frequently it is very helpful for women to learn what an orgasm feels like through masturbation. Once they are able to achieve this they can then teach their partner how to help them to achieve a climax through clitoral stimulation. In this manner sexual communication is enhanced, mutual trust is exhibited, and specific erotic desires and body areas are learned by the couple. The therapist has given permission for them to be sexual.

7. *Specific suggestions.* For some women who complain of inhibited sexual desire, erotic films are a helpful adjunct to therapy. Still others are helped by being encouraged to act out their sexual fantasies. When male premature ejaculation is found to be a problem, the so-called squeeze technique may be helpful.

Failure in the treatment of primary orgasmic dysfunction is usually caused by too much stress on the couple or a serious emotional problem in the woman, which prevents her from giving up her fears.

DRUG THERAPY. Many drugs have been advocated in the treatment of primary orgasmic dysfunction, including the administration of alcoholic beverages at bedtime. These may at times achieve the desired effect, but at best such therapy is of temporary benefit and may actually delay a more rational approach to the problem. No drug has proved to be an effective aphrodisiac.

In summary, sexual health is an integral part of total health. Fifty percent of the populace have some degree of sexual problems. The physician as an authoritative figure may be most helpful in uncovering sexual problems and providing meaningful help. A sexual history should be part of every medical evaluation, and the doctor who does this will become comfortable with the sexual feelings of his patients and their response to them and thus be a more complete physician.

REFERENCES

Bancroft, J.: Human sexuality and its problems, New York, 1983, Churchhill Livingstone.

Becker, J.V., Skinner, L.J., Abel, G.G., and Treacy, E.C.: Incidence and types of sexual dysfunctions in rape and incest victims, J. Sex Marital Ther. **8**:65, 1982.

Bell, A., and Weinberg, M.: Homosexualities: a study of diversity among men and woman. New York, 1978, Simon and Schuster, Inc.

Carson, C.C., III, Segura, J.W., and Keyes, T.W.: Psychologic characteristics of patients with female urethral syndrome, J. Clin. Psychol. **34**:312, 1979.

Dardick, L., and Grady, K.E.: Openness between gay persons and health professionals, Ann. Intern. Med. **93**(1):115, 1980.

Frank, E., Anderson, C., and Rubinstein, D.: Frequency of sexual dysfunction in ''normal'' couples, N. Engl. J. Med. **299**:111, 1978.

Good, R.S.: The gynecologist and the lesbian, Clin. Obstet. Gynecol. **19**:473, 1976.

Heiman, J., LoPiccolo, L., and LoPiccolo, J.: Becoming orgasmic: a sexual growth program for women, Englewood Cliffs, N.J., 1976, Prentice-Hall, Inc.

Hite, S.: The Hite report, New York, 1976, Macmillan Publishing Co.

Kaplan, H.S.: The new sex therapy, New York, 1974, Brunner/Mazel, Inc.

Kaplan, H.S.: Disorders of sexual desire, New York, 1979, Brunner/Mazel, Inc.

Kinsey, A.C., Pomeroy, W.B., and Motin, E.E.: Sexual behavior in the human female, Philadelphia, 1953, W.B. Saunders Co.

Masters, W.H., and Johnson, V.E.: Human sexual response, Boston, 1966, Little, Brown, & Co., Inc.

Masters, W.H., and Johnson, J.E.: Homosexuality in perspective, Boston, 1979, Little, Brown, & Co., Inc.

Money, J.: Psychosexual differentiation. In Sex research: new developments, New York, 1965, Holt, Rinehart & Winston General Book.

Munjact, D.J.: The recognition and management of desire phase sexual dysfunction. In Sciarra, J.J., editor: Gynecology and obstetrics, vol VI, Philadelphia, 1983, J.B. Lippincott Co.

Murphy, W.D., Coleman, E., Hoon, E., and Scott, C.: Sexual dysfunction and treatment in alcoholic women, Sexual. Disabil. **3**:240, 1980.

O'Connor, J.F., and Stern, L.O.: Results of treatment in functional sexual disorders, N.Y. State J. Med. **72**:1927, 1972.

Perkins, R.P.: Sexuality in pregnancy: what determines behavior? Obstet. Gynecol. **59**:189, 1982.

Riley, A.J., and Riley, E.J.: A controlled study to evaluate directed masturbation in the management of primary orgasmic failure in women, Br. J. Psychiatry **133**:404, 1978.

Sarrel, P.M., Steege, J.F., Maltzer, M., et al.: Pain during sex response due to occlusion to the Bartholin's gland duct, Obstet. Gynecol. **62**:261, 1983.

Semmens, J.P., and Wagner, G.: Estrogen deprivation and vaginal function in menopausal women (a study of menopausal vaginal physiology and the effect of exogenous estrogen therapy), J.A.M.A. **248**:445, 1982.

Shen, W.W., and Sata, L.S.: Inhibited female orgasm resulting from psychotropic drugs, J. Reprod. Med. **28**:497, 1983.

Seiss, A.M., Rosen, G.M., and Zeiss, R.A.: Orgasm during intercourse: a treatment strategy for women, J. Consult Clin. Psychol. **45**:891, 1977.

6

Kate Moffit Musello and Rebecca Jackson

Sexual assault

Rape is a crime of anger expressed as a sexual act without consent of the victim. Physicians, especially gynecologists and family practitioners, too often come unprepared to the examination of the alleged rape victim. The purpose of this chapter is to provide background information on rape and specific guidelines for those physicians involved in the care of rape victims. Let us emphasize in the beginning that, although the proof of rape must be left to the courts, competent care of the victim may provide the data with which a recovering victim and the district attorney can pursue the legal process.

It has been estimated that as many as one of every two women will be threatened with rape in her lifetime. As many as one half of all rape victims know their assailant. Although the majority of reported rapes involve one assailant, in one study approximately 30% resulted from group rape. Group rape is usually premeditated, involves street drugs and/or alcohol, and generally elicits more brutality and sexual humiliation of the victim. According to Nadelson, Notman, and Hilberman, approximately 25% of victims sustain extragenital as well as genital injury.

A significant psychologic injury to the victim's sense of self-determination should also be taken into account. Self-recrimination and guilt over one's powerlessness to avoid or deflect the attack are common reactions to rape. Appetite, sleep, and concentration disruption may be profound during the healing process. Many victims suffer from disabling fear, nightmares, intrusive recollection of the event, and even panic triggered by violence in the media. Some victims probably develop full-blown anxiety and depressive states, perhaps even psychosis, as a result of rape.

Sexual assault is an umbrella term that includes manual, oral, or genital contact by the assailant. This contact occurs without the victim's consent. Rape specifically refers to genital contact perpetrated by the assailant through some element of force. Force may be defined as anything from threats made against the victim or the victim's family now or in the future to actual display of a deadly weapon. Although resistance on the part of the victim is no longer required in most states to prove rape, evidence of force and/or resistance is very persuasive in court. A psychiatrically (for example, schizophrenic) or otherwise mentally handicapped person, including someone under the influence of drugs, is considered legally unable to offer consent.

An overview of the examination explained in lay language will help prepare the patient for its more uncomfortable aspects. During this initial contact, the physician can observe the patient's emotional state; that is, if it is one of anger, agitation, or inordinate calm. Some victims may find catharsis in recounting the rape, whereas others will relive the most terrifying and humiliating aspects of the assault. The presence of someone from a rape victim support group, as well as a friend or family member, can be an invaluable stabilizing influence on the patient in this situation. The names and affiliations of those present should be recorded on the medical record (for example, Jenny Moore present from Rape Crisis Center).

Victims of sexual assault often experience significant trauma in the form of fear of death, fear of loss of a loved one, physical injury, isolation, confusion, or mental torture. It is important that the treatment offered does not incur further trauma. Describing the available diagnostic and therapeutic techniques so that the patient can make choices for herself should be the physician's goal. Facilitating the reestablishment of the patient's sense of safety and control is a priority and yet is made difficult in the usual emergency room setting where other priorities and/or values dominate.

The following is a list of five goals of the rape examination:

1. Promotion of emotional healing
2. Evaluation and treatment of physical injury
3. Evaluation and treatment to prevent treatable sexually transmitted diseases
4. Evaluation and treatment to prevent pregnancy
5. Collection of evidence

In the first four tasks, the physician acts as the patient's advocate. In the fifth task, the physician must be a careful, impartial collector of data to be presented at a later time under the auspices of the court. All five tasks are accomplished in the usual familiar process of history taking, physical examination, laboratory testing, and treatment.

It is important to allow the patient to choose whether or not to be treated as a step in regaining control over her life and body. One way to accomplish this is through an informed consent for both the examination and the collection of evidence (see box below).

HISTORY AND PHYSICAL EXAMINATION

The physician carries the responsibility of detecting both genital and nongenital trauma. The ACOG technical bulletin "Alleged Sexual Assault" provides a standardized sexual assault history and physical that can be used instead of the usual emergency room log sheet. By standardizing the sexual assault medical record, important information will not be inadvertently omitted. If at all possible, the report of the history and physical should be dictated, since dictation facilitates recording a more detailed description. Including nonmedical explanations of medical terminology can be useful should interpretation come into question later in court. As with any legal scrutiny, the physician's and the victim's strongest ally is a comprehensive medical record.

History. *Gently* ask the patient to tell you what happened. She does not need to tell you all the details, since a sex crimes detective will go over the attack with the patient. The minimum information that the physician needs to know includes the following:

1. The sequence of accosting and assault to determine jurisdiction and to assess evidence; Where the crime began so that evidence may be collected and given to the appropriate authorities (The timing is important for assessing the likelihood of a viable specimen being present as well.)

I authorize Dr. _____ to perform a complete medical examination, including a pelvic (internal) examination on my person and to record for the proper law enforcement agency the findings as related to the prosecution of my assailant(s).
Signed_____ Date/Time_____
Witness_____ Guardian_____

2. The types of threat and injury (what the assailant actually said may be painful to recount but may give a clearer picture of the threat and the emotional/psychologic trauma).

Documentation of the history should be in the patient's own words with as little additional opinion or interpretation from the physician as possible. Many people have diffficulty describing aspects of the assault that were bizarre or unusual. Clearer descriptions of the assault may be prompted by everyday language (for example, "oral sex" may not be as clear as, "Did he force you to put his penis in your mouth?"). Although it is important that the physician not contribute to the victim's tendency toward self-blame by implying that she should not have performed such tasks as washing, the patient should be asked if she has showered, urinated, defecated, brushed her teeth, douched, or changed her appearance since the assault. A description of the assailant's behavior, the use of drugs by either the victim or the assailant, the use of foreign objects in the attack, the use of a condom, or the assailant's achievement of orgasm should be included in the history. Some conditions shown to correlate with a higher risk of sexual assault include mental retardation, alcoholism, mental illness, indigency, and transiency.

A general brief medical history should be included after the above questions have been answered. This should include a history of past or current medical conditions as well as a gynecologic history (date of last menstrual period, character of last period, gravidity, parity, cycle length, flow, previous history of infections such as herpes, syphilis, gonorrhea, condylomata, method of birth control, and the time of the patient's most recent consenting intercourse).

Physical examination. The physical examination has a dual purpose. The first is to evaluate for injury. The second is to collect evidence for future prosecution of the assailant. Most states have standardized rape evidence collection kits that should be available in the emergency room at all times. The collection of evidence and its untampered transfer to the court is extremely important. Unless there is a verifiably unbroken chain of custody and

transfer of the collected evidence (that is, evidence can be accounted for from the time of collection until it is turned over to the police) the evidence may be ruled inadmissable in court. All specimens should be signed by the person who collected them, and the amassed evidence should be labeled and locked in a police box by those who collected the evidence if it is not transferred directly to the officer in charge.

Clothing that demonstrates struggle or contains specimens from the assailant such as blood or semen should be described in the medical report and submitted with the other evidence. Foreign matter on the patient's body should also be collected and submitted. Debris beneath the nails or nail clippings may be included. If semen stains are identified, these can be collected. Some hospitals have Wood's ultraviolet lamp, which can be used to examine for semen. Because of the high histone content of semen, it will fluoresce under a Wood's lamp in a dark room.

The physical examination itself offers a healing touch to the assault victim. Doing an overall examination permits evaluation and treatment of the patient rather than of an invaded orifice alone. A good first step is to visualize the entire skin surface, the scalp, and the mucosal membranes. Nongenital injury may be important evidence. Document injuries by careful descriptions with the help of diagrams or burn sheets. Although photographs sound promising, they often do not show up well and can diminish rather than verify injury. Nongenital injuries may include choke marks, bites, scratch marks, abrasions, fractures, and hematomas. Besides possibly requiring medical attention, these injuries are objective evidence of lack of consent or resistance on the part of the victim. If the victim is examined soon after the assault, the physician may detect only tenderness. The victim should be reassured about the healing process and instructed to return if these areas of tenderness manifest visual signs of injury. If a patient returns several days after the initial examination, new evidence of injury should be documented.

After an examination of the skin, a general physical examination should be done. When this is completed, pausing to ask the patient for permission to perform the pelvic exam can give the victim a sense of control that may help her negotiate this difficult aspect of the examination. The pelvic examination should begin with the external genitalia; the physician should look for lacerations, abrasions, blood, ecchymoses, secretions, and dried semen, which looks like a whitish-yellow flaking stain. Some authors recommend applying toluidine blue to the mucosa to visualize lacerations not visible to the unaided eye.

The condition of the hymen should be described without offering an opinion as to the cause of its appearance. Hymens vary. Hymenal rupture or the lack of it is not required to prove or disprove rape. A speculum moistened with water (not lubricant, since this will interfere with the acid phosphatase and Papanicalaou test) is then gently introduced into the vagina. If a plastic speculum is used, warn the patient about the clicking sound it makes as it is opened. (In our experience, one patient responded hysterically when the physician opened the speculum because it sounded like the gun that had been placed in her vagina to play Russian roulette.) Examination of the cervix and vaginal mucosa should include a description of any trauma observed. With preadolescent children or severe injury, general anesthesia may be required to perform an adequate examination.

Two types of specimens are collected. Certain specimens will fall under the category of evidence, whereas other specimens will be used to identify the presence of disease. Swabs of the vaginal pool, anus, and oral cavities along with a wet mount should be obtained for evidence. When describing the wet mount, the physician needs to note the presence or absence of sperm and whether or not they are motile. The presence of motile sperm in the vagina has been studied and found to decrease rapidly after coitus (Soules) probably because of the pH of the vagina. Motile sperm were identified in only 50% of the women studied after 3 hours. In this group of women, however, whole sperm were identifiable for up to 18 hours, and sperm heads were identifiable for up to 24 hours. Other studies have shown that motile sperm can be seen

for as long as 28 hours after coitus, and, according to Findley, nonmotile sperm may remain for up to 48 hours. Spermatozoa may be seen later upon examination of the other specimens after special staining, even if the examining physician did not identify sperm on the wet mount. Since rape is not a crime of passion, it is not surprising to discover that some rapists suffer from sexual dysfunction and often fail to ejaculate. Other rapists will be azospermic because of any number of conditions such as inherent infertility or vasectomy. The use of condoms or coitus interruptus are other possible explanations for the absence of motile sperm on wet mount.

The vaginal swabs are used to prepare air-dried slides, which are submitted for future examinations by the forensic laboratory. After the identification of a fluid as semen with the use of either an acid phosphatase screening test or direct identification of sperm, the forensic laboratory in Albuquerque, N.M., can subject the specimen to screening for four genetic markers. These markers are phosphoglucomutase, glyoxalase I, esterase-D, and peptidase-A. Prostatic Ag can be used to identify semen from vasectomized males. All of these markers are identified with electrophoretic methods. ABO and secretor status are also determined. If ejaculation has occurred, acid phosphate will be identifiable (Wertheimer). Significant concentrations of this prostatic enzyme were seen in 50% of women 9 hours after intercourse. No acid phosphatase was seen 36 hours later. Dried acid phosphatase as found in clothing or gathered from skin may be detectable for months after an assault. The Johnson Rape Kit contains a colormetric test strip that changes from blue to dark purple when exposed to acid phosphatase. Acid phosphatase is present in a concentration of from 400 to 8000 King-Armstrong U/ml in fresh ejaculate.

Secretor or ABO status of the victim is obtained as another means of discriminating between the victim and the assailant. Approximately 80% of the population secrete blood group antigens in saliva, sweat, semen, and vaginal secretions.

Under the category of laboratory specimens a culture for gonorrhea and a Papanicolaou smear are collected and submitted. Blood may be drawn at any time that seems appropriate during the examination and should be analyzed for complete blood count, serum pregnancy test, syphilis, and alcohol/drug screening as indicated. A urine specimen should be obtained for urinalysis and toxicologic screening, if necessary.

EXAMINATION FOLLOW-UP

The victim should be offered protection against pregnancy. The pregnancy status of a woman who suspects that she might have become pregnant before the assault should be assessed before she is given protection. The patient should be counseled that efforts to prevent pregnancy after coitus must be initiated within 72 hours of the assault and are not uniformly successful. If contraception is not successful, the patient may want to consider abortion should she become pregnant as a result of a rape. One method of contraception is the administration of two Ovral birth control pills at the time of the examination if the monoclonal urine pregnancy test is negative, to be followed 12 hours later by two more Ovral birth control pills. The theory behind this therapy is that the birth control pill renders the endometrial lining relatively resistant to implantation.

The prevention of sexually transmitted disease is offered to all victims of sexual assault. This includes prevention of syphilis, gonorrhea, and chlamydia. Unfortunately, we have no preventive methods for herpetic or human papilloma virus infections. Other infections such as trichomoniasis or bacterial vaginitis should be treated when they are diagnosed. Gonorrhea is transmitted in 3% to 4% of all reported rapes, whereas syphilis develops in approximately 0.1% of all reported rapes. The patient must be counseled on the importance of follow-up syphilis serology because of potential inadequacy of prophylactic antibiotics.

The CDC recommendations for prophylaxis after rape is to give the patient tetracycline, 500 mg four times daily by mouth for a total of 7 days. Pregnant women or patients allergic to tetracycline should receive amoxicillin, 3.0 g, or ampicillin, 3.5 g, each given with probenicid, 1.0 g, as a single oral dose. A final alternative is erythomycin base, 500 mg four times daily for 7 days, or 250 mg four times daily for 14 days. The dosage of ampicillin to be given to a child is calculated as 50 mg/kg, which is also given with probenicid, 25 mg/kg orally as a single dose.

CONSEQUENCES

Each victim will respond to such an assault variously depending on coping mechanisms developed during previous events in their lives and on the circumstances of the assault. During the acute reaction, which may last from a few days to several weeks, the victim experiences a grief response expressed as shock, disbelief, or even emotional disintegration. The normal integrity of her life may be totally disrupted. The victim may become absorbed in self-recrimination or guilt. The phase resolves if the victim is able to construct an outward adjustment to being victimized, even though she has farther to go in reintegrating her anger and sense of loss of control. The long-term effects of the assault may be denied or repressed. At this time the victim may withdraw from counseling or discontinue previous contact with the rape victim support group. The third phase is characterized by integration of the assault into the victim's self-image, which may be preceded by a period of depression. Evidence of the rape trauma syndrome or posttraumatic stress disorder may be admissable in court. Successful prosecution of the assailant can be a constructive force in resolving the victim's loss of control over her life.

LEGAL CONSIDERATIONS

A physician subpoenaed to testify in a rape case should take several preparatory steps. Obtain and review records. Discuss the case at length with the District Attorney. Ask what tack the defendant's lawyer is considering to discredit the victim's charge (defamation of character, attempting to prove consent, discrediting the examiner, invalidating the evidence). A few caveats to keep in mind are: (1) rape is a legal, not a medical, definition; (2) although the physician can offer a medical opinion concerning the presence/absence of trauma, it is not his or her responsibility to prove rape or to say what caused any trauma; (3) it is admissible to state that the victim appeared to have had traumatic intercourse; (4) the word "rape," should always be preceded by the word "alleged"; (5) the physician should avoid being cornered by a defendant's lawyer into answering yes and no questions, especially those concerning situations about which no medical research exists to support the answer (for example, "Doctor, is it not true that a woman could develop a reddened vaginal opening if she had prolonged consenting intercourse?"). It is perfectly acceptable to answer, "There is no medical information with which to answer such a question," or "That question cannot be answered with an unconditional yes or no." It is important that the physician remember that he or she is not on trial and thus that he or she must remain as calm and unemotional as possible. Insults made by the defendant's lawyer are the lawyer's way of trying to unhinge the physician's reason and thereby elicit a particular response. By listening carefully, the physician can often predict and thus avoid that answer.

Cooperative efforts between medical personnel and law enforcement agencies can greatly improve a community's ability to deal effectively and compassionately with rape. There is much left to do in the way of informing both physicians and their communities that will greatly improve their response as a medical team to rape. Furthermore, rape is a crime associated with a high rate of recidivism of the rapist if untreated and a high percentage of recovery if treatment is completed; thus it behooves physicians to provide the best care of victims and most accurate collection of evidence so that a sucucessful court outcome can be obtained.

REFERENCES

1. American College of Obstetricians and Gynecologists: Alleged sexual assault, Chicago. Technical Bulletin No. 52, 1978, American College of Obstetricians and Gynecologists.
2. Breen, J.L., and Greenwald, E.: Rape. In Glass, R.H., editor: Office gynecology, ed. 2, Baltimore, 1981, The Williams and Wilkins Co.
3. Findley, T.P.: Quantitation of vaginal acid phosphatase and its relationship to time of coitus, Am. J. Clin. Pathol. **68:**238, 1977.
4. Hilberman, E.: The rape victim, Baltimore, 1976, Garmond Pridemark Press.
5. Nadelson, C.C., Notman, M.T., and Hilberman, E.: The rape experience. In Curran, W.J., McGarry, A.L., and Petty, C.S., editors: Modern legal medicine, psychiatry, and forensic science, Philadelphia, 1980, F.A. Davis Co.
6. Soules, M.R., Pollard, A.A., Brown, K.M., and Verma, M.: The forensic laboratory evaluation of evidence in alleged rape, Am. J. Obstet. Gynecol. **130:**142, 1978.
7. STD treatment guideline, 1985, U.S. Department of Health and Human Services.
8. Wertheimer, A.J.: Examination of the rape victim, Postgrad. Med. **71:**173, 1982.

7

John H. Mattox

Normal menstruation

Menstruation is the periodic discharge of blood and disintegrating endometrium after a normal ovulatory cycle. The menstrual cycle is the hallmark of reproductive function in the human adult female. Normal menstrual cycles are comprised of two phases: a *follicular* (ovary) or *proliferative* (endometrium) *phase*, beginning with the first day of menstrual flow and culminating in ovulation; and a *luteal or secretory phase,* which ends with the onset of menstruation.

PHYSIOLOGY OF THE MENSTRUAL CYCLE

Normal menstruation depends mainly on the functional integrity of three endocrine sources: the *hypothalamus*, the *anterior pituitary gland*, and the *theca granulosa cells of the ovary*. This is often referred to as the *hypothalamic-pituitary-ovarian axis*. The process is precisely coordinated, but stimuli from the cerebral cortex mediated through the hypothalamus can influence menstrual function. Examples are cessation of periods or irregular menstruation associated with fear of pregnancy or other emotional crises.

A neurochemical transmitter known as *gonadotropin-releasing hormone* (GnRH), which is produced in the hypothalamus, is liberated in a pulsatile fashion into the capillary plexus of the median eminence and is carried through the portal vessels to the anterior lobe of the pituitary gland.

The result of its neurohormonal action is the production and release of the gonadotropins FSH and LH from the anterior pituitary cells. These hormones are transmitted to the ovary, where they stimulate follicle development and ovulation. The hypothalamus becomes active before puberty as the first step in the maturation process.

The production of FSH and LH by anterior pituitary cells is not steady; rather there is a continuous secretion of pulsatile discharges of the hormones. The characteristic cyclic pattern of FSH-LH secretion during the normal menstrual cycle is governed by cyclic changes in ovarian estrogen and progesterone secretion (Fig. 7-1).

The principal modulator of hypothalamic-pituitary activity is estrogen. Estradiol (E_2) has a strong negative feedback relationship with FSH. Ovarian steroidogenesis is at a minimum during the first few days of a menstrual cycle. The low concentration of estrogen triggers secretion of GnRH with a consequent release of FSH and LH. These hormones stimulate follicle growth and an increase in E_2 production, which in itself plays an essential role in follicle growth and maturation. The increase in E_2 in conjunction with FSH increases the number of FSH receptors and granulosa cell proliferation. Intraovarian and circulating E_2 rises more steeply during the latter part of the follicular phase, reaching a maximum just before ovulation. The rising

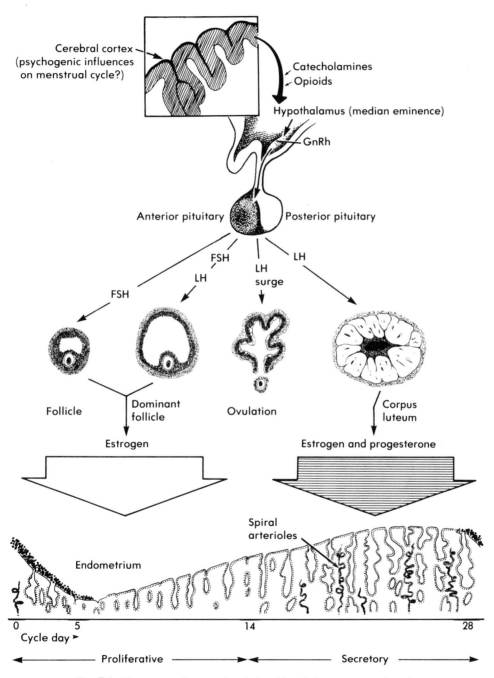

Fig. 7-1. Hormone and anatomic relationships during a menstrual cycle.

estrogen concentration inhibits FSH secretion, then a sharp peak acts on the hypothalamic-pituitary system and stimulates LH and, to a lesser extent, FSH release. *E_2 triggers the midcycle surge of LH, which must be precisely timed to induce ovulation.* The secretion of LH continues at a lower level. Its principal function is to support the growth of the corpus luteum.

The secretion of progesterone (P_4) increases rapidly after ovulation, and there is a concurrent but lesser increase in estrogen production. High levels of P_4 are maintained until about day 23 or 24 of the cycle, when the corpus luteum begins to regress if the ovum has not been fertilized. The withdrawal of hormone support of E_2 and P_4 to the endometrium is followed by its disintegration and menstruation. The low concentration of ovarian hormones permits the cycle to be reinitiated.

Hormones of menstruation (Fig. 7-2)

Hormones affecting the hypothalamus. *GnRH is a decapeptide* that was originally called LH-releasing hormone. It is produced and secreted in the hypothalamus by special neuronal tissue in the region of the median eminence. It is secreted in a pulsatile fashion becoming *circhoral* (about every 60 minutes) around the time of ovulation but less frequently during the luteal phase. The half-life of GnRH is several minutes. Although exact control mechanisms have not yet been fully elucidated, there are certain neuromodulators that are known to affect the secretory patterns of GnRH. *Endogenous opioids suppress LH* secretion presumably because of the direct effect upon the GnRH neurons. *Catecholamines* play a major role in the control of GnRH secretion. *Dopamine* generally *inhibits* LH secretion, whereas *norepinephrine* via alpha receptors *facilitates* LH secretion. The exact interrelationship of the centrally located aminergic, opioidergic, and petidergic neurons and their control is unclear. The pulsatile release of GnRH is also subject to feedback from the ovarian sex steroids E_2 and P_4.

Hormones involving the anterior pituitary. The exquisite timing of gonadotropin secretion is of paramount importance to a normal menstrual cycle.

The *gonadotrope* is a pituitary cell that is responsible for the synthesis, storage, and release of FSH and LH. Most of the pituitary gonadotropes produce both hormones. However, the cell population is heterogeneous, and some cells predominantly release one hormone or the other. The anterior pituitary is part of an endocrine unit called the *hypothalamic-hypophyseal complex*, which is subjected to numerous "messages" that result in secretion of gonadotropin hormones. The amplitude and the frequency of hormone release is determined by altering the sensitivity of this complex by making it more sensitive or less sensitive to incoming stimuli. The *negative feedback response* (E_2-inhibiting FSH and LH secretion) predominates during most of the menstrual cycle. At the time of ovulation, the *positive feedback response* (E_2-stimulating LH and FSH secretion) is the key event that ultimately results in ovum release. This stimulatory response is the hallmark of the hypothalamic-pituitary-ovarian axis.

FSH and LH are glycoproteins that have similar alpha and different beta subunits and a somewhat similar molecular weight, 33,000 and 28,000, respectively. The half-life of these hormones is contingent upon the amount of sialic acid in the molecule and is approximately 4 hours for FSH and 1 hour for LH.

The gonadotrope is stimulated by pulsatile GnRH. This intermittent GnRH stimulus induces more GnRH receptors on the gonadotrope, a self-priming effect, and makes the cells more sensitive, thereby enhancing gonadotropin secretion. The gonadotrope's responsivity is also modulated by circulating ovarian sex steroids. Although it is believed that E_2 may exert its positive feedback effect at the level of the pituitary by increasing the numbers or the sensitivity of the GnRH receptors, the exact mechanism is unknown. The preovulatory secretion of a small amount of P_4 is required for an optimum LH surge.

Prolactin (PRL) is produced by a specialized pituitary cell, the *lactotrope*, and has its physiologic role in the process of lactation. There is evidence that PRL can be released by GnRH and that intraovarian PRL secretion may have a permissive role in regulation in a normal

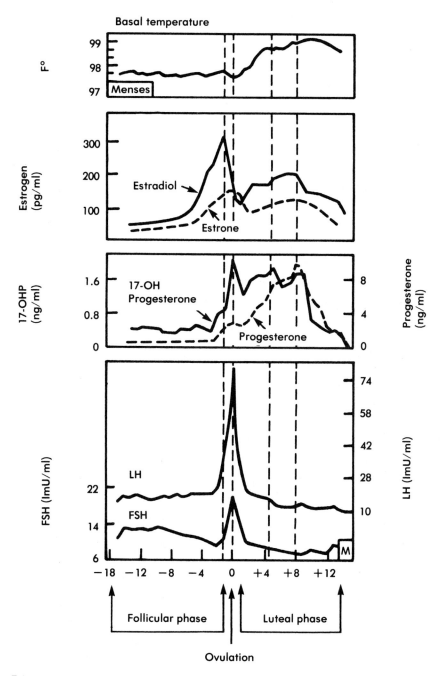

Fig. 7-2. Means of serum FSH, LH, estrone, E_2, P_4, and 17-hydroxyprogesterone during a normal menstrual cycle.

ovulatory cycle. PRL is also produced by the *endometrial decidua* and is probably stimulated by P_4 secretion. The physiologic role of decidua-secreted prolactin is also unknown.

Hormones involving the ovary. The *classic estrogens* are estrone (E_1), estradiol (E_2), and estriol (E_3). The first two hormones are elaborated by the ovary, and there is an ongoing dynamic interconversion of estrone to estradiol and vice versa; during the reproductive years the net result favors E_2 secretion. E_2 has the greater biologic potency and plays a more significant role in modulating and effecting the normal menstrual cycle. Estrogens are *18-carbon compounds* that circulate bound-to-protein *sex steroid–binding globulin*. They are inactivated at a relatively rapid rate by the liver and excreted in conjugated forms as glucuronates and sulfates by the way of the urine predominantly and the feces to a lesser extent. Estrogens are secreted as a result of the interaction of the *ovarian theca and granulosa cells*; the latter aromatizes the androgens, androstenedione, and testosterone to E_2. In a normal cycle E_2 exerts its influence on the intraovarian environment and affects the hypothalamic-hypophyseal complex. The positive-feedback response requires that E_2 concentration be at least 200 pg/ml for 48 hours in order to trigger the LH surge. During the second half of the cycle, the *luteinized granulosa cells* that comprise the corpus luteum secrete estrogen and P_4.

Although the biologically active estrogens have an important effect on the genital tissues, they also bring about the feminine habitus and have an effect on the endometrium, fallopian tubes, cervical mucus secretion, vaginal epithelium, and growth stimulation of the ductal system of the breasts. Estrogens also play a role in the long-bone growth and epiphyseal closure. The absence of estrogen after the menopause predisposes women to osteoporosis and genital and breast atrophy. A chronic excess of estrogen without the ''buffering'' effect of P_4 can result in abnormal uterine bleeding and eventually endometrial carcinoma.

Catechol estrogens. Part of the metabolic degradation of estrone is the formation of 2- and 4-hydroxy derivatives. Circulating 2-hydroxyestrone is present in very small amounts and has no known biologic activity. Ultimately, it may be found that these metabolites play some permissive role in the menstrual cycle regulation. *Catechol estrogens* compete for and are degradated by the catechol O-methyltransferase system and can bind to catecholamine receptors in the brain.

P_4 is a 21-carbon compound that is secreted by the luteinized granulosa cells of the corpus luteum and is found predominantly in the latter half of the cycle. Serum concentration of 3 ng/ml or greater is found in an ovulatory cycle. The plateau of its secretory pattern is reached about 7 days after ovulation, at which time the concentration should be at least 10 ng/ml. Just before ovulation, there is a small increase in P_4; there is significant evidence to suggest that P_4 enhances pituitary sensitivity and is necessary for an optimal LH surge. P_4 circulates bound to *cortisol-binding globulin*. For tissues to be sensitive to the action of P_4, they must first have been exposed to estrogen, since it is the estrogen that induces P_4 receptors.

The primary reproductive function of P_4 is to induce secretory activity in the endometrial glands, thereby preparing the endometrium to receive a fertilized ovum. Its other biologic effects include desensitizing the myometrium to oxytocic activity, altering the histologic appearance of the vagina, inhibiting the secretory activity of the cervical glands, stimulating development of the alvelor system of the breasts, and, because of its thermogenic property, being responsible for the increase in basal body temperature following ovulation.

Although *17-hydroxyprogesterone*, 17-OHP, is secreted during both phases of the cycle, it is generally found in greater concentrations in the luteal phase. A rise in 17-OHP occurs at about the time of the LH peak and is probably a response of the theca interna. This steroid has little progestational or other biologic activity. However, it is being investigated as a potential indicator of a subtle 21-hydroxylase deficiency of the adrenal gland in women who have been characterized as having polycystic ovary syndrome. 17-OHP concentrations are measured before and after ACTH stimulation. An exaggerated response is seen in women with the partial enzyme deficiency.

Changes in the ovary

At the time menstruation is taking place, *recruitment* of a number of primordial ovarian follicles, stimulated primarily by FSH, is initiated and continues for 5 to 7 days; LH stimulation also is required. The increased production of E_2 resulting from the increase of both FSH receptors and granulosa cells is responsible for the process of selection. The *preantral follicle* that is selected at this time will ultimately become the dominant follicle over the next 5 days. The cohorts that are excluded regress under the influence of intraovarian androgen production to undergo atresia. As the dominant follicle evolves, its lining granulosa cells become more cuboidal and multilayered; and a central cavity, the *antrum*, becomes filled with a transudate, *liquor folliculi*. The oocyte surrounded by its own granulosa cells awaits release. E_2, having played a key modulating role during this entire preovulatory process, is now at a peak. About midway in the cycle, a LH surge, produced by the positive feedback of E_2, induces follicular rupture and ovulation.

E_2 secretion in the follicular phase is thought to occur because of the interaction between the *theca* and the *granulosa* cells. LH receptors are present in the thecal cells, and small amounts of that pituitary hormone stimulate thecal cell androgen production via the second messenger c-AMP. Receptors on the granulosa cell are predominantly FSH; these cells, when stimulated by FSH, increase aromatase enzyme activity, which enables the granulosa cells to convert androgens to E_2. Hence the coordination of both cells is required for normal estrogen production.

The onset of the LH surge occurs 28 to 32 hours before ovulation; this spike also facilitates the resumption of meiosis in the oocyte, the luteinization of the granulosa cells, and the synthesis of prostaglandins required for the rhexis of the follicular wall and extrusion of the oocyte.

Oocyte maturation inhibitor (OMI) and *luteinization inhibitor* (LI) are nonsteroidal intrafollicular hormones that facilitate the entire series of events, preventing the premature release of an egg and early luteinization of the granulosa cells, respectively.

The rupture of the follicle is attended by capillary bleeding. The blood replaces the spilled follicular fluid, and a corpus hemorrhagium is formed. Through the continued action of LH, the granulosa cells soon become luteinized, and a corpus luteum results. The corpus luteum continues to grow and function, aided by the pulsatile secretion of LH, until about day 23 or 24 of the cycle, when it begins to regress. If the ovum, which was discharged at the time of ovulation, is fertilized, this regression does not take place; the corpus luteum continues to function as the corpus luteum of pregnancy being maintained by the LH effect of hCG.

In the absence of pregnancy the corpus luteum becomes progressively less sensitive to LH stimulation. As the corpus luteum regresses, it becomes hyalinized and has a characteristic convoluted structure that can be seen histologically, the *corpus albicans*.

Luteal cells become less efficient at synthesizing P_4 if the ovum is not fertilized. The luteal tissue has also been found to contain a nonsteroidal substance that prevents LH from binding to the receptor on the granulosa cells. The *LH receptor-binding inhibitor* (LHRBI) increases in concentration during the luteal phase and has been found to inhibit P_4 secretion in vitro. There is also some significant experimental evidence that suggests that E_2 plays a major role in luteolysis.

Changes in the uterus

The cervical mucosa, the myometrium, and the blood vessels of the uterus are all influenced by the cyclic changes in the levels of the hormones of ovary, but the endometrium shows the most dramatic effect of the influence of estrogen and progesterone. The changes are divided into three phases.

Proliferative phase. Immediately after menstruation the endometrium is thin, the epithelium is cuboidal, and the glands are straight and narrow. The stroma is compact. This stage lasts until the ninth day of the cycle (Fig. 7-3).

The continued stimulatory effect of estrogen brings about an increased thickness of the mucosa during the late proliferative (interval) phase. The epithelium becomes columnar. As the phase pro-

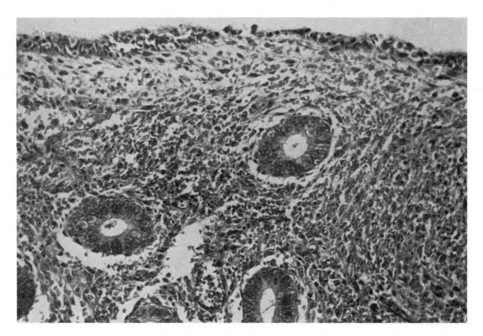

Fig. 7-3. Early proliferative endometrium. Abundant, compact, lymphoid-appearing stroma and a few small narrow, straight glands are present. (×255.)

gresses, the stroma becomes looser, more abundant, and more vascular. This phase lasts until about the fourteenth day of the menstrual cycle (Fig. 7-4).

Secretory phase. During the postovulatory premenstrual stage the progesterone from the corpus luteum stimulates the proliferative endometrium to exhibit secretory activity. The mucosa becomes thick and velvety. The glands become widened and assume a corkscrew pattern, and the stroma becomes edematous and loose. Early in the secretory phase the nuclei appear to move away from the basement membrane, leaving a characteristic area of subnuclear vacuolization (Fig. 7-5). Secretion within the lumen of the glands is maximal by the twenty-fifth day (Fig. 7-6). Special staining techniques reveal that secretions are rich in glycogen. There is an increasing coiling of arterioles.

By carefully examining the endometrial architecture with the use of well-defined criteria developed by Noyes, Hertig, and Rock, it is possible to monitor the progressive maturation. It is these dating criteria that are used to assist with the diagnosis of the luteal phase defect.

If the ovum is fertilized during the cycle and the corpus luteum persists, this phase progresses to the formation of the *decidua*, the endometrium of pregnancy.

Menstrual (bleeding) phase. In the absence of pregnancy, regression of the corpus luteum is followed by a decline in circulating estrogen and P_4. The decline in steroids initiates the process of menstruation. Although the structural changes in endometrial shedding have been observed directly in the elegant investigation of Markee, who transplanted endometrium into the anterior chamber of the eye of the rhesus monkey, the precipitating cause is unknown.

Following ovarian steroid decline, the height of the endometrium diminishes, with a subsequent reduction in blood flow and vascular stasis. The *spiral arterioles* play a special role in menstruation

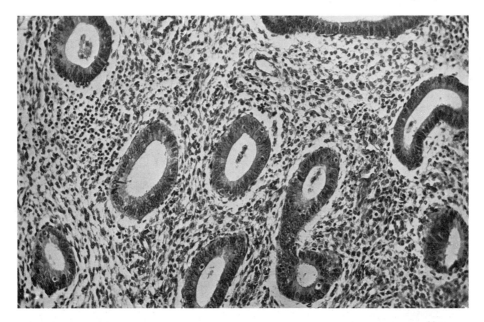

Fig. 7-4. Advancing proliferative endometrium. Note increase in number and size of glands and compactness of stroma. Although some glands are elongated, they are not tortuous. (×197.)

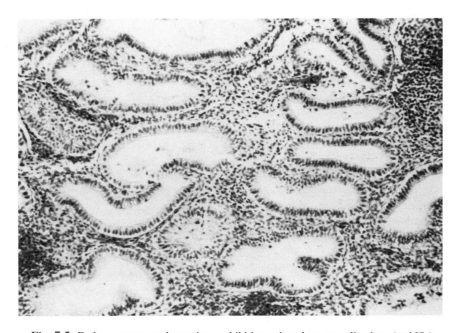

Fig. 7-5. Early secretory endometrium exhibiting subnuclear vacuolization. (×160.)

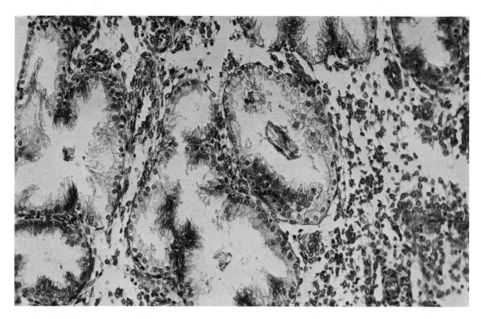

Fig. 7-6. Secretory endometrium. Stroma is scanty and loose, and dilated, tortuous glands show intraluminal tufting and secretory activity. (×220.)

by undergoing rhythmic vasoconstriction and relaxation. Ischemia is followed by tissue breakdown with cellular migration from the vascular bed; subsequently, enzymatic destruction of the endometrium occurs. The separation along the endometrial surface occurs between the layers *basalis* and the *spongiosa* and *compacta*, the latter two being discarded. Concomitantly, small vessels are being "plugged" with thrombin, and the growth of a new endometrial surface is being stimulated by estrogen. The entire event is relatively precise and uniform, occurring over the entire endometrial surface. Christiaens, Sixma, and Haspels noted that the endometrial surface diminishes from 4 mm to 1.25 mm during this phase in a course of several hours.

Concentration of prostaglandin $F_2\alpha$ increases throughout the menstrual cycle; the highest amounts are measured at the time of menstrual flow. This potent vasoconstrictor probably plays a key role in initiating spiral arteriolar spasm.

Proliferative endometrial epithelium maintains its structure by a matrix of collagen bundles held together by ground substance that is predominantly acid mucopolysaccarides. When P_4 secretion occurs in the secretory phase, a slow depolymerization process is initiated that ultimately facilitates vascular permeability.

Boutselis noted two significant periods of enzymatic activity in normal endometrium: one around the time of ovulation, which is probably E_2-dependent; and another around the secretory phase, presumably modulated by P_4. He suggested that the activity in the proliferative phase facilitates anaerobic glycolysis, whereas the secretory component promotes aerobic glycolysis. Acid hydrolases, which are identified in greater concentration and are characteristic of the secretory endometrium, presumably play a role in initiation of menstruation.

Changes in the cervical mucus during the menstrual cycle

In the immediate postmenstrual phase the cervical mucus is scant, viscid, and opaque. During the follicular phase the columnar cells become taller, and the cervical glands begin to secrete increasing quantities of thin, clear, watery mucus that exhibits the physical properties of *spinnbarkheit* (the ability to form long thin threads) and *arbori-*

zation (Chapter 2). These changes are a result of *estrogen stimulation.*

In the normal menstrual cycle the peak of estrogen activity is reached in the immediate preovulatory phase. The cervical mucus at this point is greatly increased in amount, is watery, and exhibits maximal *spinnbarkheit* and arborization. This remarkable change in the amount and character of the mucus favors sperm motility and survival and enhances its penetrability. These changes in the quality and amount of cervical mucus are a major source of information for those women wishing to practice natural family planning (Chapter 15).

After ovulation, under the influence of increasing *progesterone* production, the cervical mucus gradually decreases in amount and becomes viscid and tenacious; the arborization phenomenon disappears.

Changes in the vaginal epithelium

The adult vaginal epithelium is composed of three stratified layers of squamous cells that shed representative cells reflecting the state of hormonal stimulation. In a hematoxylin and eosin–prepared vaginal smear, cells from these layers can be identified. The *superficial cell*, the most mature cell, is large and flattened and is usually an eosinophilic staining cell with a small pyknotic nucleus. The layer below the superficial cells, the *intermediate cell* layer, is made up of medium-sized basophilic staining cells with vesicular nuclei. These are transitional cells. In an unstimulated vaginal epithelial surface that has been recently exposed to estrogen or if estrogen concentration is relatively low (for example, during the early proliferative phase of the cycle), this cell type predominates. Also, women who are in the progestational phase of their cycle will have a preponderance of these cells. The *parabasal cell* is the most immature cell and has a larger nucleus-to-cytoplasm ratio. These cells are not usually seen in the vaginal epithelial profile of a female in the reproductive age range unless infection has aided in the denudation of the surface.

In order to use the vaginal smear to assess estrogen response, special attention must be given to the preparation of the smear. There must be no evidence of infection. Information obtained from the vaginal smear can be helpful, particularly when looking for the evidence of estrogen effect in a prepubertal vagina or in the evaluation of the postmenopausal female (Chapter 2).

CLINICAL ASPECTS OF NORMAL MENSTRUATION

The length of the menstrual cycle and the duration and amount of flow vary considerably among normal women, but pronounced deviations from the accepted norms should suggest the possibility of functional or anatomic abnormality. Clinically significant characteristics of the menses are the *age at onset, periodicity, duration, amount of flow, character of flow,* and *associated symptoms.*

Age at onset. The first period usually occurs at about 12 years of age, but the menses may appear at age 10 or may be delayed until age 16 without being considered abnormal. Many factors are responsible for this wide variation. The most significant are race, heredity, the general health, nutritional status, and body mass of the individual girl. If the periods start before the age of 10 years, it is spoken of as *precocious menstruation;* if they are delayed past the age of 16 years, it is spoken of as *delayed menstruation* or *primary amenorrhea.*

Periodicity. The theoretic normal interval from the beginning of one period to the onset of the next is 28 days, but few women menstruate absolutely regularly. Intervals of 28 ± 7 days may be considered normal. The postovulatory phase is constant at 14 ± 2 days, whereas the preovulatory interval may be as short as 3 or 4 days or as long as 21 days. Cycles shorter than 3 weeks or longer than 5 weeks may indicate some disturbance of ovulation. Patients with short cycles are said to have *polymenorrhea.* If the cycle intervals are unusually long (45 to 60 days), the condition is designated as *oligomenorrhea.*

Duration. The usual length of flow is 5 ± 2 days, but periods may last as long as 8 days or stop after 2 days and yet be within normal limits. Extremely short or scant periods are designated as *hypomenorrhea,* whereas unusually long or profuse menses are referred to as *hypermenorrhea.*

Amount of flow. The amount of blood lost at each period varies greatly. The average is about 40 ± 20 ml and may be less than 20 ml; a loss of more than 80 ml is considered abnormal but may not be reflective of an ovulatory disorder.

Character of flow. The menstrual discharge consists of blood, mucus, and desquamated particles of endometrium. It is usually dark red and has a characteristic, musty odor. An interesting feature of menstrual blood is its failure to clot under normal circumstances.

Associated symptoms. A characteristic group of symptoms may appear several days before the menstrual flow. These symptoms, which include weight gain, edema, breast fullness, and discomfort, heaviness of the legs, and irritability or depression, are referred to as *menstrual molimina*. An exaggeration of these symptoms is usually termed *premenstrual syndrome* (Chapter 10).

Even though menstruation is a normal function and should be free from disturbing symptoms, most women experience some degree of discomfort during the period of bleeding. A sense of weight in the pelvic region, mild backache, and cramping are such common complaints that they may be considered as normal accompaniments of the menses. When the pain become more severe, the patient is said to be suffering from *dysmenorrhea* (Chapter 10).

HYGIENE OF MENSTRUATION

Women need not restrict their usual daily routine in any way during the menstrual flow; this includes work, social, and athletic activities. Many couples abstain from sexual intercourse during menstruation because of aesthetic reasons or because of the ancient taboo of uncleanliness. There is no medical reason for sexual abstinence during the period.

A daily bath or shower is not only permissible but most helpful in eliminating the characteristic odor that is present during the menstrual period.

External pads have been used for many years to absorb the menstrual discharge, but currently about 70% of women use intravaginal tampons. Their safety is not entirely absolute or universal. A relatively rare acute infection, *toxic shock syndrome,* although limited to neither females nor the menses, occurs far more often in women specifically at the time of the menstrual period or shortly thereafter. The organism involved is *Staphylococcus aureus;* an *endotoxin* produced by this bacterium is believed to be responsible for the clinical problem.

Tampon use has been identified as one of the risk factors. Although the incidence, estimated at 8.8/100,000 regular tampon users, is low, certain precautions have been advised. Tampons should be changed at least every 4 to 6 hours, and intermittent rather than regular use appears advantageous; for example, they may be used during the day, but external pads should replace them at night. Also, external minipads can be used when the flow is scant.

Some women prefer to douche after menses if they perceive an odor to be present. Although this practice is reasonable, there is no medical indication that it is necessary to cleanse the vagina.

REFERENCES

Boutselis, J.G.: Histochemistry of the normal endometrium. In Nomies, H.J., Hertig, A.T., and Abel, M.R.: The uterus, Baltimore, 1973, The Williams and Wilkins Co.

Christiaens, Sixma, J.J., and Haspel, A.A.: Hemostasis in menstrual endometrium: a review, Obstet. Gynecol. Surv. **37**:281, 1982.

Davis, J.P., Chesney, P.J., Wand, P.J., and LaVenture, M.: Toxic shock syndrome: epidemiologic features, recurrence, risk factors and prevention, N. Engl. J. Med. **303**:1429, 1980.

Erickson, G.F.: Normal ovarian function, Clin. Obstet. Gynecol. **21**:31, 1978.

Fritz, M.A., and Speroff, L.: The endocrinology of the menstrual cycle: the interaction of folliculogenesis and neuroendocrine mechanisms, Fertil. Steril. **38**:509, 1982.

Harris, G.W., and Naftolin, F.: The hypothalamus and control of ovulation, Br. Med. Bull. **26**:3, 1970.

McKay, D.G., Pinkerton, J.H.M., Hertig, A.T., and Danziger, S.: The adult human ovary: a histochemical study, Obstet. Gynecol. **18**:13, 1961.

Markee, J.E.: Menstruation in intraocular endometrial transplants in the rhesus monkey, Contrib. Embryol. **28**:219, 1940.

McCann, S.M.: Luteinizing hormone–releasing hormone, N. Engl. J. Med. **296**:797, 1977.

Noyes, R.W., Hertig, A.T., and Rock, J.: Dating the endometrial biopsy, Fertil. Steril. **1**:3, 1950.

Ratner, A., Dhariwal, A.P.S., and McCann, S.M.: Hypothalamic factors in gonadotropic hormone regulation. In Jaffe, R.B., editor: Hormones in reproduction, Clin. Obstet. Gynecol. **10:**106, 1967.

Rosemberg, E., and Keller, P.J.: Studies on the urinary excretion of follicle-stimulating and luteinizing hormone activity during the menstrual cycle, J. Clin. Endocrinol. **25:**1262, 1965.

Ryan, K.J., Petro, Z., and Kaiser, J.: Steroid formation by isolated and recombined ovarian and thecal cells, J. Clin. Endocrinol. Metabol. **28:**355, 1968.

Treloar, A.E., Boynton, R.E., Behm, B.G., and Brown, B.W.: Variation of the human menstrual cycle through reproductive life, Int. J. Fertil. **12:**77, 1967.

Yen, S.S.C. and Jaffe, R.B.: Reproductive endocrinology, physiology, pathophysiology, and clinical management, ed. 2. Philadelphia, 1986, W.B. Saunders Co.

8

John H. Mattox

Abnormal uterine bleeding

Excessive or inappropriately timed bleeding from the vagina is one of the most common symptoms encountered by the practitioner providing health care for women. Abnormal bleeding can be the harbinger of serious pelvic disease or denote a relatively minor problem. The source of the bleeding can be any of several sites along the menstrual outflow tract. Therefore a thorough and systematic examination is required in every patient presenting with this complaint. Blood loss of more than 80 ml during a period is called *hypermenorrhea,* whereas too frequent bleeding episodes (cycles less than 21 days) is *polymenorrhea.* Abnormal uterine bleeding between periods is called *metrorrhagia.* Another common word that denotes excessive uterine bleeding is *menorrhagia.* These descriptive terms characterize the patient's symptomatology and should not be used as the diagnosis. To understand abnormal uterine bleeding, the reader should be familiar with normal menstruation, which was discussed in Chapter 7.

ETIOLOGIC FACTORS

Most abnormal uterine bleeding is caused by a complication of pregnancy, a tumor, or hormonal dysfunction. The latter term is used to characterize a disorder of the hypothalamic-pituitary-ovarian axis, which impacts on the endometrium to produce abnormal bleeding. Women receiving exogenous hormone therapy for contraception, estrogen-progestin replacement, or as treatment for certain endocrine disorders may experience abnormal endometrial shedding as a bothersome side effect. Less commonly, a serious constitutional illness such as chronic hepatitis will be associated with abnormal bleeding. The following classification provides an overview of abnormal uterine bleeding:

I. Complications of pregnancy
II. Organic lesions
   A. Endocervical or endometrial polyp
   B. Cervical malignancy
   C. Benign leiomyoma or malignant uterine tumors
   D. Chronic endometritis
   E. Adenomyosis
   F. Endometriosis
   G. Salpingo-oophoritis
   H. Ovarian tumors
      1. Nonneoplastic cysts
         a. Follicular
         b. Lutein
      2. Functioning stromal tumors (granulosa-thecal cell type)
   I. Trauma (intrauterine device)
III. Hormonal disorders
   A. Menstrual cycle
      1. Anovulatory
      2. Ovulatory

B. Exogenous
   1. Hormone replacement therapy
   2. Contraceptive therapy
IV. Constitutional diseases
   A. Platelet disorders
   B. Liver disease
   C. Leukemia
   D. Anticoagulant therapy
   E. Thyroid disorders
   F. Adrenal disorders

Complications of pregnancy

Women of reproductive age should be suspected of being pregnant when presenting with abnormal bleeding. *Abortion* is by far the most common complication of pregnancy associated with bleeding. Other less common causes are *ectopic pregnancy* and *gestational trophoblastic diseases*. All of these topics are discussed in other chapters.

Organic lesions

Uterine leiomyomas, particularly those of the submucous variety, are the genital tract lesions that most often cause abnormal bleeding in women who are not pregnant. Other entities include *carcinoma of the vagina, cervix, uterus,* and *ovaries; adenomyosis; endometriosis;* and *chronic salpingo-oophoritis* with extensive ovarian destruction. These are discussed in other chapters.

Endometrial polyps may cause intermenstrual staining and postmenopausal bleeding, as well as menorrhagia and hypermenorrhea. Since polyps generally do not cause an appreciable enlargement of the uterus, they are frequently overlooked. Endocervical polyps may cause spotting following coitus.

Dysfunctional uterine bleeding

Definition. *Dysfunctional uterine bleeding* is abnormal endometrial bleeding caused by an endogenous endocrine dysfunction of the ovarian steroid hormones, estrogen and progesterone. The clinical manifestation is bleeding that is abnormal in amount, duration, or timing in a female of reproductive age. When this diagnosis is entertained, it is understood that the physician has ruled out other causes of abnormal uterine bleeding.

Incidence. Dysfunctional uterine bleeding may occur at any age between menarche and menopause. It is encountered most frequently at the two extremes of menstrual life, when disturbances of ovarian function are most common. More than 50% of dysfunctional bleeding occurs in premenopausal women 40 to 50 years of age, about 20% occurs during adolescence, and the remaining 30% is distributed among the other women in the reproductive period.

Pathophysiology. Dysfunctional uterine bleeding reflects a disturbance in the critical sequential hypothalamic-pituitary-ovarian interactions that are essential for induction of ovulation, normal corpus luteum function, and normal endometrial growth and development. Bleeding is caused by unopposed estrogen effects on the endometrium that results in "breakthrough bleeding" or by relative declines in circulating estrogens, causing "estrogen withdrawal bleeding."

If there is a deficiency of progesterone following ovulation, there may be abnormal bleeding, a *luteal phase defect*. If the corpus luteum fails to regress appropriately and progesterone continues to be secreted (Halban's syndrome), *"progesterone breakthrough bleeding"* occurs. Somewhat related is the chronic administration of a long-acting progestin, *medroxyprogesterone acetate*. Abnormal endometrial bleeding occurs in the absence of sufficient estrogen to maintain a structurally sound uterine lining.

Ovarian dysfunction may be caused by a primary defect or pathologic lesion within the ovary itself, or it may be a result of malfunction of other endocrine glands, notably the hypothalamus, pituitary, and thyroid. Anovulatory cycles tend be self-perpetuating. These are discussed in Chapter 9.

When the ovary is unresponsive as is the case in the aging gland of the premenopausal woman, follicles fail to develop and become luteinized, despite increased gonadotropic stimulation. Conversely, if the ovaries are healthy and responsive, the defect in ovulation may be a result of inadequate gonadotropin secretion secondary to hypothalamic-pituitary dysfunction. In either case the result is

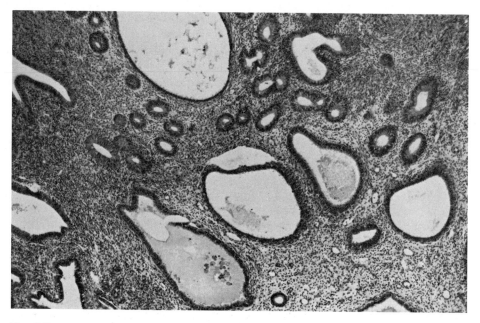

Fig. 8-1. Cystic hyperplasia. Note nonsecretory character of glands and great variation in their size, resembling holes in Swiss cheese. (×60.)

the same—absence of progesterone secretion. The granulosa-theca cell complex continues to secrete variable quantities of estrogen. This continued secretion causes a *relative excess* of estrogen that results in bleeding from the endometrium.

Pathologic findings of the endometrium. Dysfunctional bleeding is usually associated with hyperplastic endometrium, a result of long-standing, unopposed estrogen stimulation. It may also occur with normal-appearing proliferative endometrium.

Hyperplastic endometrium with dysfunctional bleeding is characteristically thickened and may be polypoid, but in some cases it may be normal in appearance. Microscopically, the typical picture is that of benign cystic (Swiss cheese) hyperplasia (Fig. 8-1). There is great disparity in the size and shape of the glands, the epithelium is cuboid or cylindric with deeply stained nuclei, and usually there is no evidence of secretion. The stroma is dense and hyperplastic. In a small percentage of patients an adenomatous pattern, closely resembling adenocarcinoma, is seen (Fig. 8-2).

Rarely, dysfunctional bleeding occurs with "mixed" endometrium, showing partial proges-

tational changes. In these instances the cycle is regular, but the bleeding period is prolonged, and the flow is irregular. This is called *irregular shedding,* a term that denotes prolongation of shrinking, shedding, involution, and epithelization of the endometrium rather than the rapid disintegrative process during the normal cycle.

The concentration of *estrogen and progesterone receptors* in endometrial cystosol varies during the menstrual cycle and is influenced by the circulating levels of the female sex steroids. Estrogen receptors and progesterone receptors reach maximum concentration during the late proliferative phase. Diamond, Aksel, and Speir measured receptor concentration in endometrial cytosol preparations in 36 women with dysfunctional uterine bleeding. Although their findings were of interest, they concluded that the *endometrial histology* rather than the concentration of receptors provided the most reliable information to determine the course of management.

Psychogenic uterine bleeding

There have been reports of irregular uterine bleeding with no evident cause other than emotional factors. The exact mechanism for the pro-

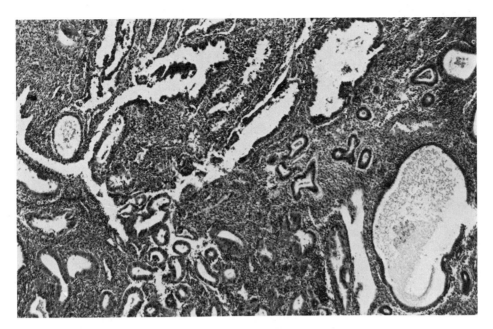

Fig. 8-2. Adenomatous hyperplasia. Glands are closely packed and back to back as result of extraluminal budding. Intraluminal budding is also present. ($\times 60$.)

duction of this type of bleeding is poorly understood.

The most likely explanation is that neurotransmitters are altered by emotional changes and adversely affect GnRH secretion of the pituitary-ovarian axis, thereby interfering with ovulation. However, Markee, Everett, and Sawyer have shown that fright will cause bleeding in endometrial transplants in the eye of the monkey. This suggests that the vasoactive substances released during acute stress could affect the endometrial arterioles and result in tissue breakdown. Even when confronted with a patient having acute psychologic distress, a thorough systematic evaluation must still be conducted by the physician.

Constitutional disease

Although these causes are uncommon, they must be considered, particularly in the female with continued, recurrent episodes of dysfunctional bleeding. Constitutional diseases most likely to cause uterine bleeding such as thrombocytopenia and leukemia interfere with the blood-clotting mechanism.

MANAGEMENT

An accurate diagnosis must be made before one can treat abnormal bleeding effectively. This implies that the physician is thoroughly aware of what constitutes normal bleeding and acceptable variations from the norm. The ultimate goal is to determine the cause of all cases of prolonged, excessive, or irregular flow. A general approach that can be applied to the assessment of most women with abnormal bleeding is found in the box on page 92.

When this outline is followed, several factors such as the age of the patient, the chronicity or recurrence of the problem, and the patient's risk of genital tract malignancy must be considered. There are also some specialized studies such as hysteroscopy or hysterosalpingography that may be helpful in diagnosing certain problems that might otherwise have been overlooked.

Adolescence

Diagnosis. In adolescent females, abnormal bleeding is almost always caused by a disturbance of ovarian function that results in anovulation. This occurs because of immaturity of the hypothalamic pituitary axis with a lack of appropriate ovarian stimulation and positive estradiol feedback. However, clinical observations suggest that fewer than 20% of postpubertal females remain anovulatory for more than 5 years after menarche.

Winter and Faiman were able to show an abnormal response to GnRH in postmenarchal adolescents who are still anovulatory. FSH dominance persisted as opposed to the normal adult pattern of FSH and LH secretion. Without an adequate LH response, luteinization of the dominant follicle cannot occur, and progesterone cannot be produced in sufficient amount.

The possibility of pregnancy, blood dyscrasia, or malignancy must be kept in mind. Adenocarcinoma of the vagina or cervix has been described in young women who were exposed to diethylstilbestrol in utero. If an acute hemorrhage occurs in the adolescent, particularly with the first menstrual flow, a blood dyscrasia or more serious illness would be suspected. Usually, a careful history will rule out the more serious conditions.

Classens and Cowell found that 28% of 79 adolescents hospitalized at the Toronto Children's Hospital from 1971 through 1980 had an underlying coagulation disorder; 10% had other pathologic conditions.

In the young female, a gentle rectal examination may suffice to evaluate pelvic structures. The use of pelvic sonography can also be considered. If the uterus and adnexa cannot be assessed readily, the physician should consider examining the patient under general anesthesia.

When ordering a *complete blood count,* interpretation of the red blood cell indices should not be overlooked. A serum ferritin level may be helpful in diagnosing iron deficiency anemia. If a *clotting disorder* is seriously considered, a platelet count, partial thromboplastin time, and bleeding time will assist in making the diagnosis.

As the risk of malignancy is remote in the adolescent female, endometrial curettage is rarely necessary. It may be required and can be useful in controlling acute hemorrhage in selected cases.

Therapy. Since most dysfunctional uterine bleeding in this age group occurs because of abnormal hormonal stimulation of the endometrium, it can usually be effectively controlled by endocrine therapy. The underlying issue with which to deal in the anovulatory patient is unopposed estrogen. This effect on the endometrium can be combated by a combined progestin-estrogen contraceptive agent or cyclic progestin therapy. Oral administration of one of the *progestin-dominant oral contraceptive steroids* for 3 to 6 months will usually regularize uterine bleeding. Periodic administration of progesterone such as *oral medroxyprogesterone acetate,* 10 mg daily for 13 days/month, will eliminate the endometrial hyperplasia caused by unopposed estrogen stimulation and regulate uterine bleeding; this is not an effective contraceptive agent. On occasion it will be necessary to control an acute episode of bleeding; *conjugated estrogens* administered intravenously, 25 mg every 4 hours for 24 hours, or a *progestin-dominant oral contraceptive steroid* such as Ovral, one tablet every 6 hours for 3 to 4 days, will usually control the acute bleeding. After the acute episode is controlled, combined estrogen-progestin oral contraceptives should be continued cyclically for 3 to 6 months. Progester-

---

DIAGNOSIS OF ABNORMAL UTERINE BLEEDING
Problem-oriented history
General physical and pelvic examination
Papanicolaou smear
Complete blood count
Serum hCG
Assessment of the endometrium

one therapy alone, orally, or intramuscularly, is not useful in controlling acute bleeding.

Bed rest, increasing oral fluid intake if a curettage is not contemplated, and iron replacement therapy are additional measures that should be instituted. In those adolescents who have a particularly heavy flow, it is prudent to continue iron therapy. If significant blood volume depletion occurs as a result of the heavy bleeding that cannot be controlled by hormone therapy and the patient is developing shock, a dilatation and curettage should be performed.

Childbearing period

Diagnosis. In women in the reproductive age range, complications of pregnancy, pelvic infections, endometriosis, leiomyomata, and neoplasia are the most likely causes of irregular bleeding. Particularly appropriate questions to be asked are: Is there intermenstrual bleeding or staining? (Suspect endometrial polyp or malignancy.) Does bleeding occur after coitus? (Suspect cervical neoplasia.) Have there been any recent periods of amenorrhea? (Suspect pregnancy or oligoovulation.) Is the patient taking any hormones? (Suspect endometrial hyperplasia.)

Again, a thorough general physical examination, pelvic examination, and Pap smear should be performed.

Women in this age range are less likely to have an unrecognized coagulopathy than are adolescents. However, *hypothyroidism* is likely, and a serum thyroid-stimulating hormone (TSH) level may be helpful. Also, for any woman with a disorder of ovulation, a *serum prolactin* should be ordered. Because uterine malignancy is uncommon before the age of 30, an endometrial sampling is not required routinely. If the physician has any reason to be suspicious of malignancy or a precursor, an in-office or outpatient endometrial sampling using an aspiration curet will usually be sufficient (Fig. 8-3). In dealing with recalcitrant or

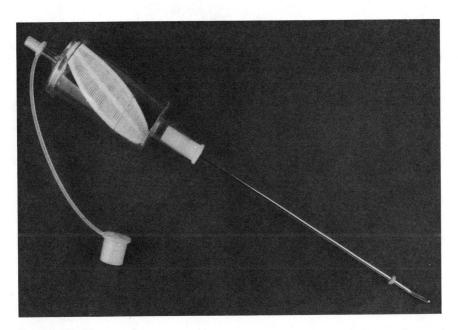

Fig. 8-3. Endometrial biopsy suction curet. Curet is attached to pump producing negative suction. Uterine cavity depth is determined, since curet is calibrated in centimeters. Sample obtained is collected in tissue trap. Preprocedure tranquilizer or paracervical block can reduce the discomfort and should be used as necessary.

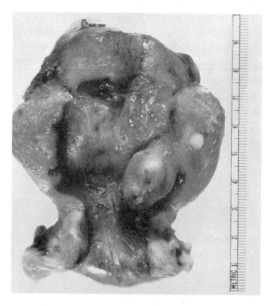

Fig. 8-4. Pedunculated submucous myoma. Uterus is normal size. Diagnosis is made by hysterogram (see Fig. 8-5).

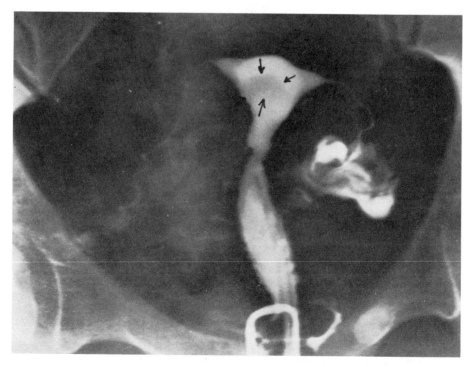

Fig. 8-5. Hysterogram showing submucous myoma. Uterine cavity is normal but has filling defect. Two previous curettages failed to disclose tumor.

recurrent dysfunctional bleeding, a *hysterogram* can be a valuable aid. Endometrial polyps and submucous myomas can be diagnosed by this procedure (Figs. 8-4 and 8-5). For those physicians who have acquired the skill, a *hysteroscopy* can often provide additional diagnostic information. The advantages of hysteroscopy include being able to perform a directed biopsy, identification and removal of endometrial polyps, and lysis of intrauterine adhesion. In a patient who has not responded to initial therapy, *dilatation and curettage* with exploration of the uterine cavity with forceps should be carried out. *Uterine curettage should generally be viewed as a diagnostic and not as a therapeutic procedure; it does not in itself correct the factors that are responsible for anovulation.* Curettage is best performed premenstrually or at the time of bleeding if it is acyclic; this will indicate whether or not there is a progesterone effect.

Therapy. In the patient with dysfunctional bleeding, if no contraindications exist, *cyclic hormone therapy* with a combination estrogen-progestin medication may be tried for 3 to 6 months. In the patient who has a long-standing history of oligo-ovulation or anovulation, *cyclic progesterone therapy,* medroxyprogesterone acetate, 10 mg; or nor-ethindrone acetate, 5 mg, for 12 days each month, should eliminate estrogen-induced endometrial hyperplasia and should produce regular withdrawal bleeding episodes. Patients with prolonged anovulation may need additional medical evaluation as discussed in Chapter 9. It is *seldom necessary to remove the uterus* because of dysfunctional bleeding. However, hysterectomy may be indicated if the bleeding cannot be controlled by hormone therapy or if there is a contraindication to its use. Some patients are unable to tolerate endocrine treatment because of side effects related to the medication, whereas others prefer hysterectomy to many years of hormonal therapy.

Nonsteroidal antiinflammatory medication has been shown to be effective in reducing uterine menstrual flow in women who have regular cyclic, but excessive, menses. An *oral iron preparation* should be administered if the patient gives a history of heavy flow; her iron stores may be depleted, but her hemoglobin may not yet have decreased enough to permit a diagnosis of anemia.

Greenberg noted that menorrhagia may be accompanied by *depression*. He diagnosed mild-to-moderate depression in 31 of 50 women being considered for hysterectomy because of excessive uterine flow.

The severity of blood loss with excessive, but regular, uterine bleeding correlates poorly with the patient's history of how many tampons or maxipads are required to contain the flow. Chimbira, Anderson, and Turnbull also found that endometrial surface area did not prognosticate the severity of flow: the larger uterine cavity, 46 cm^2, produced a mean loss of 85 ml; however, the largest mean loss, 525 ml, was found with a uterine surface area of 26 cm^2.

Tissue *prostaglandin metabolism* may provide the most significant explanation for excessive uterine bleeding associated with ovulatory cycles. Downing, Hutchon, and Poyser measured tissue uptake, in vitro, of ^{3}H-arachidonic acid (^{3}HAA) in proliferative, secretory, and endometrial tissue from patients complaining of hypermenorrhea. There was a significantly greater uptake of HAA in the endometria of patients having heavy bleeding, suggesting greater production of tissue prostaglandins.

Perimenopausal period

The assessment of women with abnormal bleeding during the *climacteric* (perimenopausal bleeding) is similar to that of women in the childbearing period. However, sampling of the endometrium should be part of the routine evaluation in this group. If the bleeding cannot be controlled easily with cyclic progestin therapy or if the patient cannot tolerate the medication, hysterectomy should be considered. The risks and benefits of estrogen replacement therapy in women over the age of 40 must be considered when discussing any surgical treatment with the patient (Chapter 50).

The patient with *postmenopausal bleeding* should be considered to have precancerous or malignant disease until proven otherwise. However, benign lesions such as atrophic vaginitis and cervical polyps are a more frequent cause of postmenopausal bleeding. *Fractional dilatation and curettage* is essential in the study of patients in this age group. Although endometrial hyperplasia may be the result of unopposed endogenous estrogen production, particularly in the obese female because of the conversion of androstenedione to estrone, the patient should still be thoroughly questioned as to whether or not she is taking estrogens. *Digoxin* has also been reported as having estrogenic activity and has been associated with endometrial hyperplasia. The possibility of an *ovarian estrogen-producing tumor* must also be considered. It is particularly important in this age group for the physician to search for an explanation of why there is excessive estrogen production at a time when it should be waning.

If anemia is diagnosed, other sources of blood loss such as *colon cancer* should be considered, and appropriate screening advised. *Hypothyroidism* is common in this age group, and the evaluation of thyroid function should be considered a routine measure.

Therapy. The treatment of irregular bleeding in the postmenopausal age group consists mainly of treating pathologic conditions of the uterus and ovaries. Endocrine therapy is less likely to be appropriate; however, *cyclic progestin therapy* (medroxyprogesterone, 10 mg daily for at least 13 days/month) may be tried after malignancy has been excluded. Progesterone prevents the replenishment of estrogen receptors in the endometrial cells and thereby reduces the growth effect of estrogen. This cellular effect is related more to the length of time progesterone is administered. In the future, it is probable that the length of progestin therapy will be increased to 14 days, whereas the daily dosage of progestogen will be reduced in the management of patients with perimenopausal dysfunctional bleeding.

REFERENCES

Aksel, S., and Jones, G.S.: Etiology and treatment of dysfunctional uterine bleeding, Obstet. Gynecol. **41**:1, 1974.

Chimbira, T.H., Anderson, A.B.M., and Turnbull, A.C.: Relation between measured menstrual blood loss and patients' subjective assessment of loss, duration of bleeding, number of sanitary towels used, uterine weight and endometrial surface, Br. J. Obstet. Gynaecol. **87**:603, 1980.

Classens, E.A., and Cowell, C.L.: Acute adolescent menorrhagia, Am. J. Obstet. Gynecol. **139**:277, 1981.

DeVore, G.R., Owens, O., and Kase, N.: Use of intravenous Premarin in the treatment of dysfunctional uterine bleeding—a double blind randomized control study, Obstet. Gynecol. **59**:285, 1982.

Diamond, E., Aksel, S., and Speir, B.R.: Endometrial estrogen and progesterone receptors in patients with dysfunctional uterine bleeding, Semin. Reprod. Endocrinol. **2**:351, 1984.

Downing, I., Hutchon, D.J.R., and Poyser, N.L.: Uptake of ³H-arachidonic acid by human endometrium: differences between normal and menorrhagic tissue, Prostaglandins **26**:55, 1983.

Fraser, L.S., Pearse, C., Shearman, R.P., Elliott, P.M., McIlveen, J., and Markham, R.: Efficacy of mefenamic acid in patients with a complaint of menorrhagia, Obstet. Gynecol. **58**:543, 1981.

Greenberg, M.: The meaning of menorrhagia: an investigation into the association between the complaint of menorrhagia and depression, J. Psychosom. Res. **27**:209, 1983.

Kroger, W.S., and Freed, S.C.: Psychosomatic gynecology, Philadelphia, 1951, W.B. Saunders Co.

Markee, J.E., Everett, J.W., and Sawyer, C.H.: The relationship of the nervous system to the release of gonadotropin and the regulation of the sex cycle, Recent Prog. Horm. Res. **7**:139, 1952.

McKelvey, J.L.: Irregular shedding of the endometrium, Am. J. Obstet. Gynecol. **60**:523, 1950.

Pritchard, J.A., and Mason, R.A.: Iron stores of normal adults and replenishment with oral iron therapy, J.A.M.A. **190**:119, 1964.

Southam, A.L., and Richart, R.M.: The prognosis for adolescents with menstrual abnormalities, Am. J. Obstet. Gynecol. **94**:637, 1966.

Speroff, L., Glass, R.H., and Kase, N.G.: Clinical gynecologic endocrinology and infertility, ed. 3, Baltimore, 1983, The Williams & Wilkins Co.

Valle, R.F., and Sciarra, J.J.: Diagnostic and operative hysteroscopy, Minn. Med. **57**:892, 1974.

Winter, J.S.D., and Faiman, C.: The development of cyclic pituitary-gonadal function in adolescent females, J. Clin. Endocrinol. Metab. **37**:714, 1973.

9

John H. Mattox

Amenorrhea

The term *amenorrhea* indicates the absence of menstruation. This is a symptom, not a disease entity, and may be caused by a variety of physiologic and pathologic processes.

Oligomenorrhea customarily refers to the occurrence of infrequent menstruation when the interval is usually 45 days or more. The term can also refer to short episodes of amenorrhea.

Amenorrhea is considered to be *primary* if a normal, spontaneous period has not occurred at age 16 years. *Secondary amenorrhea* indicates cessation of menstruation after a variable period of normal function, usually three consecutive monthly cycles.

Although a distinction concerning the evaluation of women with primary and secondary amenorrhea is no longer diagnostically relevant, some observations about these two groups of patients presenting with the *symptom* of amenorrhea may be clinically useful. Females with primary amenorrhea are more likely to have a uterovaginal anomaly, a genetic disorder, or a defective gonad.

ETIOLOGIC FACTORS

Amenorrhea can be induced by physiologic, anatomic, pathologic, or constitutional factors. Although the underlying problem may be physiologic or perhaps caused by a minor and negligible systemic or psychologic disturbance, it also may be an early symptom of a serious constitutional disease or endocrinopathy for which prompt treatment may be critical.

The following classification of the possible etiologic factors involved in amenorrhea is offered as a guide to the diagnostic study of this problem.

Causes of amenorrhea

I. Physiologic
   A. Periods during which amenorrhea occurs
      1. Adolescence
      2. Pregnancy
      3. Lactation
      4. Menopause

II. Anatomic
   A. Uterovaginal
      1. Imperforate hymen
      2. Absence of vagina/uterus
         a. Atresia
         b. Androgen insensitivity (testicular feminization)
         c. Müllerian agenesis (Mayer-Rokitansky-Kuster-Hauser syndrome)
         d. Hysterectomy
      3. Destruction of endometrium
         a. Uterine synechiae (Asherman's syndrome)
         b. Atrophy caused by irradiation or medication

c. Severe infection (tuberculosis, schistosomiasis)
B. Ovarian (gonadal)
  1. Gonadal dysgenesis
      a. 45 XO (Turner's syndrome)
      b. Mosaicism, isochromosome formation
      c. "Pure" 46 XX or 46 XY (Swyer's syndrome)
  2. Premature ovarian failure
  3. Destruction
      a. Mumps
      b. Irradiation
      c. Surgery
  4. Tumors
      a. Hormone-secreting neoplasms
          (1) Androgen (arrhenoblastoma, hilus cell)
          (2) Estrogen (granulosa-thecal cell)
          (3) hCG (dysgerminoma)
      b. Persistent corpus luteum (Halban's syndrome)
      c. Polycystic ovarian syndrome
C. Pituitary
  1. Infarction following delivery (Sheehan's syndrome)
  2. Tumor
      a. Prolactinoma
      b. Craniopharyngioma
      c. Acromegaly
  3. Irradiation
  4. Surgery
D. Hypothalamic/CNS
  1. GnRH deficiency (Kallmann's syndrome)
  2. Eating disorders
      a. Weight loss (with or without bulimia)
      b. Anorexia nervosa
  3. Stress-induced
  4. Exercise-associated
  5. Tumor
  6. Psychotropic medication
  7. Drug addiction

E. Miscellaneous
  1. Thyroid disease (usually hypothyroidism)
  2. Adrenal disease
      a. Congenital adrenal hyperplasia
      b. Cushing's Syndrome
      c. Hormone-secreting tumor
      d. Adrenal insufficiency (Addison's disease)

Physiologic causes

Amenorrhea during adolescence. The average healthy American girl usually experiences her first menstrual period at about the age of 12.5 years, but it is not at all unusual for the menarche to be delayed until 15 or 16 years of age, particularly if the young female is athletic. Similarly, although some girls bleed regularly after the onset of the first period, many exhibit considerable irregularity with frequent prolonged periods of amenorrhea during the first four years. This variation during adolescence is so common that it may be considered normal.

Failure to menstruate by age 16 warrants investigation. *Delayed menarche* is sometimes a biologic variant of maturation, but it may result from anatomic causes or serious endocrine or genetic abnormalities. The complaint of primary amenorrhea in a young woman will occasionally provide the first opportunity to uncover one of these conditions.

In women who have never menstruated, particular attention should be paid to whether or not secondary sex characteristics are present, a pivotal point that aids in the evaluation. If no *breast budding* occurs by 14 years of age, it is neither desirable nor necessary to wait until age 16, since this female is not undergoing the normal physiologic progression seen in puberty. Women with secondary amenorrhea are more likely to have a disorder of the hypothalamic-hypophyseal complex or a prolactinoma. The same algorithm (Fig. 9-5) can be followed for all women who either fail to initiate menstrual function or who develop a prolonged absence of menstruation.

Pregnancy. Pregnancy is the most common cause for amenorrhea during the reproductive years and should *always* be considered as a possible cause in all patients in the childbearing period. Instances of uterine bleeding during pregnancy are caused by a disturbance of pregnancy or by an organic lesion and not by menstrual periods.

Lactation. The first menstrual period after delivery usually occurs within 8 weeks unless the infant is breast-fed, in which event menstruation may be delayed until nursing is discontinued because of the persistence of increased levels of serum prolactin. In nonnursing and nursing mothers, basal prolactin levels can return to normal within 3 weeks after delivery. In nursing mothers, suckling can induce a tenfold or greater rise in serum prolactin. The surges decrease gradually while nursing is continued and disappear in about 80 to 100 days.

The transient hypogonadotropic hypogonadism with subsequent hypoestrogenism associated with hyperprolactinemia is caused by an inhibition of GnRH by endogenous opioids.

Hefnawi and Bodraoui reported on 340 Egyptian women who nursed infants following delivery and used no other contraceptive method for at least 1 year. Eight percent of the women menstruated during the first month, and there was a gradual increase over the next 12 months to total 61%. One fourth of the women did conceive during this time period.

In nonnursing mothers, Cronin found that ovulation occurred before the first menstrual period in one third of the cases, whereas ovulation in lactating mothers is infrequent before the tenth week after delivery. These facts underscore the importance of family planning counseling *during the pregnancy* and early in the puerperium, because occasionally ovulation and even pregnancy may occur in the lactating amenorrheic woman.

Premenopause. Variable periods of oligomenorrhea may occur for a number of years preceding the final cessation of menstruation. This is frequently a source of considerable anxiety to the middle-aged woman, who may consider the amenorrhea to be a symptom of pregnancy. Vaginal bleeding that occurs after 5 to 6 months of amenorrhea should be suspected as resulting from a cause such as cancer. Ovulatory cycles are uncommon after age 50.

Anatomic causes

Amenorrhea may be caused by congenital malformations that preclude the possibility of menstruation. These abnormalities account for about 2% of all amenorrhea not caused by pregnancy.

Atresia of the vagina and imperforate hymen (Fig. 9-1). These anatomic causes for primary amenorrhea, although not common, underscore the importance of complete examination of girls at birth and during subsequent examinations.

Absence of menstruation can result from an obstruction at some point in the vagina or cervix. An *imperforate hymen* is one of the possible congenital malformations. Since the ovaries and endometrium in these patients are perfectly normal, a discharge of blood from the uterus occurs at the time of menstruation, but it is retained and hidden in the vagina (*cryptomenorrhea*). This process is repeated from month to month and leads to *hematocolpos*, a progressive distension of the vagina with blood (Fig. 9-2). If the situation is unrecognized, the uterus and even the fallopian tubes may become filled with this material, resulting in *hematometra* and *hematosalpinx*. Periodic episodes of lower abdominal pain and backache are characteristic. Inspection of the vulva and rectal examination will readily confirm the diagnosis. A simple cruciate incision of the hymen is corrective of these disorders. In the course of the evaluation laparoscopy should be carried out, since these young females may have developed endometriosis.

Absence of the uterus and vagina. Abnormal development of the müllerian system can result in partial or complete absence of the vagina, uterine hypoplasia, or only rudimentary muscular cords. Rarely, a small functional uterine cavity may be present. Menstrual flow can be retained, resulting in periodic pelvic pain. Complete aplasia of the vagina associated with a poorly defined uterine anlage, *Mayer-Rokitansky-Kuster-Hauser syndrome*, is a relatively common cause of primary amenorrhea; about one third of these women have a renal

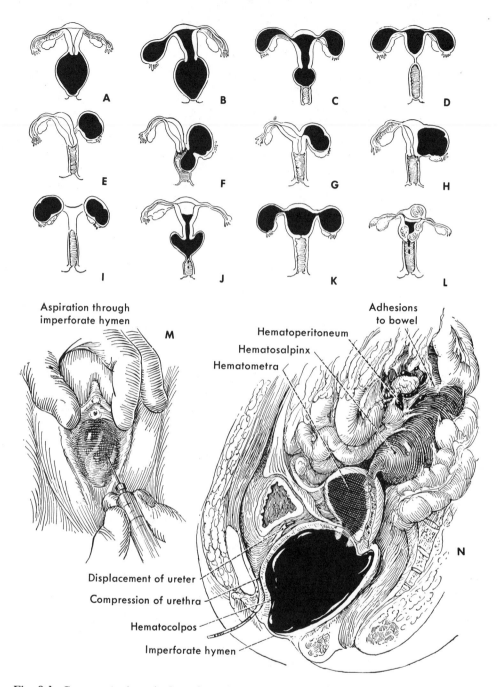

Fig. 9-1. Cryptomenorrhea. **A,** Imperforate hymen, hematocolpos. **B,** Imperforate hymen, hematocolpometra, right hematosalpinx. **C,** Congenital atresia of cervix, hematocolpometra, bilateral hematosalpinx. **D,** Congenital atresia of cervix, hematometra, bilateral hematosalpinx. **E,** Uterus bicornis unicollis, lateral hematometra in blind, rudimentary horn. **F,** Uterus didelphys, lateral hematocolpometra resulting from blind left vagina. **G,** Uterus bicornis unicollis, lateral hematometra in blind left horn. **H,** Uterus septus duplex, lateral hematometra in blind left uterine cavity. **I,** Uterus didelphys, two rudimentary horns, hematometra resulting from gynatresia. **J,** Acquired atresia of cervix, intermittent hematocolpometra. **K,** Acquired atresia of cervix, hematometra, bilateral hematosalpinx. **L,** Cervical fibromyoma, intermittent hematometra. **M,** Diagnostic aspiration through imperforate hymen. **N,** Sagittal section showing effects of cryptomenorrhea. (From Ball, T.L.: Gynecologic surgery and urology, ed. 2, St. Louis, 1963, The C.V. Mosby Co.)

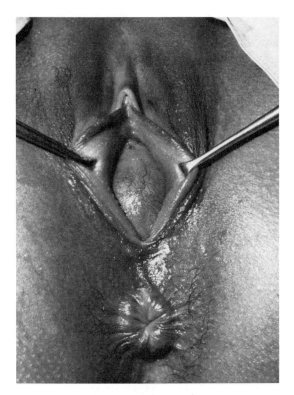

Fig. 9-2. Imperforate hymen distended by hematocolpos.

anomaly, and 12% have skeletal defects. This diagnosis should be entertained when young women with secondary sex characteristics fail to menstruate. A careful examination of the genitalia should be performed and will usually disclose a diagnosis. Androgen insensitivity, *testicular feminization syndrome,* should be included in the differential diagnosis. The latter condition should also be strongly suspected in female infants with inguinal hernias or labial masses.

Prolonged endometrial suppression following the use of injectable medroxyprogesterone acetate can result in endometrial atrophy. Although the condition is self-limiting, the uterine lining may be partially resistant to exogenous or endogenous estrogen stimulation, giving the impression that there is endometrial obliteration.

Traumatic uterine adhesions. Secondary amenorrhea may develop after repeated or too strenuous curettage, particularly in the postpartum and post-abortal uterus, *Asherman's syndrome. Postoperative endometritis* may be responsible for the development of synechiae that may partially or almost completely obliterate the endometrial cavity. The *hypoestrogenic state* seen in the early period following pregnancy is also believed to be contributory, since endometrial proliferation is less active.

The recent use of *hysteroscopy* has greatly improved both diagnosis and management of this problem. Although a hysterogram will demonstrate a filling defect, the precise locations and extent of the adhesions are far more accurately determined under direct vision. Symptoms in patients with a moderate number of adhesions are hypomenorrhea and a tendency to abort if implantation occurs. Amenorrhea occurs with extensive involvement (Fig. 9-3).

Scar tissue can be most effectively removed or lysed with hysteroscopic instruments, if available. Otherwise, a dilatation and curettage is performed, and a device such as a Foley catheter is inserted to keep the uterine walls separated during healing. Estrogen therapy should be given after surgery to stimulate endometrial growth. Return of normal ovulatory menstruation and fertility is the rule in mild-to-moderate disease.

Destruction of endometrium. Secondary amenorrhea is caused by surgical removal or irradiation of the uterus, endometrium, or ovaries. Rarely, a disease process may be destructive enough to produce a similar result. If for some reason a subtotal hysterectomy has been performed, periodic bleeding may continue from the remaining portion of the endometrium. If periods cease after subtotal hysterectomy and subsequently recur, the physician should suspect a cancer in the cervical stump rather than a resumption of menstrual function.

Irradiation of the pelvis results in either temporary or permanent amenorrhea, depending on the dose employed. This effect is produced by the destructive action on the endometrium or ovaries. If periods recur after a long period of irradiation-induced amenorrhea, an intrauterine malignancy must be ruled out as a cause of bleeding.

Gonadal factors

Gonadal dysgenesis (Turner's syndrome). Classic features of Turner's syndrome include congenital

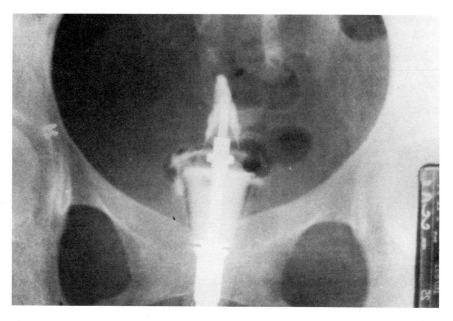

Fig. 9-3. Attempted hysterogram. Endometrial cavity obliterated following postpartum curettage. Cannula tip at cervicouterine junction, and no endometrial cavity is visualized.

webbed neck, low-set ears, cubitus valgus, short stature, shield chest, high-arched palate, increased pigmented nevi, and sexual infantilism. Other anomalies such as congenital heart disease, particularly coarctation of the aorta and renal malformation, often are present. The complete picture of this syndrome, including all the foregoing anomalies, is relatively rare, whereas sexual infantilism and short stature are consistent findings. About 30% of infants have lymphedema of the lower extremities at birth; this finding should alert the clinician to the possibility of this diagnosis.

It is not unusual for the patient to have amenorrhea as the first complaint. About 80% to 90% of these patients are chromatin negative and show a sex chromosome constitution of XO. The chromosome number therefore is 45. The chromosomal constitution in others may show *mosaicism* such as XO/XX or XO/XXX. Thus the chromosomal number of the majority is 45, whereas some have chromosomal counts of 46. An XO/XY form occurs and tends to be familial.

Turner's syndrome represents primary and complete ovarian failure. The ovaries are represented by elongated, whitish ridges or streaks on the broad ligament. They contain neither primordial follicles nor germ cells, but the stromal tissue is similar to that of the ovary. The absence of estrogen secretion is reflected by a lack of breast development, genital hypoplasia, amenorrhea, and high serum concentrations of FSH and LH.

Diagnosis is confirmed by examination of the buccal smear for nuclear sex evaluation, determination of chromosomal constitution, and detection of high gonadotropin excretion.

"Pure" gonadal dysgenesis is seen in individuals with primary amenorrhea, no secondary sex characteristics, and an eunuchoid habitus. Hypergonadotropism is present; and the karyotype can be *46 XY, Swyer's syndrome,* or 46 XX. Traditionally, no other somatic abnormalities have been associated with pure gonadal dysgenesis; however, there have been two patients reported with 46 XY gonadal dysgenesis who had renal anomalies; it is possible that these individuals may not have been sufficiently scrutinized in the past. The gonads are at risk for neoplasia, particularly if they contain Y chromosomes; the

tumors most likely to be found are a gonadoblastoma or a dysgerminoma.

The *"resistant ovary" syndrome* is a rare condition seen in women who have some secondary sexual development with associated elevation of FSH and LH levels. Their karyotype is 46 XX. Ovarian follicles can be identified in tissue obtained by an ovarian biopsy taken at laparosocopy. The cause is unknown but is thought to represent a possible gonadotropin receptor deficiency. This syndrome is not associated with other somatic abnormalities. Although pregnancy has been reported in a small number of patients identified with this problem, for all practical purposes ovulation induction has not been successful.

Premature ovarian failure is an unusual, but not rare, clinical problem presenting with secondary amenorrhea. The condition is usually permanent but can be transient. Although there are some known causal agents such as irradiation, cytotoxic drugs, genetic factors, and specific viral infection such as mumps oophoritis, the cause frequently remains a mystery. There is a significant association between premature ovarian failure of other gland systems, specifically the pancreatic beta cells and the thyroid, adrenal, and parathyroid glands, suggesting that the ovarian failure is part of an overall autoimmune disease. A high incidence of ovarian failure has been identified in women with abnormal galactose metabolism.

Nonneoplastic ovarian cysts such as a *follicular cyst* of the ovary may on occasion cause a short period of amenorrhea. As a rule, this type of ovarian cyst produces no menstrual disturbance, nor is it associated with dysfunctional uterine bleeding. A *corpus luteum cyst* (larger than 5 cm) that persists may induce a short period of amenorrhea followed by irregular bleeding. The problem is self-limiting. The symptoms and presentation of an adnexal mass may lead the physician to suspect ectopic pregnancy. With a careful history, pelvic examination, appropriate use of serum hCG levels, and ultrasound, the correct diagnosis can be reached. *Neoplastic cysts* of the ovary that may induce amenorrhea are primarily the functioning cysts of the ovarian stroma. They can be *androgen secreting (arrhenoblastomas)* or *estrogen secreting (granu-*

losa-thecal cell tumors) (Chapter 48). These possibilities must be considered in evaluation of amenorrhea; but they are exceedingly rare.

Testicular feminizing syndrome (male pseudohermaphroditism). Testicular feminizing syndrome is characterized by *androgen insensitivity.* The male tissues are partially or totally unable to respond to androgen hormone messages because of the lack of cytosol receptors. A strong familial tendency transmitted probably by an X-linked recessive mode is responsible. These individuals are chromatin negative, with a karyotype of 46 XY and thus a genotypic male; however, most are completely feminine in appearance. Breasts are distinctively developed; height is normal; and axillary, pubic, and facial hair is absent or sparse. A vaginal indentation is present, less deep than usual, but other internal female genitals are absent. The male gonads are usually found as swellings in the inguinal canal or within the abdominal cavity.

The gonad produces both estrogen and androgen. Estrogen values are higher than those found in normal males. LH levels are elevated. Inability of end-organ response to androgen is further demonstrated by the fact that serum testosterone and dehydroepiandrosterone sulfate (DHEAS) levels are in the range for normal males.

These individuals are psychologically and morphologically female and function normally in this role except that they are amenorrheic and infertile. The gonads containing a Y chromosome should be removed because of their propensity to become malignant; extirpation need not be deferred until the endogenous estrogen effects of puberty are gained. Gonadal malignancy is rare before the age of 20. *Hormone replacement* therapy (estrogen and progesterone) is indicated after gonadectomy.

Counseling of these patients and their parents and partners is a delicate matter. Artless emphasis on the genetic and chromosomal sex can be unduly traumatic. They should be considered to be and spoken of as women. The term gonad is obviously preferable to testis.

After they studied 17 families in Santa Domingo, Peterson and co-workers demonstrated the necessity of *5-*

alpha-reductase, the enzyme required to convert testosterone to dihydrotestosterone (DHT), for the formation of normal male genitalia. At birth the affected genetic males had labial-scrotal or inguinal testes, a small phallus, and a single perineal opening; they were raised as females in the society until puberty. Partial virilization with testicular descent and some penile enlargement occur, but prostatic enlargement, facial hair growth, temporal recession, and acne are absent; those biologic phenomena require dihydrotestosterone. These males undergo psychosexual reassignment and assume the role of young men.

POLYCYSTIC OVARIAN SYNDROME. The classic features of the complete symptom complex originally described by Stein and Leventhal in 1935 were amenorrhea, infertility, obesity, and facial hirsutism. The ovaries were described as oysterlike in appearance with a thick grayish capsule, numerous tiny cysts beneath the thickened tunica, and an enlargement amounting to approximately two to three times their normal size. Typical microscopic findings in polycystic ovarian syndrome are hyperplasia and luteinization of the theca interna.

It became evident later that neither ovarian enlargement nor theca luteinization was an invariable finding. Stein and Leventhal recognized that some of the symptoms were inconstant; hirsutism occurred in only about 50% of the cases, and instead of amenorrhea, menstrual irregularities with episodes of menometrorrhagia were not uncommon. The amenorrhea tends to develop gradually over a period of years. Obesity is not always present. However, ovaries with thick fibrous tunica reflecting anovulation and infertility are consistent findings.

There has been great confusion and controversy regarding the etiologic factors in the polycystic ovary syndrome. It is apparent that it represents the end result of long, uninterrupted periods of anovulation. A wide spectrum of disorders causing anovulation is associated with malfunction of the hypothalamic-pituitary-gonadal axis. Many are temporary derangements. Polycystic ovarian syndrome reflects prolonged, persistent anovulation—the development of a "steady state" in the feedback effects of estrogen on gonadotropin secretion. FSH levels fall in the low normal range with ab-

sence of the midcycle peak (negative feedback effect); LH secretion is sustained at an elevated level (positive feedback effect) with lack of an appropriate midcycle surge. In addition, there is increased sensitivity of LH to GnRH. The polycystic ovary produces an excess of androgens, mainly androstenedione and testosterone.

Persistent gonadotropin stimulation causes growth of follicles and an increase in estradiol and estrone at first, but ova are not released. The follicles arrest and become cystic or atretic, and stromal tissue is increased. The amount of estradiol produced is diminished, but estrogen precursors, androstenedione and testosterone, are significantly increased. Androstenedione can undergo conversion to testosterone within the ovary and peripherally. It also undergoes conversion to estrone by fatty tissue, and this contributes to the circulating estrogen pool. These derangements, characteristic of polycystic ovary syndrome, are thus self-perpetuating. The persistent LH excess causes some increase in adrenal and ovarian androgen secretions. However, ovarian and adrenal catheterizations performed by Kirschner and Jacobs showed that the ovary is the major source of androgens in the majority of hirsute women with polycystic ovaries.

Diagnosis. Clinical features, including menstrual irregularities—usually oligomenorrhea but occasionally menometrorrhagia—may begin in the teens or early twenties, preceding the development of secondary amenorrhea by several years. Infertility is caused by anovulation. Obesity and hirsutism may or may not be associated. Enlargement of the ovaries is a common but not essential feature. The size is within normal limits in about a third of cases. The smooth, gray, sclerotic capsule is characteristic of persistent anovulation (Fig. 9-4).

The basal body temperature is monophasic, cervical mucus displays arborization with no significant change during the cycle, and the endometrium is proliferative or hyperplastic. The secretion of estrogen is within normal limits but unopposed by progesterone.

Gonadotropin secretion assumes a relatively steady state, although the actual values vary. As a rule, FSH is in a low normal range, and LH is

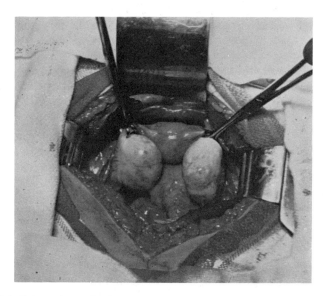

Fig. 9-4. Polycystic ovaries in young woman with polycystic ovarian syndrome.

elevated. The LH:FSH ratio is usually greater than 3:1. The urinary 17-ketosteroid level is normal or slightly elevated. The serum DHEAS is normal or mildly elevated. Plasma testosterone is usually elevated when hirsutism is associated but is usually less than 200 ng/dl.

Management of polycystic ovarian syndrome must be individualized and deserves comment separate from the overall management of amenorrhea. For the young woman who is not desirous of pregnancy, medroxyprogesterone acetate, 10 mg, may be taken daily for 14 days, beginning about the fifteenth day after bleeding begins, or at any time in women who are amenorrheic. This will produce withdrawal bleeding from the drug-induced secretory endometrium. The long-term use of medroxyprogesterone acetate will inhibit the development of endometrial hyperplasia or atypia and may protect against the development of endometrial cancer associated with unopposed estrogen stimulation. Progestins also reduce ovarian androgen secretion, but improvement in hirsutism takes many months.

If the patient is hirsute and hypertensive or if DHEAS is elevated, primary adrenal disorders must be excluded. The indicated adrenal suppression test is the administration of dexamethasone, 1.0 mg, at 11 PM. A serum cortisol drawn at 8 AM

the next morning should be less than 6 μg/dl. If mild adrenal hyperplasia is suspected, prednisone therapy may be useful.

Polycystic ovarian syndrome patients will often have associated medical problems such as diabetes mellitus, essential hypertension, and hyperlipidemia. For women who want to conceive, clomiphene citrate provides the most practical medical form of treatment. Bilateral wedge resection of the ovaries may be an alternative if repeated courses of clomiphene therapy fail.

HYPERTHECOSIS. This condition is closely related to the polycystic ovary syndrome, but hirsutism is more pronounced, temporal recession of hair is characteristic, and hypertension is usual. Hyperthecosis is not confined to the theca interna in these cases. Instead, nests of luteinized cells are found throughout the ovarian stroma. Plasma testosterone levels may be extremely high. This condition undoubtedly accounts for some failures of wedge resection performed in patients in whom an adrenal disturbance was excluded and a diagnosis of polycystic ovary syndrome was entertained.

OVARIAN NEOPLASMS. Ovarian neoplasms rarely cause amenorrhea, but they must be considered in the differential diagnosis.

Because of its malignant potential, *arrhenoblastoma* is the most important of the virilizing tumors of the ovary, all of which can cause amenorrhea. The serum testosterone is usually greater than 200 ng/dl.

Masculinizing hilus cell tumor is an exceedingly rare growth arising from the hilus cells of the ovary, which are probably the homologs of the Leydig cells of the testis. Therefore these tumors, although rather small in size, produce distinct virilization.

Pituitary gland factors. The finding of abnormally low gonadotropin values associated with either primary or secondary amenorrhea points to an anterior pituitary or hypothalamic disorder. Differential diagnosis between the two can be extremely difficult. Major advances in diagnostic radiographic techniques and new methods for dynamic testing using hypothalamic-releasing hormones have made possible greater accuracy of diagnosis.

Primary hypopituitarism with resultant amenorrhea may result from destruction of the pituitary (the anterior lobe more frequently than the posterior lobe) by tumor, irradiation, surgery, or infarction. It is estimated that 70% of the adenohypophysis can be destroyed before clinical manifestations occur. Some recovery of pituitary function following an insult can occur, and only a partial deficiency of tropic hormones may result. Following gland destruction, defective growth hormone secretion occurs in virtually 100% of patients; alteration in gonadotropin secretion is next.

Pituitary adenomas are much more common than once appreciated in the past. Three adenomas were recognized because of their dramatic clinical presentation: (1) *acromegaly* as a result of excess growth hormone, (2) hypercortisolism with sequelae caused by increased ACTH secretion *(Cushing's disease)*, and (3) amenorrhea-galactorrhea secondary to a prolactin-secreting adenoma. It has now been documented in clinically reported cases that pituitary adenomas may produce many protein hormones completely or in fragments; pituitary tumors secreting TSH, LH, FSH, and beta endorphins have been reported. Immunohistologic staining of tumor material identifies the tumor cells more appropriately than the earlier method of using histologic appearance on the basis of whether there was an acidophilic, basophilic, or chromophobic cell population.

Amenorrhea-galactorrhea represents a marked disturbance of the hypothalamic-pituitary function and often is the first clinical evidence of a small pituitary prolactinoma. The tumors are usually, but not invariably, benign. Hyperprolactinemia is found in a high proportion of these cases, and high levels tend to correlate with the tumor and its size. Normal serum prolactin values range from 3 to 25 ng/ml in women. When both amenorrhea and galactorrhea are present, prolactin values over 100 ng/ml should lead to suspicion of a functioning macroadenoma. Growth of microadenomas (below 1 cm in size) may be so insidious that hyperprolactinemia, amenorrhea, and/or galactorrhea may be present for years before an abnormality in the sella turcica is evident by x-ray film study.

Recently developed techniques in diagnostic radiology using high-resolution computerized tomography (CT) and contrast material make it possible to detect microadenomas of 4 to 10 mm with surprising accuracy. Availability of these diagnostic aids makes it apparent that pituitary adenomas are far more common than previous reports indicate.

When hyperprolactinemia in women is assessed, it should be remembered that tranquilizers and antihypertensives (phenothiazines, tricyclic antidepressants, and reserpine), oral contraceptives, and even stress situations can inhibit prolactin-inhibiting factor (PIF) through hypothalamic suppression with consequent release of prolactin. Amenorrhea-galactorrhea is therefore found in some cases of *hypothyroidism*.

Diagnostic workup of patients with amenorrhea-galactorrhea should include determination of the serum prolactin level as a screening test, since high levels tend to correlate with a tumor and indicate its size. Early pregnancy should be excluded. A careful drug history and examinations for evidence of other endocrinopathies, particularly hypothyroidism, are obviously important, since these disorders can be easily treated. Visual field measurements and a CT scan should be included.

Medical treatment can be used to treat both tumor- and nontumor-related hyperprolactinemia. *Bromocriptine mesylate (Parlodel),* a dopamine receptor agonist that is similar in action to PIF, is the most effective agent now available for treatment of a small pituitary adenoma. Ovulatory cycles and fertility are usually established within 2 to 3 months after therapy. However, favorable results are not always permanent. Recently, bromocriptine has been found to be effective in correcting the physiologic defects associated with other pituitary tumors, notably in cases of acromegaly incompletely treated with radiation or surgery.

Prolactin-secreting adenomas, particularly microadenomas, do not mandate therapy. Other variables to be considered are other findings or symptomatology such as headaches, visual field deficit, a desire for pregnancy, risk of osteoporosis, and the patient's anxiety about the tumor or hyperprolactinemia-associated depression. March and colleagues studied a group of 43 patients with radiographic evidence of tumor-associated hyperprolactinemia from 3 to 20 years. Only two patients underwent transsphenoidal surgery for tumor growth; three patients became eumenorrheic and euprolactinemic, suggesting spontaneous resolution. The remainder of the patients demonstrated no significant change in their tumor.

The *surgical method* of transsphenoidal adenectomy and *radiation* with external radiotherapy or implantation of yttrium 90 seeds have been used less often since the introduction of bromocriptine.

EMPTY-SELLA SYNDROME. Empty-sella syndrome, with similar clinical symptomatologic findings, must be differentiated from pituitary adenoma. The sellar abnormality is believed to be developmental in that the sellar diaphragm is incomplete.

The sella is filled with cerebrospinal fluid, which compresses and flattens the pituitary gland against the sellar floor. Because of the sensitivity of gonadotropin secretion, amenorrhea is likely to be the dominant symptom. Galactorrhea is occasionally associated with this syndrome, but other endocrine functions are usually normal. The main importance of this abnormality is that it must be distinguished from other more common causes of enlarged sella, such as pituitary tumors or cysts that may require surgical or radiation treatment. Prolactin-secreting adenomas have been described in women with "empty sella syndrome."

PITUITARY ADENOMA AND PREGNANCY. The pituitary gland normally increases in size during pregnancy. A preexisting pituitary adenoma likewise enlarges and may become symptomatic. Headaches occur first, and visual disturbances may follow. Magyar and Marshall studied 73 women with previously untreated pituitary microadenomas and macroadenomas during 91 pregnancies. Most experienced no complications and could be managed expectantly. In 39%, headache or visual disturbance developed during pregnancy; and in 20% of the cases, previously untreated symptoms were severe enough to require treatment during pregnancy. Delivery was usually vaginal; cesarean section was performed only as a requisite of obstetric indication. Breast-feeding was permitted.

In 78 pregnancies involving women previously treated for a pituitary tumor, headache developed in 4% and visual disturbance in 5%.

PITUITARY HYPOFUNCTION (SHEEHAN'S SYNDROME). Pituitary hypofunction is usually related to a preceding severe postpartum hemorrhage or a serious puerperal infection. The pituitary gland enlarges during pregnancy because of an increase in the number and size of the lactotropes and is more susceptible to hemorrhage, thrombosis, infarction, and resultant necrosis in the immediate period following delivery. If a considerable portion of the anterior lobe is destroyed, gonadotropic, adrenal, and thyroid functions are severely depressed, cachexia develops, and lactation is inhibited. Hormone replacement is essential to protect against adrenal insufficiency, hypothyroidism, and estrogen deficiency.

Hypothalamic factors. Since higher centers in the brain exert control over pituitary activity by affecting neurotransmitters that impact ultimately on the hypothalamus, it is not difficult to understand that "psychogenic factors" can cause disturbances in ovarian physiology. Lesions that cause destruction of or impinge on the hypothalamus can result in diminished or poorly coordinated pulsatile secretion of FSH and LH. Tumors such as craniopharyngioma, glioma, endodermal sinus tumor, or histiocytosis along with head trauma and external therapeutic irradiation have all been associated with an absence of menses.

The concept of *hypothalamic amenorrhea*

should be defined in its broadest sense as the absence of menses secondary to an alteration in psychoneuroendocrine events. Currently, not all of the biochemical pathways or interactions can be clearly connected, but that should not detract from the concept.

A striking example of the intimate relationship between the psychic and the soma is *pseudocyesis*. The condition usually occurs in emotionally unstable women who are infertile and have an intense desire for pregnancy. Current evidence indicates that there is a hypersecretion of prolactin and LH with circulating estradiol and progesterone levels comparable to those found in the early luteal phase.

Anorexia nervosa is a condition in which amenorrhea is an early and common symptom. Although the exact incidence is unknown, it was found in one out of 150 adolescent girls in Sweden. It is seen in those who are obsessed by the necessity to remain thin. Their objective is fulfilled either by restricting food or becoming *bulimic;* that is, they periodically go on eating binges, usually associated with catharsis or self-induced emesis.

These individuals are very intense and hyperactive, and frequently they are hyperachievers. They are usually members of an upper–middle class family whose parents are dominating. There may also be a history of sexual molestation. Hormonally, there is a significant inhibition of GnRH secretion similar to prepubertal state. There is also a significant effect involving the hypothalamic-pituitary-adrenal axis in that there is a hypersecretion of cortisol but diminution in adrenal androgen secretion. Although there is a wide clinical spectrum, most cases are not severe. The outcome for these individuals is usually favorable; however, death can result. Treatment centers around psychotherapy, hormone replacement therapy, and eventually regaining weight.

Psychogenic amenorrhea is seen in young women without any clinically demonstrable endocrinopathy. These are usually unmarried and weight conscious and have had previous menstrual irregularities. Often there is an antecedent event such as a stressful relationship, change in geography, or change in employment. Defective GnRH secretion, which may be modulated by beta endorphins or abnormal dopamine secretion, is probably the underlying cause. After other causes of amenorrhea have been excluded, psychologic support and, occasionally, hormone replacement therapy will suffice. This disorder is often self-limiting.

Kallmann's syndrome, hypogonadotropic hypogonadism with anosmia, was first described in males in 1944. Current understanding suggests that the primary alteration in gonadotropin secretion is related mainly to defective synthesis of GnRH; partial or complete olfactory bulb agenesis has also been documented at autopsy. Other stigmata have included color blindness, mental retardation, and congenital defects of the midline structures. It is usually inherited as an autosomal dominant trait. Patients are usually eunuchoid with no or minimal development of secondary sex characteristics; gonadotropin levels are barely detectable. Fertility is possible with menotropin or pulsatile GnRH therapy.

Miscellaneous factors

Weight. *Exercise amenorrhea* varies with different athletic endeavors. The incidence is higher in long-distance runners and ballet dancers than it is in swimmers. Although there has been some attempt to relate this to body weight, amenorrhea associated with athletic competitiveness can occur without weight loss. In a large number of women, a 15% loss of total body weight from ideal body weight will result in oligoamenorrhea. It is clear that, although the cause of the hormonal problem is mediated through deficient secretion of GnRH, it is multifactorial.

Frisch and MacArthur noted that menarche depended on the acquisition of 22% body fat. This percentage is required to maintain normal menses, and therefore diminution of percentage of body fat or an increased lean-to-fat ratio would be associated with a menstrual abnormality. Women who are obese may also have a menstrual abnormality; although the mechanism is not well understood, it is known that severely obese women have decreased sex steroid–binding globulin levels and therefore more free circulating hormone, specifically testosterone.

Thyroid gland. The thyroid gland is not directly concerned with menstruation, but ovarian function often is disturbed in women with hypothyroidism or hyperthyroidism. Amenorrhea may be associated with either mild or severe hypothyroidism and occasionally may be a symptom of Graves' disease.

Primary hypothyroidism is one of many causes for amenorrhea-galactorrhea syndrome. TRH, which is increased in this condition, induces release not only of pituitary TSH but also of prolactin. Synthetic TRH is also a potent releaser of prolactin. Thyroid substitution therapy alone is corrective of this disorder.

Adrenal gland. Amenorrhea and signs of masculinization may be produced by hyperplasia, benign adenomas, or malignant tumors of the adrenal cortex. Apart from amenorrhea, which is common to each, more specific clinical syndromes and laboratory findings reflect involvement of different components of the adrenal cortex.

Cushing's syndrome is characterized by excessive production of the major glucocorticoid, cortisol, whereas congenital adrenal hyperplasia is characterized by excessive production of adrenal androgens. Adrenal neoplasms may produce either substance, or the typcial features of each may overlap. Furthermore, adrenal hyperactivity may be secondary to excessive pituitary adrenocorticotropic hormone (ACTH) secretion.

Menstrual abnormalities, including amenorrhea, can be found in 25% of patients with primary adrenal cortical insufficiency, Addison's disease, or in a higher percentage of women with secondary deficiency related to destructive or infiltrative lesions of the pituitary or hypothalamus.

DIAGNOSIS

Often the physician can establish the cause of amenorrhea after taking a complete history, making a pelvic examination, or performing a simple laboratory procedure. On the other hand, the etiologic factors of the symptom may require extensive investigation of genetic, systemic, psychic, and endocrine factors.

A thorough physical examination, including inspection of the genitals and palpation of the pelvic organs, will enable the physician to detect gross anatomic abnormalities as well as deviations in somatic growth and genital development. Endocrine stigmas such as hirsutism, deposition of body fat,

absence of breast development, and enlargement of the clitoris are significant physical findings in the clinical evaluation of amenorrhea. Pregnancy must be excluded before the evaluation.

When the complete general examination does not provide specific clues, a practical approach as outlined in Fig. 9-5 can be followed. A baseline *serum prolactin level, a T_3 uptake and total T_4 determination,* along with the *progestin challenge* constitutes the initial assessment. If hyperprolactinemia is encountered (25 ng/ml is the upper range of normal for the nonpregnant patient in most laboratories), other causes of this problem should be investigated; a serum TSH should be part of that assessment. If a prolactinoma is strongly suspected, high resolution computerized tomography with dye enhancement will aid in the diagnosis. If androgen excess is clinically apparent, a serum testosterone and DHEA sulfate should be ordered. If the testosterone is above 200 ng/dl, an ovarian or adrenal testosterone-producing tumor should be sought. A DHEA sulfate above 700 µg/dl should make one suspicious of an androgen-producing tumor located in the adrenal gland.

If bleeding can be induced by the injection of 100 mg of progesterone-in-oil or by oral medroxyprogesterone acetate, 20 mg daily for 5 days, it may be assumed that the amenorrhea is not caused by any serious derangement of either the pituitary, ovary, or uterus, since enough estrogen is being produced to stimulate the endometrium. This would indicate a functional derangement of gonadotropic release with anovulation.

If no bleeding occurs following the progestin challenge test, either there may be failure of the ovary to secrete an appropriate amount of estrogen to prime the endometrium, or the surface may have been destroyed by surgery, medication or irradiation. To rule out *endometrial failure*, estrogen stimulation in the form of 2.5 mg/day of conjugated estrogens for 25 days followed by 7 days of medroxyprogesterone acetate, 10 mg, will assist in the differential diagnosis. If bleeding does occur, one can assume that the endometrial surface is only atrophic, perhaps because of prolonged use of medication or inactivity of the ovary. If bleeding does

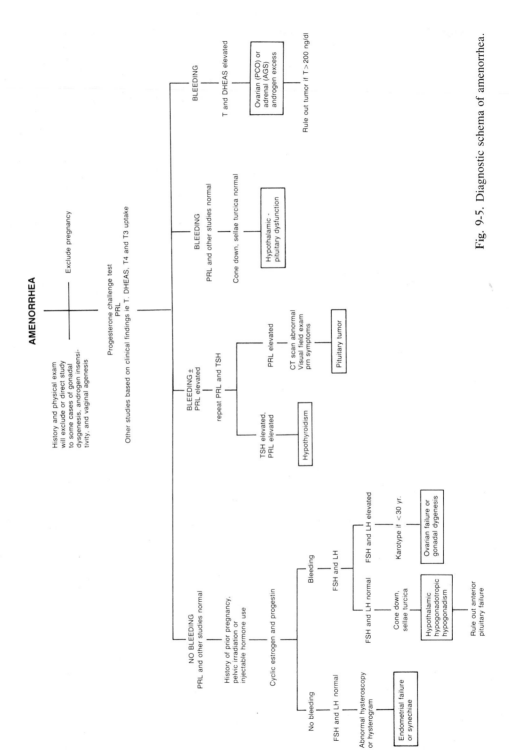

Fig. 9-5. Diagnostic schema of amenorrhea.

not occur, hysterosalpingography will provide the necessary information to diagnosis intrauterine scarring.

To differentiate these two causes for the amenorrhea it is necessary to perform an immunoassay of gonadotropins. When serum gonadotropin levels, FSH, and LH are above 50 ImU/ml, ovarian or gonadal failure is likely. A buchal smear determining the presence or absence of a Barr body and a fluorescent Y chromosome can be helpful, but a serum karyotype is often needed to ensure the accuracy of the diagnosis. Absence or low levels of gonadotropins indicate hypothalamic or pituitary failure.

TREATMENT
General principles

Appropriate therapy depends on an accurate diagnosis. With that information the physician can decide whether effective treatment is feasible or necessary. Even if no medical or surgical intervention is required, it is important that the patient be given sufficient information to ensure that she understands the problem.

Since the range of disorders found in patients with amenorrhea is extensive, an overview of therapy will be approached under four categories. Any one patient may require several treatment modalities. The physician should be continually aware of the need to address all facets of treatment, including how the patient perceives the problem, how her diagnosis may alter her relationships with friends and family, and the effect on an intimate interpersonal relationship.

Constitutional therapy

Most patients with amenorrhea will benefit from measures directed toward the improvement of their general health and well-being. One of the major considerations is *adequate nutrition*. Normal menstruation is contingent upon an appropriate body mass. When obesity is associated with amenorrhea and no other abnormalities are found, weight reduction may be corrective. It may also be desirable for a patient to gain weight to enable her hypothalamic pituitary ovarian axis to resume normal func-

tion. An increase in the amount of exercise may be a very important adjunct to an individual who is overweight; young females who participate in competitive sports or extremes of exercise such as long distance running may need to curtail these activities in order to resume menstruation. Substance abuse should be eliminated.

Psychotherapy

Psychotherapy plays an important role in the management of all patients with amenorrhea. A variable amount of anxiety and emotional distress is present in all women whose menstruation is delayed or absent. Under certain circumstances the psychologic distress may actually be the cause of the amenorrhea. Listening in a sensitive manner, providing sympathetic encouragement and a factual explanation of the mechanism of menstruation, and, at the same time, being willing to approach the patient's sexual problems are basic elements in superficial psychotherapy. Many patients will readily respond to this type of therapy. But patients with severe eating disorders like anorexia nervosa with or without bulimia, vaginal agenesis, intersex disorders, and premature ovarian failure may require more in-depth and long-range psychiatric counseling.

In patients with gonadal dysgenesis and müllerian dysgenesis other anomalies should be sought, and thorough family history should be obtained. As part of the counseling procedure a geneticist may be included to ascertain what, if any, risk is present for other members of the family.

Hormone therapy

The use of hormones should be reserved to treat specific deficiencies, reestablish periodic endometrial shedding with the hope of preventing endometrial hyperplasia, induce ovulation, or combat the adverse cosmetic effects of androgen excess. When the amenorrhea is associated with infertility, ovulation induction therapy is the obvious treatment. The administration of estrogen-progesterone combination will result in regular uterine flow, but such bleeding is unaccompanied by ovulation. The uterine response occurs only in relationship to the repeated courses of hormone therapy. Emotionally, women often feel relief by the reappearance of flow, even though the basic problem of anovulation is not being solved. Whether hormone replacement therapy has an intrinsic salutary effect on improving the state of emotional well-being remains to be answered. Estrogen-progesterone replacement is of particular value in cases of primary or secondary ovarian failure to protect the relatively young woman from developing atrophy of the genital pelvic structures, prevent osteoporosis, and reduce the incidence of cardiovascular disease.

THYROID. Hypothyroidism is an uncommon cause of amenorrhea. It is usually associated with hyperprolactinemia. The response to thyroid hormone replacement is dramatic and corrects the menstrual abnormality quickly. The empiric use of thyroid medication is not beneficial.

ADRENAL. Adrenal insufficiency is an unusual cause of amenorrhea and responds promptly to corticosteroid therapy in replacement doses. Adrenal hyperfunction is usually secondary to a congenital adrenal hyperplasia secondary to a 21-hydroxylase deficiency. Suppressive therapy with prednisone or dexamethasone is in order; the patient should be apprised of the benefits and risks of this medication and the need for additional replacement if she is involved in a serious accident or requires a major surgical operation.

Hormone replacement therapy. Conjugated estrogens, 0.625 to 1.25 mg or equivalent daily for 25 days, with the addition of a progestational agent such as medroxyprogesterone acetate, 5 to 10 mg on the fifteenth through the twenty-ninth day, will induce regular withdrawal bleeding episodes without encouraging endometrial hyperplasia. At least 0.625 mg of conjugated estrogen is required to prevent osteoporosis. Larger dosages are necessary to meet the hormone needs of younger women. Patients on this regimen should be monitored carefully by examining their weight, blood pressure, and serum lipids, as well as the patient's tolerance to the medication. FSH and LH levels are not a clinically useful parameter to assess the adequacy of treatment.

It is beneficial to induce withdrawal bleeding on a monthly basis by the use of oral progestins alone administered for at least 13 days of the cycle in those who are secreting enough estrogen to stimulate endometrial proliferation. Even though oral contraceptive steroid therapy is convenient because of its packaging, it is not the preferred hormone regimen for replacement therapy. With oral contraceptive therapy, the patient will be taking a greater amount of hormone than is necessary for her physiologic needs and assuming an attendant increase in risk and side effects.

Clomiphene citrate. Clomiphene citrate is a nonsteroid compound that is used to induce ovulation. It does require potentially functioning ovaries and production of gonadotropins. The drug acts on hypothalamic estrogen receptors and activates a negative feedback relationship between estrogen and gonadotropins. There is a resultant secretion of GnRH and ensuing FSH and LH that stimulate follicular growth that can result in ovulation. Clomiphene citrate (Clomid or Serophene) is ineffectual in the absence of endogenous estrogen, particularly when the cause is ovarian failure, anterior pituitary obliteration, or congenital absence of GnRH. Although clomiphene therapy in properly treated patients results in ovulation in a high percentage of cases, the achievement of pregnancy is only about half as successful.

Menotropins. Human menopausal gonadotropins (Pergonal) has been successful in inducing ovulation in women who have estrogen deficiency but ovaries that are capable of ovulating with the proper stimulus. Most appropriate candidates are usually women who have been unresponsive to clomiphene or who have a GnRH deficiency. Dosage of menotropin is required daily until a dominant follicle(s) is produced. The latter is determined by monitoring serial serum estradiol concentrations and follicular growth by ultrasound. When a dominant follicle is identified, an "LH surge" is produced by an intramuscular dose of hCG (Profasi, A.P.L.), 5000 to 10,000 U. Both clomiphene and menotropins can overstimulate the ovaries, give rise to multiple births, and result in severe ovarian enlargement and ascites. These effects occur more readily with menotropins.

GnRH. Synthetic GnRH (Factrel) is currently available and is approved by the FDA only for diagnostic testing, but it can be used to induce ovulation. The medicine is administered in a pulsatile fashion either subcutaneously or intravenously every 1 to 2 hours. Serum estrogen levels and ultrasound monitoring of the ovarian follicles are helpful to adjust the dosage to the proper level. The most suitable patients for this medication are those women who are GnRH deficient. Ovarian hyperstimulation and multiple pregnancies are still a possibility but are less likely with this medication.

Bromocriptine. Bromocriptine (mesylate) (Parlodel) is a dopamine agonist with similar action to PIF. It is extremely effective in inducing ovulation in those individuals with hyperprolactinemia with or without documented prolactinoma. If the patient achieves euprolactinemia, restoration of ovulatory cycles returns. During early therapy it is not unusual for the patient to have one or two cycles with an inadequate luteal phase. When pregnancy does occur, the medicine should be discontinued, although there is no information at the current time that it acts as a teratogen or is embryotoxic.

Surgery

Surgery is essential and generally curative in cases of obstruction to menstrual flow such as imperforate hymen, vaginal or cervical stenosis, and uterine synechiae. In those individuals with vaginal agenesis, self-induced pressure with vaginal dilators of increasing size can result in a pouch that is sufficient for coitus. If this method of treatment fails, an artificial vagina can be created with the use of a skin graft, the McIndoe procedure.

When there is definite evidence of pathologic changes in the ovary such as an androgen- or estrogen-secreting tumor, oophorectomy may remove the cause of the amenorrhea. Because of the risk of malignancy, any Y-bearing gonad such as would be found in a patient with Swyer's syndrome or androgen insensitivity should be removed. In selected patients, ovarian wedge resection can also be instrumental in facilitating fertility in patients with polycystic ovary syndrome. Stein and Leventhal reported an experience of 25 years with wedge resection of polycystic ovaries; of 93 patients with amenorrhea so treated, 59 subsequently became pregnant. A considerable number of the remainder of the group experienced regular cyclic bleeding over a long period of time.

REFERENCES

Baird, D.T.: Disturbances in the negative feedback loop of the pituitary-ovarian axis, Clin. Obstet. Gynecol. 3:535, 1976.

Bongiovanni, A.M., and Root, A.W.: The adrenogenital syndrome, N. Engl. J. Med. 268:1283, 1342, 1391, 1963.

Chang, R.J., Keye, W.R., Young, J.R., Wilson, C.B., and Jaffe, R.B.: Detection, evaluation, and treatment of pituitary microadenomas in patients with galactorrhea and amenorrhea, Am. J. Obstet. Gynecol. 128:356, 1977.

Cronin, T.J.: The influence of lactation upon ovulation, Lancet 2:422, 1968.

Frantz, A.G.: Prolactin, N. Engl. J. Med. 298:201, 1978.

Frisch, R.E., and McArthur, J.W.: Menstrual cycles: fatness as a determinant of minimum weight for height necessary for their maintenance or onset, Science 185:949, 1974.

Griffin, J.E., and Wilson, J.D.: The syndrome of androgen resistance, N. Engl. J. Med. 302:198, 1980.

Griffin, J.E., Edwards, C., Madden, J.D., Harrod, M.J., and Wilson, J.D.: Congenital absence of the vagina, Ann. Intern. Med. 85:224, 1976.

Hefnawi, F., and Bodraoui, M.H.H.: The benefits of lactation amenorrhea as a contraceptive agent, Fertil. Steril. 28:320, 1977.

Jewelewicz, R., and Vande Wiele, R.L.: Clinical course and outcome of pregnancy in twenty-five patients with pituitary microadenomas, Am. J. Obstet. Gynecol. 136:339, 1980.

Kase, N.: Induction of ovulation with clomiphene citrate, Clin. Obstet. Gynecol. 16:192, 1973.

Keettel, W.C., and Bradbury, J.T.: Premature ovarian failure: permanent and temporary, Am. J. Obstet. Gynecol. 89:83, 1964.

Kirschner, M.A., and Jacobs, J.B.: Combined ovarian and adrenal vein catheterization to determine the site(s) of androgen production in hirsute women, J. Clin. Endocrinol. 33:199, 1971.

Kleinberg, D.L., Noel, G.L., and Frantz, A.G.: Galactorrhea: a study of 235 cases including 48 with pituitary tumors, N. Engl. J. Med. 296:589, 1977.

Magyar, D.M., and Marshall, J.R.: Pituitary tumors and pregnancy, Am. J. Obstet. Gynecol. 132:739, 1978.

March, C.M., Isreal, R., and March, A.D.: Hysteroscopic management of intrauterine adhesions, Am. J. Obstet. Gynecol. 130:653, 1978.

March, C.M., Kletzky, O.A., Davajan, V., Teal, J., Weiss, M., Apuzzo, M.L.J., Marrs, R.P., and Mishell, D.R.: Longitudinal evaluation of patients with untreated prolactin-secreting pituitary adenomas, Am. J. Obstet. Gynecol. 139:835, 1981.

Miller, O.J.: The sex chromosome anomalies, Am. J. Obstet. Gynecol, **90:**1078, 1964.

Pearson, P.L., Borrow, M., and Vosa, C.G.: Technique for identifying Y chromosomes in human interphase nuclei, Nature **226:**78, 1970.

Peterson, R.E., Imperato-McGinley, Gautier, T., and Sturla, E.: Male pseudohermaphroditism due to steroid 5α-reductase deficiency, Am. J. Med. **62:**170, 1977.

Philip, J., Sele, V., and Trolle, D.: Primary amenorrhea: a study of 101 cases, Fertil. Steril. **16:**795, 1965.

Rolland, R., De Jong, F.H., Schellekens, L.A., and Lequin, R.M.: The role of prolactin in the restoration of ovarian function during the early postpartum period. II. A study during inhibition of lactation by bromocriptine, Clin. Endocrinol. **4:**27, 1975.

Spark, R.F., Baker, R., Bienfang, D.C., and Bergland, R.: Bromocriptine reduces pituitary tumor size and hypersecretion, J.A.M.A. **247:**311, 1982.

Speroff, L., editor: Polycystic ovary disease, Chang, R.J., guest editor, Semin. Reprod. Endocrinol. **2:**3, 1984.

Stein, I.F., and Leventhal, M.L.: Amenorrhea associated with bilateral polycystic ovaries, Am. J. Obstet. Gynecol. **29:**181, 1935.

Toaff, R., and Ballas, S.: Traumatic hypomenorrhea-amenorrhea (Asherman's syndrome), Fertil. Steril. **30:**379, 1978.

Tulandi, T., and Kinch, R.A.H.: Premature ovarian failure, Obstet. Gynecol. Surv. **36**(suppl.):521, 1981.

Vakil, D.V., Lewin, P.K., and Conen, P.E.: Value of fluorescent Y chromosome and sex chromatin tests, Acta Cytol. **17:**220, 1973.

Wachtel, S.S., Ohno, S., Koo, G.C., and Boyse, E.A.: Possible role for H-Y antigen in the primary determination of sex, Nature **257:**235, 1975.

10

Michael J. Daly and Kathy Hotelling

Dysmenorrhea and the premenstrual syndrome

In recent years, women have become employed in most areas of the work force, including the professions. Partially because of their expanding career roles, there has been a renewed medical interest in the symptoms that some women develop around the time of their menstrual periods. Dalton raised questions about women's menstrual problems in both lay and professional circles in the last 15 years. Although her stereotypic attitudes (such as viewing women as incompetent, out of control, and ruled by hormonal fluctuations) have led to much criticism, her books did identify and direct serious attention to menstrual problems. The most frequent of such symptoms is that of dysmenorrhea or "cramps." Most menstruating women have some degree of discomfort with their menstrual flow. Those women who experience pain severe enough to restrict their activities usually require medical intervention. The term "dysmenorrhea" describes the symptoms of this group. Dysmenorrhea occurs in about 50% of ovulatory women. The pain may be mild, moderate, or severe. One out of five of these women is incapacitated for 1 to 3 days each month because of pain. Dysmenorrhea is the primary cause of absenteeism in school and in the work place for women of reproductive age. This absenteeism has resulted in the loss of over 2 million working hours annually.

There are two types of dysmenorrhea, primary and secondary. *Secondary dysmenorrhea* is caused by identifiable pelvic diseases such as endometriosis, adenomyosis, pelvic infection involving the fallopian tubes and ovaries, some myomas, and certain developmental abnormalities. It is important for the physician to rule out these factors before making a diagnosis of *primary dysmenorrhea*. The identification and treatment of the problems producing secondary dysmenorrhea will be discussed elsewhere in this text.

PRIMARY DYSMENORRHEA

Primary dysmenorrhea is defined as painful menstruation that usually appears with the first ovulatory cycle after the menarche. It is not caused by pelvic disease. Dysmenorrhea, which is not associated with ovulatory cycles or which begins more than 2 years after the menarche, is probably secondary rather than primary. The pain caused by primary dysmenorrhea is usually crampy in nature, emanates from the lower abdomen, and may radiate to the back and the thighs. Of women suffering from primary dysmenorrhea, 50% also have other symptoms such as nausea, vomiting, headache, diarrhea, or fatigue. These symptoms usually begin before or shortly after the onset of the menstrual flow and persist for 12 to 36 hours. In rare instances, syncopy and collapse may occur. Childbirth and advancing age may lessen the severity of the symptoms of primary dysmenorrhea.

ETIOLOGY

There has been much speculation about the cause of primary dysmenorrhea. Most theorists today agree that it is the result of a decrease in estrogen and progesterone that causes shedding of the endometrium and release of prostaglandin $(PG)F_2\alpha$. There are various items of evidence that support this view. First, $PGF_2\alpha$, which is administered to patients for a midtrimester termination of pregnancy, produces side effects that are similar to the symptoms of primary dysmenorrhea. They include nausea, headache, vomiting, uterine cramps, and diarrhea. Second, prostaglandin levels of the endometrium and the menstrual fluid are higher in women with primary dysmenorrhea than in those who are asymptomatic. Third, $PGF_2\alpha$ metabolite levels are higher in women with primary dysmenorrhea. Last, prostaglandin synthesis inhibitors are effective in the treatment of primary dysmenorrhea.

Dawood has proposed a pathway of biosynthesis of prostaglandin. He suggested that phospholipase acts on phospholipids to produce arachidonic acid. He then further suggests that cyclooxygenase reacts with arachidonic acid to produce cyclic-endoperoxides (PGG_2, PGH_2). Then isomerase reductase brings about the synthesis of PGE_2, and $PGF_2\alpha$.

The presence of an excess amount of prostaglandin increases myometrial contractions, which causes a reduction of uterine blood flow and ischemia of the uterine muscle. This in turn results in an increased stimulation of the autonomic pain fibers from the uterus by bradykinin.

Women who suffer from primary dysmenorrhea have been shown to have an elevated uterine basal tone, greater than 10 mm hg. They also demonstrate an increased frequency of contractions and an incoordinate contractile pattern caused by prostaglandin stimulation.

As with other forms of pain, there may be associated anxiety, fear, or guilt. In addition, stress of either external or internal origin may affect the pain threshold. Slang expressions associated with menstruation such as the "curse," "falling off the roof," or "being unwell" may also have some bearing on the severity of menstrual cramps. These terms will have an obviously negative connotation. In addition to the present social attitudes toward menstruation that these terms reveal, there used to be cultural and religious beliefs that menstrual fluid was a toxic substance. Women were once excluded from Hebrew camps and assigned to a special area while they were menstruating because they were thought to be "unclean." This practice again suggests that there is something "bad" about menstruation. Such attitudes and beliefs may aggravate the pain.

In summary, the biochemical stimulation of pain fibers from the pelvis and the interpretation of this stimulation by the central nervous system are important factors in the cause of primary dysmenorrhea. Both may be affected by the emotions or may bring about an emotional response. Both physiologic and emotional responses are important considerations in patients with severe menstrual cramps.

Errors in differentiating between primary and secondary dysmenorrhea have frequently been made. Some patients have been diagnosed as having primary dysmenorrhea when they suffered from such forms of secondary dysmenorrhea as nonpalpable endometriosis. Other patients have been diagnosed as having adenomyosis, another type of secondary dysmenorrhea, when indeed they suffered from primary dysmenorrhea. The distinction is critical because the treatment of secondary dysmenorrhea requires eradication of the particular pelvic disease that is producing the pain.

Diagnosis

The patient's history should indicate that the onset of the menstrual pains began shortly after the menarche. The pain coincides with the onset of menstruation and lasts from 48 to 72 hours. The pain is cramplike in nature. A pelvic examination and a rectovaginal examination should reveal normal findings. For patients for whom the diagnosis is questionable or for those who do not respond to standard treatment, endometriosis and chronic pelvic infection should be ruled out as a cause.

Management

It is essential that there be good rapport between the physician and the patient. The physician should listen carefully to the patient's account of her symptoms. A sympathetic and understanding approach should be taken. The physician should explore any misconceptions the patient might have about menstruation. He or she should also look for any undue anxiety or guilt that might affect the patient's response to her menstrual pain.

The physician should question the patient about her general hygiene. He or she should advise her about the need for physical activity during the menstrual period; moderate exercise can help alleviate her symptoms. Careful attention to diet (such as eating more whole grains, beans, vegetables, and fruit, and less or no salt, caffeine, and sugar) have also been helpful in some women. Relaxation, massage, and biofeedback techniques have been effective in reducing pain for some women.

The physician should ask the patient if she is sexually active. If she says yes and there are no contraindications, he or she may want to prescribe *oral contraceptives*. They are quite effective in the treatment of primary dysmenorrhea. Oral contraceptives suppress ovulation and cause a reduction of endometrium and a corresponding reduction in menstrual flow. This reduction results in a decreased production of prostaglandin. Oral contraceptives will relieve the symptoms of primary dysmenorrhea for more than 90% of the women who take them. The medication should be tried for three or four cycles, and then an assessment of their effect should be made.

Women who cannot or will not use oral contraceptives or who do not respond to them should be placed on *prostaglandin synthetase inhibitors (PGSI)*. There are many types of PGSI such as aspirin, indomethacin, mefenamic acid, and ibuprofen. Others include phenylbutazone and *p*-chloromercuriben. All bring about a reduction in endometrial prostaglandin release. This reduction frequently restores normal uterine activity and eliminates pain.

Clinical trials conducted by Dawood suggest that aspirin is not much better than a placebo. Indomethacin produces a high incidence of gastrointestinal side effects and probably should not be used. The PGSI of choice are flufenamic acid, 100 to 200 mg three times a day; mefenamic acid, 250 to 500 mg three or four times a day; ibuprofen, 400 mg four times a day; naproxen sodium, 275 mg four times a day; or kepoprofen, 50 mg three times a day.

Pretreatment with PGSI is not necessary. They should be given during the first 48 hours of menstruation and may be used for the first 3 days of the menstrual flow. Contraindications for the use of PGSI include gastrointestional ulcers and hypersensitivity to the agents. The side effects are usually relatively mild. Significant complications that may occur in a few patients include indigestion, heartburn, severe abdominal pain, constipation, vomiting, diarrhea, and even bloody stools. The central nervous system also may be affected, resulting in headaches, dizziness, hearing and visual disturbances, irritability, depression, drowsiness, and sleepiness. Additionally, allergic reactions producing skin rashes, edema, bronchial spasms, hematologic abnormalities, fluid retention, and rare side effects involving the liver and kidneys have been observed.

If the patient does not respond to either oral contraceptives or PGSI, secondary causes must again be considered, and a laparoscopy is indicated. If pelvic disease is discovered, appropriate treatment should be carried out. If no pelvic pathology is found, *beta-mimetic agents* might be tried. *Calcium antagonists* such as nifedipine are being tested and may prove helpful in the future. If significant emotional stress seems to be present, a *psychiatric consultation* should be suggested.

There should be only a small percentage of patients who do not respond to this management plan. For this group, a surgical procedure such as presacral neurectomy might be considered. However, this should rarely be resorted to and should only be performed when all other avenues have been explored. Dilatation and curettage has been used in the treatment of dysmenorrhea in the past, but there is no evidence that tightness of the cervix produces painful menstruation.

In summary, in managing patients with severe menstrual pain, the physician should rule out a secondary pathologic condition within or about the pelvis. Primary dysmenorrhea, in which there is no definable pelvic pathology, will usually respond to medical treatment. Oral contraceptives are generally effective in treating primary dysmenorrhea. Patients who do not respond to or require oral contraceptives or for whom there are contraindications to their use will usually respond to PGSI. Laparoscopic examination should be done on those few patients who do not respond to either oral contraceptives or PGSI. The patient's emotional response to dysmenorrhea should be evaluated. A psychiatric consultation should be suggested for those few patients who manifest a great deal of anxiety or guilt about menstruation. A surgical procedure will be helpful only in rare cases.

PREMENSTRUAL SYNDROME

The effects of premenstrual syndrome (PMS) were first described by Frank in 1931. He suggested that women who demonstrated edema, weight gain, and emotional disturbances before the onset of menstruation had a premenstrual disease. In 1953 Dalton and other investigators suggested that women with these symptoms should be categorized under the heading PMS. The symptoms now attributed to this condition number well over 40 and are outlined in Moos' Menstrual Distress questionnaire. This questionnaire is divided into eight categories with symptoms related to (1) pain, (2) concentration, (3) behavioral change, (4) autonomic reactions, (5) water retention, (6) negative effect, (7) arousal, and (8) control.

Although premenstrual tension has been recognized for over 50 years, only recently has there been concentrated interest in the whole group of symptoms because women have become more involved in jobs outside the home and are assuming many responsible positions in the work force. Pre-

menstrual symptoms sometimes prevent women from attaining their best level of performance. In addition, PMS has occasionally been used as a legal defense in criminal cases involving charges such as murder. A great deal has been written in both the lay and professional press because of the renewed interest in this area.

Most women experience some changes in bodily sensation and mood before the onset of menstrual flow. For some women, the number and the severity of the symptoms are so extreme that they are classified as a medical disorder. Otherwise healthy women experience one or more of these symptoms in a mild-to-moderate form. It has been suggested that about 5 to 6 million women experience severe symptoms each month in the United States. Fortunately, threatening symptoms such as homicidal or suicidal ideation occur only in a very small percentage of women with PMS. More frequently, the life of the woman and significant others is disrupted, which may lead to feelings of guilt on the part of the woman.

Etiologic factors

The etiologic factors that are involved in this syndrome are *inadequate progesterone, fluid retention, nutritional problems, glucose metabolism and estrogen.* The exact cause of premenstrual tension is unknown, but its cyclic nature and timing suggest that there is a progesterone insufficiency or withdrawal in women who experience the symptoms. This insufficiency results in a relative estrogen imbalance. It has also been shown that PMS is more apt to occur in women with endometriosis or luteal phase defect, which may explain why the symptoms appear as long as a week before the onset of the menstruation, when progesterone levels are usually high.

Fluid retention. In the past fluid retention was believed to precipitate the various manifestations of PMS, and diuretics were used as part of the clinical management. Studies assessing weight change, sodium exchange, and total body water have failed to uncover a pattern of fluid retention in most women with PMS. Aldosterone levels are not significantly elevated, and there is no evidence that prolactin produces fluid retention in men. Progesterone does, however, affect the renin-angiotension-aldosterone mechanism and water metabolism by inducing a temporary natriuresis followed by fluid retention.

Nutrition. A great deal of emphasis has been placed on proper nutrition and the importance °of exercise in avoiding PMS. Deficiencies in vitamin B₆ (pyridoxine), vitamin D, and calcium have been suggested as a cause of PMS, although the supporting data are questionable. It has also been suggested that pyridoxine affects the biosynthesis of brain catecholamines that regulate mood behavior and that hypoglycemia may invoke symptoms of PMS. The relationship between the amount of carbohydrates and protein in the diet may be important. Some studies have suggested that the reduction of carbohydrates and the increase of protein may be beneficial.

Hyperprolactinemia. Hyperprolactinemia has been cited by some as another possible cause. However, some studies do not indicate that women with PMS have elevated prolactin levels. In addition, women with hyperprolactinemia rarely have symptoms of PMS.

More recently, Quigley and Yen and Reid and Yen have suggested that an endogenous opiate peptide may be responsible for the symptom in some women, especially those with the depressive symptoms. Opiate peptides do affect the amount of gonadotropin secretion and produce changes in the concentration of LH. Direct measurement of beta-endorphin concentrations in the portal-hypophyseal blood of the rhesus monkey has revealed that levels of opiate peptides are high during the midluteal phase and undetectable at the onset of menstruation. These authors postulate that progesterone, acting either alone or in combination with estrogen, can increase central endogenous opiate peptide activity. He further suggests that this may trigger the subsequent neuroendocrine manifestations of PMS. As proof of this hypothesis, he has shown that naloxone administered in high doses to normal women induces a constellation of symptoms almost identical to those of PMS. As we learn more about neutrotransmitters and/or neuromodulators, further clarification of this phenomenon should be forthcoming.

Symptomatology

Headache, nervous irritability, insomnia, and crying spells are the most common manifestations of premenstrual tension. Many women complain of backache, lower abdominal pain, and tender or painful breasts as well. These symptoms usually appear about a week to 10 days before the period is due, and they gradually increase in intensity. Usually, they disappear once the menstrual flow is well established. A weight gain of 1 to 3 kg (2 to 6½ lb) during the premenstrual phase is common. Generalized edema and oliguria occur frequently. Rapid loss of weight gained and marked diuresis usually follow the onset of menstruation, along with regression of the other symptoms. The doctor should first consider other possible diagnoses, including chronic depression, which may become aggravated before menstruation, and manic depressive illness. Schizophrenia should also be excluded as a possible cause of the symptoms.

Management

Women who suffer from PMS may experience irritability, depression, fatigue, edema, breast discomfort, and the other symptoms associated with this syndrome for quite some time before they consult a physician. Frequently, when they first seek medical help, they inform the doctor that they have the feeling they are "going crazy." *It would be helpful for physicians to inquire about the symptoms of PMS every time they take a menstrual history.* Such information provides a more complete picture of the patient. Frequently, the early diagnosis of patients with PMS can prevent many emotional difficulties within the home and on the job.

Once symptoms characterizing PMS are identified, the patient should be reassured that she is not becoming psychotic and that there are measures that can be taken to help her. Early in the management of the patient, it is usually helpful to bring the husband and other immediate family members into a discussion concerning the symptoms.

It is essential to have the patient keep a daily diary about her symptoms and behavior. She should be told that PMS is a common hormonal disorder of women in their childbearing years, that the symptoms usually disappear at menopause, and that there are a number of things that can be done to alleviate them. With treatment, the patient will learn to cope with her symptoms in a more effective manner. She should be taught the importance of a *good exercise program* such as walking regularly, and she should be put on an *appropriate diet*. The *elimination of tobacco and caffeine* has been beneficial to some patients. A diet that is low in carbohydrates but contains a reasonable amount of protein, vegetables, and fruit will help other women. Protein should be obtained primarily from fish rather than from red meat. *Pyridoxine* in doses of 100 to 400 mg/day may also be helpful.

In women with severe breast pain and swelling, *bromocriptine or danazol* has proven to be helpful. However, these medications should not be necessary for most patients.

Some patients report improvement of their symptoms with *oral contraceptives*. This form of therapy should probably be restricted to patients under the age of 35 who need contraception or who have associated dysmenorrhea. In addition, *prostaglandin inhibitors* such as mefenamic acid (250 mg) and naproxen sodium (275 mg) when taken orally every 4 to 6 hours may relieve not only dysmenorrhea but symptoms of PMS as well.

Unfortunately, diuretics are probably the most frequently used medication in the treatment of PMS. Although there is very little evidence of the contribution of fluid retention to this syndrome, 25 mg of spironolactone, to be taken orally four times a day, may be prescribed the week before menstruation when edema is severe.

Certainly, patients showing marked alteration in mood swings with manic and/or severe depressive symptoms, as well as those exhibiting psychotic behavior, should have a psychiatric evaluation before treatment. Tricyclic antidepressants have not been effective in treating this syndrome. Lithium carbonate, in dosages of 600 to 1800 mg/day taken orally, is sometimes effective in the control of manic depressive symptoms and psychotic behavior. If the patient is placed on lithium therapy, the physician needs to carefully monitor serum lithium levels because of the possibility of serious side effects from this medication.

In summary, PMS encompasses a number of symptoms that women experience before their menstrual period. Full control of these symptoms is clearly important. Patients who are prone to the syndrome should first be evaluated carefully. They should maintain a diary, itemizing their symptoms for a number of cycles. They should be reassured that they are not psychotic and that their symptoms are brought about by hormonal changes affecting their body chemistry. It is helpful to educate not only the patient but the family as well about the effects of PMS, so that the family can provide strong emotional support. With appropriate changes in life-style, which might include the start of an exercise program and a balanced diet and with certain drug therapies, most women with PMS can be helped significantly.

REFERENCES

Abraham, G.E., Elsner, C.W., and Lucas, L.A.: Hormone and behavioral changes during the menstrual cycle, Senogolia **3**:33, 1978.

Abraham, G.E.: Nutritional factors, the etiology of premenstrual tension, J. Reprod. Med. **28**:7, 1983.

Abraham, G.E., and Hargrove, J.T.: Effect of vitamin B₆ on premenstrual symptomatology in women with premenstrual tension syndrome: a double-blind crossover study, Infertility **3**:155, 1980.

Akerlund, M., Stromberg, P., and Gorsling, M.D.: Primary dysmenorrhea and vasopression, Br. J. Obstet. Gynaecol. **86**:484, 1979.

Anderson, A.N., and Larsen, J.F.: Bromocriptine the treatment of premenstrual syndrome, Drugs **17**:383, 1979.

Caspo, A.I., Pulkkinen, M.O., and Henzl, M.R.: The effect of naproxen sodium on the intrauterine pressure and menstrual pain of dysmenorrhea subjects, Prostaglandins **13**:1933, 1977.

Chan, W.Y., and Dawood, M.Y.: Prostaglandin levels in menstrual fluid of nondysmenorrhea subjects with and without oral contraceptive or ibuprofen therapy, Adv. Prostaglandin Thromboxane Res. **8**:1443, 1980.

Dalton, K.: Premenstrual syndrome, Springfield, Ill., 1964, Charles C Thomas, Publisher.

Dalton, K.: The menstrual cycle, New York, 1969, Pantheon Books.

Dalton, K.: Cyclical criminal acts in premenstrual syndrome, Lancet 2:1970, 1980.

Davies, A.J., Anderson, A.B.M., and Turnbull, A.C.: Reduction by naproxen of excessive menstrual bleeding in women using intrauterine devices, Obstet. Gynecol. 57:74, 1981.

Dawood, M.Y.: Prostaglandin, hormones, and dysmenorrhea. In Dawood, M.Y., editor: Dysmenorrhea, Baltimore, 1981, The Williams & Wilkins Co.

Dawood, M.Y.: Dysmenorrhea, Clin. Obstet. Gynecol. 26:3, 1983.

Frank, R.P.: The hormonal causes of premenstrual tension, Arch. Neurol. Psych. 26:1052, 1931.

Ganon, L.: Evidence for a psychological etiology of menstrual disorders: a critical review.

Hargrove, J.T., and Abraham, G.E.: Abnormal functions in patients with endometriosis, Fertil. Steril. 34:302, 1980.

Lundstrom, V., and Green, K.: Endogenous levels of prostaglandin $F_{2\alpha}$ and its main metabolites in plasma and endometrium of normal and dysmenorrheic women, Am. J. Obstet. Gynecol. 130:640, 1978.

Moon, Y.S., Leung, P.C.S., Yuen, B.H., and Gomel, V.: Prostaglandin F in human endometriotic tissue, Am. J. Obstet. Gynecol. 141:344, 1981.

Quigley, M.E., and Yen, S.S.C.: The role of endogenous opiates on LH secretion during the menstrual cycle. J. Clin. Endocrinol. Metab. 51:179, 1980.

Reid, R.L., and Yen, S.S.C.: The premenstrual syndrome, Clin. Obstet. Gynecol. 26:3, 1983.

Rock, J.A., Dubin, N.H., Ghogaonkar, R.B., et al.: Cul-de-sac fluid in women with endometriosis: fluid volume and prostanoid concentration during the proliferative phase of the cycle—days 8 to 12, Fertil. Steril. 37:747, 1982.

Roy, S., and Shaw, S.T.: Role of prostaglandins in IUD-associated uterine bleeding—effect of a prostaglandin synthetase inhibitor (ibuprofen), Obstet. Gynecol. 58:101, 1981.

11

John H. Mattox

Endometriosis

Endometriosis is the abnormal growth of endometrial tissue outside the uterine cavity. The disease was first mentioned in the medical literature in 1860 by the reknowned Viennese pathologist, von Rokitansky. The observations of Sampson in the 1920s focused on one of the current major theories of the origin of the disease and documented its histologic variability. Whether aberrant endometrium is located on the serosal surface of the peritoneal structures, on the ovary, *external endometriosis,* or in the tissues contiguous with the uterine mucosa, *internal endometriosis,* (adenomyosis), functioning endometrial tissue that responds to ovarian hormones, predominantly estrogen, is the prerequisite for the genesis and maintenance of this condition. Therefore it is rarely encountered before menarche and usually becomes quiescent after the menopause. *Adenomyosis* is endometriosis involving the myometrium, whereas *endosalpingiosis* is located in the fallopian tube.

It is estimated that between 1% and 2% of the female population has endometriosis, and many physicians believe that the incidence is increasing. Characteristic lesions can be recognized during at least 20% of pelvic operations, and frequently it is an unexpected finding. Some women may have asymptomatic endometriosis; it is more likely to be problematic in the third and fourth decades of life.

ETIOLOGIC FACTORS

According to the *serosal* or metaplasia theory, undifferentiated coelomic epithelial cells, like those from which the paramesonephric ducts are formed, remain dormant on the peritoneal surface until the ovaries begin to function. They respond to cyclic stimulation by ovarian estrogen and progesterone in a manner similar to that of normal endometrial cells and eventually can be identified as definite lesions on the peritoneal surface. The longer cyclic stimulation and withdrawal persist without a break such as that provided by pregnancy, the larger the lesions can become.

Sampson's investigations indicate that endometriosis can be caused by *transport of menstrual fluid from the uterus through the tubes during menstruation.* Blood often can be seen in the cul-de-sac, and endometrial tissue can be identified in the tubal lumen in women who undergo surgery during menstruation. The typical lesions of endometriosis can be produced in monkeys by diverting the menstrual flow into the peritoneal cavity. Endometriosis also occurs in young women with congenital obstructing defects in the cervix or vagina, which are associated with reflux menstruation into the peritoneal cavity.

The most tenable etiologic theory is a combination of *metaplasia* and *retrograde tubal transmission.* An irritating substance in the menstrual fluid entering the peritoneal cavity may induce the formation of endometrial glands and stroma in undifferentiated mesenchyme. This would explain the location of the lesions in the ovary and the cul-de-sac, the areas first affected by reflux menstruation.

The theory that a substance in menstrual fluid *induces* a change in certain susceptible individuals resulting in endometriosis is more tenable than is the hypothesis of the growth of transplanted endometrial cells. Endometrial cells from menstrual discharge usually do not grow in tissue culture, so it is difficult to accept cell transplantation as the most important factor in the development of a condition as common as endometriosis.

Heredity may be a factor in the development of endometriosis. Simpson and colleagues conducted genetic interviews with 123 women who had been treated for endometriosis. The incidence of the condition in female siblings over age 18 years (5.8%), mothers (8.1%), and first-degree relatives (6.9%) was considerably higher than that in the husbands' female relatives (1.0%) and mothers (0.9%). The precise genetic mechanism is not known.

PATHOLOGIC FINDINGS

Gross. The gross appearance of endometriosis is variable, depending on the stage of the disease and the length of time it has existed. Minimal lesions appear as bluish-red spots, each surrounded by a ring of puckered scar tissue, scattered over the pelvic peritoneal surfaces. Each of these small foci may grow as a result of repeated cyclic stimulation; the larger lesions are known as *endometriomas* (Fig. 11-1). As the endometriomas continue to grow, they coalesce and may completely obliterate the cul-de-sac. The tubes and ovaries become densely adherent to the posterior surfaces of the broad ligaments, and in more advanced cases the rectosigmoid adheres to the posterior surface of the uterus, further immobilizing the adnexal structures (Fig. 11-2). Eventually, the entire pelvis may be filled with a solid mass of agglutinated structures that may be completely obscured by adherent small bowel and omentum.

The adhesions produced in response to the lesions are dense and firm and can be separated only by sharp dissection. As the planes are opened, thick brown fluid escapes. This fluid, old blood, is a product of the ectopic endometrial tissue that responds, as does uterine endometrium, to the repeated rise and fall of estrogen and progesterone during normal menstrual cycles. The blood may be the irritant that initiates the peritoneal reaction, which is eventually responsible for the dense scarring.

Ovarian involvement varies from small cystic

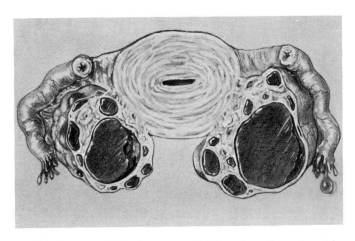

Fig. 11-1. Cross section showing uterus in center with bilateral ovarian endometriomas adherent to uterus, posterior leaves of broad ligament, and tubes.

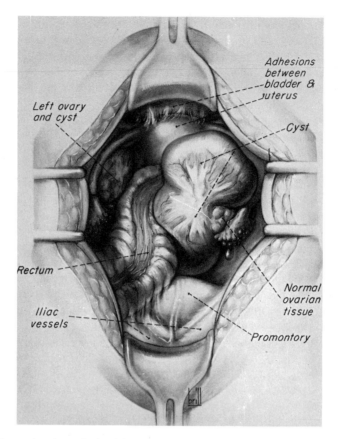

Left ovary and cyst

Adhesions between bladder & uterus

Cyst

Rectum

Iliac vessels

Normal ovarian tissue

Promontory

Fig. 11-2. Advanced endometriosis with previous rupture of endometrial cyst on right. Note adhesions and areas of normal-appearing ovarian tissue.

collections to a single loculated structure, which may measure as much as 10 cm in diameter *(ovarian endometrioma)*. Other lesions such as hemorrhage into an ovarian cyst or a corpus luteum cyst can form the "chocolate cyst" and be confused with ovarian endometriomas. Whenever possible, an exact diagnosis should be made before a definitive operative procedure is performed because the treatment of each of these lesions is different.

The rectosigmoid and urinary tract may be involved. The lesions are on the peritoneal surface and rarely penetrate the entire thickness of the wall. Occasionally, the vagina, cervix, episiotomy scars, laparotomy scars, umbilicus, round ligaments, lungs, and extremities are sites of endometrial implants. Wherever the lesion is found, its behavior is essentially the same.

A clinical classification of endometriosis based on the position and extent of the lesions is essential for comparison of the results of treatment. Several classifications have been proposed, but none has been generally accepted. One developed by a committee of The American Fertility Society is simple and informative. Points are awarded for each of several aspects of the lesions as they are seen through the laparoscope or at laparotomy. The total number accumulated is an indication of the severity of the process (Fig. 11-3).

A typical lesion of endometriosis contains glands and stroma like those of endometrium in its normal location (Fig. 11-4). The tissue responds to variations in the concentrations of ovarian hormones as does normal endometrium, except that the secretory change may be somewhat less pronounced. Often there is hemorrhage into the stroma and the surrounding tissue, a result of "menstruation" from the lesions as they disintegrate

THE AMERICAN FERTILITY SOCIETY
REVISED CLASSIFICATION OF ENDOMETRIOSIS

Patient's Name _____ Date_____

Stage I (Minimal) - 1-5
Stage II (Mild) - 6-15
Stage III (Moderate) - 16-40
Stage IV (Severe) - >40
Total_____

Laparoscopy_____ Laparotomy_____ Photography_____
Recommended Treatment_____
_____
Prognosis_____

PERITONEUM	ENDOMETRIOSIS	<1cm	1-3cm	>3cm
	Superficial	1	2	4
	Deep	2	4	6
OVARY	R Superficial	1	2	4
	Deep	4	16	20
	L Superficial	1	2	4
	Deep	4	16	20

	POSTERIOR CULDESAC OBLITERATION	Partial	Complete
		4	40

	ADHESIONS	<1/3 Enclosure	1/3-2/3 Enclosure	>2/3 Enclosure
OVARY	R Filmy	1	2	4
	Dense	4	8	16
	L Filmy	1	2	4
	Dense	4	8	16
TUBE	R Filmy	1	2	4
	Dense	4*	8*	16
	L Filmy	1	2	4
	Dense	4*	8*	16

*If the fimbriated end of the fallopian tube is completely enclosed, change the point assignment to 16.

Additional Endometriosis: _____

Associated Pathology: _____

To Be Used with Normal
Tubes and Ovaries

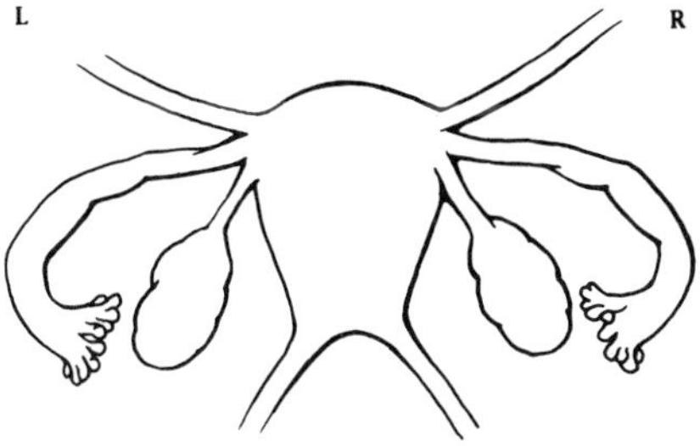

To Be Used with Abnormal
Tubes and/or Ovaries

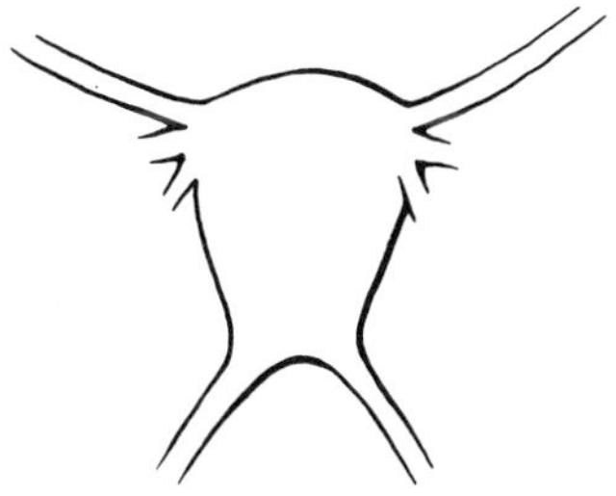

Fig. 11-3. Classification of endometriosis. (From The American Fertility Society: Revised American Fertility Society classification of endometriosis, Fertil. Steril. 43:351, 1984. Reproduced with the permission of the publisher, The American Fertility Society.)

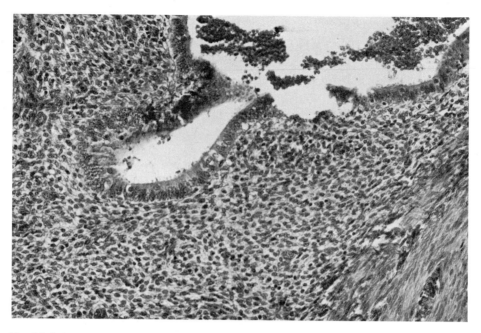

Fig. 11-4. Internal endometriosis or adenomyosis. Endometrial gland *(center)* with myometrium identified in lower right corner.

when hormone stimulation is withdrawn. Repeated episodes of bleeding within a lesion may produce enough pressure atrophy to destroy the glandular epithelium, leaving only the stroma and hemosiderin-containing macrophages. Usually a considerable amount of fibrous tissue surrounds the older lesions. During pregnancy the lesions usually exhibit a typical decidual reaction.

SYMPTOMS

Pain. Lower abdominal and pelvic pain in some form is the most common symptom of endometriosis. The cycling ectopic endometrium bleeds in conjunction with the normal menstrual flow, but the blood is contained within the involved organ or affected tissue, distending it and the surrounding peritoneum. Pain is most severe in areas of peritoneal scarring, which are stretched as the lesions expand during the bleeding phase.

As one would expect, *dysmenorrhea* is a common symptom, but dysmenorrhea in women with endometriosis is not always a result of the disease. Most women who have had painful periods since the menarche (primary dysmenorrhea) do not have

endometriosis; the pain caused by endometriosis appears at a later time (secondary dysmenorrhea).

The pain associated with endometriosis is generally severe and steady rather than cramplike. Whenever pain is caused by endometriosis, there usually is considerable involvement of the uterosacral ligaments and the cul-de-sac.

Traditionally, an attempt has been made to associate the type of dysmenorrhea with the presence or absence of endometriosis. Pelvic pain that increases in severity with the onset of menses is postulated to be indicative of endometriosis, whereas the dysmenorrhea that is relieved as menses progress is less likely to be caused by endometriosis. Although it is interesting to try to establish this clinical correlation, the character of the menstrual pain is not sufficiently discriminatory to exclude the diagnosis of endometriosis. The discomfort associated with endometriosis is usually described as deep, constant, grinding pressure in contrast to the colicky pain of primary dysmenorrhea. It often radiates to the back and down the legs. *Rectal tenesmus* and *dyspareunia* are common and severe before and during menstruation if there is considerable involvement in the cul-de-sac and uterosacral ligaments. Most women are free from pain during the first half of the cycle.

Ovarian endometriosis alone or an uncomplicated endometrial cyst of the ovary does not usually cause pain.

Disturbing features of endometriosis are that all degrees of involvement are encountered without a single symptom and that severe dysmenorrhea often occurs in women with minimal endometriosis.

Abnormal bleeding. Abnormal uterine bleeding may occur in women with endometriosis. It most often results from a considerable amount of ovarian destruction by advanced lesions.

Infertility. Many women with endometriosis are infertile. It is easy to understand why this occurs when the lesions are so extensive that the tubes and ovaries are immobilized by or even buried within the masses of endometriosis. The mechanism of infertility is not obvious when there are only scattered lesions that do not disturb tubal or ovarian function.

Several theories based on experimental findings have been proposed to explain infertility coexisting with endometriosis in the absence of a mechanical factor. It has been postulated that an *autoimmune response* is triggered in some women when endometriotic tissue is phagocytized and absorbed by the host; this results in the rejection of the embryo or disrupted sperm transport. Another theory involves the existence of the *luteinized unruptured follicle syndrome*. It is postulated that the ovarian follicle fails to release the ovum despite the occurrence of the biochemical changes that are associated with ovulation. *Increased prostanoids* have been identified in some women with endometriosis, and their presence might alter tubal smooth muscle activity, thus compromising ovum transport. Another possibility is that *increased numbers of macrophages* in the peritoneal cavity phagocytize spermatazoa.

A possible factor in infertility associated with early endometriosis has been suggested by Drake and colleagues. They observed that women with endometriosis have more peritoneal fluid than do those without the condition. They also found significant increases in thromboxane B_2 and 6-keto-prostaglandin $F_1\alpha$ in the peritoneal fluid of women with endometriosis as compared with women who were infertile from other causes and with those undergoing sterilizing operations. They have proposed that the irritating lesions of endometriosis induce the peritoneal production of a variety of metabolites of arachidonic acid that alter tubal smooth muscle activity and interfere with ovum transport.

Ruptured ovarian endometrioma. As an ovarian endometrioma increases in size because of repeated hemorrhages, its walls become progressively thinner; eventually it may rupture. The sudden prostrating pain associated with dissemination of the old blood throughout the peritoneal cavity as the cyst ruptures may be preceded by gradually increasing pain as the tumor enlarges. The treatment is prompt operation. It may be necessary to remove the ovary as well as the cyst, but ovarian tissue can often be saved even though the endometrioma is large.

Risk of cancer. Although it is rare, malignant transformation in endometriosis does occur. Sampson carefully described the qualifying criteria. These endometrioid cancers are usually adenocarcinoma and are more likely to be observed in an ovarian endometrioma. Therapy is similar to other ovarian malignancy of similar state.

Physical findings. There may be historic information suggesting the presence of endometriosis such as pelvic pain, dysmenorrhea, or infertility. There are also certain findings on pelvic examination that should raise suspicion. A fixed retroflexed uterine corpus, extreme uterosacral ligament tenderness with nodularity, bilateral fixed tender masses in the adnexa, and tender thickening of the rectal-vaginal septum are findings that have a significant association with pelvic endometriosis.

Endometriosis can only be diagnosed with certainty by direct inspection, and optimally by microscopic examination of the lesions. In some instances, histologic confirmation is impossible because both glands and stroma have been destroyed as the lesions enlarge. In this event the only remaining suggestion of endometriosis may be deposits of hemosiderin.

Laparoscopy with the use of the dual-puncture technique should be performed to confirm the diagnosis in most women suspected of having endometriosis because of the presumed characteristic history and physical findings. This is particularly true in women who cannot conceive; the extent to which the reproductive organs, particularly the tubes and ovaries, are involved can be determined only by direct inspection.

DIFFERENTIAL DIAGNOSIS

It is difficult to accurately diagnose endometriosis by history and physical examination alone. Small lesions, particularly those involving the tubes and ovaries, cannot be felt, and even those in the cul-de-sac may be missed. Endometriosis can also be confused with other conditions.

Pelvic infection. The lesions that most often simulate endometriosis are those that follow repeated attacks of salpingo-oophoritis. Both conditions may cause pain before and during menstruation and deep dyspareunia. The tubes and ovaries adhere to the posterior leaves of the broad ligaments and in the cul-de-sac in both. The residua of recurrent salpingitis are smoother as compared with a fixed nodular mass of endometriosis involving the uterosacral ligaments and the cul-de-sac. Both may be tender, but old quiescent salpingo-oophoritis is usually less so than endometriosis, except during recurring acute attacks or in conjunction with menstruation.

The history often is helpful. There is nothing in the history of a patient with endometriosis that is similar to that of recurrent attacks of acute salpingo-oophoritis; the latter is often associated with fever.

Ovarian carcinoma. Nodular cul-de-sac endometriosis may on occasion resemble ovarian carcinoma. Endometriosis usually is associated with dysmenorrhea, and pelvic examination is painful. Women with ovarian cancer usually are older, there is no associated increase in dysmenorrhea, symptoms usually are minimal and may consist only of vague gastrointestinal discomfort, and pelvic examination produces no pain.

Benign ovarian neoplasms. An endometrial cyst of the ovary cannot be distinguished from a primary benign ovarian neoplasm by pelvic examination alone. Direct inspection of the enlarged ovary is necessary.

Urinary tract lesions. Urinary tract endometriosis is suggested in women with cyclic or intermittent hematuria. This is an unusual symptom and occurs only if an endometrial lesion penetrates the bladder wall. The ureters usually are involved in extrinsic lesions, which constrict rather than penetrate. These may eventually constrict the ureter completely. Intrinsic bladder lesions can be seen and biopsied. Ureteral involvement can be diagnosed by pyelography.

Bowel lesions. Cyclic dyschezia or hematochezia is an uncommon symptom of endometriosis and usually reflects bowel mucosal involvement. Any lesion visualized at sigmoidoscopy should be biopsied. On barium enema extraluminal disfiguration or annular constriction can be seen when pelvic endometriosis involves the colon.

Other lesions. Cyclic hemoptysis has been ascribed to *bronchial endometriosis;* a well-timed bronchoscopy and directed biopsy will usually confirm the diagnosis.

Any nodular tender lesion found in abdominal scars or the perineum, particularly in association with menses, warrant investigation. A biopsy will usually confirm the diagnosis of endometriosis in such lesions.

TREATMENT
General principles

The symptoms associated with endometriosis can be relieved by surgery or a variety of hormone regimens. The treatment one chooses for a specific patient is determined by her age, the severity of symptoms, the extent of the disease, whether she wishes to become pregnant, and, if so, now or in the future. Teenagers may acquire endometriosis; therefore reproduction might be postponed for many years. An overview of the potential therapies can be seen in the box on page 129.

1. Not every women needs therapy. *Expectant management is a term that has been used to characterize the female who is not interested*

in conceiving, whose minimal endometriosis is causing no menstrual disturbance, and who has little or no discomfort.

2. Whether or not infertile patients with minimal endometriosis (American Fertility Society stage I) require therapy is currently debatable.
3. Conservative surgery is definitely more successful for moderate and severe endometriosis when improving fertility is the major objective.
4. Hormonal therapy is usually administered for at least 6 months.
5. Ovarian endometriomas larger than 3 cm in diameter are minimally responsive to medical therapy.
6. In spite of appropriate hormonal or conservative surgical therapy, a conservative estimate of recurrence over 7 years is approximately 15%.

Specific therapy

Conservative operations are those in which the most important goals are to reduce the severity of the symptoms and to retain or improve fertility. A conservative approach includes resection, or destruction by cautery, of most or all visible endometriosis; freeing tubes and ovaries that are immobilized by disease or adhesions; removing an extensively damaged tube and ovary if the other is reasonably normal; freeing and suspending a retrodisplaced uterus that is bound down in the posterior cul-de-sac; and presacral neurectomy to relieve dysmenorrhea.

Definitive operations are those in which the major goal is to relieve symptoms. They are appropriate for women who have no desire for pregnancy or when the endometriosis is so extensive that preservation or restoration of fertility is impossible. Frequently, these patients have been unsuccessfully treated with medicine or surgery. The operation most often performed is hysterectomy, bilateral salpingo-oophrectomy, and resection of at least the most prominent lesions.

Hormone therapy eliminates the repeated cyclic variations in ovarian estrogen and progesterone that stimulate periodic growth and disintegration of the

---

POTENTIAL THERAPY FOR ENDOMETRIOSIS

I. Hormonal
   A. Oral contraceptive steroid: norgestrel (Lo-Ovral)
      1. Cyclically
      2. Continuous
   B. Progestin (medroxyprogesterone acetate)
      1. Intramuscular (Depo-Provera, Amen)
      2. Oral (Provera)
   C. Androgen (Danazol)
   D. GnRH-analog
II. Surgical
   A. Conservative
      1. Laparoscopy with electrocautery or laser vaporization of lesions
      2. Removal of specific lesions and possible uterine suspension with presacral neurectomy
   B. Definitive
      1. Abdominal hysterectomy
      2. Salpingo-oophorectomy if diseased
      3. Bowel resection rarely

---

ectopic endometrium. Hormone therapy includes *cyclic low-dose combined oral contraceptives,* which produce minimal endometrial growth and scant withdrawal bleeding; *continuous high-dose estrogen-progestogen combinations* to produce a pseudopregnancy state in which uterine and ectopic endometrium is converted to decidua, which eventually undergoes necrosis; *long-acting progestogens,* which also produce decidualization, necrosis, and amenorrhea; and *Danazol.*

Indications

Patients for whom treatment must most often be planned are (1) young women who want to delay pregnancy for several years, (2) women who are infertile, and (3) those who are seeking only symptomatic relief. Each is treated differently. Laparoscopy should usually be performed to confirm the diagnosis and to determine the extent of the disease before a treatment plan is developed. This procedure can be repeated if necessary to assess the effectiveness of therapy.

Delay of pregnancy. The major concern for *young women who want to delay pregnancy* is to preserve fertility by limiting further growth of the lesions. This can be accomplished most effectively by maintaining a pseudomenopausal state with Danazol, 800 mg daily, an attenuated androgen, which is a synthetic derivative of 17α-ethynyl-testosterone. Another possibility is to create a pseudopregnancy state with a high-dose progestogen preparation or to use low-dose oral contraceptives.

Since *Danazol* suppresses gonadotropin production, the ovarian secretions of estrogen and progesterone are inhibited; and the reproductive organs, including ectopic endometrium, undergo atrophic changes. Small peritoneal implants and even larger endometriomas may disappear after 3 to 4 months, and larger lesions become much smaller. More extensive endometriosis may also disappear completely after 6 to 12 months of therapy. Normal reproductive functions are restored promptly when the drug is discontinued. Ectopic endometrium also is reactivated but less rapidly than that within the uterus. Some women remain free from symptoms for several years.

Although not permanent, Danazol's side effects may be distressing, particularly to young women. Some women develop hot flushes and vasomotor symptoms like those that occur at menopause. The anabolic activity of the drug may cause weight gain, and the androgenic effect may cause acne. These effects are reversible, and true virilism has not been reported. The side effects can be minimized by maintaining a low dosage of the drug; 400 to 600 mg a day is usually adequate.

Creation of a pseudopregnancy state with *continuous estrogen-progestogen combination* also controls the growth of endometriosis, although probably less effectively than with danazol. A product containing norgestrel can be given daily. This produces a decidual change and eventually necrosis in the ectopic endometrium and presumably limits its growth. Breakthrough bleeding is controlled by increasing the daily dosage when spotting occurs.

During the early weeks of treatment, the patient may be nauseated and is likely to feel uncomfortable because of pelvic edema and congestion. These symptoms usually disappear after decidual necrosis is established.

Another possible approach is to use *cyclic low-dose oral contraceptives*. Endometrial stimulation is minimal, and bleeding is scant; this may serve to inhibit the growth of ectopic endometrium. Buttram observed a tendency for the severity of endometriosis to vary with the duration of oral contraceptive use: the longer the use, the less advanced the lesion. Further study of this effect is necessary before a definite conclusion can be reached.

Low-dose oral contraceptives also may be considered for young women with family histories of endometriosis. The development and growth of the lesions may be inhibited or at least retarded by these preparations. The risks involved in using these substances by women in this age group are minimal.

The use of *GnRH agonists* has been shown to prevent ovarian estrogen production and thereby could be a suitable agent to treat endometriosis.

Infertility. *Women with endometriosis who are also infertile* require special consideration. The major goal in treatment is to improve fertility; hence oral contraceptives and the production of pseudopregnancy states usually should not be considered. These regimens are less effective in destroying lesions already present and in preventing the spread of endometriosis than is surgery.

These women benefit most from *conservative surgical procedures* designed to remove as much endometriosis as possible and to correct endometriosis-induced changes that reduce fertility. *Uterine suspension* may be performed if the uterus is adherent in cul-de-sac endometriosis, and *presacral neurectomy* to relieve dysmenorrhea. Pregnancy rates from 30% to 90% have been reported after surgical procedures. The major factors that affect the result are the extent of the disease and the skill of the surgeon. Buttram reported that 73% of his patients with mild, 56% with moderate, and 40% with severe endometriosis became pregnant within 15 months after their operations. The studies of Drake and colleagues, showing increased prostaglandin production associated with peritoneal endometriosis, suggest that all endometriosis, even small scattered peritoneal lesions that do not involve the tubes and ovaries, should be removed or destroyed in infertile women.

Ordinarily, *Danazol* should not be used after surgery, even though a few small areas of endometriosis are left. Since most conceptions occur during the first 12 to 15 months after surgery, the patient should be given an opportunity to use this time without suppressing ovulation. This medication may be prescribed later for patients who do not conceive or for those whose lesions recur after operation.

Danazol may prove to be as effective as conservative surgery in establishing fertility; its major disadvantage is the delay while it is being given. It may also serve an important role in preparing patients with extensive lesions for operation. If such women are pretreated for 3 to 6 months, many of the lesions will have disappeared, and those that remain will be smaller and more easily removed.

TABLE 11-1 Clinical differentiation

	Endometriosis	Adenomyosis
Approximate age when symptomatic	25-35 Years	35-45 Years
Symptomatic	Usually	Sometimes
Abnormal uterine bleeding	Yes	Yes
Dysmenorrhea	Yes	Yes
Infertility	Yes	No
Pelvic pain	Yes	Yes
Responsive to hormone therapy	Yes	No
Responsive to conservative surgery	Yes	No
Requires hysterectomy	Sometimes	Often

Pain associated with endometriosis usually is relieved during pregnancy, but the relief is temporary. Dysmenorrhea may recur when menses are reestablished. Women with endometriosis should have their children fairly close together. Endometriosis will grow during long intervals between pregnancies, diminishing the chances of conception in the future.

Relief of symptoms. When the only concern is the *relief of symptoms,* the most logical treatment is surgical, and the most appropriate operation is *hysterectomy and resection of major masses of endometriosis.* Small areas may be left in place. In women over the age of 40 the tubes and ovaries should usually be removed, but normal adnexa may be left in young women. Replacement estrogen should be prescribed for those who are castrated.

The remaining endometriosis will be troublesome in only a few women whose ovaries are left in place or who are receiving estrogen. Danazol will relieve the symptoms in the former, and the latter can be relieved by stopping the estrogen.

A *long-acting progestogen,* such as depo-medroxy-progesterone, in doses sufficient to produce and maintain amenorrhea, is effective in relieving pain. Because anovulation and amenorrhea sometimes persist for many months after it is discontinued, this drug should not be used in women who may want to become pregnant.

Other indications. Surgery is indicated for reasons other than relieving symptoms or improving fertility. An operation is indicated whenever one or both ovaries are larger than 5 cm in diameter, regardless of the age of the patient and even though she is known to have endometriosis. *Ovarian endometriomas* rarely produce symptoms, and it is impossible to differentiate them from

ovarian neoplasms by pelvic examination alone. *Oophorectomy is not often necessary, even for large ovarian endometriomas.* Individual cysts can be dissected out of the normal stroma. One can usually preserve enough ovarian tissue for normal hormone secretion and even pregnancy. A conservative approach is particularly important in young women.

Endometriosis of the rectosigmoid can cause partial or complete bowel obstruction. Bowel resection is appropriate if the lesion cannot be differentiated from cancer or whenever there is significant narrowing of the bowel lumen.

ADENOMYOSIS

Additional information concerning adenomyosis can be found in Chapter 47. Although women who have endometriosis and adenomyosis (internal endometriosis) have a disease that shares histologic similarity, the clinical pictures are different. Key points of differentiation can be seen in Table 11-1.

REFERENCES

Barbieri, R.L., and Ryan, K.J.: Danazol: Endocrine pharmacology and therapeutic applications, Am. J. Obstet. Gynecol. **141**:453, 1981.

Batt, R.E., and Naples, J.D.: Conservative surgery for endometriosis in the infertile couple, Curr. Probl. Obstet. Gynecol. **6**(1):1, 1982.

Buttram, V.C., Jr.: Conservative surgery for endometriosis in the infertile female: a study of 206 patients with implications for both medical and surgical therapy, Fertil. Steril. **31**:117, 1979.

Buttram, V.C., Jr.: Cyclic use of combination oral contraceptives and the severity of endometriosis, Fertil. Steril. **31**:347, 1979.

Dmowski, W.P.: Endocrine properties and clinical application of danazol, Fertil. Steril. **31**:237, 1979.

Drake, T.S., O'Brien, W.F., Ramwell, P.W., and Metz, S.A.: Peritoneal fluid thromboxane B_2 and 6-keto-prostaglandin $F_1\alpha$ in endometriosis, Am. J. Obstet. Gynecol. **140**:401, 1981.

Halme, J., Becker, S., Hammond, M.G., Raj, M.H.G., and Raj, S.: Increased activation of pelvic macrophages in infertile women with mild endometriosis, Am. J. Obstet. Gynecol. **145**:333, 1983.

Meldrum, D.R., Chang, R.J., Lu, J., Vale, W., and Judd, H.L.: Medical oophorectomy using a long-acting GnRh agonist. A possible new approach to the treatment of endometriosis, J. Clin. Endocrinol. Metab. **54**:1081, 1982.

Molgaard, C.A., Golbeck, A.L., and Gresham, L: Current concepts in endometriosis, West. J. Med. **143**:42, 1985.

Ranney, B.: The prevention, inhibition, palliation, and treatment of endometriosis, Am. J. Obstet. Gynecol. **123**:778, 1975.

Rock, J.A., Guzick, D.S., Sengos, C., Schweditsch, M., Sapp, K.C., and Jones, H.W., Jr.: The conservative surgical treatment of endometriosis: evaluation of pregnancy success with respect to the extent of the disease as categorized using contemporary classification systems. Fertil. Steril. **35**:131, 1981.

Sampson, J.A.: Cysts of the ovary, Arch. Surg. **3**:245, 1921.

Simpson, J.L., Elias, S., Malinak, L.R., and Buttram, V.C., Jr.: Heritable aspects of endometriosis. I. Genetic studies, Am. J. Obstet. Gynecol. **137**:327, 1980.

Strathy, J.H., Molgaard, C.A., Coulam, C.B., and Melton, L.J., III: Endometriosis and infertility: a laparoscopic study of endometriosis among fertile and infertile women, Fertil. Steril. **38**:667, 1982.

Von Rokitansky, K.: Uber uterusdausen—neubildung in uterus und ovarial-sarcomen, Ztscghr d, k k Gesellsch d aerette du Wien **37**:577, 1860.

12

Elsie Reid Carrington

The Breast

Carcinoma of the breast continues to be the most common malignant neoplasm in women. The American Cancer Society estimated that in 1984 there were 115,000 new cases in the United States and more than 38,000 deaths from the disease. Approximately 85% of cancers are detected after the age of 40, whereas occurrence in women under age 30 is only 1.5%. The death rate for breast cancer in the United States is 22.1 per 100,000 women per year. Knowledge and understanding of the nature of the various disorders of the mammary gland are essential parts of the obstetrician-gynecologist's role in providing primary health care for women of all ages.

DEVELOPMENT

The mammary glands develop from specialized skin stimulated by an induction mechanism inherent in the mammary mesenchyme underlying the epidermis. Bands of tissue gradually thicken to form the "milk line" extending from the midclavicular line to the groin. This epithelial mammary ridge is visible in the human embryo at the end of the fourth week of gestation. Regression of the caudal end and thickening of the bands limited to the region of the permanent gland become evident in the embryo of about 6 weeks. Ductal development begins at about the fifth month, and the mammary gland is fully differentiated at birth.

The normal breast hypertrophy of the newborn and secretion from the nipple, if present, regress with the decline in the levels of estrogen-progesterone of placental origin and fetal pituitary prolactin. Breast tissues are dormant until the onset of puberty when estrogen levels begin to rise. Other hormones, including growth hormone, insulin, cortisone, thyroxine, and prolactin, are involved to a lesser degree in adolescent mammary gland growth. Under these influences, differentiation and budding of ducts and an increase in fatty and connective tissues take place and are reflected in breast growth characteristic of the thelarche. The addition of progesterone accompanying ovulatory cycles is essential for optimal acinar growth.

METHODS OF EXAMINATION

Because breast cancers are so prone to metastasize while still small, early detection is essential for control. Significant strides have been made in screening techniques and in therapeutic approaches, but methodical examination at regular intervals remains a key factor in early detection. In a majority of cases the patient first discovers a mass in the breast, usually by accident and often late in the course of its development. Education of the patient in technique, timing, and reasons for self-examination should be a standard part of primary health care.

Breast self-examination. Self-examination should be carried out at monthly intervals, preferably just after the menstrual period when hormonal stimulation is at lowest ebb if the woman is premenopausal. Systematic examination begins with full inspection while sitting or standing in front of a mirror first with arms at the sides and then raised overhead; attention is directed to any change in size or shape of the breast or in appearance of the nipples or skin. The supraclavicular and axillary regions are palpated for presence of nodes. The remainder of the examination is done in the supine position using a rolled-up towel under the back to elevate the side of the chest to be examined. This flattens the breast against the chest wall. Systematic palpation with the flat of the fingers is carried out beginning at the outer margins until every part of each breast is examined. The areolar areas are similarly palpated, and the nipple base compressed and stripped for evidence of secretion. The physician's sensitivity to individual patient needs during instruction encourages self-motivation and helps allay anxieties.

The fact that properly informed breast self-examination performers gain significant advantage in survival over nonperformers following newly diagnosed breast cancer is demonstrated in the Vermont study of 1004 such patients. Death from the disease occurred in 14% of the former versus 26% of the latter during a follow-up period of 52 months.

Mammography. Techniques for breast x-ray film examination have improved in quality, and radiation dosage necessary for identification of various breast disorders has been reduced significantly. Dosages used for mammography in the 1960s ranged from 7 to 12 rad to the skin and were a cause for serious concern. Current x-ray film techniques require as little as 0.2 to 0.3 rads to the skin. This represents a dosage of 0.02 to 0.03 rad to the midbreast, which Strax considers a highly favorable risk/benefit ratio.

The sensitivity rate for these films is about 90%. The type of breast examined influences the accuracy of interpretation. The denser, more glandular breasts of young women make it more difficult to

recognize early stages of the disease. Nevertheless, mammography has the capability of detecting many cancers smaller than 1 cm, or 1 to 2 years before they would be clinically palpable. Data from the large national screening project reported by Strax revealed that a total of 2379 early cancers were found among approximately 280,000 screened women who had both clinical and mammographic examinations. Of these, 44% were detected by mammogram alone; in this group, 77% had no nodal involvement. But mammography is not infallible. It is an important complement to, but not a substitute for, clinical examination. A negative mammogram, for example, should not induce one to defer aspiration biopsy or excision of a suspicious palpable mass. Films are particularly useful for evaluating intractile papillary lesions in which microcalcifications highly suggestive of carcinoma can be seen before a mass is palpable.

Xeroradiography. Xeroradiography, a variation of mammography, uses a selenium plate that produces the breast image on paper instead of film. Some radiologists prefer this technique, but results show no real advantage of one method over the other.

Breast aspiration biopsy. Fine needle breast aspiration biopsy is a simple, safe, and cost-effective test. It is particularly useful in the management of fibrocystic disease so commonly found in young women. If the mass is cystic and the fluid is not grossly sanguinous, aspiration frequently obviates the need for radiologic procedures or surgery. Bloodstained fluids and aspirates from solid tumors require cytologic examination or cell block histology. Other particular indications include aspiration of masses in the superficial tissues or incisional areas following mastectomy and in suspicious breast masses in pregnant women, in whom delays in diagnosis are far too frequent. Complications are rare. Since even small hematomas and edema may present diagnostic difficulties in interpretation of mammography, the procedure should be deferred for 2 to 3 weeks if findings on the aspirate are inconclusive.

With the use of breast aspiration biopsy in experienced hands, indications are that false-positive results occur in less than 1% of reported cases and that false-negative results range between 10% and 20%.

Thermography. With thermography the infrared heat patterns emitted from the skin of the breast are recorded on film. Any condition that causes increased vascularization can cause changes in the thermal pattern. Consequently, the test is not specific for breast cancer. A "hot" thermogram in the absence of clinical or mammographic findings should be used only as a risk indicator.

Other techniques. *Ultrasonography* has its greatest use in evaluating breast masses in young women in whom density of the parenchyma presents difficulty for mammography and xerography because of ultrasound's ability to accurately differentiate cystic and solid masses. Early cancers are far more accurately detected by mammography. *Radioisotope scans* have not proved very practical.

The practical use of available methods of examination in relationship to the earliest possible detection of breast cancer is summarized in the American Cancer Society recommendations for breast cancer screening:

Breast self-examination monthly after age 20
Annual physician examination after age 40
Baseline mammogram between ages 35 and 40
Annual mammogram after age 50

DISORDERS
Developmental abnormalities

Supernumerary breasts or *accessory nipples* are remnants of the mammary ridge. The most common locations are just below the normal breast and in the axillary region. These are usually of no clinical significance except during pregnancy when simulation of the glandular elements, if present, causes enlargement, sometimes discomfort, and even secretion of milk.

Amastia, or failure of breast development, is extremely rare; when this condition exists, it is usually associated with deformity of the chest wall.

Minor degrees of *asymmetrical growth of the breasts* are exceedingly common. The concerned adolescent girl and her parents usually need only reassurance. Occasionally, either excessive growth or hypoplasia of one breast can be of such magnitude that cosmetic surgery is warranted. Augmentation or reduction mammoplasty should be deferred until maturation is assuredly complete.

Massive hypertrophy of the breasts, although not a common condition, is most likely to occur during puberty, less often during pregnancy. Endocrine studies are within normal limits; hence enhanced end-organ sensitivity is the apparent cause. The condition is psychologically traumatic and can also be physically debilitating. Cosmetic surgery, usually reduction mammoplasty, is indicated when full maturation is attained.

Abnormalities of secretion

Inappropriate lactation, or *galactorrhea,* is caused by a great variety of conditions, including mechanical factors that act through neural reflexes such as vigorous nipple stimulation and reactions to chest or breast surgery or disease. Certain pharmacologic agents, particularly the psychotropic drugs, tend to deplete central nervous system catecholamines and thus reduce secretion of prolactin-inhibiting factor. Occasionally, galactorrhea follows withdrawal of oral contraceptives. Thyroid and, to a lesser extent, adrenal disorders may be associated with abnormal lactation. These and the more common central nervous system and hypothalamic-pituitary disorders associated with galactorrhea are discussed in Chapter 9.

Acute infections

Localized infections. *Sebaceous cysts* arising from glands normally located in the skin of the areola frequently become infected. Similarly, *periareolar abscesses* may arise in one or more of the lactiferous ducts in association with inversion of the nipple, chronic maceration, ductal obstruction, and secondary infection. Incision and drainage may not be curative, particularly for periareolar abscess, which is prone to recur. Excision of the involved duct is advisable as a final step when the acute infection has subsided.

Puerperal mastitis. In most areas of the United States, postpartum breast infections are relatively rare, usually not exceeding 1%. Puerperal mastitis is discussed in Chapter 42.

Epidemic puerperal mastitis. Epidemic puerperal mastitis is an altogether different type of infection. The responsible agent is almost invariably a penicillin-resistant *S. aureus,* and the infection is most frequently hospital acquired. When the microorganism is present in the nursery, colonization of the nasopharynx occurs in an alarmingly high percentage of infants within 24 to 48 hours. Treatment is like that for sporadic mastitis.

Other infections. Breast lesions caused by specific pathogens such as tuberculosis, syphilis, actinomycosis, or blastomycosis occur rarely in the United States.

Mammary duct ectasia. Mammary duct ectasia (comedomastitis or plasma cell mastitis) is a benign process usually occurring at about the age of 40. The primary changes occur in the dilated subareolar ducts that become filled with inspissated breast secretions and debris. Chronic inflammation and marked periductal fibrosis develop later. Signs and symptoms include nipple discharge, recurrent pain, and often nipple retraction. The ducts, filled with thick, pastelike material and surrounded by fibrosis, are readily palpable, and the axillary glands may be enlarged. The findings during examination are, in fact, indistinguishable from breast cancer; hence excision biopsy is mandatory. No further treatment is necessary if duct ectasia is found.

Mammary necrosis. Mammary necrosis is a localized area of fat necrosis followed by the development of a firm, readily palpable mass located just below the skin. Ecchymosis may or may not be associated. It is more common in women with pendulous breasts. A history of trauma is expected, but in about half the cases the woman recalls no specific injury. Pain and tenderness are early signs. Later fibrosis and scarring occur; the mass then has a firm consistency and an irregular outline closely resembling carcinoma. Excision biopsy is necessary for diagnosis and treatment.

Mondor's disease. Mondor's disease, or *superficial thrombophlebitis of the veins of the breast and anterior chest wall,* does not occur often; however, familiarity with this condition is important because it often is overtreated. The cause is unknown. It is not necessarily associated with trauma, surgery, or oversized breasts. As a rule the first symptom is pain, although acute symptoms may not be a dominant complaint. Next, a hard, usually tender, cord appears in the superficial tissues following the course of one of the superficial veins, particularly the lateral thoracic or the superior epigastric. Retraction of the skin occurs where the vein crosses the breast and can be mistaken as evidence of infiltrating cancer. The course of the thrombophlebitis is self-limiting, although the time required for resolution varies from a few weeks to 6 months. Treatment is symptomatic during the period of pain and tenderness and includes reassurance that neither underlying breast lesions nor complications such as embolism are associated with this condition.

BENIGN DISORDERS
Fibrocystic disease

Fibrocystic changes are the most common cause of breast ''lumps.'' Typically, these are bilateral and multiple. They can be found in women throughout the reproductive years, most frequently in the thirties, and they regress after the menopause, implying hormonal dependence. Variation in response to estrogen and progesterone with estrogen dominance is believed to cause the ductal and stromal proliferations that characterize this condition. Premenstrual pain and tenderness are relatively common complaints, but the condition often is asymptomatic. Palpation of the breast may reveal a diffuse increase in consistency, shottiness, nodularity, or a fluctuant or rubbery mass. Most of the cysts are thin walled, filled with a turbid fluid, and often bluish. The stromal tissues show varying degrees of fibrosis. Although lymphocytic infiltration is common, it does not indicate mastitis.

Treatment depends on the age of the patient and on the nature of the breast changes. Patients over 25 years of age should have preoperative or baseline mammography. Readily palpable cystic masses can be aspirated. If cystic fluid is obtained and the mass disappears completely, no further treatment is needed. If the fluid is serous or bloody, or if no fluid is obtained, excision biopsy is indicated.

Medical treatment for mastodynia associated with diffuse breast involvement is mainly supportive. Oral contraceptives with low estrogen content, norethindrone acetate (Loestrin 1/20) or medroxyprogesterone can reduce pain and tenderness in about 60% to 80% of cases of severe mastodynia, but there is little effect on nodularity. Symptoms recur on cessation of treatment. The antigonadotropin Danazol given in 200 to 400 mg dosages daily, relieves pain in about three fourths of cases.

However, the side effects of menstrual irregularities and amenorrhea, acne, and weight gain, and the fact that symptoms recur after the course of treatment, seriously limit its use. Whether restriction of methylxanthines (coffee, tea, cocoa, and colas) is effective in relieving pain and to some extent reducing nodularity remains open to question.

Adenosis. Adenosis is frequently associated with fibrocystic disease and may be the dominant feature. Proliferation of ducts and acini and marked interlobular fibrosis create a firm irregular mass clinically suggestive of carcinoma. Preoperative mammography and excision biopsy are indicated.

Fibroadenomas. Fibroadenomas may occur at any age, but they are most frequently seen in women under the age of 30. They are usually solitary and asymptomatic. The tumor is firm and mobile, and the margins are well defined. When they arise in the teenage or pregnant patient, they may enlarge remarkably, presumably because of the rapid increase in hormone stimulation. All solid masses should be excised for definitive diagnosis and treatment.

Intraductile papilloma. Intraductile papilloma produces a serous or bloody discharge from the nipple, most often during the perimenopausal years. The growth is small, often less than 1 cm, and difficult to locate. Application of pressure at different points around the areola usually elicits discharge when the involved duct is pressed. In most cases a benign, friable, villous growth is found, but the possibility of papillary carcinoma must always be considered. Treatment is complete excision biopsy of the involved duct.

Galactocele. A galactocele is a cystic mass that develops in women who have recently lactated. The mass is smooth walled, movable, and filled with a thick inspissated milky fluid. Needle aspiration is curative if the fluid obtained is typical and the mass disappears thereafter. If a mass remains, excision biopsy is indicated.

Malignant lesions

The incidence and the number of deaths caused by breast cancer have increased during the past 25 years, in part because of increased aging of the population. Currently, one in 13 women will develop breast cancer in her lifetime. Certain features of the disease and identifiable risk factors of importance to the clinician are now well established. Mammary cancer tends to be multicentric and may metastasize at a relatively early stage. Five-year survival rates approach 85% in the early localized stage of the disease. The rate drops to 53% with involvement of the axillary nodes; if the supraclavicular nodes are involved, the prognosis is extremely grave. Multiple foci are frequently found with the primary lesion, and according to Leis and co-workers the overall incidence of bilateral breast involvement is between 7.5% and 10%.

Types. Mammary carcinoma is usually classified according to the site of origin in the ducts or lobules:

Intraductile carcinoma
   Scirrhous carcinoma
   Papillary carcinoma
   Colloid carcinoma
   Comedocarcinoma
   Paget's disease
Lobular carcinoma

Approximately 90% of cases arise in the ducts. Lobular carcinoma is sometimes found in an in situ stage with small, round, malignant cells filling the acini without stromal invasion. This tumor is frequently multicentric, and in about a third of cases involvement in bilateral.

Paget's disease is different because of the epidermal involvement and because delays in diagnosis are unfortunately so common. Although this is an intraductal lesion, involvement of the nipple epidermis occurs early. Itching, burning, and the gradual development of an eczematoid lesion are the first signs. The lesion may remain indolent for some time, then spread to areola and deeper into the ducts as an in situ or infiltrating carcinoma. In the absence of a palpable mass, surgical treatment is usually curative. If a mass or axillary nodes are palpable, the prognosis decreases significantly.

Any lesion confined to the nipple should raise suspicion. Biopsy reveals the characteristic Paget cells. Partly because of delay, the 5-year survival rate is only about 50%.

Inflammatory carcinoma comprises 1% to 4% and has the poorest prognosis of all breast cancers. Pain and diffuse enlargement of the breast are first evidences. The superficial tissues become indurated and pitted in appearance. A mass may or may not be palpable. Biopsy reveals dermal lymphatics plugged with neoplastic cells in most, but not all cases. This finding is sufficiently unique that controversy has arisen as to whether this disease should be considered a distinct entity. Despite the fact that fever, leukocytosis, and other systemic components of breast abscess are minimal or absent, infection is often the initial diagnosis made; and therapy may be delayed for weeks or months. Delay is critical, since the course of the disease is so virulent that metastases are almost invariably present at the time of diagnosis. Survivals rarely exceed 1 to 2 years. Grace and Cooperman emphasize the futility of surgery as the primary or sole treatment and the importance of attacking the systemic disease with appropriate courses of chemotherapy followed by surgery or irradiation, depending on the tumor bulk.

Risk factors

AGE. Breast cancer is a rarity below age 25, but its frequency increases steadily after age 35. About 85% of the total cases are in women over age 40.

FAMILY HISTORY. The risk is doubled with a positive family history and increased eightfold if the mother or sister has had bilateral breast cancer during her premenopausal years.

HISTORY OF PREVIOUS BENIGN BREAST DISEASE. Risk is increased twofold to fourfold, *but only if previously excised tissues showed atypia;* the risk rises with increasing degree of dysplasia.

PREVIOUS CANCER IN ONE BREAST. Risk of cancer in the remaining breast is five times greater than the risk of a primary lesion in the general population.

PARITY. Nulliparous women and those over age 34 at the time of their first pregnancy are twice as prone to breast cancer as are women bearing children earlier in life. Lactation presumably offers some protection against the development of breast cancer.

OTHER FACTORS. Exposure to radiation or chemical agents, the use of estrogens, and prolonged exposure to estrogens through early menarche and late menopause are less clear-cut risk factors that nevertheless belong in the patient's history.

Diagnosis. The *primary complaints* leading to suspicion of breast cancer are (1) discovery of a lump; (2) serous or bloody discharge from the nipple; (3) nipple retraction, eczema, or ulceration; and (4) skin redness, dimpling, or ulceration. Pain is not a common initial complaint for malignant breast lesions, but it does occur in some cases, mainly if the initial symptom is related to axillary or vertebral metastasis.

Details concerning these symptoms—date of onset, duration, and change in size or other features—and inquiry concerning each of the risk factors mentioned previously should be included in the history.

Systematic examination of the breast should be performed as previously described. If the patient is under 25 years of age and the mass is smooth and freely movable or obviously cystic, management as outlined for benign lesions may be most appropriate, but mammographic studies should be obtained on any woman, regardless of age, with suggestive clinical signs or symptoms or dubious findings. Mammography can identify many lesions that are not palpable because of their small size or their location in fatty tissues or within the duct. Intraductal papillary cancers, which are relatively soft and friable and may cause bloody discharge early, are frequently nonpalpable but often produce microcalcifications that are visible on film. *Aspiration biopsies* may be examined on frozen section, as well as on permanent sections. The possibility of detecting multifocal lesions, not uncommonly within the same breast and often in the opposite breast, is further reason for mammographic evaluation before biopsy. A tissue diagnosis is essential before any form of therapy is instituted.

Management of the contralateral breast in women with worrisome risk factors present remains controversial. Reports of selective biopsies of the remaining breast indicate that in situ or early cases are found in 12% to 16% of cases.

Treatment. Radical mastectomy with or without postoperative radiation remained unchallenged as optimal treatment for cancer of the breast for at least six decades. Failure to alter survival rates significantly during this period, new knowledge of the biology of breast cancers, and the larger number of cases with early occurrence of lesions of less than 2 cm were important factors in the growing trend toward conservatism and individualization. The changing concept of tumor spread is the basis for recent therapeutic approaches. There is good evidence that most mammary cancers have already metastasized by the time the tumor is clinically detectable. In patients with small breast lesions and negative axillary nodes, 75% reach a 10-year survival period without recurrence, but in 25% systemic dissemination precedes therapy. Of those with positive axillary nodes and no evidence of distant metastasis, only 25% survive for 10 years without recurrence. These results suggest differences in mammary tumor behavior and host resistance and have stimulated current studies of their interaction.

SURGICAL TREATMENT. A two-stage approach to primary surgical management is usually preferable to biopsy, frozen section evaluation, and immediate operation. The short delay has no deleterious effects, and it permits more precise pathologic assessment and participation of the patient in decisions concerning the overall therapeutic program.

The *modified radical mastectomy,* which involves total (simple) mastectomy and axillary dissection but preserves the pectoralis muscle and nerves, has practically replaced the radical procedure. The trend toward more conservative surgery for early breast cancers with better functional and cosmetic results led to a long-term study formulated by the National Surgical Adjuvant Breast Project in 1971. A total of 1665 women with a primary tumor confined to the breast or breast and axilla and movable over the underlying muscle were treated by radical mastectomy, total mastectomy without axillary dissection but with irradiation, and total mastectomy alone with axillary dissection only if nodes were subsequently positive. There were no significant differences in the 10-year survival rates related to the procedure used. In patients with clinically negative nodes, overall survival in each group was about 57%. Patients with positive nodes had a 10-year survival rate of about 38% with either modified management or radical surgery.

The estrogen receptor (ER) and progesterone receptor (PgR) status of a portion of the tumor tissue removed should be determined, since results obtained have a bearing on prognosis and also provide guidelines for subsequent therapy should recurrence arise.

PRIMARY RADIATION THERAPY. Recent interest in the use of radiation therapy as an alternative to mastectomy has gained impetus following reports showing 5-year survival rates comparable to those with surgical management. Clinical trials of longer duration are necessary and are in progress. Results from the Harvard Joint Center for Radiation Therapy reported in the 1980 National Institutes of Health Summary reveal a 5-year survival rate of 91% for stage I and 66% for stage II lesions. In most centers excision biopsy and axillary node sampling are performed for pretherapy diagnosis, but in some cases needle biopsies are used. Usual treatment includes supervoltage external beam treatments averaging 1000 rad/wk for 5 weeks aimed at treating areas of the breast; the anterior chest wall, including the internal mammary chain; and ipsilateral axillary and supraclavicular nodes; tumor site implants of iridium 192 delivering 1500 to 2000 rad are added in selected cases. Good functional and cosmetic results and a comparable 5-year outcome are the main advantages to date.

ENDOCRINE THERAPY. Hormone treatment has an important role in palliation of metastatic breast cancer. Availability of reliable methods for assay of estrogen and progesterone receptors within the tumor tissue has aided substantially in selecting therapy for individual patients. About 60% of patients with tumors that are ER positive will respond to hormonal manipulation, but only about 8% of those with ER-negative tumors will respond. Progesterone represents a critical end-step in estrogen action, and the presence of progesterone receptors appears to be more predictive of response. About 35% of estrogen receptor-positive tumors fail to respond to hormonal alterations. Numerous clinical trials have shown that women with tumors possessing both of these receptors have increased likelihood of responding to endocrine manipulation. Clark and co-workers' study of the receptor status in resectable tumors with positive axillary nodes (stage II breast cancer) showed that patients had a longer disease-free survival period when both receptors were present but that PgR levels were significantly more predictive than ER levels. The authors again stress the importance of determining both ER and PgR levels in every case of primary breast cancer and of incorporating findings into the selection of adjuvant therapy. Bilateral oophorectomy in the premenopausal patient is now usually limited to those with ER-positive tumors.

Antiestrogens such as tamoxifen have proved effective in approximately 50% of ER-positive cases; this response can be used as a predictor of patients who are likely to respond similarly to oophorectomy should drug effectiveness fail. Tamoxifen has the advantage of almost complete absence of side effects. Additive therapy of large doses of estrogens for postmenopausal patients induces tumor regression in about 30% of cases. *Adrenalectomy and hypophysectomy* also have response rates of about 30%. Patients with ER-negative tumors and those unresponsive to hormonal manipulation can still be given palliative chemotherapy.

CHEMOTHERAPY. The most recent approach to treatment of mammary cancer involves the sequential use of chemotherapy after mastectomy and axillary node dissection. The rationale for this approach is based on the concept that micrometastasis will already have occurred when positive axillary nodes are found. The 1981 National Cancer Institute report on bimodal therapy derived from studies conducted at treatment centers in the United States and Europe demonstrates that this combination significantly prolonged the disease-free intervals, as well as prolonging overall survival at 4 years by 27%. This good result occurred mainly in premenopausal patients. Further studies of bimodal therapy in terms of which drug regimens are most effective and whether patients other than those with involved axillary nodes can derive benefit from this treatment must be conducted.

Carcinoma of the breast during pregnancy. Fortunately, carcinoma of the breast during pregnancy or lactation is rare. Pregnancy does not predispose to mammary cancer; but growth, extension, and metastasis may be accelerated by the physiologic expansion of vascular and lymphatic channels and possibly by the elevated levels of estrogens.

DIAGNOSIS. Diagnosis during pregnancy or lactation is frequently delayed because a small mass in the hypertrophied breast may be difficult to detect or may be misinterpreted. Regular prenatal examinations of the breast and prompt biopsy of palpable nodes are mandatory if early lesions are to be discovered.

PROGNOSIS. The outlook for the patient with co-

TABLE 12-1 Ten-year results of radical mastectomy correlated with clinical stage, Columbia-Presbyterian Medical Center

Columbia classification	Breast carcinoma during pregnancy and lactation, 1915-1959		Personal series breast carcinoma, 1935-1959	
	Number of patients	Survival 10 years (%)	Number of patients	Survival 10 years (%)
Stage A	20	60	402	70
Stage B	11	27	154	41
Stage C	8	12.5	59	24
Stage D	9	0	11	18
TOTAL	48	33	626	54

Modified from Haagensen, C.D.: The breast, ed. 2, Philadelphia, 1971, W.B. Saunders Co.

incidental mammary cancer and pregnancy is not hopeless. The pessimistic view of inoperability of these lesions in gravid women is no longer tenable. Treatment, particularly when initiated in the early stage, is almost as effective as in the nonpregnant patient. One of the largest series of such comparisons is shown in Table 12-1.

Birks and associates reported survival rates of 57% for 5 years and 40% for 10 years, with no significant difference in patients 30 years of age and under as compared with those over 30. Within 5 years of diagnosis, 15 pregnancies occurred with no adverse consequences. Poor prognosis was related to the finding of axillary node involvement and stage of the disease rather than to coincidental pregnancy.

MANAGEMENT. The criteria of operability should be the same for pregnant as for nonpregnant patients, but the need for immediate intervention without as much as a week's delay is more imperative during pregnancy.

Subsequent pregnancies usually cause no complications if the patient is well and without evidence of recurrence after 3 to 4 years.

The value of terminating pregnancy as soon as possible after radical mastectomy is still a moot question. White found little to recommend the procedure in 78 women in whom therapeutic abortion was performed. Obviously, the management of this problem must be individualized. No benefit is derived from interference with the pregnancy in late-stage inoperable carcinoma of the breast.

REFERENCES

American College of Obstetricians and Gynecologists (ACOG) Committee on Gynecologic Practice: Needle aspiration cytology in evaluation of breast lesions, Committee Statement, June, 1984.

Birks, D.M., Crawford, G.M., Ellison, L.G., and Johnstone, F.R.C.: Cancer of the breast in women 30 years of age or less, Surg. Gynecol. Obstet. **137**:21, 1973.

Bottles, K., and Taylor, R.N.: Diagnosis of breast masses in pregnant women by aspiration biopsy, Obstet. Gynecol. **66**:763, 1985.

Clark, G.M., McGuire, W.L., Hubay, C.A., Pearson, O.H., and Marshall, J.S.: Progesterone receptors as a prognostic factor in stage II breast cancer, N. Engl. J. Med. **309**:1343, 1983.

Donovan, W.L.: Breast cancer and pregnancy, Obstet. Gynecol. **50**:244, 1977.

Fisher, B., Bauer, M., Margolese, R., Redmond, C., Fisher, E.R., Bauer, M., Wolmark, N., Wickerham, L., Deutch, M., Montague, E,. Margolese, R., and Foster, R.: Ten-year results of a randomized clinical trial comparing radical mastectomy and total mastectomy with or without radiation, N. Engl. J. Med. **312**:674, 1985.

Foster, R.S., Jr., and Costanza, M.C.: Breast self-examination practices and breast cancer survival, Cancer **53**:999, 1984.

Gallagher, H.S., Leis, H.P., Jr., Snydermann, R.K., and Urban, J.A.: The breast, St. Louis, 1978, The C.V. Mosby Co.

Grace, W.R., and Cooperman, A.V.: Inflammatory breast cancer, Surg. Clin. North Am. **65**:151, 1985.

Harper, P., and Kelly-Frye, E.: Ultrasound visualization of the breast in symptomatic patients, Radiology **137**:465, 1980.

Henderson, I.D., and Canellos, G.P.: Cancer of the breast: the past decade (part I), N. Engl. J. Med. **302**:17, 1980.

Henderson, I.C., and Canellos, G.P.: Cancer of the breast: the past decade (part II), N. Engl. J. Med. **302**:78, 1980.

Hindle, W.H., and Navin, J.: Breast aspiration biopsy: a neglected gynecologic procedure, Am. J. Obstet. Gynecol. **146**:482, 1983.

Kopans, D.B., Meyer, J.E., Cohen, A.M., and Wood, W.C.: Palpable breast masses: the importance of preoperative mammography, J.A.M.A. **246**:2819, 1981.

Leis, H.P., Jr., Merscheimer, W.L., Black, M.M., and Chabron, A.B.: The second breast, N.Y. State J. Med. **65**:2460, 1965.

Manni, A.: Hormone receptors and breast cancer, N. Engl. J. Med. **309**:138, 1983.

Marchant, D.J., and Myirjesy, I., editors: Breast disease: proceedings of an international symposium, May 13-17, 1978, New York, 1979, Grune & Stratton, Inc.

Moxley, J.H., Allegra, J.C., Henney, J., and Muggia, F.: Treatment of primary breast cancer: summary of NIH consensus development conference, J.A.M.A. **244**:797, 1980.

Pressman, P.I.: Selective biopsy of the opposite breast, Cancer **57**:577, 1986.

Sickles, E.A., Filly, R.A., and Callen, P.W.: Benign breast lesions: ultrasound detection and diagnosis, Radiology **151**:467, 1984.

Silverberg, E.: Cancer statistics 1984, Cancer **7**:23, 1984.

Strax, P.: Evaluation of screening programs for early diagnosis of breast cancer, Surg. Clin. North Am. **58**:669, 1978.

Vorherr, H.: Breast aspiration biopsy with multihole needles for histologic and cytologic examination, Am. J. Obstet. Gynecol. **151**:70, 1985.

Vorherr, H.: Fibrocystic breast disease: pathophysiology, pathomorphology, clinical picture, and management, Am. J. Obstet. Gynecol. **154**:161, 1986.

Weiss, R.B., Henney, J.E., and DeVita, V.T., Jr.: Multimodal treatment of primary breast carcinoma: analysis of accomplishments and problem areas, Am. J. Med. **70**:844, 1981.

White, T.T.: Prognosis of breast cancer for pregnant women: analysis of 1413 cases, Surg. Gynecol. Obstet. **100**:661, 1955.

13

Russell K. Laros, Jr.

Fertilization; development, physiology, and disorders of the placenta; fetal development

Successful human reproduction is dependent on an integrated sequence of physiologic mechanisms that first of all ensures normal maturation, fertilization, and growth of the ovum and then, as pregnancy advances, permits normal differentiation and adequate nutrition for the fetus.

FERTILIZATION

Union of male and female elements of procreation must be preceded by *maturation* of the germ cells. In the sexually adult male, spermatogenesis occurs continuously, whereas in the female, oogenesis is cyclic. Under the influence of hypothalamic-releasing factors and, in turn, secretion of pituitary FSH, many follicles are stimulated during the first 10 days of the cycle. Generally, only the dominant follicle is destined to reach maturity at each cycle. Its rate of growth is greatly accelerated as the ripening follicle migrates to the surface of the ovary. At present the mechanism that determines which follicle will be singled out to play a leading role in the cycle is not understood. At approximately the fourteenth day, the wall of the follicle ruptures, and the ovum with some of the surrounding granulosa cells and follicular fluid is discharged into the fallopian tube. Release of pressure allows the walls of the follicle to collapse, and blood from the congested vessels of the theca fills the cavity. The point of rupture *(blutpunkt)*

seals off. Theca cells and especially granulosa cells undergo luteinization, producing a yellow, lipid-laden body, the *mature corpus luteum*.

Final preparation of the ovum for fertilization involves the unique process of *meiosis* (Fig. 13-1). In contrast to somatic cell division, or mitosis—wherein a complete diploid chromosomal set, each chromosome an exact replica of itself, is passed to the daughter cell—gametogenesis results in reduction of the nuclear chromosomes to half the number characteristic of the species. This is accomplished by two maturation divisions, the steps involved being of utmost importance to an understanding of human chromosomal abnormalities.

Homologous chromosomes arrange themselves in pairs, and in the first *meiotic (reduction) division,* which occurs before ovulation, they separate *(dysjunction)* to form the first two daughter cells. Each daughter cell contains a haploid complement of chromosomes (23 X). Although the chromosomal material is equally divided, the oocyte retains the bulk of the cytoplasm. The other cell is the *first polar body.* The second division may begin before ovulation, but it is not completed until the oocyte is penetrated by a spermatozoon. At this time the *second polar body* is released.

Union of the ovum and the spermatozoon restores the normal diploid number with formation of the zygote, containing 44 autosomal chromo-

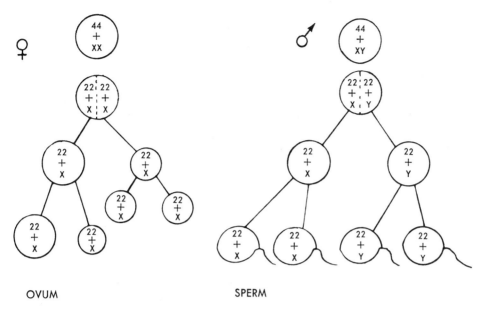

OVUM   SPERM

Fig. 13-1. Normal gametogenesis.

somes and two sex chromosomes; the zygote is female if the sex chromosomes are XX and male if they are XY (Fig. 13-2). Thus the genetic or nuclear sex is determined and fixed at fertilization.

The sex genes direct and control differentiation of the gonad and accessory structures, beginning about the sixth week of embryonic life (Chapter 3). However, the external sex is not clearly apparent until about the sixteenth week. The physical appearance of sex may be influenced by a non-physiologic hormonal environment to which the fetus is exposed. If gonadogenesis is normal, if the fetal hormonal environment is appropriate, and if there is no interference from harmful physical factors or from exogenous hormonal influences, the physical appearance of sex (phenotype) will be appropriate for the chromosomal sex (genotype).

The genetic constitution may be altered in the process of gonadogenesis by *nonassociation* or by *nondisjunction of chromosomes,* resulting in defects that are often lethal if autosomes are involved—however, there are exceptions. Nonlethal consequences are seen in developmental abnormalities that result from the number of chromo-

somes either exceeding or being less than normal (Fig. 13-3).

The normal chromosomal number of 46 is shown in the diagram in Fig. 13-4. The 22 autosomal pairs are similar in the female and the male, whereas the sex chromosomes differ in the two sexes (XX or XY, respectively).

The true genetic sex can be determined by cytologic examination of various somatic cells. The morphologic difference in the resting cell nuclei of the two sexes was first described by Barr, Bertram, and Lindsay in 1950. A dense mass of chromatin known as the *sex chromatin mass* or *Barr body* (Fig. 13-5) situated at the periphery of the nucleus just within the nuclear membrane is found in up to 90% of the somatic cell nuclei of normal females (chromatin positive) but is absent or is found in only about 1% to 3% of the nuclei of normal males (chromatin negative). The chromatin mass is derived from the female X chromosome.

The number of Barr bodies found in each nucleus equals the number of X chromosomes minus one. Thus in normal females with an XX constitution, one Barr body is seen. In females with Turner's

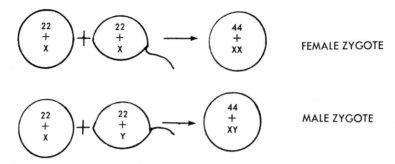

Fig. 13-2. Male and female zygotes.

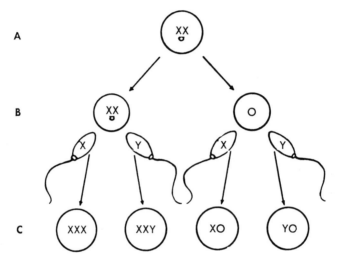

Fig. 13-3. Effects of nondisjunction during gametogenesis. **A,** Haploid daughter cell with two chromatids united by centromere. **B,** Meiosis I, nondisjunction. **C,** Meiosis II, four types of zygotes may be produced during fertilization. (From Eggen, R.R.: Am. J. Clin. Pathol. **39:**10, 1963.)

syndrome bearing the most characteristic XO pattern and in normal males with an XY constitution, the nuclear sex is chromatin negative. In Klinefelter's syndrome, individuals with an XXY or an XXXY constitution display a chromatin-one or a chromatin-two positive nuclear sex pattern, despite the fact that the phenotype is male.

Cells obtained by buccal smear are most commonly used for examination; occasionally, skin or vaginal smears are taken. Polymorphonuclear leukocytes can also be used; a characteristic mass, or "drumstick," is found in normal females in about 3% of the neutrophils. However, this may appear as an accessory lobule, and differentiation is therefore more difficult.

The *Y chromatin* of the male interphase nucleus can be identified by the characteristic fluorescent spot seen by ultraviolet microscopy after staining with quinacrine dyes.

Migration of the ovum. After release from the follicle, the ovum is surrounded by sticky cumulus cells. One long projection of the fimbria that contains muscular elements, *fimbria ovarica,* is attached to the ovary, usually at the upper pole. (1) Contraction of these and muscular elements of the parovarium approximate the fallopian tube and ruptured follicle site. (2) Motion of the *epithelial cilia* lining the fimbria promotes migration into the ostium, and, aided by *tubal peristalsis,* which is max-

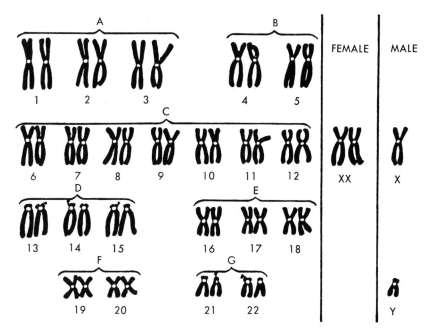

Fig. 13-4. Idiogram of human chromosomes—International System of Nomenclature (Denver). (From Eggen, R.R.: Am. J. Clin. Pathol. **39:**10, 1963.)

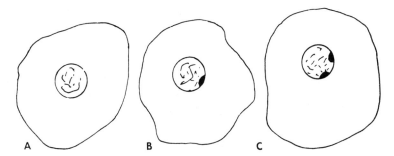

Fig. 13-5. Sex chromatin mass (Barr body) and examples. **A,** Chromatin negative XY, XO. **B,** Chromatin-one positive XX, XXY. **C,** Chromatin-two positive XXX, XXXY.

imal at this time, the ovum is carried rapidly into the ampulla of the tube. (3) The ovum is retained for about 2½ days at the ampullary-isthmic junction. The luminal fluid provides metabolic substrates and conditions suitable for survival of sperm, ovum, and zygote. (4) Cell division and cleavage continue during transport to the uterus, where implantation during the blastocyst stage occurs at 6 to 8 days after fertilization.

Using culdoscopy for 4- to 5-hour periods, Doyle reported direct observation of ovulation in three patients. He noted elongation, edema, and congestion of the tube and spread of the fimbria over the supermedial aspect of the ovary. The ovum probably is expelled directly into the ampulla of the tube. Trumpet-shaped cones of contraction developed at the fimbria at the rate of six per minute. Peristalsis continued to the isthmus, followed by a to-and-fro motion, and again peristalsis to the cornu. After about 2 hours the fimbria slid down the ovary to the cul-de-sac. Suction developed in this location may provide a means by which the tube on one side may pick up ova ruptured from either ovary (Fig. 13-6).

Fertilization. The ovum is fertilized in the outer third of the tube within a short time after ovulation, probably less than 24 hours. Viability of the ovum is somewhat less than that of spermatozoa.

The seminal fluid vehicle for transport is slightly alkaline, with a pH of 7.5. When the spermatozoa are deposited in the vagina, they are placed in an environment with a pH of 4.5. Although the buffering action of semen is to some extent capable of offsetting this difference, prompt entrance into the cervical canal is important to the continued viability of the spermatozoa. The normal pH of cervical mucus is 7.5. Tyler suggests that the difference in vaginal and cervical pH is one of the factors that favor migration of spermatozoa into the cervical canal; cyclic variations in cervical secretion further enhance their passage. At the time of ovulation the mucus is thin, abundant, rich in glycogen, and most conducive for penetration.

Active spermatozoa reach the fallopian tube within as little as 5 minutes, but the spermatozoa require a period of time within the female reproductive tract to gain the capability of fertilizing the ovum. This process, *capacitation,* is not well understood; however, it seems to involve enzymatic activity and structural alteration termed *acrosomal reaction.*

On penetration of the ovum's vitelline mem-

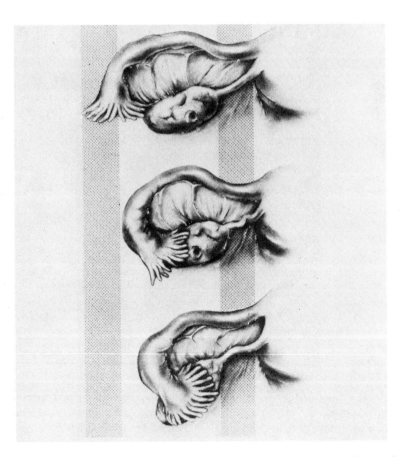

Fig. 13-6. Fimbriae enclosing rupturing follicle. (From Novy, M.I.: Am. J. Obstet. Gynecol. **137**:198, 1980.)

brane, male and female pronuclei, each with 23 chromosomes, unite to form the segmentation nucleus and restore the original 46 chromosomes.

Repeated cell divisions result in the formation of a mulberry mass, the *morula*. The outer layer of cells secretes fluid that accumulates, forming the segmentation cavity. The mass at this time is called the blastodermic vesicle or *blastocyst*.

Implantation occurs at the blastocyst stage 6 to 8 days after ovulation. Formative cells crowded to one side represent the embryonic pole or inner cell mass. The single layer of cells surrounding the vesicle is the primitive *trophoblast*.

There is much unresolved speculation regarding possible mechanisms in operation during implantation that may account for control of invasion on the one hand and prevention of immunologic rejection on the other. Just before attachment on the uterine endometrium, an aggregate of cells, the "syncytial knob," appears in the trophoblastic syncytium. These knobs are the portions

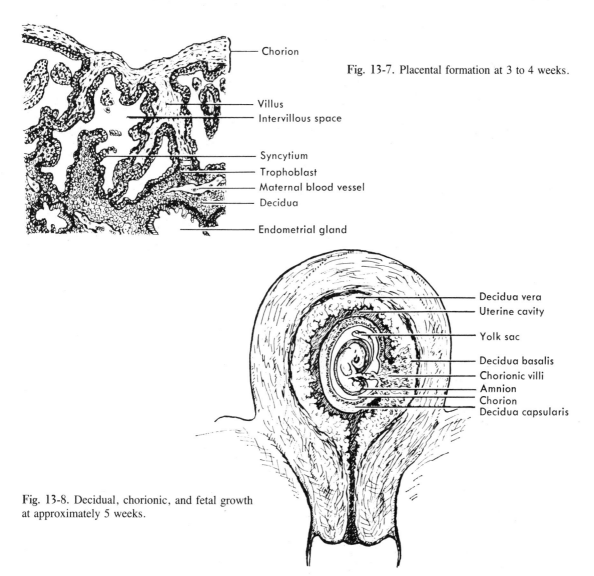

Chorion

Villus
Intervillous space

Syncytium
Trophoblast
Maternal blood vessel
Decidua

Endometrial gland

Fig. 13-7. Placental formation at 3 to 4 weeks.

Decidua vera
Uterine cavity

Yolk sac

Decidua basalis
Chorionic villi
Amnion
Chorion
Decidua capsularis

Fig. 13-8. Decidual, chorionic, and fetal growth at approximately 5 weeks.

of the trophoblast that penetrate the decidua. At the implantation site, fusion of maternal and fetal cells occurs temporarily. Behrman and Koren have speculated that such fusion of cytoplasmic and nuclear material may change the immunologic characteristics of maternal tissues and induce tolerance to fetal antigens rather than sensitization.

The pregravid endometrium is prepared to provide for nidation and nutrition of the fertilized ovum. The *decidua* develops under the influence of increasing amounts of ovarian hormones, principally progesterone. The stroma is made up of characteristic large, polyhedral decidual cells; glands become thick and tortuous; and glycogen content is high. Vascularity is greatly increased.

The trophoblast secretes proteolytic and cytolytic enzymes, which permit these cells to invade the prepared endometrium, destroying vessels, glands, and stroma locally. *Implantation bleeding* may occur. This is small in amount, is not associated with pain, and disappears within 1 to 2 days, when the aperture in the endometrium is sealed over. Decidua covering this portion of the ovum is the *decidua capsularis,* and that beneath the ovum is the *decidua basalis*. The remainder of the uterine cavity is lined by the *decidua vera*. During nidation, trophoblastic cells provide nutrition for the embryo, first by destruction and absorption of decidua and later by absorption of substances from maternal blood (Figs. 13-7 and 13-8).

DEVELOPMENTAL ANOMALIES

Normal growth and development of the fetus may be altered by a great variety of hereditary and environmental factors. These are outlined here and discussed elsewhere in the text. For a detailed description the reader may wish to refer to the work of Thompson and Thompson; Gerbie, Nadler, and Platt; or Simpson and co-workers.

It is important to realize the fact emphasized by Fraser that a minority of congenital malformations have either major environmental or genetic causes. Instead, complicated interactions between genetic predispositions and subtle factors in intrauterine environment form the basis for most malformations. Furthermore, abnormal embryogenesis can produce both gross structural alterations in any of the systems undergoing sequential interrelated actions during development of the fetus and functional derangements such as those reflected in inborn errors of metabolism or mental retardation.

Congenital defects may be classified on the basis of intrinsic factors (that is, genetic defects) and extrinsic factors. The latter may have a temporary effect on development or may cause genetic alterations of a hereditary nature.

Intrinsic factors (genetic disorders)

Human genetic disorders are generally classified as follows.

Chromosomal aberrations. Chromosomal aberrations include deviations from the normal *chromosomal number* of 46 and abnormalities in the *chromosomal structure*. Numerical aberration involving an individual chromosome is termed *aneuploidy,* which results from *nondisjunction* as shown in Fig. 13-3. Nondisjunction aberrations are related to advanced maternal age. The striking autosomal example of this phenomenon is seen in Down's syndrome (47 XXX 21, or trisomy 21). A second type Down's syndrome (D/G) involves a structural abnormality, *translocation,* with the G chromosome translocated to the D group. This condition carries a greater risk for the offspring of a maternal carrier, and it is not age dependent.

Sex chromosomal aberrations also include both numerical and structural deviations. Klinefelter's syndrome (47 XXY) is one of the most common of those containing extra genetic material. Turner's syndrome (45 XO) represents a *deletion.* Autosomal deletions are generally lethal, and the conceptus is usually aborted.

Mosaicism is found in many syndromes associated with an abnormal chromosomal number. Adjacent cells from a given individual show different chromosomal counts; for example, patients with gonadal dysgenesis do not always show a chromosomal constitution of 45 XO. A variety of mosaics are now recognized in patients with this disorder, and these findings may modify the classic clinical picture to some degree, for example, 45

XO/46 XX or 45 XO/46 XX/47 XXX. Mosaicism involving autosomal abnormalities is seen in some cases of mongolism (46/47—trisomy 21).

Aberrations in chromosome morphology include the following: *Isochromosomes* represent genetic material that is split horizontally instead of vertically. The arms on either side of the centromere therefore are identical. If the short arm is lost, the functions carried on by the genes on the short arm are also lost. Certain cases of amenorrhea are believed to result from this abnormality.

X-linked disorders. Almost all X-linked disorders occur in an *X-linked recessive inheritance* pattern with the male offspring of a female carrier being affected. Examples are hemophilia, Duchenne's muscular dystrophy, and X-linked agammaglobulinemia. *X-linked dominant inheritance* is rare because the male who has a single X chromosome is "hemizygous" rather than homozygous or heterozygous with respect to X-linked traits. Vitamin D–resistant rickets with hypophosphatemia is an example.

Single-gene disorders. Single-gene disorders represent a genetically determined biochemical disorder that results in a specific enzymatic block. These conditions are designated inborn errors of metabolism. Prenatal diagnosis can be made for a number of the 100 or more recognized disorders of this type that affect carbohydrate, lipid, amino acid, mucopolysaccharide, and other metabolic activities. Glycogen storage disease, Tay-Sachs disease, cystinuria, Hurler's disease, and thalassemia, respectively, are examples.

Extrinsic factors (multifactorial disorders)

Extrinsic factors known to affect development or genetic makeup, or both, of the fetus, include viral, parasitic, and other infections; chemicals such as drugs and hormones; and dietary deficiency. Extensive studies of all factors known to control fetal growth and development have been conducted over several years by Cheek, Greystone, and Niall; these are summarized and well referenced in their informative 1977 report. Congenital malformations representative of multifactorial inheritance include anencephaly, spina bifida, congenital dislocation of the hip, cleft lip with cleft palate, and club foot.

Antenatal diagnosis

The growing number of developmental disorders that can be diagnosed in utero has had a dramatic impact on genetic counseling. The obstetrician needs to be knowledgeable regarding the general spectrum of these conditions, the testing methods available for diagnosis, their risks, and the fact that there are options for treatment that must be fully and fairly presented by the counselor and decided on by the patient. Accuracy of diagnosis is so critical a matter that referral to a perinatal or genetic center should be advised. Methods used in diagnosis include the following.

Amniocentesis. Ultrasound-directed amniocentesis has proved to be a relatively safe procedure with a complication rate of less than 1%. Genetic amniocentesis is discussed in Chapter 2.

Chorionic villus biopsy. Chorionic villi are collected by transcervical aspiration under ultrasonic guidance. The procedure is carried out at 8 weeks of gestation and has the advantage of sampling rapidly growing trophoblast cells rather than slow-growing fibroblasts. Thus results of both chromosomal analysis and DNA probe studies are available in days rather than weeks. This technique is currently available in only selected centers and its safety is being evaluated by a national collaborative study. It is anticipated that the risk of abortion secondary to the procedure will be no greater than 3%.

Ultrasonography. Technologic advances in ultrasonography have minimized the need for x-ray film examinations. An increasing number of gross anomalies have been identified by this method, including anencephaly, limb defects, and omphalocele. Conditions such as fetal ascites and polyhydramnios that lead to suspicion of a fetal abnormality are usually readily detected with ultrasound visualization.

Fetal blood sampling. *Fetal blood sampling* can be accomplished safely under ultrasonic guidance. The umbilical vein or artery is punctured with a 25-gauge needle at its insertion into the placenta.

Fetal blood is differentiated from maternal by the size of the red cells. This technique is largely supplanting fetoscopy as the method of choice for obtaining fetal blood samples.

Fetoscopy. Studies evaluating the use of endoscopy in examination of the fetus, umbilical cord, and placenta and its safety are only now beginning to emerge. The small area of vision provided by an endoscope is a limiting factor, but several fetal deformities have been accurately detected. Fetoscopy's unique capability of obtaining skin biopsy from the fetal flank or scalp for culture and analysis and cord or placental blood samples for diagnosis of hemoglobinopathies and other disorders has generated considerable interest.

DEVELOPMENT AND PHYSIOLOGY OF THE PLACENTA

The primitive *trophoblast* proliferates rapidly after implantation. Three layers appear, all of which are believed to be derived from this structure, which first develops as typical Langhans' cells. These in turn undergo differentiation into an outer syncytial layer, the *syncytiotrophoblast,* and the proliferating Langhans' inner cell layer, the *cytotrophoblast,* underneath which is a thin layer of connective tissue, the *mesoblast.* The mesoblast provides, in effect, a supporting structure or central core of the villus and the site in which villous blood-forming elements and vascular structures make their appearance.

The outer syncytial layer is far more complex than was formerly recognized. Detailed study by electron microscopy (Fig. 13-9) reveals the so-called brush border to be a profusion of microvilli projecting from the free surface of the syncytium and of abundant highly developed structures—pinocytotic vesicles, lipoid droplets, and mitochondria—all providing structural evidence of secretory activity. This tissue is like a continuously streaming *ameboid mass* that is capable of actively engulfing substances, including maternal plasma, into the substance of the syncytium.

The fact that syncytial cells are rich in cytoplasmic ribonucleoproteins suggests that synthesis of proteins required by the growing embryo is one of the early functions of the trophoblast. Villee demonstrated that the early trophoblast has the *ability to synthesize glucose.* This function begins to decrease at about 12 weeks, when the fetal liver becomes capable of secreting glucose; in late pregnancy, placental synthesis disappears entirely. *Secretion of hormones* by the syncytiotrophoblast begins shortly after implantation, when chorionic gonadotropin appears; placental steroid hormones are secreted by cells of the syncytium.

During the first 2 to 3 weeks the chorionic villi are devoid of blood vessels. The villi project into the surrounding decidua and become filled with a core of mesoderm from the embryonal side. Islands of red blood cells develop in situ, and vascular channels appear. The villi in contact with the decidua basalis are exposed to a rich blood supply and multiply rapidly, becoming the *chorion frondosum,* or future placenta. Those in contact with the decidua capsularis become the *chorion laeve;* these eventually atrophy.

Formation of the amnion occurs while the chorion develops. Two small cavities appear in the embryonic pole. The dorsal amniotic cavity is derived from ectoderm, and the ventral yolk sac from entoderm. The amnion enlarges rapidly, causing disappearance of the extraembryonic coelom, and forces the body stalk, rudimentary blind allantois, vessels, and vitelline duct into a single pedicle, the beginning of the *umbilical cord.* The outer surface of the amnion applies itself to the inner aspect of the chorion. The two membranes are adherent but not fused. (Figs. 13-7 and 13-8.)

Immunologic properties

The placenta corresponds to a natural homograft in that it is a transplant of living tissue within the same species, yet it does not normally evoke the usual immune response reaction to homografts, resulting in destruction and rejection of the graft.

The explanation for its immunologic defense is not clear-cut. Theories have been proposed presuming the following: (1) antigenic immunity and/or immaturity of the fetus; (2) depression of maternal immune response by increasing amounts of steroid hormones; (3) mechanical blockage or absorption of antigens by the fi-

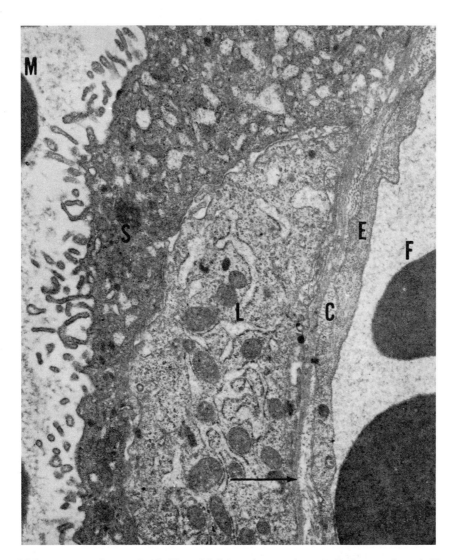

Fig. 13-9. Electron micrograph of villus of full-term human placenta. Both syncytiotrophoblast, *S*, with numerous microvilli, and Langhans' cell, *L*, persist throughout gestation. Arrow points to trophoblastic basement lamina. Connective tissue, *C*, is reduced to a minimum. Endothelium, *E*, of capillary is seen. These placental elements separate maternal, *M*, from fetal, *F*, erythrocytes. (Glutaraldehyde and osmic acid. Araldite.) (× 17,000.) (Courtesy Dr. Ralph M. Wynn.)

brinoid layer, which separates trophoblasts from endometrial cells; (4) establishment of the uterus as a "privileged site" for tissue graft; and (5) development of maternal immunologic tolerance after repeated small doses of fetal antigens. There is a reduction in T cell stimulation in early pregnancy, which may play a role in increased tolerance.

Simmons and Russell studied trophoblastic and embryonic implants in mice previously sensitized by skin grafts of the paternal type. Pure trophoblastic tissue failed to elicit the slightest cellular reaction in the host, whereas embryonic tissue was regularly destroyed by the sixth day. Thus syncytial and cytotrophoblastic cells appear to form an anatomic and immunologic buffer zone between the mother and the fetus and prevent immunologic destruction. The possibility that this protective mechanism is subject to failure and that certain cases of infertility or threatened abortion have an immunologic basis is the subject of a number of investigations. Although it is conceded that a maternal immunologic "state" exists during pregnancy, the precise mechanism is not yet known.

Circulation

By the fourteenth week the placenta is a discrete organ. Most of the villi lie free in maternal blood sinuses; anchoring villi are attached to the decidua basalis. At the point of anchorage a band of fibrin is deposited as a result of degeneration of fetal and decidual cells. This "fibrinous layer of Nitabuch" is presumed to resist overinvasion of maternal tissues by chorionic epithelium. It is absent in placenta accreta.

Circulation of the blood through the intervillous spaces (choriodecidual spaces) is dependent on (1) maternal blood pressure, with resultant gradient between arterial and venous channels, and (2) uterine contractions. The work of Ramsey and associates on placental circulation has clarified certain problems hitherto unexplained. These problems are concerned with (1) delivery of oxygenated arterial blood with suitable mixing throughout the organ, (2) an allowance of sufficient time for metabolic exchange, and (3) venous drainage through multiple channels, which Ramsey and colleagues demonstrated in the various areas at the base of the placenta, rather than through a single "marginal sinus." These authors contend that "marginal lakes" are actually the peripheral portion of the intervillous space lying within the placenta and that the course of the marginal lakes is discontinuous. This arrangement permits segmental "trapping" of blood when intervillous pressure is higher than that in endometrial veins and permits drainage when pressure is lower.

According to Ramsey and associates, arterial blood enters the placenta from the endometrial arteries under a head of pressure. The incoming stream is driven up in fountainlike jet toward the chorionic plate. The villi act as baffles, mixing and slowing the stream. The force is gradually spent, and eventually the blood that has dispersed laterally falls back on multiple orifices in the basal plate, which connects with maternal veins. Further fall in pressure in the intervillous space results in drainage through the endometrial veins. The circulatory process is enhanced by myometrial contractions. The authors demonstrated these events convincingly by x-ray film study of the circulation in the placenta of the rhesus monkey (Fig. 13-10).

Transfer mechanisms

Oxygen and substances for nutrition of the fetus must pass from the intervillous spaces through the surface epithelium of the villus, the thin stroma, and the endothelium of its capillary. Carbon dioxide and waste products from the fetus are transferred in reverse order.

Normally, there is no direct connection between maternal and fetal circulations, but damaged villa occasionally break off into the maternal lakes and allow the escape of small amounts of fetal blood into the maternal circulation. Smith and associates, with the use of maternal erythrocytes labeled with chromium 51, demonstrated passage of these cells to the cord blood of the newborn infants in 13 out of 18 instances. The rate of transfer averaged 0.3 ml in 13 hours. The authors suggest that small leaks in the barrier are responsible and are common occurrences. Certain cases of Rh sensitization in which incompatible blood has never been given the mother and instances of ABO isoimmunization are related to this phenomenon.

Fetal growth is considerably greater than that of the placenta from the twelfth or fourteenth week to term. The placenta accommodates to greater demands (1) by increasing the surface area of the villi through arborization and (2) by thinning of the villus covering. Langhans' cells become thinned out but do not disappear. Many of these cells persist and continue to function throughout pregnancy; however, reduction in their number and in the size of the cells that persist leaves, in effect, a single layer of syncytial cells, thus increasing permeability.

Numerous factors, many of which are yet unknown, influence the *rate* of transfer of substances across the placental barrier. Materials of small molecular size such as electrolytes, water, uric acid,

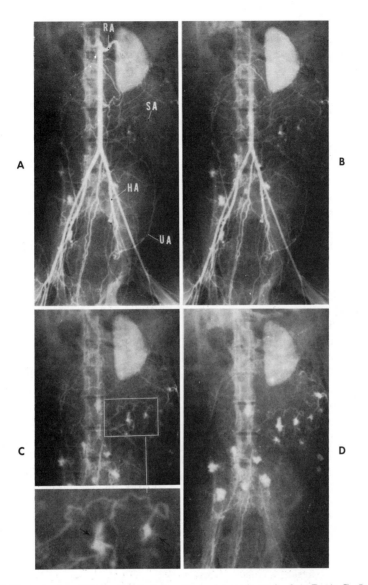

Fig. 13-10. Photographs of four of series of radiographs made at **A,** 3½; **B,** 4; **C,** 5; and **D,** 6 seconds, respectively, after injection of radiopaque dye into right femoral artery of monkey 111 days pregnant. Inset in **C** is magnification (×4) of area enclosed in box. Arrows indicate spurts of dye into intervillous space. *RA,* Renal artery; *SA,* spiral artery of endometrium; *HA,* hypogastric artery; *UA,* uterine artery. (From Ramsey, E.M., Corner, G.W., Jr., Donne, M.W., and Stran, H.M.: Proc. Natl. Acad. Sci. U.S.A. **46**:1003, 1960.)

creatine, and creatinine can but do not always pass by simple diffusion. Many drugs, notably narcotics, barbiturates, general anesthetics, sulfonamides, and antibiotics, pass readily. However, despite its obvious influence, the *size of the molecule* is not necessarily the determining factor in movement of materials in either direction. For example, the aldohexoses (glucose, mannose, and galactose) cross the placenta more readily than the ketohexoses (fructose and sorbose).

Page refers to the process of speeding up the transfer of certain molecules, such as glucose, as *facilitated diffusion*. He considers this a form of *active transfer,* carried out by carrier molecules oscillating between the boundaries of the cell. In addition, the placenta achieves active transfer of a far more complex nature by the use of *enzymatic processes* requiring expenditure of energy. In some instances large molecules are broken down by enzymatic action before passage to the fetus, and in others enzyme transport is accomplished against the concentration gradient without alteration of the molecule. Histidine is an example of rapid active transfer of amino acid to the fetus. Fats, on the contrary, do not normally cross the placenta as such. Fats are broken down into fatty acids before passage and are resynthesized by the fetal liver. The passage without structural change of certain antibodies of higher molecular weight and diphtheria or tetanus antitoxin is not readily explained by any of the mechanisms mentioned. Visualization of the ameboid motion of syncytial cells has made tenable the concept of ''droplet transfer,'' or *pinocytosis*. By this means, intact macromolecules may be transferred slowly across the membrane.

A great deal remains to be learned in regard to *selective activity* in placental transfer. It is evident that the various mechanisms operate in accordance with the particular demands of the fetus, but the placenta may act as governor. For example, after removal of the fetus, the intact placenta continues to extract iron from the maternal circulation at approximately the same rate as it did beforehand. Furthermore, in the absence of the normal fetal destination the placenta is capable of storing iron. Normally, certain substances essential for fetal growth occur in higher concentration in the fetal than in the maternal circulation. These include calcium, inorganic phosphorus, free amino acid, nucleic acid, and ascorbic acid.

Bacteria do not normally cross the placenta. Thus the danger to the fetus of pneumonia in the mother is generally related to the degree of maternal anoxia rather than infection. Tuberculosis does not endanger the fetus in utero except when complicated by placenta tuberculoma that erodes into the fetal circulation. *Spirochaeta pallida* cross the placenta, but, fortunately, penicillin administered

to the mother for treatment will also pass the barrier and provide fetal protection or treatment, depending on whether the fetus is already infected. Placental transmission of certain *viruses* has engendered justifiable cause for concern. Virus diseases are considered in Chapter 21.

Placental hormones

In addition to its function as an intrauterine organ of *respiration, nutrition,* and *excretion* for the growing fetus, the placenta functions as an *endocrine gland*. Maternal endocrine functions capable of providing a balance in the hypothalamic-pituitary-ovarian-endometrial axis to ensure ovulation and implantation are all-important in conception, but early in pregnancy endocrine regulation is taken over by the fetus and its accessory endocrine organ—the placenta. The interrelationships of fetal, placental, and maternal compartments are extremely complex, but under normal conditions the conceptus maintains regulatory control of its own private hormonal environment. Abnormal conditions arising in any of the three compartments may jeopardize the fetus. The obstetrician encounters many situations in which assessment of the fetus at risk is mandatory. Under these circumstances, a clear understanding of the physiologic and metabolic activities involved is of exceptional value.

The chief purpose of the dramatic changes in endocrine function during pregnancy is to maintain the pregnancy and to support the fetus in utero until the termination of the gestation period. Modern hormone assay techniques and methods for study of biosynthetic pathways and transfer mechanisms have evoked new concepts of endocrine activity. Several of these are of practical significance.

The classic hormone excretion curves (Fig. 13-11) still provide a valid overall view of alterations during normal pregnancy, although the excretion curves accepted as normal standards are oversimplified. Normal ranges are variable, and day-to-day changes in excretion rates are found for all measurable hormones; some of them show more pronounced deviations than do others. Means of assessing the actual amounts of the various hormones secreted by (1) maternal endocrine glands, (2) pla-

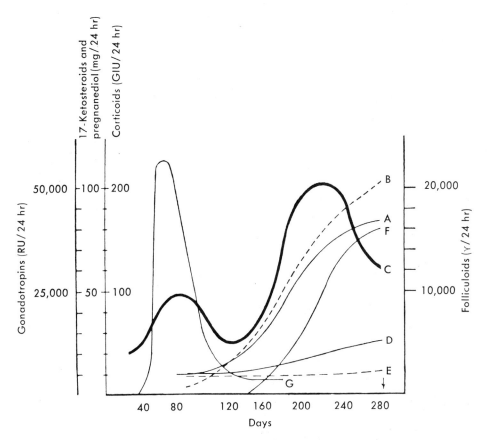

Fig. 13-11. Average values for excretion of various hormones during normal pregnancy. *A*, Pregnanediol; *B* and *F*, folliculoids; *C*, corticoids; *D* and *E*, 17-ketosteroids (depending on method); *G*, gonadotropins. (After Venning; from Selye, H.: Textbook of endocrinology, Montreal, 1947, Acta.)

centa, and (3) fetal endocrine glands are limited. Degradation, inactivation, and other metabolic changes are carried out in maternal, placental, and fetal organs. Thus excretion rates of the steroids, for instance, represent the end result of many complex actions. Furthermore, increases in one hormone may cause changes in production and metabolism of another.

From a practical point of view the fetus and placenta should be regarded as a single functional unit, with the uterus as an integral part of this unit.

Human chorionic gonadotropin. Human chorionic gonadotropin (hCG) provides the basis for biologic tests for pregnancy. Like other glycoprotein hor-

mones, hCG consists of two nonidentical subunits. The alpha subunit is similar to the alpha subunits of LH, FSH, and TSH. The larger beta subunit is hormone specific.

The precise site of production of hCG has been identified as the syncytiotrophoblast. Pierce and Midgley, using an immunohistochemical localization technique, found hCG only in the syncytiotrophoblast; they could demonstrate none in the cytotrophoblast. It is likely that the syncytium, which is derived by differentiation from the cytotrophoblast, plays an active role in production rather than simply storage and transport of this material.

hCG is present in detectable amounts by about the eighth to tenth day after conception (1 to 2 days after implantation) and reaches a peak 50 to 60 days thereafter. During this time the hormone augments and prolongs corpus luteum function and thus maintains the endometrial bed.

hCG is a glycoprotein that in highly purified form exhibits an activity of 12,000 IU/mg. One international unit represents the reaction produced by 0.1 mg of a pure standard preparation. Ideally, sensitivity of laboratory test animals (immature rats) is attained when 1 IU just induces hyperemia in the rat ovaries. Then 1 IU equals 1 hyperemia unit.

The hormone is found in all maternal tissues, blood, urine, cerebrospinal fluid, saliva, and vaginal secretions as well as in placental tissue. Appreciable amounts are found in the amniotic fluid, but only trivial amounts in cord blood. The amount transferred to the fetus directly is not known; however, since the fetus swallows amniotic fluid, differences in concentration suggest that the fetus is able to metabolize hCG and convert the hormone to compounds with little or no biologic activity.

QUALITATIVE AND QUANTITATIVE ASSAYS. The immunnoassay is exceedingly accurate in diagnosis of pregnancy and has all but replaced the less sensitive bioassay as a straightforward pregnancy test. Immunoassays are often positive by the eighth day after conception and may remain positive for 8 days or longer after delivery, although most undiluted samples are negative within 2 to 3 days.

All of the simple immunoassay methods performed with urine samples on slide or in tube tests cross-react with LH. Elevated LH levels associated with the preovulatory LH surge or with the hormonal changes of the premenopausal period may produce false-positive results if the test is sufficiently sensitive. To prevent this problem, these tests are adjusted to reliably detect levels of hCG for normal pregnancy at 2 to 3 weeks after the first missed period. The desirability of earlier, more accurate diagnosis in the management of problems in both infertility and fertility has resulted in recent development of a number of new hormone-specific tests. (See tests for pregnancy, Chapter 2.)

Progesterone. Progesterone can be formed by all steroid-producing endocrine tissues: a small amount by the adrenal, much larger amounts by the corpus luteum, the major production by the placental syncytial cells, and an undetermined amount by the fetal adrenals. In the human adrenal gland, progesterone is an intermediary in the biosynthesis of cortisone and aldosterone. It can also be converted to androgens by adrenal glands and testes. In the ovary, progesterone can be converted to estrogens (Fig. 13-12).

FUNCTIONS. The functions of progesterone are mainly the development and maintenance of the decidual bed.

METABOLISM. In late pregnancy the placenta produces about 250 to 300 mg of progesterone per day. Blood progesterone is metabolized rapidly primarily in the liver but also in the tissue at its site of action, and a considerable amount disappears into depot fat. The turnover time is approximately 3 minutes. Thus the excretion of the metabolic end product, pregnanediol, excreted in the urine as a glucuronide conjugate, averages only about 10% to 20% of the progesterone produced. On an individual basis, excretion rates of pregnanediol show a wide normal range. The mean value is about 50 mg/24 hours near term (Fig. 13-13).

Although assays of progesterone or its end products are useful in certain gynecologic conditions, they have little, if any, use during pregnancy.

Estrogens. The amount of estrogens secreted in the third trimester is enormously increased over nonpregnant levels. The gestational increase in estrone and in estradiol is approximately one hundredfold, whereas the increase in estriol is one thousandfold as compared with individual nonpregnant values. Pregnancy levels drop precipitously after delivery or after intrauterine death of the fetus.

A comparison of mean values for 24-hour urinary estrogen secretion is given in Table 13-1.

BIOSYNTHETIC PATHWAYS. In normally menstruating women the ovary produces estrogens de novo principally, if not entirely, in the biologically active forms of estradiol and estrone. Most of the estriol in nongravid women is derived from the peripheral metabolism of estrone and estradiol.

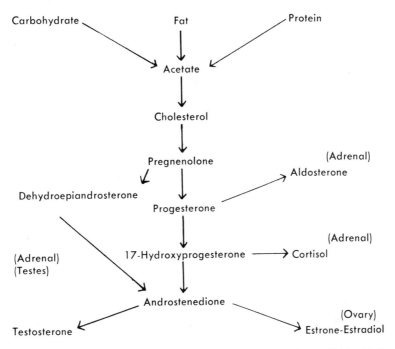

Fig. 13-12. Biosynthesis of reproductive steroid hormones. (From Carey, H.M.: Modern trends in human reproductive physiology, Washington, D.C., 1963, Butterworth & Co. [Publishers], Ltd.)

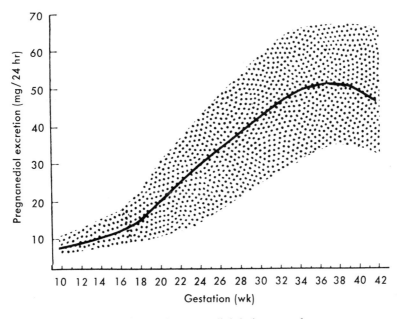

Fig. 13-13. Excretion of pregnanediol during normal pregnancy.

TABLE 13-1 Comparison of mean values for 24-hour urinary estrogen secretion

	Estrone	Estradiol	Estriol	Total
Menstrual cycle				
Early proliferative (days 1 to 7)	0 to 7*	Trace	2 to 11	3 to 20
Ovulatory peak (days 10 to 16)	15 to 27	3 to 22	8 to 120	30 to 150
Postovulatory peak (days 20 to 26)	5 to 25	2 to 11	5 to 90	15 to 100
Pregnancy				
First trimester	To 200	To 70	To 500	
Second trimester	To 1000	To 300	To 10,000	
Third trimester	To 200	To 1000	To 40,000	

From Goldzieher, J.W.: Estrogens and progesterone. In Meigs, J.V., and Sturgis, S.H., editors: Progress in gynecology, vol. 4, New York, 1963, Grune & Stratton, Inc.
*All values are expressed in micrograms.

The diagram of ovarian estrogen biosynthesis (Fig. 13-14) is based on the results of ovarian tissue incubation experiments performed by Smith and Ryan. With the use of radioactive substrates, these investigators obtained a yield of estrone plus estradiol amounting to 0.03% from acetate, 0.1% from cholesterol, 5.5% from progesterone, and 15% from androstenedione. (Note the increasing yield from intermediates closer on the pathway to the end product.)

The finding of these compounds in the incubation experiments indicates that any one or all of the biosynthetic pathways shown could be operative in human ovaries. Estradiol can be converted to estrone and vice versa, but estriol cannot be reconverted to either. Estradiol is by far the most biologically active, whereas estriol is biologically weak. The biologic activity of estriol is approximately 1/100 that of estrone and 1/500 that of estradiol.

The placenta does not synthesize estrogen de novo to any significant degree. If placental tissues were capable of producing estrogens, high excretion might be expected in cases of hydatidiform mole; however, such is not the case. Clearly, the placenta is not autonomous in this regard. Instead, a viable placenta, a healthy fetus, and an intact fetal circulation are necessary for continuous production of this steroid. When these three prerequisites exist, the placenta is highly efficient in conversion of steroid precursors to estrogens, mainly estriol. A much lower percentage of estriol is formed from conversion of estrone and estradiol in pregnant than in nonpregnant women.

Most of the estriol of late pregnancy is derived from primitive steroids such as pregnenolone and dehydroepiandroesterone. These precursors are produced by the maternal and the fetal organisms, the fetal adrenal playing a major role. This concept is supported by studies of pregnancies associated with an anencephalic fetus. Anencephaly is commonly associated with atrophy of the characteristically large fetal zone in the adrenal cortex, which may be almost absent. Frandsen and Stakemann studied 15 cases of pregnancy associated with an anencephalic fetus and found critically low levels of estriol excretion in all but one. In the only exception the infant adrenals were of normal size and contained a well-developed fetal zone. Excretion of 17-ketosteroids, 17-ketogenic steroids, pregnanediol, and hCG was normal. All fetuses were alive at the time of urine collection for assay. The placentas were normal, and there were no signs of a disturbed fetal circulation.

These investigators further demonstrated the important role played by the fetal adrenals by simultaneous injection of fetal adrenal tissue and placental tissue in castrated mice. Vaginal smears for estrogen effect were obtained daily after injection of fetal adrenal tissue alone. Smears were negative in all tests. Negative results were

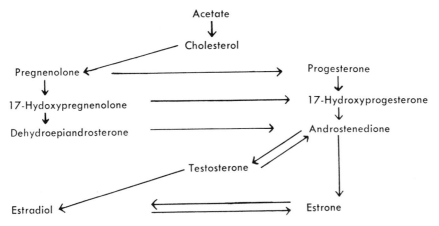

Fig. 13-14. Ovarian estrogen biosynthesis.

also obtained after injection of placental tissue alone. But when both tissues were injected intraperitoneally or subcutaneously at the same time, estrogen-positive vaginal smears were obtained in 12 of 15 cases. It was necessary to use living fetal adrenal and living placental tissues to obtain a positive response. The foregoing clinical and laboratory data point to fetal adrenals as the source of precursors and to the placenta as the organ for their metabolism to estrogens.

The importance of an intact fetal circulation in estrogen production is illustrated by the experiments of Cassmer. Therapeutic interruptions carried out by the vaginal route at approximately 20 weeks' gestation were studied as follows: The umbilical cord was brought through the cervix, ligated, and sectioned. Fetus and placenta were allowed to remain in situ for 3 days. Within 24 hours, estriol values dropped more than 70% below previous levels. Progesterone values dropped only 20%, and hCG titers remained the same.

The fetus actively conjugates estrogens, mainly as sulfates and, to a far lesser extent, as glucosiduronates. This ability is acquired at an early stage—usually by 16 weeks' gestation. Sulfurylation can be performed by fetal liver, lungs, gastrointestinal tract, and skin. By means of conjugation, biologically active compounds are converted to relatively weak compounds. The efficiency of this action suggests that it may be an important step for fetal defense against excessive estrogenization.

Some of the most precise studies of estrogen metabolism in pregnancy have come from Diczfalusy's laboratory at the Karolinska Institute in Stockholm. Results of in situ perfusion studies with various radioisotopes may be summarized as follows: The primitive steroids are produced mainly by the fetus, principally the fetal adrenal glands. The main precursor is dehydroepiandrosterone sulfate (DHAS). In the nonpregnant state, most of the urinary estradiol is derived from estrone and estradiol. During pregnancy the pathway exists within the fetoplacental unit for direct conversion of DHAS to estriol without estradiol as an intermediate. This involves the formation of 16-hydroxy-DHAS, which takes place in the fetal liver. The placenta shows little 16-hydroxylating activity but strong enzymatic activity in the final conversion to estriol, the aromatization of ring A of the steroid nucleus. The conjugates are returned to the placenta and transferred to the maternal circulation, mainly as estriol. The estrogen is metabolized and conjugated in the maternal liver mainly as a glucosiduronate and is excreted largely in this form in the urine. The 24-hour urinary estriol values therefore can serve as an indication of fetoplacental function in the gravid woman whose hepatic and renal functions are within normal limits.

One other aspect of estriol metabolism of clinical importance is the amount found in amniotic fluid in late pregnancy. Most of the free estriol returned to the fetus from the placenta is sulfurylated by various fetal organs, but a small amount is conjugated as the glucosiduronate, presumably by the fetal liver. Both the free and the sulfate forms clear the amniotic membrane rapidly, but the glucosiduronate accumulates. Compromise of fetal hepatic function, which occurs in erythroblastosis, for example, before fetal adrenal activity is affected, may be reflected in low amniotic fluid estriol values, whereas maternal urinary estriol is still in the normal range.

The range of normal urinary estriol excretion per 24 hours is wide, beginning with approximately 1 mg at 18 to 20 weeks, gradually increasing to between 4 and 8 mg at 28 to 30 weeks, and between 8 and 25 mg or more at 38 to 42 weeks. The curve for any given individual rises gradually to term and is roughly correlated with the fetal weight. Greene and Touchstone showed that when estriol output equals 12 mg/24 hours or more, the fetal weight is 2500 g or more. Daily fluctuations in estriol excretion values are common, but precipitous drops below 50% of previous peak values are warning signals. Fetal welfare is threatened when values in the range of 3 to 4 mg are found in late pregnancy, and fetal death is almost inevitable if the daily excretion is below 2 mg.

Human placental lactogen (hPL). Human placental lactogen (hPL) is a growth hormone–like substance possessing lactogenic and luteotrophic properties, which like hCG is synthesized solely by the placenta. hPL is a polypeptide and shows immunologic cross-reaction, although incomplete, with human pituitary growth hormone (hGH). Greater purification of these substances has revealed features of hPL as distinguished from hGH and elucidated their different roles in normal pregnancy.

hPL is produced by the syncytiotrophoblast and is transferred almost exclusively into the maternal circulation. Small but increasing amounts are transferred into the amniotic fluid; however, negligible amounts are passed into the fetal circulation. The hormone is detectable in maternal serum or urine as early as the sixth week of gestation. Secretion increases progressively to term, with serum values showing a tenfold or more increase in late pregnancy and prompt decrease after delivery. In contrast to the gestational increases in estriol, production of hPL is not fully dependent on the presence of a viable fetus. The hormone has been extracted from molar tissue, as well as from the serum of patients with hydatidiform mole and choriocarcinoma.

The curves for serum hPL and 24-hour urinary estriol excretion show parallel rises in normal cases. Falling serum hPL levels are directly related to reduced placental function and are therefore often predictive of fetal demise, associated with maternal hypertension, toxemia, dysmaturity syndromes, and some cases of severe diabetes. They do not reflect fetal compromise in diabetic pregnancies unassociated with vasculopathy or in other conditions in which the primary disorder is fetal in origin.

The appearance of a trophoblastic hPL early in pregnancy suggests that hPL may augment the luteotrophic effect of hCG and may be essential for full development of the corpus luteum in pregnancy. hPL shows no growth-promoting activity in itself, but it greatly increases the anabolic effects of hGH. This synergistic action is of importance in connection with nitrogen retention, essential for growth during pregnancy. New techniques have made possible critical studies of the growth hormone–like properties of hPL and its metabolic role in pregnancy. These have greatly enhanced understanding of protein, fat, and carbohydrate metabolism during pregnancy, all of which show influences of growth hormone or growth hormone–like activity.

The rate of secretion of hPL is high and, according to Grumbach and associates, far exceeds the excretion rate of any known human polypeptide hormone. During late pregnancy the concentration of hPL in the maternal circulation is approximately one thousandfold greater than that of hGH, but the hPL level in the fetal circulation is low (approximately $\frac{1}{300}$ that of the mother). In contrast, the concentration of hGH is strikingly elevated in the fetal but not in the maternal circulation.

The concept that hPL plays a key role in maternal metabolic adjustments of pregnancy, as suggested by Grumbach and co-workers, is based on these findings. Both hPL and hGH stimulate release of free fatty acids and the mobilization of fat stores, thus providing an alternate pathway of metabolism. At the same time an elevated level of free fatty acids acts as a specific peripheral insulin antagonist and results in a compensatory exaggerated production of insulin. The use of fat stores as fuel through the concerted action of hPL and insulin increases maternal capacity for protein and glucose sparing. This hypothesis is particularly convincing in light of well-established biochemical changes characteristic of abnormalities in carbohydrate metabolism during pregnancy and is further discussed in Chapter 22.

Relaxin. The nonsteroid hormone relaxin appears in the blood of women early in pregnancy and increases gradually to term. Zarrow, Holmstrom, and Salhanick found a serum level of 0.2 guinea pig U/ml at 7 weeks, a maximum of 2 guinea pig U/ml at term, and disappearance of this hormone within 24 hours after delivery. For this reason it is thought possible that the placenta may be its source during pregnancy rather than the ovary, which in the absence of pregnancy secretes relaxin during the luteal phase. A placental source has not been found, but immunoreactive relaxin has been demonstrated in ovarian vein blood at term. Relaxation of the pelvic ligaments and connective tissues in various parts of the body may represent a relaxin effect or a synergistic action with progesterone.

Adrenocorticotropic hormone. The fact that corticosteroids are normally increased as pregnancy advances indicates an increased production of adrenocorticotropic hormone (ACTH). Large quantities of ACTH have been repeatedly recovered from placental extracts, although there is some controversy as to whether the placenta acts as a repository for storage of ACTH or is the actual site of the increased gestational production.

Adrenal corticosteroid hormones. Berliner, Jones, and Salhanick have demonstrated the presence of cortisol, cortisone, 11-dehydrocorticosterone, aldosterone, and several of their degradation products in placental extracts. They contend that the increased amounts of cortisone found in these placentas can be accounted for, first, by the volume of trapped blood present and, second, by the ability of the placenta to concentrate this hormone. Their experiments in administration of radioactive cortisone to pregnant women revealed a placental concentration 2.2 times that in the peripheral blood.

The increased binding capacity of plasma globulin during pregnancy probably accounts for the fact that the high levels of 17-hydroxycorticosteroids, which equal or exceed those normally found in Cushing's syndrome, do not produce symptoms of this disease since protein-bound cortisol is biologically inactive. Aldosterone excretion begins to increase early in the second trimester and rises gradually to term.

Excretion of 17-ketosteroids shows only a slight rise during normal pregnancy. Venning found elevated values similar to those reported by several other investigators only when the method used was nonspecific and metabolites of progesterone were included in the final reading.

Placental enzymes

Given the diversity of physiologic and metabolic functions required of the placenta for maintenance and development of the fetus, it is not surprising that a large number of enzymes should be demonstrated within its substance. Attempts have been made to correlate quantitative measurements of several enzymes in maternal plasma with normal and abnormal pregnancies.

Diamine oxidase (DAO, histaminase). Diamine oxidase is an enzyme involved in the degradation of histamine and other diamines such as cadaverine and putrescine. Histamine is important in the metabolism of all growing tissues and is found in especially high concentration in fetal tissues. DAO is considered an adaptive enzyme produced by the mother in response to the increased production of the specific amine by the fetus.

Southren and co-workers studied the relative DAO activity of fetal and maternal tissues and found maximal activity in the retroplacental decidua. No significant increase in maternal DAO is induced by trophoblastic tumors. Instead, the presence of a fetus is necessary to induce enzyme production. Measurable increases in DAO can be detected within 5 to 6 weeks after the last normal menstrual period, followed by a rapid rise until approximately 20 weeks, at which time levels tend to plateau and drop sharply within 2 to 4 days after delivery. The clinical use of DAO levels in following the course of pregnancy is limited to the first half of gestation.

Oxytocinase (cystine-amino-peptidase). Oxytocinase activity increases between 50% and 100% during normal pregnancy. The source is presumed to be the syncytiotrophoblast. Serial oxytocinase levels in the maternal serum accurately reflect the functional capacity of the placenta, but they are not useful in conditions in which fetal jeopardy is caused by fetal factors per se.

Alkaline phosphatase. Maternal serum alkaline phosphatase activity increases progressively during the last trimester of pregnancy. Both maternal and fetal sources contribute to the increase. The placental alkaline phosphatase is heat stable, whereas all other alkaline phosphatase is not. Heat-stable alkaline phosphatase (HSAP) is apparently liberated during periods of placental damage similarly to the liberation of other cellular enzymes from infarcted muscle. The test is simple and inexpensive, but its reliability in predicting fetal jeopardy is limited to conditions compromising placental function (Fig. 13-15).

Term placenta

The *placenta at term* is a discoid organ, measuring 15 to 20 cm in diameter and 2 to 3 cm in thickness. Its weight is roughly 500 g, or about one sixth the weight of the infant at term except in patients with erythroblastosis or syphilis, in whom oversized placentas are characteristic. The maternal surface is divided by decidual septa into 15 to 20 *cotyledons*. The umbilical cord is usually inserted near the central portion of the smooth fetal surface. Fetal vessels fan out from the base of the

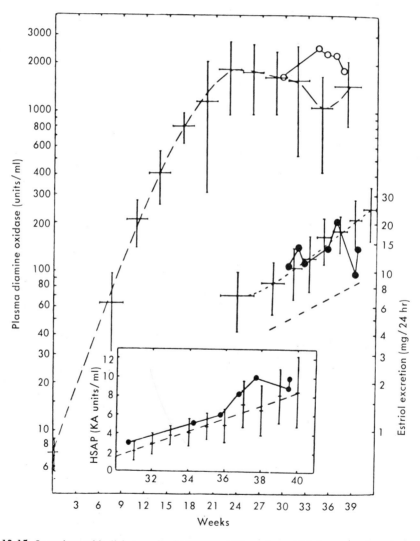

Fig. 13-15. In patient with diabetes, rise in HSAP at 37 weeks, which is suggestive of placental dysfunction, precedes fall in 24-hour urinary estriol level. Diamine oxidase (DAO) values show little change during period of fetal distress. Placental infarct found at delivery, and partial placental abruption occurred in labor. (From Carrington, E.R.: Clin. Obstet. Gynecol. **16**:1, 1973.)

cord. These disappear into the substance of the placenta near the periphery (Figs. 13-16 and 13-17).

The *umbilical cord* averages about 55 cm in length. Cord measurements, however, may vary considerably in thickness and in length. Connective tissue with high water content (Wharton's jelly) surrounds the single umbilical vein and two arteries and facilitates desiccation after the cord is tied. The vessels are usually longer than the cord, become folded on themselves, and give rise to false knots, which do not interfere with circulation.

Amniotic fluid. The volume of amniotic fluid usually averages about 50 ml at 10 weeks' gestation, 200 ml at 16 weeks', and approximately 1 L at 38 weeks, with a slight decline to term and significant decreases beyond 42 weeks. Water content is about 98%, and solids comprise 2%. Reaction is alkaline. Theories regarding its source include (1) secretion by amniotic epithelium, (2) transudation from maternal blood, (3) fetal urine, and (4) mixed origin.

Chez, Smith, and Hutchinson performed direct catheterization of the monkey fetus in utero and confirmed the fact that the kidneys contribute significantly to the quantity of amniotic fluid. In the monkey fetus near term this amounts to 5 ml/kg/hr. Scoggin and co-workers, with the use of an ingenious experimental model, demonstrated an exchange of water from mother to fetus and from amniotic fluid to maternal tissues across the placental site and the fetal membranes, respectively. According to their calculations, the total body exchange across the amniochorion amounts to 25.5 mol/hr with a net flow of 100 ml/hr from amniotic fluid to maternal circulation. The observations of Hutchinson and colleagues indicate that the umbilical cord probably plays an important role in the transfer of water from the amniotic sac, a fact not previously appreciated.

It should be clear that the amniotic fluid is not a static medium but is continuously renewed. Vosburgh and associates, with the use of radioactive sodium and deuterium oxide tracers, demonstrated a complete sodium exchange in 15 hours and water exchange in less than 3 hours.

Ultrastructure of the human amnion reveals the presence of an extensive system of canals and channels within the amniotic epithelium. Bourne and Lacy found that these channels communicate with lateral and basal vac-

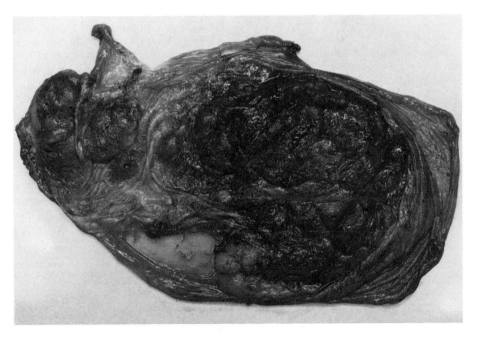

Fig. 13-16. Maternal surface of placenta showing division into cotyledons.

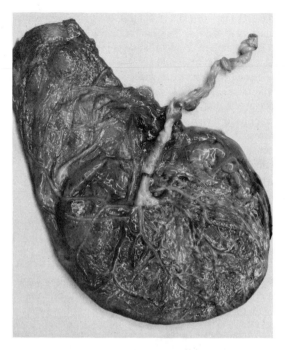

Fig. 13-17. Fetal surface of placenta with succenturiate lobe. Blood vessels disappear into substance of placenta near periphery, except those that supply succenturiate lobe.

uoles and with the extracellular space. It is a logical speculation that existence of this system is an important factor in the movement of amniotic fluid.

The rate of transfer of various substances, including drugs, is of practical importance in the management of the complications of pregnancy and in the conduct of labor and delivery of the infant. Apgar and Papper, for example, detected barbiturates in amniotic fluid, the placenta, and fetal organs within 15 minutes after intravenous injection in the mother. Since deglutition and respiration occur in utero from the fourth month on, amniotic fluid may afford an additional route for transmission of various substances to the fetus.

CONSTITUENTS. Sampling of amniotic fluid has become one of the most important diagnostic procedures for assessing the fetal status. Information regarding Rh isoimmunization, maturity, genetic disorders, and certain metabolic disturbances can

now be obtained by cytologic and biochemical examination of the fluid at various stages of pregnancy.

Genetic information can be obtained from cells found in the amniotic fluid. Such studies are usually performed at about the sixteenth week of gestation. *Prenatal sex determination* can be made accurately and is useful in counseling regarding pregnancies in women who are heterozygous for sex-linked recessive disorders such as muscular dystrophy or hemophilia. *Chromosomal aberrations* involving the number and structure of chromosomes such as Down's syndrome have been detected, as well as chromosomal breaks in fetal cells. *Biochemical studies* of cultures derived from cells contained in amniotic fluid allow prenatal diagnosis of an increasing number of hereditary metabolic disorders, including cystic fibrosis, mucopolysaccharidosis, galactosemia, glycogen storage disease, and congenital adrenal hyperplasia.

Prediction of neural tube defects can be made with a high degree of accuracy at 14 to 16 weeks' gestation by determination of amniotic fluid alpha-fetroproteins (AFP). Levels associated with fetal anencephaly, spina bifida, and myelomeningocele are approximately ten to twenty times the values found when fetal development is normal. However, high levels of amniotic fluid AFP are not entirely specific for neural tube defects, especially in late pregnancy when markedly elevated AFP values have been found in maternal serum, as well as in amniotic fluid in association with fetal death, impending fetal death, Rh isoimmunization, omphalocele, and duodenal atresia.

DIAGNOSIS OF FETAL MATURITY. The composition of amniotic fluid reflects the metabolic activity and function of various fetal structures such as lung, kidney, liver, and skin. Measurement of the following amniotic fluid constituents, all of which show characteristic changes during and beyond the thirty-fifth week of gestation, provide the most useful indices among many methods studied for prediction of fetal maturity.

Lecithin/sphingomyelin (L/S) ratio. Pulmonary maturity is dependent on the presence of sufficient amounts of surface-active phospholipids to prevent alveolar collapse with expiration. In the immature

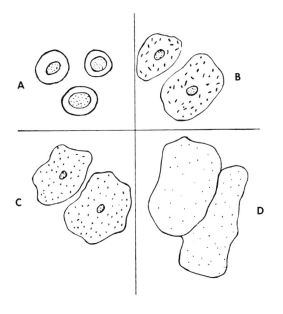

Fig. 13-18. Fetal cells from amniotic fluid: **A,** parabasal; **B,** intermediate; **C,** superficial (cornified); **D,** anucleated.

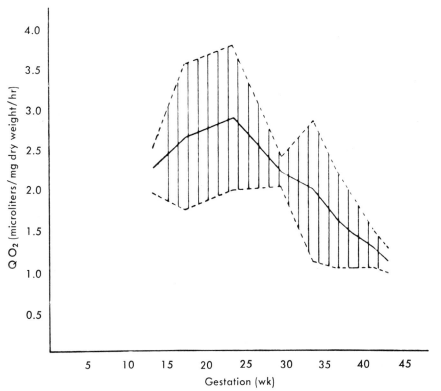

Fig. 13-19. Normal placental oxygen utilization. (From Tremblay, P.C., Sybulski, S., and Maughan, G.B.: Am. J. Obstet. Gynecol. **91:**600, 1965.)

fetal lungs, sphingomyelin concentration is greater than that of lecithin, but at 35 weeks a rapid surge in stable lecithin occurs. An L/S ratio of 2:1 or greater provides a highly reliable prediction of pulmonary maturity in normal pregnancy.

Phosphatidylglycerol (PG), a minor component of surfactant phospholipids as compared with lecithin, appears in the amniotic fluid during the thirty-fifth week of gestation. Hallman and associates demonstrated a sharp rise in this substance from 35 weeks to term when PG comprised 10% of the total phospholipids. The presence of PG correlates well with advancing fetal lung development and, with a favorable L/S ratio, provides the best assurance available of fetal pulmonary maturity.

Creatinine concentration. Creatinine concentration rises abruptly between the thirty-fourth and thirty-sixth week of gestation with increase in renal concentrating ability. Amniotic fluid creatinine values of 2 mg/dl or more are usually indicative of fetal maturity.

Amniotic fluid cytologic analysis (Fig. 13-18). Four types of fetal cells are found in late pregnancy fluid: parabasals, intermediate, nucleated squamae, and anuclear squamae. A maturation index showing 25% or more anuclear cells or the finding of over 20% ''fat cells'' stained with 0.1% Nile blue sulfate provides a simple, rough estimate of functional fetal maturity. The clinical use of biochemical and biophysical methods of assessing fetal maturity are discussed in Chapter 20.

Placental oxygen utilization (Fig. 13-19). During the first half of pregnancy the rate of oxygen uptake by the placenta is high, but according to Tremblay, Sybulski, and Maughan, there is a gradual diminution in intrinsic placental metabolic activity from a high peak at about 25 weeks to more moderate levels at term as the fetus takes on more metabolic responsibility for itself.

DISORDERS OF THE PLACENTA

Variations in shape. The outline of the placenta may appear elongated or kidney shaped, or there may be two or three incompletely separated lobes. These lobes are termed *placenta bipartita* or *placenta tripartita,* respectively. Most atypical forms occur as a result of minor alterations in the blood supply or nutritional state of the decidua early in gestation, but they have no real clinical significance.

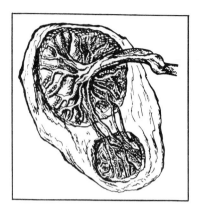

Fig. 13-20. Placenta succenturiata.

Placenta succenturiata (Fig. 13-20). One or more accessory lobes may be found at variable distances from the main placenta. Vessels from the accessory lobe traverse the fetal membranes and continue over the surface of the placenta proper. During the third stage of labor these vessels may be torn, and the succenturiate lobe retained within the uterus. Postpartum hemorrhage or infection may occur if the detached tissue is not recognized and removed. Diagnosis can be made if inspection of the fetal surface reveals an open vessel at the placenta edge.

Placenta circumvallata (Figs. 13-21 and 13-22). Occasionally, a white fibrous ring is visible on the fetal surface at a variable distance from the margin of the placenta. The ring is formed by a folding back of the amnion and of the chorion on itself, forming a double layer of fetal membranes at this site. This is presumed to occur when the early chorionic plate is relatively small. Later the villi at the periphery grow out laterally into the decidua vera. The fetal vessels do not extend to the margin of the placenta but instead terminate at the ring. In other respects the placenta is normal.

The incidence of abortion early in pregnancy and bleeding late in pregnancy or during labor may be somewhat increased in association with this condition, but in most instances the course of pregnancy and the condition of the infant are unaffected.

Placenta membranacea. Occasionally, the villi covering the decidua capsularis persist; continue to function; and form a large, thin, membranous placenta that entirely surrounds the fetal membranes. Its attachment therefore is not confined to one portion of the uterus but, instead, covers the surface completely. Separation or expulsion of a placenta membranacea during the third stage of labor may be incomplete, and consequently the danger of im-

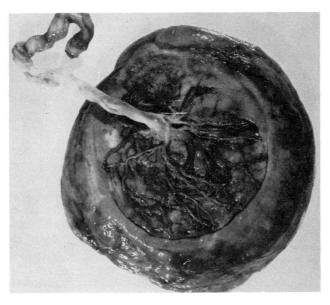

Fig. 13-21. Placenta circumvallata.

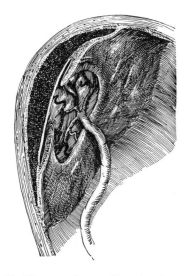

Fig. 13-22. Placenta circumvallata showing reduplication of chorionic plate and growth of villi beyond its margin.

mediate or delayed hemorrhage following delivery is increased.

Placental infarcts. Avascular areas of varying size and consistency can be found in almost all placentas at term. Many of these are not true infarcts. White or yellowish nodules are commonly *fibrin deposits,* indicative of the aging process in the placenta.

Small foci of degenerating trophoblasts may initiate localized thrombosis of the surrounding maternal blood. Fine laminations of fibrin are laid down usually parallel to the chorionic plate. These were formerly designated as "white infarcts," but the term is misleading because the process is primarily degenerative rather than vascular. Fibrin deposition is rarely so extensive as to jeopardize the fetus.

True placental infarcts are localized areas of necrosis caused by obstruction of the nutritional blood supply. Since the placenta receives its nourishment through the maternal rather than the fetal circulation, infarction occurs only when the maternal side is interrupted. On cessation of the blood flow to a cotyledon, the intervillous spaces become ischemic, and the villi deprived of nutrition undergo necrosis. The lesion may appear pale, red, or grayish, depending on its age (Fig. 13-23).

Rupture of thin-walled or brittle vessels with extravasation of blood into the decidua and subsequent hematoma formation may also cause ischemic necrosis. The placenta becomes detached in the area of bleeding, and, if separation is extensive, the fetus will die in utero. Although rupture of decidual vessels may occur without obvious cause, its occurrence is most common in patients with hypertension or chronic renal disease.

Calcification. Small areas of calcification are frequently

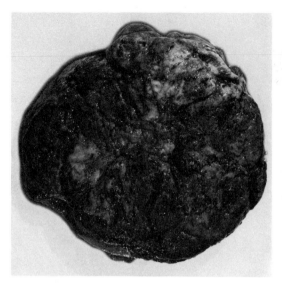

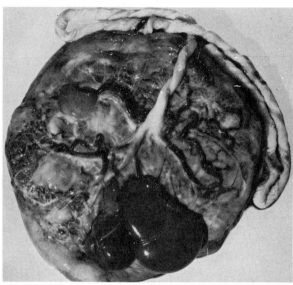

Fig. 13-23. Maternal surface of placenta showing white infarcted areas.

Fig. 13-24. Placental cyst.

found in the normal placenta. In some instances the entire maternal surface feels sandy. Occasionally, firm white plaques are found in one or more regions. Like fibrin deposits, these are the result of degeneration of the villi, a late phase in the aging process of the placenta, and have no clinical significance.

Infection. Placental infection may occur in instances of prolonged rupture of the membranes with or without prolonged labor. An *amnionitis* develops first and may spread locally to the placenta. If the process extends through the chorionic vessels, general infection may develop in the fetus. Infection of the placenta is seldom primary, and infection resulting from a *maternal bacteremia* is relatively rare.

Syphilis frequently involves the placenta, causing thickening and clubbing of the villi. The number of villous blood vessels is reduced because of endarteritic changes. Grossly, the syphilitic placenta is large in relation to the weight of the infant and presents a greasy, yellowish surface with poorly defined cotyledons. Placental *tuberculosis* is uncommon even when the disease in the mother is advanced.

Cysts (Fig. 13-24). Cysts are frequently found on the fetal surface and arise from the chorionic membrane. They vary in size up to 5 to 6 cm and are filled with yellowish or bloody fluid. Cysts found deep in the substance of the placenta usually represent advanced de-

generative changes in areas of fibrin deposition or in old infarcts.

Tumors. Neoplasms of the placenta are unusual. Of those observed, *chorioangioma* is most common. Hydramnios is often associated with these tumors.

ABNORMALITIES OF THE CORD

Variations in length of the cord between 35 and 70 cm are normal, the average length being about 55 cm. Complete absence of the cord is sometimes observed in connection with defects in the fetal abdominal wall. A *short cord* may delay descent of the fetus during labor and result in detachment of the placenta or, rarely, rupture of the cord with traction. A *long cord* predisposes to prolapse or cord entanglement. Tightening of loops about the neck or body of the infant during descent may gradually impair circulation and cause asphyxia. *True knots* are found occasionally in the cord, but unless these become tightened, fetal circulation is unimpaired.

Variations in insertion. The umbilical cord is usually inserted eccentrically but nearer the central than the peripheral portion of the placenta. A marginal insertion, designated *battledore placenta,* is relatively common and unimportant. On the other hand, *velamentous insertion* of the cord is potentially hazardous to the fetus (Fig. 13-25). Vessels separate from the umbilical cord and traverse the membranes for a variable distance before

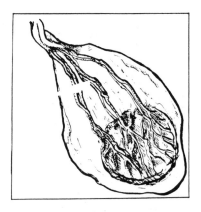

Fig. 13-25. Velamentous insertion of cord.

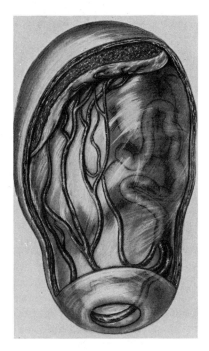

Fig. 13-26. Velamentous insertion of cord with vasa previa.

reaching the placenta. Tearing or rupture of the vessels during labor may exsanguinate the infant. If the vessels course over the dilating cervix in bulging membranes *(vasa previa)*, pressure by the presenting part may cause fetal distress or asphyxia (Fig. 13-26).

Vascular anomalies. The cord should be checked at delivery for the presence of one vein and two arteries. A single umbilical artery is found in slightly less than 1% of cases, but this abnormality is associated with a high incidence of congenital anomalies of the newborn, such as the presence of intraplacental shunts and aneurysms.

A specific type of arteriovenous shunt is seen occasionally in monozygotic twins; a fetoplacental transfusion syndrome is the result. The arterial donor twin is pale and dehydrated, whereas the venous recipient is plethoric, hypervolemic, and in greatest danger of cardiac overload.

ABNORMALITIES OF THE AMNION

Hydramnios. The accumulation of amniotic fluid in excess of 2000 ml is considered abnormal. Hydramnios usually develops gradually, but in rare instances acute hydramnios occurs, and the uterus becomes remarkably distended within the course of a few days. The cause remains obscure, although various factors associated with this condition are recognized. *Fetal anomalies,* particularly those of the central nervous system, are more common if hydramnios is present. The occurrence of anencephaly, spina bifida, duodenal atresia, or tracheoesophageal fistula has led to the theory that an increased fetal output of fluid through the spinal fluid system or the urinary tract or failure of the fetus to ingest fluid may cause hydramnios. This theory does not explain the increased incidence of hydramnios observed with *maternal diabetes* or *erythroblastosis.* An abnormality in placental transmission of fluids from the fetal circulation or an abnormally functioning amniotic membrane may be responsible.

Symptoms are more pronounced with acute than with chronic hydramnios. The patient suffers from pain caused by overdistention of the uterus and abdominal wall, edema of the lower extremities, and severe dyspnea. The accumulation may be so rapid and so enormous that prompt evacuation is necessary to prevent maternal death.

Hydramnios should be suspected if the uterus appears larger than normal for the duration of pregnancy or if the fetal parts and fetal heart tones are indistinct. The condition must be differentiated from multifetal pregnancy. Diagnosis can be made with certainty by sonogram; at the same time certain fetal deformities involving the skull and skeletal part may be detected.

Further information can be obtained by *amniography*. This technique includes amniocentesis with removal of 25 ml of amniotic fluid under sterile conditions and insertion of 15 ml or, with severe hydramnios, 25 to 30 ml of contrast media such as Renografin-60 or Hypaque-M75. These solutions are hypertonic and may initiate labor. The inclination to use larger amounts to compensate for the excessive amounts of fluid should be rejected. The fetus swallows and concentrates the material in the gastrointestinal tract. The x-ray film should be delayed and taken 1 to 2 hours after instillation of contrast material, when concentration in the gastrointestinal tract can provide information regarding gastrointestinal atresia or other soft-tissue abnormalities. This type of examination is also of great value in determining placental site, uterine deformities or tumors, intrauterine fetal death, and hydatidiform mole, in addition to providing clear-cut information regarding the degree of hydramnios.

Medical treatment of hydramnios is generally ineffectual. The patient with chronic hydramnios and only mild symptoms should be kept as comfortable as possible with rest and should be permitted to go into labor spontaneously. Since contractions are sometimes of poor quality because of overdistention of the uterus, progress in labor may be slow, and the incidence of postpartum hemorrhage is increased because of atony.

Amniotomy becomes necessary if symptoms are progressive or severe. The cervix is usually effaced because of pressure. Rupture of the membrane should be carried out under aseptic conditions, and an attempt should be made to drain the fluid slowly. Free or rapid flow may encourage prolapse of the cord or a fetal part, and sudden reduction in size of the uterus may cause placental separation.

Removal of fluid by transabdominal aspiration or insertion of polyethylene tubing into the uterus has met with little success, since the fluid reaccumulates or labor ensues shortly thereafter.

Hydramnios developing in Rh-sensitized mothers or in patients with diabetes offers an unfavorable prognosis for fetal survival. If the gestation period is sufficiently advanced, delivery is often advisable, and preparations should be made for special care of the infant.

Oligohydramnios. Marked deficiency or absence of amniotic fluid is exceedingly rare. When present, the condition is generally associated with fetal urinary tract anomalies. Potter described 49 cases of fetal renal agenesis from the Chicago Lying-In Hospital, and in none could the presence of any amniotic fluid be documented.

Relative diminution in the amount of amniotic fluid is sometimes noted late in pregnancy in connection with postmaturity and in cases of placental insufficiency and fetal dysmaturity.

FETAL DEVELOPMENT

Organogenesis is largely completed by about the eighth week after fertilization. During this period the conceptus is designated the *embryo*, after which time it is called the *fetus*. The significant features of the various developmental stages are shown in Table 13-2.

The rate of fetal growth is proportionately more rapid in the early months of pregnancy. According to *Haase's rule,* the crown-heel length of the fetus in centimeters equals the square of the lunar month during the first 5 months, and in the last 5 months the length is equal to five times the lunar month of pregnancy, as follows:

Time of measurement	Calculation of fetal length (cm)
End of third lunar month	$3 \times 3 = 9$
End of sixth lunar month	$6 \times 5 = 30$
Term	$10 \times 5 = 50$

Despite obvious difficulties in obtaining precise crown-heel measurements, the length of the fetus usually provides a more reliable index of gestation period than does the weight. The importance of an accurate estimate of fetal maturity is under-scored by follow-up studies of "small-for-date" babies, "low-birth-weight infants," or intrauterine growth retardation problems. The most common cause is intrauterine malnutrition or fetal maldevelopment. Comparison of the newborn measurements with those of standard fetal growth charts such as that developed by Lubchenco and co-workers should be routine nursery practice.

Clinical evaluation of fetal growth rate is often difficult and is discussed in Chapters 20 and 31.

The *infant at term* measures 50 cm (20 inches) and weighs 3175 g (about 7 pounds). Little lanugo

TABLE 13-2 Principle embryonal and fetal characteristics at various developmental stages

Gestation period (weeks)	Length (cm) (crown to heel)	Weight (g)	Characteristics
3			Beginning of gastrointestinal tract followed by cardiac development; appearance of limb buds
4	1		Anlage for all organs present
12	9	15	Fingers and toes visible; appearance of centers of ossification in most bones
16	16	110	Sex revealed by external genitals; appearance of respiratory movements and swallowing reflexes; meconium present
20	25	300	Fetal movements detectable
24	30	630	Skin less transparent; fine lanugo over body
28	35	1045	Fetus viable
36	45	2500	Appearance of ossification center in distal femoral epipyhysis

remains except over the shoulders. A variable amount of vernix caseosa covers the skin surfaces; this is a mixture of epithelial cells, lanugo, and the secretion of the sebaceous glands. Characteristic features of the fetal head, including suture lines, fontanels, and diameters, are of obstetric importance. The sutures and fontanels that serve as useful landmarks are the long *sagittal suture,* which separates the two parietal bones; and the *lambdoid suture,* which is between the posterior edge of the parietal bones and the occipital bone. The triangular-shaped space at the intersection of these two lines is the *posterior fontanel.* The *frontal suture* separates the frontal bones from each other, and the *coronal suture* separates the anterior edge of the parietal bones from the frontal bones. The large *anterior fontanel* is the diamond-shaped space at the junction of the sagittal, coronal, and frontal sutures (Fig. 13-27).

Respiration. Movements of the fetal chest wall have been recorded by ultrasound as early as the latter part of the first trimester of pregnancy. Rates range from 40 to 70 excursions/min. Recent studies of continuous tracings made before and during labor suggest that monitoring of human fetal breathing may be a useful adjunct to fetal heart rate monitoring. Dawes reports that fetal hypoxia and hy-

poglycemia are associated with a diminution in breathing movements and that the appearance of gasping has been noted in certain high-risk situations such as intrauterine growth-retarded babies during labor.

Circulation (Figs. 13-28 and 13-29). Initially the developing ovum derives nutrition from its own large cytoplasmic mass and then from the decidua by activity of the trophoblastic cells. The vitelline circulation is functional in the third and fourth weeks and temporarily provides nourishment for the embryo from the yolk sac. Thereafter connection is made between vessels developing in the chorion and those growing out from the fetus through the body stalk to establish the fetoplacental circulation.

Oxygen and nutrient substances pass from the maternal blood through the villi and are transported through small venules to the single umbilical vein. This divides at the liver edge. One branch empties into the portal vein, circulates through the liver, and enters the inferior vena cava through the hepatic vein. The larger portion passes directly to the inferior vena cava as the ductus venosus. In the right atrium, oxygen-laden blood coming through the inferior vena cava passes for the most part through the foramen ovale into the left atrium.

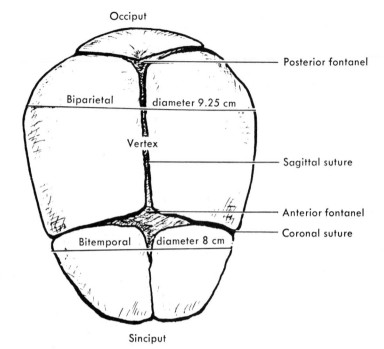

Fig. 13-27. Landmarks of fetal skull.

Occiput

Posterior fontanel

Biparietal   diameter 9.25 cm

Vertex

Sagittal suture

Anterior fontanel

Coronal suture

Bitemporal   diameter 8 cm

Sinciput

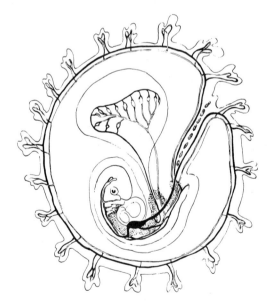

Fig. 13-28. Schema of vitelline and chorionic circulations.

Blood from the head region delivered by the superior vena cava is low in oxygen and tends to pass in a direct stream into the right ventricle. Since the lungs are not functioning, most of this oxygen-low blood entering the pulmonary artery passes through the ductus arteriosus into the aorta and is mixed with blood of higher oxygen content pumped from the left side of the heart. In the fetus the internal iliac or hypogastric arteries send out large branches on either side, which traverse the lower abdominal

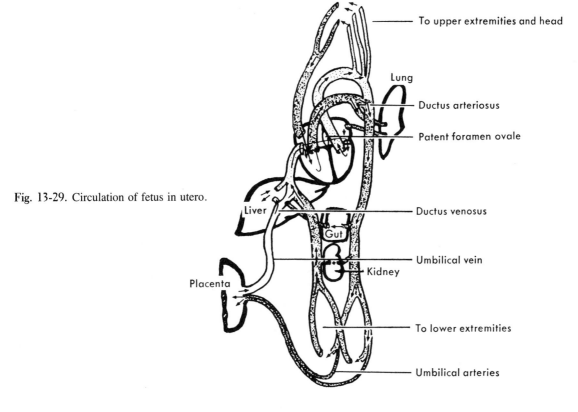

To upper extremities and head

Lung

Ductus arteriosus

Patent foramen ovale

Fig. 13-29. Circulation of fetus in utero.

Liver

Ductus venosus

Gut

Umbilical vein

Kidney

Placenta

To lower extremities

Umbilical arteries

wall to the umbilicus and continue through the cord as the paired umbilical arteries. Deoxygenated blood is thus transported back to the placenta.

Circulatory changes at birth (Fig. 13-30). As soon as respirations begin and the cord is clamped, circulatory changes occur:

1. The *ductus arteriosus* closes as the lungs begin to function. A large volume of blood is pumped by the right ventricle into the previously collapsed pulmonary arteries, thus reducing pressure within the lumen. The ductus arteriosus becomes occluded and forms the *ligamentum arteriosum*.

2. The *foramen ovale* closes as a result of increased tension in the left atrium and concomitant reduction in the right atrium. This is because of the increased volume of blood returned from the lungs as respirations are established and the diminished quantity of blood to the inferior vena cava when the umbilical cord is tied.

3. The functionless umbilical vein becomes the *ligamentum teres hepatis*.

4. The ductus venosus closes and forms the *ligamentum venosum*.

5. The obliterated umbilical arteries become the *obliterated hypogastric* or *lateral umbilical ligaments*.

Oxygenation. In the maternal circulation, arterial oxygen saturation is 96%, and venous oxygen saturation is 71%. Blood in the intervillous spaces is mixed, thus reducing the effective saturation.

In addition, oxygen diffuses through a wet membrane slowly. Oxygen passed to the fetus therefore provides only about 60% oxygen saturation. Fetal adaptation is effected by (1) high red cell count, (2) high hemoglobin values, and (3) differences in fetal hemoglobin as compared with the adult type. The oxygen dissociation curve of fetal blood is shifted to the left, and, accordingly, uptake of oxygen at low gas tension is enhanced. Studies of the oxygen and carbon dioxide pressure gradients across the placenta support the hypothesis that these gases are transferred by diffusion in accor-

Fig. 13-30. Circulatory changes in infant after birth.

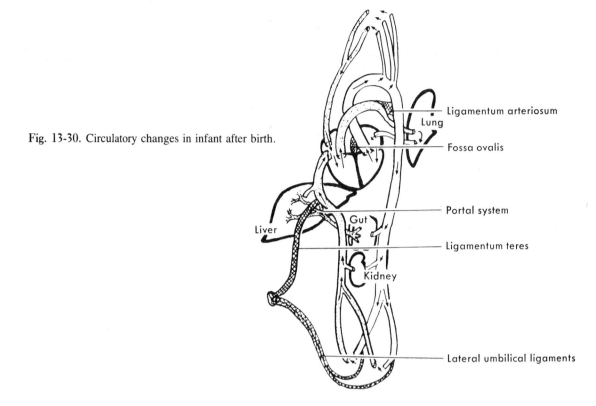

Ligamentum arteriosum

Lung

Fossa ovalis

Portal system

Liver

Gut

Ligamentum teres

Kidney

Lateral umbilical ligaments

dance with differences in pressure on either side of the membrane. Although the human placental membrane is wet and consists of three layers (syncytium, stroma, and capillary endothelium), it behaves like the lung.

Prystowsky, Hellegers, and Bruns obtained intervillous-space blood and umbilical vein and artery blood at cesarean section for comparison. They found an average oxygen tension of 47 mm Hg in the intervillous space, 30 mm Hg in the umbilical vein, and 18 mm Hg in the umbilical artery and oxygen pressure difference of approximately 24 mm Hg across the placenta. Carbon dioxide crosses the placenta more readily than oxygen and is found in higher concentration on the fetal than on the maternal side, with an average pressure gradient of 7 mm Hg.

It is important to recognize that the fetus possesses compensatory mechanisms that increase the margin of safety in coping with temporary periods of hypoxia, but even these have limitations. Glucose breakdown is the major source of energy, which under normal conditions

includes an aerobic, as well as an anaerobic, phase. If the fetus is deprived of oxygen, it has an alternate pathway, entirely anaerobic and much less efficient, to meet requirements. In the normal pathway for glucose oxidation a total of 38 high-energy phosphate bonds are produced (eight bonds in the anaerobic and 30 bonds in the aerobic phase). In the absence of oxygen, pyruvic acid is reduced to lactic acid, using six of the eight high-energy phosphate bonds so that the net result is only two instead of 38 energy sources. An increase in hydrogen ion concentration and a corresponding decrease in base is the final result. The fetal blood pH and base deficit therefore should indicate the severity of fetal hypoxia or distress, and this is the premise on which the Saling fetal scalp blood examination is based.

Fetal blood volume averages approximately 85 ml/kg or about 300 ml at term, blood pressure averages 80/40 mm Hg, cardiac rate averages 120 to 140 beats/min, and cardiac output averages 10 to 12 ml/100 g/min, which is about three times that of a normal adult.

REFERENCES

Apgar, V., and Papper, E.M.: Transmission of drugs across the placenta, Anesth. Analg. **31:**309, 1952.

Barr, M.L.: Sex chromatin and phenotype in man, Science **130:**679, 1959.

Barr, M.L., Bertram, L.F., and Lindsay, H.A.: The morphology of the nerve nucleus according to sex, Anat. Rec. **107:**283, 1950.

Behrman, S.J., and Koren, Z.: Immunology of the conceptus. In Greenhill, J.P., editor: Year book of obstetrics and gynecology, 1967-68, Chicago, 1968, Year Book Medical Publishers, Inc.

Berliner, D.L., Jones, J.E., and Salhanick, H.A.: The isolation of adrenal-like steroids in human placenta, J. Biol. Chem. **223:**1043, 1956.

Blandau, R.J., and Rummery, R.E.: Observations on the movements of the living primordial germ cells of mouse and man, Anat. Rec. **148:**262, 1964.

Blechner, J.N., Stenger, V.G., Eitzman, D.V., and Prystowsky, H.: Effects of maternal metabolic acidosis on the human fetus and newborn infant, Am J. Obstet Gynecol. **100:**934, 1968.

Bourne, G.L., and Lacy, D.: Ultra-structure of human amnion and its possible relation to the circulation of amniotic fluid, Nature **186:**952, 1960.

Carrington, E.R.: Diabetes in pregnancy, Clin. Obstet. Gynecol. **16:**28, 1973.

Carrington, E.R., Oesterling, M.J., and Adams, F.M.: Renal clearance of estriol in complicated pregnancies, Am. J. Obstet. Gynecol. **106:**1131, 1970.

Cassmer, O.: Hormone production in the isolated human placenta, Acta Endocrinol. **32:**(45):1, 1959.

Cheek, D.B., Greystone, J.E., and Niall, M.: Factors controlling fetal growth. Clin. Obstet. Gynecol. **20:**925, 1977.

Chez, R.A., Smith, F.G., and Hutchinson, D.L.: Renal function in the intrauterine primate fetus, Am. J. Obstet. Gynecol. **90:**128, 1964.

Dawes, G.S.: Breathing before birth in animals and man, N. Engl. J. Med. **290:**557, 1974.

Diczfalusy, E.: Endocrine functions of the human fetus and placenta, Am. J. Obstet. Gynecol. **119:**419, 1974.

Doyle, J.B.: Direct observations of ovulation by culdoscopy, Fertil. Steril. **5:**105, 1954.

Finn, R.: Survival of the genetically incompatible fetal allograft, Lancet **1:**835, 1975.

Frandsen, V.A., and Stakemann, G.: Site of production of estrogenic hormones in human pregnancy: hormone excretion in pregnancy with anencephalic fetus, Acta Endocrinol. **38:**383, 1961.

Fraser, F.C.: Causes of congenital malformations in human beings, J. Chronic Dis. **10:**97, 1959.

Gerbie, A.B., Nadler, H.L., and Platt, A.W.: Genetics and genetic counseling. In Romney, S.L., Gray, M.J., Little, A.B., Merrill, J.A., Quilligan, E.J., and Stander, R.W., editors: Obstetrics and gynecology: the health care of women, ed. 2, New York, 1981, McGraw-Hill Book Co.

Greene, J.W., and Touchstone, J.C.: Urinary estriol as an index of placental function, Am. J. Obstet. Gynecol. **85:**1, 1963.

Grumbach, M.M., Kaplan, S.L., Sciarra, J.J., and Burr, I.M.: Chorionic growth hormone-prolactin (CGP): secretion, disposition, biologic activity in man, and postulated function as the "growth hormone" of the second half of pregnancy. In Sonenberg, M., editor: Conference on growth hormone, Ann. N.Y. Acad. Sci. **148:**501, 1968.

Hallman, M., Kulovich, M., Kirkpatrick, E., Sugarman, R.G., and Gluck, L.: Phosphatidylinositol and phosphatidylglycerol in amniotic fluid: indicies of lung maturity. Am. J. Obstet. Gynecol. **125:**613, 1976.

Harris, R.E.: Maternal and fetal immunology. Obstet. Gynecol. **51:**733, 1978.

Hendricks, C.H., Quilligan, E.J., Tyler, C.W., and Tucker, G.J.: Pressure relationships between the intervillous space and the amniotic fluid in human term pregnancy, Am. J. Obstet. Gynecol. **77:**1028, 1959.

Hutchinson, D.L., Gray, M.J., Plentl, A.A., Alvarez, H., Caldeyro-Barcia, R., Kaplan, B., and Lind, J.: The role of the fetus in the water exchange of the amniotic fluid of normal and hydramniotic patients, J. Clin. Invest. **38:**971, 1959.

Hutchinson, D.L., Hunter, C.B., Neslen, E.D., and Plentl, A.A.: The exchange of water and electrolytes in the mechanism of amniotic fluid formation and the relationship to hydramnios, Surg. Gynecol. Obstet. **100:**391, 1955.

Lubchenco, L.O., Hansman, C., Dressler, M., and Boyd, E.: Intrauterine growth as measured by live-born birthweight: data from 24 to 42 weeks gestation, Pediatrics **32:**793, 1963.

Page, E.W.: Transfer of materials across the human placenta, Am. J. Obstet. Gynecol. **74:**705, 1957.

Page, E.W., Villee, C.A., and Villee, D.B.: Human reproduction: essentials of reproductive and perinatal medicine, Philadelphia, 1981, W. B. Saunders Co.

Pierce, G.B., Jr., and Midgley, A.R., Jr.: The origin and function of human syncytiotrophoblastic giant cells, Am. J. Pathol. **43:**153, 1963.

Potter, E.L.: Pathology of the fetus and infant, ed. 2, Chicago, 1961, Year Book Medical Publishers, Inc.

Prystowsky, H., Hellegers, A., and Bruns, P.: Fetal blood studies. XV. The carbon dioxide concentration gradient between fetal and maternal blood of humans, Am. J. Obstet. Gynecol. **81:**372, 1961.

Prystowsky, H., Hellegers, A., and Bruns, P.: Fetal blood studies. XVIII. Supplementary observations on the oxygen pressure gradient between the maternal and fetal bloods of humans, Surg. Gynecol. Obstet. **110:**495, 1960.

Ramsey, E.M., Corner, G.W., Jr., Donner, M.W., and Stran, H.M.: Radio-angiographic studies of circulation in maternal placenta of the rhesus monkey: preliminary report, Proc. Natl. Acad. Sci. U.S.A. **46:**1003, 1960.

Ross, G.T.: Clinical relevance of research on the structure of human chorionic gonadotropin, Am. J. Obstet. Gynecol. **129:**795, 1977.

Scoggin, W.A., Harbert, G.M., Jr., Anslow, W.P., Jr., Riet, B.V., and McGaughey, H.S.: Fetomaternal exchange of water at term, Am. J. Obstet. Gynecol. **90**:7, 1964.

Simmons, R.L., and Russell, P.S.: The immunologic problem of pregnancy, Am. J. Obstet. Gynecol. **85**:583, 1963.

Simpson, J.L., Golbus, M.S., Martin, A.O., and Sarto, G.E.: Genetics in obstetrics and gynecology, New York, 1982, Grune & Stratton, Inc.

Smith, K., Duhring, J.L., Greene, J.W., Jr., Rochlin, D.B., and Blakemore, W.S.: Transfer of maternal erythrocytes across the human placenta, Obstet. Gynecol. **18**:673, 1961.

Smith, O.W., and Ryan, K.J.: Estrogens in the human ovary. Am. J. Obstet. Gynecol. **84**:141, 1962.

Southren, A.L., Kolbayashi, Y., Brenner, P., and Weingold, A.B.: Diamine oxidase activity in human maternal and fetal plasma and tissues at parturition, J. Appl. Physiol. **20**:1048, 1965.

Spellacy, W.N., Teoh, E.S., and Buhi, W.C.: Human chorionic somatomammotropin (HCS) levels prior to fetal death in high-risk pregnancies, Obstet. Gynecol. **35**:685, 1970.

Thompson, J.S., and Thompson, M.W.: Genetics in medicine, ed. 3, Philadelphia, 1980, The W.B. Saunders Co.

Tremblay, P.C., Sybulski, S., and Maughan, C.B.: Role of the placenta in fetal malnutrition, Am. J. Obstet. Gynecol. **91**:597, 1965.

Tyler, E.T.: Physiological and chemical aspects of conception, J.A.M.A. **153**:1351, 1954.

Venning, E.: Adrenal function in pregnancy, Endocrinology **39**:203, 1946.

Villee, C.A.: Regulation of blood glucose in the human fetus, J. Appl. Physiol. **5**:437, 1953.

Vosburgh, G.J., Flexner, L.B., Cowie, D.B., Hellman, L.M., Proctor, N.K., and Wilde, W.S.: The rate of renewal in women of the water and sodium of the amniotic fluid as determined by tracer techniques, Am. J. Obstet. Gynecol. **56**:1156, 1948.

Wislocki, G.B., and Bennett, H.S.: Histology and cytology of the human and monkey placenta with special reference to the trophoblast, Am. J. Anat. **73**:335, 1943.

Wynn, R.M., and Davies, J.: Comparative electron microscopy of the hemochorial placenta, Am. J. Obstet. Gynecol. **91**:533, 1965.

Zarrow, M.X., Holmstrom, E.G., and Salhanick, H.A.: The concentration of relaxin in the blood serum and other tissues of women during pregnancy, J. Clin. Endocrinol. **15**:22, 1955.

14

John H. Mattox

Infertility

From the beginning of recorded time the problem of the barren marriage has played a major role in the lives of humans. Many ancient religious rites and social practices are specifically concerned with fertility and sterility. Magic potions and incantations are still used by primitive peoples to enhance the reproductive capacity of newlywed couples.

A frequently quoted estimate is that *one out of every six couples* in the United States is involuntarily childless, and there is concern that the problem is increasing in magnitude. The *fertility rate,* the number of live births per 1000 women of childbearing age, 15 to 45 years, has declined over recent decades in part because women are delaying childbearing. It was estimated that the number of females having their first child between ages 30 and 34 gradually increased to 12.1 in 1979.

Concomitantly, there have been quantum strides in the knowledge of reproductive physiology, which have served to increase the therapeutic opportunities in areas such as ovulation induction, microsurgery, and in vitro fertilization.

In order to maintain an appropriate perspective of reproductive biology, it should be recalled how inefficient the human reproductive process is. Approximately 35% to 40% of fertilized ova are lost. The generally accepted incidence of diagnosed spontaneous abortion is 15%; approximately 7% of

infants are born prematurely, and 3% to 4% have a major or minor anomaly.

DEFINITIONS

Infertility can be diagnosed if a woman has not been able to conceive during a period of 1 year of unprotected intercourse. Monthly *fecundability* (conception rate) is approximately 20%. More than 60% of normal couples who are having unprotected coitus regularly will conceive within 6 months, about 94% within 1 year, and the remainder will be pregnant by the end of the second year.

Infertility is considered to be *primary* if conception has never occurred; it is *secondary* if there has been at least one pregnancy before the present difficulty. *Sterility* implies that conception is impossible and the causative factor is irremediable. *Relative infertility* is produced by various factors that may hinder or delay conception; these are often correctable.

ESSENTIAL FACTORS FOR REPRODUCTION

Normal fertility is dependent on many factors in both the man and the woman. It is appropriate to consider the couple as the "biologic unit" of reproduction. The male must produce a sufficient number of normal, motile spermatozoa that can enter the urethra through patent pathways to be ejaculated and can be deposited at the appropriate time for fertilization. After deposition, the male gametes must be able to penetrate and be sustained in the cervical mucus. Following *capacitation,* the preparation of the spermatozoa for fertilization, they must ascend through the uterine cavity into the fallopian tube to meet the ovum.

The female must produce a healthy fertilizable ovum that enters the fallopian tube and becomes fertilized within a period of a few hours. The conceptus must be transported through the tubal lumen to the uterine cavity. There it must implant itself in endometrium that has been prepared to receive it. The embryo then must grow and develop normally.

Human sperm, while capable of existing for long periods of time in the upper genital tract of the female, maintain their fertilization potential for only about 48 hours. It is thought that a healthy ovum can be fertilized for 24 hours.

If any one of these essential processes is defective or impeded, infertility may result.

CAUSES

Although the woman of an infertile couple usually consults the physician first, it is obvious that she is not necessarily totally responsible for infertility. A male factor is either the sole cause or is an important contributing cause in about 30% to 40% of infertile marriages.

Cause of infertility (%)	
Male factor	30
Tubal factor	25
Ovulatory disorder	20
Cervical factor	15
Miscellaneous	5
Unknown	5

On the basis of available literature, these estimates may vary from clinic to clinic. In approximately 15% to 20% of couples several factors are responsible, which increase patient frustration and make therapy more complex.

Faulty spermatogenesis and insemination. Spermatogenesis is a complex and incompletely understood process. Like ovulation, the production of male gametes depends not only on the integration of hormone signals along the hypothalamic-pituitary-gonadal axis, but on the intragonadal hormone action. The intratesticular concentration of androgens and the relationship to specialized androgen-binding proteins is critical. The entire process from the formation of the primitive germ cell to the ejaculation of viable motile sperm takes approximately *3 months. Faulty spermatogenesis* may be the result of a number of congenital or acquired causes that may be apparent after taking a history and performing a physical examination. However, a significant number of infertile males have no clear antecedent information or genital abnormalities that would indicate a cause. About 25% of infertile males will demonstrate *oligospermia* (less than 20 million spermatozoa/ml); the cause is illusive, and therapy in this group of patients is disappointing. If severe oligospermia (less than 5 million sperm/ml), *azoospermia* (no sperm), or *aspermia* (no semen produced) is identified, more extensive assessment should be considered, including appropriate hormone studies, a vasogram, chromosomal analysis, and perhaps testicular biopsy.

A *unilateral or bilateral undescended testis,* regardless of the time of correction, results in semen quality lower than that produced by normal males. *Significant trauma,* which could result in a break in continuity of the testicular tubule structure, can result in the formation of sperm-agglutinating and sperm-immobilizing antibodies. Although *mumps-orchitis* experienced before puberty does not appear to affect spermatogenesis, orchitis after puberty is not unusual and can seriously damage fertility. A history of *infection* such as nonspecific urethritis and chronic prostatitis or *prior genital tract surgery* such as a hydrocelectomy, repair of torsion of a spermatic cord, or herniorrhaphy have all been associated with defective semen production.

Males with *gonadal dysgenesis* (Klinefelter's syndrome) may produce no sperm even though their Leydig cells are normal. *Hypogonadotropic hypogonadism with anosmia* (Kallmann's syndrome) and *severe hypothyroidism* are all associated with azoospermia. Certain medications may have a deleterious effect on sperm production. Males who were exposed to *DES* while in utero may have structural abnormalities of the ejaculatory system, as well as deficient spermatogenesis. *Nitrofurantoin* has been associated with deficient sperm production, and certain medicines to treat hypertension can result in impotence. Excessive use of *alcohol, nicotine,* and *marijuana* can all significantly alter the production of sperm. *Severe pyrexia* has resulted in transient oligospermia. Although great emphasis has been placed on the role of high scrotal temperature induced by constrictive underwear or long, hot baths, it is unlikely that these life habits significantly hamper fertilizing capability of an otherwise normal male. A *varicocele* has been assigned a major etiologic role in infertility. Although it is clear that reduced sperm motility may be observed and ultimately corrected following varicocelectomy, fertility is not necessarily improved. Therefore the etiologic role of the varicocele remains unclear.

Although it is essential that normal spermatozoa be present for fertilization, it is difficult to diagnose infertility accurately on the basis of sperm density alone. MacLeod found in 1951 that 5% of 1000 fertile males had counts of less than 20 million sperm/ml. There have been several additional studies to demonstrate that the normal count of fertile males is declining; the number of fertile males with counts of 20 million sperm/ml is 15% to 20%. The cause and significance of this observation is unclear.

Although sperm density, motility, and morphology are important, a major issue to be addressed is that of sperm function. Simply, can the sperm traverse the female genital tract and fertilize an ovum? *Cervical mucus penetration studies* with the use of bovine cervical mucus are presumed to complement the semen analysis. In 1976 Yanagimachi, Yanagimachi, and Rogers described a method, the *sperm penetration assay,* for evaluating human sperm penetration of specially prepared zona-free hamster ova. Cases have been described in infertile men whose semen analyses were normal but whose spermatozoa penetrated less than 10% of processed hamster ova. Holmes, Lipshultz, and Smith have investigated the possible role of *transferrin* concentrations in seminal fluid as an index of Sertoli cell function. Transferrin concentrations were significantly less in patients with oligospermia than from normospermic individuals.

Faulty sperm transmission can be a cause of infertility. *Impotence* induced by medication or for psychogenic reasons will obviously prohibit pregnancy. The number of spermatozoa and volume of the ejaculate are definitely decreased with *frequent coitus.* Optimum timing that allows for the replenishment of healthy sperm and adequate seminal plasma is approximately 36 to 48 hours. *Severe hypospadias or obstruction* caused by scarring of the epididymus, vas deferens, or urethra following infection may also interfere with insemination; the most frequent organism is *Neisseria gonorrhaeae.* If the penis is abnormally short, buried in fat, or malformed, emission may take place out of the vagina. Premature *ejaculation* may produce the same results. In the female, *dyspareunia, vaginismus,* or an *intact hymen* may prevent intromission and a normal deposition of the ejaculate.

Tubal factor. The fallopian tube is not merely a conduit. Although tubal patency is essential for fertility, the ascent of spermatozoa and the passage of fertilized ova require physiologic support. *Tubal obstruction,* either partial or complete, has been a cause in about 25% of women who fail to conceive. Although tubal closure is more likely caused by endosalpingitis that can be gonoccocal, chlamydial, or polymicrobial in origin, congenital anomalies are also a possibility. Tubal infertility is increased following *appendicitis,* particularly if rupture has taken place; *infection associated with use* of an *intrauterine device;* and pelvic surgery, particularly *ovarian wedge resection.* Peritubal scarring and immobilization of this structure can occur with *endometriosis* or *perisalpingitis* associated with a puerperal infection. Therefore mucosal damage and fimbrial compromise, as well as the kinking and mobilization that occurs from perisalpingeal involvement, can occur following infection.

After a clinically documented episode of salpingitis, a woman has an 11% to 12% chance of being infertile. After two episodes the figure increases to 23%, and after three or more episodes it is 54.3%. It has been estimated that nearly 300,000 women in the United States will be rendered sterile by salpingitis by the year 1990.

Disorders of ovulation. An abnormality of ovulation is responsible for infertility in approximately 20% to 25% of women. The finely orchestrated events resulting in the development of a normal ovum, its periodic extrusion from the follicle, and the cyclic secretion of adequate amounts of estrogen and progesterone by the corpus luteum are essential for normal fertility. In all cases of anovulation or oligo-ovulation, the underlying endocrine disorder has altered the hypothalamic-pituitary-ovarian interrelationship. Women who have complete absence of ovarian function as in *gonadal dysgenesis* or *premature ovarian failure* from whatever cause can be considered to be sterile, but with the possibility of donor ovum transfer they may have children. Although *ovarian androgen excess* (polycystic ovary syndrome) is a relatively common cause of infertility, hypothyroidism is not. *Hyperprolactinemia,* either tumor- or nontumor-related, usually produces anovulation. For a more thorough description of the disorders of ovulation, see Chapter 8. *Luteal phase deficiency* is found in 2% to 3% of infertile couples and has been discussed in Chapter 16.

Luteinized unruptured follicle syndrome (LUF) is an uncommon cause and is characterized by the biochemical events of a normal ovulatory cycle in which the ovum is not extruded from the dominant follicle. This diagnosis is relatively difficult to make except by laparoscopy; no *stigma* can be identified on the follicle that supposedly released an egg. This syndrome has been associated more commonly with endometriosis; the cause is unknown.

Cervical factor. Abnormalities in the structure or the function of the cervix are present in 10% to 15% of infertile couples. *Obstructive lesions of the cervix* such as large polyps, pedunculated leiomyomata, congenital atresia, or stenosis following cauterization or cryotherapy may interfere with ascent of spermatozoa. *Alterations in the cervical mucus* can be the result of a hormonal deficiency, a chronic infection, or medication. It is in the preovulatory cervical mucus that the sperm must undergo the process of *capacitation.* It is believed that *certain bacteria are lethal to spermatozoa. Mycoplasma hominis* infections were once thought to be an important factor in infertility. They are probably more associated with habitual abortion than a failure to conceive. Whether or not *chlamydial* infection plays any role at the level of the endocervix remains to be determined.

As ovulation approaches and the peak of estrogen production is reached, the cervical mucus secretion is increased and can be copious. Occasionally, certain women find this annoying. The mucus is thin and clear and can be drawn into threads 10 to 15 cm long, *spinnbarkheit.* Very few vaginal epithelial or white blood cells can be seen at this time, and if the mucus is allowed to dry on a slide, a pronounced *ferning* pattern is evident. Micellar channels through which sperm ascend are also formed at this point in the cycle. It is this type of mucus that permits maximum sperm survival and penetration that is essential for normal fertility. The cervix not only is a source of cervical mucus production, but forms a *reservoir* in which sperm can live for many hours after deposition and from which they can be dispatched to the upper tract to penetrate an egg. It is this concept of the reservoir that represents the basis for the postcoital test. The physical properties of normal cervical mucus during the menstrual cycle have been described by Moghissi (Fig. 14-1).

Uterine factor. Malformations, malpositions, and tumors of the uterus do not often interfere with conception, but they may occasionally be a factor in faulty nidation and early abortion. Movable, nontender retrodisplacement of the uterus is not often a factor in infertility; most of the time this should be considered a normal finding. *Submucous myomas* may obstruct the uterine ends of the tube and thus prevent fertilization or may distort the uterine cavity and interfere with nidation. Women who have been exposed to *DES* while in utero may have characteristic cervical and uterine deformities that can interfere with conception or lead to abortion or premature labor.

Miscellaneous factors. *Chronic infections, debilitating diseases,* and *severe nutritional deficiencies* may alter the function of both male and female gonads and thus reduce fertility. *Advancing age* also may play a role; in women, fertility reaches a peak between 20 and 30 years of age and then slowly declines until the menopause. Anovulatory

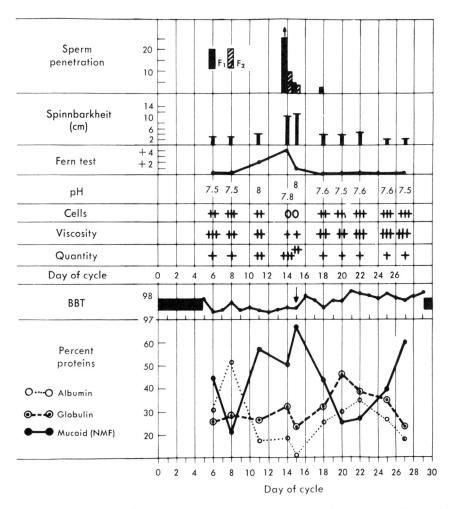

Fig. 14-1. Cyclic changes in cervical mucus. (From Moghissi, K.: Cyclic changes in cervical mucus in normal and progestin-treated women, Fertil. Steril. **17**:663, 1966. Reproduced with the permission of the author and the publisher, The American Fertility Society.)

cycles are common in the premenopausal period.

It has long been recognized that impotence, premature ejaculation, vaginismus, and dyspareunia are likely to be caused by *psychologic disturbances*. More recently our attention has been directed to the possibility of psychogenically induced tubal spasm and anovulatory cycles. Before psychogenic factors can be diagnosed, one must demonstrate conclusively that there are no detectable organic causes. An example is repeated failure to have intercourse during the fertile period because of recurrent minor illness, because the woman or

man is "too tired," or even because of periodic dyspareunia, vaginismus, or impotence. Other causes for impotence have been identified; medicine usage should be reviewed, and a prolactin level should be obtained.

Both men and women develop antibodies against the numerous antigens in seminal fluid and spermatozoa, but the importance of *immunologic factors* has not yet been determined. The fact that antibodies can be detected in serum does not mean that they are responsible for infertility; women with antisperm antibodies in serum do conceive. The antibodies must be present in cervical secretions or in the uterus or fallopian tubes where they can exert a direct influence on spermatozoa. Sperm-immobilizing antibodies are probably more important than are those that cause the sperm to agglutinate. The higher the titer of sperm antibodies, the more plausible the diagnosis of an immune factor becomes. It appears that a small percentage of cases of unexplained infertility may be caused by anti-sperm antibodies.

INVESTIGATION OF THE INFERTILE COUPLE

The investigation of infertility must be conducted systematically, according to a planned program. Since multiple factors are so common, the study of both partners should be carried out in its entirety, even though conditions that obviously would impair fertility are detected early in the investigation. Both husband and wife must be interested in the solution of their problem. The plan of study, the time, and expense involved should be explained to them during the first interview to ensure full cooperation and to prevent future misunderstandings.

The physician must not only be prepared to conduct the basic medical investigation, but be willing to expend the time and energy to deal with the couples' emotional distress. These patients, usually the females more than the males, are frustrated, angry, and depressed. On occasion, psychotherapy should be recommended. The basic studies can usually be completed within 3 or 4 months.

Optimally, the man and the woman should have their initial assessment, including the interview and physical examination, during the first appointment. However, the evaluations can be done separately at different times by a physician who is qualified and interested in the problem of infertility.

A complete history and physical examination of both partners

History. The form on p. 183 is useful in obtaining important information concerning the history of each partner.

Physical examination. A complete general physical examination should be performed on each partner. Evidence of endocrine stigmas such as abnor-

malities of body configuration or of distribution of fat and hair may suggest a cause for the infertility.

WOMAN. A systematic pelvic examination that includes careful inspection and palpation of the structures throughout the entire length of the genital tract ordinarily will indicate the residua of infections or abnormalities in development and growth that may prevent conception.

MAN. Complete physical examination, with a detailed study of the genital organs of the male partner, is essential. One should look particularly for evidence of endocrinopathy, developmental anomalies of the penis, testicular atrophy, and varicocele and for infection in the prostate, seminal vesicles, and urethra. The normal adult male testes shall be more than 4 cm in the largest diameter with a volume of at least 20 ml. The use of an orchidometer is critical to conduct an accurate examination.

Evaluation of the semen

The semen examination is one of the most important parts of the infertility study, since the male is often at least partially responsible for failure to achieve pregnancy. The simple microscopic examination of a drop of semen is utterly inadequate for accurate evaluation of fertility. A complete semen analysis and study of the effects of cervical secretions on sperm motility and survival will provide the basic information necessary for evaluating the male. A single analysis may be inconclusive because the sperm count varies from day to day and is dependent on emotional, physical, and sexual activity. Three specimens at monthly intervals should usually be examined. Previously performed sperm counts, particularly if the details of the analysis are unavailable, must be repeated, since they may not represent the current status of the male partner.

Semen analysis. The specimen should be collected by ejaculation into a clean, wide-mouthed, screw-top plastic or glass jar after masturbation following a 2- or 3-day period of abstinence from intercourse. Couples who cannot accept this method can collect the semen in a specialized condom that has been punctured in several places. A rubber condom should never be used for the collection of semen because both the sheath and the

INFERTILITY HISTORY

Woman

Age: Race: Religion:

Occupation:

Years of marriage: Previous marriage?

Duration of involuntary infertility:

Past history   *Present history*
1. Medical   1. General
   Venereal disease   Habits
   Endometriosis   Diet
   Tumors   Work and health status
   Other medical problems   Menstrual cycle
2. Surgical   2. Sexual
   Pelvic operations   Frequency of coitus
   Appendectomy   Postcoital practices
3. Obstetrics   Libido
   Full-term deliveries—complications 3. Personal
   Abortions or premature delivery   Motivation for childbearing
   Previous infertility evaluation   Attitude toward partner
4. Menstrual history   Career aspirations

Man

Age: Race: Religion:

Occupation:

Years of marriage: Previous marriage?

Past history   *Present history*
1. Medical   1. General
   Venereal infection   Diet
   Mumps orchitis   Habits
   Varicocele   Work and health status
2. Surgical   Medications
   Herniorrhaphy   2. Sexual
   Hydrocele   Frequency of coitus and technique used
   Orchiopexy   Premature ejaculation
   Injury to genitals   Adequacy of erection
                                         Timing of coitus
                                      3. Personal
                                         Motivation for childbearing
                                         Attitude toward partner
                                         Career aspirations

powder on it may be spermicidal. The jar should be tightly capped, and the specimen transported to the laboratory within 1 hour of its emission. No particular precaution need be taken to control the temperature, except that excessive heat and cold should be avoided.

Following are the standards for normal male semen analysis as determined by the World Health Organization:

Volume	2-6 ml
pH	7-8

Viscosity	Liquefaction within 30 minutes
Sperm concentration	20-250 million/ml
Sperm motility	>60% within 1 hour of collection
Mobility (quality of motility)	3-4 +
Morphology	>60% normal oval sperm

In addition, there should be no significant sperm agglutination or pyospermia. Special staining is required to differentiate between leukocytes and immature sperm. As a general guideline, a sample compatible with excellent fertility potential should be of normal volume, have at least 60 million sperm/ml, 60% motility with good mobility, and at least 60% normal morphology. The total number of live sperm in the ejaculate should exceed 100 million sperm/ml. To assess morphology accurately, a slide preparation is made, and the sperm stained by Papanicolaou technique or comparable stain before counting the different forms.

Determination of tubal patency

The usual tests for the study of tubal patency are dependent on the injection of gas or a radiopaque substance through the cervicouterine canal and the tubes into the peritoneal cavity. If properly performed, the tests provide accurate information concerning tubal structure and should, unless contraindicated, be included as a part of every infertility study. The assumption is made that patency is compatible with normal function. However, there may be some discrepancy between the two characteristics.

Tests for patency should never be performed in the presence of acute infections of the vagina, cervix, or tubes or during any episode of uterine bleeding, since at that time the gas or the contrast medium may enter the open blood vessels. If pregnancy is suspected, tests for tubal patency should be delayed until the diagnosis can be definitely eliminated.

Patency tests are best performed 4 to 5 days after the end of a menstrual period. At this time there are no open vessels; the menstrual debris, which might be forced through the tubes and into the peritoneal cavity, has all been discharged; the tubal openings are not occluded by thick secretory endometrium, and there is little chance of pregnancy.

Hysterosalpingography. X-ray film visualizaton of the uterine cavity and tubal lumina after the injection of radiopaque material is the *preferred test* to evaluate the infertile female (Figs. 14-2 and 14-3). With this procedure, the site of tubal obstruction can be located accurately, and valuable information concerning the presence of tubal abnormalities such as hydrosalpinx or fixation from adhesions is provided. It also is possible to demonstrate small submucous fibroids or other congenital or acquired defects that may be present in the uterine cavity. The principal contraindications are genital tract infections, bleeding, and the possibility of pregnancy.

If the hysterosalpingogram is normal, the patient has about a 75% chance of having normal pelvic structures and no peritubal involvement. To replace this valuable test by laparoscopy and dye instillation as a routine initial approach negates the diagnostic effect and the therapeutic value, increases the risk to the patient, and is not cost effective.

Water-soluble media are preferable to oil-soluble types because they are absorbed from the peritoneal cavity rapidly. If there are no other factors preventing conception, pregnancy often follows hysterosalpingography. The tip of the cannula is inserted about 4 mm into the cervical canal, and 1 to 2 ml of the media is injected to fill the normal uterine cavity without distending it. This may outline small irregularities that would be obscured by a larger amount. Additional contrast medium, which should distend the uterus and flow through the tubes, is then injected (Fig. 14-4).

Hysterosalpingography can be controlled more precisely if the injection is made with the help of the *fluoroscope;* the use of an image intensifier reduces the radiation hazard to a minimum.

The Rubin test (the transcervical instillation of CO_2 and subsequent measuring of the pressure caused by the egress, and listening for a characteristic sound produced by the expulsion of CO_2 associated with subdiaphragmatic pain) has been discarded by most physicians who assess fertility. The hysterosalpingogram provides a more accurate assessment of the uterine cavity and the tubes.

Laparoscopy. Direct observation of the passage of methylene blue dye from the uterus through the fimbriated ends of the tubes is possible with the

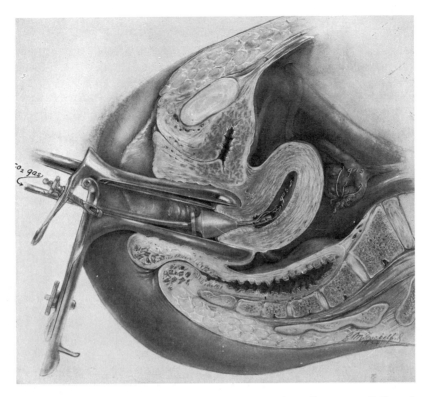

Fig. 14-2. Hysterosalpingography. Sagittal section showing technique. Contrast media flows through intrauterine cannula and out through tubes, the cervix being closed by a rubber stopper. (From Willson, J.R.: Management of obstetric difficulties, ed. 6, St. Louis, 1961, The C.V. Mosby Co.)

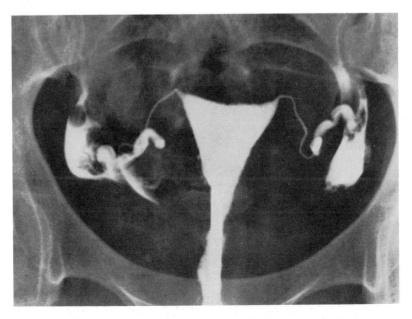

Fig. 14-3. Normal hysterosalpingogram showing passage of radiopaque material through fimbriated ends of tubes.

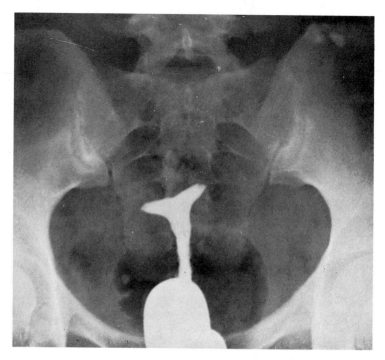

Fig. 14-4. Hysterosalpingogram. Tubes are occluded at cornual ends. (From Willson, J.R.: Management of obstetric difficulties, ed. 6, St. Louis, 1961, The C.V. Mosby Co.)

laparoscope and may be used for the determination of tubal patency by those experienced in the use of the instruments. An added advantage of this method is that it provides an opportunity for direct visualization of the pelvic structures, thus supplementing the other methods for evaluating normalcy.

In order to thoroughly assess the status of other pelvic structures and their relationships, a *dual puncture technique* with a secondary manipulating instrument placed suprapubically must be used.

Laparoscopy is an essential examination in the study of infertile women when there is no obvious cause for failure to conceive. Peterson and Behrman found unsuspected pelvic disease in 60% of 276 infertile women on whom laparoscopy was performed. Endometriosis was found in 33%, pelvic adhesion in 20%, tubal occlusion in 5%, and polycystic ovaries in 2%.

Disorders of ovulation

The production of normal ova and their release from the ovary, and pickup by the fallopian tube are primary requirements for female fertility. Women with menstrual irregularities, those with amenorrhea, and some without evidence of abnormality may not be ovulating. Documentation of when ovulation occurs is an important part of an infertility investigation. The clinical tests used to assess ovulation are indirect and determine more specifically whether or not *progesterone* is secreted in significant concentrations.

Ovulation probably is occurring if the *basal body temperature curve is typically biphasic* with a sustained rise of at least 0.6 F during the last 2 weeks of the cycle (Chapter 2). *Luteal phase deficiency* can be suspected if the thermal rise is maintained for less than 10 days. Basal body temperatures should not be taken for more than three cycles. This is long enough to learn if and when the temperature rise occurs and how long it lasts, which is all one needs to know.

The adequacy of progesterone secretion can be estimated by *an assay of serum progesterone*. At least one and preferably three assays are made between the second day after ovulation is presumed to have occurred and the onset of menses. A midluteal progesterone concentration of at least 2 ng/ml of serum suggests normal luteal function. A concentration of at least 3 ng/ml implies that ovulation has occurred.

Endometrial response to progesterone can be evaluated by determining whether the changes in the glands and stroma correspond to those that are normal for the day the biopsy was taken. Both progesterone secretion and tissue response are normal if endometrium obtained 2 days before the period begins shows normal synchronous maturation. Conversely, progesterone secretion may be inadequate if the tissue changes are *greater than 2 or more days* behind those anticipated. If the interval between the biopsy and the onset of menstruation is shorter than that expected from the histologic changes, progesterone support probably has been withdrawn too soon to provide a normal implantation site for an ovum that may have been fertilized.

It is unlikely that hormonal factors play an important role in infertility in women who ovulate regularly and whose endometria respond normally. Those with symptoms suggesting hypothyroidism, amenorrhea and hirsutism, and stigmas of other endocrine disorders need more extensive study.

Evaluation of the cervical factor

After fertility potential in the husband has been established by semen analysis, it becomes necessary to determine the effect of the vaginal and cervical secretions on the activity of the sperm. Spermatozoa can penetrate the cervical mucus during a period of only 24 to 72 hours in the entire menstrual cycle. This occurs in the ovulatory phase of the cycle when the mucus is copious, thin, and watery and exhibits maximal *spinnbarkheit* and arborization.

The *postcoital examination of cervical mucus (Sims-Huhner test)* provides information concerning the number of spermatozoa that have entered the cervical canal and the percentage that retain their motility in the cervical mucus, but it gives minimal information regarding the adequacy of the semen specimen. It is therefore not a substitute for semen analysis. It is essential that the postcoital test be performed when the secretions should be optimal for sperm penetration and survival; the day before ovulation is most appropriate. The test can only be correctly interpreted by examining the basal body temperature chart at the end of the cycle to ascertain that the timing of the examination was appropriate.

The patient is instructed to report for examination about 6 hours after coitus without having used a precoital lubricant or a postcoital douche. At least 2 days' abstinence before the test is desirable. The cervix is exposed through an unlubricated speculum, and the portio is wiped clean with saline-moistened cotton balls. Endocervical mucus is aspirated through a small plastic suction catheter or a tuberculin syringe. Negative pressure is applied as the catheter is inserted through the external os and is continued as the catheter is slowly advanced until the tip reaches the internal os. At this point the catheter is clamped and withdrawn. The material is examined for clarity, viscosity, and *spinnbarkheit*, and the pH is determined. The specimen is then spread on a clean glass slide and examined for the presence of sperm and, after it has dried, for arborization of the mucus.

The cervical reaction is clearly normal if there are 10 or more highly motile spermatozoa in mucus obtained from the uppermost part of the canal. One should repeat the test if it is not definitely normal. The most common explanation for a poor postcoital examination is the fact that the specimen is obtained at the wrong time.

TREATMENT

The treatment of infertility often begins with the first consultation, although no specific therapeutic program can be outlined until all data obtained from the complete investigation of the couple have been analyzed and correlated. A significant percentage of women conceive after the initial visit or after assessment of tubal patency; Grant reported "spontaneous" cures of primary infertility in 35% of 1415 patients. Similar results were obtained in 1166 women with secondary infertility.

Such a favorable outcome early in the investigation may be credited to helpful hints regarding the technique and timing of coitus or to the correction of a minor abnormality. However, it actually may be because of the psychotherapeutic effect of either the decision to deal with the problem actively or because of the positive transference reaction to the physician.

In general the active treatment of infertility must be directed to the factors that the investigative procedures have indicated to be responsible for the failure to conceive.

Failure of insemination. Obvious abnormalities such as an intact hymen, developmental defects, or obesity should be corrected if possible. If failure of insemination occurs because of penile abnormalities, therapeutic insemination with the husband's semen should be considered. Impotence, vaginismus, and dyspareunia are seldom of organic origin; and psychotherapy usually is necessary for their correction. Faulty sexual techniques can be corrected by discussing the coital technique with both partners and suggesting necessary modifications.

The *time at which ovulation occurs* can be estimated after the basal body temperatures have been recorded for two or three cycles. It is presumed that ovulation occurs as the temperature is falling or at the low point on the graph, since the subsequent thermal rise is a result of progesterone. If the length of the cycle is reasonably constant and if the fall in temperature occurs consistently at the same relative time, the fertile period can be calculated in advance each month without continuing the temperature recordings. The number of days between the low point preceding the thermal rise and the actual onset of menstruation is counted and subtracted from the date that menstruation presumably will begin. This will be the anticipated day of ovulation.

Coitus every 48 hours during the period starting 3 days before and ending 2 days after ovulation is anticipated should cover minor deviations from the expected ovulatory pattern. If temperatures are being recorded, the couple should have intercourse on the day the temperature falls and the day after.

Frequency of intercourse should be drastically limited if the sperm count is low, since emissions at 24-hour intervals greatly reduce the number of motile forms, thus further decreasing fertility. Ejaculation every other day affects the count less, and little change can be detected at 3-day intervals.

Failure of spermatogenesis because of *destructive testicular disease* cannot be improved, and the inability to transport the sperm because of *occlusion in the ductal system* is difficult to correct surgically. *Oligospermia* can sometimes be improved by thyroid therapy if decreased thyroid function is the responsible factor, but other endocrine preparations, with the possible exception of clomiphene, are usually ineffectual in stimulating spermatogenesis. Any *documented infection* of the male reproductive system should receive appropriate antibiotic therapy.

Failure in ascent of sperm. If *infection* is present, it must be treated because the vaginal and cervical secretions are altered by the inflammatory response and may become lethal for the sperm.

Cervical infections should be eradicated, and the cervix returned to as normal a state as possible. The treatment of benign disease of the cervix is discussed in Chapter 46.

Viscous cervical mucus, which can interfere with the ascent of the sperm through the cervical canal, may be the result of a diminished effect or production of estrogen. The administration of oral estrogen daily from the fifth to the twelfth day of the cycle may decrease the viscosity of the cervical secretions; but if the primary defect lies in the ovary, pregnancy cannot be expected to occur. Large dosages of estrogenic substance early in the preovulatory phase may delay or even prevent ovulation. Estrogen should not be given after the day of ovulation because of possible effects on the fetus if conception occurs.

THERAPEUTIC INSEMINATION. Therapeutic or artificial insemination refers to the artificial injection of semen into the cervical canal. It is termed *homologous* insemination (AIH) if the husband's semen is used and *heterologous* insemination (AID) if the semen is from a donor other than the husband.

Homologous insemination is indicated if the husband is normally fertile but is unable to ejaculate the semen over the cervix because of obesity or a penile defect or if a cervical abnormality appears to prevent the invasion of a sufficient number of sperm. AIH for oligospermia may sometimes initiate a pregnancy. Heterologous insemination may be appropriate if the husband's infertility has been proved to be irremediable. Neither type of insemination should be considered unless a complete study of the female partner proves her to be free from defects that might be partially responsible for the failure to conceive and without the expressed written consent of both partners.

Insemination with the husband's semen presents no legal problem, but heterologous insemination involves a great many emotional, ethical, legal, and religious considerations. If the male partner is solely responsible for the failure to conceive, the couple can be offered adoption, insemination, or in vitro fertilization in selected cases.

Therapeutic insemination must be timed to coincide with the ovulatory phase of the cycle. One can determine the appropriate time for insemination on the basis of several cycles of basal body temperatures and the daily examination of cervical mucus.

Healthy donors with a blood type compatible with that of the infertile husband should be selected.

Donors should be screened thoroughly for infection, including lymphotropic virus III, chlamydia, and other sexually transmitted diseases. A complete genetic history and physical examination are necessary. Routine karyotyping is not productive and is unnecessary. Fresh ejaculate is preferable for donor insemination because of a higher percentage of pregnancies, 75% to 85% after 6 months. Although frozen ejaculate can be purchased commercially, the specimens are more costly, and the number of pregnancies is less, 30% to 66% after six cycles.

Tubal abnormalities. Although restoration of tubal patency is equated with restoring tubal function, that is not necessarily the case. Attempts to force open diseased and damaged tubes with the use of contrast media, antibiotic preparations, or adrenal cortical substances have been uniformly unsuccessful and place the patient at risk for developing a serious tubal infection. Surgical procedures are preferred, but the results are not spectacular. The outcome of *tuboplasty* is determined by the cause of the occlusion, the extent of the damage, and the experience of the surgeon. It is easier to restore function in tubes that have been occluded by a sterilizing operation, *tubal reversal,* than in those that have been damaged by infection. With the use of microsurgical techniques, reversal of steriliza-

tion can result in pregnancy rates as high as 65%. Before repair of the fallopian tubes with damage secondary to infection and scarring, a diagnostic laparoscopy will be helpful in identifying the extent of the disease and will establish the likelihood of a successful repair. Fertility may also be restored by freeing tubes that have been immobilized by peritubal adhesions as part of the treatment of endometriosis. If pregnancy occurs following tubal surgery, the patient should be monitored closely since her chances of having a tubal pregnancy are increased.

Disorders of ovulation. Women who have ovarian failure, as evidenced by at least two serum FSH levels in the menopausal range, are sterile. Such patients would include those with *gonadal dysgenesis* (Turner's syndrome) and *premature ovarian failure*. There is no known way to restore ovarian function. Ultimately, it should be possible to use an ovum donor and the partner's ejaculate and, after in vitro fertilization, effect zygote transfer into the patient's uterus, which has been appropriately stimulated by estrogen and progesterone. Women who are oligomenorrheic or amenorrheic should be thoroughly evaluated before the institution of any therapy. The assessment is discussed in detail in the chapters relating to menstruation and its abnormalities. The correction of *hyperprolactinemia* with bromocriptine mesylate (Parlodel), a dopamine anagonist, restores ovulation in more than 80% of cases.

More often the cause of the ovulatory disturbance is related to hypothalamic-pituitary dysfunction, and *clomiphene citrate* is the initial drug of choice. This latter medication creates a "message" of estrogen deficiency at the level of the hypothalamus by preventing the replenishment of estrogen receptors and activates the negative feedback relationship between estrogen and gonadotropins. Because of the perceived reduction in estradiol, GnRH is secreted, stimulating the release of FSH and LH.

Clomiphene is available as a 50 mg tablet (Clomid or Serophene) and is administered initially 5 days each cycle following uterine bleeding occurring spontaneously or induced by progesterone. Most of the pregnancies occur after three consecutive ovulatory cycles, and the incidence of side effects is low. This medicine should not be used in women who have hepatic disease and should be discontinued in those who experience scotomata and severe ovarian hyperstimulation while taking the preparation.

Clomiphene is of minimal value in women who are estrogen deficient. If a pregnancy does not occur within three to six ovulatory cycles, other fertility factors should be assessed or reassessed. Individuals with *polycystic ovarian syndrome* (PCO) are often hyperresponsive to clomiphene, and a smaller dose of the medication may be required initially to induce ovulation. *Ovarian wedge resection* may result in ovulatory cycles in patients with polycystic ovarian disease who have not responded to clomiphene.

Improvement in general health and achievement of optimum weight by the patient, whether she is obese or has weight loss–associated ovulatory dysfunction, will favorably influence anovulatory cycles. Those individuals with thyroid, adrenal, and other endocrinopathies that have resulted in anovulation will normalize following appropriate corrective therapy of that specific disease.

Luteal phase defects can be treated by supplementing the deficiency of progesterone. Some clinicians use clomiphene because enhancing follicular development will result in normal corpus luteum function and progesterone output. Other individuals prefer *progesterone vaginal suppositories,* 25 mg twice a day, or *progesterone in oil,* 12.5 mg intramuscularly once a day. Treatment is started 1 to 2 days after ovulation and is continued until menstruation. If bleeding does not occur, one should order a serum pregnancy test. If the test is positive, progesterone therapy should be continued until the trophoblast assumes responsibility for progesterone production.

As a general rule, individuals who do not respond to clomiphene therapy are candidates for *menotropin therapy* (Pergonal), which contains equivalent amounts of FSH and LH, 75 IU per ampule, and is administered parenterally. This medication is expensive and needs to be monitored closely by individuals familiar with reproductive disorders and experienced with its usage. Human chorionic gonadotropin is administered to simulate the LH surge after the ovarian follicles are stimulated and a dominant follicle is developed. Ovarian hyperstimulation, multiple pregnancies, and an increased number of spontaneous abortions are a few of the complications. Before instituting this therapy, other causes of infertility should have been eliminated.

Miscellaneous. *Uterine myomas* are rarely responsible for the failure to conceive, and myomectomy is seldom indicated to improve fertility. If the myomas obstruct the cornual ends of the tubes or distort the endometrial cavity, removal should be considered if no other cause of infertility can be found. *Myomectomy* alone is valueless if other causes of infertility remain uncorrected. *Congenital fusion defects* of the müllerian system, that is, bicornuate and septate uterus, rarely cause infertility; spontaneous abortion and premature labor are more characteristic problems of these developmental anomalies. However, it is reasonable to consider *metroplasty,* a uterine reconstruction, if no other cause of infertility can be identified. It must be remembered, though, that approximately 10% of women with a uterine anomaly will have a luteal phase defect and that this should be excluded before any surgery is performed.

Infertility caused by development of *antisperm antibodies* does not occur often. The mere identification of the antibodies does not necessarily require therapy; they should be consistently present in high concentrations. Condom therapy for several months has been shown to reduce antibody concentrations but has not necessarily resulted in a greater number of pregnancies than in those individuals who are left untreated. Cyclic *corticosteroid therapy* for the male or female who is producing antisperm antibodies has resulted in higher pregnancy rates.

Although *in vitro fertilization* and *embryo transfer* (IVF-ET) is a form of therapy that was initially developed to treat women with obstructive tubal disease, it is clear that the indications are expanding. In some IVF centers severe oligospermia, disorders of ovulation, immune infertility, and unexplained fertility are considered reasonable indications after all other therapies have failed.

Emotional care. Couples with an infertility problem usually are depressed, anxious, and have decreased libido. Referral to a counselor, an appropriate support group, or RESOLVE (a national lay group that provides information and support to couples with infertility problems) and, occasionally, psychotherapy will be helpful. Although it is obvious to the practitioner that the couple is under significant stress during the fertility evaluation, the distress does not seem to have any bearing on the couple's ability to function as parents when pregnancy is achieved.

Although adoption remains a theoretic option, the number of available infants is small; thus other therapeutic modalities should be pursued as long as it is emotionally and financially feasible for the couple to do so. When it becomes apparent that all options have been eliminated, the physician has an obligation to recommend that the evaluation or therapy be discontinued and to work through this difficult time with the couple, seeking outside support if necessary. Couples who have no obvious cause for infertility still have a chance for a spontaneous conception in spite of the failure to identify a specific cause.

When pregnancies do occur, the female should be monitored carefully, since she is at great risk for spontaneous abortion, tubal pregnancy, premature labor, and perhaps perinatal mortality.

REFERENCES

Andrews, W.C.: Luteal phase defects, Fertil. Steril. **32**:501, 1979.

Babaknia, A., Rock, J.A., and Jones, H.W., Jr.: Pregnancy success following abdominal myomectomy for infertility, Fertil. Steril. **30**:644, 1978.

Beer, A.E., and Neaves, W.B.: Antigenic status of semen from the viewpoints of the female and male, Fertil. Steril. **29**:3, 1978.

Blasco, L.: Clinical approach to the evaluation of sperm-cervical mucus interactions, Fertil. Steril. **28**:1133, 1977.

Edmonds, D.K., Lindsay, K.S., Miller, J.F., Williamson, E., and Wood, P.J.: Early embryonic mortality in women, Fertil. Steril. **38**:447, 1982.

Grant, A.: Spontaneous cure rate of various infertility factors or post hoc and propter hoc, J. Obstet. Gynecol. **9**:224, 1969.

Holmes, S.D., Lipshultz, L.I., and Smith, R.G.: Transferrin and gonadal dysfunction in man, Fertil. Steril. **38**:600, 1982.

Jones, W.R.: The investigation of immunological infertility, Med. J. Aust. **2**:188, 1979.

Karahasanoglu, A., Barglow, P., and Growe, G.: Psychological aspects of infertility, J. Reprod.Med. **9**:241, 1972.

Katayama, K.P., Ju, K.S., Manuel, M., Jones, G.S., and Jones, H.W., Jr.: Computer analysis of etiology and pregnancy rate in 636 cases of primary infertility, Am. J. Obstet. Gynecol. **135**:207, 1979.

Mattox, John H.: Female infertility, J. Fam. Pract. **15**:533, 1982.

MacLeod, J., and Gold, R.Z.: The male factor in fertility and infertility. II. Spermatazoon counts in 1000 men of known fertility and in 1000 cases of infertile marriages, J. Urol. **66**:436, 1951.

Moghissi, K.: Cyclic changes in cervical mucus in normal and progestin-treated women, Fertil. Steril. **17**:663, 1966.

Naghma-E-Rehan, Sobrero, A.J., and Fertig, J.W.: The semen in fertile men: statistical analysis of 1300 men, Fertil. Steril. **26**:492, 1975.

Peterson, E.P., and Behrman, S.J.: Laparoscopy of the infertile patient, Obstet. Gynecol. **36**:363, 1970.

Rubin, I.C.: Uterotubal Insufflation, St. Louis, 1947, The C.V. Mosby Co.

Sherins, R.J., Brightwell, D., and Sternthal, P.M.: Longitudinal analysis of semen of fertile and infertile males. In Troen P., and Nankin, H., editors: New concepts of the testis in normal and infertile males, New York, 1977, Raven Press.

Timmons, M.C., Rao, K.W., Sloan, C.S., Kirkman, H.N., and Talbert, L.M.: Genetic screening of donors for artificial insemination, Fertil. Steril. **35**:451, 1981.

Verp, M.S., Cohen, M.R., and Simpson, J.L.: Necessity of formal genetic screening in artificial insemination by donor, Obstet. Gynecol. **62**:474, 1983.

Westrom, L.: Incidence, prevalence, and trends of acute pelvic inflammatory disease and its consequences in industrialized countries, Am. J. Obstet. Gynecol. **138**:880, 1980.

Yanagimachi, R., Yanagimachi, H., and Rogers, B.J.: The use of zona-free animal ova as a test-system for the assessment of the fertilizing capacity of human spermatozoa, Biol. Reprod. **15**:471, 1976.

15

J. Robert Willson

Family planning

There is little to indicate that uncomplicated pregnancy and delivery are harmful to normal women, but one cannot logically conclude that uncontrolled reproduction is desirable. The increasing social and economic demands, at both individual and community levels, make it essential that each couple reach a logical decision as to when pregnancy is appropriate and the number of children for which they can assume responsibility. Physicians, family-planning clinics, and governmental social agencies share the responsibility for making effective and appropriate contraceptive methods available to those who want them.

Physicians should always bring up the subject of contraception during premarital examinations, when they are consulted by young married couples, during any gynecologic examination, after each delivery, and with patients near the menopause. Some women hesitate to ask about contraception even though fear of pregnancy is a constant concern and a source of marital discord. Unless the subject is introduced by the physician, these problems may remain unresolved.

Physicians who choose not to provide contraception for their patients should refer them to another physician or to an agency for this essential service.

CONTRACEPTION IN TEENAGERS

A perplexing problem being encountered with increasing frequency is the teenager who seeks contraceptive advice. The importance of responding to these requests is suggested by the fact that over half of unmarried 19-year-old women are sexually active and that more than 1 million pregnancies occur every year in women between the ages of 15 and 19. Many teenagers use no contraception; in one study more than a third had used no contraceptive method during their last coital experiences.

It is difficult to ignore one's personal biases when dealing with teenage sexuality. Regardless of one's beliefs, however, such requests cannot logically be handled by a curt refusal even to consider the problem. One should learn as much as possible about the circumstances that lead to the request for contraception. Some young girls may be confused by the pressures being put on them by their peers who are already sexually active. They may be asking for help in understanding and resisting the pressures rather than for contraceptive counseling. Others who already are having intercourse need a reliable contraceptive method. It takes a great deal of courage for a young girl to ask a physician for contraception. Many feel guilty but are wise enough to want to avoid the problems inherent in pregnancy. A cold refusal, particularly when accompanied by a moralistic lecture, will be so embarrasing that many will not risk exposing themselves to similar experiences by consulting another physician. The inevitable result is preventable pregnancies.

An affirmative response to a request for contraception without exploring the relationship in some detail is also inadequate. Many girls who ask for contraceptive advice are really seeking help for the total problem. In fact the real reason for the request sometimes is that she has not yet had coitus and is being pressured to a point that she feels she must comply.

Although a 1983 Supreme Court ruling stated that minors do not need parental consent to obtain contraceptive counseling through federally funded services, there are times when it is appropriate to include parents in the decision. It is unnecessary for young women in their late teens. On the other hand, the parents of young teenagers who seek contraceptive advice should be involved. Before approaching the parents, however, one must learn all one can about the girl and her need for contraception and be ready to support her in the solution of the problem.

There is no ready answer to teenage contraception. The solution is determined by the individual problem, which will never be clarified if the physician either complies with the request or denies it without exploring the situation.

CONTRACEPTIVE METHODS

There are many contraceptive methods, ranging from relatively simple forms to operative procedures that interrupt the continuity of the fallopian tubes or of the ductus deferens. No single method is uniformly satisfactory, and the physician must be familiar with several types so that individual couples can select the one best suited to their needs after analyzing all the factors involved. Zatuchni has illustrated the factors involved in selecting a contraceptive method (Fig. 15-1).

The effectiveness of any contraceptive method is determined by its usage. *Theoretic effectiveness* refers to the protection offered by a technique under laboratory conditions or when it is used perfectly by a human couple. *Use effectiveness* refers to the protection offered to large groups of couples, many of whom may use the method carelessly or irregularly.

High use effectiveness is determined by the theoretical effectiveness of the method, how appropriate it is for an individual couple, how important it is that they prevent pregnancy, and how consistently the method is used. A method that is too difficult or complicated for a couple to use or one that is unacceptable for one reason or another will have low use effectiveness. In contrast, use effectiveness is high in couples who are strongly motivated to prevent pregnancy and who are using an effective method that is acceptable to both partners.

The use effectiveness for any contraceptive method can be calculated by determining the number of pregnancies per 100 years by use of *Pearl's formula*, which permits comparison of methods:

$$\text{Pregnancy rate}/100 \text{ yrs} = \frac{\text{Total number of conceptions} \times 1200}{\text{Total months of exposure}}$$

For example, if 100 couples use a method for a total of 3600 months and 12 pregnancies occur, the pregnancy rate is 4:

$$\frac{12 \times 1200}{3600} = \frac{14,400}{3600} = 4/100 \text{ yrs}$$

In general, contraceptive methods can be divided into (1) physiologic, (2) chemical, (3) barrier, (4) intrauterine, (5) hormonal, and (6) surgical. All attempt to prevent the union of the sperm and ovum or to interfere with nidation.

Physiologic contraception

In physiologic contraception no chemical or mechanical device is used. The two methods are coitus interruptus and avoiding coitus during the period of greatest fertility.

Coitus interruptus (withdrawal). The penis is withdrawn from the vagina just before ejaculation occurs. This method does not afford maximum protection because fertilization can occur if live sperm are present in the seminal fluid that leaks from the urethra during coitus and if the withdrawal is delayed so that part of the semen is discharged within the vagina.

Coitus interruptus is the oldest and probably the most frequently used contraceptive method throughout the world. It has been used extensively in many European countries in which birthrates have been low for years and in which other methods have not been readily available. If properly used, the pregnancy rate can be kept low, but the average is probably about 16 pregnancies/100 years of use.

Natural family planning (rhythm or safe period). Couples who use natural family planning prevent conception by confining coitus to the phases of the menstrual cycle during which conception is unlikely to occur.

The human ovum can be fertilized no later than 24 to 48 hours after it is extruded from the ovary. Although motile spermatozoa have been recovered from the uterus and the oviducts as long as 60 hours after coitus, their ability to fertilize the ovum probably lasts no longer than 24 to 48 hours. Pregnancy is unlikely to occur if a couple refrains from intercourse for 4 days before and for 3 or 4 days after ovulation *(fertile period)*. Unprotected intercourse on the other days of the cycle *(safe period)* should not result in pregnancy. The principal problems with natural family planning are that the exact

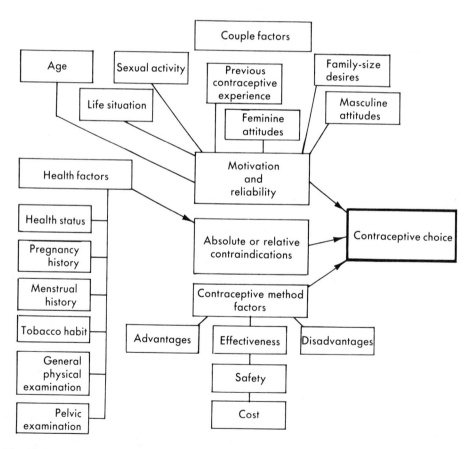

Fig. 15-1. Factors involved in selection of contraceptive method. (Modified from Zatuchni, G.I.: The Female Patient 3(5):48, 1978.)

time of ovulation cannot be predicted accurately and that couples may find it difficult to exercise restraint for several days before and after ovulation.

Ovulation usually occurs about 14 days (12 to 16) before the onset of menstruation. Therefore variations in the length of menstrual cycles are usually a result of differences in the lengths of the preovulatory phases. The fertile period can be anticipated by calculating the time at which ovulation is likely to occur by the length of the menstrual cycles *(calendar method)*, by recording the rise in basal body temperature caused by the thermogenic effect of progesterone *(temperature method)*, by recognizing the changes in cervical mucus at different phases of the cycle *(ovulation method)*, or by combinations of all three.

With the *calendar method* the fertile period is determined after accurately recording the number of days of a menstrual cycle for a year. According to the Ogino formula the first unsafe day (beginning of the fertile period) can be determined by subtracting 18 days from the length of the shortest cycle and the last unsafe day (beginning of postovulatory safe period) by subtracting 11 days from the length of the longest cycle. For example, the fertile period for a woman with 27- to 30-day cycles, extends from the ninth to the nineteenth day, and for one with 25- to 35-day cycles, from the seventh to the twenty-fourth day of each cycle (Fig. 15-2). Pregnancy rates as high as 20 to 30/100 years of use have been reported when the calendar method is used alone.

With the *ovulation method* couples are taught to recognize the characteristic changes in cervical mucus at the different stages of the menstrual cycle. Observations are made on secretions that are collected by wiping the vaginal introitus daily with white toilet tissue. During the first few days after menstruation there is little discharge and the introitus is dry. As estrogen stimulation increases, the secretions become sticky and cloudy. Ovu-

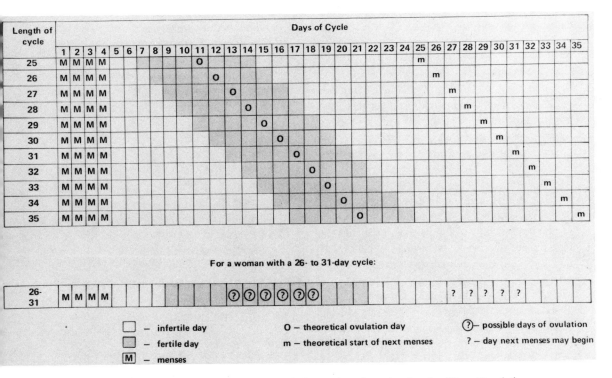

Fig. 15-2. Day of ovulation and fertile period during cycles of varying length. (From Population Reports: Periodic abstinence, series 1, no. 1, Baltimore, June 1974, Population Information Program, The Johns Hopkins University.)

lation occurs soon after the peak estrogen production, when the mucus at the introitus is abundant, clear, thin, and watery. Progesterone reduces mucus secretion, and that which is present is scant and sticky. Infertile days include those during and shortly after menstruation when the introitus is dry and those starting 3 or 4 days after ovulation when the vulva again becomes dry.

Couples should not engage in coitus after tacky mucus is first recognized and until the watery discharge characteristic of ovulation disappears. Although this method provides greater protection than does the calendar method, the average pregnancy rate may be as high as 15 to 20/100 yrs of use.

The *temperature method* is based on refraining from intercourse from the end of menstruation until 4 days after the ovulatory rise. Although this method requires the recording of basal body temperatures, at least from the tenth day until after the thermogenic shift, and a considerable amount of restraint, pregnancy rates as low as those for the best conventional methods have been reported.

Those who are unwilling to refrain from coitus during the preovulatory period can use both the ovulation and the temperature methods. This affords less protection than does postovulatory coitus alone, but it probably is better than the calendar method.

Natural family planning is satisfactory for those who cannot use other methods and for those who are planning more pregnancies sometime in the future. It is not certain enough for those in whom pregnancy must be prevented.

Chemical contraception

The chemical methods of contraception consist of the deposition of a spermicidal substance in the vagina before coitus. This material coats the vaginal wall and the cervix and collects in the fornices, thus exposing the spermatozoa to its destructive action.

This method in general affords better protection than does the calendar rhythm method but less than condoms and diaphragm with contraceptive jelly. Pregnancy rates as low as 2 and high as 39/100 yrs have been reported. The average is probably about 15 to 20.

Aerosol foams, which contain spermicidal chemicals, provide protection as good as condoms pro-

vide if they are used properly and consistently. According to Ryder, however, unintended pregnancies occurred in 31% of women using foam. The protection can be increased almost to that provided by oral contraceptives by using both a condom and aerosol foam during the few days before and after ovulation and foam alone the rest of the month.

Contraceptive sponges made of polyurethane saturated with a spermicidal substance, nonoxynol-9, were introduced in the United States in 1983. It was hoped that the barrier provided by the sponge and the additional protection from the spermicide would increase the efficacy of chemical contraception. Unfortunately, this has not proved to be true. Pregnancy rates in the United States, Canada, and the United Kingdom have varied between 16.8 and 27.3/100 women after 1 year of use. There have been several reported cases of *toxic shock syndrome* associated with the use of contraceptive sponges, but the risk seems to be slight.

Other chemical methods include the use of *foaming tablets* and *suppositories.* Neither is as effective as are aerosol foams or spermicidal jellies and creams.

An advantage of spermicidal contraception is that it appears to reduce the risk of gonococcal infections. Austin, Louv, and Alexander reported the relative risk of spermicidal users contracting gonorrhea to be 0.67 as compared with those who used no protection.

Although there has been some fear that spermicides increase the risk of spontaneous abortion and congenital malformations, Bracken's review of the available epidemiologic studies indicates that no such association exists.

Postcoital douches offer no protection against conception. Large numbers of spermatozoa enter the cervix within a few seconds after ejaculation, and there is no way they can be removed by a vaginal douche.

Barrier contraception

Before oral contraceptives were developed, the most frequently prescribed method was a combination of an *occlusive vaginal diaphragm* and a *spermicidal jelly.* A diaphragm is a dome-shaped rubber cup with a flexible rim. It fits in the vagina with its anterior edge behind the pubic bone, its lateral edges against the vaginal walls, and its posterior edge against the posterior vaginal fornix. The cervix is covered by the diaphragm, and the external os rests in a pool of spermicidal jelly, which immobilizes any spermatozoa that get past the barrier (Fig. 15-3).

It is necessary that the physician fit the diaphragm, instruct the patient in its use, and make certain, by having her return with the diaphragm in place after practicing using it at home, that she can insert it properly. For many women the insertion of a diaphragm is distasteful and too much trouble, but for those who use one regularly and properly, a diaphragm offers protection. The diaphragm must be inserted before intercourse and left in place at least 6 hours after ejaculation.

The theoretic effectiveness of this method should be comparable to that of the intrauterine device (1.5 to 3 pregnancies/100 years), and for motivated couples it is. The general use effectiveness, however, is much less; that is, between 10 and 20 pregnancies/100 years. The principal reasons for failure are inconsistent use, improper insertion, improper size, and displacement during coitus caused by expansion of the upper vagina.

Possible *side effects* in diaphragm users are irritation from the spermicidal cream or jelly and an increased incidence of urinary tract infections.

The *condom* is a common form of barrier contraceptive that offers good protection but has a number of disadvantages. It may break or slip off the penis, and it dulls sensation. It provides better protection when used in conjunction with a vaginal spermicidal jelly. The pregnancy rate with condoms can be as low as 1 to 3 pregnancies/100 years of use, but the general rate is about 15. The reasons for failure are inconsistent use, leakage of semen if the condom is put on late in coitus or as the deflated penis is withdrawn, and breakage.

The regular use of barrier methods should reduce the chance of contracting gonorrhea. To accomplish this it is essential that the condom be used throughout the entire act and that there be no unprotected contact with the female genitals.

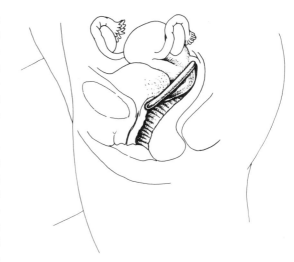

Fig. 15-3. Occlusive contraceptive diaphragm in place.

Intrauterine devices

The prototype intrauterine device (IUD) was the German silver Graefenberg ring, which was first used during the 1920s. The method was abandoned by most physicians because the rings caused ulceration of the uterine wall and infection.

In 1959 Oppenheimer reported on his use of a silkworm gut coil that effectively prevented conception with few ill effects. Since then several different plastic devices have been developed and used successfully. They are inserted into the uterine cavity and are allowed to remain in place, offering constant protection against pregnancy without need for preparing for each individual coital act. Most IUDs have a fine plastic thread that protrudes through the cervix into the vagina.

Unfortunately, IUDs are no longer available in the United States. Although the Food and Drug Administration has not withdrawn approval, manufacturers have discontinued making them because of escalating cost of defending law suits brought against them. One company (Searle), for example, spent 1.5 million dollars in the successful defense of four suits brought because of presumed injury related to the use of their Cu-7 device.

The uterus repeatedly expels the device in about 10% of women; and in another 10% to 15% it is removed because of spotting, increased menstruation, cramping, or a vague concern over the presence of a foreign body in the uterus. The continuation rate is about 70% to 80% at the end of 1 year and about 60% to 70% at the end of 2 years.

Complications that occur most often are intermenstrual spotting, increased menstrual bleeding, increased cramping during menstruation, perforation of the uterus, and infection. Because of increased bleeding, most women using IUDs should take iron regularly, and the hemoglobin should be checked periodically. *Cramping* can usually be controlled with ordinary analgesics or with prostaglandin inhibitors. Women who have had severe dysmenorrhea that was relieved by oral contraceptives will usually not continue using an IUD unless the pain can be controlled.

Perforation of the uterus probably occurs during the insertion of the device. It is unlikely that an IUD that is properly placed in the uterus will erode through the wall and enter the peritoneal cavity. The perforation may be *incomplete*, with the tip of the device protruding through the serosa and its proximal end in the uterine cavity. The tail can usually be seen coming through the cervix. Uterine contractions may eventually expel the device into the peritoneal cavity. With *complete perforation* the tip of the inserter is pushed through the uterine wall, and the device is inserted into the peritoneal cavity. Although the tail may be visible immediately after the insertion, it usually will be pulled upward as the IUD moves about.

If the tail of an intrauterine device that once was visible can no longer be seen, the device has been expelled through the cervix, it has entered the peritoneal cavity, or the tail has been drawn upward into the uterine cavity. If the device is still in the uterus, it can be located by probing the uterus, by sonography, or by a lateral x-ray film study after another IUD has been inserted or with a metal probe in the uterus. If the device is in the peritoneal cavity, it cannot be felt with the probe, and the x-ray film will demonstrate its extrauterine position as related to the second IUD or the probe. Intraperitoneal IUDs should be removed.

Perforation can almost always be prevented by careful selection of patients, care during insertion, and experience. Perforation is more likely to occur with insertion during the first 6 to 8 weeks after delivery than after the tenth.

Most *infections* are mild and localized to the uterus and the adjacent parametrium. Infection may develop soon after the device has been inserted, but more characteristically it does not appear for several months. The patient with a localized infection usually experiences low abdominal discomfort, dyspareunia, thin vaginal discharge, and perhaps low-grade fever for as long as 2 to 3 weeks. The uterus and parametria may be tender, suggesting a low-grade endometritis and cellulitis. In more severe infections, salpingitis may develop. Tubal infections related to the presence of an IUD are often unilateral in contrast to gonococcal tuboovarian abscess that usually affect both tubes. Rarely, an overwhelming bacteremia may appear soon after insertion, and this can be lethal.

The incidence of infection varies with the socioeconomic class of the user and with the number of sexual partners. Willson, Ledger, and Lovell found that 1.3% of 706 private patients who were using Lippes Loops developed infections. Of the nine, two were caused by gonorrhea and cannot be related to the device. In contrast, 8% of 623 women of the lowest socioeconomic classes developed infections; many of these were of gonococcal origin. Sandmire and Cavanaugh inserted 1504 IUDs in private patients. The infection rates per 100 years of use were one for Lippes Loops, two for copper 7's, and 2.3 for Dalkon shields. One can assume that most private patients are more likely to be monogamous and less exposed to sexually transmitted diseases than are those with many partners.

Actinomycosis colonization has been demonstrated in women using IUDs. Valicenti and co-workers report a prevalence of *Actinomyces israelii* in 1.6% of the general population and 5.3% of clinic patients who were using IUDs. No organisms were identified in women not using this type of contraception. The infections were usually local and occurred after several years of using the device. When actinomycosis is identified, the device should be removed, and the smear repeated after a menstrual period. An IUD can be reinserted after the organisms can no longer be identified.

About 50% of *intrauterine pregnancies* that occur with an IUD in place are *aborted*. Removal of the device reduces the abortion rate to 25% or less. If the pregnancy continues, a serious intrauterine infection may develop. Typically the infection occurs during the second trimester, is fulminant, and may end in septic shock and death.

When pregnancy is diagnosed, the device should be removed. If the tail is not visible, it may have been drawn upward into the enlarging uterus or extruded before conception. An IUD can often be located by sonography if there is a question as to whether it has been expelled. If the device cannot be removed, the patient should be informed of the possibility that serious infection may develop and be given the option of abortion.

Since IUDs lie outside the amniotic sac, they do not disturb embryonic differentiation and development.

IUDs prevent 97% to 98% of intrautuerine pregnancies, but *tubal* and *ovarian pregnancies* still occur. About one in 20 pregnancies in IUD users is extrauterine. Women who are at risk of developing ectopic pregnancies should use another form of contraception if possible.

The *method by which IUDs prevent pregnancy* is not completely clear. Ovulation continues, and spermatozoa can be recovered from the fallopian tubes, but there is no evidence to suggest that IUDs cause repeated abortions of normally implanted blastocysts. Segal and associates assayed blood samples for progesterone, LH, and hCG daily from the tenth cycle day until the onset of menstruation in 30 IUD users, in 30 who had had tubal sterilizations, and in 15 women who were trying to conceive. No positive hCG assays were observed during the luteal phase in IUD users. The most likely explanation is that the device creates an intrauterine environment unfavorable for implantation. The local endometrial changes, stromal edema, increased vascularity, and a sterile inflammatory reaction may alter the tissue enough so that it cannot support the blastocyst. In addition, products from the breakdown of inflammatory cells may be toxic to both spermatozoa and blastocysts.

The *pregnancy rate* is 1.5 to 3 pregnancies/100 yrs of use. Some pregnancies occur because the patient is not aware that the device has been expelled. These can be prevented if the patient feels for the thread, which is attached to the device and comes through the cervical canal to the vagina, at the end of each menstrual period (when expulsion most often occurs) and just before ovulation. If she cannot feel the thread, she should use another form of contraception until she can see her doctor.

IUDs coated with metallic copper presumably provide better protection against pregnancy than do the pure plastic types. The copper is absorbed by the endometrium and adds to the contraceptive effect of the device itself by altering local enzyme systems, DNA content, glycogen metabolism, and estrogen uptake. They must be replaced about every 3 years.

Progestin-containing devices decrease the amount of bleeding during menstruation, but they may produce annoying intermenstrual spotting. They also appear to be associated with a higher rate of ectopic pregnancies. An additional disadvantage is that they must be replaced yearly.

Although intrauterine contraceptive devices can be used by either nulliparous or multiparous women, they are more suitable for the latter. Women who have never been pregnant are more likely to experience unacceptable cramping and bleeding than are those whose uteri have been enlarged by pregnancy. Although the risk of infection is not great, it is a possibility. Salpingitis, should it occur, will reduce fertility. This is a more serious complication in nulligravidas than in women who have had several children. Daling and co-workers reported the risk of primary infertility in women who had used plastic loops to be 3.2 as compared to normal controls. The risk for women who had used only copper-containing devices was 1.3. In terms of mortality, the death rates of healthy young women using oral contraceptives is twice that for those who use IUDs. For those predisposed to developing cardiovascular disorders, the risk from oral contraceptives is three to five times that for IUDs. The risk of death from complications of pregnancy, particularly in women over the age of 30, is far greater than from IUDs.

Hormonal contraception

Variations in the production of ovarian estrogen and progesterone during the normal menstrual cycle occur in response to changing concentrations of the pituitary gonadotropic hormones FSH and LH. The normal sequence of gonadotropic hormone production is dependent on stimulation of the hypothalamic–anterior pituitary mechanism by changing concentrations of estrogen and progesterone. Interference with this sequence of events is the basis of steroid hormonal contraception.

The most popular form of steroidal contraception is provided by *oral contraceptive agents,* which are commonly, but incorrectly, called ''the pill.'' Almost all oral contraceptive preparations contain varying amounts of an *estrogen,* either mestranol or ethinyl estradiol, and a *progestin,* which usually is a 19-nor derivative of testosterone. These substances are incorporated in the available preparations in a variety of combinations; hence there are many ''pills'' rather than ''the pill.'' The progestational, estrogen, antiestrogen, and androgenic effects of the various progestins vary considerably; hence one needs to consider these, as well as the estrogen content, when prescribing oral contraceptives.

Combined oral contraceptives contain both an estrogen and a progestin. One tablet is taken each day for 21 days, starting on the fifth day of a menstrual cycle. The medication suppresses anterior pituitary secretion of gonadotropins, thereby inhibiting ovulation. It also has a direct stimulatory effect on the endometrium, so that from 1 to 4 days after the last tablet is taken the endometrium sloughs and bleeds as a result of hormone withdrawal. The bleeding usually is less profuse than that during a normal period and may last only 2 to 3 days. Some women have no bleeding at all. The patient begins another 21-day pill cycle on the eighth day after she has taken the last pill.

The contraceptive action is a combined effect of ovulation inhibition, endometrial changes, an alteration in cervical mucus, and perhaps altered tubal function.

The constant daily dosage of the estrogen-progestogen compound produces changes in the endometrium that are different from those that occur during the normal cycle in response first to ovarian estrogen alone and then to estrogen and progesterone together. Under the stimulus of an estrogen-progestogen–containing oral contraceptive, the endometrial glands are fairly widely scattered and remain straight throughout the cycle. Secretory activity can be detected in the gland cells after a few days of treatment, and it increases during the following few days, but by about the twentieth day the cells appear inactive. The stroma remains dense throughout. A predecidual effect appears as early as the seventh day but does not often advance and usually disappears in about 7 days. The reduction in menstrual bleeding is probably a direct result of the unphysiologic endometrial stimulus; the stroma remains thin, compact, and relatively avascular compared with the normal changes.

The cervical mucus remains thick as a result of the effect of the progestogen and does not provide as suitable an environment for sperm penetration and survival as does the thin viscid mucus at ovulation.

Progestin-only pills, *the minipill,* also reduce the risk of pregnancy and may be appropriate when estrogen is contraindicated. The progestin in the pills now available is either Norethindrone (0.35 g) or Norgestrel (0.075 g). The major contraceptive effects are on cervical mucus and the endometrium, but these preparations are somewhat less effective than are combined oral contraceptives. In addition, 30% to 40% of women using progestin-only pills experience irregular and even heavy breakthrough bleeding.

Complications

SIDE EFFECTS. Undesirable side effects are common but fortunately are transient, usually lasting for no more than three or four cycles. They include nausea, vomiting, breast engorgement, headache, vertigo, and fluid retention. The latter can usually be controlled by reducing sodium intake, but it is so distressing to some women that they will not continue taking the medication. Many women gain 2.7 to 4.5 kg (6 to 10 pounds) while taking oral contraceptives and cannot lose until they stop. If these disagreeable side effects do not disappear spontaneously after a few cycles, one should consider trying another pill with a different hormone distribution. Those in which estrogen is dominant are more likely to cause nausea, fluid retention, and breast tenderness than are those with a relatively high progestin content.

Depression, which may be severe and incapacitating, occurs in some women who are taking oral contraceptives. It is particularly likely to occur with progestin-dominant preparations and may sometimes be eliminated by changing to an estrogen-dominant product. Occasionally, it is necessary to discontinue oral contraceptives completely to relieve depression.

The effect of oral contraceptives on *libido* varies. Some women experience a definite increase in sexual desire and response, whereas in others, libido decreases, sometimes to a point of complete antipathy toward sexual activities. An excess of progestin may decrease sexual desire.

The total incidence of *breakthrough bleeding* is about 8% to 10%, but it occurs more often during the first few cycles than later. It also occurs more often when progestin-dominant products or those with low estrogen content are used. If the bleeding is slight and occurs only occasionally and particularly if it consists only of slight spotting during the last few days of pill ingestion, the physician should reassure the patient that it means nothing and attempt to convince her to ignore it.

Some women must discontinue oral contraceptives because of irregular bleeding that can neither be controlled nor ignored.

Most of the complications are inconsequential when compared to the ease with which pregnancy can be prevented, but others may be more significant.

Delayed resumption of menstruation

Almost all women ovulate during the first cycle after discontinuing oral contraceptives. A delay of 6 weeks before menstruation is resumed occurs frequently, and 1% to 3% are amenorrheic for several months.

There is no way to anticipate delayed resumption of menstruation. Prolonged amenorrhea may occur in nulligravid young women whose menstrual cycles were irregular before they began taking oral contraceptives, but it also occurs in women who have had several children. Amenorrhea is not related to the preparation or the length of time it is used.

Amenorrhea is caused by continuing hypothalamic suppression rather than by a local effect on the ovaries or on the endometrium. Withdrawal bleeding usually occurs in response to administering estrogen. Ovulation can be induced in many amenorrheic women with clomiphene citrate, but this should probably not be used unless the amenorrhea persists for 6 months or more.

CARDIOVASCULAR DISEASES

Thromboembolism. The relationship between oral contraceptives and an increased risk of thromboembolism was first reported from England. According to Inman and Vessey the annual mortality from pulmonary embolism and cerebral thrombosis was 1.5/100,000 oral contraceptive users between the ages of 20 to 34 as compared with 0.2 for nonusers. Comparable figures for women aged 35 to 44 years were 3.9 and 0.5.

In a study conducted by the Boston Collaborative Drug Surveillance Program, 32 of 47,000 oral contraceptive users developed venous thromboembolism. Only 11 instances of thromboembolism were diagnosed in 187,000 women of the same ages who were not using these drugs.

A more recent study of 16,638 women who had been followed in the Kaiser Foundation Health Plan of Northern California (Walnut Creek Study) also showed an increased risk of thrombophlebitis and pulmonary embolism associated with the use of oral contraceptives. They suggest, however, that the risk may be somewhat exaggerated because thromboembolism is overdiagnosed in women who are taking oral contraceptives. This concern is substantiated by Barnes, Krapf, and Hoak, who used objective methods for confirmation of clinical diagnoses. They could identify thrombi in only 16.7% of oral contraceptive users suspected of having venous thrombosis as compared with 30.7% in nonusers.

Although it appears that thromboembolism occurs more often in women who use oral contraceptives, there is no definite relationship between the length of use and the development of thrombosis. Thromboembolism appears to be related to estrogen content; the lower the estrogen level, the less likely is the complication to develop. This suggests that products with an estrogen content of no more than 50 μg should usually be prescribed.

Heart attacks. Although a relationship exists between oral contraceptives and myocardial infarction, the medication is only one of the risk factors involved; others include hypertension, obesity, diabetes, and smoking. Nonusers who smoke heavily are seven times more likely to develop heart attacks than are women who neither smoke nor use hormonal contraception. Heart attacks occur four times more frequently in nonsmokers who use oral contraceptives than in women who do neither. The risk is increased about 40 times in heavy smokers who receive contraceptive pills.

According to Rosenberg and colleagues, women whose only risk factor was the use of oral contraceptives were three times more likely to be hospitalized for myocardial infarction than were women without risk factors who used other methods of contraception. Women who smoked and used oral contraceptives were 170 times more likely to develop heart attacks. British studies report similar results.

Ory, Rosenfield, and Landman estimate the risk of women between the ages of 20 and 29 dying of heart attacks to be about 1/100,000. The risk increases to about 25/100,000 for those aged 40 to 44. The use of oral contraceptives increases the risk of dying of myocardial infarction to 3/100,000 in women aged 20 to 29 and to 75/100,000 for those aged 40 to 44.

Cerebrovascular accidents. The death rates from subarachnoid hemorrhage in the Royal College of General Practitioners Oral Contraception Study were 9.3/100,000 current oral contraceptive users and 15.9/100,000 for former users. The Walnut Creek Study, which confirms the increased risk in users, also implicates smoking. The risk of having a cardiovascular accident was much greater in those who were both smokers and users of oral contraceptives than in those who smoked but had never used birth control pills.

Slight increases in both systolic and diastolic blood pressures occur frequently in women taking oral contraceptives, and about 5% develop *overt hypertension*. The blood pressure usually rises gradually, but hypertension can develop in a few weeks. The blood pressure usually returns to normal when the medication is stopped. The mechanism appears to be a disturbance in the renin-angiotensin-aldosterone sequence. The incidence of significant blood pressure elevation is not increased in those who have had pregnancy-induced hypertension.

Plasma lipids and lipoproteins. In a study by Wallace and colleagues, plasma cholesterol, triglycerides, low-density lipoproteins, and very low–density lipoproteins in young oral contraceptive users were all increased as compared with those in control subjects. High-density lipoproteins were unchanged. The changes were more pronounced in those taking contraceptives containing more than 50 μg of estrogen than in those taking lower doses. In contrast, low-density and very low–density lipoproteins were decreased in postmenopausal

women taking estrogen alone, whereas high-density lipoproteins were significantly increased. The authors suggested that the progestin content may be equally as important as estrogen in producing the change. The relationship between these changes and circulatory diseases is not clear.

Blood coagulation. Prothrombin and factors VII, VIII, IX, and X are increased, whereas antithrombin III is decreased.

In summary, it seems quite likely that the use of oral contraceptives is associated with an increased risk of death from cardiovascular diseases. The risk is highest in older women, particularly those with other risk factors such as hypertension or obesity. Probably the most important factor is smoking. The risks for healthy, nonsmoking women between the ages of 20 and 30 are slight.

OTHER COMPLICATIONS. Oral contraceptives appear to have a *diabetogenic effect* similar to that of pregnancy. Glucose metabolism may be altered in some users. There is no indication that oral contraceptives cause diabetes, and most women with diabetes can take oral contraceptives without deleterious effects on the disease. However, there may be an increased risk of cardiovascular diseases.

Women who have had *cholestasis and jaundice* during pregnancy may respond in the same manner to oral contraceptives. The incidence of *cholecystitis and cholelithiasis* is almost doubled in oral contraceptive users. The most serious complication affecting the liver is the development of *liver tumors,* principally focal nodular hyperplasia and hepatic adenomas. The main danger is from rupture of the tumor with intrahepatic or intraperitoneal hemorrhage and death unless the blood loss is controlled promptly. Malignant liver neoplasms have not been related to the use of oral contraceptives.

There is no evidence to suggest that combined oral contraceptives increase the risk of cancer of the cervix, endometrium, breast, or any other organ. Many women who use these preparations develop a *benign proliferative adenomatous growth on the cervix* that may look like carcinoma. These have been misdiagnosed as adenocarcinoma.

There has been no increase in congenital anomalies noted in the children of women who conceive shortly after discontinuing oral contraceptives. There may be an increased incidence of abortions associated with chromosomal defects when pregnancy occurs promptly. One should recommend that women have two to three spontaneous cycles before attempting to conceive. Condoms, aerosol foam, or both may be used in the interim.

Advantages. Much has been written about the complications related to the use of oral contraceptives, but the advantages, other than protection against pregnancy, have had little publicity. Mishell lists the *noncontraceptive health benefits of oral contraceptives* as decreased menstrual blood loss and resultant iron-deficiency anemia, regulation of irregular cycles, protection against endometrial adenocarcinoma, reduced incidence of benign breast disease, protection against the development of functional ovarian cysts, protection against acute salpingitis, and possible protection against ovarian cancer and rheumatoid arthritis.

Limitations and cautions. Nevertheless, since there is still so much question concerning the physiologic effects of estrogen-progestogen combinations, it seems wise to limit their use to perfectly normal healthy young women who choose them over other methods after the risks have been described to them.

As a general rule, there is no reason why healthy nonsmoking women below the age of 35 cannot take oral contraceptives. The risk of serious complications developing increases every year thereafter. Most women over the age of 40 should be discouraged from using this form of contraception. If they choose to continue, they must be fully aware of the risks and should be advised to use low-estrogen preparations.

Each woman taking oral contraceptives should be examined before the medication is prescribed and yearly thereafter: the examination should include medical and family history, weight, blood pressure, general physical and pelvic examination, screening cervical cytologic analysis, and hemoglobin determination.

All women who take oral contraceptives should be encouraged to stop smoking. Those who continue must be made aware of the risks involved.

If contraceptive tablets are taken accordingly to the recommended schedule, the incidence of unplanned pregnancy should be close to zero. If they are taken irregularly during the cycle, ovulation and fertilization may occur.

Selection of an oral contraceptive. The estrogen and progestin contents of the oral contraceptives vary considerably. Although preparations with relatively large amounts of estrogen are available, those containing 35 g to a maximun of 50 g are appropriate for most women. The lower the amount of estrogen, the less the endometrial stimulation and growth and the greater the possibility of *amenorrhea*. This concerns both the patient and the physician because of the possibility that the failure to menstruate may be a result of pregnancy. Although it is unlikely that one who has taken her pills regularly and fails to menstruate has conceived, some women will not tolerate the uncertainty and will discontinue the method. Most, however, can be reassured if they are made aware of the reason for the amenorrhea. A pregnancy test should probably be ordered with the first episode or two of amenorrhea; but if the failure to bleed persists, repeated tests are probably not necessary.

Another problem is *breakthrough bleeding* that may occur throughout the cycle. This also is caused by low estrogen content and can be controlled by prescription of 1.25 to 2.5 mg conjugated estrogens daily, in addition to the pill, for 7 days while the bleeding is present. Often one or two cycles of additional estrogen will correct the problem.

Biphasic preparations containing varying amounts of progestin, making their effects more like those that occur during normal cycles, may also control breakthrough bleeding. The estrogen content remains constant throughout; but the progestin content, which is low during the first 10 days, is increased during the last 11 days. These preparations are designed to provide relatively low estrogen; the variations in progestin reduce breakthrough bleeding.

Triphasic preparations attempt to mimic the normal menstrual cycle by providing small amounts of progestogen during the first 11 days with an increase during the last 10 days. In contrast to biphasic preparations the estrogen content varies, being low during the first 6 days, higher during the next 5 days, and reduced during the last 10 days. These preparations provide excellent protection against conception with a low incidence of breakthrough bleeding despite relatively small amounts of both estrogen and progestogen.

Preparations that are *estrogen-dominant with relatively low progestin content* are best used in women with scanty menses, oily skin, acne, hirsutism, depression and in those who are prone to develop *Candida vaginitis. Progestin-dominant, low-estrogen preparations* are appropriate for women with heavy menses, fibrocystic breast diseases, uterine leiomyomas, and dysmenorrhea.

Contraindications to oral contraceptives. There are women for whom oral contraceptives should not be prescribed. The *absolute contraindications* include:

1. Coronary artery disease, stroke, or thromboembolism either present or in the past
2. Impaired liver function
3. Estrogen-dependent neoplasms and breast cancer
4. Suspected pregnancy
5. Smokers over age 35, particularly obese women

Relative contraindications include:

1. History of cholestasis during pregnancy
2. Migraine headaches or headaches associated with oral contraceptive use
3. Severe hypertension
4. Usually, in preparation for elective operations
5. Seizure disease
6. Diabetes mellitus
7. Sickle-cell diseases, except sickle-cell trait

Pregnancy interception. Another method of pregnancy prevention is the use of *large doses of estrogen after coitus.* This should be considered as an emergency measure to be used after unprotected coitus during the fertile period rather than as a regular method of contraception. The exact mechanism by which postcoital estrogen prevents pregnancy is not yet known, but it does produce a premature fall in corpus luteum progesterone production and changes in the endometrium, which may provide an unacceptable implantation site for the fertilized ovum.

The dosage is *DES,* 50 mg daily orally for 5 days, starting as soon as possible after exposure but certainly no later than 72 hours. Other preparations are *conjugated estrogens,* 30 mg/day, or *Ovral,* two tablets repeated once in 12 hours. Since estrogen ingested by the mother is related to the subsequent development of vaginal adenosis and clear cell carcinoma in their daughters, it is essential that each patient be examined to make certain that she is not already pregnant before the drug is prescribed. Repeat examinations to make certain that the patient did not conceive despite the drug also are essential. Abortion should be available if pregnancy occurs.

Surgical contraception

Termination of fertility by an operative procedure is the most common form of contraception in the United States. As many as 15 million couples may rely on this method. The most common medical reasons for surgical sterilization in women are chronic cardiovascular-renal disease, severe heart disease, and diabetes mellitus. It may also be performed in conjunction with vaginal plastic operations and cesarean section.

Elective sterilization is appropriate for normal women who have completed their childbearing careers and who still have several years of fertility ahead. It may be particularly important for those who cannot use an effective contraceptive method, and it usually is preferable to many years of using oral hormonal contraceptives.

The fallopian tubes can be ligated or severed in conjunction with any indicated abdominal operation or as a primary procedure. This may be accomplished by *laparoscopic tubal cautery;* by the application of *rings* or *clips,* which requires no hospitalization and a few days of disability; or removing a segment of each tube through a *vaginal* or *small abdominal incision (minilaparotomy). Puerperal sterilization,* usually during the first day or two after delivery, is easy and safe and often is an appropriate choice.

The patient should understand that it is unlikely that she will conceive after the operation but that she is being sterilized (termination of fertility), not castrated (removal of gonads).

Vasectomy can be performed in an outpatient facility with a local anesthetic. There are few complications and a minimal period of disability. Spermatozoa may remain in the reproductive tract for several weeks; consequently, an additional method of contraception should be used until aspermia has been proved. Recanalization occurs in a small percentage of cases, probably less than 5%.

One must always consider the possible emotional effects of permanent elimination of procreative ability. It is not easy, even for a woman who wants no more children, to relinquish her ability to conceive. Men who are somewhat uncertain in their masculine roles may be impotent after vasectomy. These potential effects of sterilization must be explored before the operation is performed because, even though each member of the couple may verbally agree, they may be unconsciously resisting.

Future methods

The currently available methods for controlling conception leave much to be desired. With the exception of IUDs and surgical procedures, each requires a considerable amount of motivation—particularly the taking of oral medication daily or the use of a physiologic or mechanical method consistently year after year. The current research in immunologic methods, by which it will be possible to provide temporary immunity against spermatozoa, is promising, as are hormonal methods that require single injections at long periods of time. The ideal is a method that is completely effective and without danger but reversible and that requires no preparation for individual acts of coitus.

LEGAL ABORTION

The term *legal abortion* refers to the termination of early pregnancy by a qualified physician in an approved medical facility.

Until about 1965 termination of pregnancy was considered only when it was likely that the mother would die if she remained pregnant (therapeutic abortion). Such abortions were legal in most states. Abortion was seldom considered because of fetal conditions, even if one could anticipate a fetus being born with a lethal or incapacitating condition, or for social reasons. These abortions were illegal.

Restrictive laws did not prevent women for whom pregnancy was a personal disaster from obtaining abortion. Unfortunately, they often had to seek assistance from illegal operators, and many developed serious complications or even died as a result of the procedures. Before 1970 when abortion became legal in New York, more than 50% of maternal deaths in New York City followed illegally induced abortion. During the 5-year period 1955 to 1959, 21% of maternal deaths in Michigan were attributed to illegally induced abortions. During the next 5-year period, 37% of maternal deaths followed abortion. Hospital admissions of patients with septic abortions were promptly reduced in the states that legalized abortion.

In January 1973 the United States Supreme Court declared all restrictive abortion laws unconstitutional. As a consequence, abortion is now legal in all states. The number of illegal abortions and the accompanying deaths fell precipitously after abortion became legal. During the 5-year period from 1975 to 1979, only 17 women died after illegal abortion in the United States.

The decision included directives concerning the performance of abortions, as well as decision making. During the *first trimester* the decision for abortion can be made by a patient and a physician, but the operation can only be performed by a licensed physician. States may develop regulations concerning who performs *second trimester* pregnancy terminations and where they can be done, but the decision for the procedure still rests with the patient and a physician. States may develop regulations for *third trimester* termination of pregnancy and may even proscribe termination, except to preserve the life and health of the mother.

Indications

Legal abortions include those performed because of a disorder that makes pregnancy hazardous (*medical indications*) and those performed for social or economic reasons (*nonmedical indications*).

Medical reasons (therapeutic abortion). Therapeutic abortions are performed in women with serious medical diseases that make pregnancy hazardous, fetal conditions that interfere with normal growth and development, and serious psychiatric disorders.

MATERNAL MEDICAL INDICATIONS. The *maternal medical conditions* for which abortion is most often performed are *chronic hypertension* or *renal disease,* especially when there is considerable vascular degeneration and reduced renal function; *diabetes,* especially when there are associated degenerative vascular changes; and advanced *heart disease.* These and other indications for medically indicated abortions are discussed in detail in other sections of this text.

FETAL INDICATIONS. Termination of pregnancy can be considered whenever the fetus has little chance of developing normally because of maternal disease such as rubella, when it has been exposed to teratogenic stimuli, or when it is destined to die at an early age from a lethal hereditary condition. Certain chromosomal and metabolic abnormalities that, if present, may influence a decision for abortion can be detected by appropriate amniotic fluid studies early in pregnancy.

PSYCHIATRIC CONDITIONS. Therapeutic abortion for psychiatric conditions is justified when the pregnancy interferes with necessary psychotherapy, when there is a distinct possibility of suicide, or when the psychopathologic condition of the patient and her family is severe enough to suggest that a baby reared in the atmosphere of the home would have a small chance for normal emotional development.

Nonmedical reasons (elective abortions). The *nonmedical* reasons for abortion are primarily social or economic, and the decision as to the advisability of terminating pregnancy will be one made individually by the woman and her physician.

Physician responsibility

Physicians who choose to perform *nonmedical abortions* make the decisions concerning the advisability of the procedure with individual patients. The request for the operation always originates with the patient. One important responsibility is to recognize the occasional woman for whom termination of pregnancy may not be appropriate.

It is obvious that a woman with an undesired pregnancy may think first of termination without considering other options. Therefore, it is essential that a physician not agree to perform an abortion without a thorough review of the situation with the patient. The doctor or a specially trained nurse, social worker, or counselor should discuss with the patient the advantages and disadvantages of keeping the pregnancy. An important aspect to be considered is what effect a baby will have on her life or on members of her family. Abortion is difficult for many women to accept with equanimity; hence counseling, even for those who are adamant concerning interruption, is an important part of the treatment.

The responsibility of physicians in dealing with *medical abortions* is somewhat different. They must be able, with the help of appropriate consultants, to evaluate the severity of the systemic disease and to establish the potential risk of permitting the pregnancy to continue. They therefore must recommend termination. In many instances this is difficult for the patient to accept because, in direct contrast to those who request nonmedical abortion, she wants the pregnancy.

The need for medical abortions can be kept at a minimum by *prepregnancy examinations*. If a condition that contraindicates pregnancy is found, a suitable contraceptive method can be prescribed for temporary use if the condition can be corrected, or permanently if there is no possibility of improving it.

Complications

Complications associated with abortion occur inevitably, but they can be kept at a minimum if the procedures are performed on carefully selected patients by skillful operators in properly equipped facilities. Complications most likely to occur during early abortion are perforation of the uterus, hemorrhage, and infection. Since these cannot be anticipated in advance, it is essential that provision be made to treat them promptly when they occur.

The risk of serious complications as a result of

abortion during the first 12 gestational weeks for women of all ages is about one to two per 100,000 procedures. The more advanced the pregnancy when the operation is performed, the greater the risk of serious complications. Uncomplicated induced abortion appears to have little effect on the outcome of subsequent pregnancies.

Early abortion can be performed safely in an outpatient facility that is equipped to provide supportive emergency treatment for operative complications. An arrangement must be made with a nearby hospital for immediate admission and treatment of any patient in whom a complication develops during the procedure.

At best, abortion is an unsatisfactory way of controlling reproduction. When effective contraceptive methods are used regularly, abortion is not necessary.

Technique

Blood-typing and a check for Rh antibodies are important preabortion laboratory procedures. Women who are Rh negative but who have no evidence of isoimmunization should be treated with *human anti-D gamma globulin (RhoGAM)* to prevent immunization by the fetal red blood cells that enter the maternal bloodstream during abortion.

During the first trimester of pregnancy the uterus can usually be evacuated by dilating the cervix and removing the products of conception by suction curettage. The uterus can also be emptied by extracting the fetus and much of the placenta with ring forceps followed by curettage to detach the rest of the placenta from the uterine wall. Suction usually is preferable because it takes less time and blood loss is less.

Preoperative dilatation of the cervix several hours before the uterus is evacuated will soften the cervix and reduce the need for forcible dilatation. Laminaria sticks made of seaweed that absorbs water, swells, and gently opens the cervix are inserted through the internal os the day before the operation is performed. They are removed just before the uterus is evacuated.

After the twelfth week the safest way to terminate pregnancy is by dilating the cervix and extracting the fetus and placenta with ring forceps and a large curet. This is far more difficult than is suction curettage during the early weeks and should be done only by individuals who are experienced in the technique.

Abdominal hysterotomy was used extensively in the past for second trimester abortion. Since the morbidity associated with hysterotomy is higher than for any other method of terminating pregnancy, it should be used only when other methods are inappropriate.

Prostaglandins, given by intraamniotic or intravenous infusion or by intravaginal suppositories will stimulate uterine contractions at any stage of pregnancy.

Prostaglandin $F_2\alpha$ is most often instilled into the amniotic sac, and prostaglandins E_2 and $F_2\alpha$ in the vagina. Prostaglandin analogs also appear to be effective in stimulating uterine contractions.

Most of the complications related to the use of prostaglandins are troublesome rather than dangerous. Nausea, vomiting, and diarrhea occur frequently. There are no adverse changes in the blood-clotting mechanism. The most serious complications are delayed placental delivery, transverse cervical laceration, and, occasionally, rupture of the uterus. These are common to all methods for second-trimester termination. Delayed placental delivery may lead to excessive blood loss and infection, both of which can be reduced by early removal of the placenta if it is not extruded promptly.

The uterus can also be evacuated during the second trimester by injecting *hypertonic saline solution into the amniotic cavity.* The most important *complications* accompanying intraamniotic saline injection are *infusion into the maternal bloodstream,* producing salt intoxication, and the development of *disseminated intravascular coagulation.* Laros and colleagues found consistent decreases in platelet count and fibrinogen concentration and the appearance of fibrin-split products characteristic of disseminated intravascular coagulation in 25 patients during saline abortion. Infection can also occur, particularly if there is a long interval between injection and evacuation of the uterus.

The *death rate* associated with legal abortion is determined by the stage of pregnancy, the method of induction, and the experience of the operator. Between 1972 and 1978 more than 6 million legal abortions were reported to the Centers for Disease Control. The lowest death rate, 0.5/100,000, was for abortions performed on pregnancies of 8 weeks' duration or less. The death rate increased progressively to 2.3 at 11 to 12 weeks, 6.7 at 13 to 15 weeks, and 13.9 at 16 to 20 weeks. The death rates per 100,000 procedures were one for first trimester curettage, 7.7 for dilatation and evacuation after the twelfth week, 12.3 for instillation of saline and prostaglandins, and 42.8 for hysterotomy or hysterectomy.

By 1981 the risk of death as a result of 1,300,760

legal abortions at all stages of pregnancy and by all methods had been reduced to 0.5/100,000 procedures.

When pregnancy is terminated because of a chronic condition such as heart disease, diabetes, or essential hypertension, *sterilization* should be considered, because there is little hope that the condition will improve enough to permit pregnancy in the future. This is not true of abortions performed for other reasons.

CARE OF PATIENTS AFTER ABORTION

The patient who has had an uncomplicated elective abortion and little blood loss may be discharged a few hours after the uterus has been evacuated. Those with serious medical disorders and those in whom intraoperative complications develop should remain in the hospital until they are stabilized. Normal activity may be resumed whenever the patient feels able to carry out her usual duties. Involution usually is complete with 1 month, and menstruation begins 4 to 6 weeks after the abortion has occurred.

REFERENCES

Abortion surveillance: Preliminary analysis-United States, 1981, Centers for Disease Control Morbidity and Mortality Weekly Report **33**:373, 1984.

Austin, H., Louv, W.C., and Alexander, J.: A case-control study of spermicides and gonorrhea, J.A.M.A. **251**:2822, 1984.

Barnes, R.W., Krapf, T., and Hoak, J.C.: Erroneous clinical diagnosis of leg vein thrombosis in women on oral contraceptives, Obstet. Gynecol. **51**:556, 1978.

Boston Collaborative Drug Surveillance Program: Surgically confirmed gallbladder disease, venous thromboembolism, and breast tumors in relation to postmenopausal estrogen therapy, N. Engl. J. Med. **290**:15, 1974.

Bracken, M.B.: Spermicidal contraceptives and poor reproductive outcomes: the epidemiological evidence against an association, Am. J. Obstet. Gynecol. **151**:552, 1985.

Cates, W., Jr., Schulz, K.F., and Grimes, D.A.: The risk associated with teenage abortion, N. Engl. J. Med. **309**:6211, 1983.

Cates, W., Jr., and Grimes, D.A.: Deaths from second trimester abortion by dilatation and evacuation: causes, prevention, facilities, Obstet. Gynecol. **58**:401, 1981.

Daling, J.R., et al.: Primary tubal infertility in relation to the use of an intrauterine device, N. Engl. J. Med. **312**:938, 1985.

Faich, G., Pearson, K., Fleming, D., et al.: Toxic shock syndrome and the vaginal contraceptive sponge, J.A.M.A., **255**:216, 1986.

Grimes, D.A., and Schulz, K.F.: Morbidity and mortality from second-trimester abortions, J. Reprod. Med. **30**:505, 1985.

Hatcher, R.A., et al.: Contraceptive technology 1984-85, New York, 1984, Irvington Publishers, Inc.

Hogue, C.J.R., Cates, W., Jr., and Tietze, C.: Impact of vacuum aspiration abortion on future childbearing: a review, Fam. Plann. Perspect. **15**:119, 1983.

Inman, W.N.W., and Vessey, M.P.: Investigation of deaths from pulmonary coronary and cerebral thrombosis and embolism in women of childbearing age, Br. Med. J. **2**:193, 1968.

Kelaghan, J., et al.: Barrier-method contraceptives and pelvic inflammatory disease, J.A.M.A. **248**:184, 1982.

Klaus, A.: Natural family planning: a review, Obstet. Gynecol. Surv. **37**:128, 1982.

Laros, R.K., Collins, J., Penner, J.A., et al.: Coagulation changes in saline-induced abortion, Am. J. Obstet. Gynecol. **116**:277, 1973.

Lipnick, R.J., Buring, J.E., Hennekens, C.H., et al.: Oral contraceptives and breast cancer, J.A.M.A. **255**:58, 1986.

Malhotra, N., and Chadbury, R.R.: Current status of intrauterine devices. II. Intrauterine devices and pelvic inflammatory disease and ectopic pregnancy, Obstet. Gynecol. Surv. **37**:1, 1982.

Mishell, D.R., Jr.: Noncontraceptive health benefits of oral steroidal contraceptives, Am. J. Obstet. Gynecol. **142**:809, 1982.

Nissen, E.D., Kent, D.R., Nissen, S.E., and McRae, D.M.: Association of liver tumors with oral contraceptives, Obstet. Gynecol. **48**:49, 1976.

Oppenheimer, W.: Prevention of pregnancy by the Graefenberg ring method, Am. J. Obstet. Gynecol. **78**:446, 1959.

Ory, H.W., Forrest, J.D., and Lincoln, R.: Making choices: evaluating the health risks of birth control methods, New York, 1983, Alan Guttmacher Institute.

Ory, H.W., Rosenfield, A., and Landman, L.C.: The pill at 20: an assessment, Fam. Plann. Perspect. **12**:278, 1980.

Petitti, D.B., and Wingerd, J.: Use of oral contraceptives, cigarette smoking and risk of subarachnoid hemorrhage, Lancet **2**:234, 1978.

Population Reports: Barrier methods, series H, no. 7, January-February 1984, Baltimore, Population Information Program, The Johns Hopkins University.

Population Reports: Intrauterine devices, series B, no. 3, July 1982, Baltimore, Population Information Program, The Johns Hopkins University.

Population Reports: Oral contraceptives, series A, no. 5, January 1979, Baltimore, Population Information Program, The Johns Hopkins University.

Population Reports: Periodic abstinence, series 1, no. 3, September 1981, Baltimore, Population Information Program, The Johns Hopkins University.

Ramcharan, S., Pellegrin, F.A., Ray, R.M., and Hsu, J.P.: The Walnut Creek contraceptive drug study of the side effects of oral contraceptives, J. Reprod. Med. **25**:349, 1980.

Rosenberg, L., Hennekens, C.H., Rosner, B., Belanger, C., Rothman, K.J., and Speizer, F.E.: Oral contraceptive use in relation to nonfatal myocardial infarction, Am. J. Epidemiol. **111:**59, 1980.

Ryder, N.B.: Contraceptive failure in the United States, Fam. Plann. Perspect. **5**(3):133, 1973.

Segal, S.J., et al.: Absence of chorionic gonadotropin in sera of women who use intrauterine devices, Fertil. Steril. **44:**214, 1985.

Sandmire, H.F., and Cavanaugh, M.D.: Long-term use of intrauterine contraceptive devices in a private practice, Am. J. Obstet. Gynecol. **152:**169, 1985.

Tatum, H.J., and Connell-Tatum, E.B.: Barrier contraception: a comprehensive overview, Fertil. Steril. **36:**1, 1981.

Valicenti, J.F., Jr., et al.: Detection and prevalence of IUD-associated *actinomycosis* colonization and related morbidity, J.A.M.A. **247:**1149, 1982.

Wallace, R.B., Hoover, J., Barrett-Connor, E., Rifkind, B.M., Hunninghake, D.B., Mackenthun, A., and Heiss, G.: Altered plasma lipid and lipoprotein levels associated with oral contraceptive and oestrogen use: report from the Medications Working Group of the Lipid Research Clinics Program, Lancet **2:**112, 1979.

Willson, J.R., Ledger, W.J., and Lovell, J.: Intrauterine contraceptive devices: a comparison between their use in indigent and private patients, Obstet. Gynecol. **29:**59, 1967.

Zakin, D., Stern, W.Z., and Rosenblatt, R.: Complete and partial uterine perforation and embedding following insertion of intrauterine devices. I. Classification, complications, mechanism, incidence, and missing string, Obstet. Gynecol. Surv. **36:**335, 1981.

Zakin, D., Stern, W.Z., and Rosenblatt, R.: Complete and partial uterine perforation and embedding following insertion of intrauterine devices. II. Diagnostic methods, prevention and management. Obstet. Gynecol. Surv. **36:**401, 1981.

Zatuchni, G.I.: Current methods of contraception, The Female Patient **3**(5):48, 1978.

16

John H. Mattox

Abortion

Abortion is the expulsion of the products of conception before the end of the twentieth week when the fetus weighs about 500 g. Abortions that occur during the first 12 weeks are *early abortions;* those that occur from the end of the twelfth through the twentieth week are *late abortions*. Between the twenty-first and the end of the twenty-eighth week, the fetal weight increases to about 1000 g, and some of these infants can survive outside the uterus. Termination during this period is called *immature labor*. Abortions that occur because of some maternal or ovular defect are termed *spontaneous*, whereas those that are brought on intentionally are said to be *induced*. An induced abortion is *legal* if performed by a physician in an approved facility or *illegal* if performed by an individual not approved by the law. Abortions that are accompanied by infection are termed *septic*. There are significant religious and ethical issues involved with the elective termination of a pregnancy that will not be addressed in this discussion.

Early abortions are recognized in 10% to 15% of pregnancies, but the actual rate is higher. Some occur after a slight delay in the onset of menstruation and cause so few symptoms that medical aid is not sought. In others the life of the fertilized ovum is so brief that the period is not even delayed. Miller and colleagues measured the beta subunit of hCG by radioimmunoassay during 623 cycles in 197 women who were trying to conceive; 152 were positive. Obvious abortions occurred in 14 (9.2%), whereas in 74 the pregnancies continued uneventfully. Clinical evidence of pregnancy was never detected in the other 64 in whom the tests were positive. This study suggests that almost half (43%) of all pregnancies terminate in spontaneous abortion.

SPONTANEOUS ABORTION
Etiologic factors

The causes of spontaneous abortion are multiple and include fetal, maternal, and paternal factors. A definite reason for a specific spontaneous abortion cannot always be established, because a complete analysis of all causative factors is impossible.

Zygote abnormalities. Defective growth of the ovum may include abnormalities in development and in implantation of the placenta, as well as defects in the embryo itself. Mall and Meyer were able to detect pathologic developmental changes in 48% of aborted embryos.

Many abortions of so-called blighted ova are actually a result of chromosomal aberrations. Boué, Boué, and Lazar, studying tissue from 1500 spontaneous abortions, identified chromosomal anomalies in 61%. On the basis of their material they estimate that 150 of every 1000 pregnancies will terminate in recognizable spontaneous abortion and that 100 of 150 (60%) will be caused by chromosomal abnormalities. About 52% of the latter will be autosomal trisomies; 20%, triploids; 15%, 45 X monosomies; 6%, tetraploids; and 7%, other anomalies.

Late abortions are more often associated with defective placental implantations than with defects in the embryo. However, Haxton and Bell in detailed study, including karyotyping of abortions, at 12 to 26 weeks, found major somatic anomalies in 20% and minor abnormalities in 14%. Abortion in patients with severe hypertensive cardiovascular disease may be caused in part by alterations in the circulation at the placental site secondary to the vascular abnormality.

Maternal factors. The maternal factors that may be responsible for abortion include both local and systemic conditions.

INFECTIONS. Acute febrile illnesses may be responsible for death of the embryo and abortion, but tuberculosis and other chronic diseases generally do not disturb pregnancy. Syphilis may cause fetal death, but it rarely causes abortion. Generalized peritonitis, appendiceal and pelvic abscesses, and other serious local infections often, but not invariably, cause abortion.

Ordinary cervical infections, with the possible exception of *Mycoplasma hominis* and *Ureaplasma urealyticum,* do not usually cause abortion, but genital herpesvirus infection may. Naib and colleagues reported a 33.3% abortion rate in 63 women who became pregnant after herpesvirus infection was detected. The rate in 224 pregnant women without virus infection who were matched for age with those infected was 9.4%. The abortion rate in 2791 pregnant women treated in the same hospital during a 5-month period was 11.5%.

NUTRITIONAL DEFICIENCIES. A nutritional deficiency sufficient to cause pronounced loss of weight may interfere with both fertility and the maintenance of pregnancy, but the role of subclinical deficiencies is less clear.

GENITAL TRACT ABNORMALITIES. *Cervical lacerations* that extend through the internal os may be responsible for repeated second trimester abortion and immature labor. As pregnancy advances, the support provided by the intact cervix is lacking; the internal os dilates and retracts, the membranes rupture, and labor begins.

Developmental abnormalities of the uterus, especially the more advanced duplication defects, increase the premature pregnancy termination rate severalfold if the abnormal structure cannot enlarge sufficiently to accommodate the growing fetus. Most of these are instances of immature labor rather than abortion.

The incidence of abortion associated with *uterine fibromyomas* also is increased, especially if multiple submucous tumors distort the uterine cavity and reduce the area in which normal placental implantation and growth can take place. Subserous and intramural tumors are less likely to interfere with the progression of the pregnancy. An increase in spontaneous abortion has also been documented in women with *endometriosis*.

The *position of the uterus* has little to do with abortion, except in the unusual instances in which a retrodisplaced uterus fails to rise out of the pelvis as the pregnancy advances and becomes incarcerated beneath the promontory of the sacrum.

ENDOCRINE FACTORS. Disturbances in the secretions of reproductive hormones undoubtedly are responsible for some abortions, but probably are less important than they have been considered to be. The exact role of hormonal deficiencies will be clarified when we can eliminate trophoblastic and embryonic factors that cannot yet be identified. Reduced hormone secretion may be a result of abnormal trophoblastic activity rather than a primary factor in abortion.

If the ovum is fertilized, trophoblastic hCG stimulates the corpus luteum to continue to produce estrogen and progesterone rather than to regress as it does during the normal menstrual cycle. These hormones stimulate the decidual changes necessary for implantation and for maintaining the ovum during its early growth period. The trophoblastic cells soon begin to secrete estrogen and progesterone, as well as chorionic gonadotropins. Although the ovarian corpus luteum continues to function, it becomes an increasingly less important source of estrogen and progesterone as pregnancy advances.

The trophoblast usually provides enough estrogen and progesterone to maintain pregnancy after the *tenth* gestational week.

If the secretion of progesterone by the corpus luteum is inadequate, the endometrium may be so poorly prepared for nidation and for support of the ovum that early abortion may result. It has been postulated that corpus luteum regression may be a result of defects in the trophoblast. If the trophoblast fails to develop normally, for example, when the embryo is defective, the secretion of hCG may be too low to support the corpus luteum, and production of estrogen and progesterone is inadequate to maintain normal decidua.

Normal function of other endocrine glands (for example, adrenal, thyroid, pancreas) is important for maintenance of a healthy gestation. However, it appears that only when there is a clinically serious dysfunction could one ascribe the pregnancy loss to an endocrine abnormality.

PHYSICAL TRAUMA. Surgical removal of the corpus luteum or uterine manipulation before 6 weeks' gestation increases the chances of spontaneous abortion significantly. If pelvic surgery is required, it should be postponed until early in the second trimester if it is medically feasible. Abdominal trauma rarely interrupts a normally implanted pregnancy. In many instances, pregnancy has continued despite fractures or crushing injuries to the pelvic girdle. Although a minor bump or fall can almost always be remembered to have preceded an abortion, it seems highly unlikely that injury often is a responsible factor.

EMOTIONAL FACTORS. Emotional stimuli, which do not need to be overt, shocking experiences, may precipitate abortion, but their exact role has not as yet been established.

MISCELLANEOUS CAUSES. Many of the miscellaneous causes for abortion are even less well understood than those already listed. Advanced maternal age, poor socioeconomic status and/or malnutrition, infertility, and ABO blood type incompatibility probably result in a hostile environment for an early pregnancy. The male contribution to abortion has been inadequately explored, but it may account for some instances of pregnancy failure.

Exposure to *anesthetic agents* may be a factor in abortion. Cohen, Belville, and Brown reported abortion rates of 38% among anesthetists and 30% among operating room nurses as contrasted to a rate of 10% among general duty nurses. Corbett and Ball detected significant concentrations of anesthetic gases in operating rooms and in the end-expired air of anesthesiologists for as long as 64 hours after they had administered the agent to a patient. Hemminki and co-workers reported an increased incidence of spontaneous abortion in hospital personnel involved in instrument sterilization where *ethylene oxide* was used.

Many studies suggest that *cigarette smoking* is responsible for a variety of reproductive failures, one of which may be abortion. Kline and colleagues reported that 41% of 574 women who aborted spontaneously were smokers as compared with 28% of 320 whose pregnancies continued for at least 28 weeks. Harlap and Shiono also implicated *excessive alcohol* consumption as increasing the risk of spontaneous abortion.

Mechanism

The precipitating cause of abortion is death of the embryo or its failure to develop normally. The demise usually occurs an average of 6 weeks before expulsion. The loss of the stimulus of the growing embryo results in a gradual diminution in trophoblastic production of hCG, estrogen, and progesterone. This is followed by spasm of the spiral arterioles, ischemic necrosis of the decidua, and bleeding into the decidua vera and the choriodecidual space. The accumulation of blood separates the placenta, at least partially, from its attachment to the decidua basalis. Uterine contractions, which are induced by increasing prostaglandin synthesis in the disintegrating decidua, complete the placental separation and expel the ovum completely or in part.

During the first 6 weeks after the onset of the last menstrual period, the attachment of the fetus in the decidual lining is insecure, and in most instances the fetal sac and the decidua are extruded intact. During the next few weeks, chorionic villi, which eventually form the placenta, grow and invade the underlying decidua basalis at the area of the placental site, but until about the fourteenth week the placenta is not well formed. If abortion occurs during the period of placental differentiation, portions of the immature structure are torn from the uterine wall and expelled, but some chorionic tissue usually remains adherent. A curettage following abortion is usually required during this period.

Clinical stages and types

As an abortion progresses, it advances through a series of fairly characteristic stages that can usually be recognized clinically. These are classified as *threatened, inevitable, incomplete,* and *complete* (Figs. 16-1 and 16-2). Abortion may also be *missed* or *habitual.*

Threatened abortion. The earliest stage that can be recognized clinically is spoken of as threatened abortion because the eventual outcome is uncertain and pregnancy may continue uneventfully. At some time during early pregnancy, usually after having missed one or two periods, the patient becomes aware of bleeding, which is slight and usually consists of the spotting of bright blood or of dark brown discharge. She may also experience some slight cramping pain. The symptoms may subside within a day or two, but in about half the cases both the cramps and the amount of bleeding increase. *No*

change is observed in the cervix during this stage.

Inevitable abortion. As the abortion progresses, the cramps become more severe, the cervix first becomes effaced and then begins to dilate, and more of the placenta is separated from the uterine wall. The bleeding increases and often is accompanied by the passage of clots, and the fetal membranes can be felt or seen bulging through the cervical opening before they rupture. The term *inevitable abortion* implies that the changes are irreversible and that any attempt to maintain pregnancy is useless.

In a meticulous endocrinologic assessment of women who had a spontaneous abortion, Aspillaga, Whittaker, Grey, and Lind did demonstrate that the majority of women experienced decline in estradiol, progesterone, and 17-alpha-hydroxyprogesterone levels before the pregnancy loss.

Incomplete abortion. In the majority of spontaneous abortions, particularly those that occur between the eighth and the fourteenth weeks from the last menstrual period, varying amounts of placental tissue remain within the uterus either attached to the wall or lying free in the cavity. The patient usually reports the passage of some type of

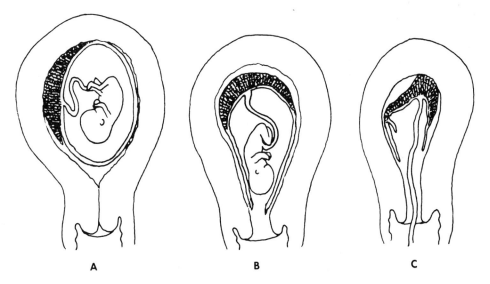

A   B   C

Fig. 16-1. **A,** Threatened abortion. Edge of placenta has separated, but cervix is closed. **B,** Inevitable abortion. Placenta has separated, cervix is effaced and partially dilated, and membranes may be ruptured. **C,** Incomplete abortion. Fetus and part of placenta have been expelled.

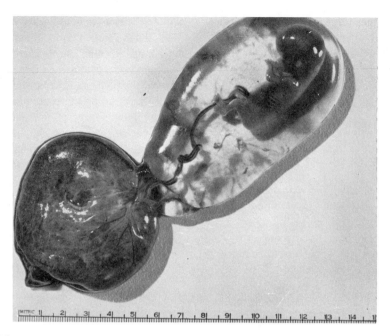

Fig. 16-2. Complete abortion. (From Willson, J.R.: Management of obstetric difficulties, ed. 6, St. Louis, 1961, The C.V. Mosby Co.)

tissue, but she rarely observes the fetus because it either has never developed or has died and degenerated some time before the contractions began. Pain associated with the cramps is severe, and the amount of bleeding may be sufficient to produce profound anemia, shock, and even death. The bleeding will continue until the remaining tissue has been removed or expelled because only then can the uterine muscle contract to compress the bleeding vessels and control the hemorrhage.

Complete abortion. A complete abortion is one in which the uterus empties itself completely of the fetus and its membranes, the placenta, and the decidual lining. This usually occurs only during the first 6 weeks and after the sixteenth week of pregnancy.

Missed abortion. Occasionally, the products of conception are retained within the uterus long after the fetus has died. Since fetal death occurs sometime before the products are expelled in the usual abortion, it has been suggested that the term *missed abortion* should not be applied unless the products

are retained for at least 8 weeks. The cause for the delay is unknown, but eventually spontaneous evacuation almost always occurs.

Missed abortion usually occurs during the early weeks of the second trimester. The clinical picture is that of a threatened abortion that seems to have subsided spontaneously or after treatment. The amenorrhea persists, but in most patients brown vaginal discharge occurs intermittently. The symptoms of normal pregnancy disappear, the breasts become smaller, uterine growth ceases, and eventually the size of the uterus diminishes. As placental production of hCG decreases, it can often no longer be detected in the urine, except by using the sensitive new monoclonal tests. Currently, with the use of serial ultrasound determinations and serum beta hCG levels to monitor early suspected abnormal pregnancies, missed abortion is diagnosed less frequently.

Habitual abortion. Although isolated instances of spontaneous abortion are fairly common and do not necessarily recur in subsequent pregnancies, repeated abortions may be the result of a permanent maternal or paternal defect and are of greater significance. The term *habitual abortion* should be reserved for patients who have lost *three* or more pregnancies *consecutively*.

Treatment

Because the treatment of each of the various stages and types of abortion is different, an accurate evaluation of the progress of uterine evacuation must be made before treatment can be planned. A properly performed pelvic examination does not adversely influence the course of the abortion and is necessary to establish the presence of a pregnancy, to eliminate tubal pregnancy as a cause of the symptoms, and to determine how far the process has advanced. The examination should include gentle digital and visual examination of the cervix and bimanual palpation of the uterus and of the adnexa. The degree of cervical effacement and dilatation can be determined by palpation. Since pathogenic organisms may be carried directly to the placental site, gloves, instruments, and materials used in the examination must be sterile.

Threatened abortion. In the patient who is destined to abort, fetal death already has occurred, and the placental production of estrogen and progesterone has diminished to a point at which the pregnancy can no longer be maintained. In these patients the initial brown vaginal discharge resulting from decidual necrosis is soon followed by bleeding and uterine cramps that ultimately expel, completely or partially, the products of conception.

In other patients a small amount of bright red bleeding begins a few days after a period is missed, when the fertilized ovum is actively invading the uterine epithelium. This is similar to implantation bleeding in monkeys, which is caused by the erosive action of the trophoblast on the vascular decidua. Later in pregnancy, bleeding may follow mechanical separation of the edge of the normally developing placenta. This type of bleeding usually is of short duration and does not recur, but occasionally it becomes progressively more severe, particularly if it is caused by separation of a placenta implanted low in the uterine cavity. Benign lesions of the cervix such as polyps and cervicitis, as well as invasive cancer, may be a source of bright red bleeding. Such lesions can be detected by visual examination of the cervix.

Since the symptoms of abortion are the result of fetal death and the consequent reduced hormone production, its progression cannot be prevented. Many women will want to go to bed because they have heard that bed rest is important whenever bleeding occurs during pregnancy. Although this need not be discouraged, one should not make patients think it is essential because bedrest will not prevent the progression of abortion. Physicians also should not permit themselves to be pressured into administering progesterone at this stage of the process; the only effect it has on the course of true threatened abortion is to delay evacuation of the uterus.

The bleeding associated with threatened abortion may be associated with uterine cramping; bleeding usually ceases in 1 to 2 days or rapidly increases in amount as other symptoms appear, whereas that from cervical or vaginal lesions is more likely to continue unchanged from day to day. Vaginal examination, including inspection of the cervix to eliminate local lesions as a cause, should be performed if the bleeding continues for more than a week.

The prognosis for continuation of the pregnancy is far better for those in whom bright red bleeding occurs initially than for those who first observe brown discharge. Most of the latter proceed to rapid termination, regardless of the type of treatment. The brown discharge is a result of decidual necrosis following decreased secretion of trophoblastic estrogen and progesterone. Conversely, a small amount of bright red blood may originate in a minor placental separation that does not affect the course of the pregnancy.

Ultrasonic scanning may be helpful in determining the probable outcome of bleeding during early pregnancy. With an intact, normal-appearing sac containing a normal embryo or fetus, the prognosis is favorable. If the sac is broken or empty, there is no chance of a normal pregnancy, and the uterus should be emptied promptly. If the sac is smaller than is anticipated for the stage of pregnancy and does not grow, missed abortion can be diagnosed.

Another test that may be helpful in predicting abortion is the radioimmunoassay involving a monoclonal antibody for the beta subunit of hCG, which is both specific and far more sensitive than ordinary pregnancy tests. *Abortion is likely to occur if the level is significantly lower than that expected for the stage of pregnancy and does not increase at the expected rate (mean doubling time 2.2 days during the first 30 days).*

A combination of serial ultrasonic screens and hCG assays provides the best prognostic information in women who bleed during early pregnancy. A favorable outcome can be anticipated if the embryo continues to grow at the anticipated rate and has normal heart action and if hCG secretion increases steadily. Conversely, low or falling concentrations of hCG coupled with inadequate embryonic growth are associated with a high probability of abortion.

Bleeding during the early weeks of pregnancy that does not terminate in abortion has little relationship to abnormal fetal development, but that occurring during the second trimester may. South and Naldrett, studying 1226 women who bled during pregnancy, noted no increase in congenital anomalies when the bleeding was confined to the early weeks. There was a significant increase in anomalies when bleeding occurred between the sixteenth and twenty-eighth weeks. In addition, the perinatal death rate was increased threefold in those who bled after the sixteenth week. Early bleeding did not affect the outcome adversely.

Inevitable abortion. Since the diagnosis of inevitable abortion implies that irreversible progress toward uterine evacuation has already taken place, treatment should be directed toward reducing blood loss and pain. *The administration of oxytocics is unnecessary* because these substances do not hasten the process and serve only to increase the discomfort. When the abortion occurs between the tenth and the fourteenth weeks, uterine evacuation will usually be incomplete whether uterine stimulants are given or not. Therefore it is preferable to empty the uterus surgically as soon as a moderate amount of cervical dilatation has occurred or earlier in the event of profuse bleeding. Intramuscular analgesia will not retard the progress of the abortion and may be given as needed to relieve the pain.

Incomplete abortion. Placental tissue remaining in the uterus after an incomplete abortion should be removed because it often becomes infected and, in addition, may be responsible for continued and excessive bleeding. The majority of clinically recognized abortions occur between the eighth and the twelfth weeks of pregnancy, and, since the passage of the products at this period is likely to be incomplete, a planned program for their management will keep complications at a minimum.

Patients with incomplete abortions are best treated in hospitals where adequate amounts of compatible blood can be obtained rapidly for those who are bleeding excessively and where major surgical procedures can be performed if they become necessary.

The patients should be examined under aseptic conditions, and any placental tissue protruding through the cervical canal should be removed gently with sterile ring forceps, since it usually interferes with uterine contraction and with control of bleeding. The instrument must not be inserted into the uterine cavity in search of loose placental tissue because of the dangers of introducing infection and of injuring the uterine wall.

Surgical evacuation of the uterus should be considered for most patients with early abortions even though the material that has been passed appears to represent the entire conceptus. Many who have had "complete" abortions between the eighth and the fourteenth weeks of pregnancy continue to bleed until the remaining placental tissue has been removed surgically.

The uterus should be evacuated promptly unless there are evidences of endomyometritis or parametritis. When infection is present the operation should be delayed, unless excessive blood loss cannot be controlled, while antibiotics are being administered.

Paracervical block usually provides adequate anesthesia, because the cervix already is dilated; but inhalation anesthesia may be required.

The remaining placenta can usually be extracted by suction curettage. If one suspects that placental tissue is still adhering to the uterine wall after the use of suction, the surface can be lightly curetted with a large sharp curette.

Loose fragments of placental tissue can also be removed by seizing them with ring or placental forceps and extracting them through the dilated cervix (Fig. 16-3). To avoid grasping and tearing the uterine wall, the surgeon should rotate the instrument slowly as the jaws are closing over a piece of tissue, and the downward traction should be slight at first until it appears certain that the uterus has not been included in the bite.

The blood loss in some patients with incomplete abortion is sufficient to require transfusion. If blood is nec-

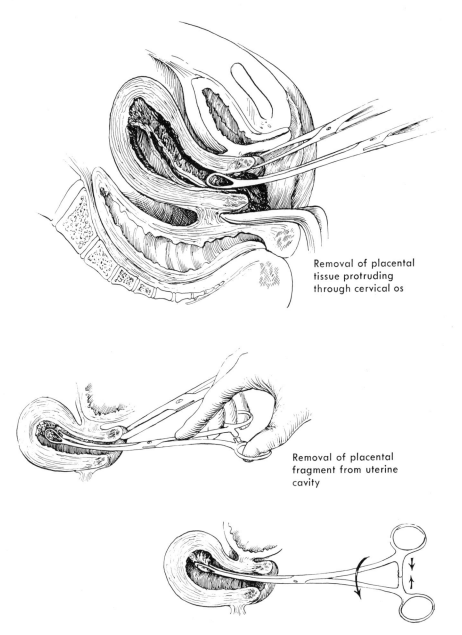

Removal of placental tissue protruding through cervical os

Removal of placental fragment from uterine cavity

Fig. 16-3. Use of ring forceps to remove placental tissue from cervix and uterus. (From Willson, J.R.: Management of obstetric difficulties, ed. 6, St. Louis, 1961, The C.V. Mosby Co.)

essary, its administration should be started before the uterus is evacuated, particularly if signs suggesting shock are evident.

Complete abortion. During the first 6 weeks after the onset of the last period, nearly all abortions are complete and require no therapy. After the sixteenth week delivery of the placenta may be delayed after expulsion of the fetus, but in most instances the placenta is passed intact, and no further treatment is required.

Missed abortion. In the past, missed abortions were generally treated expectantly until the products were expelled spontaneously, after which the uterus was curetted. It is possible to speed the process in carefully selected patients.

Before one evacuates the uterus, the diagnosis must be confirmed. Missed abortion can be suspected when the uterus is smaller than it should be for the presumed duration of pregnancy, particularly if there also has been bleeding. A definite diagnosis can be made if uterine growth ceases or if the uterus becomes smaller from week to week, when fetal heart sounds that have been clearly audible can no longer be heard, when fetal heart activity cannot be demonstrated by sonography, and when placental hormone concentrations are subnormal or decreasing.

Coagulopathy, initiated by the release of tissue thromboplastin into the maternal bloodstream from the necrotic decidua and placenta, may occur after prolonged retention of a dead fetus *(dead fetus syndrome).* Clotting defects rarely occur in association with missed abortion during the first half of pregnancy, but become progressively more likely as pregnancy advances. The defect develops slowly and is not often seen unless the dead fetus is retained for at least 4 weeks. Fibrinogen, fibrin degradation products, and platelet levels should be checked periodically after fetal death has been diagnosed because the coagulopathy usually develops without any evidence of abnormal bleeding.

A uterus smaller than that comparable to a 12-week pregnancy can usually be evacuated by suction curettage. An experienced operator can usually terminate those which are no larger than a 16- to 18-week gestation by dilating the cervix and mechanically extracting the dead fetus and the placenta. Those which are larger

should be treated by inducing labor using methods for the management of second trimester abortion when the fetus is alive.

Habitual abortion. The outlook for women who have aborted more than once is considerably less bleak than the 80% rate after three consecutive abortions that was suggested by Malpas. Warburton and Fraser calculated the risk of a repeated abortion to be about 25%. There was no appreciable increase in the risk after subsequent abortions, except for couples who had had no living children.

The etiologic factors responsible for repeated abortion include congenital and acquired structural defects in the uterus and cervix, chromosomal abnormalities, chronic infections, psychogenic factors, hormonal deficiencies, and causes such as immunologic deficiencies that are even less clearly delineated.

A significant etiologic factor or combination of factors responsible for recurrent pregnancy wastage can be identified in only 60% of couples. Although the specific mechanism of action can be speculated for the "known" entities, the exact pathogenesis is often unclear. Finally, it must be remembered that a disease associated with a single spontaneous abortion is not necessarily the explanation for habitual abortion.

Gleicher and Friberg studied four habitual aborters extensively for autoimmune diseases. These females had positive ANA titers, increased levels of lupus anticoagulant, and an IgM gammopathy. They postulated that an IgM fraction could have a deleterious effect on the growth of the fetal-placental unit.

DIAGNOSIS. Stray-Pedersen and Stray-Pedersen categorized the causes in 195 couples who had a history of three or more consecutive spontaneous abortions. A summary of their observations can be seen in Table 16-1. *Structural abnormalities* can include uterine anomalies or the presence of a leiomyoma, usually submucosal. Either condition can reduce the available endometrial surface or provide the endometrial surface with abnormal vascularization and presumably inhibit normal implantation and placentation. Some *uterine fusion defects* limit the capacity of the uterus to enlarge as the preg-

TABLE 16-1 Causes of habitual abortion—
retrospective study of 195 couples

Cause	Rate (%)
Uterine abnormalities	28.2
Corpus (15.4%)	
Cervix (12.8%)	
Infection	14.9
Endocrine dysfunction	5.1
Chromosomal disorders	2.6
Miscellaneous	5.6
Sperm disorders (4.1%)	
Systemic illness (1.0%)	
Smoking (0.5%)	
Total "known" causes	56.4
Total "unknown" causes	43.6

Modified from Stray-Pedersen, B., and Stray-Pedersen, S., Am. J. Obstet. Gynecol. **148:**140, 1984.

nancy grows. A cervix that has been injured during a prior pregnancy or surgical procedure or one that is congenitally defective may be unable to remain closed as the pregnancy advances. *Incompetency of the internal os* may be suspected by history. Characteristically, the patients have had surgery involving the cervix and have had pregnancies that have terminated in the second trimester in a characteristic manner; the cervix effaces and dilates painlessly with the membranes rupturing and labor being initiated. On the basis of the work of Danforth, it has been postulated that there are some patients who have an excessive amount of uterine muscle in the cervix and an absence of the normal concentration of fibrous tissue. This muscle relaxes, as does other smooth muscle in the body during pregnancy, and dilates prematurely. If the characteristic history is present, the diagnosis becomes more probable if a no. 8 Hegar cervical dilator can be passed through the cervical canal in the nonpregnant state without meeting resistance.

Although *chromosomal abnormalities* were identified in only 2.6% of the couples in the Stray-Pedersens' series, most authors report between a 5% to 10% incidence of chromosomal problems,

predominantly of balanced translocation. It should be remembered that if the couple has a history of recurrent pregnancy wastage and a fetus with a malformation, the probability of the chromosomal abnormality increases fivefold. Simpson has postulated that the mutant genes produce metabolic errors that interfere with some process essential to embryonic development and that polygenic factors may disturb the normal differentiation of embryonic structures.

Although *hormonal abnormalities* have long been considered to be a major cause of early pregnancy wastage, they probably are responsible for only about 5%. Diabetes mellitus and hypothyroidism receive the greatest attention. If either of these endocrinopathies is present, it would not necessarily be the only cause. Therefore an abnormality of thyroid function and carbohydrate metabolism has been consistently incriminated in most series as a probable explanation. A *luteal phase deficiency* has been suggested as a probable cause. Premenstrual endometrial biopsy that lags histologically 2 or more days behind the menstrual dates is considered the most reliable method of making this diagnosis. Serial progesterone levels have also been used. It is important that more than one cycle be studied before a diagnosis is made and therapy instituted. Once pregnancy has occurred, it is difficult to make the diagnosis of a progesterone deficiency.

Endometrial and cervical infection or, more correctly, colonization of the latter areas should probably receive greater attention. Identification of *Ureaplasma urealyticum* has been identified in up to 44% of the women with recurrent pregnancy wastage. *M. hominis* is cultured less frequently. Although significant systemic bacterial infections and viral infections have been associated with single pregnancy losses, it appears unlikely that they play a significant role in consecutive abortions.

There has been a group of *miscellaneous disorders* that have been postulated as an explanation such as systemic illness; that is, ulcerative colitis, nutritional deficiency, semen abnormalities, and excessive smoking. Although one should attempt to identify these problems and correct them if possible, again the pathogenesis remains unclear.

Recurrent abortion may be caused by *immunologic abnormality*. Couples who share HLA antigens may abort repeatedly. Women who have a high concentration of sperm agglutinating and sperm immobilizing antibodies are more likely to have a spontaneous abortion. Harger and colleagues identified a 7.5% incidence of positive ANA titers.

A summary of the assessment of the couples who have experienced repeated abortions can be seen in the box below.

THERAPY. The effective treatment of habitual abortion must be instituted before conception. It is not unusual for these couples to achieve pregnancy during the course of the workup; therefore the physician may wish to advise the couple to use some contraceptive measure for a brief period during the

course of the evaluation. The physician can approach this assessment in a positive manner. If the cause can be identified, most of the problems can be treated. If no cause can be found, the couple can be reassured that they have approximately a 75% chance of carrying the next pregnancy to completion. It seems prudent to attempt to correct any nutritional deficiencies, excessive smoking, alcohol, or drug consumption.

Surgery

Surgical procedures are seldom required to treat habitual abortion and should not be considered until the entire assessment has been completed and other potential possible causes have been corrected. More evidence is being accumulated that the *correction of a septate uterus* via hysteroscopy is feasible and offers patients satisfactory repair without metroplasty; concomitant laparoscopy is required to ensure safety of the hysteroscopic approach. In carefully selected patients, *removal of a submucous leiomyoma* may return the cavity to a normal configuration.

The *correction of cervical incompetence* is usually performed in the second trimester as the cervix shows evidence of effacement and dilatation. The risk of ruptured membranes and infection are increased during the second half of pregnancy. Although *cervical cerclage* has been recommended by several authors with a variety of suture material, the McDonald type of repair, with a large monofilament nonabsorbable suture, is commonly preferred (Fig. 16-4).

Hormone therapy

The most common entity to be treated in this category is *luteal phase deficiency*. This problem is characterized by a deficiency in progesterone, but there are several causes ranging from poor follicular development to a progesterone receptor deficiency in the endometrium. During pregnancy, estrogen and progesterone are secreted by the corpus luteum and later by the trophoblastic cells. It is more likely that progesterone is the most important for the maintenance of an early human preg-

---

EVALUATION OF THE HABITUAL ABORTER

History
   Include documentation of pregnancy loss, symptoms of systemic illness
Physical exam
   Emphasis on pelvic examination to detect leiomyomata or uterine anomaly
Hysterosalpingogram
Hysteroscopy may be used
Karyotype
   Special banding technique required to identify translocations
TSH
   If patient is symptomatic
Premenstrual endometrial biopsy
   At least two cycles assessed; collated with BBT recordings
Immune assessment
   HLA typing*
   ANA†
Cultures

---

*Applicable to the male and female.
†Recommended but significance uncertain; further immune studies warranted.

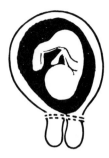

Fig. 16-4. Incompetent internal cervical os. Suture is in place.

nancy. Therefore progesterone supplementation is the recommended therapy for luteal deficiency. This drug therapy should be used only in patients who have a documented progesterone deficit on the basis of study of at least two cycles. Progesterone vaginal suppositories, 25 mg twice a day, or progesterone-in-oil, 12.5 mg IM daily, have been used. Although there is no scientific evidence to support that these substances are teratogenic, they are not currently approved for use during pregnancy by the Federal Drug Administration. Progesterone therapy should be started after ovulation and maintained until the onset of menses or through the tenth week of pregnancy. Some individuals recommend continued therapy with 17-alpha-hydroxyprogesterone caproate, but the scientific evidence to support this therapy in the patient with habitual abortion is weak. Other progestogens such as medroxyprogesterone acetate and the 19-norsteroids, norethindrone, and ethisterone should not be used. Their androgenic activity has been associated with masculinization of the external genitalia of female fetuses. Estrogen is contraindicated.

Psychotherapy

Women who undergo pregnancy loss have extremely intense grief reactions. The most significant response is characterized by self-guilt. These observations were well documented in the study conducted by Leppert and Pahlka. It is logical to assume that some compounding of this emotional distress takes place with frequent and consecutive

pregnancy wastage. Every woman who has aborted will certainly become anxious and fearful as soon as she realizes that she is pregnant again. A sympathetic approach with a special sensitivity to the problem accompanied by patience on the part of the physician are potent factors in the ultimate successful outcome of every case of repeated abortion, regardless of the cause.

There are two noteworthy studies of the treatment of women who were habitual aborters with psychotherapy. Mann studied 160 women who had aborted repeatedly. Of the 145 women who did not have a demonstrable organic cause and were treated with psychotherapy, 81% completed the pregnancy successfully. Tupper and Weil treated a group of habitual aborters, regardless of the cause, with psychotherapy and also had a similar pregnancy rate.

Other therapy

In *culture-proven infections* involving ureaplasma, an appropriate course of tetracycline therapy may result in improved pregnancy outcome. If a *male has been identified as carrying a balanced translocation,* donor insemination may be discussed as an option. In those *individuals who share major histocompatibility antigens,* immunization with or infusions of paternal leukocytes have been associated with a successful outcome. This therapeutic approach should be considered experimental, since there may be some significant risks.

INDUCED ABORTION

The exact incidence of illegal termination of pregnancy is unknown, but there are many fewer instances than there were before abortions were legalized. The death rate after illegal abortion is far higher than that after spontaneous or legal termination because infection is more likely to occur and blood loss is greater. The instrument used to induce abortion is often unclean and may carry pathogenic organisms directly into the uterus, the bloodstream, or even the peritoneal cavity if the uterus is perforated. The infection is similar to that after delivery at term but is far more serious because blood loss usually is greater, the organisms may be of a more lethal variety, and the patient may not seek treatment until the infection is advanced.

Many patients will deny having made any attempt to disturb the pregnancy, but during the examination suggestive evidence of manipulation can sometimes be detected. Tenaculum marks, fresh lacerations of the cervix or the vagina, and uterine perforations can be caused only by efforts to produce abortion, since they do not develop spontaneously.

An *infected* or *septic abortion* is one with which there is clinical evidence of genital tract infection. The term is usually applied to abortions accompanied by fever and those in which the infection has spread to the parametrium or the peritoneum. Peritonitis may be localized to the pelvic peritoneum or be diffuse, with accompanying ileus and abdominal distension. The parametritis may vary from unilateral tenderness to fully developed cellulitis that fixes the uterus in an inflammatory mass.

Pelvic examination is often unsatifactory because of pain, but the cervix almost always is open, and thin, bloody discharge, placental tissue, or profuse bleeding usually is present. The patient appears gravely ill and dehydrated. The temperature is of a septic type with peaks of at least 39.4 to 40 C (103 to 104 F), and the pulse is rapid and thready.

The organisms most often responsible for serious infections following abortion are those of the *coli-aerogenes* group, anaerobic streptococci, *Bacteroides,* enterococci, *Clostridium perfringens,* and various combinations of these and other bacteria.

Active treatment

The initial treatment of illegal abortion concerns itself primarily with evaluation of the general condition of the patient, the control of bleeding, the replacement of lost blood and fluids, and the initiation of antibiotic therapy.

Pelvic examination should be performed soon after the patient is admitted to the hospital to determine the extent of pelvic infection if present, to remove portions of the placenta that may be visible, and to obtain material from the uterus for bacteriologic study. If an IUD is present, it should def-

initely be removed; the death rates increase about seven times for IUD wearers who have a septic abortion. All unnecessary manipulations must be avoided.

A *gram-stained smear* of uterine material should be examined at once to identify the kinds of organisms present. It is particularly important to know if there are gram-negative bacteria or gram-positive bacilli, which may be clostridia. Blood culture for both aerobic and anaerobic organisms is an important diagnostic procedure.

It is well to obtain supine and standing x-ray film studies of the abdomen and pelvis. Uterine rupture is suggested by the presence of air under the diaphragm, and foreign bodies that have been pushed through the uterus may be seen. Radiolucent areas in the myometrium suggest clostridial infections.

The remaining tissue should be removed from the uterus as soon as it is practical. Antibiotic prophylaxis should be considered, especially if the white blood cell count is elevated. Compatible blood should be available for use in case excessive bleeding occurs during the operation.

Delay in completing the abortion may serve only to increase the morbidity, because the organisms proliferating in the placental tissue and the decidua have direct access to the blood vessels and thus may invade the parametrium rapidly. Early removal of the remaining placenta will eliminate this source of infection, and, in addition, will reduce the hazard from bleeding because as long as placental tissue remains in the uterus, the possibility of hemorrhage exists.

Infected induced abortion. The early treatment of infected abortion is directed toward the control of infection unless the patient is bleeding heavily enough to endanger her life. Specific treatment should include blood transfusions in a quantity sufficient to compensate for blood loss, enough isotonic electrolyte fluid to correct dehydration, and the administration of antimicrobial agents. Neither fluid nor food should be allowed by mouth, and constant suction should be instituted if the patient is vomiting (Fig. 16-5).

Details of antibiotic therapy of infected abortion are discussed in Chapter 42.

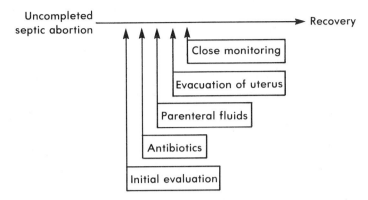

Fig. 16-5. Management of septic abortion without shock. (Courtesy R.K. Laros, Jr., M.D.)

Surgical evacuation of the uterus should usually be delayed until blood has been replaced, dehydration has been corrected, and high tissue levels of antimicrobial agents have been obtained. As soon as this has been accomplished, usually within 3 to 6 hours, the remaining placental tissue and decidua should be removed with paracervical and pudendal block anesthesia, which adds little to the risk. During the preoperative treatment period, blood pressure, pulse rate, and urine output (by indwelling catheter) should be recorded at least hourly.

Profuse bleeding accompanying incomplete abortion is usually caused by fragments of placenta that are only partially separated and are protruding through the cervical opening. The bleeding can usually be checked by removing the visible tissue with ring forceps. This is preferable to curettage before supportive treatment has been administered, but curettage should be done as soon as the general condition of the patient warrants it and whenever bleeding cannot be controlled by another method.

Complications

Most of the complications following illegal abortion are related to infection and blood loss. The majority of deaths are attributable to infection; the mortality from hemorrhage alone should be slight. *Septic shock* is one of the most lethal complications of septic abortion. Although most instances of septic shock occur as a result of infections caused by gram-negative organisms, it can also occur in conjunction with gram-positive bacteria, such as *C. perfringens*. The management of patients with septic shock is discussed in Chapter 42. *Consumptive coagulapathy* and *renal failure* are known sequalae but are less frequent occurrences in the United States at the present time.

REFERENCES

Aspillaga, M.O., Whittaker, P.G., Grey, C.E., and Lind, T.: Endocrinologic events in early pregnancy failure, Am. J. Obstet. Gynecol. **147**:903, 1983.

Batzer, F.R.: Serial β-subunit human chorionic gonadotropin doubling time as a prognosticator of pregnancy outcome in an infertile population, Fertil. Steril. **35**:307, 1981.

Boué, J., Boué, A., and Lazar, P.: Retrospective and prospective epidemiological studies of 1500 karyotyped spontaneous human abortions, Teratology **12**:11, 1975.

Cohen, E.N., Belville, J.W., and Brown, B.E.: Anesthesia, pregnancy and miscarriage: a study of operating room nurses and anesthetists, Anesthesiology **35**:343, 1971.

Corbett, T.H., and Ball, G.W.: Chronic exposure to methoxyflurane: a possible occupational hazard to anesthesiologists, Anesthesiology **34**:532, 1971.

Cousins, L.: Cervical incompetence. 1980: a time for reappraisal, Clin. Obstet. Gynecol. **23**:467, 1980.

Danforth, D.M.: The fibrous nature of the human cervix, and its relation to the isthmic segment in gravid and nongravid uteri, Am. J. Obstet. Gynecol. **53**:541, 1947.

Donald, I., Morley, P., and Barnett, E.: The diagnosis of blighted ovum by sonar, J. Obstet. Gynaecol. Br. Comm. **79**:304, 1972.

Gleicher, N. and Friberg, J.: IgM gammopathy and the lupus anticoagulant syndrome in habitual aborters, J.A.M.A. **253**:3278, 1985.

Grimes, D.A., Cates, W., Jr., and Selik, R.M.: Fatal septic abortion in the United States, 1975-1977, Obstet. Gynecol. **57**:739, 1981.

Harger, J.H., Archer, D.F., Marchese, S.G., Muracca-Clemens, M., and Garver, K.L.: Etiology of recurrent pregnancy losses and outcome of subsequent pregnancies, Obstet. Gynecol. **62**:574, 1983.

Harlap, S., and Shiono, P.H.,: Alcohol, smoking, and incidence of spontaneous first and second trimester, Lancet **2**:173, 1980.

Haxton, M.J., and Bell, J.: Fetal anatomical abnormalities and other associated factors in middle-trimester abortion and their relevance to patient counselling, Br. J. Obstet. Gynaecol. **90**:501, 1983.

Hemminki, K., Mutanen, P., Saloniemi, I., Niemi, M.L., and Vainio, H.: Spontaneous abortions in hospital staff engaged in sterilizing instruments with chemical agents, Br. Med. J. **285**:1461, 1982.

Kline, J., Stein, Z.A., Suser, M., and Warburton, D.: Smoking: a risk factor for spontaneous abortion, N. Engl. J. Med. **297**:793, 1977.

Laros, R.K., and Roberts, J.M.: Hemorrhagic and endotoxic shock: a pathophysiologic approach to diagnosis and management, Am. J. Obstet. Gynecol. **110**:1041, 1971.

Leppert, P.C., and Pahlka, P.S.: Grieving characteristics after spontaneous aboriton: management and approach, Obstet. Gynecol. **64**:119, 1983.

Mall, F.P., and Meyer, A.W.: Studies on abortions: survey of pathologic ova in Carnegie embryological collection, Contrib. Embryol. **12**:56, 1921.

Malpas, P.A.: A study of abortion sequences, J. Obstet. Gynaecol. Br. Comm. **45**:932, 1938.

Mann, E.C.: Habitual abortion, Am. J. Obstet. Gynecol. **77**:706, 1959.

Miller, J.F., Williamson, E., Glue, J., Gordon, Y.B., Grudzinskas, J.G., and Sykes, A.: Fetal loss after implantation: a prospective study, Lancet **2**:554, 1980.

Naib., Z.M., Nahmias, A.J., Josey, W.E., and Wheeler, J.H.: Association of maternal genital herpetic infection with spontaneous abortion, Obstet. Gynecol. **35**:260, 1970.

Roddick, J.W., Jr., Buckingham, J.C., and Danforth, D.N.: The muscular cervix: a cause of incompetency in pregnancy, Obstet. Gynecol. **17**:562, 1961.

Simpson, J.L.: Genes, chromosomes, and reproductive failure, Fertil. Steril. **33**:107, 1980.

South, J., and Naldrett, J.: The effect of vaginal bleeding in early pregnancy on the infant born after the 28th week of pregnancy, J. Obstet. Gyanecol. Br. Comm. **80**:236, 1973.

Stray-Pedersen, B., and Stray-Pedersen, S.: Etiologic factors and subsequent reproductive performance in 195 couples with a prior history of habitual abortion, Am. J. Obstet. Gynecol. **148**:140, 1983.

Tupper, C., and Weil, R.J.: The problem of spontaneous abortion: IX, the treatment of habitual aborters by psychotherapy, Am. J. Obstet. Gynecol. **83**:421, 1962.

Warburton, D., and Fraser, F.C.: Spontaneous abortion risks in man: data from reproductive histories collected in a medical genetics unit, Am. J. Hum. Genet. **16**:1, 1964.

17

J. Robert Willson

Ectopic pregnancy

An ectopic pregnancy is one in which an impregnated ovum implants and develops outside the uterine cavity. It is sometimes referred to as an *extrauterine pregnancy,* but this term would not apply to the occasional cornual and cervical pregnancies that are out of place but are not actually outside the uterus. An ovum may be fertilized and implanted at any point in its journey from the ovary to the uterine cavity.

SITES OF IMPLANTATION

Implantation sites of ectopic pregnancies in order of their frequency are:
1. Tubal (95% of all ectopic pregnancies)
   a. Ampullar
   b. Isthmic
   c. Fimbrial
2. Ovarian
3. Abdominal
4. Intraligamentous
5. Uterine
   a. Cornual
   b. Cervical

Twins and even triplets have been found in one tube, and bilateral tubal pregnancies have been reported. Combined tubal and intrauterine gestations are rare, occurring once in 30,000 pregnancies.

There are conflicting estimates of the incidence of tubal pregnancy because some statistics are based on total pregnancies, including spontaneous and induced abortions and intrauterine fetal deaths, whereas others are based only on deliveries. No matter how the incidence is calculated, the actual number is increasing.

Hallatt reported incidences of ectopic to intrauterine pregnancies of 1:126 in 180,079 deliveries during 1953 to 1975; 1:116 in 82,277 deliveries during 1966 to 1975; and 1:54 in 5252 deliveries for the 19-month period between January 1974 and August 1975. Data from the Centers for Disease Control (CDC) indicate that the rates for ectopic pregnancies in the United States in women aged 15 to 44 increased from 4.8/1000 live births in 1970 to 14.5 in 1980 and from 4.5/1000 reported pregnancies in 1970 to 10.5 in 1980.

Ectopic pregnancy characteristically develops in older women who previously have been pregnant rather than in teenagers. The average age, gravidity, and parity in patients reported by Schneider, Berger, and Cattell were 28.6, 3.1, and 1.8, respectively. In the CDC study the rates of ectopic pregnancies per 1000 reported deliveries were 5.1 in women aged 15 through 24, 10.5 in those aged 25 through 34, and 16 in those aged 35 through 44. The rates at all ages were higher in black than in white women.

ETIOLOGIC FACTORS

Under normal conditions the ovum is fertilized in the outer third of the fallopian tube, after which it descends through the tube and enters the uterus at the blastocyst stage. By this time the zona pellucida, which prevents implantation, has disappeared. The trophoblastic cells are now in direct contact with the decidual surface, thus initiating the implantation process.

If the progress of the fertilized ovum toward the uterus is delayed, it is still in the tubal lumen when it becomes capable of implanting. The trophoblast then invades the tubal epithelium, and implantation occurs there rather than in the uterus.

The following conditions within or around the oviduct retard or prevent the passage of the fertilized ovum and may be responsible for ectopic gestation:

1. Endosalpingitis, which may be a result of sexually transmitted infections, puerperal infections causing agglutination of the fimbria and the folds of the mucosa or diverticula, or constriction of the tubal lumen (The antibiotic treatment of acute salpingitis may prevent fimbrial agglutination but not the destructive changes in the mucosa. Vasquez, Winston, and Brosens, studying tubal epithelium by scanning electron microscopy, found the proportion of normally ciliated epithelial cells to be reduced in 25 women with tubal pregnancies as compared to tubal biopsies at the time of sterilization procedures. Ciliated cells were also reduced in eight women who had previously had tubal pregnancies and in four who developed tubal pregnancies after salpingoplasty. They proposed that the reduction in ciliated epithelial cells delayed transportation of the ovum through the tube.)

2. Scarring from tubal plastic operations performed to restore patency in tubes already damaged by infection

3. Peritubal adhesions that may kink or immobilize the tube, which may occur after infections following abortion or puerperal infections, appendicitis, or as a result of endometriosis

4. Congenital tubal abnormalities such as diverticula or atresia (Similar changes can occur as a result of intrauterine exposure to DES. Salpingitis isthmica nodosa may also be a factor.)

5. The fact that as many as 50% of pregnancies that occur after surgical sterilizations are tubal (According to Tatum and Schmidt the tubal pregnancy rate after laparoscopic coagulation alone is 42.9%, after coagulation and transection it is 14.5%, and after occlusion by loops and rings it is only 4.4%. McCausland reported 12.3% tubal pregnancies after 13,909 nonlaparoscopic sterilizations and 51% after 23,238 laparoscopic tubal coagulations.)

6. Transmigration of the fertilized ovum, a condition in which an ovum produced in one ovary enters the opposite fallopian tube (The corpus luteum is in the ovary opposite the involved tube. With *external migration* the ovum presumably is fertilized in the cul-de-sac where it begins to develop before it is picked up by the fallopian tube. With *internal migration* the fertilized ovum enters the uterine cavity but by some means crosses and enters the opposite fallopian tube. In either case the delay in entering the tube permits the ovum to develop to a point at which it can implant.)

7. The presence of an IUD, which does not appear to increase the risk of tubal pregnancy, but those that do occur are more likely to be either in the tube or in the ovary than in the uterus (According to Tatum and Schmidt, tubal pregnancy occurs five and one-half times more often in women who are using progesterone-releasing devices than with copper-bearing types. In addition, oral contraceptives containing only progesterone increase the risk of tubal implantation.)

8. Tubal spasm or altered tubal peristalsis, which can delay the progress of the fertilized ovum toward the uterus

9. Malformation of or chromosomal abnormalities in a substantial number of concep-

tuses in tubal pregnancies; may be a factor in the abnormal implantation

10. In vitro fertilization, with which the risk of tubal pregnancy is about 2% (Yovich, Turner, and Murphy reported that tubal pregnancies developed in four of 24 women in whom the embryo was placed in the uterine fundus as contrasted to only one in 56 with midcavity transfers.)

PATHOLOGIC ANATOMY

The process by which the fertilized ovum is implanted in the tube is similar to that in the uterus, but the tubal mucosa is a far less satisfactory implantation site than is the uterine decidua.

Although decidual cells can often be identified in tubal mucosa, the extensive decidual change that occurs in the endometrium is never seen.

Implantation. According to Budowick and colleagues the major growth of the conceptus occurs outside the tubal lumen. Soon after implantation the trophoblast erodes through the mucosa and grows along the length of the tube and around its circumference between the epithelium and the serosa. As it advances it destroys blood vessels; the resultant hemorrhage increases the size of the mass. The trophoblast may reinvade the tubal lumen from the outside. If this occurs, the growing conceptus and the free blood distend the tube itself.

Stock disagrees with this concept. After studying the histopathology in 110 cases of tubal pregnancy retrospectively, he concluded that the pregnancy is within the tubal lumen. He could find no evidence of deep penetration through the muscularis. As support for this theory, he suggests that unless the implantation were superficial, salpingostomy and removal of the conceptus would be impossible without damaging the tubal wall.

Pauerstein and colleagues examined 25 complete tubes that contained pregnancies and that were fixed by a technic that made them transparent so the internal anatomy could be seen in three dimensions. This permitted accurate sectioning of the tube to include the implantation site and the adjacent tubal wall. They found the trophoblastic spread to be predominantly intraluminal in 67%. In all but two of the 15 unruptured tubes the growth

was intraluminal. In seven of the ten that were ruptured the growth was predominately extraluminal.

Uterine changes. The uterine endometrium is converted to decidua similar to that of normal pregnancy even though the ovum is implanted in the tube. The decidua develops in response to the stimulus of placental estrogen and progesterone without regard for the implantation site. Decidual growth continues as long as the trophoblast is actively producing the gestational hormones, but when the placenta separates from the tubal wall or degenerates and can no longer function, the hormonal stimulation of the uterine endometrium is withdrawn, and it degenerates and sloughs. *The external bleeding that accompanies tubal pregnancy is almost entirely the result of decidual slough and indicates a failing placenta.*

The size and consistency of the uterus may change even though the pregnancy is in the tube. Both the cervix and the body of the uterus soften, and the corpus may enlarge to a size comparable to that of an intrauterine pregnancy of 6 to 8 weeks, but often it changes little. Uterine growth is caused by estrogen and progesterone.

Abdominal pregnancy (Fig. 17-1). The frequency with which abdominal pregnancy occurs is determined by the ectopic pregnancy rate. Beacham and colleagues diagnosed abdominal pregnancy in one of every 3337 births at the New Orleans Charity Hospital. In contrast, Strafford and Ragan reported an incidence of one in 7931 deliveries.

The fertilized ovum may implant directly on a peritoneal surface without entering the tube *(primary abdominal pregnancy)*. If the primary implantation site is just within the distal tubal opening, the developing placenta may grow through the ostium, attaching itself to the peritoneal covering of the pelvic viscera as it advances *(secondary abdominal pregnancy)*. If the embryo is properly nourished, the pregnancy will continue to develop, gradually extending from the tube until the entire structure is in the abdominal cavity. An abdominal pregnancy may continue to term, but the infant usually dies before the fortieth week.

The placenta may also gradually erode through the tubal wall into the broad ligament. A pregnancy that develops in this area is an *intraligamentous, or broad ligament pregnancy*. Although these are not strictly ab-

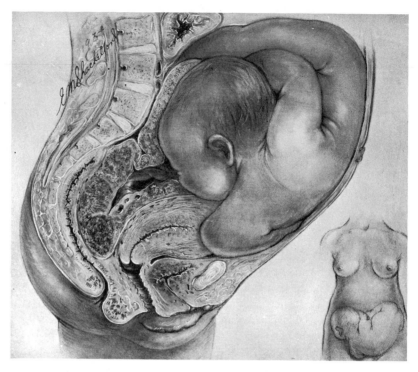

Fig. 17-1. Abdominal pregnancy near term. Placenta is attached over broad ligament, cul-de-sac, and anterior to sacrum. Delivery of living infant by laparotomy. (From Eisaman, J.R., and Ziegler, C.E.: J.A.M.A. **104**:2175, 1935.)

dominal pregnancies, their course and termination are similar to those that grow in the peritoneal cavity.

Cornual pregnancy. Cornual pregnancy occurs when the implantation site is in the interstitial portion of the tube, near the tubo-uterine junction. Characteristically, these pregnancies produce few symptoms, because the thick uterine wall in the cornual area can enlarge more before it ruptures than can the narrow tube. Eventually the uterus will rupture, but in contrast to tubal pregnancies, rupture is usually delayed until 14 to 16 gestational weeks. Since the cornual area of the uterus contains many large blood vessels, extensive intraperitoneal hemorrhage is inevitable.

Cervical pregnancy. Cervical implantations occur only once in 15,000 to 16,000 pregnancies. They often are confused with cervical malignancy because the cervix is enlarged and friable. Profuse bleeding occurs if the cervix is biopsied.

Ovarian pregnancy. With ovarian pregnancy the ovum is fertilized before it is extruded into the peritoneal cavity, and the trophoblast develops within the ovary itself.

COURSE AND TERMINATION

The duration of tubal pregnancy and the eventual outcome are determined primarily by the area of the tube in which the pregnancy is situated.

Tubal abortion (Fig. 17-2). If the ovum implants in the relatively large and distensible ampullary portion of the tube, the pregnancy will usually continue longer than it does in the narrow isthmus; however, it almost always terminates within 8 to 10 weeks after the onset of the last normal period.

Local bleeding caused by the destructive action of the trophoblastic invasion continues and increases, and eventually the hemorrhage separates the ovular sac from the tubal wall. With complete early separation, the entire sac may be extruded from the end of the tube, and, unless a major vessel is injured, the bleeding ceases.

More characteristically, however, the process is prolonged. During an episode of active bleeding,

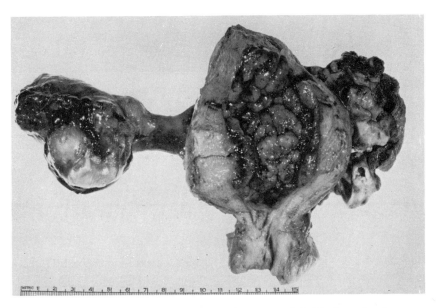

Fig. 17-2. Pregnancy in ampulla of right tube. Note pronounced decidual reaction in uterus and chronic left tuboovarian abscess. (From Willson, J.R.: Management of obstetric difficulties, ed. 6, St. Louis, 1961, The C. V. Mosby Co.)

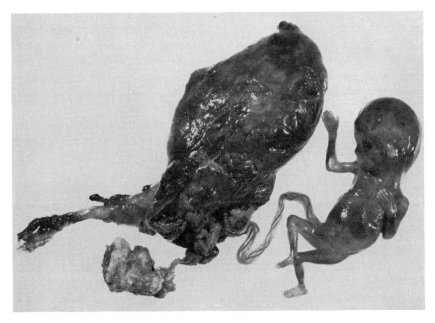

Fig. 17-3. Tubal abortion. Fetus is extruded through fimbriated end of tube, and placenta is in ampulla of tube.

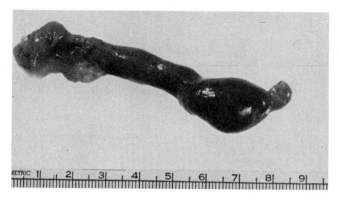

Fig. 17-4. Intact early isthmic pregnancy. Fimbriated end of tube is at left.

which soon stops temporarily, only a portion of the placenta is detached, and the remainder continues to function. The blood escapes into the peritoneal cavity and clots near the end of the tube in the cul-de-sac. After several similar episodes during which the pelvic hematoma gradually increases in size, the ovum is completely separated from its attachment and is expelled into the peritoneal cavity *(tubal abortion)*. This process may continue over a period of 2 to 4 weeks, during which time the patient becomes progressively more anemic (Fig. 17-3).

Tubal rupture. Trophoblastic cells proliferate and invade the tubal wall (Fig. 17-4). The growing conceptus and the hemorrhage caused by trophoblastic cells' destruction of the tubal tissue gradually distend the peritoneum covering the oviduct. The placenta may grow directly through the peritoneum, or the wall may become so thin and distended that it ruptures during examination or coitus or as the patient strains to defecate.

Pregnancy in the tubal isthmus usually terminates 6 to 8 weeks after the onset of the last period. The tube usually ruptures into the peritoneal cavity, and its perforation is accompanied by sudden and profuse bleeding. Occasionally, the implantation site is in the inferior wall, in which case the trophoblast erodes into the broad ligament.

Spontaneous regression. Many tubal pregnancies, probably more than become clinically obvious, must regress spontaneously. Either the ovum dies at an early stage, or it implants so close to the tubal ostium that it is soon extruded. The woman may have a slight delay in menses and mild discomfort, but one does not usually suspect tubal pregnancy, much less make an accurate diagnosis.

SYMPTOMS

The typical story of a *ruptured tubal pregnancy* is as follows. A woman who may have had a rather long period of secondary infertility *misses a period;* she may experience some of the early subjective symptoms of pregnancy but often does not. Within 2 to 4 weeks after the first missed period, she will notice a small amount of *reddish* or *brownish vaginal discharge*.

Preceding this spotting or coincident with it, she may be aware of recurrent, sharp, *fleeting pain* in the lower abdomen, which is often described as a "stitch in the side." The pain is caused by stretching of the peritoneal covering of the tube by the growing conceptus. This symptom is so evanescent that it often escapes the patient's attention and is usually elicited only after close questioning.

If the diagnosis is not made, the patient soon experiences sudden, sharp abdominal pain when the tube ruptures. The pain often is severe enough to cause her to faint. She usually reacts from the primary shock, but if the intraabdominal bleeding incident to the rupture continues, the symptoms of internal hemorrhage become progressively more severe, and the patient may lapse into profound shock.

Tubal pregnancies that rupture are usually located in the isthmus of the tube.

Tubal abortion, which produces a less dramatic clinical picture than that just described, occurs more often than does tubal rupture, and its course is more prolonged. The pain, which is located in the lower abdomen and pelvis, is cramping and intermittent and may come in attacks lasting several hours. Episodes of pain are accompanied by visible uterine bleeding; the amount varies from spotting to a flow similar to that with threatened abortion. However, profuse bleeding is unusual.

The symptoms increase in severity as ovular separation progresses. The escaping blood clots within the peritoneal cavity and forms a cul-de-sac hematoma, which enlarges with each episode of bleeding and which may press on the rectum, producing an urge to empty the bowel. The straining and increased intraabdominal pressure that accompany the patient's attempts to evacuate the rectum may dislodge the ovum and produce the final episode of internal bleeding. The patient often faints at this time; in fact, sudden, severe abdominal pain and syncope during attempts to evacuate the rectum are so common with tubal pregnancy that the diagnosis must be considered whenever a patient describes these symptoms. *Shoulder top pain* may be present if there has been enough bleeding to permit blood to collect beneath the diaphragm.

Tubal abortion is most likely to occur when the implantation site is in the tubal ampulla.

The basic symptoms that should alert one to the possibility of ectopic pregnancy are abnormal uterine bleeding and abdominal pain.

Abnormal bleeding can occur as an increase or decrease in flow during what is presumed by the patient to be a normal period, a missed or delayed period, spotting, or any other change. Many women with tubal pregnancies are unaware of having missed a period because they interpret bleeding resulting from separation of uterine decidua as normal menstruation; hence one should not discard the

diagnosis because there is no history of amenorrhea. Rather one should obtain a specific description of the timing, duration, and amount of bleeding with each of the last two or three periods in an attempt to recognize a change from the usual pattern.

Pain can vary from twinges, which may not be impressive to the patient, to a sudden, intense episode that occurs when the tube ruptures. The pain with tubal abortion is intermittent, cramping, and recurrent and may be present periodically for several days or even weeks before the final episode occurs.

The clinical course of *ovarian pregnancy* is similar to that of pregnancy in the tube.

Abdominal pregnancy can be suspected in women who have experienced repeated episodes of pain and bleeding during the early weeks if abdominal discomfort, spotting, and digestive disturbances such as nausea and gaseous distention continue despite the fact that the pregnancy appears to be developing normally.

PHYSICAL SIGNS

Pelvic examination ordinarily discloses the usual *signs of early pregnancy* such as cyanosis and softening of the cervix and slight uterine enlargement. The most important pelvic finding before tubal rupture or abortion is a *tender, sausage-shaped mass in one adnexal region.* Unfortunately, the distended tube can be detected in only about 50% of women with tubal pregnancies. In early tubal pregnancy the tubal enlargement may be so slight that it cannot be felt by a bimanual examination. One may not be able to feel a larger adnexal mass because of extreme pelvic tenderness and the consequent rigidity of the abdominal muscles.

Unilateral pelvic tenderness is a common finding. Pain in the affected tube may be induced by putting it under tension either by elevating the cervix or moving the uterus from side to side.

Bulging of the cul-de-sac can usually be detected by vaginal or rectal examination if a pelvic hematoma has formed or if the cul-de-sac is distended with fluid blood. *Signs of peritoneal irritation* and *of free fluid in the abdomen* may be present if there has been profuse or prolonged bleeding within the peritoneal cavity.

Fever is slight or absent except in the rare patient with a secondary infected pelvic hematocele. Changes in *pulse rate* and *blood pressure* are dependent on the amount of bleeding.

LABORATORY FINDINGS

The *white blood cell count* may be normal or increased to about 15,000. The *hemoglobin* concentration or *hematocrit* falls rapidly in cases of tubal rupture. The decrease is more gradual but progressive if moderate bleeding continues over a long time, as it does during tubal abortion.

Chorionic gonadotropin. Minute amounts of hCG can be detected in blood serum by *radioimmunoassay* or *radioreceptor assay;* in fact, an elevation can be measured shortly after the blastocyst implants. Radioimmunoassay and radioreceptor assay are effective aids in evaluating a patient suspected of having a tubal pregnancy because they usually are positive, even though most of the placenta has separated from the tubal wall.

Since cross-reaction with LH is possible because the alpha subunits of each are identical, the measurement of beta subunit of hCG is more specific and sensitive during early pregnancy. This test is preferable for use in patients suspected of having tubal pregnancies.

Slide or tube immunologic tests can be more confusing than helpful unless they are sensitive enough to measure minute amounts of hCG. Since insensitive immunologic tests are positive in no more than 50% of women with tubal pregnancies, a negative test does not eliminate the diagnosis. Serum receptor tests or one of the new monoclonal antibody urine tests such as the Tandem Icon hCG (Hybritech Inc.) that measure amounts of hCG as low as 40 lmU/ml should replace the less sensitive tests.

Qualitative pregnancy tests detect only the presence of hCG; hence quantitative tests are preferable in evaluating patients suspected of having tubal pregnancies. The ranges of beta hCG during the early weeks of pregnancy have been established (see Chapter 13) and can be used when tubal preg-

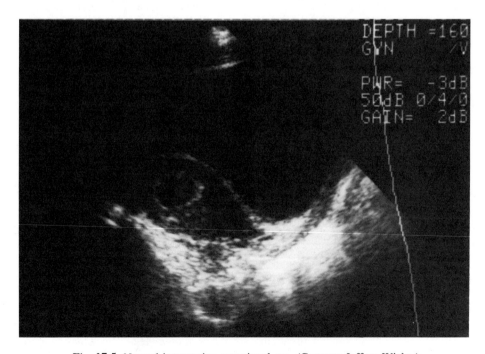

Fig. 17-5. Normal intrauterine gestational sac. (Courtesy Jeffery Wicks.)

nancy is suspected. Extrauterine trophoblast that is beginning to separate usually produces less hCG than does the normally situated placenta. In addition, during the first weeks of normal pregnancy, serum beta hCG concentrations double about every 48 hours. In a patient with symptoms suggesting ectopic gestation, the concentration of hCG may be less than that anticipated for a normal pregnancy of the same duration; and there may either be no increase in a specimen collected 2 days later, or the increase may be considerably less than that anticipated. One problem, of course, is that accurately dating an extrauterine pregnancy is more difficult than dating a normal pregnancy.

Kadar and co-workers have suggested that an intrauterine gestational sac should be evident by sonography when the level of beta hCG reaches 6000 to 6500 lmU/ml (Fig. 17-5). If the level is above 6500 and no gestational sac can be seen, the patient probably has a tubal pregnancy (Fig. 17-6).

Of course, it is only possible to delay treatment to obtain serial hormone assays if the patient's condition is stable.

DIAGNOSIS

The diagnosis of an unruptured tubal pregnancy is not too difficult to make when classic symptoms and signs are present. Unfortunately, symptoms are often atypical, and pelvic findings may be misleading. In general, the diagnosis can be made with a considerable degree of accuracy if one has a high index of suspicion for this condition and is alerted by the history.

Characteristic symptoms, abdominal pain and abnormal vaginal bleeding, should suggest the possibility of tubal pregnancy as a cause. A positive test for hCG makes the diagnosis even more likely and requires that appropriate diagnostic procedures be used promptly to confirm or eliminate the possibility of tubal pregnancy. One should not discard the diagnosis because the pelvic findings are not characteristic, particularly when a pregnancy test is positive. If the radioimmunoassay is negative for hCG, there is much less need for haste in finding the cause of the symptoms.

Special studies

Ultrasound. Sonography usually is helpful in making the diagnosis of tubal pregnancy. A direct diagnosis can be made if a typical gestational sac is identified outside the uterus. Unfortunately, this usually is not possible, so the diagnosis is most often made by exclusion. A characteristic and normally situated gestational sac within the uterine cavity virtually excludes ectopic pregnancy, except in rare instances of combined tubal-intrauterine implantation of twins.

If the scan is performed too early, the embryo may be too small to detect in the uterus. Occasionally, an image that looks like an intrauterine

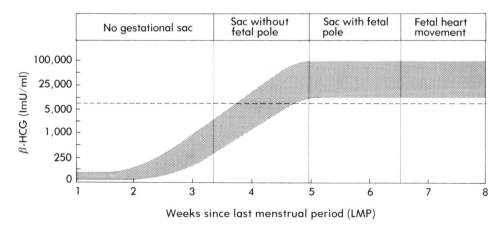

Fig. 17-6. hCG concentrations and sonogram during early pregnancy.

pregnancy or a blighted ovum can be seen in women who have a tubal pregnancy or who have aborted an intrauterine gestation. This structure, a *pseudogestational sac,* is produced by blood clots in the uterine cavity.

The combination of a positive pregnancy test without ultrasonic evidence of an intrauterine pregnancy 6 weeks or more after the onset of the last menstrual period is almost conclusive evidence of tubal pregnancy.

Diagnostic needle culdocentesis (Fig. 17-7). Intraperitoneal bleeding or a cul-de-sac hematoma can be detected by *needle culdocentesis,* which can be performed in the outpatient or hospital examining room using local infiltration anesthesia. A 15-gauge needle is inserted through the posterior fornix of the vagina about 1 cm behind the point at which the vaginal wall joins the cervix. If dark or bright red blood flows freely through the needle, the presence of intraperitoneal bleeding is confirmed. If only a small amount of bright red blood can be aspirated, the needle may have perforated a blood vessel and should be withdrawn and reinserted.

Failure to obtain blood does not rule out ectopic gestation. There is no intraperitoneal bleeding with early unruptured tubal pregnancy. Blood cannot gravitate into a cul-de-sac that is obliterated by adhesions. If the cul-de-sac is obliterated, culdocentesis is almost certain to be uninformative even though there is extensive intraperitoneal bleeding. Finally, the size of the needle may determine the result. Bits of blood clot, which may fill the cul-de-sac, can usually be aspirated through a large needle, whereas only liquid blood can be drawn through an 18- or 20-gauge needle.

If blood is aspirated from the cul-de-sac, one proceeds directly to laparotomy. If blood cannot be aspirated from the cul-de-sac in a patient with a positive pregnancy test and without sonographic evidence of an intrauterine pregnancy, it is essential that the diagnosis be confirmed or excluded by looking at the pelvic organs. This can be accomplished by *laparoscopy* or *abdominal laparotomy.*

Laparoscopy. Laparoscopy is a relatively minor and reasonably accurate procedure. One can usually see a tubal pregnancy unless it is so early that the tube is not enlarged. If a tubal pregnancy is present, one can immediately perform the operation necessary to remove it.

Laparotomy. The risks involved with opening the abdomen and the longer recovery period make abdominal laparotomy undesirable simply to make or exclude the diagnosis of ectopic pregnancy. In general, this operation should be performed to treat rather than to diagnose the condition.

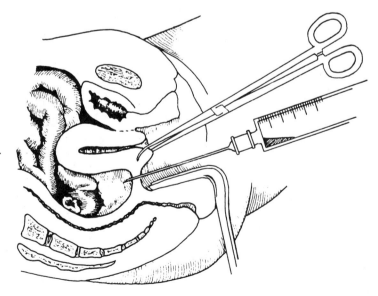

Fig. 17-7. Culdocentesis.

Dilatation and curettage. Dilatation and curettage should be performed if vaginal bleeding has been profuse and prolonged. This affords an opportunity for careful pelvic examination under anesthesia and may rule out an ectopic pregnancy if placental tissue is obtained from the endometrial cavity. If the material grossly resembles normal endometrium, further investigation, usually by laparoscopy, is indicated.

With *abdominal pregnancy* the uterus can frequently be felt as a mass separate from the extrauterine ovular sac. If uterine size remains the same while the other mass gradually enlarges, the diagnosis is more certain. However, it is difficult to outline the structures precisely, and the uterus itself is often interpreted as being an ovarian neoplasm or a fibromyoma. Later in pregnancy the fetus may be felt high in the abdomen and in an abnormal position, which changes little from week to week. Fetal echos can be seen outside the uterus by *sonography*.

X-ray film examination. If physical examination and sonography are inconclusive, an x-ray film study may help. If fetal parts can be seen lying posterior to the maternal lumbar spine in a *lateral x-ray film projection* of the abdomen, it is unlikely that the infant is in the uterus. A *hysterogram* will reveal a small uterine cavity and an extrauterine fetus.

The injection of a 0.25 to 0.5 unit of *oxytocin* intramuscularly will usually cause the uterine muscle to contract firmly, even though the pregnancy is several weeks from term. With an extrauterine pregnancy, the thick membrane surrounding the fetus, which may feel like uterine wall and even look like it on x-ray film examination, will not contract under the influence of an oxytocic agent.

DIFFERENTIAL DIAGNOSIS

Although it is usually possible to diagnose tubal pregnancy with reasonable accuracy, uterine abortion, salpingitis, appendicitis, and, more rarely, ruptured corpus luteum or follicular cysts may produce symptoms so similar that differentiation is difficult.

Threatened or incomplete abortion. The period of amenorrhea preceding the onset of symptoms usually is longer, the amount of vaginal bleeding is greater, the pain usually is less severe than in ectopic pregnancy and is in the midline and crampy in nature, and no adnexal mass and tenderness are

present. When differentiation is difficult, ultrasound will usually establish the diagnosis.

Salpingitis. The symptoms accompanying acute tubal infection usually appear at the time of menstruation rather than after a period of amenorrhea. However, with either salpingitis or ectopic pregnancy the bleeding may be irregular, prolonged, and more painful than usual. The pain, tenderness, and palpable tubal enlargement usually are bilateral. The temperature ordinarily is elevated, and leukocytosis is much greater than with ectopic pregnancy. The pregnancy test is negative.

Appendicitis. There is usually a history of digestive disturbances such as nausea and vomiting, there is no amenorrhea or abnormal bleeding, and there is no adnexal mass unless an appendiceal abscess has developed. The pregnancy test is negative.

Corpus luteum cysts. The mass in corpus luteum cysts usually is larger and more globular than in ectopic pregnancy. Unless the cyst has ruptured, there is no evidence of intraperitoneal bleeding. The pregnancy test is negative unless there is an intrauterine pregnancy.

Ruptured graafian follicle with excessive bleeding. Usually amenorrhea is not associated with ruptured graafian follicle, and the rupture occurs most often at midcycle, at the time of ovulation. The pregnancy test is negative.

Ectopic pregnancy can almost always be diagnosed accurately if one is alerted to the possibility by a typical history (abnormal bleeding and pain in a woman of childbearing age, particularly if she has had salpingitis or a previous tubal pregnancy) and by suggestive pelvic findings (unilateral tenderness, a unilateral tender adnexal mass, or distention of the cul-de-sac). Fig. 17-8 is a flowchart for managing a patient suspected of having a tubal pregnancy.

TREATMENT

The usual treatment of tubal pregnancy is surgical, but the exact procedure is determined by the duration of pregnancy and the condition of the tube. If the pregnancy has been diagnosed early, it often is possible to preserve the tube (salpingostomy or

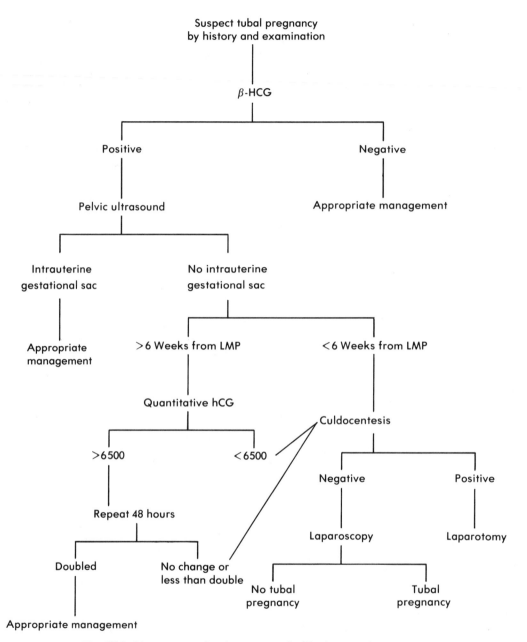

Fig. 17-8. Management of patient suspected of having ectopic pregnancy.

segmental resection). Conversely, if there has been delay in making the diagnosis, the tube may be so damaged that it cannot be salvaged and must be removed (salpingectomy).

Since Rh-negative women can be sensitized by Rh-positive blood from extrauterine embryos, they should be treated with Rh immunoglobulin as part of the treatment of tubal pregnancy. This is particularly important when the pregnancy is advanced.

The patient with ruptured tubal pregnancy and massive intraperitoneal hemorrhage must be operated on as soon as she can be transported to the hospital and the operating room can be prepared. If she is in deep shock, a surgical procedure without preliminary blood transfusion will increase the mortality. Consequently, blood must be administered while the patient is being prepared and anesthetized, even though some of it will be lost through the bleeding vessels.

An early pregnancy in the isthmus can be removed by either *linear salpingostomy* or by *segmental resection* of the involved area. In the former operation a linear incision is made through the tubal wall over the gestational sac, which is then removed. The defect can be closed or left open. With segmental resection the area of the tube containing the conceptus is removed, and the cut ends are either anastomosed immediately or at a later operation. These operations are justified when tubal distortion is slight and are particularly useful if the other tube has already been removed or is extensively damaged. However, they do increase the risk of subsequent tubal pregnancies. *Salpingectomy* may be necessary if the tube has already ruptured or is considerably distorted.

It may be possible to express the gestational sac from the ampulla without removing the tube if the diagnosis is made early; otherwise *linear salpingostomy* or *salpingectomy* may be necessary.

The treatment of abdominal pregnancy is prompt operation with removal of the fetus. Except under unusual circumstances, it is illogical to permit the pregnancy to continue to term because most of the infants are malformed and even those who are normal usually die relatively early in the pregnancy. Because the procedure usually is accompanied by excessive bleeding, particularly if an attempt is made to remove the placenta, the patient should be given blood before surgery if she is anemic, and at least 2000 ml of compatible blood must be ready for immediate administration during the surgical procedure. The placental villi often penetrate the blood vessels of the omentum and mesentery, and because there is no cleavage plane as there is in the uterus, the placenta can be removed only by tearing or cutting through its vascular bed. Unless it can be separated easily by digital manipulation or unless it is already partially detached, it is preferable to permit the structure to remain in place after trimming the membranes and severing the cord close to its fetal surface.

PROGNOSIS

Mortality. Although almost 10% of maternal deaths each year in the United States are caused by ectopic pregnancy, the death rate has decreased steadily. According to CDC statistics the death rate (deaths from ectopic pregnancy/1000 ectopics) was 3.5 in 1970, 1.6 in 1975, and 0.9 in 1980. Death rates were consistently higher for black than for white women.

Subsequent pregnancies. Many women who have had a tubal pregnancy either do not conceive again or have another pregnancy in the remaining tube. The reason is that the tubal lesions responsible for the first abnormal pregnancy may also be present in the opposite tube. Schenker, Eyal, and Polishuk studied the reproductive performance of 277 women who had been operated on for tubal pregnancy. Of these women, 114 (41.4%) had 219 pregnancies subsequent to the tubal gestation, which terminated in 114 live births, 37 spontaneous abortions, 29 induced abortions, and 39 recurrent ectopic pregnancies (16.2%).

The outlook after conservative surgery is much better than after salpingectomy. Sherman and co-workers reported an intrauterine pregnancy rate of 85% in women with normal fertility and normal pelvic organs. In patients who had had difficulty conceiving or whose pelvic organis were abnormal, the subsequent intrauterine pregnancy rates were 67% after salpingotomy and 44% after salpingectomy. He also observed more successful pregnancies in women who had been operated on when the tube was intact as compared to those in whom the tube already had ruptured.

REFERENCES

Beacham, W.D., Hernquist, W.C., Beacham, D.W., and Webster, H.D.: Abdominal pregnancy at Charity Hospital in New Orleans, Am. J. Obstet. Gynecol. **84**:1257, 1962.

Breen, J.L.: A 21 year survey of 654 ectopic pregnancies, Am. J. Obstet. Gynecol. **106**:1004, 1970.

Bronson, R.A.: Tubal pregnancy and infertility, Fertil. Steril. **28**:221, 1977.

Budowick, M., Johnson, T.R.B., Jr., Genadey, R., Parmley, T.H., and Woodruff, J.B.: The histopathology of the developing tubal ectopic pregnancy, Fertil. Steril. **34**:169, 1980.

DeCherney, A.H., and Boyers, S.P.: Isthmic ectopic pregnancy: segmental resection as the treatment of choice, Fertil. Steril. **44**:307, 1985.

Grimes, D.A., Geary, F.H., Jr., and Hatcher, R.A.: Rh immunoglobulin utilization after ectopic pregnancy, Am. J. Obstet. Gynecol. **140**:246, 1981.

Hallatt, J.G.: Ectopic pregnancy associated with the intrauterine device: a study of seventy cases, Am. J. Obstet. Gynecol. **125**:754, 1976.

Holman, J.F., Tyrey, E.L., and Hammond, C.B.: A contemporary approach to suspected ectopic pregnancy with use of quantitative and qualitative assays for the beta subunit of human chorionic gonadotropin and sonography, Am. J. Obstet. Gynecol. **150**:151, 1984.

Kadar, N., Caldwell, B.V., and Romero, R.: A method of screening for ectopic pregnancy and its indications, Obstet. Gynecol. **58**:162, 1981.

MacKay, H.T., Hughes, J.M., and Hogue, C.R.: Ectopic pregnancy in the United States, 1979-1980, Centers for Disease Control Morbidity and Mortality Weekly Report **33**:1SS, 1985.

McCausland, A.: High rate of ectopic pregnancy following laparoscopic tubal coagulation failures, Am. J. Obstet. Gynecol. **136**:97, 1980.

Pauerstein, C.J., Croxatto, H.B., Eddy, C.A., Ramzy, I., and Walters, M.D.: Anatomy and pathology of tubal pregnancy, Obstet. Gynecol. **67**:301, 1986.

Romero, R., Kadar, N., Janty, P., et al: Diagnosis of ectopic pregnancy: value of discriminatory human chorionic gonadotropin zone, Obstet. Gynecol. **66**:357, 1985.

Romero, R., Kadar, N., Copel, J.A., et al.: The effect of different human chorionic assay sensitivity on screening for ectopic pregnancy, Am. J. Obstet. Gynecol. **153**:72, 1985.

Schenker, J.G., Eyal, F., and Polishuk, W.Z.: Fertility after tubal pregnancy, Surg. Gynecol. Obstet. **135**:74, 1972.

Schneider, J., Berger, C.J., and Cattell, C.: Maternal mortality due to ectopic pregnancy, Obstet. Gynecol. **49**:557, 1977.

Seitchik, J., Goldberg, E., Goldsmith, J.P., and Pauerstein, C.: Pharmacodynamic studies of the human fallopian tube in vitro, Am. J. Obstet. Gynecol. **102**:727, 1968.

Sherman, D., et al.: Improved fertility following ectopic pregnancy, Fertil. Steril. **37**:497, 1982.

Stock, R.J.: Histopathologic changes in tubal pregnancy, J. Reprod. Med. **30**:923, 1985.

Strafford, J.C., and Ragan, W.D.: Abdominal pregnancy, Obstet. Gynecol. **50**:548, 1977.

Svensson, L., et al.: Ectopic pregnancy and antibodies to *Chlamydia trachomatis,* Fertil. Steril. **44**:313, 1985.

Tatum, H.J., and Schmidt, F.H.: Contraceptive and sterilization practices and extrauterine pregnancy: a realistic perspective, Fertil. Steril. **28**:407, 1977.

Vasquez, G., Winston, R.M.L., and Brosens, I.A.: Tubal mucosa and ectopic pregnancy, Br. J. Obstet. Gynaecol. **90**:468, 1983.

Weckstein, L.N.: Current perspective on ectopic pregnancy, Obstet. Gynecol. Surv. **40**:259, 1985.

Weiner, C.P.: The pseudogestational sac in ectopic pregnancy, Am. J. Obstet. Gynecol. **139**:959, 1981.

Yovich, J.L., Turner, S.R., and Murphy, A.J.: Embryo transfer as a cause of ectopic pregnancies in vitro fertilization, Fertil. Steril. **44**:318, 1985.

18

J. Robert Willson

Gestational trophoblastic neoplasms

Malignant diseases of trophoblastic tissue, although rare, are among the most lethal of all tumors arising in the reproductive organs. Gestational trophoblastic neoplasms are classified according to their progressive degree of histologic change. The three principal lesions are hydatidiform mole, invasive mole, and choriocarcinoma.

HYDATIDIFORM MOLE

Hydatidiform mole is a neoplastic proliferation of the trophoblast in which the terminal villi are transformed into vesicles filled with clear viscid material (Fig. 18-1). Hydatidiform mole usually is benign, but at times is has malignant potentialities and precedes the development of choriocarcinoma.

The exact frequency with which hydatidiform moles develop is not known. They are presumed to occur once in 1500 to 2000 pregnancies in the United States and much more often in Asian countries. The rate in Taiwan is said to be 1:81 pregnancies and in the Phillipines 1:200 pregnancies. The question as to the precise frequency exists because of the way rates are determined and because of differences in frequency with which pregnancy and its termination is reported. Rates based on deliveries or live births obviously ignore spontaneous and induced abortions, ectopic pregnancies, and perhaps even spontaneously evacuated hydatidiform moles. All the events of pregnancy termina-

tion are underreported in more advanced nations, and this is even truer in developing countries in which most births occur at home and may be unreported and where the number of early pregnancy terminations certainly is unknown. The reported rates include only women who were treated for hydatidiform moles in hospitals.

The generally quoted rate of hydatidiform moles in the United States probably does not represent the true incidence of molar pregnancies. This supposition was substantiated by Cohen and colleagues who identified eight hydatidiform moles among 4829 specimens from elective abortions (one in 600). Some of the moles probably would have been lost by spontaneous abortion and not diagnosed (Fig. 18-2).

Etiologic factors. Hertig and Edmonds found pathologic ova in half the specimens of tissue from spontaneous abortions they examined. Early hydatidiform placental degeneration was present in two thirds of the specimens with abnormal ova. They suggest that the vesicles develop because of the absence of fetal circulation. The physiologic activity of the trophoblast continues, but the fluid accumulates and distends the villi because it cannot be removed by the embryo.

Moles in which normal placental tissue or fetal structures can be identified are called *partial*. Those in which there are no fetal or normal placental tissues are *complete*. The latter are the more likely to become malignant.

Acosta-Sison suggested that the high incidence in Oriental women is related to *dietary protein deficiency,* since the disease occurs much more often in poor than in well-to-do Filipinas. McCorriston, studying the incidence of trophoblastic disease in Honolulu, found that Caucasians, who make up about 30% of the population, contributed only 11% of the moles. The rest occurred in women with Asian or Hawaiian backgrounds. He suggested that diet plays an insignificant role, because only 11% of the moles occurred in Hawaiians or part-Hawaiians, who represent 20% of the population and who are more likely to have inadequate diets than are the other racial groups.

Age seems to be a significant factor in the genesis of the lesion. Hydatidiform mole develops 10 times more often in women over the age of 45 than in those who are younger.

The *chromosome pattern* of most hydatidiform moles is 46 XX, and until 1977 the moles were

thought to originate from endoreduplication of the second polycyte of the ovum. Kajii and Ohama demonstrated that the entire genome of hydatidiform moles is of paternal origin. The most likely explanation is that an "empty egg," one without genetic material, is fertilized by a haploid sperm (23 X), which restores the diploid number (46 XX) by duplicating itself, and grows. Patillo and colleagues suggested that moles with 46 XY configuration occur because of fertilization with two spermatozoa, one an X and the other a Y.

Jacobs and co-workers confirmed the paternal origin of complete moles. In addition, they found a triploid chromosomal pattern in 75 of 80 partial moles. One of the remaining five was 45 X, one was 45 XX, and three were trisomic for chromosome 16.

Although these observations indicate the tissue from which the neoplasm develops, they do not account for the factors that initiate the neoplasm.

Trophoblastic disease may also have a *familial component*. Instances in monozygotic twins and a propensity for the neoplasm to develop in certain families have been reported. Parazzini and co-workers reported the interesting occurrence of two consecutive complete moles in the first two pregnancies of one woman and of a complete mole in the first pregnancy of her sister. The women's husbands were brothers. Sand, Lurain, and Brewer

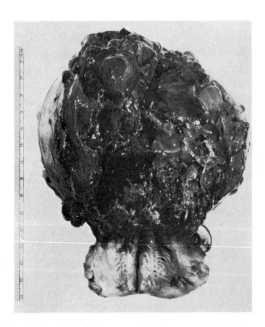

Fig. 18-1. Hydatidiform mole at approximately hundredth day of pregnancy. Note uneffaced, undilated cervix with deep molar penetration into myometrium. Patient is a 43-year-old primigravida.

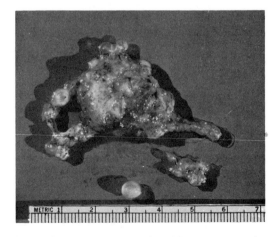

Fig. 18-2. Transitional mole found in spontaneous abortion.

reported 52 episodes of trophoblastic disease in 22 (1.33%) of 1648 women they had treated.

Pathologic findings. The trophoblast is converted into a mass of vesicles, which vary in size from a few millimeters to a maximum diameter of about 3 cm. The entire mass may be small, or it may enlarge the uterus to the size of a normal 24- to 26-week gestation. If a fetus can be identified (partial or incomplete male), it is small and malformed, although occasionally a normal baby may be born at or near term with a considerable amount of the placenta having undergone hydatidiform degeneration. These may be twin pregnancies with hydatidiform degeneration of one placenta and normal development of the other.

The histologic pattern of a benign complete mole is characterized by trophoblastic proliferation, hydropic degeneration of the stroma, and absence of blood vessels. When the mole is benign, the villous pattern is maintained, and there is neither anaplastic change nor epithelial penetration into the stroma or the myometrium.

Potentially malignant moles are characterized by more pronounced trophoblastic activity and anaplastic change. Attempts have been made to establish histologic criteria for estimating the degree of malignancy, but the most accurate method is still the clinical course.

The ovaries respond to the stimulation of the elevated levels of chorionic gonadotropic hormones by the development of *theca-lutein cysts* (Fig. 18-3). The cysts, which develop with 30% to 50% of hydatidiform moles and which usually are bilateral, vary in size from those that barely enlarge the ovary to those 20 cm or more in diameter. Definite ovarian enlargement is recognized clinically with a minority of hydatidiform moles. The change probably reflects the stage of molar development and the amount of gonadotropin being produced. After the uterus is evacuated, the ovaries gradually return to normal size as hormone levels decrease. The same change may occur during normal pregnancy.

Clinical course. After a period of amenorrhea, during which the patient considers herself to be pregnant, bright red spotting or dark brown vaginal discharge appears. This may be followed rather rapidly by cramps and expulsion of the mole, or discharge and bleeding may continue intermittently for several weeks. Patients who have bled for long periods of time may become anemic. Partial spontaneous evacuation, during which bleeding may be profuse, eventually occurs. These patients are often

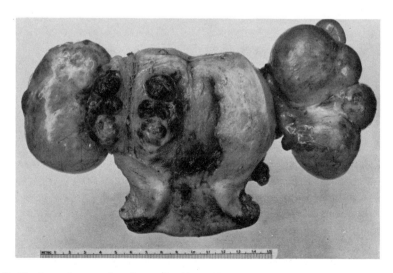

Fig. 18-3. Choriocarcinoma of uterine wall with multiple theca-lutein cysts. (From Willson, J.R.: Management of obstetric difficulties, ed. 6, St. Louis, 1961, The C.V. Mosby Co.)

diagnosed as having threatened or missed abortion until the characteristic vesicles are passed.

All the symptoms of early pregnancy may be exaggerated in women with hydatidiform mole. *Nausea and vomiting* may begin earlier, be more severe, and last longer than during normal pregnancy.

Severe *pregnancy-induced hypertension* may develop during the early part of the second trimester of a molar pregnancy; this is the only situation in which this condition is diagnosed before the twenty-fourth week. Hypertension is most likely to occur when the uterus enlarges rapidly and is considerably larger than might be expected for that stage of gestation.

Plasma thyroxine concentrations often are elevated, but obvious signs of *hyperthyroidism* occur in only about 2% of women with hydatidiform moles.

Diagnosis. Most patients with moles are treated for threatened or inevitable abortion unless typical vesicles are passed. The correct diagnosis may first be made when the physician begins to evacuate the uterus.

Hydatidiform mole can be suspected if the uterus is inappropriately enlarged for the calculated duration of pregnancy. In about half of cases the uterus is larger than expected. Usually, the discrepancy is not great, but in some the uterus may be as large as that of a 24- to 26-week pregnancy during the early second trimester. In the remainder of the cases the uterus is either appropriately enlarged or smaller than that anticipated for the gestational age. The uterus may feel firmer than one that contains a normal pregnancy. One must, of course, consider other conditions that may cause what seems to be inappropriate uterine enlargement. The most common are an uncertain date for the last menstrual period, multifetal pregnancy, and myomas.

Between the sixteenth and twentieth weeks of normal pregnancy it is almost always possible to

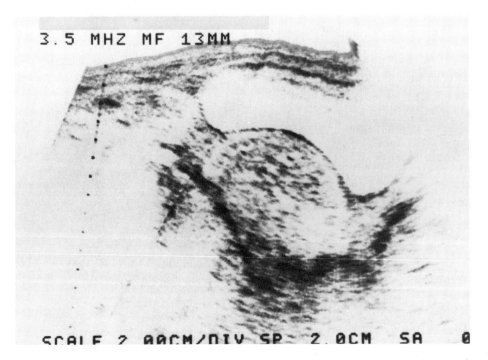

Fig. 18-4. Sonogram of hydatidiform mole, transverse view. Mottled appearance caused by cystic villi is typical. (Courtesy Jeffery Wicks.)

identify a fetus by hearing fetal heart sounds. However, the absence of these signs does not eliminate normal pregnancy.

A positive diagnosis of hydatidiform mole can be made *by sonography*. The characteristic pattern, when it is present, cannot be confused with normal pregnancy (Fig. 18-4). The pattern during early molar pregnancy may be less distinctive because the cysts are smaller. A repeat examination in 2 to 3 weeks will usually clarify the diagnosis.

Assays for hCG may be helpful in suspecting hydatidiform mole because the serum concentrations are usually much higher than during comparable stages of normal pregnancy. This alone is not a reliable diagnostic measure, however, because the levels at the time of peak secretion in normally pregnant women, at about the sixtieth to seventieth day, may be in a range consistent with a mole (Fig. 18-5).

According to Delfs the serum values of hCG rise during early normal pregnancy, reaching about 50,000 IU at 45 days and a maximum of as much as 600,000 IU at about the sixtieth day. The titer then decreases rapidly and is rarely above 20,000 IU after the hundredth day. The levels with multiple pregnancy are higher than those with a single fetus. The values for hydatidiform mole often reach 1.5 to 2 million IU, but they can also be low if the mole is regressing rather than growing.

It is evident that it would be hazardous to diagnose hydatidiform mole at the sixtieth day of pregnancy in a patient with a history suggesting threatened abortion and a uterus larger than anticipated simply on the basis of a serum gonadotropin concentration of 500,000 or even 1 million IU. On the other hand, a similar concentration after the hundredth day undoubtedly would be significant.

Romero and co-workers have suggested using *both ultrasound and hCG assay* to assist in diagnosing early hydatidiform moles. The diagnostic

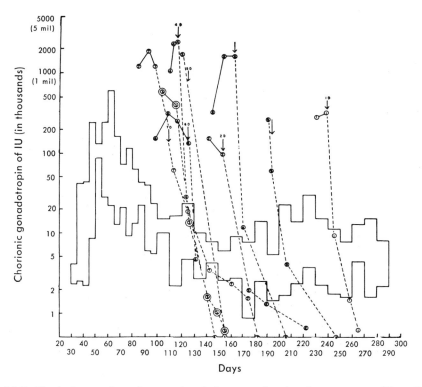

Fig. 18-5. Chorionic gonadotropin excretion during normal and molar pregnancy. (From Delfs, E.: Obstet. Gynecol. **9**:3, 1957.)

accuracy of the combined examinations is greater than that of either study alone. In 99% of normally pregnant women fetal heart activity can be detected by ultrasound when the hCG concentration is at least 82,350 lmU/ml. In their study of 36 women suspected of having molar pregnancy, the characteristic ultrasonic pattern was present in only 58.3%. When sonography was combined with hCG assay, the diagnostic accuracy rose to 90.6%. In 29 of 32 women in whom fetal heart activity could not be identified, although hCG titers were high enough to suggest that it should have been had the pregnancies been normal, complete moles were present.

Treatment. The uterus should be evacuated as soon as possible after the diagnosis is made.

The molar tissue can be removed in almost every instance by *suction curettage*. This method is appropriate even though the uterus is as large as that of a late second trimester normal pregnancy. Suction is preferable to the use of ring forceps and a standard curet because the uterus can be emptied more rapidly and its wall is less likely to be injured. An oxytocin infusion during surgery will stimulate the uterus to contract and reduce blood loss. The operation is completed by carefully curetting the uterine wall with a large, sharp curet. Tissue from the implantation site may provide more information concerning myometrial invasion and malignancy than do the vesicles.

As many as 10% of women develop *acute pulmonary complications* after curettage. These are characterized by tachycardia, tachypnea, and hypoxia. The condition is thought to result from pulmonary embolization with trophoblastic tissue combined with fluid overload, which is caused by physiologic dilutional hypervolemia and fluid administration, pregnancy-induced hypertension, and hyperthyroidism. The patient's condition can be monitored by measuring pulmonary wedge pressure, and the pulmonary symptoms are treated with administration of diuretics and oxygen and limitation of fluid administration.

Malignant potentialities of hydatidiform mole are greater in older than in younger women. For this reason it is usually wise to perform *total abdominal hysterectomy* when a mole is diagnosed in multiparous women over the age of 35 years. Hysterectomy should also be considered for nulliparas over age 40. Follow-up is identical to that for women treated by other methods.

Follow-up examinations. Between 15% and 25% of women will develop persistent trophoblastic disease after complete moles are evacuated. Although the risk of malignancy is somewhat less with partial moles, 9.9% of Berkowitz, Goldstein, and Bernstein's 81 patients developed metastatic gestational trophoblastic disease after the uterus was emptied.

Every patient treated for hydatidiform mole must be kept under observation until the physician can be certain that she does not have malignant trophoblastic disease. If the mole has been evacuated completely, uterine bleeding should cease within a week and the uterus should return to its normal size within 4 to 6 weeks. If bleeding persists and involution is delayed, another curettage should be performed in an attempt to determine whether the cause is residual benign molar tissue or a chorionic malignancy.

A more precise method for detecting continuing trophoblastic activity is by the *weekly measurement of gonadotropin concentration in the serum*. If the mole has been removed completely, the chorionic gonadotropin production will cease, and the material will gradually be excreted. It usually has all disappeared from the serum within 100 days after removal of the mole. If active molar tissue remains or if a malignant trophoblastic lesion has developed, gonadotropin secretion will persist or increase, and the concentration will plateau or rise.

A test for the beta subunit of hCG is performed at weekly intervals until the hormone cannot be detected in two consecutive specimens. If the level has fallen steadily at the expected rate, it can be rechecked every 2 to 3 months for a year. If hCG has disappeared slowly or has reached a plateau occasionally while the concentration is decreasing, it should be rechecked more often. An *effective contraceptive method* is essential during the follow-up period because hCG from a new pregnancy will mask any activity from the neoplasm. Low-dose oral contraceptives do not interfere with the interpretation of hCG assay. A *chest x-ray* film should be obtained after the mole is evacuated in search of pulmonary metastases that already may have occurred. It should be repeated during the follow-up period.

Delfs could still detect gonadotropin in 26 (21.8%) of 119 patients 60 days after evacuation of a mole. In 15 patients the concentration continued to regress and finally disappeared. The other 11 patients had an invasive mole or a choriocarcinoma.

According to Lurain and co-workers the hCG returned to normal levels in 596 (80.8%) of 738 women after hydatidiform moles were evacuated. Regression occurred in 20.8% between days 11 and 30, in 42.8% between days 31 and 60, and in 34.6% between days 61 and 170. All remained free of disease. Franke and colleagues, studying 111 patients with complete moles, found the median number of days between evacuation and return of hCG to less than 2 ng/ml to be 99.3 days. The range was 21 to 278 days.

Morrow and colleagues, testing for the beta subunit of hCG, observed a fall that was similar to those described previously. Their regression curve for the disappearance of hCG is depicted in Fig. 18-6. These studies indicate that hCG gradually disappears if the neo-

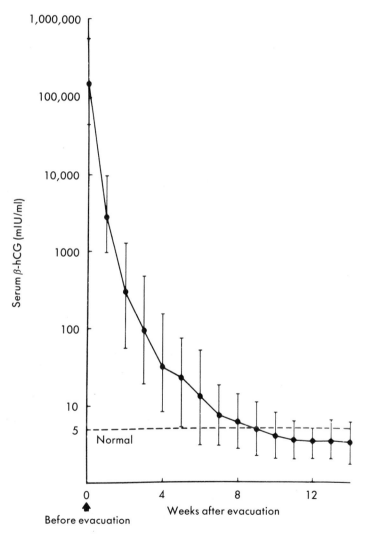

Fig. 18-6. Regression curve for hCG after evacuation of hydatidiform mole. (From Morrow, C.P., Kletzky, O.A., Disaia, P.J., Townsend, D.E., Mishell, D.R., and Nakamura, R.M.: Am. J. Obstet. Gynecol. **128**:424, 1977.)

plasm has been removed completely.

No active treatment is necessary as long as there is a progressive decline in the level of hCG. If the level plateaus or rises, one can assume that there still is active trophoblastic disease and that treatment is indicated.

Standard pregnancy tests are inadequate for following up patients who have been treated for hydatidiform mole or choriocarcinoma because only positive tests are significant. Even the most sensitive will not detect low levels of hCG, which may be present with residual active mole.

The beta-subunit radioimmunoassay is the most accurate of the assay techniques and should be used during follow-up. It is the only one that differentiates between LH and hCG; hence it measures only trophoblastic activity. It is so sensitive that it detects concentrations of hCG to which no other test responds (Fig. 18-7).

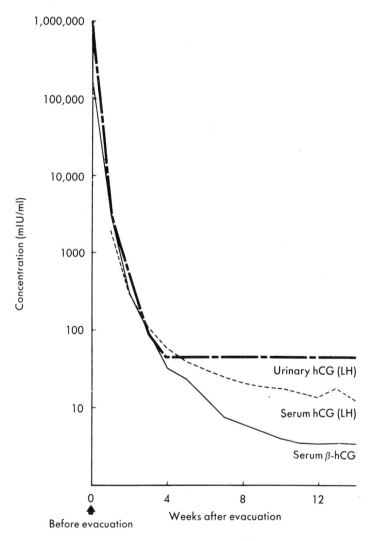

Fig. 18-7. Comparative sensitivity of test for hCG. (From Morrow, C.P., Kletzky, O.A., Disaia, P.J., Townsend, D.E., Mishell, D.R., and Nakamura, R.M.: Am. J. Obstet. Gynecol. **128**:424, 1977.)

INVASIVE MOLE

Invasive mole is similar to hydatidiform mole, from which it arises, but its malignant potentials are much greater. It invades the myometrium, in some instances penetrating the uterine wall completely and extending into the broad ligament or the peritoneal cavity. In half or more of all cases, invasive mole metastasizes through the peripheral circulation to distant sites, most characteristically the lung.

Pathologic findings. The histologic pattern is similar to that of hydatidiform mole in that the villous architecture is maintained, even in metastatic implants. The most important differences are the excessive trophoblastic proliferation and invasiveness. The degree of anaplasia is variable; in some patients the metastatic tissue looks completely benign; in others the cells are anaplastic. The preservation of the villous pattern serves to differentiate invasive mole from choriocarcinoma, which is so anaplastic that villi cannot form.

Clinical course and diagnosis. It is possible that bleeding will continue after the evacuation of a mole if the lesion is relatively superficial; there may be no blood loss if the trophoblast lies deep in the myometrium. The first evidence of the disorder may be coughing or hemoptysis from metastatic lung lesions.

Invasive mole or choriocarcinoma can be suspected if the gonadotropin titers fail to regress or continue to rise after evacuation of a hydatidiform mole. When this occurs, repeat curettage is indicated, but it may not be conclusive. If the lesion is superficial, a diagnosis may be possible; but if it lies deep in the muscle, the curet will not reach it. A chest x-ray film will reveal metastatic lesions if they are present.

The mortality from invasive mole is greater than that from benign mole but much less than that from choriocarcinoma. The primary lesion and the metastases usually respond well to chemotherapeutic agents. The main causes of death are hemorrhage, metastases, and infection.

Treatment. Treatment is identical to that for choriocarcinoma.

CHORIOCARCINOMA

Choriocarcinoma is a highly malignant trophoblastic tumor that may follow hydatidiform mole, abortion, or normal pregnancy. As many as half of choriocarcinomas are preceded by hydatidiform mole, but only about 15% to 25% of the latter have malignant propensities. About 25% follow abortion, and about 25% develop after delivery at term or ectopic pregnancy. Small foci of choriocarcinoma have been identified in otherwise normal term placentas.

Pathologic findings. The tumor appears as an irregular or circumscribed hemorrhagic growth in the uterine wall. The ulcerating surface usually opens into the endometrial cavity, but on occasion the entire tumor is embedded in myometrium (Fig. 18-3). It sometimes grows entirely through the uterus into the broad ligament or the peritoneal cavity. There may be dark red blood-filled metastases in the vagina or the vulva.

Masses of anaplastic trophoblastic cells invade the uterine wall, destroying blood vessels and muscle tissue as they grow. Necrosis and hemorrhage are prominent in the histologic appearance. The cells proliferate in masses and sheets, and villi cannot be recognized. The same pattern is retained in metastases (Fig. 18-8).

Clinical course and diagnosis. Irregular bleeding continues after the passage of a hydatidiform mole, abortion, or delivery unless the growth is situated deep in the uterine wall. Bleeding usually increases as more tissue is destroyed. Malignant tumor cells enter the circulation through open blood vessels and are transported to the lungs, brain, or other organs and soft tissues. The first evidence of an abnormality may be the appearance of symptoms caused by pulmonary or cerebral lesions or the discovery of a metastatic nodule in the vagina or vulva.

Choriocarcinoma must be suspected as a possible reason for continued bleeding after any pregnancy. A less serious lesion is more often the cause, but if each patient who bleeds is studied by curettage and tests for chorionic gonadotropin, malignant trophoblastic disease will be diagnosed as early as possible.

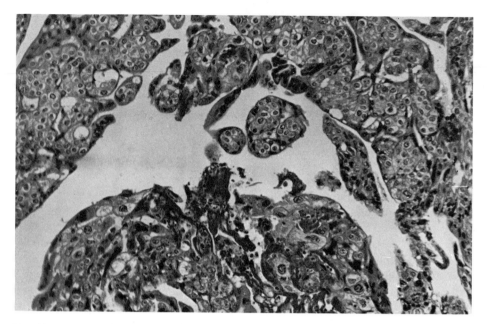

Fig. 18-8. Section through viable choriocarcinoma. Neoplastic trophoblastic cells are of both syncytial and Langhans type. There is no necrosis or hemorrhage in this field.

Curettage may be deceptive; if the tumor is situated deep in the myometrium, it cannot be reached with the curet. It may not even be possible to make an accurate histologic diagnosis from tissue curetted directly from a large ulcerating lesion because the material may represent only necrotic tissue from the surface.

The measurement of chorionic gonadotropin is the most important single diagnostic aid. Choriocarcinoma must be suspected whenever the concentration of this hormone remains high or is increasing and retained molar or placental tissue has been eliminated as its source. One can expect serum hCG to fall to less than 10 IU/L in about 30 days after induced abortion of early pregnancy, in about 19 days after spontaneous abortion, and in about 8 to 9 days after an ectopic pregnancy is removed. If the level remains elevated or continues to rise, the diagnosis is almost certain, and it is reinforced by the presence of characteristic lung lesions.

Treatment. Until chemotherapeutic drugs that specifically destroyed trophoblast became available, 80% to 85% of women with choriocarcinoma died within a year. Total hysterectomy with bilateral salpingo-oophorectomy, irradiation, and resection of local metastases were the mainstays of treatment; but they were generally ineffective because, by the time therapy was instituted, the tumor had already metastasized widely.

The prognosis for choriocarcinoma has improved considerably as a result of chemotherapeutic drugs. The response rate is determined by the extent of the lesion and the quality of treatment. The tumor can be completely eradicated in almost every patient with localized or with low-risk metastatic disease. Although the results are less satisfactory when the tumor is more extensive and is widely disseminated, 60% to 80% of those with high-risk disease respond well to treatment. The outcome will undoubtedly improve as more sophisticated chemotherapeutic regimens are developed. The best results are obtained when women with gestational trophoblastic neoplasms are treated in centers that provide the necessary diagnostic facilities and expert personnel who are experienced in administering the chemotherapeutic agents.

The drugs most often used in treating gestational trophoblastic neoplasms are *amethopterin (methotrexate)* and *actinomycin D (Dactinomycin)*. Methotrexate, a folic acid analog that interferes with normal metabolism, was the first drug to effectively eradicate abnormal trophoblast. Its principal action appears to be the prevention of synthesis of thymidylate, an essential component of DNA. Actinomycin D is an antibiotic with an action similar to that of alkylating agents. Treatment of most patients with invasive mole or choriocarcinoma can be started with one of these drugs.

Women whose hCG titers plateau or rise during postevacuation follow-up and those with invasive mole and choriocarcinoma are candidates for chemotherapy. The regimen is selected on the basis of a pretreatment survey to determine the extent of the disease. The survey includes a complete blood study with differential and platelet counts, serum biochemical determinations, liver function studies, thyroid studies, chest x-ray film examinations, an intravenous pyelogram, liver and brain CT scans, an hCG assay, and any indicated consultations.

Low-risk (good prognosis) metastatic disease includes patients who do not have brain or liver metastases or other high-risk factors. *High-risk (poor prognosis) metastatic disease* includes patients with brain or liver metastases, serum hCG concentrations above 40,000 lmU/ml when chemotherapy is started, metastatic disease that occurs after treatment with single-agent therapy, or choriocarcinoma that follows term pregnancy.

Patients with *nonmetastatic gestational trophoblastic neoplasms* are usually treated with a single agent, which is continued until the tumor has been eradicated, unless uncontrollable toxic symptoms restrict its use. Usually, the first drug is *methotrexate,* in intramuscular doses of 0.4 mg/kg body weight daily for 5 days. A second course is started after an interval of 7 days. Subsequent courses are given at the same intervals until three consecutive weekly assays for hCG are negative.

Most women suffer toxic reactions from the medication. The principal reactions are stomatitis, dermatitis, leukopenia from bone marrow depression, gastrointestinal ulceration, and alopecia. These can be kept minimal by a regimen that includes larger doses of methotrexate and folinic acid. Methotrexate, 1 mg/kg of body weight, is given on days 1, 3, 5, and 7, and 0.1 mg/kg of body weight of folinic acid on days 2, 4, 6, and 8. The effectiveness of this regimen has not yet been established.

Patients with liver or kidney dysfunction and those who cannot tolerate repeated courses of methotrexate can be treated with *actinomycin D.* This drug is given intra-

venously in doses of 10 to 13 mg/kg of body weight daily for 5 days. Daily monitoring for toxic effects is essential. Courses are repeated at 7-day intervals for as long as is necessary.

The regimen that is selected for the treatment of metastatic disease is determined by the extent of the tumor and the location of the metastases. Treatment of patients classified as *good prognosis–low risk* is begun with methotrexate or actinomycin D in the same doses as for nonmetastatic disease. Serum beta subunit hCG concentrations are determined at weekly intervals. If the tumor fails to respond, as indicated by plateauing or rising hCG titers, more vigorous treatment is necessary.

Patients classified as *poor prognosis–high risk* are usually treated with a combination of methotrexate, actinomycin D, and chlorambucil or cyclophosphamide or with a variety of combinations of other chemotherapeutic drugs.

Additional surgery or irradiation may be necessary for patients who fail to respond to the drugs. Such intensive therapy is highly toxic and must be carried out in treatment centers.

Chemotherapeutic agents have almost completely replaced surgical treatment of malignant trophoblastic disease. Not only was hysterectomy ineffective in the management of metastatic choriocarcinoma, but it eliminated all hope of future childbearing in young women. If the primary tumor and the metastases can be eradicated by drug therapy, there is no reason to remove the uterus. Menstruation will be normal, and pregnancy can occur. No evidence suggests that chemotherapeutic agents used to treat malignant trophoblastic disease will affect the growth and development of the embryo during subsequent pregnancies.

In a few patients, chemotherapeutic regimens are unsuccessful, either because the cells are unresponsive or because the drug fails to reach the primary tumor in the uterine wall. Hysterectomy to remove the local lesions may be performed. The ovaries need not be removed. Chemotherapy should be continued after surgery according to the criteria noted previously.

Hammond, Weed, and Currie have suggested that hysterectomy be an essential part of the treatment of women with localized or metastatic disease if they do not want to retain their reproductive capacities. They advocate performing the operation soon after chemotherapy is started and have found that those who are operated on require fewer courses of treatment and recover faster.

Chemotherapy is less effective in eradicating brain metastases than those in other parts of the body. Radiation therapy will sometimes destroy lesions in the brain that have not responded to drugs. Radiation therapy may also be used to treat liver metastases.

Follow-up examinations. Women who have been treated for invasive mole or choriocarcinoma should be checked at 1-month intervals for 1 year after the gonadotropin concentration has returned to normal. The essential studies are pelvic examination, chest x-ray film examination, and tests for serum chorionic gonadotropin. The pulmonary lesions usually regress slowly and, with successful treatment, disappear completely.

After the first year the examinations are repeated at 4-month intervals. If there is no evidence of recurrence by the end of the second year, one can assume that the lesion has been eradicated. An effective contraceptive method should be used during the follow-up period.

REFERENCES

Acosta-Sison, N.: Chorioadenoma destruens, Am. J. Obstet. Gynecol. **80**:176, 1960.

Berkowitz, R.S., Goldstein, D.P., and Bernstein, M.R.: Natural history of partial molar pregnancy, Obstet. Gynecol. **66**:677, 1985.

Cohen, B.A., Bruckman, R.T., Rosenshein, N.B., Atenza, M.F., King, T.M., and Parmley, T.H.: Gestational trophoblastic disease within an elective abortion population, Am. J. Obstet. Gynecol. **135**:452, 1979.

Delfs, E.: Quantitative chorionic gonadotropin, Obstet. Gynecol. **9**:1, 1957.

Eddy, G.L., et al.: Postmolar trophoblastic disease in women using hormonal contraception with estrogen, Obstet. Gynecol. **62**:736, 1983.

Franke, H.R., et al.: Plasma human chorionic gonadotropin disappearance in hydatidiform mole: a central registry from the Netherlands, Obstet. Gynecol. **62**:467, 1983.

Grimes, D.A.: Epidemiology of gestational trophoblastic disease, Am. J. Obstet. Gynecol. **150**:309, 1984.

Hammond, C.B., Weed, J.C., Jr., and Currie, J.L.: The role of operation in the current therapy of gestational trophoblastic disease, Am. J. Obstet. Gynecol. **136**:844, 1980.

Hertig, A.T., and Edmonds, H.W.: Genesis of hydatidiform mole, Arch. Pathol. **30**:260, 1940.

Hertig, A.T., and Mansell, H.: Hydatidiform mole and choriocarcinoma, Washington, D.C., 1956, Armed Forces Institute of Pathology.

Jacobs, P.A., Wilson, C.M., Sprenkle, J.A., Rosenshein, N.B., and Migeon, B.R.: Mechanism of origin of complete hydatidiform moles, Nature **286**:714, 1980.

Jacobs, P.A., et al.: Complete and partial hydatidiform mole in Hawaii: cytogenetics, morphology, and epidemiology, Br. J. Obstet. Gynaecol. **89**:258, 1982.

Kajii, T., and Ohama, J.: Androgenic origin of hydatidiform mole, Nature **268**:633, 1977.

Lurain, J.R., Brewer, J.I., Torok, E.E., and Halpern, B.: Natural history of hydatidiform mole after primary evacuation, Am. J. Obstet. Gynecol. **145**:591, 1983.

Lurain, J.R., and Brewer J.I.: Treatment of high-risk gestational trophoblastic disease with methotrexate, actinomycin D, and cyclophosphamide chemotherapy, Obstet. Gynecol. **63**:830, 1985.

McCorriston, C.C.: Racial incidence of hydatidiform mole, Am. J. Obstet. Gynecol. **101**:377, 1968.

McDonald, T.W., and Ruffolo, E.H.: Modern management of gestational trophoblastic disease, Obstet. Gynecol. Surv. **38**:67, 1983.

Morrow, C.P., Kletzky, O.A., Disaia, P.J., Townsend, D.E., Mishell, D.R., and Nakamura, R.M.: Clinical and laboratory correlates of molar pregnancy and trophoblastic disease, Am. J. Obstet. Gynecol. **128**:424, 1977.

Parazzini, F., La Vecchia, C., Franceschi, S., and Mangili, G.: Familial trophoblastic disease: case report, Am. J. Obstet. Gynecol. **149**:382, 1984.

Patillo, R.A., Sasaki, S., Katayama, K.P., Roesler, M., and Mattingly, R.F.: Genesis of 46,XY hydatidiform mole, Am. J. Obstet. Gynecol. **141**:104, 1981.

Romero, R., et al.: New criteria for the diagnosis of gestational trophoblastic disease, Obstet. Gynecol. **66**:553, 1985.

Sand, P.K., Lurain, J.R., and Brewer J.I.: Repeat gestational trophoblastic disease, Obstet. Gynecol. **63**:140, 1984.

Steir, J.A., Bergsgo, P., and Myking, O.L.: Human chorionic gonadotropin in maternal plasma after induced abortion, spontaneous abortion, and removed ectopic pregnancy, Obstet. Gynecol. **64**:391, 1984.

Yamashita, K., Wake, N., Araki, T., Ichinoe, K., and Makoto, K.: Human lymphocyte antigen expression in hydatidiform mole: androgenesis following fertilization by a haploid sperm, Am. J. Obstet. Gynecol. **135**:597, 1979.

19

Russell K. Laros, Jr.

Physiology of normal pregnancy

Profound local and systemic changes in maternal physiology are initiated by conception and continue throughout pregnancy. After expulsion of the placenta, many of these changes are rapidly reversed, although certain alterations, particularly those affecting the generative tract, are more gradual in their return to the nongravid state. For purposes of evaluating any system, whether genital, renal, cardiovascular, endocrine, or other, it is important to realize that the effects of pregnancy are not fully reversed until at least 6 weeks after the baby is born.

GENERATIVE ORGANS

Uterus. The *size of the uterus* increases five to six times (from 7 by 5 by 3 cm to 35 by 25 by 22 cm) (Fig. 19-1), the *weight* undergoes a twentyfold increase (from 50 to 1000 g at term), and the capacity increases spectacularly one thousandfold (from 4 to 4000 ml).

Uterine growth is caused almost entirely by hypertrophy of the muscle cells. In addition, an increase in the amount of elastic connective tissue adds considerably to the strength of the uterine wall, and a remarkable increase in the size and number of blood vessels provides the rapidly growing tissues with an adequate supply of oxygen and nutritive substances (Fig. 19-2).

The initial stimulus to uterine hypertrophy is hormonal. Thus in the first 6 weeks the size of the uterus is similar in either intrauterine or extrauterine pregnancy. Enlargement thereafter depends on the size of the conceptus and the actual growth of the muscle fibers.

Related uterine and fetal weights throughout gestation show that the greater part of the uterine weight is gained before the twentieth week, during which time the myometrial walls become progressively thicker. In the last half of pregnancy when the fetal growth is accelerated, the myometrium is

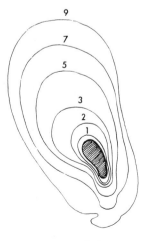

Fig. 19-1. Growth of uterus during successive months of pregnancy.

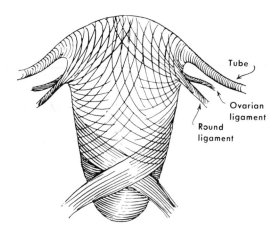

Fig. 19-2. Diagram showing interwoven pattern of uterine muscle fibers.

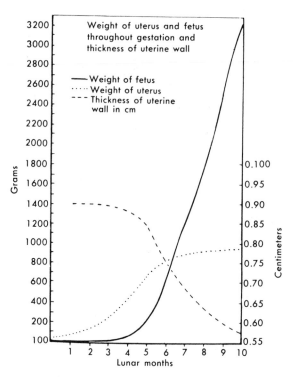

Fig. 19-3. This composite graph expresses certain weights and measurements. Note that around twentieth week uterine growth diminishes: therefore myometrium begins to thin, and fetus begins to increase rapidly in weight. (From Gillespie, E.C.: Am. J. Obstet. Gynecol. **59**:949, 1950.)

thinned out to accommodate the fetus (Fig. 19-3). Late in pregnancy and particularly during labor, myometrial contractions with shortening of the muscle fibers cause progressive thickening of the upper uterine segment as the lower segment develops.

The *position* of the gravid uterus changes as gestation advances. Early, an exaggerated anteflexion is usual; and then as the uterus rises from the pelvis, varying degrees of dextrorotation develop because the rectosigmoid occupies a relatively fixed position in the left posterior aspect of the pelvis (Fig. 19-4).

Uterine blood flow in normal term pregnancy measured during cesarean section by Metcalfe and associates averaged 500 ml/min, as opposed to 50 ml/min in the nonpregnant state. Oxygen consumption of the gravid uterus was calculated to be 25 ml/min (5 ml/kg/min), and the carbon dioxide production, 22 ml/min. On the basis of these determinations the average respiratory quotient of the uterus at term was 0.91.

Evidence for augmentation of uterine blood flow by biologically active estrogens, for alterations caused by variations in blood gas tensions and chemical substances, and for a fine control superimposed by the autonomic nervous system are discussed in detail by Lewis in a review of mechanisms involved in uterine blood flow. Elucidation of such mechanisms should have important applications in clinical practice.

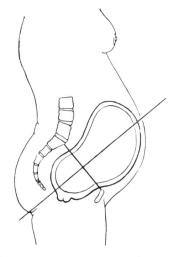

Fig. 19-4. Relationship of axis of pregnant uterus to pelvic inlet.

LOWER UTERINE SEGMENT. The uterus is differentiated into an upper and a lower segment. The wall of the upper contractile portion of the uterus becomes thicker during labor as the lower uterine segment, which must undergo circumferential dilatation to permit passage of the presenting part, becomes thinned out and about 10 cm in length. Danforth and Ivy have shown that the lower uterine segment takes its origin from the isthmic portion of the uterus and the cervix (Figs. 19-5 and 19-6).

From the beginning of the second trimester until the last few weeks of pregnancy the isthmic portion hypertrophies and becomes incorporated or indistinguishable from the rest of the uterine muscle. Late in pregnancy and most particularly during labor the lower uterine segment becomes thinned out, and its upper pole is more clearly demarcated from the thick upper segment.

UTERINE CONTRACTILITY (Fig. 19-7). The uterus contracts irregularly throughout pregnancy. Uterine activity, the increase in intrauterine pressure generated by a contraction, is measured in Montevideo units, the sum of the intensity of all the contractions in mm Hg during a 10-minute period. From early pregnancy until 30 weeks, uterine activity is less than 20 Montevideo units. Irregular, painless contractions (Braxton Hicks contractions) increase gradually thereafter from about 30 to 80 Montevideo units as the cervix ripens. At the onset of labor, intrauterine activity averages between 80 and 120 Montevideo units. At peak activity near the end of labor, when the intrauterine pressure during each contraction is increased to about 50 mm Hg and the frequency 5 contractions/10 min, an average of 250 Montevideo units is reached.

Cervix. Changes in the cervix are apparent by the sixth week. Softening and congestion are a result of increased vascularity. The glands hypertrophy (Fig. 19-8), mucus secretion is greatly increased, and the consistency is altered by steroid hormone activity. Inspissation of the water content of cervical mucus results in the formation of the thick mucous plug that acts as a barrier, protecting the conceptus against mechanical or bacterial invasion throughout pregnancy. Progesterone overshadows the effects of increased estrogen production on cervical mucus; hence ferning, or arborization, does not occur when corpus luteum activity is sufficient to support a normal intrauterine pregnancy.

The cervical epithelium is far less responsive to estrogen and progesterone than is the endometrium. The cervical stromal cells show a decidual reaction in about half of pregnant women; but aside from this change, the increased vascularity, and the edema, no alterations can be considered characteristic of specific pregnancy effects. The squamous epithelium is often thicker, and the basal layer may be increased from one- to four-cell strata. Growth of the endocervical epithelium is more pronounced, and squamous metaplasia is common. Frequently, the columnar proliferation advances beyond the external os for a variable distance on the surface of the cervix. This so-called erosion is actually a *cervical ectropion* or *eversion* of the cervical canal. Its gross appearance may be indistinguishable from pathologic conditions of the cervix. Cytologic or histologic examination is necessary.

One concern is the interpretation of basal cell hyperactivity when this change is found in the gravid cervix. Coloscopic examination can be just as informative in pregnant as in nonpregnant women, and the diagnosis of any type of epithelial abnormality must be made on the basis of changes in the cellular characteristics, particularly those of the nuclei, whether or not the patient is pregnant.

Fallopian tubes and round ligaments. The *round ligaments* are hypertrophied and elongated. Since their relationship to the uterine fundus is retained, their position in late pregnancy is almost vertical. The round ligaments help stabilize the uterus and tend to keep the heavy organ closer to the abdominal wall.

The *fallopian tubes* are also elongated and ultimately lie almost parallel to the long axis of the uterus, but unlike the round ligaments their muscular coats are not hypertrophied.

Ovaries. Because of the increased vascularity, both ovaries become somewhat enlarged and elongated. The enlargement is more pronounced in the ovary containing the corpus luteum, which reaches its maximum development during the third month.

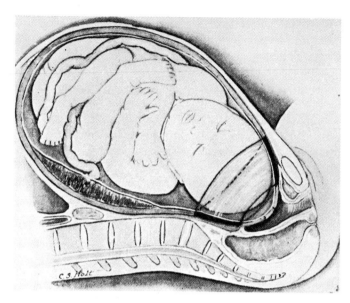

Fig. 19-5. Lower uterine segment early in labor. (From Danforth, D.N., and Ivy, A.C.: Am. J. Obstet. Gynecol. **57**:831, 1949.)

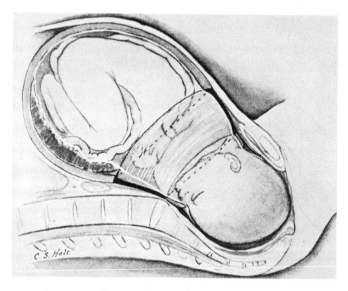

Fig. 19-6. Lower uterine segment in second stage of labor after circumferential dilatation and final elongation. (From Danforth, D.N., and Ivy, A.C.: Am. J. Obstet. Gynecol. **57**:831, 1949.)

Ovulation is suspended during pregnancy because of pituitary inhibition.

Israel and associates studied the ovary at term in patients delivered by elective cesarean section. The patchy, reddened areas and elevated ridges on the surface of the ovary proved on microscopic examination to be a decidua-like reaction of the stroma and hyperplasia of the surface epithelium, respectively. These reactions are probably related to some hormone of chorionic origin, either chorionic gonadotropin or progesterone from the same source.

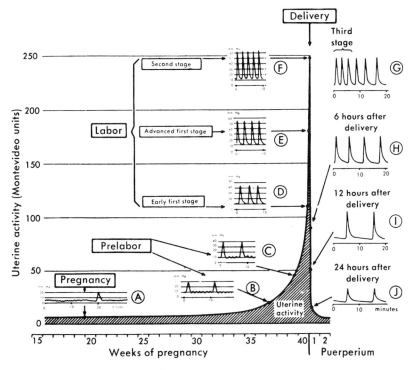

Fig. 19-7. Evolution of spontaneous uterine activity throughout pregnancy cycle is illustrated by striped area. Typical (schematic) tracings of uterine contractility at different stages of cycle are shown. (From Caldeyro-Barcia, R., and Poseiro, J.J.: Ann. N.Y. Acad. Sci. **75**:813, 1959.)

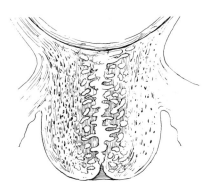

Fig. 19-8. Hypertrophy of cervical glands during pregnancy.

The infundibulopelvic ligament is enlarged during pregnancy, mainly because of the great distention of the ovarian veins. Hodgkinson found that the capacity of the veins increases more than 60 times. Such a vast change in diameter is possible because the ovarian veins are not confined within fascial sheaths as are the veins in the extremities. Compensatory hypertrophy of the smooth muscle of the vein media provides protection against spontaneous rupture.

Vagina. The vagina becomes deeply congested and cyanotic (Chadwick's sign) because of the greatly increased vascularity. In preparation for the great distention that the vagina must undergo during delivery, the mucosa thickens, the connective tissue becomes less dense, and the muscular coat hypertrophies to such an extent that the vault is considerably lengthened and the lower portion may protrude through the introitus, giving the appearance of a cystocele even in the primigravida.

Secretions present in the vaginal vault during pregnancy have a highly acid pH (3.5 to 5.5) because of the increased glycogen content of the vaginal epithelium.

GENERAL CHANGES

Abdominal walls. Tension and stretching of the anterior abdominal wall and the tissues over the outer aspect of the thighs frequently cause changes in the collagen and elastic fibers of the deep layer of the skin, producing reddish, irregular lines, the *striae gravidarum.* Poidevin did microscopic studies of stria and found that collagen and elastic fibers lost their crisscross appearance and became thinned and straightened out longitudinally but did not become disrupted. He suggested that striae are caused by the loss of the adhesive property of ground substance because of the effect of adrenocortical hyperactivity. After delivery the discoloration gradually fades, but the scarred lines do not disappear.

In the latter part of pregnancy the rectus abdominis muscles are under considerable strain, and their tone is reduced. Wide separation of the muscles *(diastasis recti)* develops when the linea alba gives way to the stress and permits abdominal contents to protrude in the midline.

Breasts. The breasts become enlarged and sensitive by the eighth week of pregnancy. The primary areola deepens in color, and a more lightly pigmented secondary areola develops at the periphery. Sebaceous glands located in the primary areola undergo hypertrophy, forming *Montgomery's tubercles.*

Colostrum can be expressed from the nipples after about the tenth week, but lactation is inhibited by the high estrogen-progesterone levels. Growth of the mammary apparatus is a direct response to hormone stimulation. Estrogen stimulates proliferation of the ducts; progesterone causes proliferation of lobule-alveolar tissue. Development is functionally complete by midpregnancy. As the breasts enlarge, the vascular supply is increased, engorged veins are frequently visible beneath the surface of the skin, and striae may appear over the outer aspects.

After delivery, anterior pituitary *prolactin* stimulates synthesis and secretion of milk (see Chapter 43).

Skin. Pigmentation of the skin in areas other than the breasts is a common finding. The *linea nigra,* a brownish black streak down the midline of the abdomen, is especially prominent in brunettes. Occasionally, pigmentation occurs in a characteristic distribution over the face, forming the "mask of pregnancy," or *chloasma,* which may persist for many months after delivery. The external genitals are similarly affected.

Palmar erythema and spider nevi or telangiectases sometimes appear over the face and upper trunk and are related to the increased concentration of estrogen.

CIRCULATORY SYSTEM

Vast alterations in hemodynamics occur as a result of (1) the increased metabolic demands of new tissue growth; (2) the expansion of vascular channels, particularly those of the generative tract; and (3) the increase in steroid hormones, which exert a positive effect on sodium and water balance.

Blood. The *total blood volume* increases approximately 30% to 40% (Fig. 19-9). The range is wide, and increases up to 50% are reported. Although the *red cell volume* and the *total hemoglobin* increase during pregnancy, the expansion of plasma volume is approximately three times greater than that of the red cell mass. Caton and colleagues, with the use of red cells labeled with radioactive iron (^{59}Fe), found an average increase in red cell mass of 495 ml at term and calculated the concomitant whole blood rise at 1800 ml. Hytten and Leitch's studies suggest that withholding of dietary iron supplements can lessen the expected red cell increase by as much as 30% to 40%.

Erythropoiesis during pregnancy is to a large extent regulated by the kidneys. Renal erythropoietic factor (REF) is produced in response to the demand by the tissues for oxygen, and this in turn activates production of erythropoietic hormone in the plasma. Human placental lactogen (hPL) and prolactin have also been shown to enhance the stimulatory effect of endogenous erythropoietin.

The disparity between the increase in fluid and cellular elements is reflected in the peripheral blood count as an apparent or dilution anemia, since both hemoglobin and hematocrit determinations are usually decreased in the third trimester as compared with the first. Cohen and Thompson showed that the average reduction in hematocrit was 15%, whereas the decrease in viscosity was 12% as a result of this dilution. True anemia is present if the

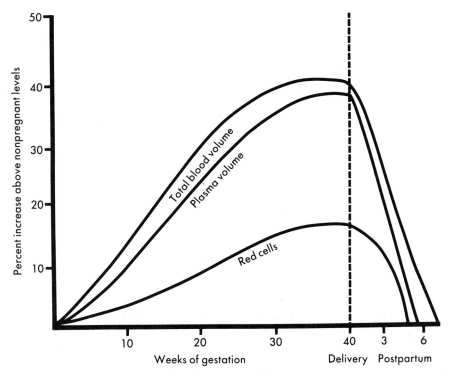

Fig. 19-9. Changes in total blood volume, plasma volume, and red cell mass during pregnancy and puerperium, based on compilation of reported data.

hemoglobin is less than 11 g, the red cell count less than 3.6 million, and the hematocrit less than 32%.

The *plasma volume* begins to increase during the first trimester, reaches a peak approximately 40% above normal at 32 to 34 weeks, and remains elevated to term. During and immediately after the third stage of labor there is a sharp temporary rise in plasma volume, followed by a rapid drop toward the normal nonpregnant range, although the original level is not actually reached until 3 or 4 weeks after delivery. On the contrary, the red cell mass continues to rise until the end of pregnancy and, according to Lund and Donovan, does not decline to its original level until the eighth postpartum week.

Most of the increase in plasma volume occurs between the sixth and the twenty-fourth week of gestation. These findings parallel the curve of in-

creases in cardiac output demonstrated by Kerr. Thus maximal risk for the patient with heart disease is reached earlier in pregnancy than previously thought and persists throughout gestation. Plasma volume correlates well with reproductive performance. Gibson found that gravid women with poor obstetric histories had lesser increases in plasma volume and smaller babies than their normal counterparts.

Interstitial fluid volume expansion is less pronounced than the plasma volume rise during the first and second trimesters. The rate is accelerated in the latter part of pregnancy and continues until term when the maximum increase of 40% is reached. Return to original levels occurs gradually by 6 to 8 weeks after delivery.

The *bone marrow* is hyperplastic throughout pregnancy and remains so for about 2 months after delivery. The white cells and the erythrocytes are increased. A *leukocytosis* in the range of 10,000 to 12,000 is normal in gravid women.

Lowenstein and Bramlage studied the peripheral blood (Fig. 19-10) and performed bone marrow aspirations in 200 normal pregnant women throughout the three trimesters of pregnancy and the puerperium and in 30 nonpregnant women of childbearing age. In the pregnant group all cellular components were shown to increase progressively, becoming maximal in the third trimester. A curious finding was that normoblastic erythropoiesis with relative increase in nucleated red cells and granulopoiesis diminished during the first week after delivery but did not return to nonpregnant normal values; activity increased again at the sixth postpartum week. These authors suggest that this late activity may be stimulated

in response to postpartum decrease in total circulating hemoglobin and red cell mass.

Serum protein concentrations are approximately 1 to 1.5 g/dl lower in pregnant than in nonpregnant women. It is not unusual to obtain values of 5.5 to 6 g/dl. The colloid osmotic pressure of the plasma is thereby reduced by about 20%. This is in part but not entirely a result of dilution. There is a significant drop in the albumin fraction that is incompletely compensated for by the rise in alpha and beta globulin. The albumin-globulin ratio is reduced from 1.5 to 0.8.

Serial studies of plasma proteins by electrophoretic fractionation during the course of pregnancy

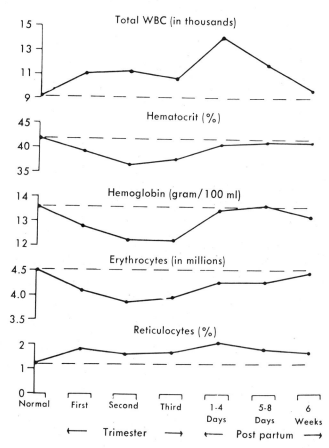

Fig. 19-10. Peripheral blood of pregnant and nonpregnant women. (From Lowenstein, L., and Bramlage, C.A.: Blood **12**:261, 1957.)

and in the puerperium have been reported by Mack (Fig. 19-11). In normal mothers, total plasma protein concentration decreases by about 13% by the third trimester. The albumin and gamma globulin concentration decrease progressively, but at the same time the alpha-1, alpha-2, beta fraction, and fibrinogen increase. The lipoproteins also increase.

Serum lipids. Total serum lipids increase by 46% during the later part of pregnancy. Total cholesterol, phospholipids, and free fatty acids are all increased. There is no change in esterified cholesterol.

Fibrinogen concentration increases progressively to term. Chemical values show an increase from 300 mg/dl to 400 to 600 mg/dl. Electrophoresis values are approximately 100 mg/dl higher.

Urea and *creatinine* are found in lower concentrations in the plasma during pregnancy because of the normal increase in renal filtration fraction.

Alpha-fetoprotein, produced by the fetal liver and yolk sac, is found in maternal serum in above normal amounts beginning at about the seventh week of gestation. Maternal serum values average 160 to 190 ng/ml at term. Newborn serum values are 100 to 150 times higher. Concentration in amniotic fluid parallels that in fetal serum in a ratio of about 1:150.

Determination of amniotic fluid alpha-fetoprotein is used in conjunction with ultrasound and other modalities in diagnosis of suspected fetal neural tube defects in which levels are elevated more than three standard deviations. Elevated values are also found in association with multiple pregnancy, fetal death, omphalocele, duodenal and esophageal atresias, and sacrococcygeal teratoma.

SERUM ENZYMES. During the prenatal period a profound change in the maternal serum enzymes is found in the increase in serum alkaline phos-

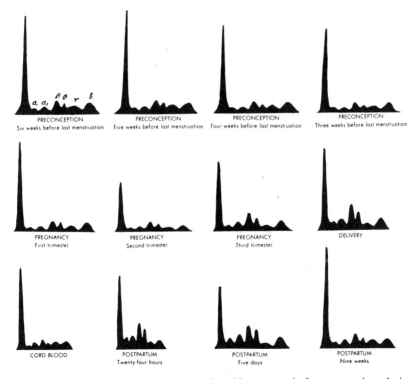

Fig. 19-11. Electrophoretic patterns of plasma of healthy woman before conception, during pregnancy, and during puerperium and of cord blood of her normal full-term infant at delivery. (From Mack, H.C.: Clin. Obstet. Gynecol. **3:**336, 1960.)

phatase. Individual variation is considerable, but in normal pregnancy values rise steadily to term. Serum glutamic oxaloacetic transaminase (SGOT) and serum glutamic pyruvic transaminase (SGPT) concentrations show significantly increased activity only during labor.

Diamine oxidase (DAO) concentrations rise in an almost linear fashion from noonpregnancy values of 3 to 4 units beginning about the fifth week of gestation to the twentieth week when values exceed 500 units in normal pregnancy. Concentrations then fluctuate but tend to continue to increase more slowly to term. Serial determinations of DAO concentrations in maternal plasma can be used as an aid in diagnosis of pregnancy or prognosis in cases of threatened abortion, but attempts to use DAO measurement to predict fetal death during late pregnancy have proved unsuccessful.

DAO is an adaptive enzyme produced primarily by maternal decidua, where its action in degradation of histamine produced by the fetus apparently provides necessary protection against transfer of histamine to the mother.

Serum cystine aminopeptidase (oxytocinase) is the primary oxytocin-inactivating enzyme of pregnancy plasma. A relatively steady rise in the enzyme is noticed beginning at about 6 weeks' gestation to term in normal pregnancies. The enzyme appears to be mainly of placental origin, but it is of limited clinical value in assessing placental function and, more particularly, fetal welfare.

Heart. Serial studies at various stages of pregnancy reveal an actual alteration in position and apparent increase in size of the cardiac silhouette. The heart is rotated slightly anteriorly and displaced upward and to the left. The factors responsible for these alterations are controversial, although recognized changes in the chest wall doubtless play an important role. The rib cage is flared out so that its circumference is increased at the base. The diaphragm is pushed up as the uterus enlarges, but it may or may not appear disproportionately elevated.

The fact that the heart appears enlarged on x-ray film examination long before the uterus is large enough to push the abdominal contents upward raises the question as to whether the cardiac muscle undergoes some hypertrophy during pregnancy. If it does so, it is likely that the hypertrophy is in proportion to the increase in total body weight. Since the cardiac output is increased by about 75 ml, it is likely that the increased blood volume is accompanied by slight cardiac dilatation.

In addition to the altered x-ray film appearance of the heart, functional changes simulating organic heart disease in nonpregnant patients must be recognized and carefully evaluated. A soft systolic *murmur* at the base or over the precordium is demonstrable in more than 50% of patients. *Extrasystoles* are common, and the *pulse rate* is slightly increased. There is a distinct change in heart rate immediately after delivery, when bradycardia is the rule, unless blood loss has been excessive. These findings and the frequent occurrence of dyspnea make the diagnosis of cardiac disease during pregnancy more difficult. Sodeman found a combination of signs and symptoms sufficient to suggest heart disease in 9.6% of 73 healthy gravid women.

Blood pressure. *Arterial blood pressure* does not increase in normal pregnancy. The level remains unchanged or may decrease during the second trimester and return to the normal range during the third trimester. Burwell found the maximal *pulse pressure* to occur during the twenty-eighth to thirty-second week, at about the time of the maximal pulse rate. *Venous pressure* measured in the antecubital region remains constant and normal. Elevated venous pressure in the upper extremity is indicative of cardiac overload. Femoral venous pressure rises 10 to 15 cm H_2O above normal in the upright or supine position as a result of increasing pressure by the enlarging uterus on the pelvic veins, a factor that contributes to the development of ankle edema and varicose veins. Femoral pressure is normal in the lateral recumbent position.

Late in pregnancy, patients often complain of feeling faint in the supine position, when venous pressure may rise to at least 20 cm H_2O. The syncope is attributed to the *vena cava syndrome*. When the heavy uterus falls back on the inferior vena cava, venous return to the heart is sufficiently impeded to cause a precipitous drop in blood pressure. The patient appears pale and apprehensive, but if she can turn on her side, which she usually does promptly, symptoms disappear almost immediately. This phenomenon is accentuated when the patient is unable to move about after an anesthetic is administered. We have seen a few patients exhibit a profound drop in blood pressure after low-dose spinal anesthesia given for cesarean section, although the level of anesthesia was no higher than the eighth or ninth thoracic segment. When pressure was exerted against the lateral abdominal wall, thus displacing the uterus to one side of the inferior vena cava, the blood pressure rose without any other aids. In such cases, delivery should be carried out without delay. If initial hypotension is caused by this condition, there is no difficulty in maintaining blood pressure once the uterus is emptied.

Capillary permeability remains unchanged except with the increased hydrostatic pressure in the lower extremities.

Cardiac output. Increased tissue demands for oxygen may be met physiologically by (1) an increase in cardiac output of oxygenated blood or (2) an increased extraction of oxygen from blood at the capillary level. Measurements of cardiac output during normal pregnancy indicate a rise, primarily in stroke volume, with the maximal increase being observed at about the twenty-eighth week. The heart rate follows the same general course but with a much lower increment of rise. In Adams' series the peak elevation in cardiac output occurred at 28 weeks and averaged 32% above nonpregnant levels. Cardiac output is increased slightly during the first stage of labor and appreciably increased during the second stage with the bearing down efforts. Immediately after delivery there is a sudden increase amounting to about 29% as the uterus contracts and forces a large volume of blood into the circulation. During these periods the patient with a diseased heart experiences further increased cardiac strain.

Kerr contends that most of the increase in cardiac output is established by the end of the first trimester and that this high level is maintained until term. Measurements of cardiac output taken in the supine position showed diminution amounting to 10% to 25% of the peak output in the last stages of pregnancy. Serial studies of cardiac output performed in the lateral recumbent position show no significant reduction of output, and therefore of ventricular work, in late pregnancy.

Since the overall increase in *oxygen consumption* is between 10% and 20% during pregnancy, it is evident that the heightened cardiac output exceeds this demand until the last trimester. Bader and associates found that the arteriovenous oxygen difference was reduced to 3.4/dl during the fourteenth to thirtieth weeks. This adjustment would appear to favor the margin of safety for fetal oxygenation. However, in the last trimester, when the cardiac output decreases, a larger percentage of oxygen must be removed at the uterine level, and the arteriovenous oxygen difference increases to values similar to or exceeding values found in nonpregnant women (4.4/dl).

RESPIRATORY SYSTEM

Functional changes in the respiratory tract are demonstrable early in pregnancy, whereas anatomic alterations become evident later when intraabdominal pressure is increased. The lower half of the thoracic cage is pushed upward and widened, and the diaphragm is accordingly elevated, especially at the periphery. The central portion may appear flattened, and its excursion reduced; hence breathing is more costal than abdominal.

The *vital capacity* remains unchanged or undergoes a slight increase. Excellent studies by Knuttgen and Emerson indicate that this increase is consistent and significant. In any case, a decrease in vital capacity should always be considered significant. In gravidas with pulmonary or cardiac disease, particularly with mitral stenosis, reduced vital capacity is one of the earliest signs of impending failure. Serial testing should be initiated early in pregnancy to permit valid interpretation of changes with advancing gestation.

Hyperventilation. The respiratory rate is slightly increased, and tidal volume rises. These changes may increase the margin of safety for the fetus. Hyperventilation lowers the carbon dioxide content of alveolar air, and, in turn, reduced carbon dioxide tension favors diffusion of carbon dioxide from fetal to maternal circulation. Thus all changes in the respiratory system during pregnancy are well compensated, and pulmonary function is not impaired in normal patients. Nevertheless, pulmonary diseases are often more serious during pregnancy when oxygen requirements of gestation are increased.

URINARY SYSTEM

Pregnancy exerts a profound influence on the entire urinary tract. The outstanding anatomic effect is a dilatation of the *ureter* and *renal pelvis* and *hydronephrosis*, all more pronounced on the right (Fig. 19-12). The capacity of a dilated kidney pelvis and ureter increases from an original 10 or 15 ml to 60 ml.

Changes appear early and are progressive until the last month or two of pregnancy. The ureter is elongated and widened, and, although it becomes curved and tortuous, actual kinking is rare. The flow of urine is reduced because ureteral peristalsis and tone are diminished. All these alterations, especially those affecting ureteral function, are basically hormonal influences, mainly of progester-

one. As pregnancy advances, pressure from the enlarged uterus may be a contributory factor. Dilatation is frequently considerably more pronounced in the right ureter than in the left, probably because of the cushioning effect of the rectosigmoid and the dextrorotation of the uterus. The muscular wall of the lower third of the ureter undergoes hyperplasia similar to that involving most structures within the broad ligament. Reduction of the lumen at this level may also contribute to dilatation of the ureter above.

Renal function. Changes in renal function during normal pregnancy follow a recognized pattern, although the extent of the alteration may vary from one individual to another. Sims and Krantz did serial studies of para-aminohippurate (PAH) and inulin clearances that demonstrated the following: (1) *effective renal plasma flow* increases approximately 25% during the first and second trimester and then falls to normal nonpregnant levels in the last trimester (600 ml/min); (2) *glomerular filtration* increases by about 50% and remains in this range until the last 2 to 3 weeks of pregnancy,

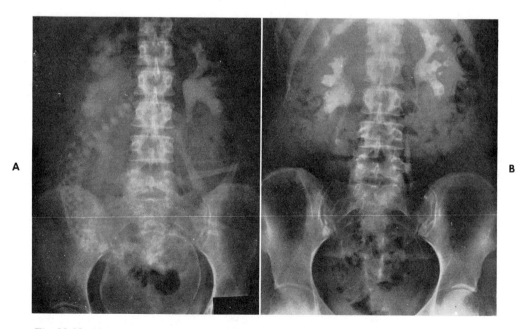

A
B

Fig. 19-12. **A,** Intravenous pyelogram demonstrating hydronephrosis and hydroureter at 34 weeks' gestation. **B,** Comparison at 6 weeks after delivery.

when the rate declines somewhat but does not fall to normal (125 ml/min) until early in the puerperium; and (3) the *filtration fraction* is elevated throughout pregnancy, particularly in the third trimester, when renal plasma flow decreases while glomerular filtration remains elevated. The filtration fraction at this time is approximately 40% above control levels.

The late pregnancy regression of renal blood flow and glomerular filtration may be related to position. Chesley, Sloan, and Wynn found that urine flow, PAH and inulin clearances, and sodium and chloride excretion were all depressed in the supine position as compared with the lateral position. Potassium excretion did not change. The fact that the lateral position is conducive to optimal function provides good reason for recommendation of programmed rest periods in this position in patients with borderline or diminishing renal function.

The alterations in renal function are most probably a result of increased maternal and chorionic hormonal secretions. Hormones capable of increasing renal function include ACTH, antidiuretic hormone (ADH), aldosterone, cortisone, growth hormone, and thyroid hormone. The part played by each of these and by the increased plasma volume of pregnancy needs further study before the final answer can be given.

The known anatomic and physiologic changes in the kidney have important clinical implications. *Glycosuria* is common because of the increase in glomerular filtration, but, before its occurrence can be assigned to a physiologic change, a glucose tolerance test is indicated. *Amino acids* are excreted in larger amounts during pregnancy. This is particularly true of histidine, the glomerular filtration of which is raised by more than 50%, whereas tubular reabsorption appears to be partially inhibited. Blood concentrations of *urea, uric acid,* and *creatinine* are lowered as a result of increased clearance rates, but the clearance of *sodium* is not significantly altered in normal pregnancy. Renal *iodide clearance* is increased, and the plasma inorganic iodine level is reduced, which increases the physiologic demands on the thyroid.

Allowances must be made for changes in the genitourinary system in the interpretation of renal function tests. The results of the *phenosulfonphthalein (PSP) test* can be misleading because the dye may be excreted normally, but dilatation of the renal pelvis and ureter and the relative stasis of this system may delay its arrival in the bladder. The test is better avoided during pregnancy. *Concentration tests,* when positive, are significant. If the urine does not show concentration, it may be related to the positive nitrogen balance, sodium retention, and low-sodium intake, particularly if the salt has been restricted for a time before the test is performed. It should be performed in the late puerperium before a final diagnosis of failure of concentrating power is made.

Serial determinations of 24-hour renal clearance of endogenous creatinine are useful and practical in evaluating renal function during pregnancy. Collection and timing of the sample are important (Fig. 19-13). Values are lower in 24-hour tests than in those performed during short test periods with fluids administered. In normal ambulatory gravid women, clearance rates ranged between 130 and 160 ml/min until the last 2 to 4 weeks of pregnancy, when values usually ranged between 100 and 110 ml/min.

The *bladder* is pulled up into the abdomen as the uterus enlarges. In the early weeks of gestation, pressure of the uterus on the bladder, traction at the vesicle neck, and hyperemia of the trigone cause frequency of urination. The vascularity of the bladder is greatly increased, and on cystoscopy engorged vessels or small varicosities are sometimes visible. Trauma that occurs late in pregnancy or during delivery may cause hemorrhage from these areas.

The hormonal influences responsible for dilatation of the structures of the urinary tract above the bladder exert a similar influence on the smooth muscle of the bladder. There is a decrease in bladder tone and a progressive increase in capacity of up to 1300 to 1500 ml during pregnancy and in the postpartum period. Overdistention of the bladder in the postpartum period is a troublesome, often protracted complication of labor and delivery in

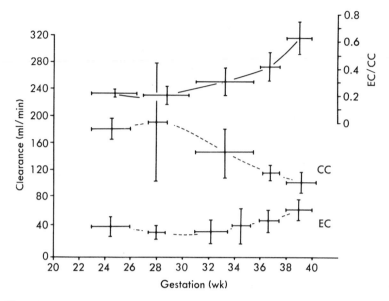

Fig. 19-13. Serial 24-hour renal clearance studies of estriol (E) and creatinine (C), and E/C ratio in 30 normal ambulatory patients during pregnancy.

which this physiologic reduction in tone plays an important role.

Renin-angiotensin-aldosterone system. The activity of the proteolytic enzyme *renin,* produced largely but not entirely by the kidney, is increased during normal pregnancy. The enzyme acts on *renin substrate, angiotensinogen,* to form *angiotensin* in two steps. Vascular reactivity to angiotensin II is reduced during pregnancy so that elevation of blood pressure does not normally occur with the increased levels of this substance, but in pregnancies complicated by preeclampsia, this relative resistance to angiotensin is lost. Angiotensin II is a major stimulus for adrenocortical secretion of *aldosterone,* which together with antidiuretic hormone favors salt and water retention during pregnancy.

GASTROINTESTINAL TRACT

An alteration in the normal *alkaline pH of the saliva* toward the acid side is common in pregnancy. It is this change rather than withdrawal of calcium that predisposes to tooth decay. The quantity of saliva is frequently increased, sometimes excessively so (hyperptyalism), but the cause of the increased secretion is not yet known. Occa-

sionally, the gums become hypertrophied and spongy and tend to bleed easily. This is attributed to a hormonal effect, although vitamin C deficiency may contribute to the disturbance. Gingivitis tends to disappear spontaneously after delivery.

Gastric acidity is usually reduced, particularly in the first trimester, although the degree of hypochlorhydria is variable. Certain cases of otherwise unexplained severe anemia are occasionally related to an exaggerated gastric hypochlorhydria.

Gastric motility is somewhat diminished throughout pregnancy, and during labor the emptying time of the stomach is so slow that oral feedings are contraindicated. Nausea and vomiting of early pregnancy may well be influenced by these functional alterations.

Reduced peristaltic activity and *diminished tone* are evident in bowel function, as well as in the stomach. These effects are a result of the same hormonal influences, mainly progesterone, that induce atony in the smooth muscle of ureters, arteries, veins, and various other structures during pregnancy. Constipation, so common in pregnant women, usually results from these functional changes, although the condition is undoubtedly ag-

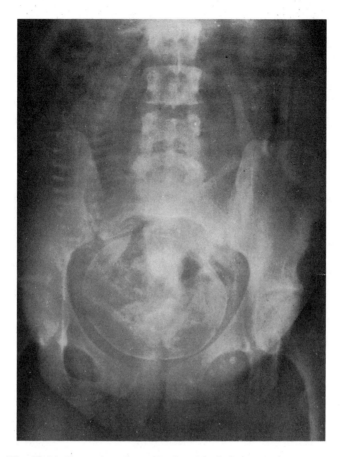

Fig. 19-14. Separation of symphysis pubis during normal pregnancy.

gravated by pressure of the uterus on the rectosigmoid.

During the last half of pregnancy the stomach is gradually pushed upward into the left dome of the diaphragm. Hormonal effects may cause relaxation or dilatation of the hiatus and predispose to the development of *hiatal hernia*. The condition is usually reversed after delivery. The cecum also undergoes a progressive upward displacement, beginning during the third month and continuing until term when the *appendix* is located out toward the right flank above the level of the iliac crest.

Gallbladder. Gallbladder emptying time is increased during pregnancy. Serum cholinesterase activity is reduced by about 25%. Relative biliary stasis and increased cholesterol levels may contribute to the formation of biliary calculi in gravid women. The ratio of women to men with calculous disease is approximately 4:1.

Liver. Measurements of liver function in human pregnancy remain in the normal range. Liver biopsies show no characteristic morphologic changes in normal mothers. However, in patients with existing liver disease, high levels of estrogens and overall added work of the liver during gestation may adversely affect hepatic function.

BONES AND JOINTS

The sacroiliac synchondroses and symphysis pubis are widened and rendered movable beginning about the tenth to twelfth week of gestation (Fig. 19-14). This alteration is believed to be almost entirely caused by the action of the hormone relaxin. Zarrow and associates demonstrated that blood concentrations of relaxin in pregnant women averaged 0.2 guinea pig U/ml of serum at 7 to 10 weeks' gestation, with a maximum concentration of 2 guinea pig U/ml at 38 to 42 weeks.

Posture changes become evident as pregnancy advances. The upper spine is thrown backward to compensate for increased size of the abdomen. Disturbances arising from altered weight bearing and from relaxation of the pelvic articulations are discussed in Chapter 27.

ENDOCRINE SYSTEM

Thyroid. The thyroid gland is palpably enlarged in more than 50% of persons during pregnancy. This is caused by a diffuse hyperplasia of glandular elements, new follicle formation, and increased vascularity.

An increase in basal metabolic rate is evident by the sixteenth week and rises 10% to 30% above the prepregnant rate during the third trimester. Since the basal metabolic rate measures total oxygen consumption rate, the growing fetal and maternal tissues logically increase the oxygen demand. The increase in thyroid activity and in the size of the thyroid gland is more likely to represent compensatory changes because of the increased renal iodine clearance and resulting reduced plasma inorganic iodine level and the protein binding of thyroxine (T_4).

Thyroid function is affected in a major way by the elevated estrogen levels of pregnancy. Estrogens increase the response of pituitary thyroid-stimulating hormone (TSH) to hypothalamic thyrotropin-releasing hormone (TRH) and also cause significant increases in thyroxine-binding globulin (TBG), the alpha globulin moiety of serum proteins. The thyroid gland secretes T_4 and small amounts of triiodothyronine (T_3). In the free form, both are biologically active hormones. Most of the circulating T_3 is derived from monodeiodinization of T_4, and a major portion of T_4 is protein bound. Hence circulating levels of free T_4 are not appreciably different from or only slightly higher than nonpregnancy levels.

The most useful means of evaluating thyroid function during pregnancy is by direct assay for T_4. This method eliminates contamination errors caused by ingested iodides or radiographic dyes. Values during pregnancy range from 5.0 to 10.5 μg/dl as compared with normal nonpregnant values of 3.0 to 7.5 μg/dl. Additional thyroid function tests are usually necessary when thyroid dysfunction is suspected. These include determination of the free T_4 index in a suspected hyperthyroid or TSH in a hypothyroid state, which are discussed in Chapter 22.

Evaluation of thyroid activity by radioactive iodine (^{131}I) uptake is contraindicated during pregnancy, since fetal thyroid follicles are differentiated by the fourth lunar month and may be damaged by ^{131}I.

Parathyroid glands. The parathyroids undergo hypertrophy as the fetal demands for calcium increase. Although more parathormone is secreted at this time, many pregnant women show a relative deficiency or a predisposition to parathyroid tetany in late pregnancy. Chvostek's sign is frequently positive in the latter part of gestation. Increasing calcium intake readily corrects relative deficiencies. One quart of milk daily is protective.

Pituitary gland. The anterior lobe of the pituitary gland increases 20% to 40% in size during pregnancy. The increase is largely in a single cell type, the "pregnancy cell," which is a prolactin-containing cell.

Serum levels of human prolactin (hPr) rise steadily from 10 ng/ml at the onset of pregnancy to about 200 ng/ml at term. Despite high, late pregnancy levels of prolactin and hPL, which also has some lactogenic activity, lactation does not occur before delivery. Friesen, Fournier, and Desjardins present good evidence that high levels of placental steroids inhibit the secretory activity of the breast by blocking the peripheral action of hPr and hPL on the breast.

The posterior lobe does not hypertrophy during pregnancy. The secretion of oxytocin and vasopressin–antidiuretic hormone is presumably increased. However, the measurements are made indirectly on the basis of increasing quantities of oxytocinase, which can be determined by electrophoresis.

Adrenal glands. Enlargement of the adrenal glands occurs progressively throughout the prenatal period because of *hyperplasia of the cortex*. A significant increase in corticosteroid secretion can be detected in the first trimester; and, according to Venning, a second higher peak reaching values similar to those found in patients with Cushing's disease normally occurs at about 200 days. The peak in corticosteroid secretion corresponds with the period during which water retention is maximal.

Not all functions of the adrenal cortex are equally stimulated during pregnancy. Corticosteroids that influence carbohydrate metabolism show the predominant and most universal rise, but, at the same time, binding protein (transcortin) is also increased as a result of the stimulus provided by increasing amounts of estrogen. As a consequence, significant amounts of otherwise excessive levels of corticosteroids are rendered biologically less active. However, there is a small actual increase in free cortisol in late pregnancy.

An increase in aldosterone levels is noted by the fifteenth week of pregnancy. Increased and fluctuant levels are attributable to the control of aldosterone secretion effected by the renin-angiotensin system.

The 17-ketosteroids associated with androgenic activity are relatively unchanged or increase only slightly in the last trimester.

Adrenal medullary activity is slightly increased in normal pregnancy. Oesterling, Tse, and Holmes report mean values for urinary-free catecholamines expressed as norepinephrine equivalents in micrograms per hour as follows: 12.5 in normal nongravid women of reproductive age, 13.2 in normal gravid women during the first and second trimesters, and 18.5 in normal gravid women during the third trimester (Fig. 19-15). Further increases in epinephrine secretion during the stress of labor might be expected. However, Israel and co-workers studied plasma epinephrine and norepinephrine during the third trimester, in labor, and after delivery and found no significant change in either catecholamine. The mean plasma value of epinephrine was 0.1 μg/L and of norepinephrine, 1.5 μg/L.

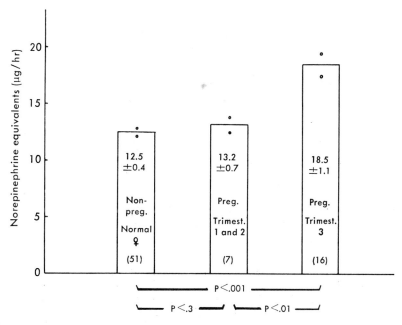

Fig. 19-15. Excretion of urinary-free catecholamines (epinephrine, norepinephrine, and dopamine) in normal nongravid women of reproductive age and in normal gravid women. (Courtesy M.J. Oesterling.)

METABOLISM

Proteins. A positive nitrogen balance demonstrable early in gestation increases progressively through the third trimester when fetal requirements are greatest. Macy and Hunscher and other investigators have repeatedly shown an accumulation of nitrogen during pregnancy far beyond the needs of the conceptus. Nitrogen accumulation during the last half of pregnancy totaled 446 g. Net gain after delivery was 310 g. A negative balance continues in the puerperium with blood loss, lactation, and involutional changes in the uterus and other maternal tissues. Maternal protein intake should be at least 65 g/day throughout pregnancy.

Another means of estimating protein alterations in pregnancy is by measuring total body water, since this space and lean body mass are normally increased proportionately. Seitchik and Alper studied changes in body composition by measuring total body water (antipyrine) and extracellular water (mannitol) (Fig. 19-16). The expansion of both spaces paralleled one another, and the average increase was 40% for each. The gain in lean body mass of mother and fetus exceeded the maternal weight gain, and thus the authors contend that some solid (fat) must be lost or exchanged in favor of the increased

active protoplasmic mass. They suggest that the excess nitrogen accumulation of pregnancy implies that synthesis of lean body mass must occur during pregnancy and that this is associated with the use of body fat stores. The process is reversed in the puerperium, when lean body tissue is lost and fat is apparently gained.

Good maternal protein nutrition plays a key role in providing for normal fetal growth and development and may well be related to the actual condition of the newborn. Beydoun and co-workers have used spot and 24-hour urinary urea nitrogen/total nitrogen (UN/TN) ratios as an index of maternal protein nutrition. When prenatal dietary protein intake is adequate, the UN/TN ratio is in the range of 60 to 80. On low-protein diets, the ratio usually ranges between 20 and 40. Birth weight of babies born to mothers with high UN/TN ratios averaged more than 1 pound higher than the weight of babies born to mothers with low UN/TN ratios. The differences in well-matched subjects are highly significant. The test is relatively simple and provides a tool for identifying the protein-deficient mother and assessing her response to dietary therapy.

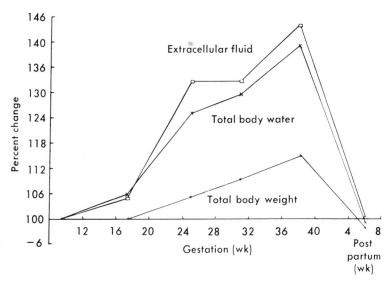

Fig. 19-16. Percentage change of total body and extracellular water in pregnancy. Average of 5 normal patients; 100% equals average value found at initial study in early pregnancy. (From Seitchik, J., and Alper, C.: Am. J. Obstet. Gynecol. **71**:1165, 1956.)

Carbohydrates. Reducing substances can be found in the urine at some time or other during pregnancy in about 30% of persons. In most instances the reducing substance is glucose. The presence of lactose in the urine is unusual except for the 2- to 3-week period preceding the onset of labor, although during the puerperium lactosuria is common.

The renal threshold for glucose may be reduced from normal nonpregnant levels, which range between 150 and 200 mg/dl, to a range of 100 to 150 mg/dl because of the increased glomerular filtration that normally occurs during pregnancy. Chesley, Sloan, and Wynn state that renal tubular reabsorption of glucose may fail to increase proportionately. This phenomenon accounts for many cases of glycosuria and may contribute to the relatively low fasting level of blood sugar found in gravid women. However, in some instances glycosuria during pregnancy provides the first evidence of a diabetic state. Fasting blood sugar determination alone is not sufficient for diagnosis. Instead a glucose tolerance test is essential for differentiation of physiologic and abnormal glycosuria of pregnancy. These problems are discussed in detail in Chapter 22.

A maternal glucose sparing effect noted in pregnancy is related to the demands of the fetus. Although secretion of insulin during pregnancy is increased, resistance to insulin by elevated free fatty acids and destruction of insulin by the placenta is also increased. The level of growth hormone per se is not appreciably increased, but its counterpart, chorionic hPL, is greatly elevated and is probably responsible for the elevated free fatty acids (FFA) and increased insulin resistance. Increases in corticosteroid and T_4 levels in normal gravid women may have some effect on carbohydrate metabolism, but protein binding of these substances is sufficiently increased so that actual biologic activity related to the free form of each is only slightly elevated during pregnancy. Plasma insulin antagonists are found in latent and overt diabetic women during pregnancy, but no such antagonists are detectable in the plasma of normal pregnant women.

Fats. Fat metabolism is altered during pregnancy in concert with the changes in carbohydrate metabolism just described. Metabolic alterations include an increase in maternal use of fat stores and a related increase in insulin resistance. hPL plays an important role in mobilization of FFA. The elevated level of FFA exerts an antiinsulin effect by interfering with peripheral use of glucose. Oxidation of fats provides an alternate maternal source of energy, and glucose sparing ensures that the critical needs of the fetus for this energy source are met.

Estrogen is known to increase the production of the alpha globulins, including lipoproteins, and the glucocorticoids are known to increase serum cholesterol. The lipoproteins are significantly increased during pregnancy, particularly the beta lipoproteins. Neutral fats are approximately doubled. The level of free cholesterol progressively increases until the thirtieth week of pregnancy. Ketonuria occurs more readily in pregnant than in nonpregnant women when carbohydrate production is reduced or when dietary fat is increased.

The normal values for maternal and cord plasma glucose and nonesterified fatty acids (NEFA) have been established by Whaley, Zuspan, and Nelson in a group of rigidly controlled normal pregnancies. Maternal values average 92.9 mg/dl for glucose and 881.8 mEq/L for NEFA; umbilical cord values average 61.9 mg/dl and 536.0 mEq/L, respectively. The differences in maternal-to-newborn ratios of glucose (1.3:1) and NEFA (1.7:1) suggest independent homeostasis in this biologic system. Because various metabolic diseases are known to influence blood glucose and NEFA levels, alterations in the ratio of these substances may provide a useful tool in investigation of these disorders.

Minerals. Demands for inorganic substances necessary for growth rise sharply at about the fourth lunar month when the fetus begins to increase rapidly in weight. Materials used for blood and skeletal formation continue to increase progressively to term.

CALCIUM AND PHOSPHORUS. Requirements for calcium and phosphorus are approximately doubled during pregnancy. These demands are satisfied by the daily intake of 1.5 g of calcium and 2 g of phosphorus. Total storage during the course of pregnancy is approximately 50 g and 35 to 40 g, respectively. Only about half of these amounts are used by the fetus; the remainder is stored in maternal tissues. Total serum calcium levels fall in the last half of pregnancy as a result of the decrease in serum albumin to which calcium is bound. However, free ionized calcium level remains within the normal range unless there is a relative or actual deficiency in parathyroid function. Since most of the fetal calcium deposition takes place in the latter part of pregnancy, relative deprivation or a deficiency in parathyroid function will cause a decrease in concentration of ionized calcium.

During pregnancy, calcium is more rapidly exchanged between the maternal circulation and bone. The bone therefore can be considered part of the metabolic calcium pool and can be drawn on when calcium supplies are low. The skeletal system is protected by a delicate balance in the rise of parathyroid hormone, which causes withdrawal of calcium from bone in response to hypocalcemia, and the rise in thyroid secretion of calcitonin during pregnancy, which inhibits this response when circulating calcium levels are elevated.

Osteomalacia, a condition in which softening and distortion of the long bones occurs as a result of excessive mobilization of calcium, is almost never found in the United States. Dentin does not contribute to the metabolic pool, and thus dental caries associated with pregnancy are not caused by the removal of calcium from the teeth but by local changes in pH and oral bacteria flora.

FOLIC ACID. Folates play an essential role in the metabolism of several amino acids and in the synthesis of nucleic acids. During pregnancy, rapid tissue growth of trophoblastic, maternal, and fetal origins creates an increased demand for folic acid. The undisputed example of maternal folic acid deficiency is seen in the development of megaloblastic anemia resulting specifically from inadequacy of folate and not from vitamin B_{12} deficiency. Association of less severe depletion of folic acid with other obstetric complications has been suggested. These include spontaneous abortion, placental abruption, premature deliveries, preeclampsia-eclampsia, and fetal abnormalities.

The daily requirement of folic acid during pregnancy is about 300 to 500 μg. Green vegetables, some fruits, liver, and kidney are the principal sources.

IRON. The demand for iron is increased, especially in the last trimester of pregnancy, because fetal absorption is far greater at that time. In addition, the hemoglobin mass continues to increase until term, and a small amount is necessary for other maternal tissues such as the uterus. Total body iron in the normal female ranges from 3.5 to 4 g. Holly estimates a net loss of iron to the mother of approximately 400 mg throughout pregnancy and delivery, or about one eighth of her total supply. Many women in apparently good nutritional state have less than the normal 1 g of available iron in storage, and therefore iron supplements are necessary in most to prevent a nonanemic iron deficiency state or an obvious iron deficiency anemia.

Acid-base balance. Maternal plasma bicarbonate and total base are normally reduced during pregnancy. According to Kydd, the values for total base averaged 146 mEq/L in normal gravid women as compared with 154 mEq/L in nonpregnant control subjects. At term the average carbon dioxide combining power value is about 45 ml/dl as compared with the nonpregnant average of approximately 60 ml/dl or plasma bicarbonate values of 22 to 25 mmol/L, respectively. Since the blood pH is unchanged, the alkali deficit is well compensated. The specific cause for this alteration remains unknown. It is probable that the normally increased ventilation effects the change, but whether the hyperventilation of pregnancy is of sufficient magnitude to reduce the carbon dioxide and induce the compensatory increase in renal excretion of sodium is as yet uncertain.

REFERENCES

Adams, J.Q.: Cardiovascular physiology in normal pregnancy: studies with dye dilution technique, Am. J. Obstet. Gynecol. **67:**741, 1954.

Assali, N.S., Douglass, R.A., Baird, W.W., Nicholson, D.B., and Suyemoto, R.: Measurement of uterine blood flow and uterine metabolism, Am. J. Obstet. Gynecol. **66:**248, 1953.

Bader, R.A., Bader, M.E., Rose, D.F., and Braunwald, E.: Hemodynamics at rest and during exercise in normal pregnancy as studied by cardiac catheterization, J. Clin. Invest. **34:**1524, 1955.

Bartter, F.C., Casper, A.G.T., Delea, C.S., and Slater, J.D.H.: On the role of the kidney in control of adrenal steroid production, Metabolism **10:**1006, 1961.

Beard, R.W., and Nathanielsz, P.W.: Fetal Physiology and Medicine, Philadelphia, 1976, W.B. Saunders Co.

Beydoun, S.N., Cuenco, V.G., Evans, L.P., and Aubry, R.H.: Maternal nutrition. I. The urinary urea nitrogen/total nitrogen ratio as an index of protein nutrition, Am. J. Obstet. Gynecol. **114:**198, 1972.

Bleicher, S.J., O'Sullivan, J.B., and Freinkel, N.: Carbohydrate metabolism in pregnancy. V. The interrelationships of glucose, insulin and free fatty acids in late pregnancy and post partum, N. Engl. J. Med. **271:**866, 1964.

Burwell, C.S.: Circulatory adjustments to pregnancy, Bull. Johns Hopkins Hosp. **95:**115, 1954.

Caldeyro-Barcia, R., and Poseiro, J.J.: Oxytocin and contractility of the pregnant human uterus, Ann. N.Y. Acad. Sci. **75:**813, 1959.

Carrington, E.R., Frishmuth, G.J., Oesterling, M.J., Adams, F.M., and Cox, S.E.: Gestational and postpartum plasma diamine oxidase values, Obstet. Gynecol. **39:**426, 1972.

Carrington, E.R., Oesterling, M.J., and Adams, F.M.: Renal clearance of estriol in complicated pregnancies, Am. J. Obstet. Gynecol. **106:**1131, 1970.

Caton, W.L., Roby, C.C., Reid, D.E., Caswell, C.J., Maletskos, C.J., Fluharty, R.G., and Gibson, J.G., II: The circulating red cell volume and body hematocrit in normal pregnancy and the puerperium, Am. J. Obstet. Gynecol. **61:**1207, 1951.

Chesley, L.C., Sloan, D.M., and Wynn, R.M.: Effects of posture and angiotensin 2 upon renal function in pregnant women, Am. J. Obstet. Gynecol. **90:**281, 1964.

Cohen, M.E., and Thompson, K.J.: Studies on the circulation in pregnancy, J.A.M.A. **112:**1556, 1939.

Danforth, D.N.: The fibrous nature of the human cervix and its relation to the isthmic segment in gravid and non-gravid uteri, Am. J. Obstet. Gynecol. **53:**541, 1947.

Danforth, D.N., and Ivy, A.C.: The lower uterine segment: its derivation and physiologic behavior, Am. J. Obstet. Gynecol. **57:**831, 1949.

Friesen, H.G., Fournier, P., and Desjardins, P.: Pituitary prolactin in pregnancy and normal and abnormal lactation. Clin. Obstet. Gynecol. **3:**25, 1973.

Gibson, H.M.: Plasma volume and glomerular filtration rate in pregnancy and their relation to differences in fetal growth, J. Obstet. Gynaecol. Br. Commonw. **8:**1067, 1973.

Gillespie, E.C.: Principles of uterine growth in pregnancy, Am. J. Obstet. Gynecol. **59:**949, 1950.

Hendricks, C.H., Quilligan, E.J. Tyler, C.W., and Tucker, G.J.: Pressure relationships between the intervillous space and the amniotic fluid in human term pregnancy, Am. J. Obstet. Gynecol. **77:**1028, 1959.

Hibbard, B.M., and Hibbard, E.D.: Folate metabolism and reproduction, Br. Med. Bull. **24:**10, 1968.

Hodgkinson, C.P.: Physiology of the ovarian veins during pregnancy, Obstet. Gynecol. **1:**26, 1953.

Holly, R.G.: Dynamics of iron metabolism in pregnancy, Am. J. Obstet. Gynecol. **93:**370, 1965.

Hytten, F.E., and Leitch, I.: The physiology of human pregnancy, ed. 2, London, 1971, Blackwell Scientific Publications, Ltd.

Israel, S.L., Rubenstone, A., and Meranze, D.R.: The ovary at term. I. Decidua-like reaction and surface cell proliferation, Obstet. Gynecol. **3:**399, 1954.

Israel, S.L., Stroup, P.E., Seligson, H.T., and Seligson, D.: Epinephrine and norepinephrine in pregnancy and labor, Obstet. Gynecol. **14:**68, 1959.

Jepson, J.H.: Endocrine control of maternal and fetal erythropoiesis, Can. Med. Assoc. J. **98:**844, 1968.

Kerr, M.G.: Cardiovascular dynamics in pregnancy and labour, Br. Med. Bull. **24:**19, 1968.

Knuttgen, H.G., and Emerson, K., Jr.: Physiologic responses to pregnancy at rest and during exercise, J. Appl. Physiol. **36:**549, 1974.

Komins, J.I., Snyder, P.J., and Schwarz, R.: Hyperthyroidism in pregnancy: a review, Obstet. Gynecol. Surv. **30:**527, 1975.

Kydd, D.M.: Hydrogen ion concentration and acid-base equilibrium in normal pregnancy, J. Biol. Chem. **91:**63, 1931.

Laros, R.K., Jr.: Blood disorders in pregnancy, Philadelphia, 1986, Lea & Febiger.

Lewis, B.V.: Uterine blood flow, a review, Obstet. Gynecol. Surv. **24:**1211, 1969.

Lowenstein, L., and Bramlage, C.A.: The bone marrow in pregnancy and the puerperium, Blood **12:**261, 1957.

Lund, C.J., and Donovan, J.C.: Blood volume during pregnancy: significance of plasma and red cell volumes, Am. J. Obstet. Gynecol. **98:**393, 1967.

Mack, H.C.: The plasma proteins, Clin. Obstet. Gynecol. **3:**336, 1960.

Macy, I.G., and Hunscher, H.A.: Evaluation of maternal nitrogen and mineral needs during embryonic and fetal development, Am. J. Obstet. Gynecol. **27:**878, 1934.

Metcalfe, J., Romney, S.L., Ramsey, L.H., Reid, D.E., and Burwell, C.S.: Estimation of blood flow in normal human pregnancy at term, J. Clin. Invest. **34:**1632, 1955.

Milunsky, A., and Flyate, E.: Prenatal diagnosis of neural tube defects: problems and pitfalls. Analysis of 2495 cases using the alpha-fetoprotein assay, Obstet. Gynecol. **48:**1, 1976.

Oesterling, M.J., Tse, R.L., and Holmes, H.M.: Spectrophotometric determination of catecholamine excretion in the free and conjugated forms, Fed. Proc. **21:**192, 1962.

Page, E.W., Villee, C.A., and Villee, D.B.: Human reproduction: essentials of reproductive and perinatal medicine, ed. 3, Philadelphia, 1981, W.B. Saunders Co.

Pitkin, R.M.: Calcium metabolism in pregnancy: a review, Am. J. Obstet. Gynecol. **121:**724, 1975.

Poidevin, L.O.S.: Histopathology of striae gravidarum, J. Obstet. Gynaecol. Br. Commonw. **66:**654, 1959.

Reynolds, W.A., Williams, G.A., and Pitkin, R.M.: Calcitropic hormone responsiveness during pregnancy, Am. J. Obstet. Gynecol. **139:**855, 1981.

Rose, D.J., Bader, M.E., Bader, R.A., and Brunwald, E.: Catheterization studies of cardiac hemodynamics in normal pregnant women with reference to left ventricular work. Am. J. Obstet. Gynecol. **72:**233, 1956.

Seitchik, J., and Alper, C.: The estimation of changes in body composition in normal pregnancy by measurement of body water, Am. J. Obstet. Gynecol. **71:**1165, 1956.

Seitchik, J., and Alper, C.: The body compartments of normal pregnant, edematous pregnant, and preeclamptic women, Am. J. Obstet. Gynecol. **68:**1540, 1954.

Sims, E.A.H., and Krantz, K.E.: Serial studies of renal function during pregnancy and the puerperium in normal women, J. Clin. Invest. **37:**1764, 1958.

Sodeman, W.A.: Cardiac changes in pregnancy unrelated to the usual etiological types of heart disease, Am. Heart J. **19:**385, 1940.

Venning, E.A.: Endocrine changes in normal pregnancy, Am. J. Med. **19:**721, 1955.

Whaley, W.H., Zuspan, F.P., and Nelson, G.H.: Glucose and nonesterified fatty acid levels in maternal and cord plasma, Am. J. Obstet. Gynecol. **92:**264, 1965.

Yen, S.S.C.: Endocrine regulation of metabolic homeostasis during pregnancy, Clin. Obstet. Gynecol. **16:**130, 1973.

Zarrow, M.X., Holmstrom, E.G., and Salhanick, H.A.: The concentration of relaxin in the blood serum and other tissues of women during pregnancy, J. Clin. Endocrinol. **15:**22, 1955.

20

J. Robert Willson

Diagnosis and duration of pregnancy and prenatal care

Prenatal care can be defined as a program of examination, evaluation, observation, treatment, and education of pregnant women directed toward making pregnancy, labor, and delivery as normal and as safe as possible for mothers and their infants. Physical abnormalities and emotional disturbances that might alter the course of pregnancy can be detected and often corrected so that the mothers will approach the time for delivery in as perfect health as possible.

The current program of prenatal care, which was developed early in the twentieth century, was designed to help reduce maternal, fetal and neonatal deaths by giving the physician an opportunity to diagnose conditions such as preeclampsia-eclampsia soon after their onset rather than in their terminal stages. The effectiveness of systematic prenatal care is evidenced by the reduced mortality from such disorders.

The general improvement in health, particularly of middle-class women, has permitted a change in the emphasis of prenatal care. One important objective of prenatal care is to identify women who have unusual emotional responses to reproduction and to support them in their areas of need.

Educational programs relating to general health care can be made available to prenatal patients. Most women return for prenatal visits periodically for 5 to 6 months, which provides time for a fairly extensive program. Appropriate subjects for discussion include nutrition, infant and child care, general health care, and contraception.

Conditions that may constitute temporary or permanent contraindications to pregnancy can be detected by *prepregnancy examination*. Every woman who is contemplating pregnancy should be examined completely before she attempts to conceive. At this time the physician should also attempt to evaluate her emotional reactions toward pregnancy and to initiate an educational program that may help her learn more about reproduction and her own responses to it. The *premarital examination* can serve as the initial prepregnancy examination if it is properly structured.

Several systems have been designed to quantitate the risks that individual women assume when they become pregnant. A variety of medical and obstetric conditions are scored numerically according to their potential for placing either the mother or the fetus in jeopardy; the higher the score the greater the risk. Actually, one does not need a numerical score to recognize a patient with a *high-risk pregnancy*. Any condition that is known to interfere with normal growth, development, and delivery of the fetus or any maternal disease that may be present at conception or develop during pregnancy increases the risk. Many of these conditions can be recognized during a prepregnancy

273

examination or at the first prenatal visit, and others that develop during pregnancy at subsequent visits. A special program of care should be developed for each patient with a high-risk pregnancy. Following are the most important risks:

I. Sociodemographic risks
   A. Age and parity
      1. Under age 15
      2. Age 30 to 40, birth order 1 and 5 +
   B. Lowest social classes
   C. Illegitimacy
II. Medical-obstetric risks
   A. Conditions present at conception
      1. Previous abortion, ectopic pregnancy, fetal death, neonatal death, or congenital anomaly
      2. Previous low-birth-weight infant
      3. Less than a year since last pregnancy terminated
      4. Difficulty in conceiving
      5. Chronic cardiovascular-renal or collagen diseases
      6. Diabetes mellitus
      7. Malnutrition and anemia
      8. Chronic urinary tract infection
      9. Congenital malformation of reproductive organs
     10. Syphilis
     11. Herpes virus and papilloma virus infections
     12. Tuberculosis
     13. Tobacco, drug, or alcohol addiction
     14. Abnormal pelvis
     15. Uterine or ovarian neoplasms
   B. Conditions developing during pregnancy
      1. Pyelonephritis
      2. Preeclampsia-eclampsia
      3. Bleeding
      4. Acute infectious diseases
      5. Malnutrition
      6. Sexually transmitted diseases
      7. Multifetal pregnancy
   C. Conditions during labor and delivery
      1. Premature labor
      2. Premature rupture of membranes
      3. Abnormal labor
      4. Abnormal fetal position
      5. Cesarean section
      6. Hemorrhage following delivery

Neither prepregnancy nor prenatal care can be expected to compensate for inferior care during labor and delivery. To achieve the lowest maternal and perinatal morbidity and mortality, the responsible physicians and their associates must maintain careful supervision of the entire pregnancy and delivery.

Too often prenatal "care" consists of a series of visits during which a patient is weighed, the blood pressure is recorded, and an abdominal examination is performed. She is told that her weight gain is just right (which she knows) and that the baby is alive and growing (which she also knows) and is directed to return in 2 weeks. She hesitates to ask questions because she knows there are many other women to be seen. As a consequence she may make 10 to 15 prenatal visits and learn little about pregnancy, labor, delivery, and infant care and nothing about general health measures.

Since the healthy women with a normal pregnancy needs little medical care, it seems appropriate that health professionals other than obstetrician-gynecologists play a major role in providing pregnancy care. An appropriate method for accomplishing this is through an *obstetric team,* consisting of a physician and one or more nurse midwives or obstetric nurse practitioners. Each patient is evaluated at the first prenatal visit to determine the level of care she needs. Thereafter responsibility is divided; the physician concentrates on women with problems, and the nurses provide most of the care for those who are normal and the educational program for all patients.

With such a distribution of responsibilities, it is possible to provide appropriate care for every woman. Nurses will have sufficient time to spend with healthy women, and physicians can concentrate their efforts on women who need special medical care.

INITIAL EXAMINATION

Ideally, each patient should be examined as soon as it is reasonably clear that she is pregnant, usually about 2 weeks after she has missed a menstrual period. Unfortunately, the initial examination often is delayed either because the patient does not call or because the first open appointment is several weeks in the future. This presents no great problem for the healthy woman, but it may have serious consequences for those with complicated medical conditions or those who may need or want an abortion.

The problem can be solved by scheduling each initial prenatal visit with an obstetric nurse, usually within a few days of her first call. The nurse obtains a complete history, records the weight and blood pressure, determines the approximate duration of pregnancy, and orders the necessary laboratory studies. If the patient is normal, the nurse schedules the next visit with a physician who will have all the necessary information available. If any problem is suspected or if the patient wants an abortion, consultation is obtained before the patient leaves.

The *obstetric history* includes a general medical and social review with particular reference to diseases or conditions in the patient or her family that might affect the course of pregnancy and a detailed analysis of gynecologic function. The details of alcohol, tobacco, and drug use should be noted.

One should record the *date of onset and the duration of at least the last two periods*. It is particularly important to determine specifically whether the last period of bleeding was normal and came at the expected time. Many women report any bleeding, even spotting, as a "menstrual period" unless questioned in detail. One should also record the *contraceptive method* the patient was using before she conceived. Ovulation is often delayed for some time after birth control pills are discontinued. The "last period," the episode of withdrawal bleeding, may have preceded conception by several weeks.

Information concerning *previous pregnancies* should include their duration at delivery; the length of labor; the type of delivery; the size, condition, and subsequent development of the infant; the occurrence of complications; and the patient's emotional reaction to the event. Previous pregnancy failures such as abortion, ectopic pregnancy, and fetal and neonatal deaths should be recorded also.

A *general medical examination* is performed after the patient has been interviewed. The *pelvic examination* includes bimanual palpation of the reproductive organs and inspection of the external genitals, the vagina, and the cervix. Manual measurements of the bony pelvis are obtained during the initial pelvic examination. If the patient is unusually tense, this can be postponed until later in pregnancy.

Basic laboratory studies in the normal patient include determinations of the hemoglobin level or hematocrit, blood type, and Rh; a serologic test for syphilis; urine tests for protein and sugar; and a screening cytologic examination for cervical abnormalities.

A *screening antibody test,* which is nonspecific in that it indicates the presence of any abnormal antibody not the precise type, should be run. If it is positive, further tests are necessary to identify the specific factor involved. A *rubella antibody titer* should also be obtained if it has not already been done.

A *chest x-ray film examination* need not be performed on every pregnant woman, but it should be a part of the prenatal examination for patient groups in whom the incidence of pulmonary tuberculosis is high, for individuals who have had pulmonary diseases, for those whose tuberculin tests have converted from negative to positive, or if there is any question as to the presence of a disease process. The abdomen and pelvis must be properly protected. *Skin tests for reaction to tuberculin* are appropriate for women who are ordinary risks for infection.

It is unnecessary to *examine the urine sediment* in every prenatal patient, but when such an examination is indicated, it is best done on a specimen obtained by catheter to eliminate contamination by vaginal or vulvar secretions. Since about 7% of all pregnant women have asymptomatic bacteriuria, and since most urinary tract infections before and after delivery occur in women with bacteriuria, it is wise to obtain a *urine culture* early in the second trimester in all pregnant women. This is particularly important in women who have had urinary tract infections.

Fasting and *2-hour postprandial blood sugar*

concentrations should be determined on women whose history suggests the possibility of diabetes.

Genetic amniocentesis is recommended for women whose fetuses are likely to have chromosomal or biochemical abnormalities (Chapter 2).

After the examination has been completed and the diagnosis of pregnancy has been established, the findings are discussed with the patient. This portion of the interview should be unhurried and presented in words that she can understand easily. The physician first confirms the fact that she is pregnant, if this is possible, and indicates the date at which delivery can be expected. Unless there is some abnormality, she should be assured that her physical condition is satisfactory, that her pelvis is adequate, and that no complications are anticipated.

In the past it was customary to give a detailed description of what to expect during pregnancy, precise instructions concerning diet, general activities, what to do when labor starts, and numerous other directions at the time of the first visit and to believe that this needs to be done only once. Unfortunately, patients heard little of such monologues because they were so excited or disturbed by the confirmation of the pregnancy that they failed to listen.

It is impossible for most women to understand the full implication of pregnancy and to realize that they are going to have a baby, in contrast to being pregnant, until they actually can feel fetal activity. As a consequence, it is preferable to discuss specific problems at appropriate times during the pregnancy when the patient has some interest in them and when they are applicable. It usually is helpful to have printed instructions to which the patient can refer.

DIAGNOSIS OF PREGNANCY

The diagnosis of pregnancy is made on the history of the *subjective symptoms,* which are the sensations experienced by the patient, and the detection of the *objective signs,* which are evident to the examiner. It may be difficult to establish an accurate diagnosis early, but the physician who uses all available aids will make few mistakes.

Subjective symptoms

It is not possible to make a diagnosis of pregnancy on the basis of symptoms alone. Each of the characteristic symptoms can be associated with conditions other than pregnancy, and some gravid women have none of them except amenorrhea.

Amenorrhea. Cessation of menstruation should always suggest the possibility of pregnancy, but it should not be concluded that the patient is pregnant only because amenorrhea is present. A few women bleed at irregular intervals throughout pregnancy because of some abnormality, and others may cease menstruating for reasons other than pregnancy. Regular cyclic menstruation cannot occur during pregnancy because ovarian function is suspended.

Morning nausea and vomiting. Morning nausea and vomiting usually appear a week or two after the period is missed and continue until about the tenth or twelfth week. The severity varies from mild nausea, which is easily relieved by ingesting food, to persistent vomiting, which depletes fluid and electrolytes (Chapter 24).

Although some degree of nausea and vomiting is experienced by more than half of all pregnant women, it is not diagnostic of pregnancy. Women who are not pregnant, as well as husbands of women who are, may have morning nausea and vomiting.

Bladder disturbance. Frequency of urination is caused by pressure or tension on the bladder by the enlarging uterus.

Breasts. Enlargement, tingling, or actual discomfort in the breasts is the result of hormonal stimulation of alveolar and ductal structures. This may also occur premenstrually.

Quickening. Quickening is a term that indicates the perception of fetal motion by the mother. Multiparas first feel the infant at about the seventeenth week, and primigravidas about 2 weeks later. Women with pseudocyesis also experience ''quickening.''

The first sensation is usually described as a slight fluttering or a feeling similar to gas passing through the bowel. As the fetus grows and becomes more active, the sensation becomes stronger and may even be painful.

Objective signs

Breasts (Fig. 20-1). The breasts are firm and distended, and Montgomery's glands are prominent. The nipple and areola become darker as pregnancy advances and are surrounded by an area of increased pigmentation in the normal skin, the *secondary areola*. Colostrum can be expressed from the nipples; but it is not a reliable sign, since it may also be produced in pseudocyesis, with anterior lobe pituitary tumors, and in multiparas between pregnancies.

Genitals. The most remarkable changes take place in the genital organs.

VAGINA. The vaginal wall becomes cyanotic and congested (Chadwick's sign). This may also be detected before menstruation or with increased local congestion from any cause.

CERVIX. Softening in the tip of the cervix (Goodell's sign) can be detected soon after the onset of pregnancy. The entire cervix eventually is softened.

UTERINE ISTHMUS (Fig. 20-2). The isthmus of the uterus is soft at 6 to 8 weeks and can be compressed between the fingers on bimanual examination (Hegar's sign). Within a few weeks the entire cervix and the corpus become much softer, and the difference can no longer be detected.

UTERUS (Fig. 20-2). The consistency and shape of the firm, pear-shaped nonpregnant uterus change as pregnancy advances. Soon after the fertilized ovum implants, a soft bulge can be detected in half of the uterus, usually fairly high in the fundus, whereas the other side remains firm. The softened area probably indicates the implantation site.

The consistency of the uterus becomes soft and doughy rather than firm as pregnancy advances, and a progressive increase in size can be detected by repeated examinations. Intermittent, painless uterine contractions (Braxton Hicks contractions) can sometimes be felt during the second trimester. Later they become stronger, and the patient may be aware of them.

Demonstration of the fetus (Fig. 20-3). The fetal parts can usually be *palpated* by the twentieth week of pregnancy unless the patient is too obese, the abdomen is tender, or there is an excessive amount of amniotic fluid (hydramnios). It may be possible to feel the fetus slightly earlier by *ballottement* through the vagina. The examining fingers in the vagina push the anterior vaginal wall and lower

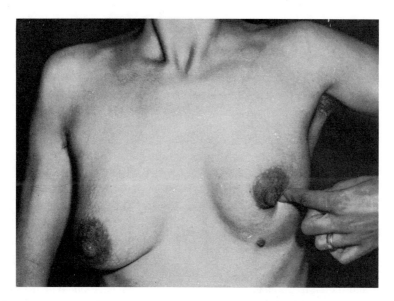

Fig. 20-1. Breast changes. Montgomery's glands are prominent, and nipples and areolae are deeply pigmented. Accessory nipple beneath left breast is also pigmented.

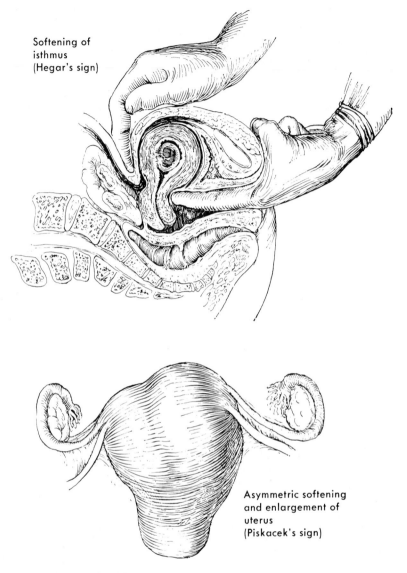

Softening of
isthmus
(Hegar's sign)

Asymmetric softening
and enlargement of
uterus
(Piskacek's sign)

Fig. 20-2. Uterine changes in early pregnancy.

uterine segment sharply upward, and the fetus first rises and then falls back, bumping against the fingertips.

Fetal motion can usually be seen, felt, or heard by the physician after the eighteenth week. Quickening is subjective and therefore unreliable.

The *fetal heart tones* can be heard first with an ordinary stethoscope at about the eighteenth to twentieth week low in the midline. The normal rate varies from 120 to 160 beats/min, and usually it is not difficult to differentiate the double beat of the fetal heart from the maternal pulse. The sounds may be obscured by obesity, hydramnios, or an unusual fetal position. With the Doppler apparatus, one can detect the fetal heart consistently by the twelfth week and sometimes a week or two earlier.

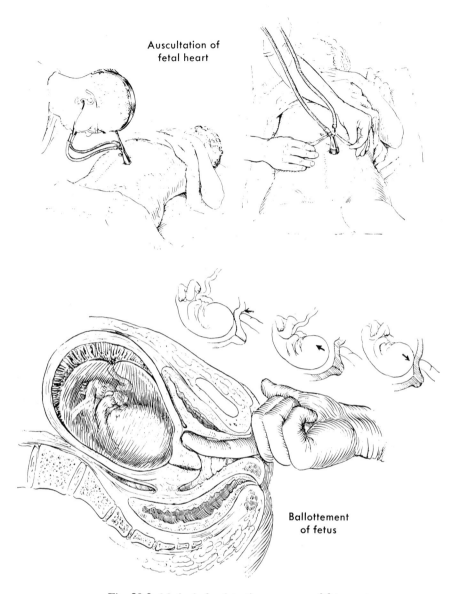

Fig. 20-3. Methods for detecting presence of fetus.

Obesity, fluid, and other barriers do not alter the accuracy of the instrument.

Pregnancy can be confirmed much earlier by sonography than by physical examination. A *gestational sac* can usually be identified 5 to 6 weeks after the beginning of the last period, a *fetal pole* can be seen by about the eighth week, and the *skull and thorax* can be identified by about the fourteenth

week. With real-time ultrasound techniques *fetal heart motion* can be detected by about the seventh week.

The *fetal skeleton* can be detected by x-ray film examination after some calcification has taken place. Under favorable conditions it may be seen at about 14 weeks and almost always after 16 to 18 weeks. X-ray film studies at this stage of pregnancy are best not used unless it is essential to attempt to demonstrate the presence of a fetus and no other method is available.

Pregnancy tests. The laboratory tests for pregnancy are based on the identification of chorionic gonadotropic hormones. Since similar hormones are produced by certain teratomas of the ovary and testes, choriocarcinoma, and hydatidiform mole, as well as by normal placenta, a positive test does not necessarily indicate the presence of normal pregnancy. Conversely, a negative result does not necessarily eliminate pregnancy. Some of the immunologic tube and slide tests are not sensitive enough to detect low levels of hCG during early pregnancy (Chapter 2).

It usually is not necessary to order a pregnancy test unless there is need to diagnose pregnancy before the characteristic changes in the cervix and uterus can be appreciated; for example, when ectopic pregnancy is suspected. If a normal patient is examined before the physical changes can be identified, pregnancy can usually be diagnosed by repeating the examination in 2 or 3 weeks.

Positive diagnosis

A positive diagnosis of pregnancy can be made only if the fetus is identified by palpating its parts, by hearing its heart, by palpating motion, or by sonography. This can be accomplished during the first trimester of pregnancy only by sonographic techniques.

Differential diagnosis

Typical uterine changes must make the physician suspect pregnancy even though the patient denies the possibility. Repeated pelvic examination will clarify the problem because the size, shape, and consistency of the pregnant uterus will undergo the characteristic changes as pregnancy advances (Chapter 19).

Cystic ovarian neoplasms situated either in the posterior cul-de-sac or in the anterior pelvis may simulate a pregnant uterus. Ovarian neoplasms alone do not often cause amenorrhea. They usually can be separated from the uterine fundus, and they do not increase in size as rapidly as the pregnant uterus.

Sonography may be helpful. If the patient is not pregnant, one can expect to see an adnexal mass separate from a normal uterus without any evidence of pregnancy.

Uterine fibromyomas, particularly a large single tumor situated in the fundus of the uterus, may be almost impossible to differentiate from a normal pregnancy. Uterine tumors do not cause amenorrhea; and, since they grow slowly, one can detect little or no change in the uterus by repeated examinations at intervals of 2 to 3 weeks.

Other disorders such as *hematometra* caused by imperforate hymen or congenital malformations of the vagina are uncommon and can usually be diagnosed by history and examination.

Pregnancy and fibromyomas or ovarian tumors often occur simultaneously. In situations of this kind it may be necessary to use every possible diagnostic aid. Pregnancy must be considered in women who have missed one or more periods and in those whose periods have been normal but who are now bleeding irregularly, even though an ovarian cyst, a fibroid tumor, or another obvious lesion is present. In such women, pregnancy tests and sonography may be particularly helpful in diagnosing early pregnancy.

PSEUDOCYESIS (Fig. 20-4)

Pseudocyesis (spurious or pseudopregnancy) is an outstanding example of emotional control of physiologic function. Women with pseudocyesis may be amenorrheic or have significantly reduced menstrual flow, and the breasts may become firm, enlarge, and secrete colostrum. The abdomen enlarges, but, in contrast to pregnancy during which the umbilicus becomes flattened or even everted, the navel retains its normal depression. The abdominal enlargement is in part caused by weight gain, which often is greater than that during normal pregnancy. Patients with pseudocyesis experience all the symptoms of normal pregnancy; in fact they may be exaggerated. They also report "quickening" but frequently earlier than one would anticipate if the pregnancy were normal.

The exact mechanism responsible for the changes in women with pseudocyesis has not been determined, and there have been few recent studies of the hormonal status of women with pseudocyesis. Starkman and co-workers, studying two women, found elevated plasma testosterone and estradiol and low progesterone concentrations. Pro-

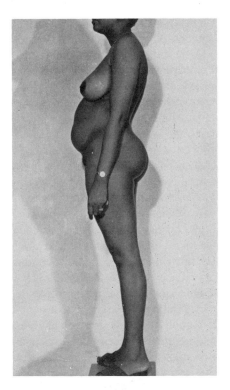

Fig. 20-4. Pseudocyesis. Protrusion of abdomen, increased lordosis, and posture are typical of pregnancy.

lactin was normal and fell rapidly after the administration of dopamine. Growth hormone changed little during sleep and did not respond to dopamine. In one patient LH was elevated and FSH was normal; in the other both LH and FSH were normal. They postulated that the hormone levels were like those of the late follicular phase of the normal cycle and that the amenorrhea might be caused by persistence of this state.

Pseudocyesis may appear at any age but is more common in older women. It usually represents an emotional need for an infant in an attempt to maintain a failing marriage, proof for herself that she can conceive, or a similar psychologic reason.

The diagnosis can be suspected if the physician cannot detect characteristic pregnancy changes in the pelvic organs and can be confirmed if the pregnancy test is negative, by sonography, or if the uterus does not enlarge progressively.

Because of the emotional factors involved, it does no good and in fact may be harmful simply to tell the patient that she is not pregnant. An attempt must be made to uncover the underlying emotional problem that makes

pregnancy necessary to her. In some instances she should be interviewed several times before she is even told that she is not pregnant. Intensive psychotherapy may be necessary.

SIGNS OF LIFE OR DEATH OF THE FETUS

During the first 16 to 18 weeks of pregnancy the physician must rely on progressive uterine growth, detection of fetal heart activity by an ultrasonic instrument, or sonography to determine whether the fetus is alive and growing. Later the heartbeat can usually be heard with an ordinary stethoscope, and fetal motion can be felt or heard.

If *fetal motion suddenly ceases* and cannot be detected by the mother or the physician and if the *fetal heart can no longer be heard,* the fetus may have died. Occasionally, the fetal heart cannot be heard with an ordinary stethoscope because the fetus has assumed an unusual position and its chest wall is not in contact with the anterior uterine wall. A positive answer can be obtained by real-time ultrasonography; if fetal heart motion can be detected, the fetus is alive.

If the fetus has died, *uterine growth ceases,* or the size of the uterus may even regress. When placental function is disturbed, the breasts become softer and smaller.

Estriol production ceases when the fetus dies, and the change can be detected by repeatedly determining the level of this estrogen fraction. A fall in estriol excretion will occur more rapidly than a *reversal of pregnancy test* because estriol production is a function of both fetus and placenta, whereas the chorionic gonadotropins are produced entirely by the placenta. The placental cells may continue to survive and function, and the pregnancy test may remain positive for some time after the fetus dies.

DURATION OF PREGNANCY

The duration of pregnancy extends over an approximate period of 280 days from the first day of the last normal menstrual period or 268 days from fertilization. The duration of pregnancy therefore is about 40 weeks when calculated from the onset of the last period and 38 weeks when calculated from conception.

The exact time of fertilization can only be determined accurately by women who are recording basal body temperatures or by those who conceive by artificial insemination; consequently, the first day of the last normal menstrual period is used as a starting point. The thirteenth week of pregnancy therefore is the thirteenth week after the onset of the last normal period, not the thirteenth week after conception. Since most women do not keep calendar records of menstruation, this calculation is far from precise, but it is acceptable for clinical use.

There is no accurate method for determining exactly when labor will begin; however, the patient will want some day toward which to point—*the expected date of confinement, or EDC*—and this may be provided by the following methods:

1. The date of the first day of the last normal menstrual period minus 3 months plus 7 days gives the day of expected delivery. Since the date of the last menstrual period often is unreliable, and since the last period of bleeding recognized by the patient may or may not have been true menstruation, this date does not necessarily indicate the day delivery will occur, but it usually is within 2 weeks on either side.

This calculation often is inaccurate in women with irregular cycles and when conception occurs after discontinuing oral contraceptives. Ovulation and conception may not occur for several weeks after the last withdrawal bleeding.

2. The EDC may also be calculated by adding 268 days to the day of ovulation as determined by basal temperature recordings or to the date of presumed fruitful coitus. The latter may well be inaccurate.

Unless there is a point of reference such as the date of the last menstrual period or an isolated coitus, the physician may find it difficult to determine when a patient is approaching term. The size of the uterus is helpful, but it is more important to determine, if possible, the age of the fetus.

The physician can eliminate much confusion concerning the accuracy of the EDC of women who are first seen early in pregnancy by means of the following:

1. Comparing uterine size with the presumed duration of pregnancy on the basis of menstrual history at the first examination
2. Comparing uterine size with dates at specific weeks of pregnancy when the size of the uterus can be determined reasonably accurately (Fig. 20-5) (At the end of the twelfth week the uterine fundus can usually be felt above the upper border of the pubis; by the sixteenth week it is about halfway between the pubis and the umbilicus; and by the twentieth week it has reached the level of the umbilicus. Between 20 and 30 weeks the height of the fundus in centimeters, measured from the top of the uterus around the curve of the abdomen to the upper border of the symphysis pubis, approximates the week of gestation. This measurement becomes less accurate during the last weeks of pregnancy.)
3. Recording the exact date of quickening and the uterine size when fetal motion was felt
4. Recording the date when the fetal heart was first heard with an ordinary stethoscope

Andersen and colleagues, studying 418 patients who were delivered of infants weighing at least 3000 g, found the date the last normal menstrual period began to be the most reliable determinant of when to expect delivery. The mean number of days between the first day of the last period and delivery was 283.5 for primigravidas and 285 for multiparas. Next in reliability was the time at which the top of the fundus reached the level of the umbilicus; the mean interval to delivery was 142 days in primigravidas and 137.5 days in multiparas. The dates at which the mother first experienced quickening and at which the physician first heard the fetal heart with an ordinary stethoscope were less reliable. If, however, the date at which the last period began was not known, a combination of the dates at which the fundus reached the umbilicus, the mother first felt the fetus move, and the obstetrician first heard the fetal heart provide a reasonably reliable baseline on which the EDC can be calculated.

When this information is not available (for example, when conception occurs before the menses

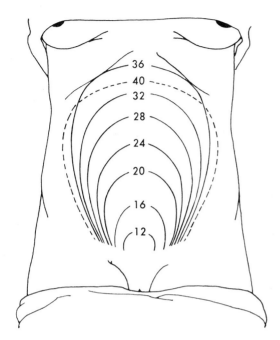

Fig. 20-5. Height of uterus above pubis at various weeks of pregnancy.

have returned after abortion or delivery, before a patient has had a normal period after discontinuing oral contraceptives, or when her periods are grossly irregular), it still is possible to arrive at a reasonable approximation of fetal age and maturity by using *sonography* and *amniotic fluid analysis*.

Sonography. During the first trimester, fetal age can be estimated with reasonable accuracy after the seventh or eighth week by *measuring the crown-rump length of the embryo*. After the sixteenth week one can measure the *biparietal diameter of the fetal skull*. At 16 weeks the average variation between gestational age on the basis of an accurate menstrual history and that calculated from the biparietal diameter is ±7 days. This increases to about ±10 days between weeks 17 and 26, to ±14 days during weeks 27 and 28, and to as much as ±21 days after week 29.

Amniotic fluid analysis. An amniotic fluid examination may be helpful in determining fetal age.

LECITHIN/SPHINGOMYELIN (L/S) RATIO. The concentrations of lecithin and of sphingomyelin in am-

niotic fluid are about equal before the thirty-fifth week of pregnancy. After that time the lecithin concentration rises rapidly until term, whereas the sphingomyelin concentration decreases. High-lecithin concentration indicates fetal lung maturity. Consequently, if the L/S ratio is at least 2:1, the lung is probably mature, despite fetal size, and there is little likelihood that serious respiratory distress will develop.

PHOSPHOTIDYLGLYCEROL. The presence of the surfactant activity of this substance gives evidence of lung maturity and provides reasonable reassurance that the infant, if delivered, will not develop respiratory distress syndrome. Its absence, however, is a less positive indication that respiratory distress syndrome will occur. The test for phosphotidylglycerol is not influenced by the presence of blood, meconium, or amniotic fluid.

These tests are more sensitive indicators of pulmonary maturity and the risk of the newborn infant developing respiratory distress syndrome than are other evaluations of amniotic fluid.

FETAL CELLS. Shed fetal cells, presumably from sebaceous glands, stain orange with Nile blue sulfate, whereas squamous cells stain blue. The number of orange-staining cells in amniotic fluid increases as the fetus matures and can be used as a rough determinant of fetal age. Bishop and Corson state that when the count of orange cells is less than 2%, the prematurity rate is 85%; but when more than 20% of the cells in amniotic fluid are of the orange-staining type, the infant will weigh at least 2500 g.

CREATININE. The fetal kidneys become progressively more active as maturity advances. One evidence of improving renal function and of the increasing fetal muscle mass is the amniotic fluid creatinine concentration. The infant is presumed to be mature when amniotic fluid creatinine concentration is more than 2 mg/dl.

DIET AND WEIGHT GAIN

Weight gain. An increase of about 9 kg (20 pounds) over the prepregnancy weight can be accounted for by the products of conception and physiologic changes in the maternal organs. The weight of these components averages as follows:

	Kilograms	Pounds
Fetus	3600	7.5

Placenta	720	1.5
Amniotic fluid	960	2
Uterus	960	2
Breasts	480	1
Plasma volume	1440	3
Extracellular fluid	1440	3

Maternal weight gain		Birth weight
(kilograms)	(pounds)	(grams)
0-4.8	0-10	3278
5.3-9.6	11-20	3301
10.1-14.4	21-30	3426
14.9-19.2	31-40	3562
+19.7	+41	3636

Most women gain more than this, the *average weight gain during normal pregnancy* being about 11.5 kg (24 pounds). Those who gain an average amount usually return to their prepregnancy weights after involution is complete. According to Naeye the lowest perinatal mortality occurs when the weight gain is about 20 pounds in normally proportioned women and about 30 pounds in those who are underweight.

Gains greater than 11.5 kg (24 pounds) can usually be accounted for by the ingestion of a diet too high in calories, the result of which is a residual increase in fat stores, or by the accumulation of fluid in the extravascular spaces. The former is responsible for many of the overweight women who find it difficult to lose the excess fat later and who repeat the same process during each of several pregnancies.

Excessive storage of fluid is not likely to be a cause of obesity but has a more serious immediate significance because it is one of the warning signs that preeclampsia may be developing. Excessive weight gain per se is not a cause of toxemia, but most women with preeclampsia do gain abnormally because of fluid retention. Conversely, the majority of women who store an excessive amount of fluid during pregnancy do not develop preeclampsia.

There is a definite relationship between maternal weight gain and the weight of the baby. Eastman and Jackson studied the records of 6675 white women and 5236 black women who were delivered of normal, living, single infants between the thirty-ninth and forty-second weeks of uncomplicated pregnancies. The mean weight gain for white women was 10.6 kg (22.1 pounds) and for black women, 9.8 kg (20.5 pounds). The mean birth weight of white infants was 3395 g, and progressive increases in maternal weight gains were accompanied by progressive increments in infant birth weights. The mean infant birth weights and maternal weight gains were as follows:

An interesting finding is that the mean birth weights of 61 infants whose mothers had lost weight during pregnancy was 3360 g.

The incidence of babies weighing 2500 g or less decreased progressively from 4.4% if the mothers gained 0 to 4.8 kg to 0.5% in 202 women who gained more than 19.7 kg. Of the mothers who lost weight, 3.3% were delivered of low-birth-weight infants.

The infants of black women followed a similar pattern but weighed less in each group than did the white babies.

Nyirjesy, Lonergan, and Kane, studying 12,569 primigravidas who were delivered at term, also noted progressively increasing infant weight and a decreasing incidence of low-birth-weight babies with increasing maternal weight gains.

It is illogical to recommend that the mother gain excessively solely in an attempt to increase the size of the baby. It also is illogical to try to restrict the infant's weight by drastically curtailing the mother's caloric intake. This can only lead to impaired fetal development.

The *rate of gain* may have prognostic significance. The weight gain during the first trimester of normal pregnancy may be no more than 0.7 to 1.4 kg (1.5 to 3 pounds), even though there is no nausea. During the last two trimesters the gain usually is fairly steady at a rate of less than 0.48 kg (1 pound) per week. Excessive weight gain that begins during the first trimester and continues throughout pregnancy is almost always a result of excessive caloric intake. During the last 16 weeks of pregnancy, sudden increases in weight or gains of more than 1 kg (2 pounds) weekly are almost always an indication of excessive fluid accumulation.

Women who are *underweight* may be malnourished. Whenever possible, the nutritional deficit should be corrected before pregnancy, but generally, these patients are not seen until the first prenatal visit. At this time each underweight patient should be impressed with the importance of altering her diet to one that is suitable for pregnancy. Underweight patients can gain more than 11.5 kg (24 pounds), but the diet must provide the ingredients necessary for fetal growth. Naeye calculated that the lowest perinatal mortality for infants born to underweight women occurs when the weight gain is about 30 pounds.

Overweight women are also likely to be malnourished; their diets may be deficient in everything except calories. The pregnancies of obese women are more often complicated by hypertension and abnormal glucose metabolism than are those of more normal-weight mothers. Overweight women have a higher incidence of excessively large babies; conversely, they deliver fewer low-birth-weight infants.

It would appear that the weeks of pregnancy when a woman is under regular medical observation might be an appropriate time for controlled weight reduction, but this is not true. The primary nutritional objective should be to prevent excessive weight gain rather than to reduce or even to maintain weight. Excessive caloric reduction may require elimination of some essential nutrients, interfere with use of protein, produce ketonuria caused by catabolism of stored fat, and restrict fetal growth. Naeye calculated that the lowest perinatal mortality in infants who are born to overweight women occurs when the weight gain is about 16 pounds.

Some pregnant women gain at an excessive rate because they become progressively less active as pregnancy advances and continue to ingest the same amount of food. Pregnant women should be encouraged to remain active and to exercise.

Compulsive eating leading to excessive weight gain during pregnancy and subsequent obesity can have an emotional basis. The possibility of a psychogenic cause should always be considered, particularly in women with unusual reactions toward their pregnancies and those who are depressed.

One can predict with reasonable certainty that the diets of most *teenagers* are deficient and that many of them are malnourished. Nutrition may be one of the most important factors determining the outcome of pregnancy in young girls.

The adolescent girl who conceives before she has reached maximum longitudinal growth is at even greater risk of malnutrition than are those who become pregnant several years later. The dietary intake of the young pregnant teenager must include the nutritional requirements for her own continuing growth as well as for the pregnancy.

The caloric content of the diet influences fetal growth. Delgado and associates supplemented the inadequate basic diets of two groups of mothers: one with an increase in both calories and protein and one with an increase in calories alone. The weights of the newborn infants were similarly increased in both groups. One can conclude from this study that calories are essential for fetal growth but that the birth of a large baby does not indicate conclusively that the mother's diet was optimal.

It is particularly important that the pregnancy diet contain an *adequate amount of good-quality protein* because it is essential for fetal development and for many of the basic maternal changes during pregnancy. There is no information, however, to suggest that a high-protein diet is essential for either maternal or fetal well-being. Zlatnik and Burmeister could find no differences in birth weight and anthropometric indices of infants born to mothers with mean protein intakes of 0.7 g/kg/day as compared to those of mothers whose mean intake of protein was 1.5 g/kg/day.

Many women survive on *vegetarian diets* that may be either vegan, which exclude fish, meat, poultry, eggs, and milk; or ovolacto, which exclude only fish, meat, and poultry. The former may be quite inadequate for pregnancy, whereas the latter may provide the necessary food elements.

Protein deficiencies may alter brain development. The brains of rats born of mothers who are maintained on diets inadequate in protein are qualitatively and quantitatively inferior to brains of rats whose mothers are well nourished before and during pregnancy. Brains of the experimental rats' offspring contain fewer neurons than do the brains of the control rats' offspring, and each cell contains less protein.

In humans, maximal neuron growth occurs during pregnancy and the first year of life. That protein deprivation during these periods may alter the brain is suggested by the fact that brain cellularity is reduced in infants who die of malnutrition during the first year of life but not necessarily in those who become malnourished and die later. Functional impairment can also be demonstrated in malnourished children.

Normal pregnancy diet. The fetus has the remarkable ability to acquire whatever it needs for its growth and development in utero. If the necessary ingredients are not supplied in the mother's diet, they will be obtained at the expense of her tissues. During the winter of 1944-1945 the caloric intake of the population of the Netherlands was reduced to as little as 450 kcal/day. The median birth weight of infants born to mothers who were pregnant during this time was reduced by about 240 g, but perinatal mortality was not increased. A diet that provides the materials required for fetal growth prevents depletion of maternal tissue.

The daily dietary requirements for women of various ages and the additions necessary during pregnancy and lactation are listed in Table 20-1.

To provide these requirements, each day's food intake should include the following:

Protein
Lean meat, fish, chicken—2 servings
Eggs—at least 1
Milk—1 liter; 150 ml (10 tablespoons) of dried skim milk powder provides an equivalent amount of protein
Additional protein—112 g cottage cheese, additional meat or eggs

Vegetables
Potato—1 serving
Cooked vegetables (preferably colored such as carrots, spinach, or greens)—2 servings
Raw vegetables (cabbage, lettuce, carrots)—1 serving

TABLE 20-1 Recommended daily dietary allowances for mature women with added allowances for pregnancy and lactation

	Recommended daily allowances for nonpregnant women	Recommended daily allowances added for pregnancy	Recommended daily allowances added for lactation
Calories (kcal)	2100	300	500
Protein (g)	44	30	20
Vitamin A (RE)	800	200	400
Vitamin D (μg)	7.5	5	5
Vitamin E (mg equiv)	10	2	3
Ascorbic acid (mg)	60	20	40
Folacin (mg)	0.4	0.3	0.1
Niacin (mg equiv)	14	2	5
Riboflavin (mg)	1.3	0.3	0.5
Thiamine (mg)	1.1	0.4	0.5
Vitamin B (mg)	2	0.6	0.5
Vitamin B_{12} (μg)	3	1	1
Calcium (g)	800	400	400
Phosphorus (g)	800	400	400
Iodine (μg)	150	25	50
Iron (mg)	18	Supplement	0
Magnesium (mg)	300	150	150
Zinc (mg)	15	5	10

Based on data from Recommended dietary allowances, ed. 9, Washington, D.C., 1979, National Academy of Sciences.

Fruits
Fresh fruit or fruit juice—2 servings, one of which should be tomatoes, oranges, or grapefruit

Bread and cereal
Whole grain cereal (oatmeal, enriched grits, whole wheat cereal)—1 serving
Bread—2 slices whole wheat or rye bread

Other foods
Sugar—small amount as desired
Butter or margarine—45 ml (1 tablespoon)
Fluids—water or other nonfattening liquids may be taken in any quantity; 8 to 10 glasses daily are desirable

Supplements
A multivitamin preparation and iron

Total parenteral nutrition. The nutritional needs of pregnant women who cannot ingest adequate diets can be met parenterally, at least until they can eat again. Seifer and co-workers provided parenteral nutrition to ten women for from 7 to 27 days. There were no obstetric or fetal complications attributable to the therapy, and the infants were at or above the tenth percentile of expected weights.

Pica. The term pica indicates the ingestion of materials not ordinarily considered as foods. The most common are laundry starch, clay, and coal. Pica is more prevalent in black than in white women and is usually increased during pregnancy. The ingestion of large amounts of these materials often leads to malnutrition, iron deficiency anemia, and even bowel obstruction. Pregnant women from population groups in which pica is common should be questioned in detail about their eating habits.

Low-sodium diets. Low-sodium diets have been used extensively in an attempt to prevent or to control edema during pregnancy and in the treatment of preeclampsia-eclampsia. The accumulated evidence suggests that sodium restriction during pregnancy, even in women with edema and preeclampsia-eclampsia, may be harmful. As a consequence, low-sodium diets are usually not appropriate for pregnant women.

PRENATAL INSTRUCTIONS

In addition to needing advice concerning diet, the patient must know what she is permitted to do and what she should avoid doing during her pregnancy. The normal individual does not need to alter her activities much because she is pregnant.

Exercise. The amount of physical activity permitted is determined by the tolerance of the individual patient and what she is used to doing. Any usual activity, including walking, jogging, golf, tennis, and cycling can be continued by normal pregnant women. They become less agile as pregnancy advances and must consider the possibility of injury with more strenuous activities. Women who gain weight excessively should be encouraged to increase physical activity.

Swimming is an excellent form of exercise that can be continued throughout pregnancy. Snorkeling in reasonably calm water is permissible, but *scuba diving* should be avoided. The effects of diving on fetal development have not yet been determined.

Most of the studies on the effects of exercise on the fetus have been performed on animals. Although uterine blood flow is decreased and maternal temperature is increased during strenuous activity, there is no evidence to suggest that maternal exercise, within the tolerance of the individual, has a deleterious effect on the fetus.

Work. Pregnant women can continue working until term if the pregnancy is normal and if the environment in which they work and the physical activity involved pose no threat to the fetus or to the pregnancy. Women who develop complications and those with multiple fetuses usually should stop working.

Naeye and Peters reported that women who continue to work throughout pregnancy, particularly those who must stand for long periods of time, have more placental infarcts and babies whose weights are reduced by 150 to 400 g than do women who do not work. The overall maternal weight gain did not correspond to newborn weights. This suggests that women whose jobs require prolonged periods of standing, repeated stooping and bending, climbing ladders or stairs, and heavy lifting might be advised to stop working several weeks before term. It is not certain, however, whether the outcome is primarily a result of working or whether socioeconomic factors that require women to work are responsible.

Travel. The only danger in travel for the normal patient is that she may abort or go into labor while away from home. Those who have aborted previously or who have abnormal pregnancies should not travel. Train, airplane, or automobile trips are permissible. The normal patient may drive a car or ride in buses or trolleys until term.

Intercourse. Although there is conflicting information concerning the effects of coitus during pregnancy, it seems likely that normal women can continue intercourse without fear of injury or infection. The desire for intercourse may be reduced during pregnancy, but it usually returns after delivery.

Some women are aware of uterine contractions that occur after orgasm, and fetal bradycardia has been reported. Chaven and associates recorded fetal heart patterns during intercourse in two normal pregnant women between the twenty-eighth and fortieth gestational weeks. Both mothers were aware of uterine contractions and increased fetal movements after orgasm. Fetal heart patterns included late decelerations, loss of short-term variability, periods of bradycardia lasting from 5 to 7 minutes, and periods of tachycardia lasting as long as 10 minutes. Since contractions occur with orgasm, produced either by coitus or masturbation, it seems likely that orgasm rather than prostaglandins from the ejaculate stimulates the uterine activity.

Bathing. Tub or shower baths are permitted throughout pregnancy. As pregnancy advances, the patient must take care not to lose her balance as she climbs into and out of the tub.

Bladder. Pubococcygeus exercises, if performed daily and if continued after delivery, will aid in preventing urinary incontinence after delivery.

Bowel. Constipation, which is probably caused by the physiologic decrease in peristalsis during pregnancy, can usually be corrected by adding bulky foods to the diet, an adequate fluid intake, and the judicious use of prune juice, milk of magnesia, and stool softeners.

Breast care. The nipples may be massaged and stretched with fingers lubricated with cocoa butter if the patient wishes, but this probably will not influence their response to nursing. She must be careful not to injure the nipples, particularly if they are inverted or abnormal. During the last weeks of pregnancy, nipple stimulation may induce uterine contractions.

Clothing. No special clothing is necessary, but all clothes should be loose and hang from the shoulders. *Circular garters* may promote the development of varicose veins. *Low-heeled shoes* increase stability and decrease backache. High heels rotate the body forward, thereby increasing the normal pregnancy lordosis and strain on the back muscles to balance the protuberant abdomen. A *maternity brassiere* that may be used after delivery should be worn if breast support is required. A *maternity girdle* is necessary only to control unusual discomfort caused by backache, pelvic pressure, or a pendulous abdomen.

Dental care. The teeth should be examined and any necessary repairs performed at least twice during pregnancy. Necessary extractions are permissible. Only local anesthesia should be used.

Alcohol. Fetal alcohol syndrome has been described in the offspring of human alcoholics. The affected infants have a variety of craniofacial, limb, and neurologic anomalies. They are below normal in intelligence, and they may develop behavioral problems. The estimate of overall prevalence of the fetal alcohol syndrome in the United States is 1 to 2/1000 births. For alcohol abusers the risk is increased to 23 to 29/1000 births. The effects of high blood alcohol levels may be enhanced by excessive smoking, drug use, and malnutrition, all of which may accompany alcoholism.

There is as yet no exact correlation between the amount of alcohol ingested and fetal growth and development, but the offspring of heavy drinkers are in greater jeopardy than are those whose mothers drink moderately. Mills and co-workers, from data collected prospectively from 31,604 pregnancies, found that the risk of small-for-date babies, as compared to nondrinkers, increased from 1.11 for women who had less than one drink daily to 1.96 for those taking three to five drinks a day. Rosett and associates found weight in the tenth percentile or less in 32%, length in the tenth percentile or less in 20%, head circumference in the tenth percentile or less in 12%, and morphologic abnormalities in 12% of 25 heavy drinkers. There was little evidence of growth retardation in those who drank moderately or rarely or in those who reduced alcohol consumption before the third trimester. However, 11% of the offspring of the latter group, had morphologic abnormalities as compared to 1% of those who drank moderately and 3% of those who drank rarely.

It seems prudent to suggest that pregnant women refrain from drinking, particularly during the early weeks when fetal anomalies can be produced. If possible, women who abuse alcohol should be identified before they conceive and be encouraged to stop drinking, at least during pregnancy.

Tobacco. The babies of women who smoke heavily are smaller than those of nonsmokers. According to Underwood and co-workers, the mean birth weight of babies of 4856 nonsmokers was 3395 g; that of women who smoked one to 10 cigarettes daily, 3286 g; that of women who smoked 11 to 30 cigarettes daily, 3196 g; and that of even heavier smokers, 3182 g. Other studies confirm the decreased birth weights associated with maternal smoking.

Perinatal death rates among infants born to smoking mothers also are increased. Butler, Goldstein, and Ross reported a 30% increase in late fetal mortality and a 26% increase in neonatal death rate in infants born to mothers who smoked after the fourth month of pregnancy. Rush and Kass concluded that perinatal mortality is increased by 34.4% in infants of smoking mothers and that smoking rather than socioeconomic status is the cause.

The effect on the fetus may result from hypoxia caused either by reduced placental perfusion from the vasoconstrictive effects of nicotine or because carbon monoxide reduces oxygen capacity of both maternal and fetal hemoglobin. Another possible factor is that smoking reduces appetite and may be responsible for decreased maternal caloric intake.

One can only conclude that smoking is harmful to the fetus and that it may represent the difference between life and death when other factors that may influence survival also are present.

Drugs. It has long been known that fetal anomalies can be produced experimentally by the administration of certain drugs at appropriate times during embryonic development. Drugs such as thalidomide, methotrexate, and testosterone, together with many other presumably innocuous preparations, are known to produce anomalous development of the human fetus.

As a general rule, no drugs should be prescribed during the first trimester of normal pregnancy. Only medications that are essential to the health of the patient should be permitted. One may even logically question the advisability of prescribing vitamins for well-nourished women whose diets adequately supply the dietary needs of pregnancy. The use of drugs during pregnancy is discussed in detail in Chapter 34.

SUBSEQUENT VISITS

Although the adequacy of care cannot be gauged by the number of visits to the physician, frequent observation is necessary. For many years it has been customary to space prenatal visits at 3- to 4-week intervals during the first 28 weeks, at 2-week intervals between the twenty-eighth and thirty-sixth weeks, and then weekly until delivery. This schedule may be appropriate for the primigravida who has little responsibility at home, who will have many questions concerning the pregnancy, and who may need a considerable amount of support and reassurance. It generally is completely inappropriate for healthy multiparas whose previous pregnancies have been uncomplicated. These women have little to learn about the course of pregnancy, and their prenatal visits often are social calls rather than significant medical consultations.

If one can be assured after the first two or three visits that there are no abnormalities and that the fetus is growing at a normal rate, the subsequent examinations can be scheduled at 6- to 8-week intervals until the twenty-eighth or thirtieth week, at 3- to 4-week intervals until the thirty-sixth week, and at 2-week intervals until delivery. One should schedule a visit for about the twelfth week and another for about the twentieth week because these are good times to compare uterine size and duration of pregnancy. In addition, one should be able to hear the fetal heart at the twentieth week and can also record the quickening date. Such a schedule is appropriate only if the patient is comfortable with it and understands that she can see the obstetrician whenever she thinks it necessary and that she must call at once if there is any question of an abnormality.

At each visit the following are done:

1. The patient is weighed, and not only the total gain but the gain since the last visit are calculated. The diet is reviewed and any necessary adjustments made.
2. The blood pressure is recorded and compared with the previous readings.
3. A urine specimen is examined for protein and sugar.
4. The patient is questioned regarding symptoms.
5. Any change in treatment indicated by the findings is suggested.

The *pelvic examination* may be repeated if the first was inconclusive, if any abnormality was encountered, or if pelvic symptoms appear. *Vaginal examinations* may be performed in the office at any time during normal pregnancy. During the last weeks or whenever there is a question of early labor, one should use sterile gloves and instruments to decrease the possibility of introducing pathogenic bacteria.

The *abdomen is usually examined* at each visit. During the first 30 weeks the principal information one can gain from abdominal examination is the rate at which the uterus is enlarging. The fetal heart can be heard with an ordinary stethoscope after 20 weeks, and the position and presentation can be determined with reasonable accuracy in normal women after 30 weeks. During the final weeks before labor starts, one can chart the descent of the presenting part into the pelvic inlet.

The *breasts* should be examined at least once during the last trimester of pregnancy. This provides a good opportunity to discuss breast-feeding.

Certain *laboratory examinations* should be repeated even though they were normal during early pregnancy. The hemoglobin, hematocrit, and antibody screen should be ordered between 26 and 30 weeks. A 2-hour postprandial blood sugar test

should be obtained at the same time. Serologic tests for syphilis and cervical cultures for gonorrhea should be repeated in late pregnancy when exposure to venereal disease is likely.

The administration of 300 μg of Rh immunoglobulin to unsensitized Rh-negative women at 28 to 32 weeks of pregnancy will aid in preventing Rh sensitization during late pregnancy.

Symptoms that appear during the prenatal period must be thoroughly investigated, making use of any physical or laboratory test that may be indicated. The problems most often encountered during pregnancy (nausea, vomiting, heartburn, backache, separation of the symphysis, and varicosities of the legs and vulva) are discussed elsewhere.

High-risk pregnancy. Women with proven or suspected abnormalities that may interfere with the course of pregnancy must be seen more often than normal women. The spacing of visits is determined by the complication. It usually is advisable to see *high-risk patients* on a special day when the efforts of all the office staff can be directed toward them and their specific problems.

Patient education. Too many obstetricians consider only the medical aspects of prenatal care and think little of *patient education*. Healthy women need a minimum of medical attention during pregnancy, and the outcome for most normal middle- and upper-class women would probably be changed little if prenatal care were unavailable to them. This is not true for those with medical conditions that may complicate pregnancy or for women of lower socioeconomic classes; for these individuals a well-designed prenatal program may be essential in determining the outcome of pregnancy. Unfortunately, those who need the least medical care (that is, healthy middle- and upper-class women) usually make the greatest number of prenatal visits and gain the least from them.

Too little effort is made to use the prenatal period as an educational experience. Prenatal "education" too often consists of the physician outlining at the first visit what the patient can expect during pregnancy or recommending a book to read. Later in the pregnancy the physician may advise the patient and her husband to attend a prenatal class, which often is nothing more than a large group lecture given by a house officer who is assigned the task. Such lectures are often contracted courses in obstetrics and are inappropriate for an individual patient with personal problems. These problems are usually not covered in the lectures, and the patient may be given no opportunity to discuss them with her busy obstetrician.

The most effective educational programs are those conducted in an office or a clinic that are designed to meet individual as well as group needs. Since obstetricians are generally too busy to devote adequate time to teaching sessions, they are best conducted by nurse midwives or trained obstetric nurses. The essential information concerning reproduction, motherhood, nutrition, and general health care can be considered in small group discussions led by the nurse. Individual problems are often brought up by patients and discussed by the group. Much can be learned of the reactions of a patient to pregnancy by her interaction with other members of the group. Individual counseling sessions for patients who need them can be arranged.

The nurse can perform prenatal examinations on women in the educational groups on the days they meet, thus relieving the obstetrician of this responsibility.

Each obstetrician should conduct two prenatal programs, one for healthy women and one for those at risk. The major responsibility for the examination and education of healthy women can be delegated to nurse midwives or trained obstetric nurses. The obstetrician should assume immediate responsibility for all women with complications and serve as consultant to the nurses for well women, whom the physician can also see occasionally. Such a program can meet individual needs of all patients while making appropriate use of the skills of the professionals who are conducting it.

REFERENCES

Andersen, F.H., Johnson, T.R.B., Jr., Barclay, M.L., and Flora, J.D., Jr.: Gestational age assessment. I. Analysis of individual clinical observations, Am. J. Obstet. Gynecol. **139:**173, 1981.

Andersen, F.H., Johnson, T.R.B., Jr., Flora, J.D., Jr., and Barclay, M.L.: Gestational age assessment. II. Prediction from combined clinical observations, Am. J. Obstet. Gynecol. **140:**770, 1981.

Barman, M.R.: (Work during pregnancy) Candid views on how to improve the system, Contemp Obstet. Gynecol. **23:**95, 1984.

Bishop, E.H., and Corson, S.: Estimation of fetal maturity by cytologic examination of amniotic fluid, Am. J. Obstet. Gynecol. **102:**654, 1968.

Butler, N.R., Goldstein, H., and Ross, E.M.: Cigarette smoking in pregnancy; its effect on birth weight and perinatal mortality, Br. Med. J. **2:**127, 1972.

Chaven, B., et al.: Fetal heart rate changes during coitus (Abstr. 22). Las Vegas, 1985, Society of Perinatal Obstetricians.

Delgado, H., et al.: Maternal nutrition: its effects on infant growth and development and birth spacing. In Moghissi, K.S., and Evans, T.N., editors: Nutritional impacts on women, New York, 1977, Harper & Row, Publishers.

Eastman, N.J., and Jackson, E.: Weight relationships in pregnancy. I. The bearing of maternal weight and pre-pregnancy weight on birth weight in full-term pregnancies, Obstet. Gynecol. Surv. **23:**1003, 1968.

Gross, T., Sokol, R.J., and King, K.C.: Obesity in pregnancy: risks and outcome, Obstet. Gynecol. **56:**446, 1980.

Henderson, G.I., et al.: Fetal alcohol syndrome: overview of pathogenesis, Neurobehav. Toxicol. Teratol. **3:**73, 1981.

Lotgering, F.K., Gilbert, R.D., and Longo, L.D.: Maternal and fetal responses to exercise during pregnancy, Physiol. Rev. **65:**1, 1985.

Mahan, C.S., and McKay, S.: Let's reform our antenatal care methods, Contemp. Obstet. Gynecol. vol. 147, 1984.

Mills, J.L., et al.: Maternal alcohol consumption and birth weight. How much drinking during pregnancy is safe. J.A.M.A. **252:**1875, 1984.

Naeye, R.L.: Weight gain and outcome of pregnancy, Am. J. Obstet. Gynecol. **135:**3, 1979.

Naeye, R.L., and Peters, E.C.: Work during pregnancy: effects on the fetus. Pediatrics **69:**724, 1982.

Nyirjesy, I., Lonergan, W.M., and Kane, J.J.: Clinical significance of total weight gain in pregnancy. Obstet. Gynecol. **32:**391, 1968.

Reamy, K., and White, S.E.: Sexuality in pregnancy and the puerperium: a review. Obstet Gynecol Surv. **40:**1, 1985.

Rosett, H.L., et al.: Patterns of alcohol consumption and fetal development, Obstet. Gynecol. **61:**539, 1983.

Rush, D., and Kass, E.H.: Maternal smoking: a reassessment of the association with perinatal mortality, Am. J. Epidemiol. **96:**183, 1972.

Ryan, G.M., Jr., Sweeney, P.J., and Solola, A.S.: Prenatal care and pregnancy outcome, Am. J. Obstet. Gynecol. **137:**876, 1980.

Sabbagha, R.E.: Diagnostic ultrasound applied to obstetrics and gynecology, New York, 1980, Harper and Row, Publishers.

Seager, K.G.: The onset of labor in relation to the length of the menstrual cycle, J. Obstet. Gynecol. Br. Commonw. **60:**92, 1953.

Seifer, D.B., et al.: Total parenteral nutrition in obstetrics, J.A.M.A. **253:**2073, 1985.

Shiono, P.H., Klebanoff, M.A., and Rhoads, G.G.: Smoking and drinking during pregnancy: their effects on preterm birth, J.A.M.A. **255:**82, 1986.

Starkman, M.N., et al.: Pseudocyesis: psychologic and neuroendocrine interrelationships, Psychosom. Med. **47:**46, 1985.

Underwood, P.B., Kesler, K.F., O'Lane, J.M., and Callagan, D.A.: Parental smoking empirically related to pregnancy outcome, Obstet. Gynecol. **29:**1, 1967.

van der Velde, W.J., Copius Peereboom-Stegeman, J.H.J., Treffers, P.E., and James, J.: Basil lamina thickening in the placentae of smoking mothers, Placenta **6:**329, 1985.

Zlatnik, F.J., and Burmeister, L.F.: Dietary protein in pregnancy: effect on anthropometric indices of the newborn infant, Am. J. Obstet. Gynecol. **146:**199, 1983.

21

William J. Ledger

Infectious diseases during pregnancy

Pregnant women are susceptible to and can contract any infectious disease as readily as nonpregnant women. In most instances, infectious diseases neither affect the infant nor alter the course of pregnancy. However, certain notable exceptions are discussed in this chapter.

ACUTE INFECTIOUS DISEASES

Measles (rubeola). Measles probably do not cause congenital defects, but they increase the incidence of abortion and premature labor. The infant may be infected in utero and may even be born with a typical rash or develop it during the first few days of life.

Rubella (German measles). Gregg reported a high incidence of congenital defects in the eyes of infants whose mothers had contracted rubella during early pregnancy. Swan later calculated that 74.4% of infants would develop a congenital malformation if the maternal infection occurred during the first 4 months of pregnancy.

Cooper and Krugman, studying 344 infants with congenital rubella diagnosed during the first 18 months of life, found 73 to be normal and 271 abnormal. Defects diagnosed included congenital heart disease (142), hearing loss (140), cataract or glaucoma (107), psychomotor retardation (109, of which 65 were severe or moderate), and neonatal purpura (58). Thirty-five infants died. Other man-ifestations of congenital rubella found in 58 infants with neonatal purpura included hepatomegaly (72%), splenomegaly (69%), congenital heart disease (67%), eye lesions (45%), adenopathy (22%), bone lesions (22%), hepatitis (19%), anemia (17%), and genitourinary defects (7%). Progressive sclerosing panencephalitis has been reported to occur during the second decade of life as a late complication of congenital rubella.

Many infants who survive have prolonged active viral infections. Rubella virus has been cultured from infected infants well past the second year of life. It is obvious that an infant who sheds virus can serve as a source of infection for others. Susceptible nurses who are or who might become pregnant should not care for infants with congenital rubella.

Other effects of rubella during early pregnancy are abortion, premature delivery, and intrauterine fetal death.

Therapeutic abortion is justifiable whenever unquestioned rubella is contracted during the first 20 weeks after the onset of the last menstrual period, unless the parents are willing to accept the risk of the infant's being affected.

Distasteful as it may seem, termination should also be considered for women who acquire infections late in the second trimester. Hardy and co-workers found only seven of 22 children whose

293

mothers had had rubella between the thirteenth and thirty-first weeks to be normal. Two others died. Only four of 11 infants of women who had rubella after the twentieth week were normal. Four of the seven abnormal infants had psychomotor disturbances (three of these were retarded), two others had congenital anomalies, five had small heads, and all nine infants who were examined shed virus.

Before abortion is approved, one must be certain that the patient actually had rubella. An exact clinical diagnosis, particularly in retrospect, is difficult because the course of rubella is much like that of several other viral infections. A precise diagnosis can be made on the basis of antibody studies. Hemagglutination-inhibition (HI) antibodies are not present in susceptible persons, but they can be detected within 48 hours after the appearance of the rash and reach a peak within 2 weeks.

HI titers can be used to differentiate rubella from other nonteratogenic virus infections only by demonstrating a rise in titer after the acute infection. It is essential therefore that the titer be determined within 2 to 3 days after the appearance of the rash and again about 2 weeks later. A significant increase in titer on the second test indicates that the infection actually was rubella. If the titer is unchanged, the patient did not have rubella.

A high HI titer on a single test 1 to 2 weeks after a presumed rubella infection is of no diagnostic significance; there is no way to determine from such a single examination whether the elevated titer occurred in response to an infection years or days before the study.

A test for *complement-fixing antibodies* may provide an answer. These antibodies appear a few days after the onset of the rash and reach peak levels 3 to 5 weeks later. If both HI and complement-fixing antibodies are elevated, the infection was a recent one. An elevated HI titer without complement-fixing antibodies suggests a remote infection that will not affect the embryo. *Rubella-specific IgM antibody response* can be demonstrated shortly after the rash appears. Since the response rises and falls fairly rapidly, the absence of response several weeks after exposure or illness does not eliminate rubella.

A rubella antibody study should be performed at the first prenatal visit. If the titer is 1:8 or more, the woman is immune. If it is less than 1:8, she is susceptible, and the appearance of antibodies after an acute illness will be diagnostic of rubella. The serum used for the test during early pregnancy should be frozen and stored. It can then be used for comparison of antibody titer if an acute illness like rubella occurs later.

Gamma globulin, given in an attempt to prevent infection after exposure or to modify the course of the disease, only obscures the issue. It may prevent only the rash without affecting the viremia and fetal involvement. Gamma globulin should not be given, even with definite exposure. If infection does not occur, nothing needs be done; if rubella develops, abortion can be considered.

Approximately 10% of women of childbearing age in this country are susceptible to rubella. If unprotected women are discovered and vaccinated before they become pregnant, the chances of their developing clinical rubella are minimal. Although rises in HI and complement-fixing antibody responses occur in as many as 80% of vaccinated persons during rubella epidemics, the clinical evidence is that the fetuses of the vaccinated women are protected.

Rubella antibody testing should be a part of every premarital and prepregnancy examination if it has not already been done. Those who are susceptible can then be immunized. It is essential that the possibility of pregnancy be eliminated before a woman is vaccinated.

Rubella vaccinelike virus has been recovered from fetal tissues after vaccination during pregnancy, but the danger of serious fetal infection is not great. Preblud and colleagues determined the outcome of the pregnancies of 633 women who were vaccinated between 4 weeks before and 16 weeks after the estimated date of conception. The immune status of two thirds of the women was not known, 27.6% were susceptible, and 5.7% were immune when they were vaccinated. Of the total, 24 aborted spontaneously, abortion was induced in 197, and the outcome was unknown in 48. There were not congenital anomalies in any of the 364 liveborn infants, including the 112 whose mothers were known to be susceptible to infection when they were vaccinated.

Although these results suggest that the vaccine virus is less teratogenic than the wild virus, there is a definite risk that the fetus will be infected because the virus does cross the placenta.

One should recommend that a patient not become pregnant for 3 months after vaccination. If she does, abortion can be offered even though the risk of congenital defect is small. One of the best times to immunize a woman whose susceptibility has been discovered during pregnancy is while she is still in the hospital after delivery.

Physicians, nurses, and others who work with pregnant women should be checked for the presence of rubella antibodies. Those who are susceptible should be vaccinated. This is necessary not only for their own protection, but to protect susceptible pregnant women who will see these people during the antepartum period.

Chickenpox. The pregnant woman who develops chickenpox may be seriously ill with the disease and may die from the complications. The infant can be infected in utero, but the total fetal loss does not appear to be increased. A specific syndrome of fetal malformation characterized by low birth weight, Horner's syndrome, limb defects, and skin scars has been reported. If the woman acquires the infection just before the delivery, specific varicella-zoster globulin (VZIG) may be life saving for the fetus.

Scarlet fever. The serious effects of scarlet fever can be reduced by the early administration of penicillin, but abortion occurs frequently. Because the infecting organism is a hemolytic streptococcus, infected women should not be treated or delivered in an obstetric unit.

Mumps. Hyatt found approximately a 15% incidence of abortion and fetal death and a similar incidence of congenital anomalies in the infants of 94 pregnant women with mumps (four of his patients and 90 collected from the literature). The high rate of anomalies has not been confirmed by others. Garcia and colleagues, studying tissue from one spontaneous and two induced abortions in women with mumps, described diffuse necrotic villitis and viral inclusions in both chorionic and fetal tissues.

Whooping cough. Pertussis is rare in adults. If the mother has pertussis at the time she delivers, the child should be isolated from her until she is no longer infectious.

Typhoid fever. Typhoid fever is uncommon in the United States, but if it occurs, it can be treated with ampicillin.

CYTOMEGALOVIRUS DISEASE

Cytomegalovirus disease is one of the most common and the most destructive of all congenital infections. About 10 of 1000 newborn infants excrete cytomegalovirus, and characteristic immediate or remote changes caused by infection with the virus can be recognized in at least one of 1000. The most serious effects include microcephaly, hydrocephaly, cerebral calcification, deafness, chorioretinitis, hepatosplenomegaly and jaundice, thrombocytopenia, hemolytic anemia, and convulsions. Some of those in whom the initial infection was mild and not recognized have impaired intelligence and hearing defects.

The precise mechanism by which the fetus or newborn infant is infected is not known. At least 60% of the general population have acquired antibodies to the virus by the age of 35 to 40. The virus may be transmitted across the placenta to the fetus as a result of a new maternal infection or, rarely, by persisting activity of an old infection. The virus is present in the cervical secretions of at least 5% of all women during pregnancy, and the recovery rate increases as pregnancy advances; hence the infant may become infected during delivery. The virus can be recovered from breast milk, urine, tears, and saliva; so infection can also occur during the neonatal period.

Griffiths, Campbell-Benzie, and Heath found complement-fixing antibodies in 57% of 5575 women at the first prenatal examination. Repeat studies in 1608 who had been seronegative at the first test indicated that 14 (0.87%) had experienced a primary infection during pregnancy. Although all 14 infants appeared normal at birth, one subsequently developed a hearing defect, and one was microcephalic. Studies from Alabama indicate that maternal antibody is not totally protective for the fetus, but the most serious newborn outcome occurs in those women who have a primary infection during pregnancy. There is a significant acquisition of cytomegalovirus among mothers with infants in day care centers. Susceptible pregnant women should be aware of this danger.

Since acute cytomegalovirus infections in adults may cause only minor symptoms, there is no good way to anticipate the birth of an affected fetus. It may be worthwhile to evaluate pregnant women for the presence of antibodies to cytomegalovirus in the first trimester and repeat the testing in the third trimester in susceptible women. There is no effective treatment for either the mother or an infected newborn infant.

Toxoplasmosis. The parasite *Toxoplasma gondii,* which causes toxoplasmosis, can be transmitted to humans in raw meat or from cat feces, which contain infective oocysts. The symptoms of an acute infection can be similar to adult influenza, but toxoplasmosis is accompanied by lymphadenopathy. In 90% of the adult cases, there is no symptomatology.

In most instances the fetus is infected as a consequence of parasitemia during the initial acute attack. Fetal infection does not occur as a result of chronic maternal infection.

Abortion occurs frequently when the infection is acquired during early pregnancy. If the infection occurs during the later weeks of pregnancy, approximately half the fetuses will be affected. Perinatal mortality is increased, and the prognosis for those who survive is poor. Affected infants have combinations of encephalitis, microcephaly, hydrocephaly, chorioretinitis, convulsions, hepatic splenomegaly, jaundice, and mental retardation.

Pregnant women should avoid eating raw meat and exposure to infected cats.

Toxoplasmosis is diagnosed in humans by the appearance of antibodies in the serum. Generally, a single study is uninformative because the presence of antibody may indicate only a previous acute infection. A rising titer when checked at 2- to 4-week intervals suggests an acute infection. Complement fixation tests can be very helpful. They appear after an acute attack and do not persist. Abortion is justifiable for acute infections that occur during early pregnancy.

Herpes. Genital herpes infection can be a threat to the fetus. Unlike other viral infections, transplacental infection early in pregnancy occurs rarely. Instead, nearly all newborn infections occur from newborn contact with the virus during labor or after membranes have been ruptured.

The presence of maternal antibody to herpes is not protective to the baby. The care of women with genital herpes requires periodic culturing of the mother, particularly during the third trimester. If the mother remains culture negative, a vaginal delivery can be attempted. If the woman has active lesions or has a positive culture, cesarean section should be performed.

Immunizations during pregnancy. The decision as to whether a pregnant woman should be immunized against an infectious disease is influenced by several factors: susceptibility to the disease, the possibility of exposure, the effect on mother and fetus if the disease is contracted, and the risk to the fetus from immunization.

Although information about the effects of acute infectious diseases on the course of pregnancy and the fetus is incomplete, it is evident that any risk involved can be eliminated by preventive immunization. An important part of premarital and prepregnancy examinations therefore is to learn which infectious diseases the patient has had, to test for susceptibility to diseases known to be teratogenic, and to vaccinate susceptible women before they conceive.

Pregnant women with chronic cardiac, pulmonary, or metabolic diseases should be considered candidates for immunization against influenza and pneumonia; however, as a general rule, immunization is best avoided during pregnancy. Immune globulins, toxoids, and vaccines made from inactivated organisms are usually safe for pregnant women, but, except in emergencies, those made from live organisms should be avoided; they may infect the fetus.

CHRONIC INFECTIOUS DISEASES

Malaria. Intrauterine infection of the fetus with malaria is rare because the parasites do not often cross the placenta. Quinine and other antimalarial drugs can be administered without hesitation to pregnant women.

REFERENCES

Amstey, M.S.: Varicella in pregnancy, J. Reprod. Med. **21**:89, 1978.

Cooper, L.Z., Green, R.H., Krugman, S., Giles, J.P., and Mirick, G.S.: Neonatal thrombocytopenic purpura and other manifestations of rubella contracted in utero, Am. J. Dis. Child. **110**:416, 1965.

Cooper, L.Z., and Krugman, S.: Clinical manifestations of postnatal and congenital rubella, Arch. Ophthalmol. **77**:434, 1967.

Desmonts, G., and Couvreur, J.: Congenital toxoplasmosis: a prospective study of 378 pregnancies, N. Engl. J. Med. **290**:1110, 1974.

Garcia, A.C.P., Pereira, J.M.S., Vidigal, N., Lobato, Y.Y., Pegado, C.S., and Branco, J.P.C.: Intrauterine infection with mumps virus, Obstet. Gynecol. **56**:756, 1980.

Gregg, N.M.: Further observations on congenital defects in infants following maternal rubella, Trans. Opthalmol. Soc. Aust. **4**:119, 1946.

Griffiths, P.D., Campbell-Benzie, A., and Heath, R.B.: A prospective study of primary cytomegalovirus infection in pregnant women, Br. J. Obstet. Gynaecol. **87**:308, 1980.

Grossman, J.H. III, Wallen, W.C., and Sever, J.L.: Management of genital herpes simplex virus infection during pregnancy, Obstet. Gynecol. **58**:1, 1981.

Hanshaw, J.B., Scheiner, A.P., Moxley, A.W., Gaev, L., Abell, V., and Scheiner, B.: School failure and deafness after "silent" congenital cytomegalovirus infection, N. Engl. J. Med. **295**:468, 1976.

Hardy, J.B., McCracken, G.H., Gilkeson, M.R., and Sever, J.L.: Adverse fetal outcome following maternal rubella after the first trimester of pregnancy, J.A.M.A. **207**:2414, 1969.

Horstmann, D.M., Liebhaber, H., LeBouvier, G.L., Rosenberg, D.A., and Halstead, S.B.: Rubella, reinfection of vaccinated and naturally immune persons exposed in an epidemic, N. Engl. J. Med. **283**:771, 1970.

Hume, O.S.: Toxoplasmosis and pregnancy, Am. J. Obstet. Gynecol. **114**:703, 1972.

Hyatt, H.W.: Relationship of maternal mumps to congenital defects and fetal deaths, and to maternal morbidity and mortality, Am. Pract. **12**:359, 1961.

Mann, J.M., Preblud, S.R., Hoffmann, R.E., Brandling-Bennet, A.D., Hinman, A.R., and Herrmann, K.L.: Assessing risks of rubella infection during pregnancy: a standardized approach, J.A.M.A. **245**:1647, 1981.

Preblud, S.R., Stetler, H.C., Frank, J.A., Jr., Greaves, W.L., Hinman, A.R., and Herrmann, K.L.: Fetal risk associated with rubella vaccine, J.A.M.A. **246**:1413, 1981.

Raine, D.N.: Varicella infection contracted in utero: sex incidence and incubation period, Am. J. Obstet. Gynecol. **94**:1144, 1966.

Reynolds, D.W., Stagno, S., Hosty, T.S., Tiller, M., and Alford C.A., Jr.: Maternal cytomegalovirus excretion and perinatal infection, N. Engl. J. Med. **289**:1, 1973.

Riggall, F., Salkind, G., and Spellacy, W.: Typhoid fever complicating pregnancy, Obstet. Gynecol. **44**:117, 1974.

St. Geme, J.W., Jr., Noren, G.R., and Adams, P., Jr.: Proposed embryopathic relation between mumps virus and primary endocardial fibroelastosis, N. Engl. J. Med. **275**:339, 1966.

Stagno, S., Pass, R.F., Dworsky, M.E., Henderson, R.E., Moore, E.G., Walton, P.D., and Alford, C.A.: Congenital cytomegalovirus infection, N. Engl. J. Med. **306**:945, 1982.

Swan, C.: Rubella in pregnancy, an etiologic factor in congenital malformations, stillbirths, miscarriages, and abortions, J. Obstet. Gynecol. Br. Commonw. **56**:591, 1949.

Syphilis trends in the United States, Centers for Disease Control Morbidity and Mortality Weekly Report **30**:441, Sept. 11, 1981.

22

Russell K. Laros, Jr.

Endocrine disorders during pregnancy

Physiologic alterations in secretions of the endocrine glands are so essential to the reproductive process that even minor abnormalities in pituitary, ovarian, thyroid, placental, or other hormone production may seriously affect fertility, nidation, or the maintenance of pregnancy.

DIABETES MELLITUS

The steady increase in the number of patients with diabetes complicating pregnancy is the result of (1) insulin therapy, (2) improved management of the obstetric problems peculiar to diabetic mothers, and (3) the hereditary tendency of the disease. In the preinsulin era the reproductive potential of women with diabetes was incredibly poor. Menstrual disturbances were common, and sterility was the rule. The maternal mortality in the few patients who did conceive was 25% to 30%, and the fetal loss was as high as 60% to 70%. At present the perinatal mortality is at least 10% throughout the United States, but it is much lower in perinatal centers where women with diabetes can be given special attention. The danger to the mother is no different from that for nondiabetic mothers.

Incidence. Frank diabetes occurs in about one in 300 deliveries. O'Sullivan and Mahan screened 20,070 pregnancies and found abnormalities in carbohydrate tolerance that met the criteria for diagnosis of gestational diabetes in one in 116 prenatal registrants. Progression to frank diabetes occurred in 28.5% of these patients within 5½ years.

Diagnosis. Pregnancy may precipitate rapid onset of diabetic symptoms, leading to acidosis in women with undiagnosed diabetes. Consequently, *the presence of reducing substances in the urine of gravid women should be regarded as abnormal and suggestive of diabetes.* Lactosuria is rare during pregnancy, but it is not uncommon after delivery. The renal threshold for glucose is reduced during pregnancy, in part at least, from the physiologic increase in glomerular filtration rate. This accounts for many instances of glycosuria, but the exact cause can only be determined by glucose tolerance tests.

Influence of pregnancy on diabetes. Metabolic control of diabetes is more difficult during pregnancy. *Vomiting* disturbs chemical balance, and acidosis may develop with little warning. *Lowering of the renal threshold for glucose* is variable; a large amount of sugar may be excreted, even though the blood glucose concentration is only slightly elevated; hence urine tests for sugar may fail to provide an accurate index on which to base insulin dosage. *Carbohydrate tolerance is altered,* but the direction and the degree of change is unpredictable. As a rule, glucose tolerance is reduced in the latter half of pregnancy. In relatively few patients the status is unchanged or improved.

Insulin requirements are increased in approximately 70% of patients, beginning about the twenty-fourth gestational week. Speculations regarding the mechanism by which this diabetic challenge is evoked have been logically focused on the hormonal changes of pregnancy. Studies of fetoplacental function indicate that the fetus and placenta are specifically implicated. Anabolic and diabetogenic properties of a lactogenic growth hormone–like substance (human placental lactogen, hPL) are now well recognized. Contrainsulin effects of hPL and, in addition, active degradation of insulin by placental proteolysis may well account for the increased insulin demands of pregnancy.

Evidence for placental degradation of insulin is clearcut. Freinkel and Goodner localized a proteolytic enzyme (insulinase) in the soluble cytoplasm of placental elements and demonstrated its ability to cleave insulin into constituent peptide and amino acid residues. Inactivation or increased destruction of insulin is only part of the picture. hPL plays a key role in the metabolic adjustments of pregnancy. Large amounts of hPL secreted by the syncytiotrophoblast pass unidirectionally into the maternal circulation. The rise in plasma free fatty acids (FFAs) is at least in part induced by hPL. Gustafson and associates have shown that hyperprolactinemia produces a hyperglycemic hyperinsulinemia similar to that seen in pregnancy when serum prolactin levels rise from prepregnant levels of 10 ng/ml to 200 ng/ml at term. This and other factors related to insulin receptors and insulin transport, the roles of which have not yet been clarified, may contribute to the characteristic pancreatic islet cell hypertrophy and hyperinsulinemia. In normal pregnancy, mobilization of fat stores provides an alternate pathway of metabolism so that the needs of the conceptus for glucose and gluconeogenic precursors can be met. Elevated FFAs act as a specific peripheral antagonist to insulin in normal gravid women, but in diabetic mothers insulin resistance is exaggerated. Glucagon levels rise slightly during pregnancy, but this small increase plays little if any role in maternal gestational insulin resistance, and no significant amount reaches the fetus.

In normal pregnant women, fasting glucose levels are approximately 20 mg/dl lower than in nonpregnant subjects, a reflection of the increased glucose space and the mandate of the fetus, in addition to the maternal brain, for glucose.

A decrease in peripheral use of glucose is indicated by a diminution of the normal degree of hypophosphatemia after an intravenous glucose load. Plasma FFA levels are considerably higher in the maternal circulation during late pregnancy, whereas fetal plasma FFA levels are low. Concurrently, an increase in maternal insulin resistance is clearly evident in lower reactivity to both insulin and tolbutamide tests.

Reduction in insulin requirements after delivery can be anticipated because the contrainsulin effects of hormones and placental destruction are halted abruptly. *Hypoglycemic shock* occurs more often in the immediate period following delivery than at any other time in pregnancy. This reaction can be prevented by appropriate reduction in insulin dosage and by frequent chemical and clinical observations.

Influence of diabetes on pregnancy. The adverse effects of diabetes on pregnancy can be greatly reduced but not entirely prevented by good chemical control. Maternal *acidosis* is frequently disastrous to the fetus. Although chemical derangement may occur at any stage, particularly if vomiting or infection develops, it is most common during the last half of pregnancy when insulin demands are increased. Although severe acidosis is still a major cause of fetal loss, it is a preventable complication.

Water balance is readily disturbed. Both fetal and maternal edema are common complications. *Hydramnios* occurs in 10% of diabetic mothers— an incidence twenty times that observed in nondiabetic mothers.

The incidence of *hypertensive disorders of pregnancy* may be as high as 50%. The risk from preeclampsia to the mother with severe diabetes is greatly increased if vascular sclerosis or renal damage already exists. Fetal loss associated with preeclampsia-eclampsia per se is increased in diabetic pregnancies.

The harmful effects of diabetes may be demonstrable in the fetus of the patient exhibiting the earliest manifestations of the disease. *Excessive size of the infant is so common a finding that unrecognized maternal diabetes should be suspected in patients who deliver babies weighing more than*

4320 g (9 pounds). There is an actual increase in both splanchnic and somatic growth.

The cause for macrosomia in the infant of a diabetic mother is not yet fully understood. Bergquist believes that it may well be related to an increased insulin production by the fetus acting independently or in synergism with fetal growth hormone. Insulin is capable of promoting growth in experimental animals, and *hyperplasia of the islets of Langerhans* is a consistent finding in postmortem examinations of affected infants. The combination of increased human growth hormone (hGH) common to all newborns and the fetal islet cell hyperplasia with a significant hyperinsulin response to glucose in the newborn infant of a diabetic mother bears certain similarities to the situation found in studies of growth hormone and serum insulin levels demonstrated by Karam, Grodsky, and Forsham in obese subjects.

In the human, insulin does not pass the placental barrier freely; therefore it is unlikely that the increased fetal insulinogenesis is of much significance to the diabetes of the mother. On the contrary, glucose is readily transferred, and thus hyperglycemia in the mother probably serves as an important stimulus for pancreatic islet cell hyperplasia in the fetus.

Stillbirth and *neonatal death rates* are increased, even with mild maternal diabetes. The risk of intrauterine fetal death rises sharply after the thirty-sixth week.

It is difficult to predict impending fetal death on the basis of clinical evidence alone. A mother may notice a *reduction in activity of the fetus* as its metabolic disturbance increases. In addition, a *rapid increase in the amount of amniotic fluid* and *decreasing insulin requirements* suggest that the condition of the fetus and placenta, respectively, are deteriorating. Any of the maternal complications arising in late pregnancy may jeopardize the fetus.

The newborn infant of a diabetic mother exhibits certain characteristic signs. *Excessive size* and *a puffy, plethoric, "Cushinglike" appearance* is most common. However, the more advanced the diabetes, the smaller the baby is likely to be. *Newborn infants of mothers with diabetic vasculopathy may actually exhibit intrauterine growth retardation.*

Until recently, *respiratory distress syndrome* posed the greatest threat to infants of diabetic mothers. The large study conducted by Robert and associates at Harvard in 1976 showed that the risk for these infants was 5.6 times greater than the risk for infants of nondiabetic mothers when corrected for gestational age and route of delivery. This has been greatly reduced by the many advances in prenatal management that permit individualization of the time for delivery and by advances in neonatal intensive care for the sick infant who must be delivered before maturity is complete. Perinatal mortality caused by birth asphyxia and trauma, particularly in vaginal delivery of the oversized infant, has also decreased and should be largely preventable.

Liveborn infants who subsequently become ill show *evidence of acidosis at birth* as demonstrated by high PCO_2 and low pH of arterial cord blood and a *hypoglycemia at 2 to 4 hours of birth* that is more profound and more persistent than the hypoglycemia common to infants of normal mothers. There is an increased incidence and intensity of *hyperbilirubinemia* and hypocalcemia. The occurrence of *congenital anomalies,* particularly those affecting the skeletal, cardiac, and central nervous systems, is increased. The anomaly rate is approximately three times higher when vascular complications of maternal diabetes exist than in insulin-dependent mothers without vascular disease. In the large survey reported by Pederson, the anomaly rates were 18% and 5%, respectively. This is similar to the reports from the Joslin Clinic and from several other large clinics in the United States. Half of the perinatal losses in diabetic pregnancies are now attributable to major congenital anomalies.

Because the critical period for the teratogenic effects of diabetes is very early in pregnancy, a number of investigators have focused on this time period. The concentration of hemoglobin A_{1c} reflects the blood glucose concentrations during the preceding 4 to 12 weeks. Several studies have measured maternal hemoglobin A_{1c} in early pregnancy and found a significant increase in the rate of congenital anomalies if the level was above 10%. Thus, to decrease the incidence of anomalies, it will be necessary to achieve excellent glucose control in the earliest weeks of pregnancy. In view of the currently available data, diabetic women and their partners should be counseled **before** pregnancy about the risks of birth defects and the importance of good glucose control. A number of ongoing studies hope to demonstrate the efficacy of a program of preconceptual counseling on reduction in the rate of congenital anomalies.

Other alterations include a more frequent occurrence of *renal vein thrombosis, enlargement of the liver and spleen* with extramedullary erythropoiesis, *cardiomegaly,* and a *higher than average incidence of hyaline membrane disease for gestational age. Beta cell hyperplasia of the pancreatic islets* is the most common pathologic finding in infants who fail to survive. The islet cell hyperplasia with infiltration of eosinophils is the most consistent evidence of diabetic embryopathy. Its appearance is identical in stillborn infants of mothers with diabetes irrespective of the mildness or severity of the disease.

Management. Principles of management of diabetic pregnancies now widely recognized as the major factors responsible for the remarkable improvement in outcome for both mother and baby are (1) experienced team care; (2) accurate diagnosis, preconceptual counseling, and risk assessment; (3) rigid metabolic control with home glu-

cose monitoring; (4) screening for congenital anomalies including maternal serum alpha-fetoprotein determination at 16 weeks' gestation and level three ultrasonic evaluation of the fetus at 18 to 20 weeks; (5) fetal surveillance; (6) allowing the pregnancy to continue until fetal lung maturity is demonstrated, unless contraindicated by deterioration of mother or fetus; and (7) neonatal intensive care.

The importance of adhering to these principles is underscored by the results reported by Gabbe from several centers capable of carrying out such programs (Table 22-1). Even in the diet-controlled class A, perinatal mortality can be three or more times higher if gestational diabetes is ignored. The 1.6% perinatal mortality achieved by these groups is not different from that of nondiabetic pregnancies. In classes B and C and today even in class D, successful outcomes can be achieved in 90% or better when optimal team management and facilities are available.

Study of each patient early in pregnancy should include the laboratory tests essential to metabolic regulation and those necessary for detection of cardiovascular or renal disease and retinopathy. The blood pressure record, 24-hour urine protein determination, and funduscopic examination are requisite baseline studies of the vascular system. Electrocardiographic study is indicated when evidence of vascular disease is found or in

TABLE 22-1 Current perinatal mortality in diabetic pregnancies in relation to class (White classification of diabetes in pregnancy)

Class	Age of onset (yr)	Duration (yr)	Vascular disease	Insulin		
A	Any	Pregnancy	0	0	No. Class	
B	>20	<10	0	†		
C	10-19	or 10-19	0	†	830 A	16
D	<10	or >20	Benign retinopathy	†	555 B	48
F	Any	Any	Nephropathy	†	314 C	79
R	Any	Any	Proliferative retinopathy	†	268 D	100
H	Any	Any	Heart disease	†	59 F-R	186

PNM/1000: 0 — 100 — 200

From Gabbe, S.G.: Semin. Perinatol. **2:**361-371, 1978, by permission.

any case of long-standing diabetes. Renal function tests are mandatory in women with kidney disease because the prognosis is determined in large measure by the ability of the kidney to respond to the demands of pregnancy. The outlook for the diabetic patient with severe renal damage is so unfavorable that termination of pregnancy may be advisable. Retinopathy may be revealed and intensified, and vision may be threatened during pregnancy.

All prenatal patients with diabetes should be examined by the obstetrician and the internist at least every 2 weeks during the first half of pregnancy and weekly thereafter.

DIET. Total caloric allowance must be adjusted in accordance with the patient's nutritional status. A diet containing 30 to 35 kcal/kg of ideal body weight with a lower limit of 1800 kcal and an upper limit of 2600 kcal is prescribed. Approximately 125 g (500 kcal) of protein are included with the remainder of the calories equally divided between fat and carbohydrate. Four feedings per day are advised. Supplementary vitamin and mineral preparations should be prescribed.

INSULIN. In the past few years many studies in the United States and abroad have demonstrated that stricter metabolic control than was previously considered acceptable is a major factor in improving perinatal morbidity and mortality. Rigid control aims at maintaining euglycemia between 60 and 120 mg/dl whole body glucose levels. Karlsson and Kjellmer reported a perinatal death rate of 3.8% in 95 diabetic patients when the mean maternal glucose levels were 100 mg/dl or less as compared with 28.6% perinatal mortality in diabetic pregnancies when the mean blood glucose levels were above 150 mg/dl. Furthermore, rigid control apparently results in a significantly lower incidence of macrosomia and neonatal hypoglycemia. This is evident in Roversi and co-workers' study of 242 tightly controlled diabetic pregnancies with the remarkably low perinatal mortality of 2.5% and the occurrence of macrosomia in only 6% and hypoglycemia in 15%.

Better techniques have been developed to achieve good metabolic control even on an ambulatory basis. A steadier state is obtained by combining intermediary NPH and regular insulin for both the prebreakfast and the predinner doses, using two thirds of the total in the morning in the ratio of 2:1 and the other third in the evening in the ratio of 1:1. Some patients will require a third dose consisting of preprandial regular insulin at lunch time.

Regulation of insulin dosage is greatly enhanced by the use of glucose oxidase reagent strips and a small reflectance meter either in the clinic or by the patient at home. The 2-hour postprandial blood sample is more informative than the preprandial, which is generally well below the peak.

FETAL SURVEILLANCE. Techniques for monitoring maternal metabolic control and fetal welfare and maturity have made possible individualization of prenatal care and timing of delivery and in many cases reduced the need for long hospitalizations. However, monitoring of the fetus does not minimize the importance of clinical observations and judgment. The threat to the fetus is greatly increased at any stage of pregnancy by neglect or by development of any of the complications commonly associated with maternal diabetes: ketoacidosis, hypertensive disorders of pregnancy, progressive hypertension, pyelonephritis, or polyhydramnios.

Ultrasound scanning is useful in detecting abnormalities in fetal growth, gross anomalies, placental site, and polyhydramnios. The first scan should be done at about 20 weeks as a baseline to permit a meaningful interpretation of growth later in pregnancy.

Maternal *estriol determinations,* using either the 24 hours estriol/creatinine ratio or the unconjugated plasma estriol described by Distler and associates, provides the best of the various biochemical tests of both fetal and placental metabolic activities. Early baseline values should be obtained beginning at about 28 weeks and repeated at weekly intervals until the thirty-fourth week if estriol production is steadily increasing. The test may need to be repeated much more frequently thereafter depending on clinical conditions, the preceding estriol level, and the results of electronic fetal monitoring.

Electronic fetal monitoring should begin at 30 weeks. Fetal heart rate testing using the *nonstress test (NST)* provides a good and relatively simple screening method for predicting fetal distress or morbidity. The *contraction stress test (CST)* is positive if decelerations occur with contractions. Alternatively, the biophysical profile can be used. Abnormal results for the various tests of fetal surveillance are summarized in Table 22-2, and the sequence of monitoring in Fig. 22-1.

LABOR AND DELIVERY. The loss of the infant of an insulin-dependent mother when delivery has been carried out needlessly early is a disaster that should rarely occur today. If one can be certain of the gestational age and adequate fetal pulmonary maturity, problems related to prematurity are not an issue after 38 weeks. An amniocentesis performed during weeks 37 to 38 should reveal an *L/S ratio* of 2 or greater and the presence of *phosphatidylglycerol.* The latter substance represents

TABLE 22-2 Tests of fetal well-being useful in managing the pregnant diabetic

Test	Abnormal result
Kick counts	Decreasing count day-to-day or absence of movement for three 20-min periods in one day
Urinary estriol	Decline of 35% over the previous three highest values
Plasma estriol	Decline of 40% over previous three highest values
Nonstress test	Fewer than four fetal movements with accelerations of the fetal heart of at least 10 beats per minute in a 20-min period
Contraction stress test	Persistent late decelerations in the fetal heart rate

Biophysical profile	Nonstress test
	  Interpreted as above
	Fetal breathing
	  Absence of a 1-min episode of fetal breathing in a 30-min time span
	Fetal body movement
	  Less than three movements in a 30-min time span
	Fetal tone
	  Less than one episode of extension in a 30-min time span
	Amniotic fluid volume
	  Less than a 1 cm pocket of fluid

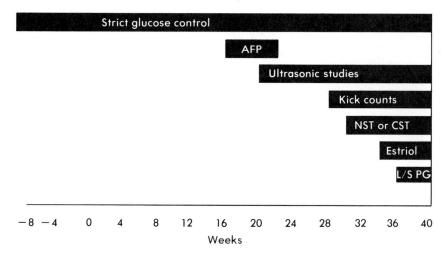

Fig. 22-1. Serial monitoring in surveillance of diabetic pregnancies. *AFP*, α-fetoprotein; *NST*, Nonstress test; *CST*, Contraction stress test; *L/S*, lecithin/sphingomyelin ratio; *PG*, phosphatidyl-glycerol.

the final step in maturation and is a particularly useful addition to the L/S ratio in diabetic pregnancies.

More well-controlled, uncomplicated diabetic pregnancies can now continue to term if all monitoring techniques indicate fetal well-being. On the other hand, it is not uncommon for signs of fetal distress to appear in some apparently uncomplicated diabetic pregnancies; intervention then is essential. Maternal complications that cannot be readily reversed, fetal distress, or both frequently mandate delivery well before term. Fetal pulmonary maturation often appears to be accelerated in connection with certain maternal complications, particularly hypertension, but meticulous neonatal intensive care is the critical factor for intact survival in these cases.

Vaginal delivery may be both difficult and dangerous because of the size and fragility of the infant and the need for early intervention. Delivery by the normal route is feasible if the diabetes is uncomplicated, if the pelvis is normal, if the size of the infant is not excessive, and if the cervix is favorable for induction. A normal oxytocin challenge test provides a measure of assurance that vaginal delivery is appropriate and safe. Electronic monitoring should be continued throughout the labor.

Cesarean section is indicated if the disease is severe, if pregnancy complications exist, if induction is unsuccessful, or if the progress in labor is poor. *Regional anesthesia* is preferable, and narcotics should be withheld until the baby is delivered.

Readjustment of insulin dosage is required during labor, delivery, and the period following delivery. It is best to withhold long-acting insulin on the day of delivery and administer all insulin as a drip. The patient is given an intravenous infusion of 5% glucose in normal saline, and the insulin dosage is regulated on the basis of regular blood sugar determinations. The usual requirement will be from 0.5 to 2 U/hour. Because the insulin requirement will frequently drop dramatically during the first few days after delivery, long-acting insulin should be reinstituted with care and a significantly decreased dosage.

Subsequent course. Despite the difficulties encountered during the course of pregnancy and the immediate puerperium, frank maternal diabetes is generally not made worse by pregnancy. Furthermore, a previous intrauterine or neonatal loss should not discourage the mother from attempting another pregnancy unless her diabetes is complicated by cardiovascular renal disease. Although perinatal losses may be repeated, meticulous management of the prenatal course, optimal timing of delivery, and skillful care of the newborn infant can provide the diabetic mother with a reasonably good prognosis.

Management of the newborn patient. Infants of diabetic mothers are often of necessity subjected to the cumulative effects of prematurity, delivery by cesarean section, and acidosis and hypoglycemia. Since the incidence of hyaline membrane disease is increased, every effort should be made to prevent or reduce respiratory distress. Treatment begins at delivery and consists of aspiration of mucus and other material from the respiratory passages, administration of oxygen, removal of the gastric contents by suction through a small tube, and treatment in an intensive care nursery.

Intensive care and laboratory and clinical support measures are essential. Correction of acid-base abnormalities are maintenance of optimal hydration, glucose levels, and oxygenation are often critical matters. Observations for development of hyperbilirubinemia and hypocalcemia must be made, and appropriate treatment initiated if dangerous levels are reached.

SUBCLINICAL DIABETES

The following classification of progressive stages of diabetes mellitus is based on the extensive work of Conn and Fajans in this field and modified in accordance with our experience.

1. The *prediabetic stage* is the period in which the disease process is not manifested in any way. The predisposition to diabetes is genetically determined and present from conception. There is no evidence of reduced carbohydrate tolerance during this period.

2. *Subclinical diabetes* is the term applied to temporary derangements in which hyperglycemia is found only during stress such as pregnancy, infection, emotional crises, or after cortisone administration.

3. *Chemical diabetes* is a more advanced stage in which the glucose tolerance test is abnormal in the absence of stress.

4. *Overt, or clinical, diabetes* is the stage in the dynamic disease process in which hyperglycemia is permanent and symptoms arise. The interval between the appearance of subclinical diabetes and the development of clinical diabetes may be short or make take many years. Some apparently susceptible individuals may escape metabolic deterioration altogether during their lifetime.

Women who subsequently develop diabetes tend

to produce oversized infants and to suffer a high fetal loss for many years before their disease becomes apparent. In 1944 Miller and associates analyzed 252 such pregnancies and found that the incidence of stillbirths and neonatal deaths was 19.8% during the 20 years preceding the onset of diabetes; the loss of viable infants rose to 35.4% in the 5 years immediately before the onset of clinical disease. Perinatal mortality can be reduced to approximately the rate for nondiabetic pregnancy if the metabolic disorder is recognized and treated and if good pediatric care is given.

Infants born during the maternal latent diabetic years may exhibit embryopathy identical to that found in infants born of true diabetic mothers, indicating that the abnormal environment for the fetus is similar in both groups. The newborn infant may be large, edematous, and plethoric. Respiratory disturbances are common. Infants who die show hyperplasia of the pancreatic islets, hematopoiesis of the immature type (Fig. 22-2), and a tendency to form hyaline membrane.

The factors contributing to excessive size of infants and intrauterine fetal deaths during these years before maternal hyperglycemia, acidosis, or other evidence of diabetes appears are unknown. It is becoming increasingly clear that diabetes is a generalized process and that the time relationship between the appearance of hyperglycemia and the development of retinopathy or vascular changes, for instance, can vary widely. A characteristically affected offspring can be the earliest manifestation of the maternal disease process.

Diagnosis. Because diabetic symptoms in the

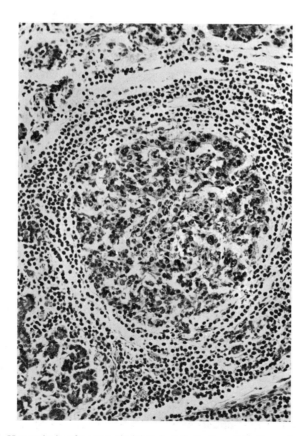

Fig. 22-2. Hyperplasia of pancreatic islets in infant of prediabetic mother ($\times 231$.)

mother are virtually absent in the early stages of the disease, a glucose screening test should be performed in patients whose records include one or more of the following: (1) a family history of diabetes, (2) previous stillbirth or unexplained neonatal loss, (3) oversized infants, (4) glycosuria during pregnancy, (5) hydramnios, and (6) repeated abortions. The presence of obesity in a patient with any of these disorders is often significant.

Many authors now recommend glucose screening in all pregnant women. Women who have not been found to have glucose intolerance before the twenty-fourth week should be screened between the twenty-fourth, and twenty-eighth weeks. The screen consists of a 50 g oral glucose load given without regard to the time of the last meal or the time of day. Venous plasma glucose is measured 1 hour later; a value of greater than 140 mg/dl is abnormal and dictates the performance of a standard glucose tolerance test.

The glucose tolerance test should follow the recommendations of O'Sullivan and Mahan. The test is performed in the morning after an overnight fast of 8 to 14 hours and after at least 3 days of an unrestricted diet containing at least 150 g of carbohydrate. A 100 g oral glucose load is given, and the venous plasma glucose measured fasting and at 1, 2, and 3 hours. An abnormal test requires that two or more of the following glucose values be exceeded: fasting, 105 mg/dl; 1 hour, 190 mg/dl; 2 hours, 165 mg/dl; and 3 hours, 145 mg/dl.

The abnormality improved rapidly after the uterus is emptied in the same way that insulin requirements are decreased after delivery in the patient with clinical diabetes. Hence glucose tolerance tests obtained during the puerperium are usually uninformative of conditions existing during pregnancy. However, postpartum measurement of glycohemoglobin, which reflects the mean blood glucose level during the 2 months or so before testing, may be more informative. Hemoglobin A_{1c}, the most abundant of the minor hemoglobins, is formed by slow glycosylation of hemoglobin A. The process is relatively irreversible and persists throughout the life span of the cell. Normal values range from 3% to 6%. A clearly elevated value is significant in detection of previously unrecognized maternal diabetes, but a normal value would not rule out the diagnosis.

In general, an abnormality in carbohydrate metabolism found during one pregnancy tends to become increasingly abnormal in a subsequent pregnancy.

The cortisone glucose tolerance test performed in the nonpregnant state may confirm the existence of subclinical diabetes. Plasma insulin levels in response to glucose loading are also significantly increased during the early stages of diabetes (Fig. 22-3).

Management. The condition of many patients can be controlled by dietary restrictions alone during the early stages of diabetes. Insulin should be added if the 2-hour blood glucose level cannot be kept within normal range on the prescribed diabetic diet.

Oral hypoglycemic agents, which in contrast to insulin pass the placental barrier with ease, should be avoided. Severe and protracted hypoglycemia of the newborn has been encountered, particularly with use of the long-acting agents, a situation that carries considerable risk of death or cerebral damage in surviving infants.

Many patients with subclinical diabetes can be carried to term uneventfully and delivered normally. Early delivery is justifiable in patients with a previous poor obstetric history, those in whom obstetric complications arise that cannot be readily reversed, and those in whom a significant fall in estriol levels or abnormalities in fetal monitoring tests or both give evidence of failing fetoplacental function.

DIABETES INSIPIDUS

Diabetes insipidus is seldom associated with pregnancy because the disease is relatively rare. However, the reproductive capacity of patients with this condition is not necessarily reduced. Symptoms may be aggravated, improved, or unchanged during pregnancy. But for the most part these alterations can be met by adjusting the dosage of antidiuretic hormone. The disease may appear transiently during the course of pregnancy and must be differentiated from psychogenic polydipsia. Labor and delivery do not differ significantly from normal pregnancies, and there is no increase in fetal loss.

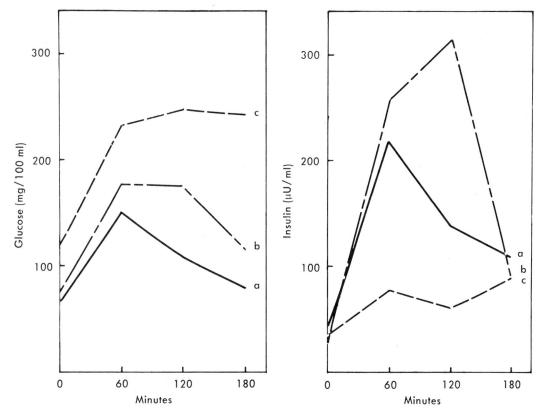

Fig. 22-3. Comparisons of serum glucose and insulin responses to 100 g oral glucose during normal pregnancy, *a;* pregnancy complicated by subclinical diabetes, *b;* and untreated overt diabetes, *c.* *(From Carrington, E.R.: Clin. Obstet. Gynecol.* **16:**31, 1973.)

Vasopressin (Pitressin) should be used for treatment throughout pregnancy instead of pituitary extract because vasopressin lacks the oxytocin principle. If the mechanism of labor proves faulty, oxytocin (Pitocin) can be given as indicated.

DISEASES OF THE THYROID GLAND

Thyroid disease occurs four times more often in women than in men. The female reproductive functions can be adversely affected by any of the various types of thyroid disorders. Fortunately, effective treatment is available for hypothyroid and hyperthyroid states, including those complicating pregnancy. However, special problems in diagnosis and management are encountered during pregnancy that must be taken into account in the interest of both the mother and her offspring.

Simple colloid goiter

The basic disturbance in simple goiter is an iodine deficiency resulting in reduced transport of thyroxine to the tissues. In response, thyrotropic stimulation is increased, and the thyroid undergoes hypertrophy followed by involution and increased storage of colloid. As a rule, thyroid function remains within normal limits, and neither the pregnancy nor the condition of the infant at birth is affected, although the gland frequently undergoes further enlargement during pregnancy when iodine intake is borderline. If thyroid function tests reveal thyroid deficiency, patients with colloid goiter should receive thyroid substance and iodine supplement throughout pregnancy to prevent congenital goiter or frank cretinism in the infant.

Hypothyroidism

Menstrual disturbances, sterility, and repeated abortions are common in women with thyroid deficiency. In some cases, conception and maintenance of the pregnancy proceed uneventfully, but untreated hypothyroidism in the mother is a potential cause for cretinism or congenital goiter in the infant. Preconceptional diagnosis and replacement therapy continued throughout the prenatal period are highly effective in preventing pregnancy complications because of thyroid deficiency.

Accurate evaluation of thyroid activity may be difficult during pregnancy. Levels of thyroxine (T_4) and triiodothyronine (T_3) are elevated during pregnancy as a result of increases in specific binding proteins induced by high levels of estrogen. T_3 resin uptake (T_3RU), which measures the unoccupied sites on the circulating thyroid-binding proteins, is decreased. The free thyroxine index (FTI) should therefore remain in the normal range. The FTI can be estimated by the following formula:

$$FTI = \frac{T_3RU}{T_4 \times 100}$$

In hyperthyroid patients the index is elevated, and in hypothyroid patients it is decreased in relation to the normal range of 1.0 to 3.5. Measurement of thyroid-stimulating hormone (TSH) is highly significant if the values are well above the top normal of 10 μU/ml. Borderline values are not definitive, since TSH cross-reacts with chorionic gonadotropin in pregnancy testing.

Thyroxine-binding globulin (TBG) can now be measured directly, and values obtained throughout pregnancy confirm the fact that the fraction of bound hormone is significantly larger as the binding globulin concentration increases. The need for an increased production of thyroid hormones is evident by 6 weeks' gestation. Abortion is likely in patients with antecedent borderline hypothyroidism who fail to compensate for this demand. Substitution therapy with T_4 is indicated and highly effective if given before the rise in TBG occurs.

Myxedema

Infertility rate is so high that only a few cases of pregnancy in women with proven myxedema have been reported. The outstanding features of six offspring of a myxedematous mother described by Hodges and co-workers were multiple congenital anomalies and mental retardation.

Hyperthyroidism

The incidence of hyperthyroidism complicating pregnancy is about 0.2%. Views concerning the influence of pregnancy on the development of this disorder differ. In Mussey, Harris, and Ward's series the initiation of hyperthyroidism during the gestation period was rare. Dailey and Benson, on the other hand, reported the onset of symptoms concurrent with pregnancy in 12 of their 21 patients. In either event the course of hyperthyroidism is essentially the same in gravid and in nongravid patients, but the pregnancy may be affected. Fetal loss is higher, particularly in early pregnancy, if the disease is untreated.

Diagnosis. The recognition of mild degrees of hyperthyroidism may be difficult. Nervousness, some increase in pulse rate, and thyroid enlargement are frequently found in normal pregnant women. A serum T_4 value above 12 μg/dl with a normal T_3RU will best establish the diagnosis.

Since amenorrhea is not an uncommon symptom of hyperthyroidism, radioactive iodine should not be used for diagnosis of this condition until pregnancy has been ruled out. Fetal tissues have higher avidity for ^{131}I than do maternal tissues. Ill effects in fetal life have resulted not only in hypothyroidism and mental retardation but also in increased incidence of congenital anomalies and in the occurrence of thyroid carcinoma during childhood.

Treatment. Thyrotoxicosis can be adequately controlled during pregnancy and therefore does not provide an indication for therapeutic abortion. Certain safeguards must be observed in the interest of the fetus. Generally, these are concerned with avoidance of overtreatment, causing myxedema in the mother and thus increasing the risk of abortion or of inducing goiter in the infant. On the contrary, hyperthyroidism in the mother does not produce permanent effects on the fetus, although the newborn infant may exhibit symptoms or hyperthyroidism at birth and may require antithyroid treatment temporarily.

Thyroidectomy after medical preparation with iodine or antithyroid drugs seldom affects the pregnancy, par-

TABLE 22-3 Normal values for thyroid function tests in nonpregnant and pregnant women and in cord blood*

	Nonpregnant women	Pregnant women	Cord blood
T_4 ($\mu g/dl$)			
By displacement	5-12	9-15	6-13
By column	3-7.5	5-10.5	
T_3 (ng/dl)	50-175	140-200	40-60
TBG (mg/dl)	3-5	7-9	
T_3RU (percent)	25-35	>20	10-15
Free T_4 (ng/dl)		1.6-2.4	1.5-3
PBI ($\mu g/dl$)	4-8	6-11	4.5-5

*Values in various laboratories may differ, but the relationship should remain the same.

ticularly if surgery is performed during the second trimester. Postoperative deficiency should be anticipated and corrected by the administration of desiccated thyroid.

Antithyroid drugs such as propylthiouracil may be used during pregnancy without resorting to surgery, but they must always be used with caution. These drugs cross the placental barrier with ease. This treatment consists of administering antithyroid drugs until normal pregnancy levels of T_4 are reached.

Thyroid hormone does not cross the placental barrier to any significant degree. Hence if a maternal level of T_4 appropriate for pregnancy is maintained during treatment, the addition of thyroid substance to the maternal antithyroid therapy provides no added benefit to the fetus.

Poorly controlled hyperthyroidism of a pregnant woman risks development of a thyroid crisis with tachycardia, cardiac arrhythmia, fever, sweating, widened pulse pressure, and tremulousness. An excessively high T_4 level is the usual finding, but in a small percentage T_3 is remarkably elevated with not much change in T_4. Occasionally, both are elevated. In addition to intravenous fluids, antithyroid therapy, cooling, and intravenous propranolol may be necessary for control. Although the condition and the treatments put the fetus in some jeopardy, stabilization must be fully achieved before any thought of delivery is considered.

Breast-feeding is inadvisable in patients taking antithyroid compounds or iodine, since these drugs are secreted in maternal milk.

The clinical diagnosis of mild or moderate degrees of hypothyroidism and mental retardation is admittedly difficult in the newborn infant. Cord blood or blood levels

of thyroid hormones should be obtained in any newborn infant in whom potential depression exists. These levels should be only slightly lower than those obtained in the mother (Table 22-3). Several states have instituted required screening programs for detection of neonatal hypothyroidism.

DISEASES OF THE PARATHYROID GLANDS
Hypoparathyroidism

During normal pregnancy circulating levels of calcium are lowered mainly in the protein-bound fraction because of the decrease in serum albumin concentration. The ionized calcium that controls parathyroid hormone secretion is essentially unchanged.

Changes in calcium metabolism during pregnancy and lactation may predispose to *parathyroid tetany*. Calcium requirements are doubled after the fourth month of gestation, and consequently the need for parathyroid hormone is increased. Relative deficiency of parathyroid hormone may interfere with phosphorus excretion and permit the serum level of ionized calcium to drop below 6 mg/dl. Latent tetany is aggravated by inadequate intake or low absorption of calcium and by hyperventilation, which causes a diminution in ionizable calcium through alkalosis.

Treatment consists of regulation of the intake with a high-calcium, low-phosphorus diet supplemented by calcium lactate, 2 to 4 g daily. Aluminum hydroxide can be used to reduce the absorption of phosphorus from the gastrointestinal tract. During an acute attack, 10 to 20 ml of 10% calcium gluconate given intravenously will effect prompt temporary control.

An increase in fetal morbidity and mortality is associated with this disease. The major problems of the newborn are tetany and convulsions and occasionally heart block with electrocardiographic changes characteristic of hypocalcemia. All of these symptoms are reversed with prompt calcium replacement.

Hyperparathyroidism

This condition has been considered relatively rare, although it does occur in women of child-bearing age, usually because of a single parathyroid adenoma. In recent years hypercalcemia has been observed after renal transplantation. Renal stones are common, and pregnancy losses are frequent in patients with hyperparathyroidism. Neonatal tetany occurs in at least 50% of the infants and may be the first evidence of unrecognized maternal hyperparathyroidism. The tetany is thought to result from suppression of the fetal parathyroid glands by the high levels of calcium that readily cross the placenta. Mild cases can be treated medically with oral phosphates to create a calcium-phosphorus balance, but most require parathyroid surgery.

DISEASES OF THE ADRENAL GLANDS
Adrenal insufficiency (Addison's disease)

In 1953 Plotz collected data on maternal mortality in 72 women with Addison's disease complicated by pregnancy. Maternal death occurred in 78% when no hormonal treatment was given, in 29% when early adrenocortical extracts were used, and in 11% when potent adrenocortical extracts and desoxycorticosterone acetate were used. The outlook is much improved with cortisone therapy.

Difficulties in control are encountered early in pregnancy if nausea and vomiting ensue and again during labor and delivery. However, adrenal crisis occurs most frequently in the period immediately following delivery. Acute vascular collapse at this time is caused by a combination of several factors, including poor tolerance to the stress of labor or cesarean section, depletion of carbohydrate reserves, blood loss superimposed on low blood volume, and removal of placental hormones.

Treatment is by substitution therapy with special provision made for salt and carbohydrate replacement during labor and delivery. Because of the specific salt- and water-retaining properties of deoxycorticosterone acetate, cortisone plus additional salt in the diet is preferable for control during the prenatal period. A daily maintenance dose of 30 mg of cortisone is usually sufficient. At the onset of labor, 200 mg of cortisone should be given orally, since administration by this route is more rapid than intramuscular injection, and 100 mg of hydrocortisone should be given intravenously at delivery.

Patients with hypoadrenalism have an exceedingly low tolerance to analgesics and anesthetics. Oversedation occurs if more than half the usual dosage of narcotics is administered. An intravenous drip of 5% or 10% glucose in physiologic saline solution offers protection against hypoglycemia and dehydration common to these patients under stress. Cortisone should be reduced gradually after delivery until the maintenance dose is reached on the sixth or seventh day. The infant is unaffected by the maternal disorder.

Acute adrenocortical failure

Sudden collapse, persistent shock, and finally death can occur as a result of acute adrenal failure during pregnancy or in the puerperium. This rare condition should be considered when severe obstetric shock occurs, since death can be prevented by recognition and prompt treatment of adrenal failure. The pathologic lesions found in 53 women who died of adrenal insufficiency were hemorrhage, necrosis, or infarction of the adrenal glands. Preeclampsia, late vomiting, hemorrhage, and infection frequently were precipitating causes, but at autopsy each of these 53 deaths proved to be primarily of adrenal origin. In addition to treatment with hydrocortisone and with other measures, as outlined in the discussion of Addison's disease, it may be necessary to administer dopamine intravenously by slow drip as a temporary measure to maintain blood pressure.

Adrenal atrophy

The administration of adrenocortical hormones may suppress adrenal function and induce adrenal atrophy presumably through inhibition of pituitary production of ACTH. Impairment of adrenal function persists for varying periods of time after hormone therapy is discontinued. The increasing use of cortisone and similar drugs for many varied disorders is cause for concern. Suppression of the patient's own adrenal function may be sufficient to prevent a normal response to sudden stress. Death has followed relatively simple operations in patients with induced adrenal atrophy. Patients who have taken cortisone-like drugs for a protracted period, even if discontinued within 3 months, should be treated prophylactically with 200 mg of cortisone at the onset of labor; and treatment should be continued in gradually decreasing dosage after delivery.

Adrenal hyperfunction

Adrenocortical hyperplasia (Cushing's syndrome). Although patients with adrenocortical hyperplasia are relatively infertile, Hunt and McConahey reported seven pregnancies in four patients with this disturbance. The primary threat to pregnancy was chronic hypertension, and the resultant fetal loss was high (43%).

Medullary hyperfunction (pheochromocytoma). Maternal and fetal mortalities associated with pheochromocytoma are appalling. Peelen and De Groat reviewed 30 pregnancies in 20 patients with this condition. Of the 20 women, 10 died; one died undelivered, and the other nine died within 72 hours after delivery. There were eight stillborn and three nonviable fetuses. Hypertension is extreme, may be paroxysmal or persistent, and is likely to progress during pregnancy. The usual symptoms are headache, anxiety, substernal pain, and nausea and vomiting, followed by exhaustion and profuse sweating. Profound and irreversible vascular collapse is the great threat and occurs most commonly soon after delivery.

When symptoms are found in late gestation they are usually confused with those of a severe hypertensive disorder of pregnancy; and, since pheochromocytoma is generally a benign tumor, it is important to make the diagnosis before its effects are disastrous. Pharmacologic tests are helpful but not definitive. Histamine vasopressor test and phentolamine tests are associated with severe side reactions, particularly in pregnancy. However, side reactions are not severe with tyramine test, and false-positive reactions are rare, although false-negative reactions sometimes occur. Final diagnosis is dependent on increased production of catecholamines or their major metabolites, and metanephrines (MN) or vanillylmandelic acid (VMA). Accuracy of diagnosis is so important that specific tests for these substances must be used; no reliance should be placed on some of the crude screening tests currently available. Values must be elevated distinctly above the normal pregnancy levels for these substances.

REFERENCES

Bergquist, N.: The influence of pregnancy on diabetes, Acta Endocrinol. 15:166, 1954.

Carrington, E.R.: Biochemical monitoring of the fetus. In Bolognese, R.J., and Schwarz, R.H., editors: Perinatal medicine, Baltimore, 1977, The Williams & Wilkins Co.

Carrington, E.R.: Diabetes in pregnancy: symposium on high-risk pregnancy with emphasis upon maternal and fetal well-being, Clin. Obstet. Gynecol. 16:28, 1973.

Conn, J.W., and Fajans, S.S.: The prediabetic state: a concept of dynamic resistance to a genetic diabetogenic influence, Am. J. Med. 31:839, 1961.

Dailey, M.E., and Benson, R.C.: Hyperthyroidism in pregnancy, Surg. Gynecol. Obstet. 94:103, 1952.

Distler, W., Gabbe, S.G., Freeman, R.K., Mestman, J.H., and Goebelsmann, U.: Unconjugated and total plasma estriol in the management of diabetic pregnancies, Am. J. Obstet. Gynecol. 130:424, 1978.

Fisher, D.A.: Maternal-fetal thyroid function in pregnancy, Clin. Perinatol. 10:615, 1983.

Freinkel, N., and Goodner, C.J.: Carbohydrate metabolism in pregnancy. I. Metabolism of insulin by human placental tissue, J. Clin. Invest. 39:116, 1960.

Gabbe, S.G.: Application of scientific rationale in the management of the pregnant diabetic, Semin. Perinatol. 2:361, 1978.

Gabbe, S.G.: Definition, detection, and management of gestational diabetes, Obstet. Gynecol. 67:121, 1986.

Gabbe, S.G., and Quilligan, E.J.: General obstetric management of the diabetic pregnancy, Clin. Obstet. Gynecol. 24:91, 1981.

Gustafson, A.B., Banasiak, M.F., Kalkhoff, R.K., Hagen, T.C., and Kim, H.J.: Correlation of hyperprolactinemia with altered plasma insulin and glucagon: similarity to effects of late human pregnancy, J. Clin. Endocrinol. Metab. 51:242, 1980.

Hodges, R.E., Hamilton, H.E., and Keettel, W.C.: Pregnancy in myxedema, Arch. Intern. Med. 90:863, 1952.

Hunt, A.B., and McConahey, W.: Pregnancy associated with diseases of the adrenal glands, Am. J. Obstet. Gynecol. 66:970, 1953.

Jovanovic, L., Peterson, C.M., Saxena, B.B., Dawood, M.J., and Saudek, C.D.: Feasibility of maintaining normal glucose profiles in insulin-dependent diabetic women, Am. J. Med. 68:105, 1980.

Karam, J.H., Grodsky, G.M., and Forsham, P.H.: The relationship of obesity and growth hormone to serum insulin levels, Ann. N.Y. Acad. Sci. 131:374, 1965.

Karlsson, K., and Kjellmer, I.: The outcome of diabetic pregnancies in relation to the mother's blood sugar level, Am. J. Obstet. Gynecol. 112:213, 1972.

Kitzmiller, J.L., Cloherty, J.P., Younger, M.D., Tabatabaii, A., Rothchild, S.B., Sosenko, I., Epstein, M.F., Singh, S., and Neff, R.K.: Diabetic pregnancy and perinatal mortality, Am. J. Obstet. Gynecol. 131:560, 1978.

Komins, J.I., Snyder, P.J., and Schwarz, R.H.: Hyperthyroidism in pregnancy, a review, Obstet. Gynecol. Surv. 30:527, 1975.

Kjaergaard, J.J., Hansen, P., Madsen, H., and Ditzel, J.: Hemoglobin A_{1c} as an indicator of long term glucose levels in diabetes with special reference to diabetic pregnancy, Acta Endocrinol. **94**(Suppl. 238):25, 1980.

Lemons, J.A., Vargas, P., and Delaney, J.J.: Infant of the diabetic mother: review of 225 cases, Obstet. Gynecol. **57**:187, 1981.

Lewis, S.B., Murray, W.K., Wallin, J.D., Coustan, D.R., Daane, T.A., Tredway, D.R., and Navins, J.P.: Improved glucose control in nonhospitalized pregnant diabetic patients, Obstet. Gynecol. **48**:260, 1976.

Mennuti, M.T.: Teratology and genetic counseling in the diabetic pregnancy, Clin. Obstet. Gynecol. **28**:486, 1985.

Miller, H.C., Hurwitz, D., and Kuder, K.: Fetal and neonatal mortality in pregnancies complicated by diabetes mellitus, J.A.M.A. **124**:271, 1944.

Montoro, M.N., Collea, J.V., and Mestman, J.H.: Management of hyperparathyroidism in pregnancy with oral phosphate therapy, Obstet. Gynecol. **55**:431, 1980.

Mussey, R.D., Harris, S.F., and Ward, E.: Hyperthyroidism and pregnancy, Am. J. Obstet. Gynecol. **55**:609, 1948.

O'Sullivan, J.B., and Mahan, C.M.: Criteria for the oral GTT in pregnancy, Diabetes **13**:278, 1964.

Parer, J.T.: Handbook of fetal heart rate monitoring, Philadelphia, 1983, W.B. Saunders Co.

Peacock, I., Hunter, J.C., Walford, S., Allison, S.P., Davison, J., Clarke, P., Symonds, E.M., and Tattersall, R.B.: Self-monitoring of blood glucose in diabetic pregnancy, Br. Med. J. **2**:1333, 1979.

Pedersen, J.: Assessors of fetal perinatal mortality in diabetic pregnancy: analysis of 1332 pregnancies, Diabetes **23**:302, 1974.

Pederson, L.M.: Pregnancy and diabetes: a survey, Acta Endocrinol. **94**(suppl. 238):13, 1980.

Peelen, J.W., and De Groat, A.: Pheochromocytoma complicated by pregnancy, Am. J. Obstet. Gynecol. **69**:1054, 1955.

Plotz, J.: Nebenniereinsuffizienz und Schwangerschaft, Klin. Wochenschr. **31**:831, 1953.

Ramsay, I., Kaur, S., and Krassas, G.: Thyrotoxicosis in pregnancy: results of treatment by antithyroid drugs combined with T_4, Clin. Endocrin. **18**:73, 1983.

Robert, M.F., Neff, R.K., Hubbell, J.P., Taeusch, H.W., and Avery, M.E.: Association between maternal diabetes and the respiratory distress syndrome in the newborn, N. Engl. J. Med. **294**:357, 1976.

Roversi, G.D., Gargiulo, M., Nicolini, U., Pedretti, E., Marini, A., Barbarani, V., and Peneff, P.: A new approach to the treatment of diabetic pregnant women: report of 479 cases seen from 1963 to 1975, Am. J. Obstet. Gynecol. **135**:567, 1979.

Selenkow, H.A., Birnbaum, M.D., and Hollander, C.S.: Thyroid function and dysfunction during pregnancy, Clin. Obstet. Gynecol. **16**:66, 1973.

Sugrue, D., and Drury, M.I.: Hyperthyroidism complicating pregnancy: results of treatment by antithyroid drugs in 77 pregnancies, Br. J. Obstet. Gynecol. **87**:970, 1980.

Widness, J.A., Schwartz, H.C., Zeller, W.P., Oh, W., and Schwartz, R.: Glycohemoglobin in postpartum women, Obstet. Gynecol. **57**:414, 1981.

White, P.: Diabetes mellitus in pregnancy, Clin. Perinatol. **1**:331-347, 1974.

Zucker, P., and Simon, G.: Prolonged symptomatic neonatal hypoglycemia associated with maternal chlorpropamide therapy, Pediatrics **42**:824, 1968.

Russell K. Laros, Jr.

Diseases of the respiratory system, the circulatory system, and the blood during pregnancy

Diseases affecting the lungs, the heart, the blood vessels, and the hematopoietic system are encountered in only a small percentage of pregnant women, but they are potentially more serious than are many other complications. Most disorders affecting the cardiovascular system are not difficult to recognize and can be detected by the usual prenatal studies.

DISEASES OF THE RESPIRATORY SYSTEM

Pulmonary function is not impaired during pregnancy in women of normal health, even though functional and anatomic changes occur that produce significant alterations in respiration (Chapter 19). However, both the mother and the fetus can be compromised if pulmonary function is decreased significantly.

Pulmonary tuberculosis. Pregnancy does not alter the clinical course of pulmonary tuberculosis. The effect of tuberculosis on the mother is determined by the extent of the lesion rather than the fact that she is pregnant. The risk is slight with small lesions, particularly if they are diagnosed and treated properly. Mortality may be high with advanced lesions, but it is comparable to the death rate in nongravid women with similar lesions.

Physical examination alone is inadequate for the detection of all cases of pulmonary tuberculosis, even for lesions that are moderately advanced.

X-ray film examination provides a more precise diagnostic method, but the number of cases that will be detected by routine chest screening during early pregnancy is so small that it does not justify even the slight risk from radiation. This is particularly true of women of upper and middle socioeconomic classes who are not likely to have tuberculosis.

Tuberculin skin testing should be performed early in pregnancy as a screening procedure for patients believed to be at high risk. Patients of low socioeconomic status and recent immigrants from Southeast Asia should be screened. If the tuberculin test is positive, a chest x-ray film should be performed if the patient is known to have a negative reaction in the past or if the time of conversion to positive cannot be determined. Patients with either a history or physical findings suggestive of active pulmonary tuberculosis should have an x-ray film made, regardless of the outcome of the tuberculin test.

Treatment of tuberculosis during pregnancy need not differ from that in nonpregnant individuals. Isoniazid, ethambutol, and rifampin can be used safely; as far as is known, none of these drugs has a deleterious effect on the infant.

MANAGEMENT DURING LABOR. There is no need to induce labor because of pulmonary tuberculosis, but certain precautions are necessary during labor and delivery.

Sedation. Caudal or epidural analgesia can be used to advantage in relieving pain during labor.

Delivery. Low forceps delivery to eliminate the perineal phase of labor will prevent the increased intrapulmonary pressure and possible dissemination of infection that may result from violent voluntary bearing-down efforts. Difficult operative deliveries should be avoided whenever possible, and blood loss must be kept at a minimum. Cesarean section need be performed only for obstetric indications.

THERAPEUTIC ABORTION. Abortion need not be considered for women with tuberculosis when the lesion is small and stationary and when adequate treatment and follow-up is possible. Abortion should be considered for women with actively progressing lesions, those with several children who must add the care of a new baby to their multiple responsibilities, and those with advanced or terminal disease.

CARE OF THE INFANT. Tubercles are often found in the placenta, but intrauterine infection of infants of tuberculous mothers is unusual. In almost every instance the baby is infected by contact with the mother after delivery. Consequently, the baby and the mother should be separated immediately after birth, and contact should be prohibited until it seems certain that the mother is not infectious. Nursing, of course, should be prohibited.

Asthma. Bronchial asthma is encountered in between 1% and 2% of pregnant women. Reports on the effects of pregnancy on asthma differ, but in about a third of women the asthma improves during pregnancy, in about a third it is unchanged, and in another third it becomes worse. Bronchial asthma does not alter the course of pregnancy significantly, and the fetal and neonatal mortality and morbidity are not affected.

With few exceptions the patients' usual medications can be continued during pregnancy. It is important to remember that the volume of distribution for agents such as theophylline increases significantly during pregnancy. Serum theophylline levels should be obtained periodically, and the dosage adjusted as required. There is no contraindication to corticosteroids when they are necessary to control asthma. Medications containing *iodine* should be avoided; the iodine crosses the placenta, interferes with normal fetal thyroid hormone synthesis, and may cause congenital goiter. Abortion may be appropriate in women with severe asthma,

but *prostaglandin induction* is contraindicated. These preparations are potent bronchoconstrictors. Women with asthma who want no more children should be offered sterilization.

Acute respiratory infections

Upper respiratory disease. Pregnant women are somewhat more susceptible to the development of the common cold, and upper respiratory infections tend to last longer than in nonpregnant women. The usual symptomatic treatment can be administered.

Although there is no evidence to suggest that the usual viruses that presumably cause the common cold have a teratogenic effect, some viral diseases that are characterized by respiratory symptoms may. Brown and Evans found a significant increase in congenital heart lesions in the infants of mothers who had coxsackievirus B, types 3 and 4, infections during pregnancy.

Pneumonia. Pneumonia is far less serious since the development of the antibiotic drugs than it was in the past; but when it occurs during pregnancy, it may prove fatal to the mother or her fetus. The choice of an antibiotic is determined by the responsible organisms.

Influenza. During the 1918 influenza pandemic, the total maternal mortality was 27%, and the infant mortality was 26%. If the mother also had pneumonia, the figures rose to 50% maternal and 52% infant mortality. The prognosis for uncomplicated influenza is good.

Chemotherapeutic agents have no effect on the influenza virus, but they reduce the severity of the complications. *Immunization* may be considered if an epidemic is anticipated.

Asian influenza. Gravid women appear to contract Asian influenza more frequently than do those who are not pregnant, and the infection is more severe. Of the women of childbearing age who died of Asian influenza and its complications in Minnesota during the 1957 epidemic, 50% were pregnant, and the deaths accounted for 19% of the maternal mortality for that year. All had fulminating pneumonitis, many dying within 24 hours of the onset of symptoms. Treatment was ineffective. There was no evidence to suggest that the fetus was affected.

Reduced pulmonary function

Pregnancy is not necessarily contraindicated in women who have had pulmonary resections if there is enough normal lung tissue to meet the requirements for pregnancy. Even women who have had pneumonectomies may be able to tolerate pregnancy with little difficulty. The principal risk for those with limited capacity is the possibility of losing much of the remaining function from an acute attack of pneumonitis; hence respiratory infections should be treated vigorously.

DISEASES OF THE CIRCULATORY SYSTEM
Heart disease

About 1% of all pregnant women have organic heart disease. In the past almost all were of rheumatic origin, but improvements in the treatment of rheumatic fever have decreased the incidence of significant valvular lesions. As a consequence, there has been a reduction in the total number of pregnancies complicated by heart disease, but the proportion caused by congenital malformation has increased.

Diagnosis. The diagnosis of heart disease is made on the basis of clinical history and examination, electrocardiographic recordings, echocardiography and cardiac x-ray film examination. A more precise diagnosis can be made with cardiac catheterization. It may be difficult to make an accurate diagnosis of heart lesions during pregnancy by clinical examination alone. At least half of all women develop systolic murmurs during pregnancy; and the heart sounds, particularly those of the apex, are altered. The changes, which are caused by the increase in plasma volume and cardiac output, altered viscosity of the blood, and changes in the shape of the heart, begin during the early second trimester and reverse rapidly after delivery.

Patients suspected of having a cardiac lesion should be treated as are those who actually have one, even though a precise diagnosis cannot be made until after delivery. The lesions are classified according to the functional classifications of the New York Heart Association as follows:

Class I: Patients with cardiac disease that does not limit activity. Ordinary physical activity does not cause discomfort. The patients have neither symptoms of cardiac insufficiency nor anginal pain.

Class II: Patients with cardiac disease that produces slight limitation of activity. They are free from symptoms while at rest, but ordinary activity is accompanied by undue fatigue, palpitation, dyspnea, or anginal pain.

Class III: Patients with cardiac disease that produces marked limitation of activity. Less than ordinary activity is accompanied by undue fatigue, palpitation, dyspnea, or anginal pain.

Class IV: Patients with cardiac disease that prevents them from carrying out any activity without discomfort. Symptoms of cardiac insufficiency or anginal pain are present at rest, and any activity increases them.

Prognosis. The prognosis for a patient with cardiac disease is determined by the functional capacity of the heart and its ability to meet the increased demands placed on it by the normal physiologic changes of pregnancy, the most important of which are the expanded plasma volume and the great increase in the total vascular bed in the enlarging uterus. Another physiologic change that adds to the cardiac load is a gradual rise in heart rate, with a maximum increase of 10 to 15 beats per minute near term. Additional factors that influence the outcome are the ability of the patient to adhere to the physical restrictions necessary during pregnancy, the quality of the medical care available to her, and the possibility that added complications such as serious infections may develop.

To maintain an adequate circulation, the cardiac output begins to rise at about the tenth week and reaches a maximum, at least 30% above that of nongravid women, between the twenty-eighth and thirty-second weeks. It remains elevated until term. The changes in output occur mostly in response to alterations in stroke volume. The curve for cardiac output roughly parallels that for plasma volume. Plasma volume, however, continues to increase until at least the middle of the third trimester and often until term. If an adequate output can be maintained, the patient will progress through pregnancy and delivery without difficulty, but if cardiac reserve is limited, the heart will be unable to respond to the increasing demands.

Maternal mortality is approximately 0.4% in class I or II and 6.8% in class III or IV of the New

York Heart Association's classification. Patients with pulmonary hypertension appear to be at greatest risk. *Most deaths are caused by heart failure.* Although this can occur at any time, it is most common when the maternal blood volume is at a maximum. The normal heart has no difficulty in increasing its output as the plasma volume expands, but, if there has been significant valvular damage, the heart may be unable to respond to this and other demands.

Ueland, Novy, and Metcalfe studied cardiac response to light exercise during and after pregnancy in 21 women with valvular lesions. Resting cardiac output in all 21 was less than that of pregnant women with normal hearts. Cardiac output increased less during exercise in those with valve lesions than in normal women. The inability to respond was most pronounced in women with mitral lesions.

Plasma volume and cardiac output decrease slightly, if at all, during the last weeks of pregnancy, and general physical demands increase. Failure can occur at this time if cardiac reserve is limited.

Heart failure also occurs during labor, when the demands are greater than are those during pregnancy. Hendricks and Quilligan observed a 30% increase in cardiac output during each first-stage uterine contraction. The systolic blood pressure increased 10 to 20 mm Hg during each contraction, and there were consistent changes in heart rate and stroke volume. The heart rate rose at the onset, decreased below the resting level at the peak of the contraction, and returned to normal as the uterus relaxed. Stroke volume first fell and then rose significantly at the peak of the contraction.

Ueland and Hansen described similar changes but also noted alterations caused by position. Cardiac output during a contraction increased 24.8%, and stroke volume increased 33.1% with the patient in the supine position; when the patient was on her side, these values increased only 7.6% and 7.7%, respectively. Ueland and Hansen attribute the change to compression of the vena cava and aorta by the heavy uterus and the consequent alterations in venous return and in arterial pressure when the patient lies on her back.

The changes that occur may be because 250 to 300 ml of blood is forced from the uterine vessels into the general circulation during a uterine contraction. Comparable changes in cardiac output, arterial pressure, and pulse rate can be produced by the rapid infusion of blood or plasma expanders into experimental animals.

According to Ueland and Hansen, cardiac output reaches a maximum during labor and delivery but declines somewhat, although it is still well above the prelabor level, during the first few hours following delivery. The changes in stroke volume are similar. This probably can be attributed to the expanded plasma volume resulting from the drastic reduction in uterine circulatory capacity at delivery and the consequent redistribution of blood in the general circulation.

Parity is far less important than age as a causative factor in decompression; a sharp increase in deaths from heart disease in pregnancy occurs after the age of 35 years. There is a high incidence of heart failure and death in women who have experienced previous episodes of decompensation or atrial fibrillation.

If the patient survives the pregnancy, the course of her heart disease and her life expectancy should not be altered. Chesley could detect no evidence that pregnancy altered either the course of the heart disease or the life expectancy of 134 women with functionally severe rheumatic heart lesions who were delivered in the Margaret Hague Maternity Hospital, Jersey City, New Jersey, between 1931 and the end of 1943 and who were followed until 1975 when all but 9 had died.

Maternal heart disease alone does not increase *perinatal mortality,* but intrapartum death from hypoxia may occur from circulatory changes accompanying decompensation, paroxysmal tachycardia, and similar complications. Infants born of mothers with heart disease are likely to weigh less than those whose mothers are normal. This suggests that the heart lesion and the reduced ability to increase cardiac output in response to exercise may reduce uterine perfusion and interfere with fetal growth.

Treatment during pregnancy. The patient with heart disease should be examined before she becomes pregnant so that the lesion can be accurately diagnosed and cardiac function evaluated. A patient with a serious lesion, certainly one in functional class III or IV, should usually be advised against pregnancy. If a patient with heart disease is first seen during pregnancy, it often is wise to admit her to a hospital for study; this is particularly important with severe lesions. In most instances consultation with a cardiologist is indicated, but the fact that the cardiologist offers a good prognosis should not alter the physician's care of the patient. She may decompensate during pregnancy even though the lesion seems relatively innocuous.

With proper treatment, the mortality should be minimal, even in those with advanced lesions; but if the cardiac abnormality is ignored or if she cannot or will not follow instructions, the death rate will be high.

Acute infections, particularly those of respiratory origin, often precipitate failure; consequently, most women with active infections other than uncomplicated upper respiratory infections should be treated in the hospital until they have recovered.

It is usually recommended that patients with class IV heart disease be admitted 10 to 14 days before delivery is anticipated for controlled rest in preparation for labor.

Rest is of utmost importance, and a specific plan should be developed for each individual. Rest periods each morning and afternoon and at least 10 hours in bed each night are advisable. Although light tasks around the home are permissible if they do not produce symptoms, unusual activity such as stair climbing, shopping, and heavy cleaning should be avoided; this is particularly true after the middle of pregnancy. Patients who have decompensated or those in whom slight exertion causes symptoms should remain in bed or in a chair at the bedside almost all the time. If the cardiac reserve is limited, coitus should be avoided after the twentieth week.

There is no need to reduce salt intake or to prescribe diuretics unless they are essential to the management of the heart lesion. A reduced salt intake may limit the normal expansion of plasma volume that is essential for adequate circulation.

An *iron supplement* is important because anemia

increases the demands on the heart. *Digitalis* is used when indicated. Women with class III lesions must be considered to be partially decompensated; consequentely, they, as well as those with class IV lesions, usually should take digitalis throughout the pregnancy.

THERAPEUTIC ABORTION. Termination of pregnancy is unnecessary in women with milder lesions and even in those of classes III and IV if they can be provided proper care during the entire pregnancy. Unfortunately, this is not always possible, and if a patient cannot or will not follow advice, the risk from continuing pregnancy may offer a serious threat to her life. If proper treatment cannot be administered, termination of pregnancy and tubal sterilization are justifiable for the following patients.

1. Those who have decompensated previously, particularly those who have been in failure between pregnancies (about two thirds of these will decompensate during pregnancy)
2. Those with atrial fibrillation
3. Those in functional classes III and IV (the incidence of failure is high, particularly with the more advanced lesions)
4. Those over age 35 years with serious lesions
5. Those with pulmonary hypertension

Interruption should be performed as early as possible because a major operative procedure may prove too much for the heart already burdened with gestational demands. In fact, the operation may actually contribute to the patient's death. Interruption should never be performed in a patient who is already in failure; the decompensation should be corrected first.

VALVULOTOMY AND HEART VALVE PROSTHESES. Operations to correct heart lesions are seldom necessary during pregnancy, as is indicated by the excellent results that can be obtained by medical treatment alone. Occasionally, however, mitral commissurotomy is warranted in a woman with stenosis if the constricted opening prevents the necessary increase in blood flow through or from the heart. The mortality is less than 3%, and there should be no effect on the fetus if all phases of the operative procedure are managed properly. Whenever possible, the operation should be performed during the first trimester; but, when necessary, it can be done later.

Valvulotomy, even that performed between pregnancies, does not always permit cardiac function that is adequate for normal gestation. Schenker and Polishuk, reporting on 182 patients who had mitral valvulotomies, found increased rates of spontaneous and therapeutic abortions and of intrauterine and neonatal deaths. In addition, 10 of 18 deaths (55%) occurred as a result of pregnancy and delivery. Decompensation occurred in 42% of patients who delivered for the first time after the operation. Atrial fibrillation developed in 35 patients (18%) during pregnancy; five patients (14.2%) died, 48.8% developed congestive failure, and 20% had thromboembolic phenomena.

Although the experience in treating women with heart valve prostheses is limited, it appears that they are poor candidates for pregnancy and require even more care than do other women with heart disease. Most of them must be treated with antibiotics and maintained on heparin throughout pregnancy. Warfarin (Coumadin) sodium crosses the placenta, is teratogenic, and should not be used during pregnancy.

Care during labor. Induction of labor for heart disease alone is contraindicated. If the patient is allowed to start labor spontaneously, the physician can be assured that labor will more likely be short and normal than if induction is attempted early. Heart disease does not alter the length of labor.

Although failure usually does not occur during labor, it may set in soon after delivery; in most instances there is adequate warning that cardiac function is deteriorating. The best index of the condition of the heart during labor is offered by the pulse and respiratory rates; which, with the blood pressure, should be checked and recorded every 15 minutes. Failure is likely to occur if the pulse rate increases above 110 and the respiratory rate above 24 during the first stage. If there are any signs of beginning decompensation, oxygen should be administered, and the patient should be given digitalis rapidly unless she already is receiving an adequate dosage of digitalis. A pulmonary artery catheter (Swan-Ganz) and a radial artery catheter should be placed at the onset of labor in patients with hemodynamically significant heart disease and in all cases of pulmonary hypertension. A number of clinically significant cardiovascular parameters can then be monitored continuously, and pharmacologic agents used to alter preload, afterload, and contractility as needed.

Pain, anxiety, and muscular activity add to the burden on the heart, and the physician should try to eliminate them. This is best achieved with a caudal or epidural anesthetic if it can be administered safely. These techniques usually have little effect on blood pressure; therefore oxygenation is maintained. The anesthetic is started when the patient becomes uncomfortable, if she is making satisfactory progress in labor; and; can be continued for delivery.

If caudal or epidural anesthesia is not available, the discomfort can be relieved with morphine sulfate, 0.01 to 0.016 g, or meperidine (Demerol), 75 to 100 mg, as needed. Scopolamine may increase both heart rate and muscular activity and is contraindicated. Phenothiazine derivatives should be used with caution because they may cause hypotension, particularly when a general anesthetic agent also is administered.

The American Heart Association no longer recommends prophylactic antibiotics to prevent subacute bacterial endocarditis in uncomplicated vaginal deliveries. Broad spectrum coverage with penicillin and an aminoglycoside (vancomycin for women with penicillin allergy) are indicated for operative vaginal deliveries and cesarean sections. However, in view of the simplicity of prophylaxis and the serious consequences of subacute bacterial endocarditis, many cardiologists and perinatologists continue to recommend prophylaxis in all cases of congenital or acquired heart disease.

Delivery. Vaginal delivery is usually preferred to cesarean section unless there is an obstetric reason for the latter. A test of labor is ordinarily contraindicated for patients with moderate or severe cardiac disease because it increases the risk of infection or decompensation if labor is prolonged or if cesarean section becomes necessary after several hours of ineffectual labor.

The choice of anesthesia is one of the most important considerations when cesarean section must be performed on women with heart disease. Ueland, Gills, and Hansen found that cardiac output increased 52%, stroke volume increased 67%, and heart rate decreased 11% when cesarean section was performed with spinal anesthesia. When epidural anesthesia was used, cardiac output increased 25%, stroke volume increased 20%, and heart rate changed little. One can conclude from these findings that epidural anesthesia is the preferred form of conduction anesthesia for cesarean section in women with heart disease.

Bearing-down efforts raise intravascular pressure and increase the possibility of decompensation; consequently, they should be prevented by eliminating the perineal phase of labor as completely as possible. This can be accomplished by low forceps extraction soon after the head begins to bulge the perineum and should be performed in most primigravidas. It is not necessary in multiparas, who usually will deliver with a few second-stage contractions. Caudal, spinal, or pudendal block anesthesia will obliterate the perineal sensation, thereby eliminating bearing-down efforts, and they do not interfere with oxygenation.

Ergonovine maleate (Ergotrate) sometimes produces transient but severe hypertension and should not be used. If it is necessary to stimulate uterine contractions, oxytocin can be given safely.

Postpartum care. The heart is more likely to decompensate during the early puerperium than during labor, but the incidence can be kept low by meticulous care during pregnancy and labor. Those with cardiac symptoms should usually remain in bed until the symptoms have disappeared.

Ambulation for those in classes I and II usually need not be delayed. Antibiotics are continued until it seems certain that the danger from infection is past. Women with heart disease may nurse their babies if they have no cardiac symptoms and if nursing is not too tiring. The patient may be discharged whenever the physician is certain the danger from decompensation is past. Most patients should remain in the hospital longer than normal women, particularly if they must assume complete responsibility for care of the child and the home.

Reproduction in women with heart disease should usually be limited, the size of the family being determined by the functional capacity of the heart and the desires of the patient and her husband. The patient should be instructed about a reliable contraceptive method before she leaves the hospital. Tubal sterilization may be considered if the parents desire no more children and if the operation can be performed with only slight risk.

Subacute bacterial endocarditis

Pedowitz and Hellman analyzed the pregnancies of 85 women who conceived after they had recovered from subacute bacterial endocarditis and 35 who were pregnant when this complication developed. The mortality was 3.5% and 14.2%, respectively. They concluded that if the endocarditis is well healed, the prognosis for pregnancy depends almost entirely on the heart lesion and its effect on cardiac function. The treatment of active endocarditis is not altered because of pregnancy.

Coronary artery disease

Coronary occlusion or thrombosis does not occur often during pregnancy, but when it does, the mortality is high. Pregnancy usually is contraindicated in women who have had coronary occlusion, particularly if the blood pressure is elevated; therefore therapeutic abortion can justifiably be advised. Acute coronary occlusion in a gravid woman should be treated as though she were not pregnant. In most instances vaginal delivery is permissible if precautions are taken to prevent pain, unusual muscular activity, and hypoxia during labor and delivery.

Peripartum idiopathic cardiomyopathy

There is a clinical entity characterized by peripartum heart failure of obscure cause. Women with this disease are more commonly older, multiparous, and black and have hypertension. In most patients the heart returns to normal size soon after delivery. Most authors advise against subsequent pregnancies for women with this disorder because it often recurs.

Congenital heart lesions

Most women with the milder forms of congenital heart disease have little difficulty during pregnancy, but the prognosis is less favorable for those with reduced cardiac function, particularly if they are cyanotic. The highest mortalities are associated with Marfan's syndrome (50%), Eisenmenger's syndrome (30% to 35%), uncorrected tetralogy of Fallot (10% to 15%), and coarctation of the aorta (10%). The mortality associated with these lesions is so high that therapeutic termination of early pregnancy often is justifiable. Abortion need not usually be considered for other congenital lesions unless cardiac reserve is so limited that decompensation can be anticipated as pregnancy advances.

The most frequent causes of death are heart failure and, in women with septal defects and patent ductus arteriosus, bacterial endocarditis; rupture of the aorta is common in women with coarctation.

The basic principles of management are similar to those for women with other types of heart disease.

Most women with mild congenital heart lesions can be delivered vaginally unless cesarean section is indicated for obstetric reasons. Abdominal delivery frequently is safer for those with advanced coarctation because the changes in circulatory dynamics accompanying uterine contractions and bearing down are likely to rupture the defective or recently repaired aorta. Cesarean delivery may also be selected when women with more serious lesions must be delivered prematurely.

Pregnancy should offer less hazard if disturbed cardiac function has been corrected by surgical repair of the defect. In most instances, cardiac operations should be performed between pregnancies.

Congenital heart lesions in the mothers may be duplicated in their offspring. Infants born to mothers with congenital heart disease, particularly those with cyanosis, are likely to be small, presumably as a result of intrauterine growth retardation.

Kyphoscoliotic heart disease

The collapsed rib cage in women with kyphoscoliosis reduces vital capacity by compressing the lungs and limiting their ability to expand. The enlarging uterus exaggerates the difficulty. The right ventricle hypertrophies to maintain an adequate pulmonary circulation, and cardiac failure may occur if the heart is unable to meet the increased demands as pregnancy advances.

Since the pelvis, as well as the spine, usually is deformed, cesarean section may be necessary. Therapeutic abortion is justifiable for those with limited cardiac reserve.

Varicose veins

Venous varicosities in the legs and vulva are common during pregnancy and are particularly likely to occur in women whose general supporting tissues are weak. In many women a history of similar defects in other members of the family can be elicited. The veins begin to distend during the first trimester and become progressively larger as pregnancy advances. The engorgement of the pelvic veins and delayed circulation through the lower part of the body exert increasing pressure on the vein walls; if the walls are not strong enough to resist the internal force, they stretch, producing the typical large tortuous veins of pregnancy.

Some women have no symptoms related to the enlarged veins, but many complain of heaviness and discomfort that become progressively worse the longer they remain in an upright position. Vul-

var varicosities are particularly uncomfortable. The veins begin to improve within a few days after delivery and may disappear completely, only to recur and become worse with the next pregnancy. In many women the vulvar varicosities remain but become smaller between pregnancies.

The treatment during pregnancy is to compress the distended vessels with elastic stockings, which are best applied before the patient arises in the morning while the veins are collapsed and empty. It is more difficult to compress vulvar varicosities, but supporting pads and garments are available in surgical supply stores. It is seldom necessary to operate on varicose veins during pregnancy.

Nosebleeds

Mild nosebleeds occur frequently during pregnancy and can usually be controlled with pressure. Occasionally, it may be necessary to pack the nose or cauterize the bleeding area.

Other vascular changes

Spider nevi and palmar erythema are common during pregnancy and disappear after delivery. Both are thought to result from the elevated estrogen level.

DISEASES OF THE BLOOD

Unlike the normal nonpregnant individual whose blood picture remains relatively stable, the blood of pregnant women undergoes both qualitative and quantitative alterations. The *plasma volume* increases, reaching its maximum during the third trimester. The *red blood cell mass* and, as a consequence, the *total blood volume* also increase. If iron intake is adequate, the *total hemoglobin* content increases; and serum iron, erythrocyte protoporphyrin, and iron-binding capacity remain normal (Fig. 23-1).

The body of a normal woman contains about 4 g of iron; 60% to 70% of this is carried in hemoglobin; about 30% is stored in the liver, spleen, bone marrow, and other cells; and most of the rest is carried as transport iron in the iron–beta globulin complex. During pregnancy approximately an additional gram of iron is required: at least 400 mg

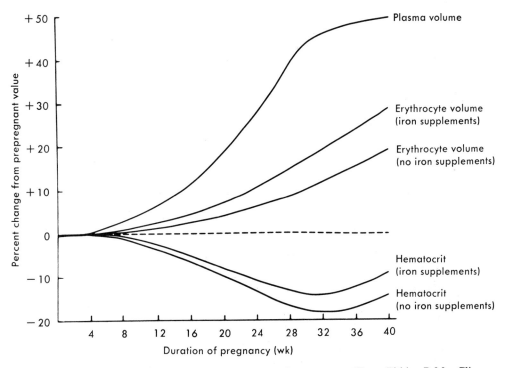

Fig. 23-1. Physiologic changes in blood during normal pregnancy. (From Pitkin, R.M.: Clin. Obstet. Gynecol. **39**:489, 1976.)

for the expanded red cell mass, 300 or 400 mg for fetal hemoglobin, and at least 100 mg to replace that lost through bleeding during and after delivery. Although iron is absorbed from the intestinal tract more readily during pregnancy, the usual dietary intake provides less than that required; the estimated deficit averages about 400 mg.

The *white blood cell* count is slightly increased during pregnancy, but it seldom exceeds 12,000 in normal women. The differential cell count is unaltered except for a slight decrease in eosinophils.

Iron-deficiency anemia. Iron-deficiency anemia is the most common form of anemia in pregnant women. It is caused by an iron deficit from rapidly recurring pregnancies, abnormal blood loss, or nutritional inadequacies.

The hemoglobin concentration falls during pregnancy, even though iron stores are adequate, because the increase in plasma volume is proportionately greater than the increase in red blood cell mass. The lowest hemoglobin concentration is reached when the plasma volume is expanding most rapidly between the twenty-sixth and thirty-fourth weeks. Hemoglobin concentration increases slightly during the last few weeks. Most authorities agree that *the lower limit of normal hemoglobin during pregnancy is 11 g and that anemia can be diagnosed when the hemoglobin is less than that amount or the hematocrit is less than 32%* (Fig. 23-1).

In women who are anemic the serum iron is reduced, whereas iron-binding capacity and protoporphyrin are increased. Red blood cells are normocytic and hypochromic with mild anemia, but the characteristic abnormalities associated with iron deficiency can occur with the more profound degrees of deficiency.

Whenever possible, iron-deficiency anemia should be corrected before conception. As a general rule, supplemental iron should be prescribed for all menstruating women, because the cumulative iron loss from month to month is significant.

An effective iron preparation should be prescribed for all pregnant women even when the diet is considered adequate. A daily dose of about 200 mg of elemental iron will be more than adequate to meet the needs during pregnancy. This can be supplied in 1 g of ferrous sulfate or 2 g of ferrous gluconate daily. Gastrointestinal disturbances can be kept at a minimum if the preparation is ingested in small amounts three or four times each day.

Parenteral administration of iron is seldom necessary, but it may be considered for those who cannot take iron orally. Blood transfusions also are seldom necessary, particularly if the patient is several weeks from term, because the anemia can be improved by the ingestion of iron. In those at term or in labor with hemoglobin readings below 7 or 8 g, compatible blood should be available to compensate for excessive bleeding during delivery.

Iron-deficiency anemia can also follow *blood loss during pregnancy* (abortion, placenta previa, or abruptio placentae). This is treated by transfusion when large amounts of blood have been lost and iron therapy until the blood has returned to normal. *Anemia associated with chronic infections and malignancy* is uncommon in pregnant women. The response to iron therapy is limited.

Megaloblastic anemia. Megaloblastic anemia is far less common than that caused by iron deficiency, but it is usually much more severe. It is also called *pernicious anemia of pregnancy* or *macrocytic anemia.*

The cause of megaloblastic anemia is folic acid deficiency. Folic acid requirements increase during pregnancy, and a deficiency may develop in individuals whose diets are deficient in animal protein and in uncooked fresh vegetables and those in whom there is diminished intestinal absorption of folic acid. Vitamin C deficiency may interfere with folic acid metabolism.

The earliest cellular change in peripheral blood resulting from folic acid deficiency is hypersegmentation of neutrophils. This is followed by increased urinary excretion of formiminoglutamic acid and by anemia and macrocytosis; eventually a few megaloblasts may be seen in peripheral blood smears.

The diagnosis is made by demonstrating a low serum folate and a normal vitamin B_{12} level, a megaloblastic marrow, and a prompt reticulocyte response to folic acid therapy.

Mild degrees of folic acid deficiency occur frequently during pregnancy, even in women with the potential for adequate nutrition. According to Avery and Ledger, 21% of presumably normal prenatal patients in the University of Michigan Hospital had low serum and RBC folate levels during the last weeks of pregnancy. None had clinical symptoms of megaloblastic anemia. Folic acid deficiencies can develop in pregnant women with hemoglobinopathies, those with multiple fetuses, and those who are alcoholic.

Megaloblastic anemia develops late in pregnancy and can be suspected whenever the hemoglobin falls progressively despite adequate iron intake. The most advanced clinical stages, which are characterized by extreme pallor, dyspnea, edema, and hemoglobin readings as low as 4 or 5 g, are not often seen in the United States.

Folate deficiencies in pregnant women can be prevented by the ingestion of 300 µg of folic acid daily. This and a prophylactic dose of iron should prevent anemia. Adequate amounts of both substances can be supplied in multivitamin preparations that include both drugs.

Anemia caused by folate deficiency can be treated with 1 mg of folic acid three times daily. Nutritional deficiencies should also be corrected.

Folic acid deficiencies have not been implicated in the origin of pregnancy complications other than anemia. Perinatal mortality and morbidity are not increased as a result of folic acid deficiencies.

Hemoglobinopathies. For many years, sickle-cell anemia was recognized as a serious complication of pregnancy, but the various types were not appreciated until electrophoresis became available. This test differentiates normal hemoglobin A from sickle hemoglobin S, fetal hemoglobin F, hemoglobin E, and hemoglobin C. *Sickle-cell trait* occurs with an S-A pattern, *sickle-cell anemia* with homozygous S-S pattern, and *sickle-cell hemoglo-*

bin C disease with the heterozygous S-C combination. *Sickle-cell beta-thalassemia* is characterized by decreased proportions of hemoglobin A and increased proportions of hemoglobin A_2. Hemoglobin F and hemoglobin S can also be identified. *Sickle-cell hemoglobin F disease* (S-F) and homologous *hemoglobin C disease* (C-C) occur infrequently. Homozygous beta-thalassemia is characterized by a pattern of elevated hemoglobin F and A_2, whereas the heterozygous individual shows only an elevation of hemoglobin A_2. Alpha thalassemia occurs in four forms, depending on how many alpha genes are missing. The four-gene deletion state is characterized by an elevated level of hemoglobin H, and individuals with the one- or two-gene deletion state have no electrophoretic abnormality. All forms of thalassemia are characterized by microcytic, hypochromic red cells.

The various sickle hemoglobinopathies are seen almost exclusively in blacks. Hemoglobin E is most frequent in Southeast Asians, and thalassemia is found most commonly in individuals of Mediterranean, Asian, or black ancestry.

Sickle-cell trait (S-A), the sickling of red blood cells with an S-A electrophoretic pattern, is present in about 10% to 12% of black women, but the outlook for pregnancy is much more favorable than with S-S or S-C disease. According to Whalley, Pritchard, and Richards, the incidence of pyelonephritis is significantly increased in women with sickle-cell trait; but abortion, toxemia, prematurity, and perinatal mortality occur with a frequency similar to that in a comparable group of normal black women. *Sickle-cell anemia* (S-S) has usually been diagnosed well before the woman has a pregnancy. Current data show that the spontaneous abortion rate is not increased and that the prepregnancy course of the disease is a good index to the anticipated course during pregnancy. The principles of care include avoidance and early detection of infection, symptomatic treatment of crises when they occur, and the prevention of a crisis by a program of prophylactic transfusion. The most common infections are pyelonephritis and pneumonia.

Prophylactic transfusion is usually begun at 22 to 26 weeks of pregnancy and continued until term.

Sufficient volumes of packed red blood cells are given to achieve a hemoglobin A level of more than 40% and a hematocrit of more than 35%. The transfusions are repeated when the hemoglobin A level falls below 20%, if the hematocrit falls below 25%, or if labor or crisis occur. Reports by Cunningham, Pritchard, and Mason and Morrison, Schneider, and Whybrew indicate that such a program coupled with meticulous prenatal care and antepartum and intrapartum fetal surveillance will produce an excellent perinatal result.

Sickle cell hemoglobin C disease (S-C) usually has a fairly benign course with most individuals having few crises and living a normal life span. However, during pregnancy up to 50% of these women will develop a clinical course similar to individuals with sickle cell disease. In contrast, however, they experience severe anemic crises caused by splenic sequestration and bone marrow infarction with subsequent marrow emboli that can be fatal.

These individuals should be followed closely, and prophylactic transfusions begun if they become symptomatic. Although such an approach has significantly improved maternal and fetal outcome, the incidence of intrauterine growth retardation still remains elevated.

Most women with the sickle-cell diseases can be permitted to deliver normally unless cesarean section is warranted because of an obstetric complication. Excessive blood loss should be replaced promptly. *Tubal ligation* for multiparas with sickle-cell disease, particularly those with an S-C pattern, is justifiable.

In all these hemoglobinopathies, the involved genes may be considered recessive. Although the heterozygote is either normal or has a mild anemia, the homozygous or double heterozygous individual is severely affected. The development of in utero diagnostic techniques now allows the obstetrician to give parents definite answers rather than statistical probabilities. Couples at risk can avoid having a homozygous child without remaining childless.

However, to make this technology available, one must first identify the asymptomatic, heterozygous individuals. Each patient registering for prenatal care should have a complete blood count, including red blood cell indexes. Additionally, each black patient must have a screening hemoglobin electrophoresis done. If the mean corpuscular volume is found to be less than 80 femtoliter or if hemoglobin S or C is detected, complete evaluation is carried out that includes a definitive diagnosis of hemoglobin type for both partners. When both are found to be heterozygous carriers, the couple is referred for antenatal diagnosis.

Leukemia. The outlook for leukemia does not appear to be altered by pregnancy; hence there is no reason to consider abortion. Treatment is the same as that in nonpregnant women; but the effects on the fetus of x-radiation and antimetabolites, particularly antifolic acid compounds, must be considered. Teratogenesis is less likely to occur with treatment after 16 to 20 weeks than during early pregnancy.

Hodgkin's disease. Pregnancy does not alter the course of Hodgkin's disease, neither does the condition have any effect on pregnancy or the growth of the fetus. If x-ray film therapy is administered, the uterus must be shielded. Abortion is not necessary.

Thrombocytopenic purpura. *Idiopathic (autoimmune) thrombocytopenic purpura* is rarely encountered in gravid women. The bleeding tendency and the reduced platelet count are not affected by pregnancy. The infant may have a transient thrombocytopenia, which can usually be corrected by the administration of fresh blood or of adrenal corticosteroids. The mother is usually best treated with adrenal corticosteroids during pregnancy. If this medication does not correct the bleeding tendency, splenectomy is indicated. Some authors have suggested that delivery should always be by cesarean section. The operative route is chosen in the hope that avoiding labor and vaginal delivery will decrease the incidence of intracranial bleeding in those few infants who are profoundly thrombocytopenic. Because the available literature does not support this recommendation, the obstetric service at the University of California, San Francisco allows labor and vaginal delivery unless there is an obstetric indication for cesarean section.

Disseminated intravascular coagulation (DIC). DIC is really a syndrome produced as part of an underlying disease process that in some way leads to activation of the coagulation mechanism. DIC is seen in association with placental abruption, gram-negative sepsis, amniotic fluid embolism, the dead fetus syndrome, and severe preeclampsia and eclampsia.

The signs and symptoms are basically those of the underlying disease plus hemorrhage and, on occasion, microvascular obstruction. The hemorrhage occurs because of consumption of procoagulants and the production of fibrin/fibrinogen split products that are themselves anticoagulants. The obstructive symptoms are produced by large numbers of microthrombi being formed faster than they are removed by the fibrinolytic system.

The diagnosis is confirmed by demonstrating a low level of platelets and fibrinogen, elevated levels of circulating fibrin/fibrinogen split products, and the presence of fragment red blood cells. The most important step in therapy is the recognition and treatment of the underlying disease process. If the levels of procoagulants are reduced and the patient is clinically bleeding, replacement therapy with cryoprecipitate and platelet concentrates is begun. In the rare circumstance of significant, clinically evident microvascular obstruction (acute cortical necrosis or gangrene of skin or digits), the patient should also be anticoagulated with heparin.

Thrombotic thrombocytopenic purpura is a rare and serious condition characterized by thrombocytopenia, microangiopathic hemolytic anemia, fever, central nervous system manifestations, and renal impairment. It can be confused with severe preeclampsia accompanied by hemolytic anemia and thrombocytopenia. The most effective treatment is plasma infusion, vincristine, corticosteroids, and oral antiplatelet agents. These modalities should be used sequentially, and, if a response is not achieved, splenectomy and PGI_2 infusion should be tried.

REFERENCES

Alger, L.S., Golbus, M.S., and Laros, R.K., Jr.: Thalassemia and pregnancy: results of an antenatal screening program, Am. J. Obstet. Gynecol. **134:**662, 1979.

Avery, B., and Ledger, W.J.: Folic acid metabolism in well-nourished pregnant women, Obstet. Gynecol. **35:**616, 1970.

Benedetti, T.J., Valle, R., and Ledger, W.J.: Antepartum pneumonia in pregnancy, Am. J. Obstet. Gynecol. **144:**413, 1982.

Brown, G.C., and Evans, T.N.: Serologic evidence of Coxsackievirus etiology of congenital heart disease, J.A.M.A. **199:**183, 1967.

Catanzarite, V.A., and Ferguson, J.E.: Acute leukemia and pregnancy: a review of management and outcome, 1972-1982, Obstet. Gynecol Survey **39:**663, 1984.

Chesley, L.C.: Severe rheumatic cardiac disease and pregnancy: the ultimate prognosis, Am. J. Obstet. Gynecol. **136:**552, 1980.

Chesley, L.C.: Rheumatic cardiac disease in pregnancy: long-term follow-up, Obstet. Gynecol. **46:**699, 1975.

Cunningham, F.G., Pritchard, J.A., and Mason, R.: Pregnancy and sickle cell hemoglobinopathies: results with and without prophylactic transfusions, Obstet. Gynecol. **62:**419, 1983.

Cutforth, R., and MacDonald, C.B.: Heart sounds and murmurs during pregnancy, Am. Heart J. **71:**741, 1966.

Gililland, J., and Weinstein, L.: The effects of cancer chemotherapeutic agents on the developing fetus, Obstet. Gynecol. Survey **38:**6, 1983.

Greenberger, P.A., and Patterson, R.: Management of asthma during pregnancy, N. Engl. J. Med. **312:**897, 1985.

Hendricks, C.H., and Quilligan, E.J.: Cardiac output during labor, Am. J. Obstet. Gynecol. **71:**953, 1956.

Jacobs, C., Donaldson, S.S., Rosenberg, S.A., and Kaplan, H.S.: Management of the pregnant patient with Hodgkin's disease, Ann. Intern. Med. **95:**669, 1981.

Kagan, R., and Laros, R.K., Jr.: Immune thrombocytopenia, Clin. Obstet. Gynecol. **26:**537, 1983.

Laros, R.K., Jr.: Acquired Coagulation Disorders. In Laros, R.K., Jr., editor: Blood disorders in pregnancy, Philadelphia, 1986, Lea & Febiger.

Laros, R.K., Jr., Hage, M.L., and Hayashi, R.H.: Pregnancy and heart valve prostheses, Obstet. Gynecol. **35:**241, 1970.

Laros, R.K., Jr., and Kalstone, C.E.: Sickle cell beta-thalassemia and pregnancy, Obstet. Gynecol. **37:**67, 1971.

Lowenstein, L., Pick, C., and Philpott, N.: Megaloblastic anemia of pregnancy and puerperium, Am. J. Obstet. Gynecol. **70:**1309, 1955.

Mendelson, C.L.: Cardiac disease in pregnancy, Philadelphia, 1960, F.A. Davis Co.

Milner, P.F., Jones, B.R., and Döbler, J.: Outcome of pregnancy in sickle cell anemia and sickle cell-hemoglobin C disease, Am. J. Obstet. Gynecol. **138:**239, 1980.

Morrison, J.C., Schneider, J.M., and Whybrew, W.D.: Prophylactic transfusion in pregnant patients with sickle hemoglobinopathies, Obstet. Gynecol. **48:**274, 1980.

Pedowitz, P., and Hellman, L.M.: Pregnancy and healed subacute bacterial endocarditis, Am. J. Obstet. Gynecol. **66:**294, 1953.

Perkins, R.P.: Thrombocytopenia in obstetric syndromes: a review, Obstet. Gynecol. Surv. **34:**101, 1979.

Pitkin, R.M.: Nutritional support in obstetrics and gynecology, Clin. Obstet. Gynecol. **39:**489, 1976.

Powars, D.R., Sandhu, M., Niland-Weiss, J., Johnson, C., Bruce, S., and Manning, P.R.: Pregnancy in sickle cell disease, Obstet. Gynecol. **67:**217, 1986.

Pritchard, J.A., Scott, D.E., Whalley, P.J., Cunningham, F.G., and Mason, R.A.: The effects of maternal sickle cell hemoglobinopathies and sickle cell trait on reproductive performance, Am. J. Obstet. Gynecol. **117:**662, 1973.

Schaefer, G., Zervoudakis, I.A., Fuchs, F.F., and David, S.: Pregnancy and pulmonary tuberculosis, Obstet. Gynecol. **46:**706, 1975.

Schenker, J.G., and Polishuk, W.Z.: Pregnancy following mitral valvulotomy, Obstet. Gynecol. **32:**214, 1968.

Sullivan, J.M., and Ramanathan, K.B.: Management of medical problems in pregnancy—severe cardiac disease, N. Engl. J. Med. **313:**304, 1985.

Ueland, K., Akamatsu, T.J., Eng, M., Bonica, J.J., and Hansen, J.M.: Maternal cardiovascular dynamics, Am. J. Obstet. Gynecol. **114:**775, 1972.

Ueland, K., Gills, R.E., and Hansen, J.M.: Maternal cardiovascular dynamics, I. Cesarean section under subarachnoid block anesthesia, Am. J. Obstet. Gynecol. **100:**42, 1968.

Ueland, K., and Hansen, J.M.: Maternal cardiovascular dynamics, II. Posture and uterine contractions, Am. J. Obstet. Gynecol. **103:**1, 1969.

Ueland, K., and Hansen, J.M.: Maternal cardiovascular dynamics, III. Labor and delivery under local and caudal analgesia, Am. J. Obstet. Gynecol. **103:**8, 1969.

Ueland, K., Novy, M.J., and Metcalfe, J.: Hemodynamic responses of patients with heart disease to pregnancy and exercise, Am. J. Obstet. Gynecol. **113:**47, 1972.

Weinstein, R.A., Boyer, K.M., and Linn, E.S.: Isolation guidelines for obstetric patients and newborn infants, Am. J. Obstet. Gynecol. **146:**353, 1983.

Weinstein, A.M., Dubin, B.D., Podleski, W.K., Spector, S.L., and Farr, R.S.: Asthma and pregnancy, J.A.M.A. **241:**1161, 1979.

Whalley, P.J., Pritchard, J.A., and Richards, J.R., Jr.: Sickle cell trait and pregnancy, J.A.M.A. **186:**1132, 1963.

Whittemore, R., Hobbins, J.C., and Engel, M.A.: Pregnancy and its outcome in women with and without treatment of congenital heart disease, Am. J. Cardiol. **50:**641, 1982.

24

J. Robert Willson

Digestive tract disorders during pregnancy

The structural and functional changes that occur in the digestive organs during pregnancy may account for many disturbing symptoms. In the majority of gravid women the secretion of free hydrochloric acid and pepsin decreases, and gastric motility is reduced. The stomach is pushed upward and to the left by the enlarging uterus, and the tone of the entire intestinal tract is reduced.

CARE OF THE TEETH

Pregnancy does not induce or hasten tooth decay, but pregnant women should make regular visits to their dentists.

Dental operations do not cause abortion or other pregnancy complications. On the contrary, it is to the patient's advantage to have dental disorders corrected, regardless of the gestation period. Local anesthesia should be used when an anesthetic is necessary.

GINGIVITIS

In about 50% of pregnant women the gums hypertrophy and become inflamed, spongy, and friable. The cause is not known, but it appears to be related to poor oral hygiene and the hormonal changes associated with pregnancy. The condition regresses spontaneously after delivery. Astringent mouthwashes may provide symptomatic relief for gingivitis.

PTYALISM

Excessive salivation is occasionally encountered. It usually corrects itself spontaneously by the middle of the second trimester, but during the peak of saliva production more than 1 L may be secreted daily. Although tincture of belladonna, atropine, and other drugs may be prescribed, they alter the salivary secretion only slightly.

NAUSEA AND VOMITING

The nausea and vomiting experienced by at least half of all women during the first trimester of pregnancy varies in degree from mild, transient morning nausea to severe, constant vomiting that endangers the life of the patient. The symptoms usually appear within 2 weeks after the period has been missed, reach a maximum in about 2 more weeks, and then begin to regress by the tenth to twelfth week of gestation. They usually disappear completely by the fourteenth week, but in a few women, nausea persists throughout the pregnancy. Nausea and vomiting usually reappear and, in fact, may become worse with each pregnancy.

Nausea and vomiting that begin after the tenth to twelfth week are more likely to be caused by a medical or surgical condition than by pregnancy alone.

The nausea is most likely to occur when the stomach is empty, on arising in the morning or before meals, and it may be precipitated by certain odors or foods. In many women, it is present on awakening and may persist until they have eaten breakfast. In others the symptoms are somewhat more pronounced; a few will be nauseated all day, and an occasional patient develops true *hyperemesis gravidarum,* with constant nausea and frequent vomiting that may seriously affect health.

Brandes found that about 75% of 7027 pregnant women experienced nausea and vomiting during the first trimester; there was an even higher incidence with multifetal gestations. The perinatal mortality rate was increased in those without nausea (39.2 versus 33.4); the rate of small babies and early delivery was also increased in those who were free from symptoms.

The less severe degrees of nausea do not interfere with nutrition, and weight loss is slight; but hyperemesis may produce serious physiologic disturbances. The patient may lose 20 or more pounds and become severely dehydrated. The pulse increases to 110 to 120, and the temperature rises to 38 to 38.3 C (100.5 to 101 F). The serum electrolyte concentrations are reduced because of the unreplaced loss of sodium, chloride, and potassium in the vomitus. Blood urea nitrogen increases, and a metabolic acidosis develops. The degree of change is determined by the duration and severity of the vomiting and the food and fluid ingestion.

The histopathologic changes in women who die of hyperemesis are like those that occur with starvation and include centrilobular fatty infiltration of the liver, sometimes with necrosis; degenerative changes in the renal tubules; punctate hemorrhages in the brain and retina; and degenerative neuritis in the peripheral nerves.

Etiologic factors. The underlying causes responsible for nausea and vomiting during pregnancy are not completely clear, but it seems likely that the disturbance is caused by the addition of some substance new to the patient rather than by the sudden development of a deficiency of vitamins, hormones, or other substances. The symptoms appear at a time during which the trophoblastic tissue is actively invading and destroying the decidua and when the function of the endocrine organs and hormone production are being drastically altered. Nausea is most pronounced when gonadotropin production reaches a maximum during the first trimester of normal pregnancy and is likely to be more troublesome with hydatidiform mole and multiple pregnancy, with which gonadotropin levels are even higher.

Soules and co-workers found no relationship between the levels of chorionic gonadotropin and the severity of nausea in women with normal pregnancies and those with hydatidiform moles. Conversely, Kauppila, Huhtaniemi, and Ylikorkala reported higher titers of serum gonadotropins between 7 and 14 gestational weeks in women with hyperemesis as compared to those whose pregnancies were uncomplicated by excessive vomiting.

It is not likely that nausea is initiated by an emotional disturbance, but women with such disturbances are more likely to vomit, and the nausea can certainly be aggravated by psychologic stimuli. In all probability most instances of severe nausea and vomiting (hyperemesis gravidarum) develop as a result of an emotionally stimulated increase of the "normal" pregnancy nausea. Psychiatric studies indicate that many women with hyperemesis unconsciously wish not to be pregnant, even though they may profess to want children. Some have even undergone extensive studies and treatment for infertility, whereas others have experienced orgasmic dysfunction, dyspareunia, and aversion to coitus.

Treatment. Since the basic cause for nausea and vomiting during pregnancy has not yet been established, treatment must of necessity be directed toward reducing the severity of the symptoms. Each patient should understand that the symptoms are temporary and that they not only can be improved but should disappear within a short time.

Nausea that appears in the morning when the stomach is empty can usually be eliminated by having the patient eat two or three soda crackers as soon as she awakens and before she gets out of bed. After 15 to 20 minutes she arises and eats a light breakfast, and, if there is no recurrence of the nausea during the day, no other treatment is necessary.

Nausea that is constant throughout the day often can be controlled by frequent small feedings, keeping something in the stomach at all times. The patient is directed to eat in small amounts at least every 2 hours from the time she awakens until bedtime. Dry foods such as crackers, toast, baked potato, white meat of chicken, and cereal are preferable because they are more likely to control the nausea. Hard candy frequently is effective. Liquids should be taken between feedings rather than with solid food; tea, ginger ale or other carbonated beverages, or anything else the patient can retain are permitted. It usually is not possible for these patients to adhere to a full pregnancy diet.

Many types of medication have been used in patients with nausea and vomiting during pregnancy, but none is uniformly effective. The mild symptoms can usually be controlled with diet alone, so drugs are unnecessary. If, however, the symptoms are more severe and do not respond to diet therapy, some sort of medication may be prescribed. Bendectin (doxylamine succinate and pyridoxine hydrochloride) was the most effective of these; but even though there is no evidence to suggest that the preparation interferes with early fetal development, it has been withdrawn from the market because of many lawsuits alleging that it caused anomalies.

The patient who has lost considerable weight and is dehydrated because of hyperemesis must be admitted to the hospital. The important factors in the treatment of hyperemesis are (1) to control the vomiting, (2) to replace the fluid, (3) to replace water-soluble vitamins, and (4) to restore electrolyte balance. Interruption of pregnancy, which has been resorted to frequently in the past, is almost never necessary.

The type and amount of *intravenous fluid* necessary to hydrate the patient and restore chemical balance will be determined by the urine volume and serum electrolyte and creatinine concentrations, which should be repeated daily. Ascorbic acid and vitamin B complex should be administered in the parenteral fluids; a protein hydrolysate solution can also be given if the patient is seriously depleted. Parenteral administration of fluids is continued until the patient is able to retain food and fluids.

Prochlorperazine dimaleate (Compazine) can be administered intramuscularly in doses of 5 to 10 mg every 6 to 8 hours. If prochlorperazine alone does not control the vomiting, it may be necessary to reinforce its *sedative action* with intramuscular injections of amobarbital (Amytal) sodium, 0.4 to 0.6 g every 6 to 8 hours. It is seldom necessary to continue heavy sedation for longer than 48 to 72 hours.

The *diet* must be limited until the vomiting is controlled, after which small amounts of food can be ordered. One should proceed slowly with the addition of foods because the vomiting may recur if the progression toward a normal diet is too rapid.

Once the vomiting has been stopped and chemical balance has been restored, the pregnancy usually progresses without a recurrence of the symptoms. Occasionally, the vomiting does recur when the patient leaves the protective environment of the hospital, only to be easily controlled by readmittance. In such instances an emotional cause is likely, and an attempt should be made to identify the responsible factor in the patient's life situation.

HEARTBURN

Heartburn is a common complaint during pregnancy and varies in severity from occasional mild discomfort to constant incapacitating pain accompanied by nausea and vomiting. It is caused by regurgitation of stomach contents into the lower esophagus and, according to Lind and co-workers, is a result of changes in the pressure relationships in the stomach and in the esophagus at the level of the gastroesophageal sphincter. Reflux of acid stomach contents can occur if the pressure in the stomach is considerably higher than that in the esophagus.

In normal nonpregnant subjects the mean resting intragastric pressure was 12.1 cm H_2O, the sphincter pressure was 34.8 cm H_2O, and the stomach-to-sphincter gradient was 22.7 cm H_2O. In pregnant women without heartburn the mean intragastric pressure was 17.2 cm H_2O, the maximum sphincter pressure was 44.8 cm H_2O, and the stomach-to-sphincter gradient was 27.6 cm H_2O, the latter being comparable to the control subjects. There was a striking difference in the pregnant women with heartburn; the intragastric pressure was unaltered, being 16.5 cm H_2O, but the maximal sphincter pressure was only 23.8 cm H_2O. The stomach-to-sphincter gradient of 7.3 cm H_2O was obviously not high enough to prevent reflex of stomach contents.

The management of heartburn is similar to that described for hiatus hernia.

HIATUS HERNIA

Hiatus hernia can be demonstrated in about 12% of women during the last half of pregnancy. It is more often present in multiparas than in primigravidas and may produce annoying or even serious symptoms. Heartburn, which usually begins before the middle of pregnancy, is almost always present with hiatus hernia. It is usually made worse by lying down; therefore it often is noted at night and may interfere with sleep. Belching, hiccoughing, and regurgitation of sour material into the mouth also occur, but nausea and vomiting are somewhat less characteristic.

Since the hernias almost always disappear after delivery, treatment should be directed toward controlling symptoms; surgical correction is almost never necessary. The regimen should include frequent small bland feedings, antacids such as aluminum hydroxide or magnesium trisilicate tablets taken whenever necessary. Elevation of the head on several pillows when the patient lies down will reduce regurgitation through the relaxed esophagogastric junction.

JAUNDICE

Although no definite histopathologic changes can be observed in liver cells by light microscopy, there are evidences of altered liver function. *Sodium sulfobromophthalein (BSP) excretion* is reduced; *serum alkaline phosphatase* may be doubled, probably from a source in the syncitiotrophoblast; and *plasma albumin concentrations* and *plasma cholinesterase activity* are reduced. *Serum cholesterol* is slightly increased, and *spider nevi* and *palmar erythema* may develop. The changes are thought to be caused by the increase in circulating estrogens. The usual liver function tests aspartate aminotransferase (AST, formerly serum glutamic–oxaloacetic transaminase [SGOT]) and alanine aminotransferase (ALT, formerly serum glutamic–pyruvic transaminase [SGPT]) are usually within the normal range. Jaundice develops in about one of 1500 pregnant women.

Intrahepatic cholestasis of pregnancy. A small percentage of women become jaundiced during the last trimester of pregnancy without having definite evidence of viral hepatitis or other liver disease. Icterus usually is preceded by anorexia, nausea with or without vomiting, and pruritus. Liver function tests are altered: *serum alkaline phosphatase*

is elevated above the normal concentration for pregnancy, *AST activity* may be normal or slightly increased, and the *serum bile acids* (cholic acid, chenodeoxycholic acid, and deoxycholic acid) are consistently elevated. Histopathologic changes, which are characteristic of *intrahepatic cholestasis,* include centrilobular bile staining of the liver cells, canalicular bile plugs, and occasionally slight parenchymal cell necrosis. This condition, which is known as *idiopathic intrahepatic cholestasis of pregnancy,* clears promptly after delivery, and there is no demonstrable residual.

Reid and Ivey observed one neonatal and five intrauterine deaths between 33 and 34 weeks in 56 women with cholestasis. There were 18 spontaneous premature deliveries, and eight infants developed severe bradycardia during labor. Postpartum hemorrhage occurred in 10 of the 50 vaginal deliveries, and five women lost more than 2000 ml of blood.

Pruritus gravidarum, with which there is generalized itching that is difficult to relieve by any form of medication, is probably the same basic condition but with less impairment of hepatic function, since there is no accompanying jaundice.

Cholestyramine, a bile acid–exchange resin agent, relieves the itching. It may be less effective in well-established cases of cholestasis than in mild pruritus gravidarum.

Cholestasis and pruritus gravidarum occur during late pregnancy and are thought to be caused by the response of the liver cells to estrogen, which reaches its maximal concentration during this period of gestation. Kreek and co-workers treated a group of nonpregnant women who previously had pruritus or cholestasis during pregnancy with large doses of ethinyl estradiol and reproduced the symptoms they had experienced. Normal control subjects experienced only mild morning nausea or had no symptoms during the treatment period.

ACUTE FATTY LIVER OF PREGNANCY

Acute fatty liver of pregnancy is a rare but potentially lethal disease that appears to be peculiar to pregnancy, during which it develops without obvious cause. A similar condition can occur when severe pyelonephritis is treated with large doses of tetracycline and in patients with Reye's syndrome. The symptoms, malaise, persistent vomiting, abdominal pain, and jaundice usually begin after the thirtieth week of pregnancy. Often disseminated intravascular coagulation is associated with these conditions. Characteristic histologic changes include infiltration of liver cells with fine fat droplets with minimal evidence of necrosis or inflammatory response. The only known treatment is delivery, by either induction of labor or cesarean section (despite the risks caused by the coagulopathy), after which the process subsides. With medical therapy the maternal mortality is at least 75%.

VIRAL HEPATITIS

Acute viral hepatitis occurs during pregnancy with the same frequency that it does in nonpregnant women and is a cause for at least 40% of the cases of jaundice. It is equally distributed throughout the three trimesters. Infections are caused by hepatitis A (HAV) or hepatitis B (HBV) viruses. The former, infectious hepatitis, is transmitted by contaminated food or water; and the latter, serum hepatitis, by innoculation with blood, blood products, saliva, or semen or vaginal secretions. Another form, non-A-non-B, is usually transmitted by blood transfusions. Hepatitis can also be caused by cytomegalovirus and by Epstein-Barr virus infections.

Hepatitis A infections are usually relatively innocuous and may not be diagnosed unless jaundice develops. There is no specific treatment. The risk to the fetus is not great; there is no evidence of teratogenicity, and the virus does not appear to be transmitted to the fetus. There may be an increased incidence of preterm delivery.

Hepatitis B infections occur more often and offer more risk than do those caused by HAV. The incidences of anomalies and fetal death are not increased, but that of premature delivery is. In addition, the fetus may be infected during or after delivery if the mother has active disease, is a carrier, or has chronic active hepatitis. This is known as *vertical transmission*. HBV is a DNA virus containing a surface antigen (HB_sAG), a core antigen (HB_cAG), and HB_EAG, all of which stimulate antibody production. During the ususal infection the antigens disappear as the infection clears, but the induced antibodies remain.

In patients with chronic active hepatitis B, HB_sAG and HB_EAG remain; HB_c antibody can be detected, but antibodies to the other antigens are absent. In asymptomatic chronic carriers HB_sAG and anti-HB persist, but HB_EAG is replaced by HB_E antibody.

The infants of mothers with chronic active HBV infections and of those who are carriers can be infected from ingesting maternal secretions, blood or amniotic fluid and from nursing. Some affected infants are asymptomatic, some develop fulminating disease and eventually die from cirrhosis, and others become chronic carriers.

The initial symptoms of viral hepatitis consist of anorexia, nausea, vomiting, headache, lassitude, and fever. Jaundice becomes evident in about 1 week and may last as long as 4 to 6 weeks. The recovery period may extend over a 2- to 3-month period.

The mortality is low for those who were in good health at the time they contracted the disease and who are provided with adequate diets and rest as they recover. Both maternal and perinatal mortalities are increased in poor, undernourished women who do not receive proper medical attention.

Treatment is primarily of a supportive nature and includes a diet high in carbohydrate, protein, and vitamins and the prevention of dehydration. If the patient is vomiting or has severe anorexia, nutrition can be maintained temporarily by intravenous administration of these substances. Termination of pregnancy is not necessary.

Immune globulin preparations should be administered to pregnant women who are at risk of developing hepatitis through their work or because of travel in areas where the disease is endemic. Infection of the newborn infant can usually be prevented by injection of hepatitis B immune globulin soon after birth, followed by hepatitis B vaccine.

PEPTIC ULCER

The symptoms of peptic ulcer often subside during pregnancy, since gastric acidity and motility are reduced. Clark reported that 44.8% of 118 women with peptic ulcer were free from symptoms during 313 pregnancies, whereas 43.4% were improved; pregnancy had no effect on 11.8%. Perforation and hemorrhage are rare, but either may occur. Medical treatment can be continued during pregnancy, but it may be necessary to alter the diet to meet the added nutritional requirements.

PANCREATITIS

Acute pancreatitis is rare in pregnant women, and, when it occurs, it often is not diagnosed. The clinical course is similar to that in nonpregnant women, but the presence of an advanced pregnancy may prejudice the medical attendants. The basic confirmatory study, elevated activity of serum amylase, is as valid during pregnancy as in nonpregnant women.

Pancreatitis may occur in pregnant women being

treated with thiazide preparations and tetracycline and should be considered when a patient receiving treatment with these preparations develops abdominal pain, nausea, and vomiting.

The treatment is supportive, and operation is contraindicated if the diagnosis of pancreatitis is confirmed.

INFLAMMATORY BOWEL DISEASE

The outcome of pregnancy in women with inflammatory bowel disease is often determined by the activity of the disease at conception. Those who conceive during periods of activity appear to be at greater risk of aborting or of delivering prematurely. If either ulcerative colitis or Crohn's disease is inactive at conception, the risk of exacerbation is not great. Conversely, exacerbation occurs more often when the disease is active or has recently undergone remission when pregnancy is initiated.

Mogadam and colleagues studied 531 pregnancies in women with inflammatory bowel disease in an attempt to determine whether the diseases or the medications used to treat them had any effect on the outcome of pregnancy. Of the 531 women, 287 (172 with ulcerative colitis and 115 with Crohn's disease) were treated with corticosteroids, sulfasalazine, or both. A second group of 244 women (137 with ulcerative colitis and 107 with Crohn's disease) received neither drug. There were no significant differences in the rates of abortion, premature delivery, congenital defects, perinatal loss, and maternal death among the women in the study groups and between the women with bowel disease and the general population. The patients with Crohn's disease who needed both drugs had more complications than did those who were untreated and those taking only sulfasalazine. There were no differences in patients with ulcerative colitis.

Diseases requiring surgery

Acute surgical emergencies involving the gastrointestinal organs occur no less frequently in gravid than in nongravid women of a like age and must be treated in the same manner. With prompt diagnosis and surgical intervention, the operative risk is not increased because of the pregnancy; but complications develop rapidly, and the prognosis is more serious in the pregnant woman if a necessary operation is deferred.

Physiologic changes associated with pregnancy can increase the difficulty of early diagnosis. *"Physiologic" nausea and vomiting may be pres-*ent during the early weeks, but they never begin after the first trimester and are not associated with abdominal pain.*

A leukocytosis of 12,000 or 14,000 is not uncommon during pregnancy, but granulocytosis with an increasing percentage of nonsegmented forms is abnormal. The *sedimentation rate* is increased in pregnancy and is of no value in differential diagnosis.

Pain must be distinguished from discomfort related to the enlarging uterus, the pelvic ligaments, the corpus luteum, or urinary tract disturbances.

The choice of anesthetic is the joint responsibility of the anesthesiologist and the obstetrician, with major considerations being freedom from pain, adequate relaxation, safety, and prevention of fetal hypoxia.

Endocrine therapy for prevention of abortion after operative procedures is rarely necessary. The incidence of abortion is low if the uterus is not manipulated and its serosa is not involved in an infectious process. If progesterone is used at all, particularly after surgical procedures that disturb the corpus luteum, the dosage should be adequate. At least 250 mg should be given daily for the first few days and the amount reduced gradually thereafter. Beta-adrenergic drugs may also be used to inhibit contractions.

Antibiotic therapy is neither necessary nor desirable as a prophylactic measure simply because of the pregnancy. However, these drugs may be lifesaving when an operation must be performed in a contaminated field or when the problem is already complicated by infection. They should then be used in full amounts for a sufficient time and in accordance with the culture and sensitivity patterns.

APPENDICITIS

Acute appendicitis occurs with the same frequency in pregnant as in nonpregnant women, but the diagnosis is more difficult, and delay in treatment is hazardous. In 373 cases of acute appendicitis during pregnancy, Black found no maternal deaths when appendicitis developed during the first trimester, 3.9% in the second trimester, 10.9% in the third trimester, and 16.7% during delivery.

The enlarged uterus may obscure the appendix, which tends to be displaced upward and laterally in the direction of the right iliac crest (Fig. 24-1). Its ultimate position, however, is variable.

Suppuration of the acutely inflamed appendix is rapid, and rupture occurs early. Diffuse spreading peritonitis results because the increased vascularity, reduced omental protection, and motion of the uterus hinder localization. Abortion or premature labor may occur if the infection involves the uterine serosa. Uterine contractions stimulated by the infection are frequently tetanic and predispose to fetal hypoxia and intrauterine fetal death.

Diagnosis. Nausea and vomiting, epigastric pain localizing in the right side of the abdomen, and tenderness anywhere from McBurney's point to the right flank are suggestive. Evidences of infection including elevated temperature and, more particularly, an increased pulse rate are usually present. A single white blood count is of doubtful value in the questionable case because a slight leukocytosis is physiologic during pregnancy. Serial studies at hourly intervals that reveal an increase in both total count and in young polymorphonuclear cells indicate the presence of an acute infectious process.

Differential diagnosis. Urinary tract infection or ureteral stone presents the greatest difficulty in the differential diagnosis. Examination of a catheterized urine sample is indicated in every case and should be repeated in an hour or two if the diagnosis is questionable. In the last trimester appendicitis must be differentiated from abruptio placentae or uncomplicated premature labor.

Treatment. Appendicitis complicating pregnancy requires surgery as soon as the diagnosis can be established.

Technical difficulties are increased late in pregnancy because of the large uterus and the position of the appendix. Tilting of the patient to the left side is helpful. If leakage or perforation has occurred, the peritoneal cavity should be lavaged with large quantities of warm saline solution, and large dosages of broad-spectrum antibiotics should be administered parenterally. Since abortion or premature labor after appendectomy is not related

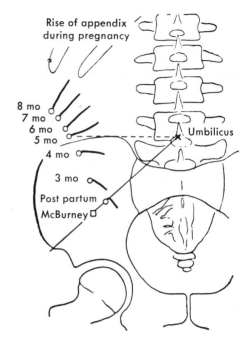

Fig. 24-1. Rise of appendix at various stages of pregnancy. (From Baer, J.L., Reis, R.A., and Arens, R.A.: J.A.M.A. **98**:1359, 1932.)

to changes in hormone levels, the administration of progesterone after surgery is of little value.

If labor ensues soon after surgery and cannot be stopped, it should be conducted according to usual obstetric principles, but elimination of the second stage by low forceps delivery to prevent voluntary bearing-down efforts is advisable. Caudal or epidural anesthesia during labor and delivery can be a valuable aid in such circumstances.

Maternal mortality is no higher in gravid than in nongravid patients if there is no delay. After perforation the threat to the pregnant woman increases because a large uterus may prevent adequate localization of the infection. Fetal loss associated with peritonitis is high.

INTESTINAL OBSTRUCTION

Intestinal obstruction should be suspected in any pregnant woman with a history of previous abdominal surgery or infection in whom abdominal pain is accompanied by nausea, vomiting, and constipation. Changes in size and shape of the uterus, which then exerts tension on intraperitoneal adhesive bands, or kinking and constriction of adherent bowel are the usual causes. Volvulus accounts for 15% to 25% of all cases of intestinal obstruction.

Early in pregnancy, valuable time may be lost if the symptoms are regarded as physiologic nausea and vomiting, but examination of the patient should clarify this problem, since pain, tenderness, and distention are not characteristic of any physiologic process. *Vomiting that makes its first appearance after the first trimester must be considered to be caused by some condition other than pregnancy itself.* During late pregnancy recurrent colicky pains must be differentiated from labor.

Decompression and correction of blood volume deficits with fluid, electrolytes, and plasma as indicated are essential first steps in management, but the necessary surgery should be performed as soon as possible thereafter. Operation should be aimed at removing the cause of obstruction without disturbing the pregnancy, even though labor ensues within a few hours; however, if exposure cannot be otherwise obtained, the uterus must be emptied irrespective of the gestation period.

RECTAL OPERATIONS

Hemorrhoids. Because of pressure from the enlarging uterus and the predisposition to constipation during pregnancy, the hemorrhoidal veins are frequently dilated. Medical treatment is preferable during the prenatal and puerperal periods, except for the acutely painful thrombotic hemorrhoid, which can be incised and the clot evacuated with local anesthesia. Hemorrhoidectomy is indicated only in the rare instance in which bleeding is persistent and depleting despite conservative therapy.

Rectal carcinoma. Cancer of the rectum is an unusual but serious complication of pregnancy. In Bacon and Rowe's experience, therapeutic abortion is not essential during the first trimester; they advise radical surgical removal of the cancerous rectum with regional lymph node dissection but without hysterectomy if the patient does not want the pregnancy terminated. During the second trimester the enlarged uterus interferes with visibility and should be removed. After the twenty-eighth week,

definitive operation is preceded by cesarean section. Of 21 cases involving surgery during pregnancy, the fetal salvage was 85%, and the maternal mortality 10%.

GALLBLADDER DISEASE

Physiologic changes during pregnancy alter gallbladder function. Real-time ultrasonographic studies by Braverman, Johnson, and Kern revealed that after the first trimester the gallbladder volume, during fasting and after contraction, was twice that of nonpregnant control subjects. Delayed emptying time and incomplete evacuation permits the retention of cholesterol crystals. This may account for the increased incidence of cholelithiasis in parous women. Similar changes did not occur in women who were using oral contraceptives.

Symptoms usually appear in the latter half of pregnancy during the period corresponding to physiologic or gestational biliary stasis, but they may be encountered at any stage. In early pregnancy, pain and jaundice, if present, serve to differentiate cholecystitis and cholelithiasis from simple nausea and vomiting. In late pregnancy, gallbladder disease must be differentiated from severe preeclampsia, in which vomiting, upper abdominal pain, tenderness over the liver, and occasionally jaundice may be present. Gallstones can be demonstrated by ultrasonographic examination.

Medical management is preferred during pregnancy, and, in most cases, regulation of the diet and antispasmodic drugs provide adequate control. Operation should be performed if medical treatment fails or in patients with impacted common-duct stone or empyema.

HERNIA

Hernias may appear or increase in size during pregnancy. Inherently weak fascial structures are further weakened by the pressure of the enlarging uterus and by the effects of pregnancy hormones.

Inguinal or *femoral hernias* rarely give rise to serious complications. The enlarging uterus pushes the bowel upward and tends to occlude the defect.

Umbilical hernias are most common. If the ring is small, adherent omentum may fill the sac. Tension often produces pain, but obstruction is unusual. Large umbilical defects and ventral hernias are more likely to contain bowel, but these can be readily reduced. During labor the use of an abdominal support adds to the patient's comfort and prevents the uterus from protruding through a large ventral defect. Except in the rare instance in which strangulation occurs, herniorrhaphy should be delayed until after delivery.

JEJUNOILEAL BYPASS

Grossly obese women who have had jejunoileal bypass operations are usually young and are likely to become pregnant. The information on pregnancy after bypass operations is limited, but the infants appear to do well, although they may weigh slightly less than average. Most of the mothers experienced no metabolic disturbances during their pregnancies. The diet should be supplemented with iron, folic acid, vitamin B_{12}, and other vitamins. Ketosis should be prevented.

REFERENCES

Bacon, H.E., and Rowe, R.J.: Abdominoperineal proctosigmoidectomy for rectal cancer complicating pregnancy, South. Med. J. **40**:471, 1947.

Black, W.P.: Acute appendicitis in pregnancy, Br. Med. J. **1**:1938, 1960.

Brandes, J.M.: First trimester nausea and vomiting as related to outcome of pregnancy, Obstet. Gynecol. **30**:427, 1967.

Braverman, D.Z., Johnson, M.L., and Kern, F., Jr.: Effects of pregnancy and contraceptive steroids on gallbladder function, N. Engl. J. Med. **301**:362, 1980.

Cohen, M. and Cohen, H.: Dealing with viral hepatitis during pregnancy, Contemp. Obstet. Gynecol. **22**:29, 1983.

Donaldson, R.M., Jr.: Management of medical problems in pregnancy-Inflammatory bowel disease, N. Engl. J. Med. **312**:1616, 1985.

Douvas, S.G., et al.: Liver disease in pregnancy, Obstet. Gynecol. Surv. **38**:531, 1983.

Fairweather, D.V.I.: Nausea and vomiting in pregnancy, Am. J. Obstet. Gynecol. **102**:135, 1968.

Heikkinen, J., Mäentausta, O., Ylöstalo, P., and Jänne, O.: Changes in serum bile acid concentrations during normal pregnancy, in patients with intrahepatic cholestasis of pregnancy and in pregnant women with itching, Br. J. Obstet. Gynaecol. **88**:240, 1981.

Johnston, W.G., and Baskett, M.B.: Obstetric cholestasis, Am. J. Obstet. Gynecol. **133**:299, 1979.

Kaplan, M.M.: Acute fatty liver in pregnancy, N. Engl. J. Med. **313**:367, 1985.

Kauppila, A., Huhtaniemi, I., and Ylikorkala, O.: Raised serum human chorionic gonadotropin concentrations in hyperemesis gravidarum, Br. Med. J. **1**:1670, 1979.

Kreek, M.J., Weser, E., Sleisenger, M.H., and Jefferies, G.H.: Idiopathic cholestasis of pregnancy, N. Engl. J. Med. **277**:1391, 1967.

Lind, J.F., Smith, A.M., McIver, D.K., Coopland, A.T., and Crispin, J.S.: Heartburn in pregnancy: a manometric study, Can. Med. Assoc. J. **98**:571, 1968.

Mixson, W.T., and Woloshin, H.J.: Hiatus hernia in pregnancy, Obstet. Gynecol. **8**:249, 1956.

Mogadam, M., Dobbins, W.O., Ill, Korelitz, B.I., and Ahmed, S.W.: Pregnancy in inflammatory bowel disease: effect of sulfasalazine and corticosteroids on fetal outcome, Gastroenterology **80**:72, 1981.

Nielsen, O.H., et al.: Pregnancy in ulcerative colitis, Scand. J. Gastroenterol. **18**:735, 1983.

Reid, R., and Ivey, K.J.: Fetal complications of obstetric cholestasis, Br. Med. J. **1**:870, 1976.

Sherlock, S.: Acute fatty liver of pregnancy and the microvesicular fat diseases, Gut **24**:265, 1983.

Soules, M.R., et al.: Nausea and vomiting of pregnancy. Role of human chorionic gonadotropin and 17-hydroxy progesterone, Obstet. Gynecol. **55**:696, 1980.

Varner, M., and Rinderknecht, N.K.: Acute fatty metamorphosis of pregnancy, J. Reprod. Med. **24**:177, 1980.

Wilkinson, E.J.: Acute pancreatitis in pregnancy: a review of 98 cases and a report of 8 new cases, Obstet. Gynecol. Surv. **28**:281, 1973.

Wong, V.C.W., Lee, A.K.Y., and Ip, H.M.H.: Transmission of hepatitis B antigens from symptom free mothers to the fetus and infants, Br. J. Obstet. Gynaecol. **87**:958, 1980.

Woods, J.R., Jr., and Brinkman, C.R., III: The jejunoileal bypass and pregnancy. Obstet. Gynecol. Surv. **33**:697, 1978.

25

J. Robert Willson

Urinary tract disorders during pregnancy

The structure and function of the urinary organs are altered considerably during pregnancy, but unless the tissues are seriously damaged by infection or direct injury, they return to normal during the puerperium. It is important that physicians be completely familiar with the structural and functional changes that occur during pregnancy; otherwise they will be unable to assess the risks of pregnancy for women with renal diseases, and they may interpret physiologic alterations as abnormalities.

The outstanding anatomic change is *dilatation of the ureters and the renal pelvis*. The changes begin late in the first trimester and are progressive throughout pregnancy. They are more pronounced in primigravidas than in multiparas and on the right side than on the left. The reason for the hydronephrosis is presumed to be pressure from the enlarging uterus. The right side is more often involved than the left because of greater pressure caused by the normal dextrorotation of the uterus. One reason why the left side is spared may be that the sigmoid colon acts as a cushion between the ureter and the uterus. The high levels of progesterone may decrease ureteral tone and inhibit contractions.

The major functional effects of these normal physiologic changes are reduced ureteral tone and peristalsis, resulting in delayed flow of urine through the upper tract.

The *glomerular filtration rate* and *renal plasma flow* in normal women begin to increase as early as the tenth week of pregnancy. Glomerular filtration may increase as much as 50% by the twentieth week; it continues to rise somewhat more slowly and remains elevated until delivery. Effective renal plasma flow also begins to rise early in pregnancy, but it increases less than does glomerular filtration, and it decreases during the third trimester.

Some of the discrepancies in studies on renal function may be related to the position of the subjects during the tests. Renal plasma flow, glomerular filtration, and sodium excretion may be much lower in the supine than in the lateral recumbent position during late pregnancy.

The *specific gravity* of urine during pregnancy often is as low as 1.01, and the kidney may be unable to concentrate urine to more than 1.02 or 1.022 during a standard concentration test. The concentrating ability returns to normal after delivery.

Diurnal changes in concentrating ability must also be recognized. In normal nonpregnant women, urine volume is decreased, and specific gravity is increased during the night. The reverse is true during pregnancy. The extravascular fluid volume is

335

expanded during the day as a result of leakage from the plasma caused by the upright position. The excess tissue fluid returns to the bloodstream and is excreted during the night when the woman is in a horizontal position. This accounts both for nocturia and for the low specific gravity of early morning specimens.

The normally functioning kidney does not permit the passage of more than *500 mg of protein daily.*

Renal function tests such as phenolsulfonphthalein, which are dependent on measuring the amount of a foreign substance excreted in the urine during specific time periods after a single injection, are not reliable during pregnancy. Although the kidneys excrete the material at a normal rate, its passage to the bladder may be delayed because of pyeloureteral dilatation, reduced ureteral peristalsis, and the resultant stasis of urine; hence the results may fall into an abnormal range. This is less likely to occur when one measures excretion rates of a substance such as *endogenous creatinine,* which is produced at a relatively constant rate, or of a foreign substance such as *inulin* when a high plasma concentration is maintained by constant infusion.

When 2- or 3-hour clearance studies are run, it is essential that (1) the urine volume be at least 2 ml/min, (2) the bladder be emptied completely by catheter at the end of each accurately timed collection period, and (3) the patient be in the lateral recumbent rather than the supine position to obtain maximal renal perfusion and function. Although less accurate than well-controlled inulin clearances, 24-hour creatinine clearances are adequate for clinical use.

The sustained increase in glomerular filtration during normal pregnancy allows for more efficient excretion of the products of nitrogen metabolism. The concentration of *urea nitrogen* in the serum is generally between 8 and 12 mg/dl, and that of *creatinine,* about 0.5 mg/dl. Urea nitrogen concentrations greater than 15 mg/dl and concentrations of creatinine much greater than 1 mg/dl must be considered as abnormal.

Cystoscopy can be performed throughout pregnancy, but during the last 4 to 6 weeks it may be relatively uninformative. At this period of gestation the bladder is pulled upward, and the presenting part descends, making insertion of the instrument and inspection of the interior of the bladder difficult.

X-ray film studies of the urinary tract should rarely be performed because of possible ill effects on the fetus. Heavy exposure during the first few weeks may disturb embryonic development. If an x-ray film study is essential, it should be performed with the smallest amount of radiation that will provide the information needed. Urography can usually be delayed until after delivery.

INFECTION

Urinary tract infections occur frequently during pregnancy and after delivery, but almost all of them can be prevented. From 2% to 10% of all pregnant women have a significant but *asymptomatic bacteriuria* (more than 100,000 colonies/ml of a single organism in a catheterized or clean, voided urine specimen). The probability that a woman will develop bacteriuria is determined by her parity, race, and socioeconomic status. The lowest incidence is in white, primigravid, private patients, and the highest is in black multiparas with sickle-cell trait.

Of those with asymptomatic bacteriuria, 30% will develop symptomatic urinary tract infections during late pregnancy or the puerperium. Whalley, Martin, and Pritchard found bacteriuria in 13.9% of 475 pregnant women with sickle-cell trait as compared with 6.9% of a control group. A third of the bacteriuric women with sickle-cell trait developed symptomatic infections during pregnancy, and 13.6% after delivery. Comparable figures for control bacteriuric patients were 18.7% and 12.3%. Of 33 women with sickle-cell trait, 19 had radiographic evidence of chronic pyelonephritis.

The bacteria are usually present during the first trimester, and there usually is no accompanying pyuria. The reason for the bacteriuria is not always obvious, but chronic pyelonephritis or lower tract infections can be demonstrated in some women, particularly those who have had repeated symptomatic urinary tract infections. *Escherichia coli* and *Enterobacter* species are the responsible organisms in most acute infections, but others may be present in women with chronic or recurring infections.

It has been suggested that premature labor is more prevalent in women with asymptomatic bacteriuria, but most investigators have not found this to be true. However, severe, acute pyelonephritis with high fever may be a factor in inducing labor prematurely.

Naeye found a perinatal death rate of 42/1000 births in women with urinary tract infections during pregnancy as compared with 21/1000 in those who were not infected. The excess mortality, most of which was related to maternal hypertension and ketonuria, amniotic fluid bacterial infections, abruptio placentae, and hydramnios, occurred with urinary tract infections that were diagnosed within 15 days of delivery. Further study is necessary to determine whether the deaths were related to the urinary tract infections or to an associated complication, such as chronic renal disease.

Symptomatic infections can generally be prevented if pregnant women with bacteriuria are identified and treated. Whalley, Martin, and Peters found that bacteriuria persisted after delivery in 90 (81%) of 111 women who had positive cultures during pregnancy but who were not treated; it persisted in only 45 (39%) of 115 women who were treated for bacteriuria.

Since asymptomatic bacteriuria is so important in the genesis of symptomatic urinary tract infections during pregnancy or after delivery, it is advisable to screen all obstetric patients for the presence of bacteria. This is particularly important in patient populations in which urinary tract infections occur frequently. Urine culture early in the second trimester detects almost all women with bacteriuria. A diagnosis of bacteriuria should not be made on the basis of a single positive culture, particularly if the colony count is less than 100,000/ml. A positive diagnosis can be made if the same organism is grown on repeat culture, even though the colony count is less than 100,000/ml. The diagnosis is in doubt if repeat culture is negative or if different bacteria are grown. The latter probably represents contamination rather than infection.

An attempt should be made to eradicate the infection. Whalley and Cunningham treated 300 women with asymptomatic bacteriuria during pregnancy with standard doses of sulfamethizole; nitrofurantoin, 200 mg daily for 14 days; or nitrofurantoin, 100 mg daily continuously. The urine was sterilized for the rest of the pregnancy in 65% of those treated for 14 days; most of those who relapsed responded to second or third courses. Of those treated continuously, 88% remained abacteriuric during the pregnancy. Harris reduced the incidence of acute pyelonephritis during pregnancy from 4% to 0.8% by treating patients with asymptomatic bacteriuria actively.

Appropriate treatment for most women with asymptomatic bacteriuria is sulfisoxazole (Gantrisin), 1 g four times daily, or ampicillin, 1 g daily, for infections caused by usual organisms. Nitrofurantoin (Macrodantin), 50 to 100 mg three or four times daily, may be used if the other drugs fail. Treatment should usually be continued for 10 days. Harris, Gilstrap, and Pretty treated 86 pregnant women with single doses of ampicillin, cephalexin (Keflex), nitrofurantoin, or sulfisoxazole and were able to eradicate the infection in 69%. They suggested that this regimen might be appropriate for noncompliant patients.

Repeat urine cultures should be obtained during pregnancy and after delivery in all women who have had either asymptomatic bacteriuria or symptomatic infections during pregnancy.

Urologic study, including pyelograms, is indicated for women who have had repeated infections or those in whom bacteriuria persists after delivery.

URETHROCYSTITIS

Acute lower urinary tract infections occur in 1% to 2% of women during pregnancy and more often after delivery. About one third of those who develop acute infections have had asymptomatic bacteriuria; detection and treatment of the latter would prevent most overt infections.

The principal symptoms are frequency, dysuria, and suprapubic pain and tenderness. The temperature may be normal. Many pus cells, red blood cells, and bacteria can be seen in the urine.

Sulfisoxazole, 1 g, nitrofurantoin, 50 to 100 mg, or ampicillin, 500 mg every 6 hours will eradicate most infections. Treatment should usually be continued for 10 days, although single-dose therapy, as described above, may be sufficient. In addition to antibiotics, patients who have had urinary tract infections should be advised to void at least every 2 hours. Voluntary retention of urine and overdistention of the bladder predisposes to infection.

Pyelonephritis

Infection of the upper urinary tract may develop initially during pregnancy, or women with chronic pyelonephritis may conceive.

Acute pyelonephritis. Acute upper urinary tract infections may develop during pregnancy, usually late in the second trimester, early in the third, or after delivery. They occur in from 1% to 3% of all pregnant women, and although they are treated intensively, they may recur in subsequent pregnancies. Approximately two thirds occur in women who have asymptomatic bacteriuria.

The usual symptoms are chills, fever, flank pain, dysuria, and nausea and vomiting. The temperature may swing from high levels of 40 to 41 C (104 to 106 F) to as low as 34 to 36 C (93 to 97 F). Patients with acute pyelonephritis look ill and usually are dehydrated. Palpation of the kidney area produces severe pain, and there may be tenderness along the course of the ureter and over the bladder. The right kidney is most often involved, but the infection frequently occurs bilaterally.

The diagnosis is confirmed by examination of a catheterized or clean, voided specimen of urine, which will contain many pus cells (single or in clumps), red blood cells, and bacteria. At the peak of the infection the white blood cell count may be as high as 20,000 to 30,000.

The *differential diagnosis* can be difficult, particularly in the recently delivered patient. The pain may begin in the right lower quadrant, and, since nausea and vomiting are frequently encountered in association with urinary tract infections, appendicitis may be suspected. In urinary tract infections there is no muscle spasm, and the urine is infected. Puerperal infection must also be ruled out as a cause in patients who have the symptoms following delivery.

TREATMENT. Undelivered patients with acute pyelonephritis are best treated in the hospital with parenteral antibiotics until the infection is brought under control. Most will respond to ampicillin given intravenously in doses of 1 g every 6 hours for from 48 to 72 hours after which it can be given orally. The temperature usually returns to normal within 3 to 5 days, but the medication should be continued for at least 14 days. If there is no response, another antibiotic, as determined by sensitivity studies, should be ordered. A subsequent urine culture should be taken after the course of treatment is completed.

The patient should be encouraged to ingest at least 3000 ml of fluids daily unless she is vomiting, in which case an equivalent amount of 5% dextrose should be given intravenously. Urinary output should be checked carefully, because renal function is significantly reduced during the acute phase of the infection. Although septic shock is uncommon, it may develop during the first few days of the infection.

Recurrences usually mean that treatment has been discontinued before the infection is eradicated or that the fundamental cause of the infection is still present. If the infection recurs or if bacteriuria persists, an antibiotic or chemotherapeutic agent should be continued until after delivery.

It is seldom necessary to terminate pregnancy because of repeated episodes of pyelonephritis, but occasionally if the patient has several attacks in spite of adequate antibacterial treatment, the physician should consider the possibility of inducing labor as soon as it can be accomplished safely after the fetus has matured. This may prevent permanent damage to the kidney.

The urine should be examined for the presence of infection during the early puerperium and again after involution in all women who have had acute pyelonephritis during pregnancy. If the infection has been recurrent or if bacteriuria persists, pyelograms should be made 2 to 3 months after delivery in an attempt to demonstrate a lesion that could have caused the attacks or any damage that may have been produced by the infection.

Chronic pyelonephritis. If acute pyelonephritis is inadequately treated, the symptoms may subside, but the infection may never be completely eradicated. In time there may be enough tissue damage to impair kidney function and, occasionally, even to cause hypertension and renal insufficiency. However, at least half the women with chronic pyelonephritis have no history of antecedent urinary tract infections.

Chronic infection does not necessarily preclude pregnancy if kidney function is normal, but acute attacks are likely to occur. Women with chronic urinary tract infections can be treated prophylactically with small daily doses of medications throughout pregnancy to prevent acute recurrences. If renal function is impaired and the blood pressure is elevated, pregnancy may be contraindicated. The outcome depends on the ability of the kidney to respond to the demands of pregnancy.

Toxic effects of drugs

The physician must be aware that certain drugs used to treat urinary tract infections may cause undesirable reactions in either the mother or the fetus.

Tetracyclines. Several instances of acute toxic reactions and even death after the administration of tetracycline to pregnant women with pyelonephritis have been reported. In most of them, vomiting persisted, or it first appeared after treatment was started, and azotemia and jaundice developed. Whalley, Adams, and Combes found fine-droplet fatty metamorphosis of the liver and pancreatitis in five patients, one of whom died. The toxicity may be a result of reduced renal function, allowing accumulation of high concentrations of tetracycline in the tissues. This can be prevented by using smaller doses and by stopping the medication if urinary output is reduced, if the blood urea nitrogen concentration increases progressively, or if there are other evidences of renal failure.

Tetracycline may also affect the infant because of its propensity to accumulate in embryonic bone. Tetracycline hydrochloride added to cultures of embryonic bone of experimental animals is deposited throughout the calcified area, preventing normal mineralization. Maldeveloped bones result.

Tetracycline can also be deposited in the enamel

of fetal teeth, giving them a permanent yellow, mottled, fluorescent appearance.

Sulfonamides. Sulfonamides enter the fetal circulation freely and are potentially dangerous if they accumulate in fetal tissues and are not eliminated promptly. Sulfonamides dissociate bilirubin from its binding to albumin, permitting bilirubin to circulate freely and to diffuse into fetal tissues. The most serious complication that may occur from high concentrations of unconjugated bilirubin is kernicterus, particularly in premature infants. This is not likely to occur while the fetus remains in the uterus, because the bilirubin is transferred across the placenta, but it is a problem in newborn infants.

Because of this possibility, sulfonamides should be used with caution during late pregnancy and particularly in women who may deliver prematurely. They should not be used during labor.

Chloramphenicol. Chloramphenicol may depress maternal bone marrow; total white blood cell and differential counts should be obtained twice weekly in an attempt to detect the first evidence of depression. This drug probably has no harmful effect on the fetus in utero, but in large doses it causes the ''gray syndrome'' in newborn infants.

Nitrofurantoin. Nitrofurantoin may cause hemolysis of red blood cells and megaloblastic erythropoiesis in pregnant black women with glucose-6-phosphate dehydrogenase deficiency.

Renal tuberculosis

Tuberculosis of the kidney occurs rarely during pregnancy and may produce no symptoms unless the bladder is involved.

Antituberculosis drugs can be administered safely during pregnancy. Nephrectomy, when indicated, can be performed. It usually is not necessary to terminate pregnancy because of renal tuberculosis.

URINARY CALCULI

Calculi occur infrequently in pregnant women, the incidence of renal stones being about 0.04% and of ureteral stones about 0.08%, despite urinary stasis, which occurs regularly, and infection. These changes, which often influence the development of calculi, are transient in pregnant women, being present only until delivery.

Another factor is that calculous disease occurs most often in women older than 35 years of age, and most pregnancies occur in women younger than age 35.

Ureteral and renal calculi may produce fewer symptoms in pregnant than in nonpregnant women because of the decreased muscle tonus and dilatation in the urinary tract. Small stones in the ureter may be passed spontaneously as the pregnancy changes develop.

Treatment depends on the size and position of the stones and the symptoms they cause. It may be necessary to remove obstructing calculi or those producing severe pain. It is rarely necessary to terminate pregnancy in women with stones.

HEMATURIA

Blood in the urine can come from a lesion at any level of the urinary tract. The possible causes of hematuria are severe infection, rupture of small varicosities of the bladder, calculi, acute glomerulonephritis, tuberculosis, tumors, and other rare lesions.

Although it is essential to attempt to determine the cause of hematuria, the usual urologic examination must be modified during pregnancy. Cystoscopy can be performed at any stage, but it is more difficult and less accurate during late pregnancy when the bladder is drawn upward and the presenting part is entering the pelvis. X-ray film examination should usually be avoided; but if it is essential, if should be modified to reduce the amount of radiation to the minimum necessary to make a diagnosis. The progression of ureteropelvic dilatation can be monitored by ultrasound. In most instances, particularly when hematuria occurs late in pregnancy, complete examination can be deferred until after delivery.

NEPHRITIS
Acute glomerulonephritis

An initial attack of glomerulonephritis is uncommon in gravid women, but, when it occurs, the pregnancy adds a complicating factor. Urinary output is diminished or ceases completely; and the urine is smoky or bloody, is of high specific gravity, and contains large amounts of protein and many cellular casts. The blood pressure usually is elevated, there is generalized edema, and the patient feels and looks sick.

Spontaneous abortion, intrauterine fetal death, or premature delivery may occur during the acute phase. The place of therapeutic abortion is not clearly defined, but it is not often necessary, since the acute process usually subsides within 2 or 3 weeks.

Chronic glomerulonephritis

Fortunately, the combination of chronic glomerulonephritis and pregnancy is seldom encountered. The abnormal renal function and the accompanying changes in the cardiovascular system increase the hazards for both mother and baby considerably.

The prognosis depends in a large measure on whether the kidney is able to respond to the increasing demands as pregnancy advances. Bear, studying 44 pregnancies in 37 women with chronic renal disease, divided the patients into two groups; 36 pregnancies in 29 women with serum creatinine concentrations less than 1.5 mg/dl and eight pregnancies in eight women with serum creatinine concentrations greater than 1.6 mg/dl. Of the first group, 28 were delivered of normal infants by vaginal delivery, and six by cesarean section, two because of increasing hypertension, and two because of abruptio placentae. There was one spontaneous abortion. The pregnancies of all eight patients with more severe renal disease were complicated. It was difficult to control hypertension, and renal function often deteriorated. One was aborted therapeutically, and four were delivered prematurely by cesarean section. In four the disease progressed rapidly to death or renal failure after delivery.

Minimal basic studies when chronic glomerulonephritis is suspected should include (1) history and physical examination; (2) examination of the retinal vessels; (3) blood pressure determinations at least twice daily; (4) determination of hemoglobin or hematocrit, white blood count, and red blood cell count; (5) measurement of blood urea nitrogen and creatinine concentrations; (6) complete examination of several urine specimens; (7) determination of daily urinary protein excretions; and (8) creatinine clearances.

If renal impairment is minimal and blood pressure is normal or only slightly elevated, pregnancy may be allowed to continue as long as the patient remains reasonably normal, but if the blood pressure rises progressively or if renal function diminishes as pregnancy advances, termination should be considered.

The *perinatal mortality* is much higher than that for normal pregnancy, the principal causes of death being abruptio placentae, growth retardation caused either by an unusually small placenta or extensive infarction—which is characteristic of hypertensive cardiovascular disease—and premature labor. Since babies born of mothers with chronic glomerulonephritis are often smaller than the infants of normal women at a comparable stage of pregnancy, a relatively small uterus should not influence the physician to delay delivery if the vascular renal status is deteriorating. Unless the baby is delivered, it may die in utero.

Therapeutic termination of early pregnancy is advisable if renal function is significantly impaired. Since the kidney lesions are irreparable, pregnancy will be no less hazardous in the future; consequently, sterilization should also be advised.

Abnormal menses and infertility, which occur frequently with chronic renal insufficiency, often are corrected by hemodialysis. Successful pregnancies have been reported in women who must rely on regular dialysis to survive, but as a general rule pregnancy should be prevented, and abortion should be made available to those who conceive.

CONGENITAL POLYCYSTIC KIDNEY DISEASE

Congenital polycystic kidneys are only rarely encountered in pregnant women. Landesman and Scherr reported that the diagnosis was made in 114 of 390,000 patients admitted to the New York Hospital. Only 28 were pregnant. The diagnosis is often overlooked in young women, because clinical signs and symptoms usually do not appear until after the age period in which most women bear children.

Congenital polycystic kidney disease is an autosomal dominant trait, so 50% of the offspring of a parent with polycystic kidneys will inherit the gene. It is important that the diagnosis be made as early as possible so that young women with the disorder can consider the problems associated with childbearing. Milutinovic and colleagues, with the use of excretory urograms with nephrotomography and radionuclide imaging, diagnosed polycystic kidneys in about 50% of suspected cases in which the patient was older than 20 years (95% of those at risk) but in only 30% (60% of those at risk) between the ages of 15 and 19. Although the diagnosis should be made early, negative studies in young women may provide a false sense of security.

Unless renal function is depressed, women with polycystic kidneys usually do well during pregnancy. Blood pressure elevation alone does not contraindicate pregnancy, but if proteinuria is present and renal function is depressed, prompt termination usually is warranted.

SINGLE KIDNEY

The lack of a kidney is no contraindication to pregnancy if the function in the remaining one is normal. Renal function should be evaluated before pregnancy is contemplated, as soon as possible after conception, and periodically during pregnancy. Therapeutic abortion should be considered only if renal function is impaired, if there is a large calculus with infection, or if the patient has chronic pyelonephritis or repeated urinary tract infections that cannot be controlled.

KIDNEY TRANSPLANTS

A kidney transplant is not necessarily a contraindication to pregnancy if kidney function is normal, but the prognoses for both mother and infant must be guarded. The changes in renal function are like those that occur in normal women. As pregnancy advances, mothers with renal transplants are more prone to develop both bacterial and viral infections, particularly urinary tract infections, than are normal women because of the immunosuppressive drugs they must take. They also are likely to develop hypertension and reduced kidney function during late pregnancy. This may lead to kidney failure and eventually even death. Labor begins prematurely more often than in normal women, but the abortion rate is not increased significantly.

Congenital anomalies caused by immunosuppressive drugs may occur more often in human fetuses, and adrenocortical deficiency has been reported. The newborn infant who has been exposed to immunosuppressive drugs may not be able to cope adequately with infections.

The disturbed menstrual function, which often occurs with chronic renal insufficiency, is usually corrected by kidney transplantation; hence women who were infertile before the operation are likely to conceive when normal menstrual function is resumed.

The prescription of a reliable contraceptive method is essential in the care of transplant patients. Pregnancy should be delayed until kidney function is normal and until the dosages of immunosuppressive drugs have been reduced to maintenance levels.

Women who are considering pregnancy after kidney transplantation, even when kidney function is normal, should be informed of the immediate hazards of pregnancy and of the long-term outlook. The life of a transplanted kidney is limited, so the mother will eventually need another operation or permanent dialysis. Her life expectancy also is limited, she may be chronically ill, and the chances of her leading a normal, healthy life until the child is grown are small.

Care during pregnancy is similar to that for normal women except that particular attention must be paid to monitoring kidney function and to the detection and treatment of urinary tract infection. Decreasing kidney function or the inability to eradicate infection are indications for termination. Sterilization following delivery should be considered even though kidney function has remained normal throughout pregnancy.

Women with transplanted kidneys can deliver normally unless the position of the kidney obstructs the pelvic inlet, in which event elective cesarean section is indicated.

REFERENCES

Baird, D.: Anatomy and physiology of the upper urinary tract in pregnancy: relation to pyelitis, J. Obstet. Gynecol. Br. Commonw. **38**:516, 1931.

Bear, R.A.: Pregnancy in patients with renal disease, Obstet. Gynecol. **48**:13, 1976.

Coe, F.L, Parks, J.H., and Lindheimer, M.D.: Nephrolithiasis during pregnancy, N. Engl. J. Med. **298**:324, 1978.

Davison, J.M.: The kidney in pregnancy: a review, J. R. Soc. Med. **76**:485, 1983.

Davison, J.M.: The effect of pregnancy on kidney function in renal allograft recipients, Kidney Int. **27**:74, 1985.

Davison, J.M., and Lindheimer, M.D.: Pregnancy in renal transplant recipients, J. Reprod. Med. **27**:613, 1982.

Dunlop, W.: Serial changes in renal haemodynamics during normal human pregnancy, Br. J. Obstet. Gynaecol. **88**:1, 1981.

Gabert, H.A., and Miller, J.M., Jr.: Renal disease in pregnancy, Obstet. Gynecol. Surv. **40**:449, 1985.

Gilstrap, L.G., III, Cunningham, F.G., and Whalley, P.J.: Acute pyelonephritis in pregnancy: an anterospective study, Obstet. Gynecol. **57**:409, 1981.

Harris, R.E.: The significance of eradication of bacteriuria during pregnancy, Obstet. Gynecol. **53**:71, 1979.

Harris, R.E., Gilstrap, L.C., III, and Pretty, A.: Single-dose antimicrobial therapy for asymptomatic bacteriuria during pregnancy, Obstet. Gynecol. **59**:546, 1982.

Hou, S.: Pregnancy in women with chronic renal disease, N. Engl. J. Med. **312**:836, 1985.

Kass, E.H.: Bacteriuria and pyelonephritis of pregnancy, Arch. Intern. Med. **105**:194, 1960.

Kline, A.H., Blattner, R.J., and Lunin, M.: Transplacental effect of tetracycline on teeth, J.A.M.A. **188**:178, 1964.

Klein, E.A.: Urologic problems of pregnancy, Obstet. Gynecol. Surv. **39**:605, 1984.

Landesman, R., and Scherr, L.: Congenital polycystic kidney disease in pregnancy, Obstet. Gynecol. **8**:673, 1956.

Milutinovic, J., Fialkow, P.J., Phillips, L.A., Agoda, L.Y., Bryant, J.I., Denney, J.D., and Rudd, T.G.: Autosomal dominant polycystic kidney disease: early diagnosis and data for genetic counselling, Lancet **1**:1203, 1980.

Naeye, R.L.: Causes of the excessive rates of perinatal mortality and prematurity in pregnancies complicated by maternal urinary-tract infections, N. Engl. J. Med. **300**:819, 1979.

Penn, I., Makowski, E.L., and Harris, P.: Parenthood following renal transplant, Kidney Int. **2**:221, 1980.

Saxen, L.: Tetracycline: effect on osteogenesis in vitro, Science **149**:870, 1965.

Schaefer, G., and Markham, S.: Full-term delivery following nephrectomy, Am. J. Obstet. Gynecol. **100**:1078, 1968.

Wallach, E.E., Brody, J.I., and Oski, F.A.: Fetal immunization as a consequence of bacilluria during pregnancy, Obstet. Gynecol. **33**:100, 1969.

Whalley, P.J., Adams, R.H., and Combes, B.: Tetracycline toxicity in pregnancy, J.A.M.A. **189**:357, 1964.

Whalley, P.J., and Cunningham, F.G.: Short-term versus continuous antimicrobial therapy for asymptomatic bacteriuria in pregnancy, Obstet. Gynecol. **49**:262, 1977.

Whalley, P.J., Martin, F.G., and Peters, P.G.: Significance of asymptomatic bacteriuria detected during pregnancy, J.A.M.A. **193**:879, 1965.

Whalley, P.J., Martin, F.G., and Pritchard, J.A.: Sickle cell trait and urinary tract infection during pregnancy, J.A.M.A. **189**:903, 1964.

26

William J. Ledger

Genital tract disorders during pregnancy

Pathologic conditions originating in the genital tract may complicate the course of pregnancy, labor, or delivery. These disturbances include (1) local infections or infestations, (2) neoplasms, (3) uterine malpositions, and (4) congenital malformations. Some of these disorders become evident for the first time during pregnancy, particularly if gestation is threatened or if growth of the uterus and other local physiologic changes result in the development of symptoms. Careful prenatal pelvic examination, preferably during the first trimester, offers the best opportunity for diagnosis of genital tract disturbances and makes possible timely planning for the management of these conditions.

VULVOVAGINAL DISORDERS

Mucoid secretion from the vagina is increased during pregnancy because of vascularity and increased activity of the cervical glands. In the absence of symptoms or evidence of inflammation, treatment of vaginal discharge is unnecessary. These changes are conducive to the development of persistent local disturbances.

Vulvitis. Local irritation and itching frequently are caused by some form of vaginitis. During pregnancy, this is most commonly caused by *Candida* organisms. The diagnosis can be made by microscopic examination of vaginal secretions. The vulva may become swollen, red, and edematous. Intertrigo extending over the inner aspect of the thighs is common in obese women. Treatment consists of diagnosing and treating the vaginitis. Occasionally, local antifungal cream applied to the area will be helpful.

Condylomata. Condylomata acuminata may increase in size during pregnancy, occasionally attaining proportions sufficient to interfere with vaginal delivery (Fig. 26-1).

Tiny isolated lesions can be eradicated by touching them with 25% podophyllin, but if they are more numerous another method of treatment is preferable. Podophyllin may be teratogenic and has been reported to cause both maternal and fetal death. Treatment with laser can be very effective in these cases, but some form of anesthetic will be necessary.

Infection of Bartholin's glands. Acute lower genital tract infection caused by pyogenic microorganisms may occur during pregnancy and involve the vulvovaginal glands. An abscess that develops despite antibiotic therapy should be drained, even during the last few weeks of pregnancy. Drainage prevents the inevitable rupture and genital tract contamination during delivery. An asymptomatic Bartholin's cyst usually should not be excised during pregnancy because of the great increase in vulvar vascularity.

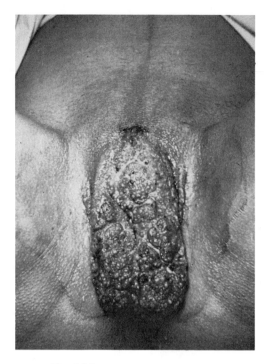

Fig. 26-1. Condylomata acuminata.

Sexually transmitted diseases

Gonorrhea. Pregnancy offers no protection against lower genital tract gonorrhea, but the infection is usually limited to the lower genital tract. Extension of a newly acquired infection upward to the tubes is uncommon during pregnancy, but upper genital tract infection may develop in the first trimester or during the puerperium if the disease is not eradicated beforehand. During labor and delivery, infected cervical, Skene's, or Bartholin's glands may cause *ophthalmia neonatorum* as a result of *Neisseria gonorrhea* in the infant. The diagnosis and treatment of gonorrhea are discussed in Chapter 42.

Syphilis. Syphilis is an uncommon disease in pregnant women. In 1979, only 331 cases of congenital syphilis were reported from over 3 million deliveries.

Syphilis is as difficult to diagnose clinically in the pregnant woman as it is in the nonpregnant woman. Any punched out painless lesions on the vulva or cervix should be subjected to dark-field examination.

The effect on the infant is determined in part by the age of the infection. If the syphilis has recently been acquired and is active, the child is almost certain to be affected and may die in utero or be born prematurely. If the infection is old and inactive, the infant may escape the disease completely. If the infection has been acquired shortly before delivery, the infant may be entirely normal unless it is inoculated from local primary lesions in the birth canal. In this event its initial blood serologic reaction may be negative, and evidences of infection may not appear for several weeks.

Spirochetes have been found in fetal tissues as early as the eighth week of pregnancy, but there is little host reaction before the twentieth week. This is the basis for the misconception that the placenta is impervious to spirochetes before the sixteenth to eighteenth gestational week. The earlier maternal syphilis is diagnosed and treated, the greater the protection afforded the fetus.

DIAGNOSIS. Almost every case of syphilis can be diagnosed by determining the blood serologic reaction. These reagin tests are nonspecific and should be accompanied, if positive, by a specific test, a fluorescent treponemal antibody-absorption test (FTA-ABS).

The disease may be acquired during pregnancy; therefore even though the screening test is negative, it should be repeated in high-risk patients during the final weeks.

TREATMENT. An adequate course of treatment begun during the first half of pregnancy will afford almost complete protection for the infant. Regardless of the duration of pregnancy, however, treatment should be started as soon as the diagnosis is established. Even though the infant is already infected, its disease can be controlled, and further damage prevented by treating the mother.

Following are the treatment regimens recommended by the Centers for Disease Control:

1. *Pregnant women with gonorrhea who may also have syphilis.* Treatment is as for early

syphilis alone. The blood serologic reaction should be checked 2 to 3 months after treatment is completed.

2. *Primary or secondary syphilis or disease of less than 1 year's duration.*

   a. A single injection of benzathine penicillin G: 2.4 million units, half in each buttock.

   b. For patients who are allergic to penicillin: oral erythromycin 500 mg four times daily for 15 days, a total of 30 g. *Erythromycin offers less protection to the fetus than does penicillin; hence the newborn infants should be treated as through they have congenital syphilis.*

3. *Latent syphilis or disease of more than 1 year's duration.*

   a. Benzathine penicillin G: 2.4 million units at weekly intervals for 3 weeks, a total of 7.2 million units.

   b. Erythromycin: 500 mg four times daily for 30 days, a total of 60 g.

   c. Quantitative serologic tests (reagin) should be made every month until delivery.

The mother's serologic reaction may still be positive at delivery although the infection has been eradicated. The baby's serologic reaction may also be positive at birth because maternal IgG immunoglobulins are transferred across the placenta from maternal to fetal blood.

Genital herpesvirus infections. Disseminated herpesvirus infections may develop in infants born of mothers with active genital herpetic lesions. The infant is almost always infected by direct contact during delivery. The virus may also reach the infant in utero if the membranes are ruptured and possibly by transplacental transmission, even though the amniotic sac is intact. Bolognese and co-workers were able to identify antibodies against herpesvirus in the sera of 35.7% of 985 pregnant women. They also isolated herpesvirus type 2 from cervical cultures in 0.65%, a recovery rate almost identical to that reported by Nahmias and co-workers for pregnant women without genital lesions. No virus was identified in 211 samples of amniotic fluid.

Nahmias and co-workers diagnosed genital herpes in 140 (1.2%) of 13,766 pregnant women, and 43 (0.58%) of 7357 women following delivery at the Grady Memorial Hospital. Typical herpetic genital lesions were present in only 36% of prenatal patients; 43% had no symptoms of the infection.

In 37 women the infection was diagnosed before the twentieth week of pregnancy: 12 (34%) aborted, four (16%) delivered prematurely, and 21 delivered at term. The premature delivery rate (16% of the 25 patients who did not abort) was similar to the general premature rate in that hospital. No pathologic evidence of herpes infection was detected in the placentas or embryos of the 12 abortion specimens.

Amstey and Kobos inoculated the vaginas of pregnant mice with herpesvirus type 2; 26% of the newborn mice delivered through the infected vaginas acquired disseminated herpesvirus infections. In contrast, only 4% of newborn mice whose mothers had been inoculated with herpesvirus subcutaneously died.

Amstey and Monif studied 29 patients with acute genital herpes infections during pregnancy; 15 were free of virus at the time of delivery, and 14 had active genital tract infections. All who were virus free were allowed to deliver vaginally, and all the infants were normal. Infections occurred in two of 14 who were shedding virus at delivery, two who delivered vaginally were normal, two of the 12 who were delivered by cesarean section developed herpesvirus infection, and one died. The two affected babies were delivered 24 and 70 hours after the membranes had been ruptured.

In 101 of Nahmias and associates' patients the infection was diagnosed after the twentieth week. Of these women, 20% delivered prematurely, and 80% delivered at term. Five of nine premature babies and four of nine term babies whose mothers had genital herpes infections at the time of delivery developed herpes infections after vaginal delivery. The two premature infants and the two term babies who were delivered by cesarean section 6 or more hours after the membranes had ruptured were infected. In contrast, none of four infants (two premature and two term) who were delivered by cesarean section before the membranes ruptured or within 4 hours of rupture was infected.

The presence or absence of antibodies transferred to the fetus from the mother has little effect in the infant infection rate. The most important factor is the presence of a primary genital infection.

The possibility that the infant will be infected as it passes through the birth canal is approximately 40%.

It seems appropriate therefore to obtain cervical cultures at weekly intervals after the thirty-sixth week on all women who have had genital herpesvirus infections. If there are no visible lesions and the cultures are negative, one can plan for vaginal delivery. If there are lesions, or if the cultures are positive, elective cesarean section when the fetus becomes mature or emergency cesarean section if labor begins or the membranes rupture is appropriate. Cytologic examination of cervical secretions, although less accurate, may be helpful if culture is not available or when a decision as to management must be made promptly because labor has begun or the membranes have ruptured. The demonstration of characteristic intracellular inclusions indicates the presence of virus.

If the pregnancy is of less than 26 weeks' duration, or if the membranes have been ruptured 12 or more hours, vaginal delivery is usually preferable to cesarean section.

Chlamydial infections. These infections are caused by an obligatory intracellular parasite, *Chlamydia trachomatis*. *C. trachomatis* has been isolated mainly from the lower genital tract of both males and females and is one of the most common sexually transmitted diseases. Chlamydial cervicitis, like gonorrhea, can be asymptomatic; in fact, the two are often found concomitantly in the cervix. Acute and chronic chlamydial infections in the female involve the cervix and fallopian tubes. In the male nongonococcal urethritis and epididymitis are usual effects. Maternal chlamydial cervicitis poses a risk to the neonate or newborn infant. *Inclusion conjunctivitis* of the newborn, an acute mucopurulent infection, is now several times more often the cause of ophthalmia than is gonorrhea. *Neonatal pneumonia* caused by *C. trachomatis* does not occur as frequently, and symptoms tend to develop insidiously after discharge from the hospital. Infections usually respond to treatment with tetracycline or erythromycin.

Laboratory diagnosis is difficult, but new techniques hold promise. Rapid evaluation using a

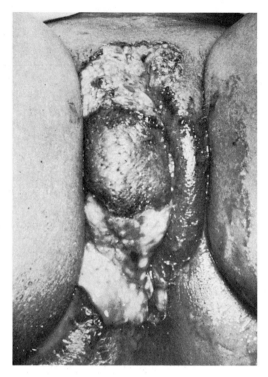

Fig. 26-2. Granuloma inguinale.

monoclonal antibody technique provides an accurate diagnosis in most cases and has replaced cell culture techniques in most hospitals.

Lymphogranuloma venereum, also called lymphopathia, is a rare venereal disease caused by *C. trachomatis*. The disease itself has no effect on the pregnancy or vice versa, but the dense pelvic fibrosis may make vaginal delivery hazardous. It must be differentiated from another rare venereal disease, *granuloma inguinale* (Fig. 26-2), in which the primary infection tends to remain more superficial. Diagnosis of this disease is confirmed by the demonstration of Donovan bodies in scrapings obtained directly from the surface of the ulcers (Fig. 26-3). The treatment of lymphogranuloma venereum and granuloma inguinale is discussed in Chapter 26.

Haemophilus vaginitis. Designation of this type of vaginitis has been changed first to *Corynebacterium* and currently to *Gardnerella* vaginitis, indicating the tendency of microbiologists to rename organisms. Recent data indicate that anaerobes are important in the production of foul-smelling discharge. Infection is charac-

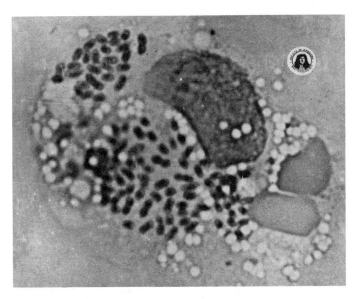

Fig. 26-3. Donovan bodies—direct ulcer scrapings. (S.A.B. No. 292.) (From Dougherty, J.M., and Lamberti, A.J.: Textbook of bacteriology, ed. 3, St. Louis, 1954, The C.V. Mosby Co.)

terized by a malodorous, grayish discharge that is often profuse and commonly found in sexual partners. The odor suggests a symbiosis with anaerobic organisms. In other respects the disturbance is generally asymptomatic, and its presence during labor and delivery has shown no deleterious effects on the newborn. Diagnosis and treatment are discussed in Chapter 45.

Molluscum contagiosum. Molluscum contagiosum is a venereally transmitted disease that appears as papules with depressed centers filled with a cheesy material. If is often asymptomatic. Its main importance is that it be differentiated from more frequently encountered lesions. Clusters of small papules may resemble herpes simplex. Larger lesions may look like basal cell carcinoma. Scrapings from the center of the lesion reveal typical viral inclusion bodies.

Trichomonas vaginalis vaginitis. The presence of vaginal trichomoniasis is a source of great annoyance throughout the prenatal period.

Metronidazole (Flagyl) is a singularly effective trichomonocidal agent, particularly since the drug can be administered orally to both male and female partners, but its use during the first trimester of pregnancy has been questioned. Diagnosis and treatment are discussed in Chapter 45.

Mycotic vulvovaginitis. *Candida (Monilia) albicans* frequently is a cause of vaginitis in pregnant women. The vaginal environment during pregnancy is conducive to the development of candidiasis. Intense itching is usually the first symptom. Vaginal discharge may be scant, but thick white plaques are often visible over a reddened mucous membrane. *Candida* organisms transferred to the infant during delivery are a usual cause of thrush in the newborn. The diagnosis and treatment are discussed in Chapter 45.

NEOPLASTIC GROWTHS

Various benign neoplasms involving the generative organs and occasionally malignant tumors are found in gravid women. Their existence during pregnancy presents certain diagnostic and therapeutic problems. Opinions have been divided as to whether pregnancy has an accelerating effect on the rate of neoplastic growth, but certainly early diagnosis serves the best interest of the mother and usually her unborn child as well.

Cervical polyps. Cervical polyps tend to increase in size during pregnancy because of edema. The usual symptom is bleeding.

If the polyp is growing and/or the patient is bleeding, the polyp should be carefully excised and sent to the laboratory for tissue examination. Polypectomy is unlikely to cause abortion. Bleeding can be a problem, and the physician should have instruments, including sutures, and anesthetic available. Usually the bleeding can be controlled by the application of a hemostatic agent such as Surgicel or the use of a tampon kept firmly in place for several hours.

Cervical carcinoma. Speculum examination and vaginal smears are innocuous, regardless of the stage of gestation. Screening cervical cytologic analysis is an essential part of the first prenatal examination. All suspicious or positive smears found during pregnancy require investigation. Colposcopic examination is a valuable aid in delineating abnormalities of visible areas of the cervix and vagina. The diagnosis and management of in situ and invasive carcinoma of the cervix complicating pregnancy are discussed in Chapter 46.

Uterine fibromyomas. The coexistence of uterine fibromyomas and pregnancy is relatively common (Fig. 26-4). Small tumors are of little consequence unless their location is submucous, in which case the abortion rate is almost doubled. Although tumors of any size may produce symptoms of pain or pressure, surgical intervention is rarely necessary during pregnancy. Complications are principally related to the size and location of the tumors, to degenerative changes in the fibroid, or to torsion of a pedunculated tumor.

DIAGNOSIS. The main problem in diagnosis is the recognition of the existence of pregnancy in a fibroid uterus. This is particularly difficult when implantation bleeding or threatened abortion complicates the early course. An accurate menstrual history is an important early guide. Delayed or abnormal bleeding, symptoms of early pregnancy, softening of the cervix, or recent increase in size of a fibroid uterus should suggest the possibility of pregnancy in every case. If any doubt remains, a pregnancy test or sonography should be done before an ill-advised laparotomy is performed.

When a symmetrically enlarged uterus is inadvertently discovered during operation, the differential diagnosis

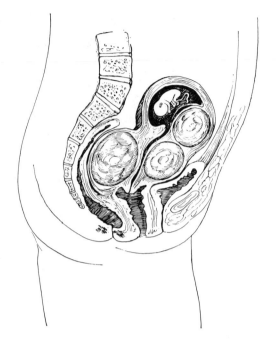

Fig. 26-4. Pregnancy in myomatous uterus.

must be made between a soft myoma and an intrauterine pregnancy (Fig. 26-5). If the enlargement results from pregnancy, the consistency is different because of the thin wall and the amniotic fluid. In addition, the tubes and round ligaments are elongated, since the relationship of their attachments to the fundal portion of the uterus is retained. The tubes and round ligaments are usually attached low on the uterus if the symmetric enlargement results from a soft, fundal leiomyoma. If these evidences are inconclusive, needle aspiration can be done in an attempt to detect amniotic fluid. Neither laparotomy nor needle aspiration is likely to disturb pregnancy if the uterus is not unduly manipulated.

COMPLICATIONS. Uterine fibroids tend to enlarge during pregnancy and diminish again as involution takes place. Their apparent growth results mainly from edema and to a lesser extent from the hormonal stimulation of pregnancy.

Degenerative changes are likely to occur during pregnancy, the hemorrhagic variety *(red degeneration)* being the most common. Pain, local tenderness, and slight elevation of temperature are the usual symptoms. The pathologic process is ordinarily limited to the substance of the fibroid proper and tends to subside spontaneously in 2 to 3 days.

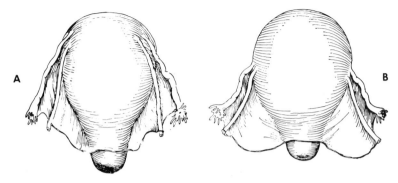

Fig. 26-5. Relationship of insertions of round ligaments and tubes to fundus in **A,** gravid uterus, and **B,** nongravid uterus, with symmetric enlargement caused by fundal fibroid.

Hence conservative treatment with bed rest, local application of heat, and mild analgesics such as Tylenol and codeine will control the symptoms in most instances.

Myomectomy is rarely necessary and is frequently followed by abortion if the uterine wall is incised. Occasionally a hysterectomy will be necessary to control bleeding. An exception is a *pedunculated tumor,* which may twist and become necrotic as the uterus enlarges and rises out of the pelvis. If torsion occurs, laparotomy is imperative before gangrenous changes and general peritonitis develop. Fortunately, this type of tumor can usually be removed with impunity if wedge incision through the pedicle and imbrication of the cut edges can be accomplished without invading the myometrium.

The major complications resulting from fibroids arise during labor and delivery: (1) obstruction of the birth canal, (2) an increased incidence of dysfunctional labor, (3) fetal malpositions, (4) faulty placental separation, and (5) hemorrhage following delivery.

Tumors blocking the inlet may make cesarean section necessary. Those situated low in the anterior wall are usually pulled up out of the pelvis as the lower uterine segment lengthens, but if the tumor is situated posteriorly, elevation may be prevented by the promontory of the sacrum. Vaginal examination should be performed early in labor before deciding on the route of delivery. If the birth canal is not obstructed and the fetal position does not preclude vaginal delivery, a trial of labor should be given. Occasionally, the presence of fibroids alters uterine contractility and induces dysfunctional labor or hemorrhage following delivery. In rare instances the placenta is attached over a submucous or deep intramural fibroid, which may interfere with the normal process of separation and expulsion.

Despite the various potential hazards, vaginal delivery is frequently uneventful even in the presence of multiple uterine fibroids. If cesarean section is necessary because of pelvic obstruction or abnormal labor, hysterectomy may or may not be indicated, but myomectomy should generally not be done. Except in the instance of the removal of a pedunculated tumor, cesarean section followed by myomectomy is attended by higher mortality and morbidity than cesarean section alone or cesarean section followed by hysterectomy.

During the puerperium the blood supply to uterine myomas may be reduced suddenly. Red degeneration is more common in the period following than at any other time. Laparotomy is indicated if symptoms of degeneration develop and persist during the stage of uterine involution.

Ovarian neoplasms. Ovarian neoplasms occur once in every 500 to 1000 pregnancies. Their existence may be unsuspected before the prenatal examination, at which time the finding of an ovarian enlargement may present considerable diagnostic and therapeutic difficulties.

DIAGNOSIS. The ovary containing the corpus luteum may be enlarged during the first trimester, but on reexamination at 2- or 3-week intervals it becomes progressively smaller after the eighth to tenth week of pregnancy. *True ovarian neoplasms* are usually larger than 5 cm in diameter and do not decrease in size on repeated examinations. Discovery of an adnexal mass is much easier if the first prenatal pelvic examination is performed in the first trimester. As pregnancy advances, an ovarian cyst is displaced by the enlarged uterus. If it is displaced laterally or is trapped in the cul-de-sac, it is still palpable by bimanual examination, but frequently the cyst is carried upward above the uterus. In this case it is felt only by abdominal examination. In most instances the diagnosis can be made clinically, and the treatment is operative. Radiography is rarely necessary, but sonography may be helpful.

COMPLICATIONS AND MANAGEMENT. Ovarian tumors in pregnant women cannot be viewed with complacency because the incidence of malignancy in women with an ovarian neoplasm is approximately 5%. Small cysts found early in pregnancy should be reevaluated at 2- or 3-week intervals. Those larger than 5 cm that do not regress and all solid ovarian tumors require laparotomy. The most favorable time in pregnancy for their removal is during the early weeks of the second trimester for the following reasons: (1) nausea and vomiting of pregnancy are less likely to complicate the postoperative course, (2) the uterine size does not interfere with whatever surgery is necessary, (3) a corpus luteum cyst will have shown regression, and (4) placental hormone production is adequate to support the pregnancy. How long the corpus luteum is essential for maintenance of the pregnancy is debatable. There have been numerous instances of its removal in early pregnancy without abortion ensuing. Pratt reported two cases of women in whom the corpus luteum was removed at 21 and 30 days after the last normal menstrual period without disturbing the pregnancies. Delivery occurred at 272 and 279 days, respectively, verifying the history and clinical findings of early gestations at the time of surgery. Grimes and coworkers reported 28 cysts removed in the first trimester; 16 contained the corpus luteum, and one abortion occurred.

Immediate removal of the cyst is necessary, regardless of the stage of pregnancy if symptoms of torsion or hemorrhage arise or if rapid growth of the mass is detected. If the neoplasm is diagnosed late in pregnancy and the birth canal is not obstructed, vaginal delivery is preferable, but cystoophorectomy should be carried out in the immediate period following delivery. Torsion of the elongated pedicle is common as the uterine size decreases. If the cyst obstructs the pelvis (Fig. 26-6), it or the uterus may rupture during labor. No attempt should be made to evacuate the cyst by cul-de-sac aspiration or drainage, since leakage into the periotoneal cavity may result in widespread peritonitis, shock, or dissemination of malignant cells. Cesarean section and cystectomy are preferable. Since ovarian lesions are frequently bilateral, examination with biopsy of the opposite ovary is indicated in every case in which the ovary appears abnormal.

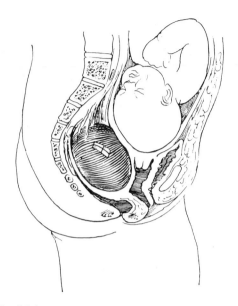

Fig. 26-6. Obstruction of birth canal by ovarian cyst.

MALPOSITIONS OF THE UTERUS

Anterior displacement. Early in pregnancy the uterus is anteflexed, but it straightens as the uterus arises from the pelvis and meets the resistance of the anterior abdominal wall. Significant anterior displacement occurs during the last few weeks of pregnancy if the rectus abdominis muscles are widely separated or extremely lax. The uterus falls directly forward, producing sharp angulation at the cervicouterine junction.

Apart from the patient's discomfort, effects on the pregnancy are minimal until labor begins. Dystocia is common if the position is uncorrected, since the force of uterine contractions is misdirected, driving the presenting part toward the sacrum rather than into the pelvis. In addition, the anterior portion of the cervix is compressed; hence retraction and dilatation may be impaired. These difficulties can be overcome by application of a good support during pregnancy and a firm abdominal binder during labor.

Ventrofixation. Ventrofixation of the gravid uterus to the rectus fascia is relatively rare, since fixation operations for the correction of uterine retroversion during the childbearing years have fortunately become obsolete. Occasionally, firm adhesions develop between the uterus and anterior abdominal wall after myomectomy or cesarean section. Abortion may occur because the growing uterus is incapable of uniform distention. If the pregnancy continues, the uterus enlarges almost entirely by stretching of the posterior uterine wall. This becomes remarkably thin, forming a *posterior sacculation* of the uterus. Cesarean section is usually necessary for delivery.

Retrodisplacement. Some degree of uterine retroversion or retroflexion is observed in at least 20% of normal women. Ordinarily, fertility is not affected if the retroversion is uncomplicated. Spontaneous correction is the rule as the uterus gradually enlarges and rises out of the pelvis. This is true even in instances in which posterior adhesions resulting from previous infection or endometriosis are present. Adhesions of this type usually stretch or undergo dissolution, permitting spontaneous restitution by the twelfth week of pregnancy. Once the fundus rises above the sacral promontory, there is no danger of recurrence.

Occasionally, the retrodisplaced uterus fails to rise out of the pelvis and becomes impinged beneath the sacral promontory as it grows. Abortion occurs if the uterine circulation is significantly reduced by compression. Pressure symptoms may develop acutely if the condition is uncorrected by the thirteenth or fourteenth week, and the pregnant uterus becomes incarcerated in the pelvis (Fig. 26-7). The rectum is compressed posteriorly, whereas the cervix is pulled sharply forward, exerting pressure against the urethra and vesicle neck. The patient may have difficulty urinating and may even develop urinary retention with overflow.

Manual replacement is indicated early in pregnancy if symptoms arise or after the twelfth week if spontaneous correction has not taken place. This is more easily accomplished with the patient in the knee-chest position. Should gradual bimanual manipulation alone fail to elevate the fundus, simultaneous traction against a tenaculum applied to the cervix is generally effective. A pessary should then be inserted to maintain the correction. This can be removed by the sixteenth week. Anesthesia may be necessary to dislodge and elevate the uterus, but laparotomy is seldom indicated.

Prolapse. Descensus of the gravid uterus may be present before conception or may develop after pregnancy is established. Spontaneous correction will sometimes occur at about the sixteenth week when the uterus becomes too large to enter the pelvis, but mechanical replacement will provide earlier relief and prevent progressive elongation, edema, and congestion of the cervix. If the enlarging prolapsed uterus becomes incarcerated in the pelvis, abortion is likely to occur. Obviously, ulceration and infection increase the hazard of delivery, but, if treatment

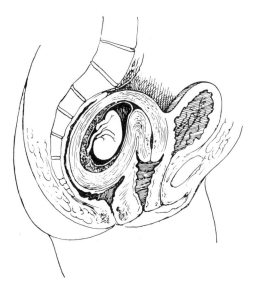

Fig. 26-7. Incarceration of gravid uterus.

has been instituted beforehand, labor and delivery should be relatively uncomplicated.

MANAGEMENT. Replacement of the uterus is indicated at whatever stage of pregnancy prolapse appears. Bed rest in a slight Trendelenburg position is advisable for a few days if cervical edema is severe. If prolapse occurs during the first trimester, a properly fitting pessary can be introduced and left as long as necessary.

CONGENITAL ANOMALIES

The müllerian ducts make their first appearance by the sixth week of embryonic life. Growth of the paired ducts and fusion of their lower portions forming the uterus and vagina should be complete by the sixteenth week. Failure of development on the one hand or failure of fusion on the other will result in absence or reduplication of related structures. Because of the close embryonic association, anomalies of the genital tract are frequently accompanied by malformations of the urinary apparatus. For example, when a double uterus is observed, absence of one kidney is common (Fig. 26-8). Minor deviations may have no effect whatever on reproductive function, and, as a consequence, many remain undetected. On the contrary, the patient with pronounced uterine malformation is subject to many complications of pregnancy, la-

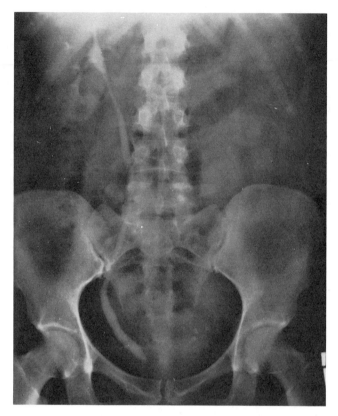

Fig. 26-8. Pregnancy at 6 weeks' gestation in patient with uterus didelphys and congenital absence of one kidney.

bor, and delivery and consequently suffers a higher fetal loss. Early recognition, regardless of the gradation of the abnormality, is the best preventive measure.

Types. Various types of uterine malformations are graphically demonstrated according to a modification of Jarcho's classification (Figs. 26-9 to 26-12):

1. Uterus didelphys bicollis with septate vagina (complete duplication of uterus, cervix, and vagina)
2. Uterus duplex bicornis bicollis (vagina simplex)
3. Uterus bicornis unicollis (vagina simplex)
4. Uterus septus (complete)
5. Uterus subseptus (partial)
6. Uterus arcuatus (concave fundus)
7. Uterus unicornis

Early complications. Genital malformations ordinarily do not reduce fertility. Although many pregnancies continue uneventfully, spontaneous abortions and premature labors are significantly increased. These accidents occur because the deformed uterus is less likely to provide a normal implantation site or to supply adequate nutrition for the early conceptus. In addition, the influence of underdeveloped uterine musculature may become apparent by lack of distensibility or accommodation, with premature contractions and early rupture of the membranes, or by ineffectual contractions after labor begins in women approaching term.

Pregnancy in one side of a double uterus is frequently associated with vaginal bleeding during the first trimester (Fig. 26-13). Philpott and Ross encountered this symptom in more than 50% of their 56 reported cases. This bleeding can be associated with either a threatened abor-

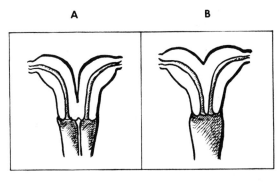

Fig. 26-9. **A,** Uterus didelphys bicollis (septate vagina).
B, Uterus bicornis bicollis (vagina simplex).

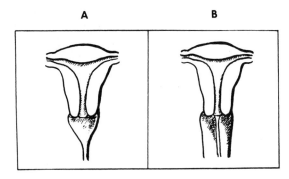

Fig. 26-10. **A,** Congenital stricture of vagina. **B,** Septate
vagina.

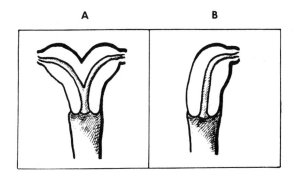

Fig. 26-11. **A,** Uterus bicornis unicollis (vagina simplex). **B,** Uterus unicornis.

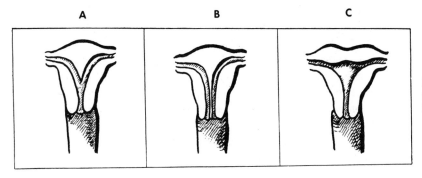

Fig. 26-12. **A,** Uterus subseptus. **B,** Uterus septus. **C,** Uterus arcuatus.

tion or with the casting off of decidua from the nonpregnant side. Recognition is important to avoid unnecessary medical treatment or surgical interference.

Late complications. Vaginal delivery can often be accomplished with little or no difficulty, and the opportunity should be afforded as long as conditions during labor remain satisfactory. Nevertheless, close observation is necessary because *malpositions,* particularly transverse lies, and *uterine inertia* are not uncommon

complications. Occasionally, the birth canal becomes obstructed by the nonpregnant portion of a double uterus, and abdominal delivery is necessary. *Obstructed delivery* caused by vaginal septa requires nothing more than local excision. The third stage of labor is often complicated by *retained placenta* requiring manual removal.

Diagnosis and management. Early diagnosis is difficult at best and becomes more so if the first pre-

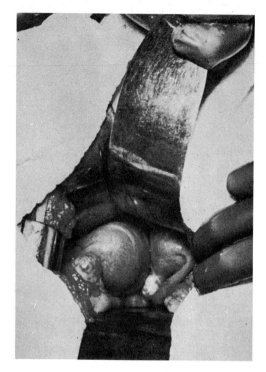

Fig. 26-13. Double uterus showing pregnancy in right uterus.

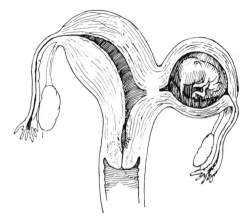

Fig. 26-14. Pregnancy in rudimentary horn.

natal examination is done after the fourteenth week of gestation. Discovery of a vaginal septum should arouse suspicion of other genital and urinary tract anomalies. Intravenous pyelography is indicated, except during pregnancy, whenever a malformation of the reproductive tract is discovered. Patients in whom preconception examination is suggestive and those with histories of repeated unexplained abortions, premature labors, or fetal deaths deserve further study by hysterosalpingography before another pregnancy is attempted.

A sterile vaginal examination should be carried out early in labor. Vaginal delivery can be expected if the fetal position is normal, if there is no obstruction from an accessory organ, and if the mechanism of labor is not faulty. Division of a vaginal septum is necessary only if descent of the presenting part is delayed. Bleeding from this procedure is usually minimal. Manual removal of the placenta is frequently necessary, and as a result of defective musculature, poor uterine contractions after the

third stage increase the likelihood of hemorrhage following delivery.

Delivery by cesarean section because of congenital malformations is necessary when vaginal delivery is impossible. Malformations of the uterus do not provide an indication for therapeutic abortions or sterilization.

A unification operation is highly effective in the treatment of double uterus, provided no other cause for pregnancy losses can be found. If these factors are normal, the occurrence of two or more consecutive abortions or pregnancy failures is ample indication for surgery.

Pregnancy in the rudimentary horn of uterus didelphys presents a rare but urgent problem in which early diagnosis is of utmost importance (Fig. 26-14). This condition differs from other uterine malformations in that the rudimentary horn may have an inadequate opening into the more developed uterine cavity. The clinical course resembles that of ectopic pregnancy except that the musculature, although defective, may permit a more advanced gestation than implantation in the fallopian tube. As a consequence, rupture may occur somewhat later and incite more profuse intraabdominal hemorrhage and shock.

Differential diagnosis usually rests between uterine myoma, ovarian cyst, and ectopic pregnancy. Treatment is surgical with complete removal of the rudimentary horn.

REFERENCES

Amstey, M.S., and Kobos, K.: An experimental model for disseminated herpesvirus infection of the neonate, Am. J. Obstet. Gyneecol. **125**:40, 1976.

Amstey, M.S., and Monif, G.R.G.: Genital herpesvirus infection in pregnancy, Obstet. Gynecol. **44**:394, 1974.

Annual Summary 1979; reported morbidity and mortality in the United States, Centers for Disease Control Morbidity and Mortality Weekly Report **28**:83, 1980.

Bolognese, R.J., Corson, S.L., Fuccillo, D.A., Traub, R., Moder, F., and Sever, J.L.: Herpesviris hominis type II infections in asymptomatic pregnant women, Obstet. Gynecol. **48**:507, 1976.

Evans, T., and Poland, M.L.: Vaginal malformations, Am. J. Obstet. Gynecol. **141**:910, 1981.

Fenton, A.N., and Singh, B.P.: Pregnancy associated with congenital abnormalities of the female reproductive tract, Am. J. Obstet. Gynecol. **63**:744, 1952.

Fenton, L.J., and Light, I.J.: Congenital syphilis after maternal treatment with erythromycin, Obstet. Gynecol. **47**:493, 1976.

Grimes, W.H., Jr., Bartholomew, R.A., Colvin, E.D., Fish, J.S., and Lester, W.M.: Ovarian cyst complicating pregnancy, Am. J. Obstet. Gynecol. **68**:594, 1954.

Gupta, P.K., Lee, E.F., Erozan, Y.S., Frost, J.K., Geddes, S.T., and Donovan, P.A.: Cytologic investigations in *Chlamydia* infection, Acta Cytol. **23**:315, 1979.

Jarcho, J.: Malformations of the uterus, Am. J. Surg. **71**:106, 1946.

Josey, W.E.: The sexually transmitted infections, Obstet. Gynecol. **43**:465, 1974.

Lamb, E.J., and Greene, R.R.: Microscopic study of growth of leiomyomas of the uterus during pregnancy, Surg. Gynecol. Obstet. **108**:575, 1959.

Nahmias, A.J., Josey, W.E., Naib, Z.M., Freeman, M.G., Fernandez, R.J., and Wheeler, J.H.: Perinatal risk associated with maternal genital herpes simplex virus infection, Am. J. Obstet. Gynecol. **110**:825, 1971.

Philpott, N.W., and Ross, J.E.: Congenital uterine anomalies and associated complications of pregnancy, Am. J. Obstet. Gynecol. **68**:285, 1954.

Piver, M.S., and Spezia, J.: Uterine prolapse during pregnancy, Obstet. Gynecol. **32**:765, 1968.

Pratt, J.P.: Corpus luteum in its relation to menstruation and pregnancy, Endocrinology **11**:195, 1927.

Rock, J.A., and Jones, H.W., Jr.: The clinical management of the double uterus, Fertil. Steril. **28**:798, 1977.

Schachter, J.: Chlamydial infections, N. Engl. J. Med. **298**:428, 1978.

Schneider, G.T.: Sexually transmissible vaginal infections in pregnancy. I. Common infections, Postgrad. Med. **65**:177, 1979.

Schneider, G.T.: Sexually transmissible vaginal infections in pregnancy. II. Less common infections, Postgrad. Med. **65**:185, 1979.

Syphilis-CDC recommended treatment schedule, Centers for Disease Control Morbidity and Mortality Weekly Report **25**:101, 1976.

Tawa, K.: Ovarian tumors in pregnancy, Am. J. Obstet. Gynecol. **90**:511, 1964.

Wilkin, J.K.: Molluscum contagiosum venereum in a woman's outpatient clinic: a venereally transmitted disease, Am. J. Obstet. Gynecol. **128**:531, 1977.

Elsie Reid Carrington

27

Disorders of the nervous system, the skin, and the bones and joints during pregnancy

With the exception of puerperal psychosis, disorders of the nervous system do not differ appreciably in pregnant and nonpregnant women either from the standpoint of their incidence or their prognosis. However, symptoms may be temporarily exaggerated when the mechanical and physiologic burdens of pregnancy are added to chronic disease of the nervous system. In general, skin diseases also affect gravid and nongravid women similarly. On the contrary, disturbances of the bones and joints are most frequently related to the physiologic changes of pregnancy that are responsible for separation and increased mobility especially affecting the pelvic joints.

DISORDERS OF THE NERVOUS SYSTEM
Seizure disorders

Among the various forms of epilepsy, only the idiopathic type poses a risk of *hereditary transmission,* which amounts to less than 2% affected offspring. There is an *increased incidence of congenital anomalies of various types in infants born of mothers on a regimen of anticonvulsant drugs.* In Lowe's series, the difference in incidence in offspring of epileptic mothers with and without these drugs was 6.7% to 2.7%, respectively. Cleft palate, cleft lip, and heart anomalies predominate. *Growth retardation* is likely to occur.

Symptoms. Temporary effects of pregnancy are wholly unpredictable. In the majority of epileptic mothers, symptoms remain unchanged or become aggravated; but, in some, seizures are reduced throughout the prenatal period and return with their usual frequency after delivery. Rarely, grand mal attacks make their first appearance during pregnancy or in the puerperium and must be distinguished from eclampsia. Positive water balance associated with pregnancy can increase epileptic attacks, presumably as a result of cerebral edema.

Treatment. Phenytoin (Dilantin), phenobarbital, or other anticonvulsant drugs obviously need to be continued throughout pregnancy. A single rather than a multiple anticonvulsant drug regimen is advisable when possible. Folic acid deficiency is known to occur in patients on long-term anticonvulsant therapy, and the drug also interferes with vitamin K absorption, leading to a coagulation disorder in the fetus or newborn and, to a lesser degree, to maternal bleeding before or after delivery. The use of folic acid throughout pregnancy and vitamin K once weekly during the last month will usually be protective.

Attacks during labor occur, but fortunately these are rare. Lactation does not increase convulsions, but nursing should be restricted or supervised to prevent injury to the baby if an attack occurs while it is at breast.

Status epilepticus. Repetitive seizures constitute a medical emergency. Slow intravenous injection of diazepam (Valium), 5 to 10 mg, and establishment of an airway are the first steps. Resuscitative measures may be necessary. In refractory cases intravenous diazepam may be repeated once in the first hour, and anticonvulsant therapy instituted with intravenous phenytoin given at the rate of 50 mg/min as a maximum for a total of 200 mg.

Sterilization is advisable for epileptic women who show progressive mental retardation and those with a history of status epilepticus.

POLIOMYELITIS

Incidence. Acute poliomyelitis during pregnancy has almost been eliminated by immunization.

Management. The treatment of poliomyelitis should not be altered because of the pregnancy. Since the uterine muscle is not involved, normal labor can be anticipated. Local anesthesia or pudendal block is preferable for delivery.

Fetal effects. Only a few cases of neonatal poliomyelitis have been reported, generally as a result of contamination with the mother's virus at the time of delivery.

Immunization. Travelers in underdeveloped countries and otherwise susceptible pregnant women can be given Salk vaccine. The immunologic response is comparable to that of nonpregnant individuals. There is no increase in abortion rate in women vaccinated during the first trimester, and no known teratogenic effects attributable to the administration of vaccine have been encountered.

Polyneuritis and polyradiculopathy (Guillain-Barré syndrome)

Polyneuritis as a result of dietary deficiencies has all but disappeared in the United States. It is occasionally found in connection with severe hyperemesis gravidarum. Deaths have occurred with polyneuritis as a result of cardiac or phrenic nerve involvement and respiratory failure.

Polyneuritis attributable to other causes such as diabetes, alcohol, drugs, and heavy metals must be differentiated from the foregoing, the cause removed, and substitution therapy instituted promptly.

Guillain-Barré syndrome, or polyradiculopathy, simulates poliomyelitis or polyneuritis with multiple peripheral and cranial nerve involvement, including bulbar paralysis, which is reported in one third of cases. The fetus in utero is not afflicted with the disorder per se but is at risk if maternal pulmonary support is inadequate. Diagnosis is made by examination of the cerebrospinal fluid in which there is a significant elevation of protein without pleocytosis. This is a temporary disorder, although remissions and exacerbations are known to occur. Recovery rate is high if appropriate supportive therapy is applied.

Chorea gravidarum

Chorea is now a rare complication of pregnancy. It is a form of Sydenham's (rheumatic) chorea associated with pregnancy. Its occurrence has decreased dramatically as a result of antibiotic and other medical therapy in control of acute rheumatic carditis. The primary attack is most common in young primagravidas, but it may occur at any parity. Except in severe cases, pregnancy and labor are unaffected.

At present other disorders known to manifest choreaic movements such as parathyroid or basal ganglia disturbances, systemic lupus erythematosis, and genetic types of chorea should be excluded.

Myasthenia gravis

Myasthenia gravis is a neuromuscular disorder that is now recognized as an autoimmune disorder. An immunologic attack upon the acetylcholine receptors at the neuromuscular junction with resulting receptor loss has been demonstrated by Fambrough, Drachman, and Satyamurtis. This loss, which produces interference or block of normal neuromuscular function, is responsible for muscle weakness and fatigue characteristic of the disease.

Ptosis of the eyelids is usually an early symptom with progressive weakness of skeletal muscles and difficulty in swallowing, in speaking, and in respiratory functions. The thymus gland may be enlarged, and thymomas have been found in 10% of cases. In these patients the disease is more serious, and the course more rapidly downhill. For this reason Genkins is convinced that, in addition to anticholinesterase drugs, thymectomy is advisable early in the course of the disease, even before pregnancy is contemplated, because of its favorable effect on the overall course of the disease.

The clinical course of myasthenia is one of remissions and exacerbations. Although the effect of childbearing is not entirely predictable, in most instances the pregnancy is tolerated well, and normal vaginal delivery can be anticipated. The disease rarely provides an indication for abortion. The dosage of anticholinesterase medication frequently must be adjusted during pregnancy and the puerperium.

Ten percent to 20% of infants of mothers with this

disease show evidence of neonatal myasthenia. Anticholinesterase drugs cross the placental barrier freely. The effects are usually transitory and tend to disappear within 2 to 4 weeks. Prompt treatment with neostigmine (Prostigmine) is essential for survival and should be continued for as long as muscle weakness persists. If there is doubt regarding the cause of respiratory difficulty in the newborn, parenteral injection of 0.05 ml edrophonium chloride (Tensilon) should be given. If the cause is transient myasthenia, improvement is evident immediately, and anticholinesterase drug therapy is required for at least a week or 10 days. Although the disease can be familial, congenital myasthenia gravis is exceedingly rare.

Multiple sclerosis

There is no evidence that exacerbations are increased or that the progress of multiple sclerosis is accelerated during pregnancy. The fetus is not affected.

Normal labor and delivery can usually be expected. Because this disease is progressive and ultimately incapacitating, childbearing should be limited.

Subarachnoid hemorrhage, cerebral aneurysm, and occlusive cerebral disorders

Spontaneous subarachnoid hemorrhage and rupture of a cerebral aneurysm may occur during pregnancy, but the incidence is not increased in gravid women as compared with others of similar ages.

Etiologic factors. The usual cause is a bleeding aneurysm or angioma, and only rarely are cardiovascular or other disturbances such as blood dyscrasias, tuberculosis, or tumors responsible. Occasionally, there is no discoverable disease.

Diagnosis. The onset is generally sudden with severe headache, vomiting, paralysis, and eventually coma. The blood pressure may be elevated, but the characteristic findings of nuchal rigidity, increased intraspinal pressure, and grossly bloody spinal fluid differentiate this lesion from coma of intracerebral or metabolic origin. The clinical course is determined by the size of the vessel involved and the extent of the hemorrhage. The mortality rate associated with spontaneous subarachnoid hemorrhage is high, amounting to almost 50%, whether the victim is pregnant or not. About half of fatalities occur within the first 24 hours.

Treatment. Initial medical treatment is aimed to gaining control of bleeding, convulsions, and associated symptoms. Cerebral arteriography can be done when symptoms have subsided. Pregnancy is not a contraindication to the procedure. If an aneurysm is found and its location is accessible, surgical correction is advisable to prevent recurrence.

The method of delivery should be individualized, but if the vaginal route is chosen, the second stage of labor should be eliminated, and forceps delivery carried out as soon as the cervix is fully dilated. Cerebrospinal fluid (CSF) pressures are not much changed with uterine contractions alone but rise significantly when the patient bears down with contractions. If any delay or difficulty is anticipated, delivery by cesarean section is preferred.

Nonhemorrhagic stroke is also seen in gravid women. Cross, Castro, and Jennet at the Institute of Neurological Sciences at Glasgow found that strokes occurring in association with pregnancy were more frequently a result of occlusive cerebral arterial disease than cerebral venous thrombosis. They reported 31 cases of carotid artery ischemia, all with hemiplegia and 16 with dysphasia. The onset was abrupt in 23 women. Prodromal headache, visual disturbances, epilepsy, and paresthesias were often noted. Since five of these patients had occlusion of the internal carotid artery in which surgery might have been corrective, and since the clinical features per se do not distinguish between these two types of cerebral vascular disease, definitive diagnosis by angiography should not be deferred.

Pseudotumor cerebri

This disorder, also referred to as *benign intracranial hypertension,* is characterized by papilledema, headache and increased intracranial pressure. Cerebral edema is present, but there are no focal neurologic lesions. The CSF pressure is elevated, and, except for low protein levels, laboratory findings are normal. If pressure becomes high enough to cause loss of visual acuity, nausea and vomiting, and constant severe headache, lumbar puncture and removal of CSF fluid is necessary and may need to be repeated.

The cause is unknown but is presumed to be a hormone-related fluid retention process. Symptoms usually disappear after pregnancy although some loss of vision may persist. Recurrences in subsequent pregnancies are reported in about one third of cases.

Peripheral neuropathies

Neuritic disturbances of varying severity are observed during pregnancy. Manifestations range from sensory effects such as paresthesia and pain, which are common, to sensory and motor changes, which are rare.

Etiologic factors. Neuritis may be caused by:

1. Inadequate intake of vitamin B complex, which is responsible for most symptoms of numbness and tingling of the hands and feet and for the most severe form of polyneuritis

2. Mechanical factors, which are largely responsible for sciatic and traumatic neuritis

PARESTHESIAS. Paresthesias often persist throughout pregnancy despite therapy and disappear slowly thereafter.

Acrodysesthesia. Acrodysesthesia (brachialgia statica dysesthetica), or numbness, tingling, and stiffness of the upper extremities, may appear and persist during pregnancy. Symptoms are caused by stretching of or pressure on the brachial plexus when relaxation of the ligaments allows greater motion of the shoulder girdle in both forward and backward direction. Discomfort is greatest when steady traction is exerted, and for this reason the patient usually complains of numbness—sometimes almost complete anesthesia of the hands, particularly in the distribution of the ulnar nerve—on awakening from sleep. Since this is purely a mechanical problem, relief can be obtained by supporting the shoulder in a favorable midposition by use of pillows at night and by assuming proper posture in the daytime. There is no permanent motor or sensory damage.

Carpal tunnel syndrome. Carpal tunnel syndrome is not an uncommon occurrence during pregnancy. Numbness, tingling, and sharp pain radiating up to the elbow region result from compression of the median nerve under the carpal ligament at the wrist. Edema of the perineural structures resulting from water retention during pregnancy is believed to be the cause. The symptoms can be severe. Diagnosis is confirmed by eliciting symptoms: with hyperextension and hyperflexion of the wrist or by the tourniquet test. Symptoms can be relieved by splinting the wrist or by local-steroid injection, but they disappear spontaneously after the pregnancy.

SCIATIC NEURITIS. Pain and tenderness over the sciatic and, occasionally, the femoral distribution

result from relaxation of the sacroiliac joints and subsequent tension or trauma to the nerves involved. Immobilization of the sacroiliac joints by use of a firm back support and bed boards offers relief, but some discomfort may persist for several weeks after delivery.

TRAUMATIC NEURITIS OR MATERNAL OBSTETRIC PARALYSIS. Pain, paresthesia, or muscle weakness developing in the lower extremities during labor or soon afterward suggests the syndrome of traumatic neuritis or maternal obstetric paralysis. Dorsiflexors of the foot are most frequently affected. Compression of the lumbosacral trunk by the fetal skull is the usual cause. This may occur spontaneously with arrest of the fetal head at the pelvic brim, particularly in the platypelloid pelvis with reduced anteroposterior diameter, or as a result of a difficult forceps delivery. In some women, protrusion of a lumbar intervertebral disc is the cause.

The *peroneal nerve* can be injured by undue pressure against the stirrups during delivery. Footdrop is the result. Since the nerve is superficial as it passes laterally around the fibular neck, this area should be protected by padding when the patient is positioned and by avoiding pressure against the knee when the patient is anesthetized.

Treatment of traumatic neuritis consists of splinting, active and passive exercises, and galvanic stimulation of the affected muscles. Prognosis for recovery within several weeks after delivery is good.

The incidence of Bell's palsy is increased in pregnant women. Facial paralysis, pain, taste disturbance, and decreased tearing usually disappear gradually after delivery.

POLYNEURITIS. Fortunately, polyneuritis is a rare complication. Actual degenerative nerve changes that occur result in diminished sensation, paralysis, and muscular atrophy. The process may be limited to a single nerve but can become generalized and rapidly fatal with bulbar involvement. Manifestations are similar to those of Landry's ascending paralysis.

Treatment is preventive. Deficiency states developing in the course of severe hyperemesis or other depleting disorders should be prevented by early replacement of fluid, electrolytes, water-soluble vitamins, and carbohydrates. When nerve damage characteristic of poly-neuritis develops, changes may be irreversible.

SKIN DISORDERS

With few exceptions, no cutaneous diseases occur only during pregnancy. Any of the *acute skin eruptions* can occur coincidentally, but their course and treatment are not appreciably altered in gravid women. *Chronic skin diseases,* however, are frequently influenced by pregnancy. Eczema, psoriasis, and various allergic skin manifestations may be improved in some patients and aggravated in others. Acne and hypertrichosis may be more apparent during pregnancy than otherwise.

Herpes gestationis

This vesicobullous disease of pregnancy, also termed *pemphigoid gestationis,* is an autoimmune process believed to be induced by certain hormones of pregnancy, since similar lesions have been encountered in patients with hydatidiform mole and choriocarcinoma. Eruptions, usually beginning in the periumbilical region, consist of superficial vesicobullous or pustular lesions with an erythematous base. These occur in patches that may be distributed over the entire body. An intense pruritus usually persists throughout pregnancy and disappears gradually after delivery. Blood counts show marked eosinophilia. Occasionally constitutional symptoms of chills and fever occur with periods of exacerbation.

Diagnosis can be established with certainty by direct immunofluorescence of lesional and normal skin.

Treatment with antihistaminics provides minimal relief of symptoms. Daily administration of corticosteroids has resulted in significant improvement of both symptoms and pregnancy outcome and is the mainstay of treatment of severe cases.

Maternal mortality is not increased. Risk to the fetus is debated. Holmes and Black found no increase in perinatal deaths in 33 cases but a significant increase in low-birth-weight and "small for gestational age" infants. Only two newborns showed minor bullous eruptions, and they resolved within 1 week.

Impetigo herpetiformis

Impetigo herpetiformis is a rare inflammatory disease of the skin that occurs mainly in association with pregnancy but has also been found in patients with hypoparathyroidism. The cause is unknown, but lesions are so similar to those of psoriasis, both grossly and microscopically, that it may well be a form of that disease. Characteristic lesions are miliary pustules arranged in irregular or circinate clusters. The pustules spread peripherally as the centers undergo desiccation. Usual sites are the inner aspects of the thighs and genitocrural areas. Mucous membranes of the oral cavity may be involved with lesions that appear as grayish-white plaques.

Symptoms include severe burning and itching of the skin, chills, fever, vomiting, diarrhea, and prostration. Mortality in reported cases has been high and often associated with septicemia. Antibiotic therapy, correction of dehydration, and corticosteroid therapy have greatly improved the outcome. Termination of pregnancy is rarely indicated.

Pruritus

Generalized pruritus is not an uncommon occurrence during pregnancy. Skin manifestations other than scratch marks are frequently absent, but occasionally urticarial reactions are visible. When there is no associated jaundice and no increase in blood bilirubin levels, a neurogenic cause is most likely. In some patients the itching is related to *idiopathic cholestasis.*

Symptoms range from mild discomfort to intolerable itching, restlessness, and fatigue. Treatment consists of antihistaminics, mild sedation, and local analgesic applications.

A relatively rare and intensely pruritic lesion is designated *pruritic folliculitis* or *papular dermatitis of pregnancy* and is characterized by the appearance of erythematous papules over the trunk and forearms. Lesions become excoriated with scratching. The cause is unknown, and treatment symptomatic. The disturbance disappears after delivery but tends to recur with subsequent pregnancies.

Pruritic urticarial papules and plaques of pregnancy (PUPPP) is a more common distinctive skin lesion of pregnancy. The incidence is underreported because of its relatively benign nature. The eruption appears first on the abdomen in late pregnancy as erythematous papules that blanch on pressure and urticarial plaques. Lesions spread, covering thighs, buttocks, and arms. Biopsy shows lymphocytic infiltration, edema, and local spongiosis. The cause is unknown, but immunofluorescent staining is negative for complement and immunoglobulins. There are no maternal or fetal complications. Treatment is symptomatic, and the eruption disappears after delivery.

Lupus erythematosus

Lupus erythematosus is of interest because it occurs most frequently in women during the reproductive years; although the spontaneous abortion rate is increased particularly in those in whom *lupus anticoagulant factor* can be identified, it does not otherwise affect fertility. The disease is serious and unpredictable at best.

The outcome in puerperal women depends more on the organ involved and severity of the disease than the existence of pregnancy. With the *discoid type,* neither mother nor baby is much affected. *Systemic lupus erythematosus* poses far greater risks for both mother and baby. Although patients with disseminated lupus experience remissions, those with renal involvement (which constitute over 50% of patients with systemic disease) are prone to exacerbations and progressive renal impairment. Maternal mortality is increased, and in survivors life expectancy is significantly shortened when active lupus glomerulonephritis is associated with pregnancy. Fetal death often occurs, particularly in the presence of lupus anticoagulant factor.

Since systemic lupus erythematosus can no longer be considered a rare disease, the diagnosis should be considered in otherwise unexplained proteinuria during pregnancy, especially in patients with fever, arthralgia, alopecia, or rashes.

Corticosteroid therapy provides the most effective form of treatment, and it can be administered during pregnancy without endangering the fetus. In McGee and Makowski's series, high dosages of corticosteroids that were continued during labor and after delivery in patients receiving prenatal therapy appeared to reduce the possibility of postpartum exacerbation. No form of maternal treatment was effective in improving the excessive prematurity and stillbirth rates.

Abortion is of little value in improving the prognosis of severe systemic lupus. Mortality following abortion is in the range of 25%, and few instances of postoperative improvement have been reported.

Bridge and Foley showed that the lupus erythematosus factor crosses the placental barrier. These and other investigators have found lupus erythematosus cells in cord and peripheral blood of infants whose mothers had systemic disease, although the babies appeared normal and healthy in each case. The lupus erythematosus cells are not demonstrable in the offspring after 7 weeks of life.

Melanoma

Pigmented moles frequently become more obvious during pregnancy, just as increased pigmentation of other areas of the skin may be observed at that time. The question of which of these innumerable lesions, most of which are benign, should be removed often arises. On the basis of their wide experience with 1050 patients with malignant melanoma, including 32 cases complicated by pregnancy, Pack and Scharnagel recommend removal of pigmented moles in the following circumstances: (1) those on the trunk that are subject to irritation and all those on the genitals and feet where true melanomas are disproportionately more common; (2) moles that are smooth and blue-black; and (3) those exhibiting growth, ulceration, or pain. These should be excised wide of the lesion and never removed by desiccation, since each specimen requires microscopic examination.

Malignant melanoma is a highly malignant tumor, whether associated with pregnancy or not. Overall 5-year survival rates are not significantly different, especially in the early stage when chance of surgical cure is likely. Endocrine manipulation, including termination of pregnancy, ovarian ablation, or administration of hormones has no benefits. Although not usual, placental metastasis and transmission to the fetus can occur.

BONE AND JOINT DISORDERS

The bones forming the pelvic girdle are solidly united in the adult woman except during pregnancy, when hormonal effect on the sacroiliac joints and the symphysis pubis permits varying degrees of motion. Radiographic evidence of relaxation can be observed as early as the first trimester, becoming maximal by the beginning of the third trimester.

Sacroiliac relaxation

Sacroiliac relaxation is the most common cause of low back pain in pregnant women. Backache may be limited to the lower lumbar region or radiate down the back of the legs in the distribution of the sciatic nerve. Occasionally, pain follows the course of the femoral nerve over the anterior aspects of the lower abdomen and thighs. Although symptoms may be transitory, they frequently persist throughout pregnancy and for several weeks after delivery. Tenderness can be elicited by palpation over the posterior surface of the sacroiliac joint or by pelvic palpation below and lateral to the sacral promontory. X-ray film examination is generally contraindicated.

Complete immobilization is impractical, if not impossible, during pregnancy, and accordingly few persons are cured; however, relief can be obtained by the use of a firm sacroiliac support, bed boards, and increased periods of rest.

Symphyseal separation

Widening of the symphysis occurs regularly during pregnancy, and, although the increase is sometimes remarkable, symptoms arise less frequently than might be expected. It is likely that acute or chronic trauma to the periosteum is necessary before characteristic signs appear. These may occur during the course of pregnancy but are far more common after a difficult forceps delivery or the birth of a large baby.

The patient experiences severe pain over the pubic and lumbar regions on walking or in attempting to turn in bed. Efforts to reduce motion of the pelvic girdle result in a typical waddling gait. Motion of the pelvic bones can be demonstrated on direct palpation of the lower border of the symphysis while the patient transfers her weight from one extremity to the other. The degree of disability, however, is not necessarily related to the amount of separation.

Treatment. Immobilization of the pelvic girdle by an encircling elastic binder or tight maternity support will permit gradual ambulation. In most cases, symptoms disappear within 2 to 3 weeks after delivery, although some persist for months.

Spinal fusion

Patients who have had orthopedic problems involving the spinal column, particularly those requiring spinal fusion, need special management during pregnancy and delivery. A detailed survey of these problems conducted by Trelford showed that a high proportion of patients who had fusion before pregnancy experienced exacerbation of symptoms and in nine of 17 instances required repeat fusion after delivery. This complication can usually be prevented by use of a support or brace that provides three-point fixation (symphysis pubis, lower sacrum, and upper lumbar–lower rib cage) and, often, hospitalization during the prenatal period.

Spondylolisthesis

The stress directed at the fifth lumbar and first sacral segments during late pregnancy may be a factor in the initiation or aggravation of spondylolisthesis in women. The lithotomy position can be detrimental. The use of human leg holders or delivery in the dorsal or lateral position is preferable in the conduct of vaginal delivery. Trial of labor should not be protracted. If progress is not satisfactory after 6 to 8 hours, operative delivery is advisable.

Ankylosis of the sacrococcygeal joint

Fusion or injury resulting in ankylosis of the sacrococcygeal joint may be suspected during prenatal pelvic examination if the configuration is unusual or the joint rigid. No difficulties arise until the patient is in labor and then only if the coccyx is angulated anteriorly. Descent of the presenting part is delayed, but fracture of the coccyx during forceps extraction usually permits vaginal delivery. In this event, pain during sitting or straining can be expected for several weeks.

Dislocation of the coccyx

Dislocation of the coccyx may cause excruciating pain that makes its appearance immediately after the parturient recovers from anesthesia. Replacement by rectal manipulation with the patient under morphine analgesia or light anesthesia affords startling and prompt relief.

Osteogenesis imperfecta

Osteogenesis imperfecta has a strong hereditary tendency, since it is transmitted by an autosomal dominant gene. The underlying process is a diffuse mesenchymal hypoplasia manifested by severe osteoporosis with fracture caused by minimal trauma, blue sclerae, and middle ear deafness. The disorder may be early in onset or latent. Neonatal osteogenesis imperfecta is often considered incompatible with life, but the outlook is not always so hopeless. We have delivered three infants of a family with paternal osteogenesis imperfecta. Fractures were demonstrable by x-ray film examination before delivery. All infants survived.

As ultrasound techniques have improved, accurate diagnosis is now possible in some, but not all, cases. This method should be used first, but, if findings are dubious, x-ray film examination is still warranted. The risk of fracture and hematoma formation is greater with vaginal delivery. Cesarean section is indicated if predelivery examination shows involvement of the fetus in utero.

REFERENCES

Benson, R.C., and Inman, V.T.: Brachialgia statica dysesthetica in pregnancy, West. J. Surg. **64**:115, 1956.

Bridge, R.G., and Foley, F.E.: Placental transmission of the lupus erythematosus factor, Am. J. Med. Sci. **227**:1, 1954.

Cohn, S.L., Schreier, R., and Feld, D.: Osteogenesis imperfecta and pregnancy, Obstet. Gynecol. **20**:107, 1962.

Cross, J.N., Castro, P.O., and Jennett, W.B.: Cerebral strokes associated with pregnancy and the puerperium, Br. Med. J. **3**:214, 1968.

Digre, K.B., Yarner, M.W., and Corbett, J.J.: Pseudotumor cerebri and pregnancy, Neurology **34**:721, 1984.

Fambrough, D.M., Drachman, D.B., and Satyamurtis, S.: Neuromuscular junction in myasthenia gravis: decreased acetylcholine receptors, Science **182**:293, 1973.

Foldes, F.F., and McNall, P.G.: Myasthenia gravis: a guide for anesthesiologists, Anesthesiology **23**:837, 1962.

Genkins, G.: Myasthenia and pregnancy. In Rovinsky. J.J., and Guttmacher, A.F.: Medical, surgical, and gynecologic complications of pregnancy, ed. 3, Baltimore, 1985, The Williams and Wilkins Co.

Hertz, K.C., Katz, S.I., Maize, J., and Ackerman, A.B.: Herpes gestationis: a clinicopathologic study, Arch. Dermatol. **112**:1543, 1976.

Hill, R.M., Verniaud, W.M., Horning, M.G., McCulley, L.B., and Morgan, N.F.: Infants exposed in utero to antiepileptic drugs: a prospective study, Am. I. Dis. Child. **127**:645, 1974.

Holmes, R.C., and Black, M.M.: The fetal prognosis in pemphigoid (herpes) gestationis, Br. J. Dermatol. **110**:67, 1984.

Horn, P.: Obstetric management of poliomyelitis complicating pregnancy, Clin. Obstet. Gynecol. **1**:127, 1958.

Lawley, T.J., Hertz, K.C., Wade, T.R., Ackerman, A.B., and Katz, S.I.: Pruritic urticarial papules and plaques of pregnancy, J.A.M.A. **241**:1696, 1979.

Lookingbill, D.P., and Chez, R.A.: Herpes gestationis, Clin. Obstet. Gynecol. **26**:605, 1983.

Lowe, C.R.: Congenital malformations among infants born to epileptic women, Lancet **1**:9, 1973.

Massey, E.W., and Cefelo, R.C.: Neuropathies of pregnancy: a review, Obstet. Gynecol. Surv. **34**:489, 1979.

McGee, C.D., and Makowski, E.L.: Systemic lupus erythematosus in pregnancy, Am. J. Obstet. Gynecol. **107**:1008, 1970.

Morrow, C.P., and DiSaia, P.J.: Malignant melanoma of the female genitalia: a clinical analysis, Obstet. Gynecol. **31**:233, 1976.

Pack, G.T., and Scharnagel, I.M.: The prognosis of malignant melanoma in the pregnant woman, Cancer **4**:324, 1951.

Robinson, J.L., Hall, C.J., and Sedzmir, C.B.: Subarachnoid hemorrhage in pregnancy, J. Neurosurg. **36**:27, 1972.

Smith, D.W.: Teratogenicity of anticonvulsive medications, Am. J. Dis. Child. **131**:1337, 1977.

Trelford, J.D.: Spondylolisthesis in pregnancy, Am. J. Obstet. Gynecol. **91**:320, 1965.

Zegart, K., and Schwartz, R.: Chorea gravidarum, Obstet. Gynecol. **32**:24, 1968.

Zoberman, E., and Farmer, E.R.: Pruritic folliculitis of pregnancy, Arch. Dermatol. **117**:20, 1981.

Zurier, R.B.: Systemic lupus erythematosus: management during pregnancy, Obstet. Gynecol. **51**:78, 1978.

28

Russell K. Laros, Jr.

Hypertensive disorders during pregnancy

Hypertensive disorders that occur during pregnancy are similar in that they are all characterized by elevated blood pressure. Some are specifically related to pregnancy and occur only when the uterus contains trophoblastic tissue. With others, pregnancy adds a complication to an already existing disease. Hypertensive disorders account for about one sixth of all maternal deaths and are significant factors in perinatal mortality. Many deaths can be prevented by early recognition of the condition and by treating it appropriately.

CLASSIFICATION AND DIAGNOSIS

In the past, hypertensive disorders were designated by the nonspecific term *toxemia of pregnancy*. A more accurate classification, proposed by the Committee on Terminology of the American College of Obstetricians and Gynecologists, follows:

1. Preeclampsia
2. Eclampsia
3. Gestational hypertension
4. Gestational proteinuria
5. Gestational edema
6. Chronic hypertensive disease
7. Chronic hypertensive disease with superimposed preeclampsia

Hypertension indicates a rise in systolic blood pressure of at least 30 mm Hg and in diastol-ic pressure of at least 15 mm Hg or of a systolic pressure of at least 140 mm Hg and a diastolic pressure of at least 90 mm Hg. The levels must occur on two occasions at least 6 hours apart.

Proteinuria is defined as a concentration of protein greater than 0.3 g/L/24 hr or a concentration greater than 1 g/L in two or more random urine samples collected at least 6 hours apart.

Edema is the generalized accumulation of fluid that accounts for a weight gain of at least 2.4 kg (5 pounds) in a week or when there is 1 plus pitting edema after 12 hours of rest in bed.

The patient with *preeclampsia* appears normal during early pregnancy, but hypertension, proteinuria, and edema appear after the twentieth week. The exception is that certain women with hydatidiform moles can develop typical preeclampsia during the first half of pregnancy.

One can diagnose *eclampsia* when convulsions occur in a woman with preeclampsia if there is no other reason for the seizures.

Gestational hypertension refers to hypertension that develops during the last half of pregnancy or during the first 24 hours after delivery if there are no evidences of preeclampsia or of chronic hypertensive disease and if the blood pressure returns to normal within 10 days after delivery. Some of these women may have preeclampsia; in others the rise in blood pressure may be evidence of chronic hypertensive disease.

Gestational proteinuria is proteinuria occurring during pregnancy in women who have no evidence of acute or chronic hypertension or of renal disease.

Gestational edema is edema that fits the criteria for the diagnosis of edema, which have already been listed.

Chronic hypertensive disease is diagnosed if hypertension was present when the patient became pregnant, is found before the twentieth week of gestation, or persists beyond the forty-second day after delivery.

In some patients with chronic hypertensive disease the blood pressure will rise at least 30/15 mm Hg during the second half of pregnancy, and the rise will be accompanied by proteinuria and edema. This is *chronic hypertension with superimposed preeclampsia.*

INCIDENCE

About 5% of all pregnancies are complicated by preeclampsia. The incidence may be as high as 10% in indigent women and as low as 2% in those who are more affluent.

PREECLAMPSIA-ECLAMPSIA

Since preeclampsia and eclampsia are phases of a single disorder and differ only in severity, they will be discussed as a single progressive process, preeclampsia-eclampsia.

Preeclampsia-eclampsia occurs only in pregnant human beings; it has no exact counterpart in the hypertensive states in nonpregnant persons. The signs appear after the twentieth week of pregnancy except in the rare instances in which it is associated with hydatidiform mole. It is more common in both young and older primigravidas than in multiparas and is characterized by *edema, proteinuria,* and *hypertension.*

Clinical course. The first evidence of an abnormality is usually an excessive gain in weight, more than 1 kg (2 pounds) a week (Fig. 28-1). After a period of abnormal weight gain, the other signs appear together or one slightly in advance of the other. If the condition is untreated, it may progress

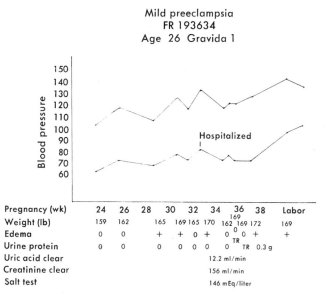

Fig. 28-1. Course of mild preeclampsia. Abnormal weight gain is evident early, whereas blood pressure, although gradually rising, is still within normal range. (From Willson, J.R.: Med. Clin. North Am. **39**:1781, 1955.)

until the patient develops eclampsia, which is the most advanced stage of acute pregnancy-induced hypertension.

EDEMA. Total body water is increased by 6 to 8 L during normal pregnancy. This requires the retention of enough sodium and other electrolytes to maintain an isotonic concentration.

The physiologic high levels of both total body water and exchangeable sodium are increased even more when a pregnant woman develops preeclampsia-eclampsia. Whether this represents an exaggeration of the normal mechanism or is a new process has not yet been determined. Nonetheless, a rapid increase in body weight usually precedes the other clinical signs of preeclampsia by days or weeks.

Fluid and sodium are retained by normal pregnant women despite changes that favor increased sodium excretion: (1) the remarkable increase in glomerular filtration; (2) a high concentration of circulating progesterone, which favors natriuresis; (3) reduced resistance in renal blood vessels; and (4) decreased plasma oncotic pressure. Obviously, sodium depletion would occur rapidly if tubular reabsorption were not increased enough to compensate for these changes. The result is retention of fluids and electrolytes, which is responsible for the expanded plasma volume and for the accumulation of fluid in the extravascular compartments. During most of pregnancy there is a positive sodium balance that reaches at least 20 to 25 mEq/week during the last weeks. The total excess is about 1000 mEq, or 60 g, of sodium chloride for the entire pregnancy.

The pathophysiologic changes with preeclampsia that may favor excessive sodium and fluid retention are (1) depression of glomerular filtration, (2) increased renal vascular resistance, and (3) reduced plasma volume. Because of decreased glomerular filtration, a smaller sodium load reaches the tubules. In addition, altered rates of secretion of aldosterone, desoxycorticosterone, and other substances may be important factors, but their roles have not yet been clearly defined. The changes in fluid and electrolyte exchange and in renal function are results, not the cause, of preeclampsia. The disorder is not induced by the ingestion of salt, but an excessive sodium intake can exaggerate the pathophysiologic changes.

The end result of this alteration in salt metabolism can be demonstrated by injecting hypertonic saline solution intravenously and measuring the urinary output of sodium and chloride (Dieckmann salt test) (Fig. 28-2). The excess electrolytes and water are eliminated less rapidly in normal pregnant women than in nonpregnant women, but there is a further delay in those with preeclampsia. In normal pregnant women the sodium excretion during the first 2 hours after the administration of 1000 ml of 2.5% salt solution averaged 267 mEq/L. Of the normal women, 88% eliminated the excess fluid rapidly, returning to the pretest weight within 48 hours; 70% of those with preeclampsia had not returned to the pretest weight within 96 hours.

HYPERTENSION. The most important pathophysiologic change with preeclampsia-eclampsia is widespread arteriolar spasm, which is the direct cause of hypertension that characterizes preeclampsia-eclampsia. Hypertension is seldom the initial sign of the disorder. The height of the blood pressure in itself does not indicate the overall severity, the average systolic blood pressure in preeclampsia being only about 160 mm Hg. The rise in diastolic pressure may be disproportionate to that of the systolic pressure, thereby *narrowing the pulse pressure*. Diastolic pressures of 110 to 120 mm Hg are not unusual.

Although any blood pressure over 140/90 mm Hg is considered to be abnormal, the physician should not wait for the blood pressure to reach this level before suspecting that something is wrong. Since the blood pressure during normal pregnancy usually is below the prepregnancy level, a gradual but persistent rise should arouse one's suspicions. An increase of more than 30 mm Hg in systolic pressure or of more than 15 mm Hg in diastolic pressure or both, even if they remain within the limits of normal, is suggestive that preeclampsia is developing.

The vascular changes can be seen in the retinal and conjunctival vessels and can be measured in the kidney and in the brain. *Renal blood flow* becomes progressively more reduced as preeclampsia progresses. The alteration is a result of increased resistance in the afferent glomerular arterioles and narrowing of the lumina of the glomerular capillaries. McCall observed *increased vascular resistance in cerebral vessels,* although blood flow and cerebral oxygen consumption remained normal.

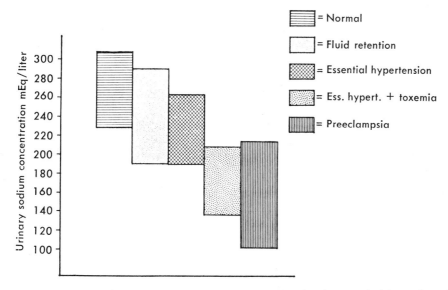

Fig. 28-2. Results of Dieckmann salt test. Urinary excretion of sodium is reduced with preeclampsia and essential hypertension with acute toxemia superimposed.

Uterine blood flow also is reduced, although precise methods for measuring it in humans are not yet available.

The mechanism by which arteriolar spasm is initiated and maintained is not as yet clearly understood, but it probably has no relationship to changes in the autonomic nervous system. The blood pressure in pregnant women with essential hypertension will fall, sometimes precipitously, in response to ganglionic blocking agents. These drugs have little effect on the hypertension associated with preeclampsia.

The arteries in women with preeclampsia are much more responsive to pressor substances, such as norepinephrine and angiotensin, than are those of normal pregnant women. This may be, at least in part, a result of the increased sodium concentration in the arteriolar walls, which increases vascular reactivity in isolated vessels. *Prostaglandins,* or prostaglandin-like substances, may play a role in this reaction. Prostaglandin, which is synthesized in the vascular wall, may prevent the vessel from responding to the stimulus of angiotensin. This reaction can be eliminated by prostaglandin inhibitors.

PROTEINURIA. The third important sign of preeclampsia is the excretion of protein in the urine. This makes its appearance at about the same time as the hypertension and increases in severity as the disease progresses.

The examination of the urine in patients with early preeclampsia reveals no abnormality except for the presence of protein. The amount increases with the severity of the condition, and eventually as much as 10 g may be excreted daily.

One of the important prognostic signs is the amount of urinary protein. A qualitative measurement of protein is likely to be misleading because a given amount of protein diluted in a large amount of urine may be read 1 plus, whereas the same amount in a small quantity of urine may give a 3 or 4 plus reaction. By measuring the total excretion in successive 24-hour periods, the physician has an accurate means of evaluating changes in renal function. This simple test should be part of the study of every pregnant woman with hypertension.

URINE MICROSCOPY. As the disease progresses, the urinary findings increase; in the severe case, large amounts of protein, red blood cells, white blood cells, and all kinds of casts may be found. At this stage the urine examination is of little value in the differential diagnosis of the condition.

RENAL FUNCTION. The renal function in early preeclampsia is slightly reduced as shown by inulin, creatinine, and uric acid clearances that are below those for normal pregnancy. *A pregnant woman must always be in the lateral recumbent position during clearance studies to obtain an accurate result.* Glomerular filtration and sodium excretion are significantly lower in the upright and dorsal positions than in the lateral.

As the disease becomes severe, there is progressive diminution both in renal function, as shown by a further depression in the excretion of the various testing substances, and in urine volume. Women with severe preeclampsia and eclampsia may excrete only 100 to 200 ml of urine in a 24-hour period or may even be completely anuric.

That the decreased function is not directly related to the elevated blood pressure is suggested by the fact that after delivery the renal function is reestablished, with the blood pressure at a level that usually is at least as high as in the predelivery period.

PLASMA VOLUME. A progressive *hemoconcentration,* the result of the abnormal flow of fluid from the bloodstream into the tissue spaces and cells, accompanies severe preeclampsia. As the blood volume decreases, so does the amount of urine excreted; the patient with severe preeclampsia or eclampsia may be anuric. There can be no diuresis without a reversal of the flow of fluid back into the bloodstream from the tissue spaces and reestablishment of blood flow through the glomerular capillaries.

URIC ACID. Uric acid metabolism also is disturbed. As preeclampsia becomes more severe, the renal clearance of uric acid becomes progressively more reduced, and subsequently the serum concentration rises. The maximum normal serum uric acid concentration is 6 mg/dl, and the minimum normal uric acid clearance is 10 mg/min. The increase in serum uric acid is probably a result of decreased renal excretion.

SEVERE PREECLAMPSIA. Progression of the pathophysiologic changes is reflected in changes in physiologic functions and physical findings. Severe preeclampsia can be diagnosed when any of the following develop:

1. Systolic blood pressure of at least 160 mm Hg or diastolic pressure of at least 110 mm Hg on two or more occasions at least 6 hours apart with the patient resting in bed
2. At least 5 g of protein in a 24-hour urine specimen (qualitative 3 or 4 plus)
3. Less than 400 ml urinary output in 24 hours
4. Cerebral or visual symptoms
5. Pulmonary edema or cyanosis
6. Epigastric pain
7. Abnormalities in liver function or coagulation

ECLAMPSIA. Eclampsia represents a progression of preeclampsia with the addition of convulsions or coma or both.

The physiologic changes are simply a continuation of those found in severe preeclampsia. There is a further increase in blood pressure, but this need not be to exceedingly high levels; the systolic blood pressure is often below 200 mm Hg except during the actual convulsions, but the diastolic pressure may be 120 to 130 mm Hg. The oliguria increases to anuria, and there is a further increase in the hemoconcentration, the hematocrit at times reaching 45 or 50. A retention of nitrogenous and material accompanies the depression of kidney function, and for the first time a rise in blood urea nitrogen may be observed.

Eclampsia may develop before the onset of labor, during labor, or within the first 24 hours after delivery.

Etiologic factors. The cause of preeclampsia-eclampsia has not been clearly established, but it is evident that the condition can develop only in women with active trophoblastic tissue. One important factor appears to be the amount of placental tissue. Preeclampsia occurs more often during pregnancies with multiple fetuses and with hydatidiform mole; in both there is a greater volume of trophoblastic tissue than with a single fetus. The incidence is increased in patients with chronic cardiovascular renal disease, diabetes mellitus, fetal hydrops, and severe anemia.

The role of *dietary deficiency* in the development of preeclampsia-eclampsia is not clearly defined, but it is presumed to be an important factor. Pregnancy-induced hypertension develops more often in women of the lower socioeconomic classes than in middle- and upper-class women. This has been attributed to chronic malnutrition, particularly to an inadequate intake of protein; but the precise role of diet is not clear. If malnutrition were the sole cause of preeclampsia-eclampsia, the disease would occur in multiparas, particularly those who had been affected in previous pregnancies, as often as in primigavidas, but it does not. It is unlikely that dietary, economic, and environmental conditions will change enough between pregnancies to account for the reduction in incidence in parous women.

The possibility of an *immunologic factor* being responsible for the development of preeclampsia has been proposed. This is an intriguing suggestion because the development of the disorder during the first exposure to trophoblast apears to provide protection against its recurrence in subsequent pregnancies. Much more information is necessary before such a mechanism can be confirmed.

Many attempts have been made to correlate geographic and climatic conditions with its development. So far no convincing evidence has been advanced.

The most tenable current theory is that of *uterine ischemia*. A reduction in blood flow to the choriodecidual space could alter placental function, permitting the trophoblast or the decidua to produce thromboplastin or thromboplastin-like material, pressor polypeptides, or other substances that might initiate the characteristic vascular changes. The basic theory has much in its favor. Preeclampsia-eclampsia occurs most often in young primigravidas, particularly those with twins, and in women with hydatidiform moles, particularly those in whom the uterus is larger than that expected for the duration of pregnancy. In each of these the uterus tends to be either tense or more distended than usual. This could cause a reduction in blood flow through the smaller vessels. The incidence in women with preexisting hypertensive disorders and with diabetes, particularly those with vascular degeneration, also is high. In these women, too, uterine blood flow is reduced.

Cavanagh and associates have developed a model of preeclampsia in the pregnant baboon.

Relative uterine ischemia is produced by constriction of the aorta below the level of the renal vessels. The animals developed hypertension, a decrease in plasma renin activity, an increase in renal resistance, an increase in serum uric acid and glomerular changes consistent with those seen in human preeclampsia. McKay has reported blood changes that resemble those of *disseminated intravascular coagulation* in women with preeclampsia. Some of his findings have been confirmed by others.

Clinically significant disseminated intravascular coagulation (DIC) is rare, occurring in only 10% of patients with severe preeclampsia or eclampsia. Pritchard and co-workers demonstrated thrombocytopenia in 29% and a prolonged thrombin time (an indicator of circulating fibrin/fibrinogen split products) in 50% of 95 eclamptic women. Directly measured fibrin/fibrinogen degradation products were only elevated in 3%, and circulating fibrin monimer in 5% of the cases. However, if sensitive tests of procoagulant consumption are used such as the ratio of factor VIII activity/factor VIII antigen or beta thromboglobulin, changes are almost always found. Deposits of fibrin have been reported by some, but not all investigators in liver, kidneys and other organs. Fibrin deposition is invariably present in the intravillous space. This suggests that focal deposition at the placental site rather than generalized DIC may be the pathophysiology of procoagulant consumption.

The more severe the toxemia, the more pronounced the changes. Some women with advanced preeclampsia-eclampsia develop a full-blown coagulation defect.

Weinstein has presented data that define a unique group of preeclamptic women. These individuals develop hemolysis, elevated liver enzymes, and thrombocytopenia; the so-called HELLP syndrome. This is probably not a unique syndrome, but rather a variant of severe preeclampsia that may develop either before or after delivery.

Chesley, Annitto, and Cosgrove studied the toxemia rate in the daughters of women who had had eclampsia in an attempt to determine if there is a *familial factor*. The incidence of first-pregnancy toxemia in the daughters was 26% and of toxemia in subsequent pregnancies, 22%. The incidence of first-pregnancy toxemia in daughters-in-law of the same women was 8%. Daughters-in-law were selected as control subjects because their ages and social status were comparable to those of the study group. Sutherland and colleagues confirmed this observation by repeating the study in reverse. Fourteen percent of the mothers of women with severe preeclampsia, as compared with 3% of control subjects and 4% of mothers-in-law, had had a similar condition.

Prediction. One can always anticipate that preeclampsia may develop in primigravid women who have diabetes or chronic cardiovascular renal disease, those who are poor and malnourished, and those with multiple pregnancies. It is more difficult to predict that it will occur in presumably normal women.

Gant and associates developed a test that may indicate many of those who are likely to develop preeclampsia. Blood pressures are recorded between 28 and 32 weeks after stabilization first in the lateral recumbent position and then in the supine position. In the study a rise in diastolic pressure of more than 20 mm Hg occurred on assuming the supine position in 93% of normotensive multiparas who later developed pregnancy-induced hypertension. In addition, most of the same women demonstrated a rise in blood pressure in response to angiotensin. Conversely, 91% of those with minimal blood pressure elevation with a change in position and with little response to angiotensin remained normal throughout pregnancy. Although not absolutely accurate, this simple test may indicate most women who are in danger of developing preeclampsia.

Prophylaxis. It will not be possible to prevent the development of acute pregnancy-induced hypertension until more is known about its basic cause. The serious advanced stages with their high perinatal and maternal mortality can be prevented if the alert physician detects the earliest evidence of preeclampsia and institutes appropriate treatment.

Primigravid women and those who have conditions that predispose them to the development of preeclampsia-eclampsia should be seen more often than normal multiparas during the last half of preg-

nancy. The signs of developing preeclampsia can be detected in almost every instance if the patient is examined every other week between the twenty-eighth and thirty-fifth weeks of pregnancy and weekly thereafter.

Treatment. Dieckmann divided the signs and symptoms of preeclampsia into groups that indicate progressive severity of the condition. The list has been expanded to include laboratory changes and may be used as an aid in guiding treatment.

Group A
Edema (weight), hypertension, proteinuria

Group B

Cerebral	*Visual*
Headache	Diplopia
Dizziness	Scotomas
Tinnitus	Blurred vision
Tachypnea	Amaurosis
Tachycardia	*Renal*
Fever	Oliguria
Gastrointestinal	Anuria
Nausea	*Laboratory*
Vomiting	Evidence of DIC
Epigastric pain	Evidence of hepatocellular disease
Hematemesis	Hematuria
	Hemoglobinuria

The only evidences of preeclampsia before its immediate preconvulsive stage are those in group A, which the physician must recognize. The patient usually has no symptoms as the condition is developing; in fact, she may have none with severe preeclampsia. The presence of group B signs and symptoms suggests that eclampsia is imminent.

OFFICE TREATMENT OF PREECLAMPSIA. The earliest evidence of pregnancy-induced hypertension can be recognized by an alert observer, but whether treatment influences the course of preeclampsia is questionable.

Excessive weight gain associated with exaggerated fluid retention is often the earliest warning that preeclampsia may be developing. A diagnosis cannot be made on the basis of weight gain or edema alone, however, because most women have dependent edema during the last weeks of pregnancy and few develop preeclampsia. The other signs, hypertension and proteinuria, will appear in those whose edema is caused by early preeclampsia.

Women who gain weight suddenly, those who gain more than 1 kg (2 pounds) per week, and those with obvious edema must be seen more often than patients who gain at an anticipated rate. In those with preeclampsia the blood pressure will rise and proteinuria will appear. These changes will not occur in the others.

Since blood pressure generally rises slowly as preeclampsia is becoming evident, examinations approximately every 3 days are adequate to recognize the changes. Abrupt blood pressure rises, which sometimes occur, will also be detected promptly with this schedule.

The only *laboratory studies* that may be helpful in differentiating early preeclampsia from excessive fluid retention are uric acid and creatinine clearances, which may be reduced slightly in women with early preeclampsia. Serum uric acid concentrations, which rise as clearance is reduced, will probably be in the normal range at this stage.

There is no *treatment* that will effectively reverse the pathologic processes of preeclampsia. It has been customary to recommend low-sodium diets for edematous women and for those with preeclampsia, but this is not appropriate. Sodium is necessary, even in women with preeclampsia, to supply tissue needs and to prevent contraction of plasma volume and the fluid volume in the extravascular compartments. Bed rest in the lateral recumbent position will enhance excretion of excess fluid, but diuretics are contraindicated. Of course, adequate nutrition is essential, but improving an inadequate diet at this late stage will not solve the immediate problem.

Because the placental site is one of the target organs in preeclampsia, less than optimal placental function should be anticipated. This can be evidenced by intrauterine fetal growth and evidence of diminished placental reserve. When preeclampsia is mild, fetal well-being should be assured with biweekly nonstress tests (NSTs) and/or contraction stress tests (CSTs) and biweekly ultrasonic evaluation of fetal growth and amniotic fluid volume. If the preeclampsia is severe, the NSTs or CSTs should be performed daily.

If the blood pressure rises and proteinuria appears during the period of observation, a diagnosis of preeclampsia can be made, and the patient should be admitted to the hospital even if the changes are slight. Those with exaggerated physiologic edema can be observed as outpatients without specific treatment, but they must be seen frequently.

HOSPITAL TREATMENT OF PREECLAMPSIA. The initial hospital treatment of preeclampsia concerns itself primarily with the classification of severity of the condition and the initiation of a regimen designed to control the signs and symptoms. With the exception of an evaluation of the duration of pregnancy, the size and position of the fetus, and the adequacy of the pelvis, the pregnancy is, at the onset, ignored.

The *blood pressure* should be checked four times daily, and the patient *weighed* each morning at the same time. The *fluid intake* and *urine output* are carefully measured and recorded daily, and the amount of edema is evaluated. Daily quantitative determination of the *total urinary protein excretion* likewise is of prognostic significance. A steady increase or a constant excretion of more than 3 to 5 g daily is a grave sign. Daily protein excretion greater than 5 g is associated with a definite increase in intrauterine fetal death. The *serum uric acid* and the *uric acid and creatinine clearances* should be checked twice a week. The *retinal vessels* should be examined at regular intervals for evidence of increasing spasm and alterations in the vessel walls.

Women with preeclampsia should remain in bed much of the day, since bed rest enhances sodium and water excretion. The lateral recumbent position is preferable to the supine because renal function is further reduced in the dorsal position. A *house diet* can usually be ordered, unless there is a reason other than preeclampsia for a special diet. There is no need to limit *fluid intake*.

Success is determined by stabilization or reversal of the abnormal signs (weight, blood pressure, and proteinuria) and by the absence of symptoms. If the response to this regimen is favorable (that is, if an adequate urine output (at least 1500 ml) is maintained, the proteinuria does not increase, the clearances do not fall to dangerous levels, the blood pressure is controlled, and the weight is stabilized), the regimen may be continued until the cervix is "ripe," at which time labor can be induced.

Advance in severity of the condition is characterized by increasing weight and edema, a progressive diminution in urinary output with an increase in total protein, an increase in serum uric acid and creatinine, a decrease in uric acid and creatinine clearances, further elevation of blood pressure, hemoconcentration as indicated by an increase in hemoglobin and hematocrit, progressive change in the retinal arterioles, and, in many cases, the appearance of symptoms that become progressively more pronounced.

It is important to recognize that weight loss and regression of edema can occur, even though the other signs indicate an increasingly severe process; hence evaluation on the basis of a change in one sign alone is inappropriate.

Stimulation of renal function. The maintenance or promotion of urinary output is desirable in treating severe preeclampsia, but it cannot always be achieved. It is essential that the patient not be overloaded with fluid that she cannot excrete. Reduction of vasospasm may be helpful, but diuretics are usually contraindicated because they are ineffective in stimulating urine output.

Sedation. Sedatives are important in the management of severe or progressing preeclampsia but are unnecessary during the mild phases of the condition. Oversedation should be avoided because, if too much is given, hypoxia may be increased and it may be difficult to differentiate the lethargy or coma produced by the drug from that attributable to the disease.

The cerebral depressant action of *magnesium sulfate* produces general sedation; this and its ability to decrease vascular tone tend to lower blood pressure, promote excretion of urine, and help prevent convulsions. McCall, studying cerebral hemodynamics in pregnancy toxemia, found that magnesium sulfate not only lowers blood pressure but relieves cerebral vasospasm, increases cerebral blood flow, and increases oxygen use by brain tissue. All these tend to reverse the changes of preeclampsia-eclampsia.

Magnesium sulfate can be given intramuscularly as a 50% solution or intravenously in a 20% or 25% solution. Intramuscular injection has the disadvantages of being painful and of the unpredictable absorption rate because of vascular spasm. When given intravenously, an initial dose of 4 to 6 g is administered during a period of 4 to 5 minutes. The maintenance dosage is about 1 g/hr using an infusion pump. Calcium gluconate, which counteracts the effect of magnesium promptly, should be kept at the bedside where it will be readily available if needed.

Magnesium intoxication is possible but is unlikely to occur if the patient is being observed properly. Magnesium is excreted in the urine; consequently, an adequate urinary output is essential. If the urine volume decreases below 30 ml/hr, the dosage of magnesium sulfate must be reduced. Magnesium sulfate also decreases hyperactive reflexes, thereby decreasing the possibility of convulsions. The reflexes can be used to monitor dosage; as long as the patellar reflexes are present, there is no immediate danger of magnesium toxicity. Reflexes should be checked about every 30 minutes.

In many institutions serum magnesium levels are monitored. Certainly they are required if one is to administer magnesium in cases in which the patellar reflexes initially are depressed or in which the patient is oliguric. Table 28-1 shows the clinical effects anticipated at various magnesium levels.

Control of blood pressure. Unless the blood pressure is greatly elevated, hypotensive drugs ordinarily are unnecessary in the treatment of severe preeclampsia because the magnesium sulfate will usually depress the blood pressure to a reasonably safe level. If the pressure falls to an unusually low level or sometimes even to the normal range, the output of urine may be greatly reduced.

If the systolic blood pressure is rising rapidly or is over 160 to 180 mm Hg or if the diastolic pressure is higher than 110 mm Hg, a definite effort should be made to control it. *Hydralazine (Apresoline)*, 10 to 20 mg diluted to 20 ml and given slowly intravenously, will often lower the blood pressure and maintain it at a safe level for several hours. This is particularly effective during labor. The effect of hydralazine on cerebral blood vessels and blood flow is similar to that of magnesium sulfate but more pronounced. When given by mouth, the drug has much less effect.

Termination of pregnancy. The decisive cure for preeclampsia-eclampsia is termination of pregnancy at a carefully chosen time. In most women with severe preeclampsia any response to medical

TABLE 28-1 Clinical effects of various magnesium levels

Clinical condition	Serum magnesium level	
	(mg/dL)	(mEq/L)
Normal	1.8-3	1.5-2.5
Therapeutic	6-8	5-6.7
Loss of patellar reflex	12	10
Respiratory depression	18	15
Cardiac arrest	36	30

treatment is temporary, and the progression of the disease cannot be halted. Delivery after a preliminary period, during which attempts are made to stabilize the process, is the only way to prevent eclampsia with its increased maternal and perinatal mortality. Women with mild preeclampsia that progresses despite treatment and those with severe preeclampsia, even though it responds to medical therapy, should usually be delivered regardless of the duration of pregnancy. Delaying delivery in an attempt to increase infant survival by permitting the fetus to become more mature is usually ineffective. This is particularly true when the pregnancy has advanced to at least 30 to 32 weeks and facilities for intensive neonatal care are available. As discussed above, fetal growth retardation is common with severe preeclampsia because of compromised uteroplacental circulation, and the fetus may die in utero.

Labor can often be induced in these women, even though the cervix may feel unfavorable; hence in most instances the membranes should be ruptured and oxytocin given as an initial procedure. Cesarean section can be performed if labor has not begun within 6 to 12 hours.

HOSPITAL TREATMENT OF ECLAMPSIA. If the patient develops convulsions, the prognosis at once becomes grave.

Unless the natural tendency to overtreat the patient with eclampsia is curbed, the mortality may be increased by the treatment administered. Before any medication is ordered for a convulsing patient, she must be examined to be certain that she actually has eclampsia and to evaluate her general condition. If she is comatose, as most women with eclampsia are, large doses of sedative drugs may be harmful.

The aims in the treatment of eclampsia are (1) to control convulsions, (2) to lower blood pressure, and (3) to terminate pregnancy.

General treatment. The patient is placed in a dimly lighted, quiet room with an attendant constantly present. A *mouth gag*, prepared by wrapping gauze around a tongue blade, should be available to insert between the teeth during convulsions to prevent injury to the tongue. Facilities for *aspiration of mucus* from the pharynx and trachea should be available. Recordings of *blood pressure, urine volume, temperature, pulse, respirations,* and *response to treatment* should be made every 30 minutes. Nothing is given by mouth until after delivery, and the stomach should be aspirated if the patient is vomiting. An *intravenous infusion of 5% dextrose* is run at a rate of about 100 ml/hr.

Since hypoxia always is associated with hemoconcentration, the administration of *oxygen* is a valuable aid in therapy. Copious pulmonary secretions may fill the bronchi and lower trachea, thereby obstructing the airway. Oxygenation can be improved by performing *endotracheal intubation* whenever pulmonary edema is diagnosed, when respirations are labored, or when there is a suggestion of cyanosis.

Renal function. An indwelling catheter is inserted into the bladder, and hourly urine outputs are recorded. The ordinary diuretic preparations are completely valueless, because the anuria is a result of decreased glomerular filtration and most diuretics act at a tubular level. Since the decrease in glomerular filtration is at least in part a result of glomerular arteriolar spasm, the most important part of the treatment is to decrease peripheral vasospasm, which can best be accomplished with magnesium sulfate and other antihypertensive agents.

Control of convulsions. Sedation and control of convulsions are important steps in treatment. Magnesium sulfate, administered as described for severe preeclampsia, will usually provide adequate sedation and control the convulsions. If the convulsions continue, one should suspect that the dose of magnesium sulfate is inadequate. Sibai and colleagues, studying women who continued to convulse despite what was considered to be adequate doses of the drug, found that blood levels often were below those that usually are effective (6 to 8 mg/dl).

Convulsions that continue despite adequate magnesium sulfate therapy can often be controlled by the intravenous administration of diazepam (Valium), 1 mg, or amobarbital sodium (Amytal), 300 mg. These drugs should not be necessary often and should be used with caution, since they are powerful cerebral depressants.

Control of blood pressure. It is not necessary to lower the blood pressure to a normal level; in fact, in some patients even a moderate fall in blood pressure will reduce the renal output of urine. If the diastolic pressure remains above 100 mm Hg, an antihypertensive agent should be administered. *Hydralazine*, 10 to 20 mg diluted to 20 ml, can be given slowly intravenously. The blood pressure should be checked several times as the drug is being injected to detect precipitate drops, which sometimes occur. If the diastolic pressure remains above 110 mm Hg, an additional dose can be given in about 20 minutes. Hydralazine can be repeated if a significant rise in diastolic blood pressure occurs.

Cardiovascular monitoring. Pulmonary edema occurs in patients with severe preeclampsia or eclampsia because of increased intravascular pressure, decreased oncotic pressure, increased capillary permeability or a combination of the three. Because of the threat of pulmonary edema and the difficulty of its management without continuous evaluation of cardiopulmonary function, many clinicians advise the placement of a pulmonary artery (Swan-Ganz) and radial artery catheter in all cases of eclampsia and in many cases of severe preeclampsia. Minute-to-minute monitoring allows appropriate and timely use of preload and afterload reduction and inotropic stimulation.

Termination of pregnancy. Termination of the pregnancy is the decisive step in the treatment of both preeclampsia and eclampsia, but ill-advised attempts at delivery at an inopportune time may result in the death of a patient who otherwise might have survived. Initial treatment by delivery by any method without a preliminary period of medical treatment of the disease is accompanied by an alarming maternal mortality; hence control of convulsions and hypertension must precede delivery. Ordinarily, patients with eclampsia should be delivered soon after convulsions are controlled.

Vaginal delivery from below is preferred if there are no contraindications. Cesarean section is to be considered only for those in whom there is a contraindication to vaginal delivery or for those in whom labor cannot be induced by rupturing membranes and administering oxytocin.

Care following delivery. Any patient with severe preeclampsia may develop eclampsia during the first 24 hours after delivery. During this time, diuresis should begin; if this occurs, it is unlikely that the condition will progress. Should the anuria continue, however, the patient is in danger of convulsing. The same careful observations and the same treatment given the undelivered, severely preeclamptic patient are continued after delivery until the disease process has reversed itself. The urine output is carefully measured at hourly intervals. Sedation should be continued for about 48 hours after delivery but in diminishing amounts. These patients should not be allowed out of bed until the process has definitely reversed itself.

Pathologic changes. The morphologic changes are mostly the result of the characteristic circulatory changes. Fibrin emboli and the acute degenerative changes that can be observed in the small vessels and the hemoconcentration of eclampsia certainly disturb the blood flow through the tissues and may lead to local anoxia and functional or anatomic disruption.

KIDNEY. Acute degenerative changes and fibrin deposition may be observed in the smaller vessels. The size of the glomerular capillary lumina is reduced by swelling of the endothelial cells, by the deposition of amorphous material beneath the normal basement membrane of the capillaries, and by proliferation of the intercapillary cells that lie between the vascular loops. These changes, called *glomerular endotheliosis*, which formerly were thought to be from thickening of the capillary basement membrane, have been clarified by electron microscopy. The tubular cells appear to be degenerated, but the changes probably are caused by excessive absorption of protein. *Cortical necrosis* may occur in women with severe abruptio placentae.

Histologic identification of the precise kidney lesion will establish the diagnosis more accurately than will the clinical signs alone. Spargo, McCartney, and Winemiller found changes characteristic of chronic renal disease in renal biopsies from 16 of 62 primigravidas in whom a diagnosis of preeclampsia had been made and in 32 of 152 multiparas diagnosed as having chronic hypertension with superimposed preeclampsia.

ADRENAL GLANDS. Adrenal hemorrhage and necrosis may occur, particularly in patients who die in a state of vascular collapse.

LIVER. Fibrin thrombi in the vessels and exudates and hemorrhage or actual tissue necrosis in the periportal areas may be found with severe preeclampsia-eclampsia. Extensive subcapsular hemorrhage often occurs when a coagulation defect develops. Liver involvement is minimal or absent with mild preeclampsia.

BRAIN. The same vascular changes may be observed in the brain as elsewhere. Hemorrhage from the rupture of large cerebral vessels is the cause of death in about 15% of women with eclampsia. Cerebral edema may be a postmortem change.

RETINAL VESSELS. Narrowing of the vessels and retinal edema may be observed relatively early. As the toxemia advances, hemorrhages and complete retinal detachment may occur. Recovery usually is complete.

Mortality. The maternal mortality for preeclampsia is low in general, and in the early stages there should be no mortality from the disease itself. As it progresses in severity, there may be mortality from the disease and also from the treatment. The maternal mortality for properly treated eclampsia should be less than 5%. Pritchard, Cunningham, and Pritchard have treated 245 women with eclampsia with only one death.

Principal causes of death are congestive heart failure, cerebral hemorrhage, and liver necrosis. Others are infection and adrenocortical necrosis with vascular collapse. Hemorrhage is even more lethal than with normal delivery because of hemoconcentration, which is so characteristic of eclampsia; much more hemoglobin is lost in concentrated than in an equal amount of normal blood.

The perinatal mortality also is high, averaging 20% to 25%. The principal causes of death are intrauterine anoxia, the complications of prematurity, toxemia, and infection.

Relationship of eclampsia to chronic hypertension. There has been much discussion concerning the relationship between eclampsia and the subsequent development of chronic vascular disease. Most studies have suggested that there is no direct relationship, but the numbers of women who could be included in such studies are small, because so frequently the immediate prepregnancy blood pressure is unknown. Chesley, Annitto, and Cosgrove traced 267 of 270 women who had been treated for eclampsia in the Margaret Hague Maternity Hospital, Jersey City, New Jersey, between 1931 and 1951. They found that women who had eclampsia in the first pregnancy carried to viability had the same prevalence of hypertension more than 20 years later, as did an unselected control group of the same ages. The remote mortality for white women who had eclampsia in the first pregnancy carried to viability was like that of the control group, but death rates were increased two to five times in all black women who had eclampsia and in white women whose eclampsia occurred after the first pregnancy. The authors suggest that this represents an increased basic tendency to the development of vascular disease rather than an effect of eclampsia and conclude that there is no relationship between eclampsia and the subsequent development of chronic vascular disease.

An unexpected finding in this study was that diabetes was increased two and one-half times in women who had eclampsia during the first pregnancy and four times if eclampsia developed in multiparous women.

CHRONIC HYPERTENSIVE DISEASE IN PREGNANCY

Essential hypertension may be present in a woman who becomes pregnant or may first manifest itself during pregnancy. It may become a serious complication jeopardizing the lives of both mother and infant.

Diagnosis. If the patient has a history of hypertension either between pregnancies or repeatedly during pregnancy, it is likely that the present episode is a chronic vascular disease. The blood pressure elevation usually is present before the twentieth week of pregnancy, and there may be other evidences of chronicity of the condition such as organic changes in the retinal vessels. Cardiac enlargement and serious renal pathologic findings are seldom encountered in hypertensive pregnant patients because they are usually young women who have not had severe hypertension long enough to produce these changes. If the elevation in blood pressure is not accompanied by edema (abnormal weight gain) and proteinuria, a diagnosis of essential hypertension is likely.

Effect of pregnancy on hypertension. Pregnancy often has no effect on the hypertension, but this cannot be relied on. In about a third of all pregnant women with essential hypertension, acute preeclampsia is superimposed on the chronic condition. This presents a much more serious problem than preeclampsia in the otherwise normal patient, and the incidence of both fetal and maternal death is increased. In another third of patients with chronic hypertension the blood pressure falls during the second trimester; it may reach normal levels, but this is the exception rather than the rule. Generally, it rises to at least its prepregnancy level during the last few weeks. In the remaining patients the blood pressure is unchanged throughout the entire pregnancy.

Effect of hypertension on pregnancy. In most women with essential hypertension the pregnancy progresses uneventfully, but the complications that can develop are severe.

The principal danger from essential hypertension during pregnancy is to the fetus, but the mother's life may also be endangered. The infant almost always weighs less than do those born after normal pregnancies of the same duration. The cause of the *growth retardation* is altered placental function. The placenta usually is smaller than expected, and its functional capacity may be further reduced by *multiple small infarcts* as a result of hemorrhage into the decidua from maternal arterioles supplying the choriodecidual space. The placental tissue overlying the area of hemorrhage separates. If enough placental tissue is involved, the placenta's ability to maintain normal function is reduced; fetal growth may be compromised, or the fetus may even die in utero. *Early abortion*, which occurs frequently, adds to the fetal loss. A patient who begins pregnancy with a systolic blood pressure higher than 200 mm Hg and a corresponding rise in diastolic pressure has no more than a 50% chance of delivering a normal baby.

ABRUPTIO PLACENTAE. About half of all cases of severe premature separation of the placenta occur in women with vascular disease. This is associated with a high fetal and an increased maternal mortality.

ACUTE PREECLAMPSIA. Of all women with vascular disease, 30% to 40% will develop signs characteristic of preeclampsia during pregnancy. The complication usually appears late in the second trimester at about the period of viability and is associated with a high fetal and maternal mortality. The signs appear earlier, and the disease progresses more rapidly than does the similar process in normal women. The blood pressure may rise to alarming heights in a few days, and renal function deteriorates rapidly. The condition is even less responsive to treatment than is preeclampsia in women with normal vascular function.

CEREBRAL HEMORRHAGE. Intracranial hemorrhage is a more common cause of death in chronic hypertensive disease than in preeclampsia because the vessels may have undergone an organic degen-

erative change and because the arterial blood pressure usually is much higher.

RENAL CORTICAL NECROSIS. Renal cortical necrosis is sometimes encountered in women with hypertension and premature placental separation.

Treatment. Patients with severe hypertension should be quickly and completely evaluated when first seen. The examination should include (1) general physical examination; (2) frequent blood pressure recordings; (3) eye examination for evidence of retinitis; (4) renal function studies such as fluid intake and urine output measurements, creatinine and uric acid clearances, quantitative protein determinations, and microscopic urine examination; (5) blood urea nitrogen determination; and (6) cardiac evaluation. A baseline is thus established for repeat examinations during pregnancy, and a decision can be made as to whether pregnancy should continue.

INTERRUPTION OF PREGNANCY. Pregnancy is dangerous, and interruption should be recommended if the systolic blood pressure is higher than 180 to 200 mm Hg or the diastolic pressure is 110 mm Hg or more and remains elevated after a period of bed rest, if there are degenerative changes in the retinal arterioles, if the patient has had a previous cerebral hemorrhage or preeclampsia during a previous pregnancy, or if renal function is reduced.

TEST OF PREGNANCY. If the pregnancy is allowed to continue, the patient is informed of her condition and advised of the possibilities. She is told to be prepared to enter the hospital at any time and to remain in the hospital for a long period. As long as the pregnancy remains uneventful, it is to be allowed to continue; but should the patient develop superimposed preeclampsia that does not respond to treatment, interruption must be considered.

PRENATAL CARE. Patients with chronic hypertension should be examined at least every 2 weeks and often more frequently. They should rest every morning and afternoon and spend at least 10 hours in bed each night.

Antihypertensive drugs may serve a useful purpose, particularly if the blood pressure is already being maintained at a normal level when conception occurs. If treatment is started during pregnancy, the initial drug should be a thiazide diuretic. If adequate control is not achieved, additional agents are added in a stepwise manner. Table 28-2 summarizes the effects of various antihypertensive agents.

Any prenatal patient with hypertension should be ad-

TABLE 28-2 Antihypertensive agents in pregnancy

Drug	Mechanism of action	Cardiac output	Renal blood flow	Side effects
Thiazide	*Initial:* Decreased plasma volume	Decreased	Decreased	*Maternal:* Electrolyte depletion, increased uric acid, thrombocytopenia, pancreatitis
	Later: Decreased peripheral vascular resistance	Unchanged	Unchanged	*Neonatal:* Thrombocytopenia
Methyldopa	False neurotransmitter	Unchanged	Unchanged	*Maternal:* Lethargy, fever, hepatitis, hemolysis, positive Coombs' test
Reserpine	Depletes norepinephrine from sympathetic nerve	Unchanged	Unchanged	*Maternal:* Nasal stuffiness, depression *Neonatal:* Nasal congestion, increased respiratory tract secretions, cyanosis
Hydralazine	Direct peripheral vasodilator	Increased	Unchanged	*Maternal:* Flushing, headache, tachycardia, palpitations, lupus syndrome
β-blockers	β-adrenergic blockade	Decreased	Decreased	*Maternal:* Increased uterine tone with possible decreased placental perfusion *Neonatal:* Depressed respirations
Prazosin	Direct peripheral	Unchanged	Unchanged	*Maternal:* Hypotension with initial dose; little data on use in pregnancy
Clonidine	CNS effect	Unchanged	Unchanged	*Maternal:* Rebound hypertension; little data on use in pregnancy
Ganglionic blockers	Decrease in peripheral resistance by adrenergic ganglionic blockade	Decreased	Decreased	*Maternal:* Marked sensitivity with secondary hypotension *Neonatal:* Meconium ileus

mitted to the hospital at once if (1) the blood pressure rises, (2) protein appears in the urine, (3) weight gain is abnormal or edema develops, or (4) symptoms appear.

TERMINATION OF PREGNANCY. If the patient with hypertension develops superimposed preeclampsia that cannot be controlled with medical treatment, the pregnancy must be terminated even though the infant is not yet viable. Indications for termination of pregnancy are (1) rising blood pressure that fails to respond to treatment, (2) increasing evidence of retinal vascular damage, or (3) decreasing renal function. Since these women usually are multiparas, labor often can be induced by amniotomy if the cervix is effaced; otherwise, cesarean section may be necessary.

If the blood pressure remains stable throughout the pregnancy or falls slightly and if preeclampsia does not develop, the prognosis is reasonably good. It usually is advisable to induce labor as soon as conditions for induction are favorable and if amniotic fluid examination indicates fetal maturity because the fetal death rate increases after approximately 39 weeks.

CARE DURING LABOR. Magnesium sulfate is less effective in lowering blood pressure in essential hypertension than in preeclampsia-eclampsia. Hydralazine may be given if the blood pressure is unusually high or rises during labor.

POSTPARTUM CARE. During the immediate period after delivery the blood pressure must be taken at regular intervals because it may either rise rapidly or fall precipitously, and the output of urine must be recorded every hour until diuresis has been established.

Special problems. Special problems involve fetal death, abruptio placentae, and future pregnancies.

PREVIOUS FETAL DEATH. Some of the women may have had previous intrauterine fetal deaths at about the same time in each pregnancy. If the infant can be delivered either vaginally or by cesarean section while it is still alive, it may survive, even though it is premature. Tests for fetal well-being and continuing growth (indicating adequate placental function) are *periodic fetal activity, contraction stress tests, nonstress tests,* and *periodic sonographic measurement of various fetal diameters* to determine if they are increasing (Chapter 34).

ABRUPTIO PLACENTAE. Placental separation usually is severe and may be associated with a high mortality. The prompt transfusion and delivery of such patients will reduce the maternal mortality.

FUTURE PREGNANCIES. Tubal sterilization should be considered for any patient with essential hypertension who has evidence of degenerative vascular changes in the retinal vessels, decreased renal function, or cardiac enlargement. Those whose blood pressure is higher after each pregnancy and those who have had repeated intrauterine fetal deaths and premature placental separation also are poor risks for further pregnancy. If more pregnancies are not contraindicated, the deliveries should be spaced about 18 months apart to complete childbearing while the patient is young and before the degenerative vascular changes appear.

Mortality. The maternal mortality is increased ten to twenty times over that of the normal patient, and the fetal loss is as high as 30% to 40%. The principal causes of death are abruptio placentae, eclampsia, cerebral hemorrhage, postpartum collapse, renal cortical necrosis, and infection. The mortality can be reduced by recognition of the fact that hypertension is a serious complication of pregnancy requiring special attention. Careful prenatal care and interruption of pregnancy at any time the vascular signs progress and fail to respond to treatment will contribute most to this reduction in deaths.

REFERENCES

Benedetti, T.J., Kates, R., and Williams, V.: Hemodynamic observations in severe preeclampsia complicated by pulmonary edema, Am. J. Obstet. Gynecol 152:330, 1985.

Cavanagh, D., Papineni, S.R., Knuppel, R.A., Desai, U., and Balis, J.U.: Pregnancy-induced hypertension: development of a model in the pregnant primate, Am. J. Obstet. Gynecol. 151:987, 1985.

Chesley, L.C., Annitto, J.E., and Cosgrove, R.A.: The remote prognosis of eclamptic women, Am. J. Obstet. Gynecol. 124:446, 1976.

Chesley, L.C., Annitto, J.E., and Cosgrove, R.A.: The familial factor in toxemia of pregnancy, Obstet. Gynecol. 32:303, 1968.

Chesley, L.C., and Duffus, G.M.: Preeclampsia, posture and renal function, Obstet. Gynecol. 38:1, 1971.

Dieckmann, W.J.: The toxemias of pregnancy, St. Louis, 1952, The C.V. Mosby Co.

Gant, N.F., Chand, S., Worley, R.J., Whalley, P.J., Crosby, U.D., and MacDonald, P.C.: A clinical test useful for predicting the development of acute hypertension in pregnancy, Am. J. Obstet. Gynecol. 120:1, 1974.

Hughes, E.C., editor: Obstetric-gynecologic terminology, Philadelphia, 1972, F.A. Davis Co.

Kraus, G.W., Marchese, J.R., and Yen, S.C.: Prophylactic use of hydrochlorothiazide in pregnancy, J.A.M.A. 198:1150, 1966.

Lindheimer, M.D., and Katz, A.I.: Sodium and diuretics in pregnancy, N. Engl. J. Med. 288:891, 1973.

Lindheimer, M.D., and Katz, A.I.: Pathophysiology of preeclampsia, Annu. Rev. Med. 32:273, 1981.

Lindheimer, M.D., and Katz, A.I.: Hypertension in pregnancy, N. Engl. J. Med. 313:675, 1985.

McCall, M.L.: Cerebral blood flow and metabolism in toxemias of pregnancy, Surg. Gynecol. Obstet. 89:715, 1949.

McKay, D.G.: Chronic intravascular coagulation in pregnancy and preeclampsia, Contrib. Nephrol. 25:108, 1981.

Pritchard, J.A., Cunningham, F.G., and Pritchard, S.A.: The Parkland Memorial Hospital protocol for treatment of eclampsia: evaluation of 245 cases, Am. J. Obstet. Gynecol. 148:951, 1984.

Pritchard, J.A., Cunningham, F.G., and Mason, R.A.: Coagulation changes in eclampsia: their frequency and pathogenesis, Am. J. Obstet. Gynecol. 124:855, 1976.

Roberts, J.M., and Perloff, D.L.: Hypertension and the Obstetrician-Gynecologist, Am. J. Obstet. Gynecol. 127:316, 1977.

Rubin, P.C.: Beta-blockers in pregnancy, N. Engl. J. Med. 305:1323, 1981.

Sibai, B.M., Lipshitz, J., Anderson, G.D., and Dilts, P.V., Jr.: Reassessment of intravenous MgSO₄ therapy in preeclampsia-eclampsia, Obstet. Gynecol. **57:**199, 1981.

Spargo, B., McCartney, C.P., and Winemiller, R.: Glomerular capillary endotheliosis in pregnancy, Arch. Pathol. **68:**593, 1959.

Speroff, L., Haning, R.V., Jr., and Levin, R.M.: The effect of angiotensin II and indomethacin on uterine artery blood flow in pregnant monkeys, Obstet. Gynecol. **50:**611, 1977.

Sutherland, A., Cooper, D.W., Howie, P.W., Liston, W.A., and MacGillivray, I.: The incidence of severe pre-eclampsia amongst mothers and mothers-in-law of pre-eclamptics and controls, Br. J. Obstet. Gynaecol. **88:**785, 1981.

Weinstein, L.: Preeclampsia/eclampsia with hemolysis, elevated liver enzymes, and thrombocytopenia, Obstet. Gynecol. **66:**657, 1985.

Willson, J.R., Williams, J.M., and Hayashi, T.T.: Hypertonic saline infusions for the differential diagnosis of the toxemias of pregnancy, Am. J. Obstet. Gynecol. **73:**30, 1957.

29

J. Robert Willson

Bleeding during late pregnancy

At least half of the women who bleed from the vagina during late pregnancy do not have a serious lesion, but, since bleeding of any type is abnormal, the physician should attempt to determine its source whenever it occurs.

PLACENTA PREVIA

About once in every 200 deliveries (0.4%) the entire placenta or part of it is implanted in the lower portion of the uterus rather than in the upper active segment. This is called *placenta previa*.

Types (Fig. 29-1). The types of placenta previa are determined by the relationship of the placenta to the internal cervical os. In *complete placenta previa* the entire cervical os is covered by placental tissue; in *incomplete placenta previa* the os is only partially covered. *Marginal placenta previa* is one in which the edge of the placenta extends to the margin of the cervical opening. With a *low-lying placenta*, a portion of the placenta is implanted in the lower uterine segment, but the placental edge may be several centimeters above the internal os.

The classification is made on the basis of findings at the initial examination and may change as labor advances (Fig. 29-2). For example, the placenta may encroach only slightly on the cervical opening when the cervix is dilated no more than 2 to 3 cm. As labor progresses and as the lower segment retracts, the inferior portion of the placenta will be separated from the uterine wall. When the cervix is 6 to 8 cm dilated, as much as half of the opening may be covered by placenta. Conversely, if the border of the placenta extends just across the opening when labor begins, one cannot feel the edge, and complete placenta previa is diagnosed. As the cervix dilates, the placenta will be drawn upward with the retracting lower uterine segment; late in labor the placenta covers only part of the opening. If the first examination is made at this time, the diagnosis will be incomplete placenta previa.

Etiologic factors. The reasons that the ovum implants in the lower segment are not always obvious. Placenta previa occurs more often in multiparas than in primigravidas, in women who are pregnant late in their reproductive lives, and in those who have been delivered previously by cesarean section. Clark, Koonings, and Phelan found that 0.26% of 92,917 women with intact uteri developed placenta previa, whereas the incidence after cesarean section increased progressively to 10% in those who had had four or more abdominal deliveries. McShane, Heyl, and Epstein found that 22% of 100 multiparous women with placenta previa had had cesarean sections. In addition, 15% of all 147 of their patients had had elective pregnancy terminations, and 31% had had previous spontaneous abortions.

Signs and symptoms. Bleeding is the most reliable

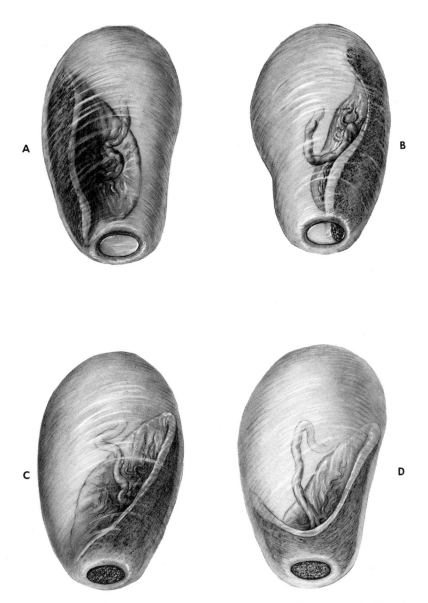

Fig. 29-1. Types of placenta previa. **A,** Marginal. **B,** Incomplete. **C** and **D,** Total. (From Willson, J.R.: Atlas of obstetric technic, ed. 2, St. Louis, 1969, The C.V. Mosby Co.)

single sign of placenta previa. Characteristically, the bleeding is painless, and the blood bright red because it flows directly into the vagina from the open sinuses just above the internal cervical os. The first bleeding occurs late in the second trimester or early in the third, usually before the thirty-second week. A few patients may have had bleeding, suggesting threatened abortion during the first half of pregnancy; others will have aborted. The initial episode usually consists of spotting or a gush of bright red blood. Overwhelming hemorrhage rarely occurs at the onset, unless the placental edge

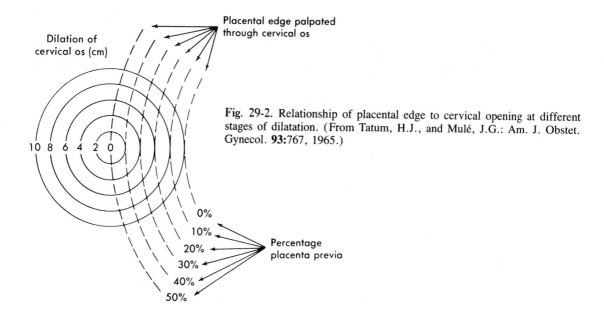

Fig. 29-2. Relationship of placental edge to cervical opening at different stages of dilatation. (From Tatum, H.J., and Mulé, J.G.: Am. J. Obstet. Gynecol. **93**:767, 1965.)

is separated from the uterine wall by digital examination or during coitus.

Each bleeding episode generally subsides, only to recur in a few days or at the most after a week or two. Subsequent bleedings are likely to become progressively heavier until, finally, profuse hemorrhage may occur. Occasionally, placenta previa produces no symptoms until late in pregnancy or even until labor begins.

The source of bleeding is maternal blood from the choriodecidual spaces, and the cause is the mechanical separation of a portion of the placenta from its uterine attachment as the lower segment lengthens during late pregnancy.

Diagnosis. Placenta previa can be suspected from a history of painless bleeding that begins during the last part of pregnancy.

EXAMINATION. The reason for bleeding can be determined only by examining the patient.

Abdominal examination. An exact diagnosis cannot be made by abdominal examination alone, but it may provide suggestive information. *Transverse lie and breech positions occur frequently with placenta previa. If the presenting part is high above the inlet and deviated anteriorly or laterally and cannot be pushed into the pelvic inlet, the placenta*

may be preventing its descent. The location of the placental souffle is of little value in determining placental site.

Vaginal examination. A digital examination must be made at some time on almost every patient suspected of having placenta previa to confirm the diagnosis and to determine the degree of involvement. If the patient is bleeding profusely, vaginal examination should be performed as soon as arrangements can be made in the operating room because it undoubtedly will be necessary to deliver her regardless of the stage of the pregnancy.

Immediate vaginal examination for those who are several weeks from term and are bleeding only slightly is usually contraindicated. The manipulations necessary to make an accurate diagnosis may separate enough placenta to cause an alarming hemorrhage and force the delivery of a premature baby who may not live. Under such circumstances it is preferable to obtain a placental localization study and to withhold digital examination until the baby has matured enough to survive outside the uterus. A sterile speculum examination should be performed to eliminate a cervical lesion as the source of the bleeding, but the cervix should not be manipulated.

Vaginal examination should be performed when it is appropriate to terminate pregnancy, either because of hemorrhage or when pulmonary maturity has been documented. The following precautions are necessary:

1. The examination must be performed in an operating room that is ready for any type of treatment necessary to control the bleeding and deliver the patient.

2. Compatible blood, 1000 ml, should be available before the examination is made.

3. An operating team of obstetricians, anesthesiologists, and nurses must be available.

4. A pediatrician, an anesthesiologist, or an obstetrician should be available to resuscitate the infant if its respirations are depressed.

If the cervix is soft and patulous, the index finger is carefully introduced in an attempt to feel the cotyledons of a complete placenta previa covering the opening or the edge of an incomplete variety. If the fetal membranes and the presenting part are felt directly above the cervical os, the examining finger is swept gently around the lower segment in an attempt to reach the edge of the placenta. The finger is withdrawn as soon as the placenta is felt; vigorous manipulation will certainly separate more of it and initiate bleeding.

If the cervix is closed, no attempt should be made to force the finger through it.

Placental localization. If the implantation site can be located, one can either implicate or eliminate placenta previa as a likely cause of bleeding.

Placental localization studies are usually contraindicated if bleeding is profuse, because it probably will be necessary to deliver the patient and a decision as to the most appropriate method for delivery can only be made after the patient has been examined. Placental localization studies are also unnecessary after the thirty-seventh week of pregnancy. Women who bleed at this stage should generally be delivered promptly; hence diagnostic vaginal examination is appropriate.

Ultrasonography is the most accurate (95%) of all the methods of placental localization. It can be performed any time after the end of the first trimester, when the placenta can first be identified. Nei-

ther the mother nor the fetus is exposed to ionizing radiation. The entire placenta and its relationship to the uterine wall and the cervical os can be seen in the sonogram (Fig. 29-3); hence the degree of placenta previa can be estimated. In contrast to other methods, posterior wall implantation can usually be seen clearly.

The concept of "placental migration" must be considered in ultrasonic evaluation. During the second trimester the placenta may cover as much as half the surface of the uterine cavity, and before the thirtieth week it often appears to be implanted near or over the cervix. As pregnancy advances, the lower uterine segment lengthens, and the placenta is drawn upward with the enlarging uterus. The placenta will be normally situated at term in almost all patients in whom an ultrasonic diagnosis of placenta previa is made during the early part of pregnancy. This is true even when the first study was made because of bleeding. Comeau and co-workers found placenta previa at delivery in 3.2% of those in whom low implantation was identified between 20 and 25 weeks, in 5.2% when it was first seen between 25 and 30 weeks, and in 23.9% when it was first seen between 30 and 35 weeks. It seems likely that the change in position is a result of enlargement of the uterus rather than an actual change in the implantation site.

Differential diagnosis. Bleeding like that resulting from placenta previa can also be produced by benign or malignant lesions of the cervix, rupture of placental vessels, premature labor, premature separation of the normally implanted placenta (abruptio placentae), bladder or bowel lesions, and other causes. These can be excluded during the course of the examination.

Treatment. To maintain a low maternal and infant mortality, the treatment of placenta previa must be planned individually for each patient.

DELAYED TREATMENT. Under certain circumstances, termination of the pregnancy may be delayed in the interests of the fetus. Since placenta previa manifests itself as early as 30 gestational weeks, immediate delivery is associated with a high fetal loss. This can be reduced if the pregnancy is allowed to continue until a later date. It is seldom appropriate to delay termination if the fetus is mature.

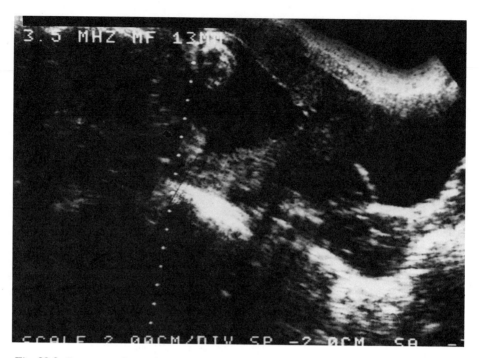

Fig. 29-3. Sonogram of complete placenta previa, longitudinal view. (Courtesy Jeffery Wicks)

A placental localization study is obtained, and the cervix is inspected with a sterile speculum. No digital examinations are performed: the examining finger can separate the placental edge and precipitate bleeding profuse enough to require immediate delivery. If a lower segment implantation site is identified and the bleeding ceases or is slight, active treatment can be delayed until it is made necessary by a progressive increase in bleeding or by the onset of labor. When the pregnancy reaches the thirty-seventh week, the patient should usually be delivered if the L/S ratio indicates that the fetus is mature.

Delayed treatment is feasible only if the bleeding is slight and if compatible blood and facilities for rapid treatment of hemorrhage are constantly available. Blood transfusions can be given if the hematocrit falls significantly after repeated small bleeds. Delay is contraindicated if the bleeding is profuse, if the fetus is dead or abnormal, or if the fetus is mature. If treatment facilities are inadequate, the patient should be transferred to a perinatal center for care.

ACTIVE TREATMENT. When the patient is to be delivered, vaginal examination, performed with the precautions outlined previously, will indicate the condition of the cervix and type of placenta previa so that the proper method for delivery can be selected.

Incomplete placenta previa. Cesarean section is the best method for terminating pregnancy in most women with placenta previa.

If the fetus is dead, the cervix is soft and patulous, only an edge of placenta can be felt, and bleeding is minimal, vaginal delivery may be possible. This is particularly true if labor has already started. Induction of labor is hazardous but occasionally is a logical choice. Cesarean section is justifiable, even though the baby is dead, if bleeding is profuse and cannot be controlled.

Vaginal delivery may also be possible in an occasional multipara with a soft, effaced, and partially dilated cervix and a minor degree of placenta previa. If the membranes are ruptured, the fetal head will descend, exert pressure against the placenta, and compress the bleeding uterine sinuses beneath it.

Vaginal delivery usually increases the hazard for the infant because compression of the placenta by the pre-

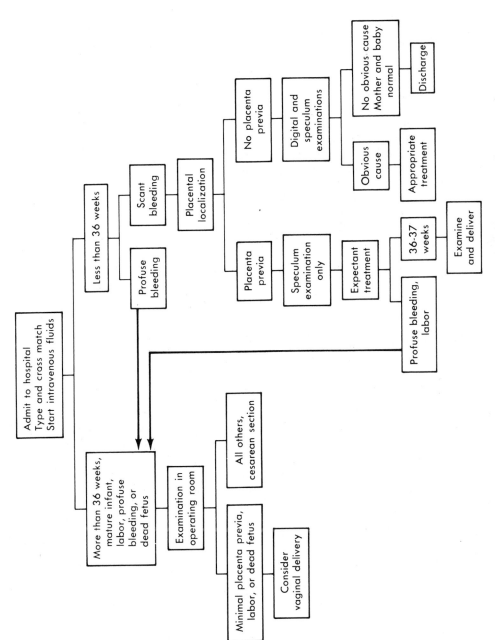

Fig. 29-4. Steps in diagnosing and management of bleeding during late pregnancy placenta previa.

senting part obstructs fetal vessels. If a large enough area of fetal circulation is eliminated, the infant will die of anoxia. Electronic fetal monitoring is essential in patients who are allowed to labor.

Vaginal delivery is most appropriate before the twenty-eighth week, when the baby has little chance of surviving. Under these circumstances, if labor can be induced and bleeding controlled until the infant is delivered, the potential problems of a uterine scar during subsequent pregnancies will be prevented.

When vaginal delivery is selected, there are several possible methods for reducing maternal blood loss, but all are appropriate only when the baby is dead or has little chance of surviving. *Scalp traction* with a long Allis forceps or a tenaculum may be used if simple rupture of the membranes does not suffice. The force necessary to compress the maternal sinuses is supplied by manual traction on the forceps or a weight. When the breech presents and the cervix is partially dilated, one or both legs can be pulled down, permitting the *buttocks to tamponade the placenta.*

Whenever the placenta is implanted in the lower segment, the tissues in that part of the uterus and in the cervix are far more vascular and friable than in normal pregnancy. They are easily torn by manipulations designed to control bleeding from the placental site, and many deaths have occurred as a result of ill-advised attempts to effect delivery through the vagina simply to avoid cesarean section.

Complete placenta previa. The patient with complete placenta previa should be delivered by cesarean section, even though the fetus is dead.

SUPPORTIVE TREATMENT. Lost blood must be replaced with blood. No other fluid will do. Maternal mortality will be high if blood is not replaced promptly and adequately. Plasma, glucose, or saline solution may be used only as a temporary measure while blood is being obtained.

The steps in the diagnosis and management of women suspected of having placenta previa are shown in Fig. 29-4.

Effect of placenta previa on mother and infant. Low implantation of the placenta can be responsible for *early abortion. Postpartum hemorrhage* occurs more often because the lower segment does not contract and control bleeding as well as the upper part of the uterus.

Maternal deaths are mostly from blood loss and

should be rare with adequate fluid therapy and blood replacement. The *perinatal death rates* in the Collaborative Perinatal Study were 176.06 for 142 white women and 190.91 for 110 black women with placenta previa. In the group of white women the stillbirth rate was 70.42 and the neonatal death rate, 113.64. For black women the stillbirth rate was 63.64 and the neonatal death rate, 135.92. Comparable perinatal death rates for pregnancies not complicated by placenta previa were 26.17 for white women and 33.20 for black women. Silver and co-workers reported a perinatal mortality rate of 42/1000; and McShane, Heyl, and Epstein a rate of 81/1000 in 147 cases.

The principal causes of perinatal mortality are *prematurity, intrauterine anoxia* as a result of placental separation and prolapsed cord, *respiratory distress syndrome, injury,* and occasionally *exsanguination from placental injury. Developmental anomalies* are more common with placenta previa.

ABRUPTIO PLACENTAE

The term *abruptio placentae,* or *premature separation of the normally implanted placenta,* indicates a complication of late pregnancy in which the placenta separates from its normal implantation site in the upper segment of the uterus before the birth of the baby. The mild types that ordinarily occur during labor are at least as common as placenta previa. The more severe ones, however, usually occur before the onset of labor and are encountered approximately once in 500 deliveries. If the placenta is completely detached from the uterine wall, *complete separation* can be diagnosed, but, if a portion of it retains its connection, it is termed *partial separation.*

Etiologic factors. The cause of placental separation is not always obvious, but *trauma* and *short umbilical cord* play a minor role in its production.

Premature separation occurs more often in woman of *high parity* than in those who have had no more than five children.

Hypertension is often associated with abruptio placentae, the reported incidence varying from about 11% to about 65%. Elevated blood pressure is more likely to be present in women with complete placental separation than in those with minor degrees. Abdella and colleagues diagnosed abruptio placentae in 23.6% of 55 women with eclampsia, in 10% of 290 with chronic hypertension, and in 2.3% of 2320 with preeclampsia.

The *supine hypotensive syndrome*, in which the vena cava is compressed by the weight of the uterus, has been suggested as a cause of premature placental separation. The increased venous pressure below the block may produce bleeding in the choriodecidual space and placental separation. Although this may occur, it probably does not do so often. Vena caval ligation during pregnancy does not necessarily interfere with uterine circulation.

Severe abruptio placentae *recurs* in about 10% of patients, probably because the factors causing the initial separation are still present.

ACCIDENTS OF LABOR. Any sudden decrease in size of a uterus overdistended by hydramnios or multiple pregnancies may produce partial placental separation.

Mechanism of separation and clinical course. Bleeding into the decidua basalis from disruption of an abnormal blood vessel separates an area of placenta from its attachment to the uterus. The extent of placental separation is determined by the amount of decidual bleeding. If the area is small and the bleeding is readily controlled by the pressure from the surrounding tissues, a small infarct may develop. If the bleeding is more extensive, part or all of the placenta may be dissected off the uterine wall.

As the bleeding continues, the blood may remain in the retroplacental area, gradually dissecting the placenta off the uterine wall without any visible hemorrhage at the onset. This is known as *concealed bleeding*. The blood may also remain concealed if it dissects upward between the membranes and the uterus rather than downward toward the cervix and if the fetal head occludes the internal os so completely that the blood cannot escape into the vagina. In most instances, the blood escapes from beneath the placenta, dissects the membranes off the uterine wall, and flows through the cervix, producing *external hemorrhage*.

The physiologic effects of hemorrhage are di-

rectly related to the volume of blood lost, but the signs may not correlate with the amount of *visible* bleeding. This occurs in part because a large volume of blood may be retained within the uterine cavity *(concealed hemorrhage)*, but there are other reasons. Blood is also lost through hemorrhage into the uterine wall *(Couvelaire uterus or uteroplacental apoplexy)*, through extrauterine hematoma formation, and through bleeding beneath serosal surfaces and mucous membranes if a *clotting defect* develops. An overt clotting defect is most likely to occur with complete placental separation, but alterations in the clotting mechanism may develop with less serious varieties (Fig. 29-5).

The clotting defect is caused by activation of the normal coagulation mechanism. Thromboplastin from abnormal subplacental decidua, the disrupted placenta, and serum in the subplacental clot enters the bloodstream through the open vessels at the placental site and initiates an exaggerated intravascular clotting process. Fibrinogen is converted to fibrin, which may occlude small vessels throughout the body, producing local tissue anoxia. As more thromboplastin is introduced into the circulation, more fibrinogen and consumable clotting factors are used and become seriously depleted. The blood then becomes incoagulable, and abnormal bleeding is evident.

Since the coagulation defect is a *consumption coagulopathy*, or *disseminated intravascular coagulation*, factors other than fibrinogen are involved. Factors V, VIII, and XIII and platelets are consumed. A fibrinolytic process that disintegrates the fibrin emboli is initiated; as a consequence, *fibrin degradation (split) products* form. They inhibit platelet aggregation and have a direct antithrombin effect that interferes with fibrin conversion and the production of normal fibrin threads in the clot.

Patients with severe abruptio placentae may develop anuria because of *acute tubular necrosis* or *bilateral renal cortical necrosis*. Those with tubular necrosis will recover if the damage is not too extensive, but they may need renal dialysis. Most patients with cortical necrosis die. These lesions seem to develop because of intrarenal vasospasm,

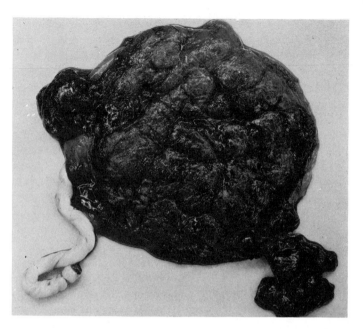

Fig. 29-5. Abruptio placentae. Note organized clots and dark, depressed areas of separation involving more than half of total placental surface.

and their severity is probably determined by the amount of blood lost and the depth and duration of hypovolemic shock. The outcome appears to be related directly to how rapidly and completely blood is replaced.

The less severe types of placental separation usually occur during labor and may be the result of mechanical separation of a portion of placenta. This can be suspected if the patient develops more pain than she has been experiencing, particularly if the fetal heart tones become a bit irregular, the vaginal bleeding increases, and the labor becomes tumultuous. This type of separation ordinarily does not affect maternal or infant mortality.

Page, Fulton, and Glendenning have divided abruptio placentae into three grades: mildly severe, moderately severe, and severe. With the *mild* forms, bleeding is minimal and none may be obvious; the uterus is slightly tender and irritable but not tetanically contracted. The conditions of the mother and infant are good, and the clotting mechanism is undisturbed. With *moderately severe*

types, bleeding usually is heavier and may be concealed. The uterus is hypersensitive and may be tetanically contracted. The maternal pulse rate is elevated, and the infant may be dead. A soft clot forms, but it may disintegrate within an hour. With the *severe* types, bleeding frequently is excessive but may be concealed. The uterus is tender to light pressure and firmly contracted. The mother is in shock, and the infant is dead. An overt clotting defect has developed.

Signs and symptoms. *Bleeding* associated with *pain* that varies in severity is characteristic of premature separation of a normally implanted placenta. Hurd and colleagues noted vaginal bleeding in 78% of 59 cases, uterine tenderness or back pain in 66%, fetal distress in 60%, high-frequency contractions in 17%, uterine hypertonus in 17%, premature labor in 22%, and dead fetus in 15%.

The pain may come on suddenly and be severe and constant when there is a major separation or milder and intermittent with a less severe lesion.

The blood may be dark or even clotted if it is

retained within the uterine cavity for a time before it is discharged into the vagina. This is in contrast to the bright red blood with placenta previa, which comes from the placental site just within the cervical opening. Discharge may consist only of blood-stained serum, which is squeezed out of the retroplacental clot. If there is a considerable amount of concealed bleeding, the pain will increase in severity as the uterus becomes distended and the muscular wall is infiltrated with blood.

Diagnosis. Ordinarily, it is not difficult to recognize the severe forms of abruptio placentae, but milder degrees may be less obvious.

CLINICAL EXAMINATION. In most instances the diagnosis can be made by history and clinical examination of the patient.

Abdominal examination. The abdominal findings change as the condition progresses in severity, but, in general, the *uterus feels firm and is tender to the touch.* At the onset the tenderness may be confined to a small area of the uterine wall, but eventually the gentlest palpation at any point produces pain.

If there is a considerable amount of concealed bleeding, the uterus will gradually enlarge as the blood collects within its cavity and infiltrates the muscular wall.

At the onset, intermittent uterine contractions can usually be palpated, but eventually they may no longer be discernible. The uterus is hard and tetanically contracted, and one may not be able to outline fetal parts because of tenderness and the contracted uterus. Odendaal recorded uterine contractions in 63 patients with abruptio placentae severe enough to cause fetal death. The rate varied from two to 14 contractions per 10-minute period, the average number being 8.4. This is considerably higher than the rate during normal labor. Although tonus is elevated, the pressure rise generated by uterine contractions is comparable to that during normal labor.

Fetal heart rate. The fetal heart tones may be normal if only a small amount of placenta is separated, or may be completely absent in the more severe forms. Slow and irregular fetal heart tones suggest severe intrauterine hypoxia.

Vaginal examination. Vaginal examination should usually be performed in the delivery or operating room as an aid in diagnosis and to determine how delivery will be effected. In contrast to placenta previa, placental tissue will not be felt within the cervical canal, and the presenting part may be deep in the pelvis rather than high, as it is with an abnormally implanted placenta.

Ultrasound examination. A subplacental blood clot can sometimes be detected, but failure to identify a clot does not eliminate abruptio placentae. Sonography is appropriate only for minor degrees of separation as an aid in clinical diagnosis.

Laboratory examinations. The hemoglobin may be reduced, the level depending on the amount of bleeding. The white blood cell count often is elevated to 20,000 or 30,000, whereas in placenta previa it is more likely to be within the normal range.

A *clotting defect* can be demonstrated by the Lee-White clotting time and by observing the type of clot and its stability. Blood, 5 ml, is placed in a clean test tube, and the time required for a clot to form and the quality of the clot are recorded. Further observation will indicate whether the clot remains intact or is lysed *(clot observation test).* If the blood fails to clot or if a clot forms but is lysed, a coagulopathy has developed. Conversely, a firm clot that forms promptly and remains intact indicates a normal coagulation process.

Coagulation studies in women with abruptio placentae and DIC will reveal depletion of consumable coagulation factors V, VIII, and XIII and of fibrinogen and platelets and the presence of fibrinolysin and fibrin degradation products. Complete coagulation study is not particularly important in the immediate management of the patient but will provide baseline studies if the clinical problem cannot be resolved promptly. The clot observation test repeated at hourly intervals continues as the most readily available method for following the course of the defect.

Differential diagnosis. Abruptio placentae can be confused with placenta previa, but in most instances it is possible to differentiate between them as follows:

Placenta previa

1. The bleeding is painless unless labor has started.
2. The blood is bright red.
3. Observed bleeding and signs of shock usually are comparable.
4. The bleeding is usually slight at the onset.
5. The uterus is soft, not tender, and may be contracting if labor has started.
6. The fetus can be felt easily, and fetal heart tones usually are present.
7. The placenta may be felt.
8. There usually is no hypertensive disease.
9. The urine usually is normal.
10. The blood usually clots normally.

Abruptio placentae

1. The bleeding usually is accompanied by pain.
2. The blood usually is dark.
3. Signs of shock may be out of proportion to visible bleeding.
4. The first bleeding often is profuse.
5. The uterus may be firm, tender, and tetanically contracted.
6. The fetus may be difficult to feel, and fetal heart tones may be absent or irregular.
7. The placenta cannot be felt.
8. The patient may have acute or chronic hypertensive disease, but the blood pressure may be low because of excessive bleeding.
9. The urine may contain protein, or the patient may be anuric.
10. A clotting defect may be present.

Treatment. Each patient must be carefully evaluated before a plan for treatment is evolved.

COMPLETE PLACENTAL SEPARATION. Complete placental separation usually occurs before the onset of labor. The infant often is dead, and the patient is in poor condition from blood loss. The first step in treatment is to improve the general condition by treating shock with oxygen and intravenous fluid, followed as rapidly as possible by large amounts of compatible blood.

Whenever the diagnosis of abruptio placentae is suspected, blood is drawn for a *clot observation test* and for *basic coagulation studies*. If the blood fails to clot or if an unstable clot forms and disintegrates, a clotting defect can be diagnosed, and treatment should be started. The clot observation test does not detect falling levels of fibrinogen. The normal concentrations of plasma fibrinogen during pregnancy range between 300 and 700 mg/dl, and the clotting test does not change until the concentration is less than 150 mg/dl. The actual concentration of fibrinogen and numbers of platelets should be measured at intervals in women with abruptio placentae who do not have an overt coagulation defect.

Whole blood transfusion is essential to replace the blood lost as a result of placental separation and that associated with a coagulation defect. It also helps correct the deficiency of consumed clotting factors, particularly fibrinogen and platelets. Many patients with placental separation are given inadequate amounts of blood. This may contribute to the development of renal failure and delay reversal of the abnormal coagulation mechanism. Some patients may need as much as 6 L or more to replenish the blood adequately. The amount of blood and fluid required to correct hypovolemia and to maintain a normal volume is best determined by continuous *central venous pressure* or *pulmonary wedge pressure measurement*.

Adequate blood replacement and prompt delivery will usually correct the coagulopathy. Extremely low levels of fibrinogen can be corrected temporarily, for example, just before cesarean delivery, by the administration of *cryoprecipitate*.

DELIVERY. Patients with severe abruptio placentae should be delivered as soon as possible. Prompt delivery will prevent the development of abnormal clotting if the mechanism has not already been disturbed. If a coagulation defect is present, delivery will remove the source of thromboplastin, which initiates clotting, and the abnormal mechanism will reverse itself promptly. In addition, delivery will allow the uterus to contract and control bleeding.

Even though the cervix is uneffaced, vaginal delivery may be possible. Therefore a sterile vaginal examination should be performed *to rupture the membranes* soon after emergency treatment has been started. Dilute *oxytocin* solution can also be administered intravenously to stimulate uterine contractions. Oxytocin solution must be given with even more than the usual care because the uterus can rupture if it is infiltrated with blood.

Vaginal delivery is more often possible in multiparas than in primigravidas, but one may be surprised by the rapidity with which many primigravidas deliver. If labor has already begun, amniotomy may hasten its progress. Electronic fetal monitoring is essential, and cesarean section should be performed promptly if evidence of fetal distress is detected.

Cesarean section, in the interest of the fetus, should be considered with the milder forms of abruptio placentae if bleeding and uterine tenderness are increasing and delivery is not imminent. Conversely, cesarean section performed solely in the interest of the fetus is contraindicated if the fetal heart monitor tracing indicates irreversible damage. In cases in which profuse bleeding continues even though the fetus has died, cesarean section should be performed if early vaginal delivery cannot be anticipated.

Uteroplacental apoplexy is caused by the coagulation defect, and the bleeding into the uterine wall and from serous surfaces should respond to its treatment. Hysterectomy should seldom be necessary to control bleeding.

INCOMPLETE PLACENTAL SEPARATION. Incomplete placental separation usually occurs during labor and is much less severe than the complete variety. The only treatment usually necessary is to hasten labor by rupturing the membranes, to administer oxygen to the mother, and to complete the delivery as soon as it can be done safely. Fetal heart rate should be monitored continuously. If the fetal heart pattern remains normal, no particular haste is necessary, but, if the infant shows signs of hypoxia, delivery as soon as it can be accomplished safely usually is advised. The uterus almost always contracts well, and bleeding is not excessive because clotting defects rarely, if ever, occur with milder types of premature separation.

Perinatal mortality. The perinatal mortality reported by the Collaborative Perinatal Study was 144.61 in 408 white women and 295.73 in 328 black women with partial abruptio placentae. The rates for complete separation were 862.07 in 29 white women and 826.09 in 46 black women. Perinatal mortality rates in white women without abruptio placentae was 23.88 and in black women, 28.94.

Hurd and co-workers reported a fetal mortality of 17% and neonatal mortality of 14% in 59 cases. The perinatal mortality of infants alive on admission was 18%. Mortality for those delivered vaginally was 20%, and for those delivered by cesarean section it was 15%. The principal causes of death are anoxia from placental separation, the complications of prematurity, and maternal toxemia.

Maternal mortality. The maternal death rate should be about 1%. It has been suggested that results with vaginal delivery are better than those with cesarean section, but this is not borne out by experience in most clinics. Most patients with more serious abruptio placentae are delivered by section, whereas those with the less severe forms are delivered vaginally, thus weighing the statistics in favor of vaginal delivery. Patients who are given liberal blood transfusions and in whom coagulation defects are recognized and corrected are most likely to survive.

Anuria may follow abruptio placentae. This occurs most often in association with the severe lesions occurring in hypertensive patients. Failure to produce urine may result from renal cortical necrosis, in which event treatment appears to be valueless, or from *tubular necrosis*, the course of which may be influenced by adequate care. It may be possible to prevent renal complications by prompt recognition and treatment of coagulation defects and by early and adequate blood replacement.

OTHER CAUSES OF BLEEDING

Cervical lesions. Benign or malignant lesions of the cervix may bleed during late pregnancy, particularly if the cervix is manipulated. The cervix should be inspected as part of the examination of any pregnant woman with bleeding. Tissue should be taken for biopsy from any suspicious-looking cervical lesion. Lesions other than carcinoma ordinarily need not be treated.

Rupture of a placental vessel. In the rare abnormality of rupture of a placental vessel, the blood comes from the fetus. This is most likely to occur with vasoprevia, and, unless the patient is delivered promptly, the fetus will be exsanguinated. The diagnosis is not often made, but if the blood is examined, one will be able to identify fetal red blood cells.

Bladder and bowel lesions. The source of the bleeding may not always be obvious to the patient and may come from bladder or bowel lesions. Hemorrhoids often bleed during pregnancy, and occasionally a pregnant woman will bleed from benign or malignant rectal lesions. Bladder hemorrhage can be detected by examining a catheterized specimen of urine.

REFERENCES

Abdella, T.N., et al.: Relationship of hypertensive disease to abruptio placentae, Obstet. Gynecol. **63:**365, 1984.

Chervenak, F.A., et al.: Role of attempted vaginal delivery in the management of placental previa, Obstet. Gynecol. **64:**798, 1984.

Clark, S.L., Koonings, P.P., and Phelan, J.P.: Placenta previa/accreta and prior cesarean section, Obstet. Gynecol. **66:**89, 1985.

Comeau, J., et al.: Early placenta previa and delivery outcome, Obstet. Gyneco. **61:**577, 1983.

Cotton, D.B., Read, J.A., Paul, R.H., and Quilligan, E.J.: The conservative aggressive management of placenta previa, Am. J. Obstet. Gynecol. **137:**687, 1980.

Crenshaw, C., Jr., Jones, D., and Parker, R.T.: Placenta previa: a survey of twenty years' experience with improved perinatal survival by expectant therapy and cesarean delivery, Obstet. Gynecol. Surv. **28:**461, 1973.

Hurd, W.W., et al.: Selective management of abruptio placentae: a prospective study, Obstet. Gynecol. **61:**467, 1983.

Knab, D.R.: Abruptio placentae: an assessment of the time and method of delivery, Obstet. Gynecol. **52:**625, 1978.

McShane, P.M., Heyl, P.S., and Epstein, M.F.: Maternal and perinatal mortality resulting from placenta previa, Obstet. Gynecol. **65:**176, 1985.

Niswander, K.R., and Gordon, M.: The women and their pregnancies: the Collaborative Perinatal Study of the National Institute of Neurological Diseases and Stroke, Philadelphia, 1972, W.B. Saunders Co.

Odendaal, H.J.: Uterine contraction patterns in patients with severe abruptio placentae, S. Afr. Med. J. **57:**908, 1980.

Page, E.W., Fulton, L.D., and Glendenning, M.B.: The cause of the blood coagulation defect following abruptio placentae, Am. J. Obstet. Gynecol. **61:**1116, 1951.

Pritchard, J.A., and Brekken, A.L.: Clinical and laboratory studies on severe abruptio placentae, Am. J. Obstet. Gynecol. **97:**681, 1967.

Pritchard, J.A., Mason, R., Corley, M., and Pritchard, S.: Genesis of severe placental abruption, Am. J. Obstet. Gynecol. **108:**22, 1970.

Sher, G., and Statland, B.E.: Abruptio placentae with coagulopathy: a rational basis for management, Clin. Obstet. Gynecol. **28:**15, 1985.

Silver, R., Depp, R., Sabbagha, R.E., Dooley, S.L., Socol, M.L., and Tamura, R.K.: Placenta previa: aggressive expectant management, Am. J. Obstet. Gynecol. **150:**15, 1984.

Tatum, H.J., and Mulé, J.G.: Placenta previa: a functional classification and a report on 408 cases, Am. J. Obstet. Gynecol. **93:**767, 1965.

30

J. Robert Willson

Determination of position and lie

The position of the fetus within the uterine cavity is of no importance during pregnancy, but it must be favorably situated if labor and delivery are to progress normally.

The term *lie* refers to the relationship between the long axis of the mother and the long axis of the infant. In a *transverse lie* the infant's spine crosses that of the mother at a right angle, whereas in a *longitudinal lie* the fetal and maternal spines are parallel. In an *oblique lie* the baby's spine crosses the mother's at an acute angle.

The *presenting part* is the portion of the fetus that descends first through the birth canal. It is therefore the part that can be palpated through the cervix with the examining finger. *Presentation*, which has been used as a synonym of lie, is now generally used to indicate the intrauterine situation of the fetus somewhat more accurately and simply. For example, the term *face* or *breech presentation* is used to indicate a longitudinal lie in which the face or the breech is the presenting part.

The exact fetal *position* is determined by the relationship of some definite part of the baby (the guiding point) to a fixed area of the maternal pelvis. The guiding point may be directed anteriorly toward the symphysis, posteriorly toward the sacrum, laterally toward the acetabula, obliquely anteriorly toward the area between the symphysis and the acetabula, or obliquely posteriorly toward the area between the sacrum and the acetabula. The possible positions clockwise around the pelvis are therefore direct anterior (A), left anterior (LA), left transverse (LT), left posterior (LP), direct posterior (P), right posterior (RP), right transverse (RT), and right anterior (RA) (Fig. 30-1).

Attitude refers to the relationship of the parts of the fetus to each other. This, ordinarily, is one of complete flexion with the chin resting on the chest, the spine flexed in a smooth curve, the arms folded across the chest, and the hips and knees flexed. With the *deflexed* attitude the head is extended, and the curve of the spine is reduced (Fig. 30-2).

The position and presentation vary considerably during pregnancy because the fetus can move freely within the amniotic cavity, particularly when there

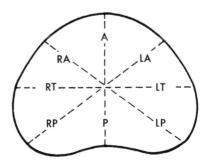

Fig. 30-1. Directions of fetal position in maternal pelvis from below.

393

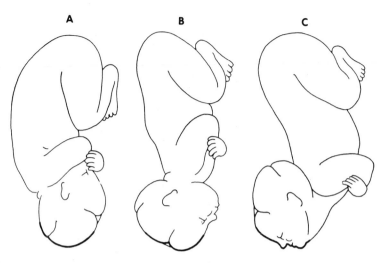

Fig. 30-2. Degrees of deflexion of head. **A,** Flexed (occiput position). **B,** Partially deflexed (brow position). **C,** Completely deflexed (face position).

is a relatively large amount of fluid. During the last 8 weeks of pregnancy the fetal mass expands rapidly, and the volume of amniotic fluid is relatively decreased. As a consequence, the fetus fills the uterine cavity more completely, it can no longer move freely, and its position becomes more stable. Some portion of the fetal head is the presenting part in about 96% of women at term, but this is not true during the earlier weeks. Breech presentation can be diagnosed in about a third of all women at the middle of pregnancy, but the incidence gradually decreases to 3% or 4% at delivery. Transverse lies are encountered in only 0.25% to 0.5% of deliveries at term, but the total incidence at some time during pregnancy is far greater.

Of all the reasons that have been advanced to account for the preponderance of vertex positions, the most logical is that the infant can accommodate itself most comfortably to the shape of the uterine cavity with its head down. The buttocks, thighs, and feet are more bulky than the head and fit better in the comparatively wide uterine fundus than in the lower segment.

DIAGNOSIS OF FETAL POSITION

The physician can usually determine position by clinical examination alone, particularly if the preg-

nancy is well advanced. Until about the thirtieth week, however, diagnosis is less accurate because the fetus is small and there may be a relatively large amount of amniotic fluid. Fortunately, precise diagnosis of position is of little importance before the last 8 weeks because it changes frequently and because abnormalities in presentation are far less formidable complications of labor during early pregnancy than they are later, when the infant is much larger.

Abdominal palpation. A reasonably accurate diagnosis of the position of the infant can be made by abdominal palpation unless the abdominal wall is unusually thick or resistant, the uterus is tender or irritable, or there is an excessive amount of amniotic fluid. Any of these may prevent the physician from outlining the fetal structures.

Abdominal examination should be performed systematically and gently with the patient in the dorsal position on the examining table (Fig. 30-3). The examiner first determines which fetal pole occupies the fundus of the uterus. The head is round, firm, and smooth and can be ballotted between the fingers if there is enough fluid; the breech is softer, less regular, more pointed, and not ballottable. The back is located by palpating through the sides of the uterus with the palmar surfaces of

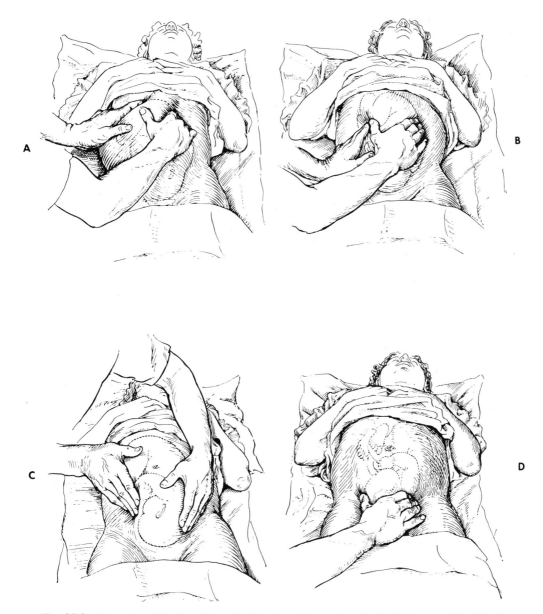

Fig. 30-3. Diagnosis of fetal position. **A,** Palpation of superior pole. **B,** Palpation of fetal back and small parts. **C,** Palpation of cephalic prominence. **D,** Ballottement of presenting part.

the fingers of each hand. The fetal spine presents a smooth convex curve in contrast to the ventral surface, which is concave, soft, and irregular; the motion of the extremities can be felt on the side opposite the back.

The fetal pole that lies over the inlet should be felt next to identify the presenting part; the fetal pole is easier to identify if it has not yet entered the pelvic inlet than if it is deeply engaged. If the vertex is presenting, one can usually palpate the *cephalic prominence*, which is, as the name implies, the part of the fetal head that is most readily felt. This area, which is opposite the back if the head is flexed and on the same side as the back in deflexed attitudes, can usually be felt without difficulty unless the face is pointed almost directly posteriorly (Fig. 30-3, *C*). The examiner can tell how deeply the head has descended through the inlet by grasping it between the fingers of one or both hands and attempting to move it back and forth or by palpating the anterior shoulder to determine how far it has descended toward the pubis.

Auscultation of the fetal heart. This method is not accurate for determining position, although the heart is usually heard best above the level of the umbilicus with breech positions and in the lower quadrants when the head presents. The heart sounds are transmitted through the area of the fetal chest wall that lies in contact with the uterine wall and are usually loudest about a third of the distance from the mother's umbilicus to the anterior superior iliac spine in occipitoanterior positions and more laterally in the occipitoposterior positions. The heart may be inaudible in obese women or those with hydramnios or if the infant's position is unfavorable.

Vaginal examination. Identification of the presenting part by direct digital palpation will aid in establishing position. For greatest accuracy the cervix must be open enough to permit the insertion of the finger; consequently, this method is more often used during labor than earlier in pregnancy. The landmarks on the presenting part may be obscured by edema or intact membranes, and if there has been little descent, the physician may be unable to insert the finger deeply enough to reach it.

The principal identifying structures on the fetal skull are the diamond-shaped *anterior fontanel (bregma)*, the triangular *posterior fontanel*, and the *sagittal suture*, which connects the two (Fig. 30-4).

The posterior fontanel is located at the juncture of the sagittal suture and the two lambdoidal sutures. The anterior fontanel is located at the juncture of the sagittal suture, the frontal suture, and the two coronal sutures.

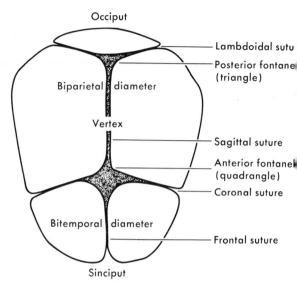

Fig. 30-4. Landmarks on fetal skull.

The anterior fontanel is usually the larger of the two, but, if the head is molded, the differences in size and shape may not be appreciable. It usually is possible to identify a fontanel by sweeping the examining finger around it and counting the sutures that enter it, four anteriorly and three posteriorly.

LONGITUDINAL LIE

In longitudinal lies, some portion of the head is almost always the presenting part.

Occiput positions. In the occiput positions, which comprise about 95% of all vertex presentations, the fetal head is flexed, and its occipital portion becomes the presenting part or guiding point (Fig. 30-5). On abdominal examination the breech is felt in the fundus, the back on the right or left side of the uterus, and the head in the inlet in a flexed attitude, with the cephalic prominence on the side opposite the back. The landmarks on the fetal skull and their relationships to the bony pelvis as they would feel on vaginal examination are illustrated in Fig. 30-6.

The possible occiput positions are also shown in Fig. 30-7. Their abbreviations are as follows:

Occipitoanterior	OA
Left occipitoanterior	LOA

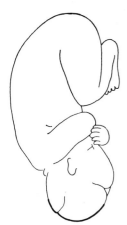

Fig. 30-5. Occiput position. Note smooth curve of flexed spine and head. Cephalic prominence (forehead) is on same side as fetal small parts.

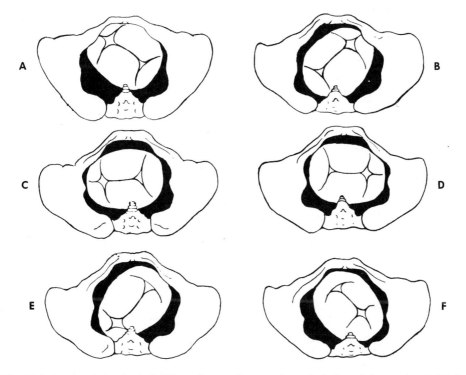

Fig. 30-6. Landmarks on fetal skull in various occiput positions. **A,** Left occipitoanterior. **B,** Right occipitoposterior. **C,** Left occipitotransverse. **D,** Right occipitotransverse. **E,** Left occipitoanterior. **F,** Right occipitoanterior. (From Titus, P., and Willson, J.R.: The management of obstetric difficulties, St. Louis, 1955, The C.V. Mosby Co.)

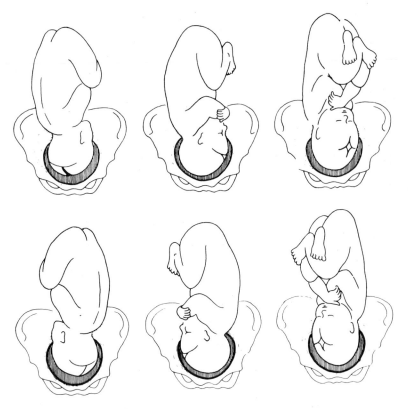

Fig. 30-7. Varieties of occiput positions. *Left to right: above*, right occipitoanterior, right occipitotransverse, and right occipitoposterior; *below*, left occipitoanterior, left occipitotransverse, and left occipitoposterior.

Left occipitotransverse	LOT
Left occipitoposterior	LOP
Occipitoposterior	OP
Right occipitoposterior	ROP
Right occipitotransverse	ROT
Right occipitoanterior	ROA

Of these, approximately 60% are occipitotransverse, 15% to 20% are oblique anterior or posterior, and the rest are direct anterior or posterior positions when labor begins. The position is determined by the shape of the bony pelvic canal. The long anteroposterior axis of the oval fetal skull tends to accommodate itself to the long axis of the pelvic inlet, which is most often the transverse, thus accounting for the predominance of occipitotransverse positions. In the direct occipitoanterior or posterior positions the anteroposterior axis of the bony pelvis is usually longer than the transverse.

Brow positions. If the head is partially extended, some part of the vertex anterior to the occiput becomes the presenting part (Fig. 30-8). The position is designated as a brow or frontum when the area of the head between the anterior fontanel and the supraorbital ridges descends first through the cervix. The possible brow positions and their abbreviations are as follows:

Frontoanterior	FA
Left frontoanterior	LFA
Left frontotransverse	LFT
Left frontoposterior	LFP
Frontoposterior	FP
Right frontoposterior	RFP
Right frontotransverse	RFT
Right frontoanterior	RFA

Face positions. If the head is completely deflexed to a point at which its occipital region lies in contact with the infant's back, the face descends through the birth

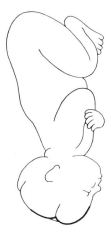

Fig. 30-8. Brow position. Note deflexion of head, extension of spine, and cephalic prominence on each side.

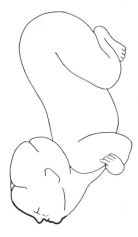

Fig. 30-9. Face position. Note extension of spine and complete deflexion of head with cephalic prominence on same side as fetal back.

canal first, and the chin (mentum) becomes the presenting part (Fig. 30-9). The possible face positions and their abbreviations are as follows:

Mentoanterior	MA
Left mentoanterior	LMA
Left mentotransverse	LMT
Left mentoposterior	LMP
Mentoposterior	MP
Right mentoposterior	RMP
Right mentotransverse	RMT
Right mentoanterior	RMA

Breech positions. If the breech or buttocks present at the pelvic inlet, the sacrum becomes the guiding point, and the possible positions and their abbreviations are as follows:

Sacroanterior	SA
Left sacroanterior	LSA
Left sacrotransverse	LST
Left sacroposterior	LSP
Sacroposterior	SP
Right sacroposterior	RSP
Right sacrotransverse	RST
Right sacroanterior	RSA

TRANSVERSE LIE

A transverse lie or shoulder presentation is one in which the long axis of the fetus lies at a right angle to that of the mother. The position is designated according to the quadrant of the pelvis toward which the scapula is directed. The possible positions and their designated abbreviations are as follows:

Left scapuloanterior	LScA
Left scapuloposterior	LScP
Right scapuloposterior	RScP
Right scapuloanterior	RScA

REFERENCES

Hughey, M.J.: Fetal position during pregnancy, Am. J. Obstet. Gynecol. **153**:885, 1985.

Scheer, K., and Nubar, J.: Variation of fetal presentation with gestational age, Am. J. Obstet. Gynecol. **125**:269, 1975.

31

William J. Ledger

Labor and delivery

Labor is the mechanism by which the products of conception are expelled from the uterus and vagina and the beginning regression of the pelvic organs is initiated. This is accomplished almost entirely by the activity of the uterine muscles.

Certain definitions that are essential to an understanding of labor and delivery are based on the duration of pregnancy. Pregnancies are dated from the first day of the last normal menstrual period, even though fertilization does not occur until later. *Abortion* is the expulsion of the products of conception before 20 completed weeks. Termination between the beginning of the twenty-first week and the end of the twenty-seventh week is called *immature labor*. Delivery between the beginning of the twenty-eighth week and the end of the thirty-sixth week when the infant weighs about 2500 g is called *premature labor*. The difference between prematurity based on weight and on duration of pregnancy will be discussed later. *Delivery at term* occurs between the beginning of the thirty-seventh week and the end of the forty-second week. *Post-term birth* occurs after the forty-second week.

A woman is a *parturient* when she is in labor and a *puerpera* after delivery. The term *gravida* refers to the total number of pregnancies, regardless of their type, location, and time or method of termination. For example, a woman who has had two normal intrauterine pregnancies, one tubal pregnancy, one abortion, and one hydatidiform mole is a gravida 5. A *primigravida* is pregnant for the first time, and a *nulligravida* has never been pregnant.

Parity refers to the number of deliveries of viable infants. In the past a *viable infant* was considered to be one weighing 1000 g, which corresponds to about the twenty-eighth week of pregnancy. However, because of obstetrical and neonatal advances, infants weighing less than 1000 g survive. The survival rate for infants above 800 g is significant, and obstetricians intervene with a cesarean section if it is necessary to avoid the stress of labor and vaginal delivery in infants estimated to be this weight or greater.

A fetus weighing 400 g can theoretically live an independent existence; this corresponds to a pregnancy of about 20 weeks. *Para* therefore indicates the number of pregnancies, regardless of the method of delivery, which terminate after the twentieth week. A *nullipara* has never carried a pregnancy beyond the twentieth week, a *primipara* has carried one pregnancy beyond the twentieth week, and a *multipara* has carried more than one. Parity refers to the number of deliveries, not the number of babies born; for example, the delivery of quadruplets at the thirty-fourth week by a primigravida makes her a para 1. A woman who has had five pregnancies, including one abortion, one ectopic pregnancy, one infant delivered normally at 26 weeks, one set of twins delivered normally at 36 weeks, and a single infant delivered by cesarean section at 41 weeks, is a gravida 5 para 3.

A more complete description of past pregnancies can be indicated by summarizing their outcomes by a series of numbers indicating, in order, term deliveries, premature deliveries, abortions, and presently living children. For example, 4-2-0-1 means four term deliveries, two premature deliveries, no abortions, and one living child.

CHANGES PRECEDING THE ONSET OF LABOR

According to Reynolds, the growth of the uterus during pregnancy is divided into three phases.

1. The first is a short period of preparation during which the progestational changes necessary for nidation develop.

2. The second phase is a period of uterine enlargement characterized by hypertrophy of muscular and connective tissue elements, producing a rapid increase in the weight of the uterus. In humans this phase ends at about the twentieth week.

3. This is followed by a period of uterine stretching during which the rate of growth, as indicated by a slower increase in weight, is much less rapid. The progressive enlargement of the cavity to accommodate the rapidly growing fetus is accomplished primarily by longitudinal stretching and thinning of the muscular walls so that the uterus becomes elongated rather than spherical. The uterus also becomes wider as the infant grows, but the lateral expansion is less than the longitudinal (Fig. 31-1).

Until about the twentieth week of pregnancy the human uterus is spherical in shape, and its walls are thick. During the last half of pregnancy the wall becomes progressively thinner, and the increase in size of the uterus is predominantly a result of elongation. Uterine weight increases from 60 to 80 g at conception to about 800 g by the twentieth week and about 1000 g at term (Fig. 31-2).

Certain other changes take place in the uterus

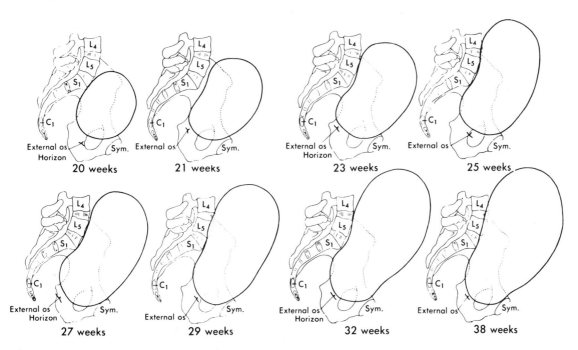

Fig. 31-1. Change in shape of uterus during pregnancy. (From Gillespie, E.C.: Am. J. Obstet. Gynecol. **59:**949, 1950.)

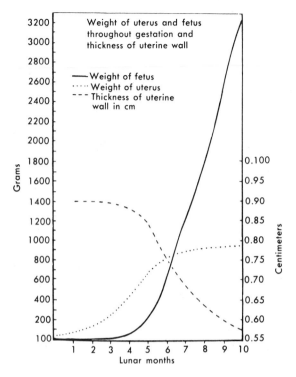

Fig. 31-2. Composite graph expressing certain weights and measurements. Around twentieth week uterine growth diminishes; myometrium therefore begins to thin, and fetus begins to increase rapidly in weight. (From Gillespie, E.C.: Am. J. Obstet. Gynecol. **59:**949, 1950.)

during pregnancy. These consist of the demarcation of the uterus into two separate divisions: the *upper uterine segment,* which is composed of the active contracting muscle tissue that supplies the force necessary to complete delivery; and the thin, passive *lower uterine segment,* through which the presenting part passes into the pelvic cavity.

According to Danforth and Ivy, the lower uterine segment is derived principally from the isthmus of the uterus—the area of the muscular corpus that is situated immediately superior to the histologic internal os of the cervix. The muscle tissue of the isthmus is indistinguishable from that of the rest of the body of the uterus, which is a predominantly muscular organ. In contrast, the stroma of the cervix contains fibrous connective tissue with some

elastic tissue and only a few smooth mucle cells. Less than 15% of total mass is muscular.

Until about the sixteenth week of pregnancy it is almost impossible to identify the isthmus as a distinct entity, but at about that time the area of the isthmus beings to lengthen, or *unfold,* as an aid in providing room to accommodate the rapidly growing fetus. The entire fibrous portion of the cervix below the isthmus remains closed (Fig. 31-3).

Uterine muscle fibers have certain characteristics that are essential for normal pregnancy and successful delivery. They must be able gradually to *elongate* to permit the progressive increase in uterine size necessary to accommodate the growing fetus. As pregnancy advances, the length of individual muscle cells increases from an original 50 μm to about 500 μm. They must be *elastic* so they can return to their normal length after periods of uterine distention. Since labor and delivery are accomplished by the force generated by uterine muscle activity, they must be able to *contract* and force the products of conception from the uterus. It is evident that unless the uterus remains closely approximated to the fetus as it is gradually expelled from the cavity, the effect of each successive contraction will be diminished. As labor advances and the fetus descends through the birth canal, the uterine cavity gradually becomes smaller so that effective force is maintained. This is accomplished by *brachystasis,* the unique ability of uterine muscle fibers to become progressively shorter and thicker while they retain their power to contract forcibly.

Muscular activity, which is present throughout pregnancy, has been studied extensively by recording the effects of the contractions on amniotic fluid pressure. The *uterine tonus,* the amniotic fluid pressure between contractions, is from 3 to 8 mm Hg during normal pregnancy. *Two types of spontaneous contractions can be identified:* small contractions that occur in localized areas of the uterine wall and that increase the pressure by 2 to 4 mm Hg, and *Braxton Hicks contractions,* which involve more uterine muscle and which increase pressure by 10 to 15 mm Hg. Both are painless, and only

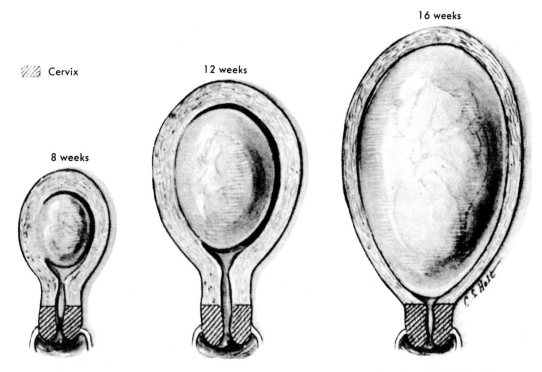

Fig. 31-3. Development and expansion of the isthmus of the uterus. (From Danforth, D.N.: Am. J. Obstet. Gynecol. **53:**541, 1947.)

the latter can be felt by the pregnant woman. Braxton Hicks contractions occur irregularly during early pregnancy but become stronger and closer together as pregnancy advances.

Uterine activity increases during the last 8 to 10 weeks of pregnancy. The Braxton Hicks contractions gradually become stronger, and the small contractions can no longer be identified. By the time labor begins, the intrauterine pressure during a contraction averages 28 mm Hg. *The increased muscle activity is responsible for the characteristic prelabor changes in the uterine corpus and cervix* (Fig. 31-4).

Since the fibers in the active upper segment shorten during each contraction, it is obvious that this portion of the uterine wall must become shorter and thicker during periods of muscle activity. Such a change would reduce the capacity of the uterine cavity unless a compensatory expansion of some other area of the uterus occurred during a contraction. This is in fact what happens. As the muscle fibers of the upper active segment shorten during a contraction, the inferior border of this portion of the uterus is drawn upward, exerting tension on the lower uterine segment. In response, the relatively passive fibers in the wall of the isthmus elongate as they are pulled upward because the relatively firm cervix remains closed. The wall of the lower part of the uterus therefore becomes thinner during each contraction.

As the muscle of the upper segment relaxes at the end of the contraction, the individual fibers lengthen, the lower border of the upper segment returns almost to its original position, and the isthmus shortens and its wall thickens. Each individual contraction produces no perceptible permanent change, but the upper segment gradually becomes shorter and shorter and its wall thicker and thicker

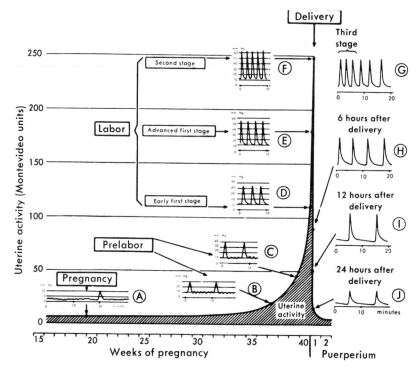

Fig. 31-4. Evolution of spontaneous uterine activity throughout pregnancy cycle is illustrated by striped area. Typical (schematic) tracings of uterine contractility at different stages of cycle are shown. (From Caldeyro-Barcia, R., and Poseiro, J.J.: Ann. N.Y. Acad. Sci. **75:**813, 1959.)

from progressive retraction of individual muscle fibers. Simultaneously, the lower segment gradually becomes longer and thinner.

During this initial period of preparation for labor, the increased length of the lower segment is almost entirely a result of elongation of the isthmus; the cervix remains closed until the last 2 to 3 weeks and in many cases remains closed until labor begins. Eventually, however, the cervix is *effaced,* or *taken up,* by a process similar to that by which the isthmus is lengthened. As the isthmus is stretched by the contraction and retraction of the muscle fibers in the active segment, the internal cervical os begins to open, being gradually pulled upward around the membranes and the presenting part and incorporated with the isthmus in the lower segment (Fig. 31-5).

As a result of the upward traction on the internal os against the resistance of the presenting part of the fetus, the cervical component of this cervical

uterine complex lengthens, becomes thinner (this becomes apparent on vaginal examination), and assumes a funnel shape; as effacement continues and the internal os is pulled higher and higher, the cervical canal becomes shorter and shorter, until finally it is completely obliterated.

The completely developed lower uterine segment is about 10 cm long; the thinned-out, elongated isthmus and the effaced cervix each make up approximately half its length. The area of demarcation between the thick, upper contractile portion of the uterus and the thinner, passive, lower segment has been called the *retraction ring.* The junction can be appreciated by palpating the interior of the uterus, but it is not visible on the external surface.

In primigravidas the cervix is usually well effaced before the contractions of true labor begin (Fig. 31-6), but preparation of the cervix in multiparas differs slightly. In multiparas the cervix

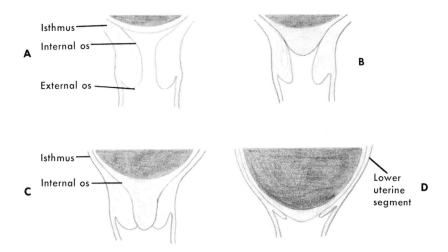

Fig. 31-5. Cervical effacement. **A,** Uneffaced cervix with definite cervical canal. **B,** Internal os retracting upward around bag of water, which precedes head (black area). **C,** Further upward retraction of internal os, expansion of isthmus, and descent of head. **D,** Completely effaced cervix incorporated into lower uterine cervix.

may be incompletely effaced when labor starts. The isthmus of the uterus elongates, and the internal os is retracted and opened. The cervical canal is wide, patulous and considerably shortened; it usually is possible to insert two fingers through it without difficulty. In many multiparas, however, the cervical canal is completely obliterated when labor begins (Fig. 31-7).

TABLE 31-1 Method for predicting success of induction of labor

Physical findings	Rating			
	0	1	2	3
Cervix				
Position	Posterior	Midposition	Anterior	
Consistency	Firm	Medium	Soft	
Effacement (%)	0-30	40-50	60-70	≥80
Dilatation (cm)	0	1-2	3-4	≥5
Fetal head				
Station	−3	−2	−1	

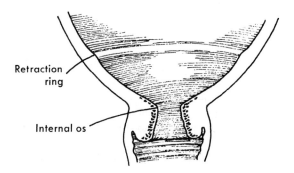

Fig. 31-6. Ripe cervix in primigravida. Retraction ring is at junction of isthmus and active upper segment.

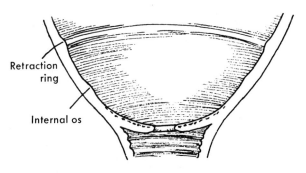

Fig. 31-7. Ripe cervix in multipara.

The changes in the cervix can be felt most accurately by vaginal palpation, and the physician should become thoroughly familiar with them to be able to recognize the *prepared,* or *ripe, cervix.* The changes noted on examination can be characterized by a grading system, the Bishop score. See Table 31-1. The higher the score, the more likely an indicated induction will be successful.

FORCES IN LABOR

Labor occurs as a result of the force of muscular contractions. The *primary force,* produced by the involuntary contractions of uterine muscle, is more important than the *secondary force,* produced by voluntary increase in intraabdominal pressure. Labor can often be completed by the primary forces alone, but the secondary powers are effective only during the second stage. The secondary forces play no part in dilating the cervix.

Primary force. Uterine muscle contractions during labor have certain distinctive characteristics. They are *involuntary* and *recur intermittently* and *rhythmically,* and they usually *produce discomfort.* The amount of perceived discomfort varies greatly among patients and can be different in the same patient in subsequent labors. At the onset of labor they may come irregularly and last only a few seconds, but they soon recur at shorter and shorter intervals, last longer, and produce more discomfort. Each uterine contraction is slight at its onset but can be palpated or recorded several seconds before the patient is aware of it; the intensity gradually increases until the uterus becomes hard and cannot be indented with finger pressure applied through the abdominal wall to the fundus. At this time the patient feels pain, which probably is caused by pressure of the presenting part against the cervix and the other structures in the pelvis. After reaching its acme, the force of the contraction gradually subsides. Between contractions the uterus in normal labors is soft and relaxed.

Caldeyro-Barcia, Alvarez, Reynolds, Hendricks, and others have studied the effects of uterine muscle contraction during pregnancy and labor by measuring changes in amniotic fluid pressure or by recording the force of muscle contractions directly by means of recording devices placed within the myometrium.

During the prelabor period, Braxton Hicks contractions recur more often and become progressively stronger. They involve more and more uterine muscle as term approaches. Uterine contractions during labor are presumed to be initiated by one of two *pacemakers* situated in the cornual areas of the fundus. One predominates, and during normal labor each contraction is initiated by a single pacemaker. The contraction is propagated downward from its site of origin at a speed of about 2 cm/sec; in about 15 seconds the entire uterus is contracting. The contraction mechanism is so well coordinated that the peak of contraction is reached in all parts of the uterus simultaneously. This means that the systolic phase of the contraction is longest in the region of the pacemaker and that it becomes progressively shorter in areas more distant from the fundus of the uterus. There is more muscle in the fundus than in the lower part of the uterus; hence the intensity of the contraction in this area is approximately twice that in the isthmus.

During early normal labor the contractions recur irregularly, but as labor advances they come at intervals of 2 to 4 minutes. The intrauterine pressure ranges between 35 and 55 mm Hg at the peak of a normal contraction. Between contractions the resting intrauterine pressure, or *tonus,* is from 4 to 12 mm Hg.

The exact duration of each contraction is difficult to determine without using precise recording devices. The uterus can be felt to contract after an increase in amniotic fluid pressure to about 20 mm Hg, but the patient will feel no discomfort until the pressure rises to about 25 mm Hg. The uterine fundus can usually be indented until the pressure has increased to about 50 mm Hg, after which it is too firm to depress. After reaching its acme, the force of the contraction gradually diminishes, and the uterus softens. By clinical observation a normal contraction may last 90 seconds, but the pressure changes can last as long as 200 seconds (Fig. 31-8).

The ultimate effect of the three principal characteristics of a normal labor contraction—propa-

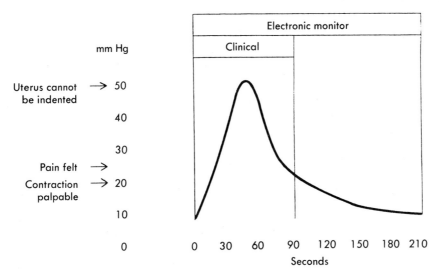

Fig. 31-8. Duration of normal uterine contraction.

gation of the wave downward from a fundal source, a prolonged fundal systolic phase, and a maximal fundal intensity—is a gradient of force directed from the fundus to the least active and weakest area of the uterus, the cervix. This is called *fundal dominance*. The force generated by each contraction is applied to the amniotic fluid and directly against the pole of the infant that occupies the upper segment. Therefore each time the muscle contracts the uterine cavity becomes smaller, and the presenting part of the infant or the forebag of waters lying ahead of it is pushed downward into the cervix. This tends to force it to open, or *dilate* it.

A more potent factor in cervical dilatation, however, is the *retraction of the upper segment*. As this area of the uterus becomes shorter and thicker, it pulls the lower segment and the dilating cervix upward around the presenting part at the same time the uterus contracting directly against the infant tends to push it through the cervical opening (Fig. 31-9). The cervix opens or is dilated by a combination of these two factors, but retraction is probably more important than the pressure of the presenting part, since dilatation will occur even though the presenting part does not descend into it. This can be observed with a transverse lie, with which

the cervix may dilate completely even though the presenting part, the shoulder, cannot enter the pelvis. A *completely dilated cervix* that will permit a term infant to pass through it has a diameter of about 10 cm.

The total uterine work necessary to dilate the cervix completely has been measured by Cibils and Hendricks using an intrauterine recording apparatus during prelabor and throughout the first stage. *Uterine work* is defined as the sum of the peak intensities of all uterine contractions from the onset of labor until the cervix is completely dilated. *Efficiency of uterine work* is determined by relating the total uterine work to the time required to dilate the cervix completely. Cibils and Hendricks' important work provides objective evidence not only that less work is required to dilate the multiparous cervix but also that the uterus works more effectively; the time required to dilate the cervix completely is less for multiparas than for primigravidas. Efficiency is significantly improved by rupture of the membranes and by anterior position of the fetal head, both of which provide better mechanical adaptation to the birth canal and to the lower segment and dilating cervix.

Secondary force. Voluntary contractions of the abdominal muscles with the diaphragm fixed after forced inspiration increase intraabdominal and,

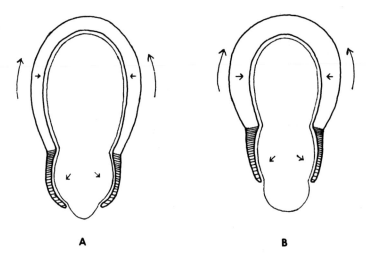

Fig. 31-9. **A,** Cervix is partially dilated and has not yet retracted around presenting part. **B,** Cervical dilatation is complete, and cervix is being pulled upward as presenting part descends.

secondarily, intrauterine pressure. *The secondary forces have no effect on cervical dilatation, but they are of considerable importance in aiding the expulsion of the infant from the uterus and vagina after the cervix is completely dilated.* Contractions of the abdominal muscles can begin involuntarily when the patient feels the presenting part pressing on the rectum and distending the perineum. When the pressure sensation is eliminated by analgesic drugs or by anesthesia, the *bearing-down* efforts cease, and the second stage may be prolonged indefinitely if the primary forces are not strong enough to expel the infant.

CAUSE OF LABOR

Why labor begins is not definitely known, but changes in the amniotic fluid, placenta, fetus, myometrium, cervix, and pituitary gland all seem to be important.

The uterus is active throughout pregnancy, but during the last 8 to 10 weeks the contractions increase in frequency and duration and in the immediate prelabor period are similar to those of the normal first stage. The effects of changing concentrations of estrogen, progesterone, and prostaglandins on uterine muscle activity have not been clearly defined, but it seems likely that altered con-

centrations of these substances are important factors in muscle contraction.

The contractile ability of uterine muscle fibers is dependent on *actomyosin*, the contractile protein; *adenosine triphosphate*, which supplies the energy necessary for contraction; and *adenosine triphosphatase*, the enzyme that splits adenosine triphosphate to release the energy. The role of estrogen in uterine muscle contraction is suggested by the fact that the concentrations of contractile elements are greater in the pregnant than in the nonpregnant uterus, and, in fact, they increase as pregnancy advances and estrogen production rises. The lowest concentrations of these substances are found in the uteri of castrates and postmenopausal women, but normal amounts can be restored by the administration of estrogen.

Of course, other chemical substances, enzymes, and electrolytes are essential for muscle contraction. Changes in the relationships of these substances alter membrane potential, thereby determining uterine activity. Recently, there is increasing evidence that oxytocin receptors on uterine muscle cells increase as term approaches. Membrane potential in uterine muscle cells is increased to -60 mV during pregnancy. As term approaches, the membranes become progressively less polarized and more responsive to the stimuli that initiate contractions.

The inciting changes that alter membrane potential to a point at which contraction is triggered include a decreased intracellular sodium concentration, an increased intracellular potassium concentration, and mobilization of calcium ions from binding sites on sarcoplastic reticulum. The effect of progesterone is to fix calcium at its binding sites; release occurs with a decreasing concentration of progesterone.

Estrogen is thought to enhance the orderly propagation of muscle contractions by providing a cell-to-cell electrical coupling mechanism. Conversely, progesterone inhibits contraction by a reverse mechanism that inhibits intracellular conduction.

The progesterone concentration is not equal throughout the uterus. Progesterone is elaborated by the fetoplacental unit and is transmitted to the mother from the fetal circulation through the placenta; as a consequence the concentration in maternal blood in the intervillous spaces is greater than in the peripheral circulation. The concentration of progesterone in subplacental myometrium is greater than in the rest of the uterine muscle, and the sodium-potassium ratio in muscle cells reflects this difference.

These findings suggest a reason why the placenta does not separate from the uterine wall as the uterus becomes more active. The placenta is rather loosely attached to the decidua and is easily separated at the completion of normal labor by firm contraction of the underlying myometrium. The placenta presumably remains attached during pregnancy because the high concentrations of progesterone in this area prevents muscle activity. The muscle in the rest of the uterus, where progesterone concentration is lower, contracts.

According to the *progesterone theory*, labor begins because of the difference between the amount of area of the subplacental myometrium and that of the rest of the uterus and because of differences in progesterone concentration. The area of uterine wall beneath the placenta remains relatively unchanged during the last weeks of pregnancy, whereas that of the rest of the uterus increases as the fetus grows; thus the ratio between subplacental and extraplacental area changes. If progesterone production decreases, an excess will still accumulate in the subplacental muscle, but the concentration in the periphery will be reduced, permitting uterine activity to increase. At some critical point, labor begins. There is clinical evidence to suggest that this theory may have validity. The overdistended uterus of patients with multiple gestations or hydramnios is associated with premature labor.

Oxytocin, when properly administered, stimulates physiologic uterine contractions. The uterus may not re-

spond even to high concentrations of oxytocin during early pregnancy, but it becomes progressively more responsive as term approaches. This seems to be related to the increasing number of oxytocin receptors in the uterus as the patient nears term. Another attractive theory can be constructed to explain the onset of labor on the basis of the relationship of oxytocin production to that of placental oxytocinase, which destroys it; however, until recently this hypothesis could not be tested. The development of a sensitive, reproducible radioimmunoassay for oxytocin has provided more information concerning the secretion of this substance. Oxytocin concentration in maternal blood rises gradually throughout pregnancy and the first stage of labor and reaches peak levels during the second stage. The concentration of oxytocin is higher in blood from the umbilical artery than that from the umbilical vein; this suggests a fetal source for at least some of the increase. Oxytocin stimulates prostaglandin production in the uterus; this may be its most important activity.

Prostaglandins E_1, E_2, $F_1\alpha$, and $F_2\alpha$, all of which will induce uterine contractions at any stage of pregnancy, are present in amniotic fluid during labor or abortion, but almost none can be identified during pregnancy. These substances can also be identified in increasing amounts in maternal venous blood during labor. Unlike oxytocin, which is most effective at term, prostaglandins E_2 and $F_2\alpha$ stimulate uterine contractions at any stage of pregnancy. They are effective when administered intravenously, intraovularly, extraovularly, or vaginally. The effect appears to be a result of their ability to inhibit calcium binding by the sarcoplastic reticulum.

Bejar and co-workers have postulated that labor is initiated by amniotic and chorionic phospholipase A_2, an enzyme that liberates arachidonic acid esters from the phospholipids of the placental membranes. The subsequent synthesis of prostaglandins would stimulate the uterus to contract. Of particular interest to clinicians is that the bacteria associated with intrauterine contamination that is occasionally noted with premature labor have high concentrations of phospholipase A_2.

Manipulation of the cervix may stimulate the onset of labor. Labor will often begin several hours after the membranes have been digitally stripped away from the lower uterine segment or when an operative procedure such as cone biopsy is performed on the cervix. This suggests that *neurogenic factors* play a part in normal labor. Stretching of the cervix stimulate uterine activity, but it probably is not related to the release of oxytocin from the posterior pituitary. There is a concentration of adrenergic nerve endings in the cervix and lower segment, and it seems likely that the adrenergic nervous system is an important factor in uterine activity.

The role of the *fetus* in initiating labor is not clear, but many animal studies suggest that biochemical or hormonal stimuli from a mature fetus and placenta are an important factor in initiating labor at an appropriate time.

Destruction or removal of the hypothalamus, pituitary, or both adrenal glands of a single sheep fetus will prolong pregnancy indefinitely. If the operation is performed on only one of twins, labor will begin at the usual time. The operations prevent the increased fetal cortisol secretion that precedes the onset of labor in sheep and goats. The increasing concentration of cortisol presumably causes decreased progesterone and increased estrogen secretion and a consequent stimulation of prostaglandin synthesis, which results in uterine contraction.

A similar reaction occurs in human pregnancies with anencephalic fetuses. The hypothalamus fails to develop; hence the anterior pituitary is hypoplastic and produces no hormones. The absence of ACTH results in fetal adrenal hypoplasia and reduced cortisol secretion. Pregnancy is likely to be prolonged unless there is associated hydramnios.

MECHANISM OF NORMAL LABOR

The *mechanism of labor* is a term applied to the series of changes in the attitude and position of the fetus that permits it to progress through the irregularly shaped pelvic cavity. A complete understanding of how this is accomplished is fundamental to the practice of intelligent obstetrics and is an absolute necessity for safe operative delivery, since the normal mechanism must be followed as closely as possible. Physicians who have a clear understanding of the basic concepts of the mechanism of normal labor for the occiput positions can determine what to expect during any labor and what the probable mechanism will be for any position the fetus can assume.

The steps in the mechanism of labor for the occiput positions are *descent, flexion, internal rotation, extension, restitution,* and *external rotation.* These do not occur as separate processes but are combined. For example, descent through the pelvis, flexion, and internal rotation may all occur more or less simultaneously.

The progress of labor is the result of the tendency for each uterine contraction to push the fetus downward through the pelvis, of the resistance of the soft tissue and the bony pelvis to its descent, and of the shape of the fetal head, which must conform to the different shapes of the pelvic cavity at its various levels. The infant itself is entirely passive. With each uterine contraction the fetus is pushed lower into the pelvic cavity, and its position gradually is altered to accommodate it to the shape of the part of the pelvis through which it must pass.

Descent. In occiput positions the longest diameter of the infant's head, the anteroposterior, enters the normal pelvis in the longest diameter of the inlet, the transverse, in almost every instance. If the sagittal suture is equidistant from the symphysis and the sacral promontory, the head is said to be entering the inlet in a *synclitic* manner. Some degree of *asynclitism* generally is present (Fig. 31-10). If the sagittal suture lies closer to the sacrum than to the pubis and the anterior parietal bone lies over the inlet, an *anterior parietal bone presentation* can be diagnosed. If the sagittal suture lies closer to the pubis and the posterior parietal bone lies over the inlet, it is a *posterior parietal bone presentation.* The latter is usually present at the onset of normal labor (Fig. 31-11).

When labor begins, the area of the infant's head just below the parietal eminence rests on the sacral promontory, the opposite parietal eminence lies above the superior border of the pubis anteriorly, and the sagittal suture is in the transverse diameter of the inlet, closer to the pubis than to the sacrum (Fig. 31-11, *A*). As uterine contractions become more effective, the anterior parietal bone is slowly forced downward behind the pubis. During this process the sagittal suture gradually moves posteriorly as the head assumes a synclitic position in the inlet (Fig. 31-11, *B*). The head *descends* through the inlet with its biparietal diameter approximately parallel to the plane of the inlet (Fig. 31-14, *C*).

Generally, some degree of *molding of the fetal head* is correlated with descent through the inlet. The term *molding* describes the changes in the shape of the head that are necessary to permit it to

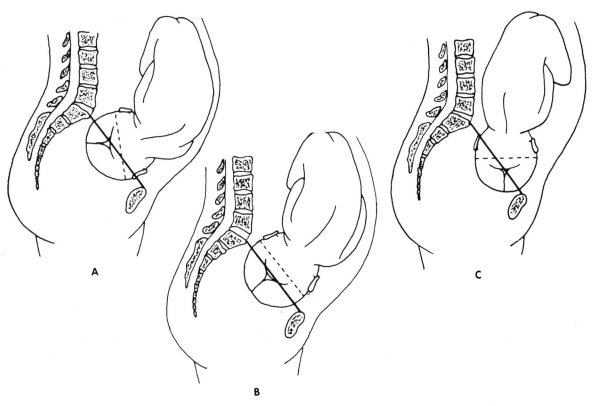

Fig. 31-10. Descent through inlet. **A,** Anterior parietal bone presentation. Sagittal suture is in posterior segment of inlet. **B,** Synclitism. Sagittal suture is equidistant from sacrum and pubis. **C,** Posterior parietal bone presentation. Sagittal suture is in anterior segment of inlet.

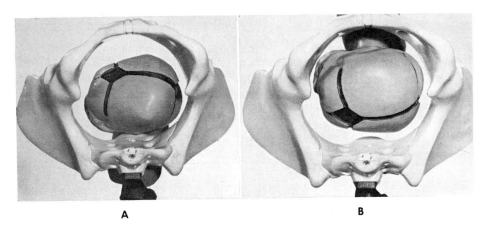

Fig. 31-11. Asynclitism. **A,** Posterior parietal bone presentation. **B,** Sagittal suture rotates posteriorly with descent.

adapt itself to the size and shape of the maternal pelvis through which it must pass. Molding is accomplished by gradual elevation or depression of the parietal, frontal, and occipital skull plates made possible by the mobility of these bones, which are not yet fused to each other. Rearrangement of the relationships between the skull plates alters the transverse, anteroposterior, and vertical measurement of the fetal skull. Molding is a dynamic process: the shape of the head changes constantly throughout labor. Little molding is necessary to permit a normal-sized fetus to pass through a normal pelvis; however, if pelvic diameters are reduced, considerable change in the shape of the head may be necessary to permit vaginal delivery.

The head is said to be *engaged* after the widest transverse diameter, the biparietal, has passed the plane of the inlet. In the normal unmolded head the distance between the occiput and the plane of the biparietal diameter is less than the distance between the ischial spines and the inlet; hence, if the occiput is the presenting part, engagement occurs as the head passes the level of the spines. *However, the fact that the lowest portion of the head is at the level of the spines does not always mean that engagement has occurred.* If there has been considerable molding and elongation of the head to permit it to pass an inlet with reduced measurements, the biparietal diameter may still not have entered the true pelvis when the lowest portion reaches the level of the spines. When the head is completely deflexed, as in face positions, the biparietal diameter does not pass the pelvic inlet until the presenting part reaches the pelvic floor.

Descent can be delayed by an incompletely dilated cervix; resistant soft tissues; disproportion between the size of the head and the size or shape of the pelvic cavity; and weak, ineffective uterine contractions. Descent usually occurs more gradually in primigravidas than in multiparas because the cervix dilates more slowly and the soft-tissue resistance is greater.

The degree of descent is gauged by the *station* of the presenting part (Fig. 31-12), which is its relationship to the plane of the ischial spines. If the lowest point of the presenting part is at the level of the spines, it is at station 0; if 1 cm above the spines, at station minus 1; if 2 cm above the spines,

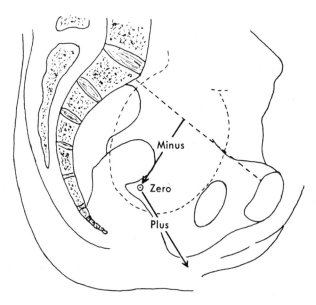

Fig. 31-12. Stations of birth canal. Presenting part *(dotted lines)* is just below station zero. Biparietal diameter has passed plane of inlet.

at station minus 2, and so on. If the lowest level of the presenting part is above the plane of the pelvic inlet, it is said to be *floating*. If the presenting part is 1 cm below the plane of the spines, it is at station plus 1, and so on. When the presenting part reaches station plus 3, it usually has just reached the pelvic floor.

Flexion. The head usually lies in the pelvic inlet during late pregnancy in a partially flexed attitude. The degree of flexion increases during descent, particularly if the pelvis is small. The purpose of flexion is to substitute the suboccipitobregmatic diameter of 9.5 cm for the occipitofrontal diameter, which measures 10.5 to 11 cm (Fig. 31-13). Descent of the head through the inlet and upper pelvis is illustrated in Fig. 31-14.

Flexion occurs because the force applied by the resistance of the maternal bone and soft tissues to the anterior portion of the head is greater than that applied to the posterior portion. If the anteroposterior diameter of the infant's head is considered as a lever with its fulcrum at the foramen magnum, where the spinal column joins the skull, one can

see how this might occur. The anterior arm of the lever is longer than the posterior arm; consequently, when equal force is applied to each, the resultant force anteriorly is greater, and the head flexes (Fig. 31-13). The smaller the pelvis, the greater the resistance and the more complete the flexion. The head may flex only slightly if the pelvis is large and the baby is small.

Internal rotation. Rotation of the long axis of the fetal head from the transverse diameter in which it descended through the upper pelvis to the anteroposterior diameter at the outlet is essential. The transverse diameters of the normal middle and lower pelvis are too short to permit the head of a normal-sized infant to descend further without rotating. Rotation begins at the level of the ischial spines but is not completed until the presenting part reaches the lower pelvis.

The bispinous diameter is too short to permit a normal-sized head to pass in the transverse diameter; consequently, it is rotated slightly by simple pressure from one of the protruding spines. In an occiput left transverse position, for example, the

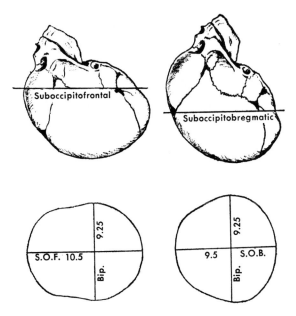

Fig. 31-13. As flexion increases, anteroposterior diameter of head, which must pass through pelvis, becomes shorter. (From Beck, A.C.: Obstetrical practice, Baltimore, 1955, The Williams & Wilkins Co.)

occiput is directed to the left as it descends through the upper pelvis. As flexion increases, the occiput is lower than the frontal portion of the head and will reach the spine first. The spine lies slightly posterior and therefore will contact the posterior portion of the occipital area. Each time the uterus

contracts and the head descends slightly, the occiput will be pushed anteriorly a bit more by the pressure of the ischial spine. As the occiput rotates anteriorly, the face rotates posteriorly. When the anteroposterior diameter of the head coincides with a diameter of the pelvis in which it can descend,

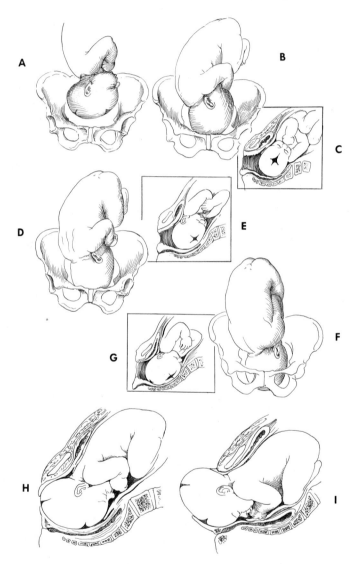

Fig. 31-14. **A,** Position of head in inlet when labor begins. **B,** Flexion as head descends. **C,** Head descends to midpelvis in transverse position. **D** and **E,** Partial anterior rotation as head passes spines. **F** and **G,** Further anterior rotation as occiput reaches lower pelvis. **H** and **I,** Complete anterior rotation and extension of head. (From Willson, J.R.: Atlas of obstetric technic, ed. 2, St. Louis, 1969, The C.V. Mosby Co.)

the head will pass the midpelvis (Fig. 31-14, *D* and *E*).

Rotation is completed because the bony side walls of the lower pelvis slope anteriorly and slightly inward and because the levator ani muscles form a double-included plane, the resultant slope of which is anterior. As the flexed head descends, its presenting part, the occipital portion that already has been rotated slightly anteriorly by the spine, strikes the bony pelvis and the levator sling anteriorly and with each uterine contraction slides further up the muscle plane until it lies in the midline beneath the pubic arch (Fig. 31-14, *F* and *G*).

Both the levators and the bony pelvis are important for anterior rotation. This is illustrated in a negative sense in multiparas in whom the head fails to turn anteriorly when muscular support has been compromised by previous childbirth injury and in women with normal levator slings that have been paralyzed by continuous regional anesthesia. In a few women the shape of the bony pelvis is so altered or the diameters are so shortened that they present a mechanical obstruction to rotation.

Extension. The upper half of the pelvic canal is directed posteriorly toward the sacrum and the lower half anteriorly, making the canal a curved rather than a straight tube. The course of descent of the presenting part must therefore change to conform to the pelvic architecture. After the occiput has rotated to an anterior position, the suboccipital area impinges beneath the pubis, and the parietal bossae impinge on the levators and the descending pubic rami, where they remain while the forehead slides up the inclined plane formed by the perineum as the head extends. The forehead, face, and chin progressively emerge from the introitus, and the face then falls posteriorly, freeing the occiput. At this stage of labor the fetal spine is no longer flexed but is extended to conform to the contour of the birth canal (Fig. 31-14, *H* and *I*).

Restitution. After the head is free from the introitus, it rotates 45 degrees to the right or left of the midline to assume its normal relationship to the back and shoulders. If the fetal back is on the left, the occiput rotates in that direction; and if on the right, it rotates to that side.

External rotation. As the shoulders descend and rotate within the pelvis, the occiput rotates further externally; thus external rotation of the head actually indicates a change in position of the undelivered body of the fetus.

With an occiput left position the shoulders pass the inlet after the head is delivered and descend with the long bisacromial diameter in the left oblique diameter of the pelvis. The anterior shoulder, the right one, meets the levator sling first as descent continues and, like the occiput, is rotated 45 degrees anteriorly to a position beneath the pubic arch. The left shoulder then lies directly over the sacrum in the muscular gutter formed by the two levator muscles. The anterior shoulder remains impinged beneath the pubic arch, and the fetal spine bends laterally as the posterior shoulder is forced up over the perineum. When the posterior shoulder is free, it falls backward, and the opposite one is pushed out from beneath the pubic arch. The body of the infant is delivered without any particular mechanism (Fig. 31-15).

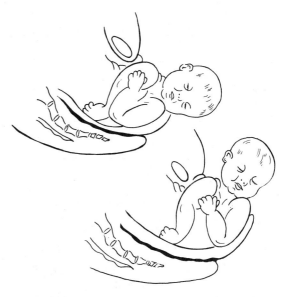

Fig. 31-15. Anterior shoulder remains beneath pubic arch, as posterior shoulder is forced anteriorly over distended perineum.

The mechanisms for occiput right and occiput left positions are identical except that in the former the occiput and back descend down the right side of the pelvis and rotate from right to left.

CLINICAL COURSE OF LABOR

Prodromes. Certain symptoms and objective signs precede the onset of labor.

ENGAGEMENT. In primigravidas the fetal head begins to settle into the upper pelvis from 2 to 3 weeks before labor begins. This coincides with the period of elongation of the lower segment and the progressive effacement of the cervix, which permits the head to descend. In multiparas, development of the lower segment and effacement is less complete, and the head usually remains high until early in labor. If engagement fails to occur with the first pregnancy, the physician should consider the possibility of a contraction of the bony pelvis, placenta previa, a pelvic tumor, abnormal fetal position, or anything else that might prevent the head from descending.

As the infant "drops," the pressure on the diaphragm is reduced; consequently, the patient breathes more easily, but she experiences more pelvic pressure, frequency of urination, and discomfort as the presenting part presses on the pelvic organs.

VAGINAL DISCHARGE. As the cervix effaces and the pressure on it increases, the patient may note more mucous discharge. Labor often begins a few days after this is observed.

PASSAGE OF MUCOUS PLUG. The thick mucus in the canal, the *mucous plug,* and portions of the hypertrophied crypts are expelled from the obliterated cervix. This often is blood streaked and is called the *show.*

Onset and diagnosis of labor. The contractions of labor produce discomfort and thus differ from the Braxton Hicks contractions during pregnancy. They occur irregularly at the onset of labor but usually increase until they recur every 2 to 3 minutes and last from 60 to 90 seconds. *The contractions of true labor produce progress such as thinning of the cervix, dilatation of the cervical opening, or descent of the presenting part.*

The principal criterion necessary for the diagnosis and evaluation of labor therefore is progress rather than the character of the contractions. In some patients, labor progresses rapidly, although the contractions recur irregularly and feel weak. In others no progress can be detected despite contractions that are regular, feel forceful, and are painful. This is called *false labor.* The contractions of false labor usually stop after a few hours and can almost always be controlled by the administration of a barbiturate. False labor can be diagnosed, therefore, if no progress is made and if the contractions cease spontaneously or with medication.

Stages of labor. *Labor begins when the patient first experiences recurring painful uterine contractions, which terminate in delivery.*

FIRST STAGE. The first stage of labor lasts from its onset until the cervix is completely dilated. The membranes usually rupture during the latter part of the first stage. They may remain intact until delivery.

SECOND STAGE. The second stage begins when the cervix is completely dilated and ends with the delivery of the baby.

Neither the first nor the second stage can be timed accurately unless the patient is examined frequently; during normal labor the exact duration of each of the two stages is not particularly important.

THIRD STAGE. The third stage begins when the baby leaves the uterus and ends with the delivery of the placenta.

COURSE AND DURATION OF LABOR

One of the most critical of several variables that influence the calculated length of labor is the decision as to when labor began. The progression of uterine activity from prelabor to real labor, when recognizable changes in the cervix occur, is difficult to pinpoint, even though the contractions are monitored continuously. A record of the time at which the patient first became aware of the contractions and the time at which changes in the cervix are first appreciated is helpful in deciding how to manage abnormal labor.

The decision as to when labor began is made by

the physician who admits the patient to the labor-delivery unit and is recorded on the labor graph. If this is not done, the time of onset may be modified if subsequent progress is not normal. Cesarean section for an "arrest" in the active phase of cervical dilatation may be justified if the hours of prelabor are included; this can be interpreted as an abnormally prolonged total labor. Conversely, one can justify permitting the labor to continue in the hope that the fetus can be delivered vaginally if the latent phase is not considered to be an integral part of the entire process. *Such arbitrary modifications can be avoided if the time at which the patient first felt uterine contractions, even though they may have been irregular and short at the beginning, is considered to be the time at which labor began and is recorded in the labor record when the patient is admitted.* Errors are inevitable. Some women thought to be in early labor will be discharged later with a diagnosis of false labor, whereas cervical dilatation in others thought not to be in labor will progress rapidly.

Friedman made a major contribution to the understanding of labor by graphing the progress of cervical dilatation against time (Fig. 31-16). He divided the first stage of labor into the *latent phase*, during which effacement is completed and cervical dilatation begins, and the *active phase*, during which cervical dilatation is completed. His complex description of cervical dilatation is difficult to reproduce with prospective graphing of dilatation on a labor unit. The *acceleration phase* cannot be documented unless the frequent vaginal examinations necessary to demonstrate the changes are made. The *deceleration phase* may be a measure only of the vagaries of clinical observation. The recognition of a deceleration phase, if it occurs regularly, requires almost constant observation during the terminal portion of the first stage.

There are no absolute values for the normal length of the first stage of labor. "Normal" lengths in four separate groups of women are depicted in Fig. 31-17. All of these statistical evaluations show variations that may reflect differences in the patient populations or in clinical practice.

The second stage can be evaluated more closely. Calkins states that the second stage is concluded with no more than 20 contractions in primigravidas

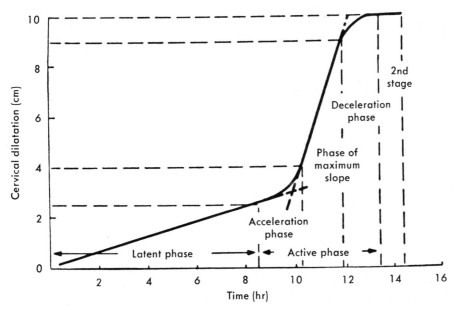

Fig. 31-16. Phases of labor in primigravida. (From Friedman, E.A.: Obstet. Gynecol. **6:**567, 1955.)

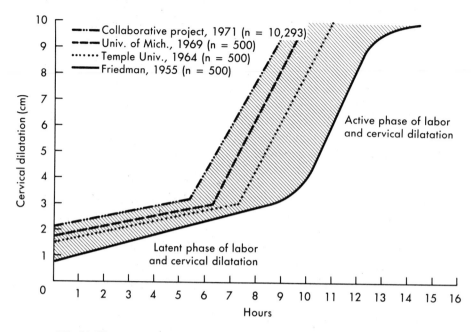

Fig. 31-17. Cervical dilatation graphs from four populations of nulliparas.

and with 10 or fewer in multiparas. This corresponds well with a median duration of 50 minutes for primigravidas and of 20 minutes for multiparas reported by Hellman and Prystowsky.

The duration of labor in any individual is determined by parity, the size and position of the fetus, the shape and capacity of the pelvis, the consistency of the cervix, the efficiency of the uterine contractions, and the patient's attitude toward pregnancy and motherhood.

PREPARATION FOR LABOR

During the prenatal period, physicians and their associates should make every effort to eliminate misunderstandings and fears and to instill confidence in their patients. The primigravida, who has not yet experienced labor, is certain to be apprehensive, particularly if she has acquired a considerable amount of misinformation from her friends and relatives. As the weeks go by, much can be learned about the patient's attitudes by simple questions, and many of her fears can be allayed.

The principal concerns are about the length of labor, how much pain there will be and how it will

be relieved, anesthesia, the welfare of the baby, what happens in the hospital, and who will be responsible for her care. These and many other questions can be considered during the office discussion periods described in Chapter 18. It often is helpful to take the patient and her partner on a tour of the maternity unit during the last weeks of pregnancy. This will give them an opportunity to learn about admitting procedures, to see the labor-delivery area, to meet some of the personnel, and to ask questions.

The parents should have an opportunity to participate in childbirth education courses if they are interested. Those that concentrate on the complications of pregnancy and how they are recognized and on the mechanics of delivery are not particularly helpful. The most effective childbirth education courses are designed to provide couples with an understanding of what actually will happen physiologically during labor and delivery and of the part each can play to make childbirth safe and satisfying.

Instructions to the patient. Some time during the last month the patient must be instructed as to how to recognize the onset of labor and what to do when the contractions begin.

WHEN TO ENTER THE HOSPITAL. The normal primigravida should usually enter the hospital when the contractions are recurring regularly at about 5-minute intervals, but multiparas must come in earlier because so many have rapid labors.

RUPTURE OF MEMBRANES. Rupture of the membranes should be reported because the physician will usually want to examine the patient to be certain that a serious complication such as prolapse of the umbilical cord has not occurred.

BLEEDING. Any vaginal bleeding, no matter how slight, should be reported.

FOOD. The gastric emptying time is prolonged during labor, and food may be vomited and aspirated during delivery. *Patients should be warned against ingesting either solid food or liquids after the contractions begin or the membranes rupture.*

Each patient should be examined as soon as she arrives at the hospital. Her prenatal record should be available for review. A brief interval history is recorded, and a physical examination is made. The fetal position and presentation, the location, rate, and regularity of the fetal heart tones, the height of the fundus, and the frequency and the duration of the uterine contractions are determined by *abdominal palpation* and *ausculation*. Unless there is bleeding a *vaginal examination* is next made to confirm fetal position and to determine the amount of cervical dilatation and the station. The *blood pressure* is recorded, a *urine specimen* is examined for protein and glucose, and a *hemoglobin* or *hematocrit* determination is made.

Unless the patient is about to deliver, an external recording device should be applied to the maternal abdomen, and a 30-minute recording of fetal heart rate made. More intensive monitoring will be required if baseline fetal heart rate is flat, if decelerations are observed, if labor appears to be abnormal, or if the patient is classified as "high risk."

If the patient actually is in labor, orders to *shave the perineum* are at the discretion of the obstetrician, but are not necessary. The pubic hair should not be removed in any case. An *enema* need not be given if the rectum is empty. *An enema should never be administered to a patient who is bleeding until serious lesions such as placenta previa or abruptio placentae are eliminated as causes.* Patients in early labor may take *showers.*

CARE DURING LABOR

Patients in labor, even though they are multiparas, are usually apprehensive and uncomfortable, and every effort must be made to allay fear and to make the entire experience as rewarding as possible. The attendants must refrain from laughing, joking, and loud conversation near the labor rooms because these are all annoying to the patients. The discussion of other patients and particularly of obstetric problems must be strictly avoided if there is any chance that the conversation can be overheard.

Under ideal conditions, an experienced labor nurse or a physician should remain with each patient throughout her labor, but practically this is not always possible. As an alternative, nurses and physicians should visit each patient every few minutes to make certain that labor is progressing normally. No laboring patient, particularly one who is unusually apprehensive, should be left alone for any appreciable period of time.

The father should remain in the room if he and the patient so desire. He may be particularly helpful and supportive if he and the patient have had a childbirth education course. His presence should not influence close observation of the patient by professional attendants. If the father is not present, the mother should be able to have some person with her during labor to offer support.

Observations during labor. The following observations will indicate the condition of the mother and her infant and the progress of labor.

FETAL HEART. In term pregnancies the fetal heart sounds are an index of the condition of the fetus and should be counted and recorded at least every 15 minutes during the first stage and more often during the second stage of normal labor. More complete evaluation can be done with an external recording of fetal heart sounds made during labor. This technique is of great help in identifying fetuses at risk. Even though the preliminary monitor strip is normal, observations of the fetal heart must be continued throughout the labor. One can either continue using the external monitor or follow the heart sounds with a stethoscope. If the latter is used, the heart rate is checked during or immediately after a contraction as well as in the interval between contractions because changes caused by interference with fetal oxygenation are usually heard first during the period of uterine activity.

Electronic monitoring of the fetal heart is indicated during premature labor and whenever the pregnancy is complicated. This provides a more accurate assessment of heart rate and permits continuous rather than intermittent evaluation. Fetal heart monitoring is discussed in detail in Chapter 34.

The fetal heart tones should be counted during several contractions after the membranes rupture, and vaginal examination should be performed because the cord may be washed through the cervix with the gush of fluid.

BLOOD PRESSURE. The blood pressure is recorded at 30-minute intervals because it may rise to alarming levels during labor.

CONTRACTIONS. The length, duration, and intensity of uterine contractions and the interval between them are recorded at 30-minute intervals. The length is determined by palpation rather than by the patient's statements because she cannot feel the contraction until several seconds after it has begun and the discomfort disappears before the uterus is relaxed. Intensity is estimated by the firmness with which the muscle contracts.

Electronic monitoring of uterine contractions is probably not necessary during normal labor at term if there are no fetal heart rate abnormalities. The equipment and someone familiar with its use and with the interpretation of the tracings should be available in the labor-delivery area of hospitals that provide obstetric services. Monitoring of the uterine contraction pattern and of the fetal heart rate is essential during abnormal labor, if fetal heart rate abnormalities are present and whenever labor is induced or stimulated.

Examinations. The progress of labor is determined by various examinations.

ABDOMINAL EXAMINATION. Abdominal examinations are performed to evaluate the uterine contractions and to follow the descent of the presenting part into the pelvis. As descent occurs, the cephalic prominence and the anterior shoulder, which can be palpated above the pubis, move downward. When the head is deep in the pelvis, the cephalic prominence can no longer be felt, and the shoulder lies just above the pubis.

PERINEAL PALPATION. The presenting part can be palpated through the perineum after it has reached the pelvic floor. A bit later, perineal bulging and crowning can be seen.

VAGINAL EXAMINATION. The progress of cervical dilatation and of descent can be determined by vaginal palpation. Since bacteria inevitably are carried on the fingertips from the introitus and the vagina to the interior of the uterus, it is essential that vaginal examinations be performed properly and that they be limited in number. As a general rule no more than three or four are necessary during a normal primigravid labor: one when the patient is admitted, one when it appears that she may need sedation, and one or two more as labor advances.

Examinations made simply to determine position, station, and cervical dilatation can be performed in the labor bed with the patient in dorsal position. The examiner wears sterile gloves, and an antiseptic solution is used to cleanse the vulva and act as a lubricant. The labia are separated with the fingers of one hand, and the index and second fingers of the other are inserted into the vagina, palpating the fetal head and the cervical rim (Fig. 31-18). If more information must be obtained, for example, if there is a question of cephalopelvic disproportion or of placenta previa or if an abnormal presentation is suspected, the examination must be performed with the patient in the lithotomy position.

It is essential that physicians' examinations and nurses' observations and treatment be recorded accurately in the labor record. The progress of labor is best appreciated if cervical dilatation, descent, and position are plotted on a labor graph (Fig. 31-17). On such a graph, deviations from the normal

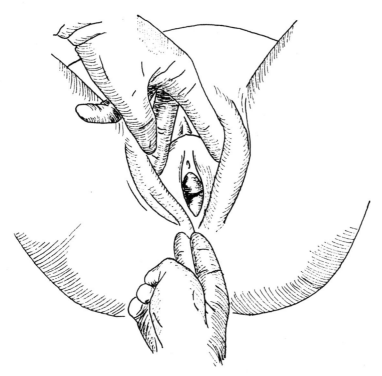

Fig. 31-18. Vaginal examination. Labia are separated to prevent them from being rolled into vagina as fingers are inserted.

are obvious and can be appreciated much earlier than by other recording methods.

General care. General nursing care during labor is directed toward making the patient as comfortable as possible and protecting her from infection and injury.

POSITION. Patients in early labor may be out of bed if they wish, but they usually prefer to lie down when labor is advanced. Most are more comfortable on their sides than on their backs, and in fact the lateral position has many advantages, the most important of which are that the force of uterine contractions, uterine perfusion, and fetal gas exchange are greater in the lateral position. Presumably this is a result of enhancing vena caval blood flow, which may be impeded by pressure from the uterus in the dorsal position. Those who have been sedated should be confined to bed.

FOOD. The gastric emptying time is delayed during normal labor, and the administration of anal-gesic and sedative drugs decreases it even more. Fluids and food should not be ingested orally during labor. Glucose solution can be administered intravenously if labor is prolonged.

BLADDER. As the lower segment lengthens and the cervix is retracted, the bladder is pulled upward. This and the pressure from the descending presenting part may make spontaneous voiding impossible. The distended bladder can be seen and felt as a fluctuant mass in the lower abdomen. If the patient cannot void during labor, she should be catheterized at intervals.

Transfer to delivery room. Patients should be taken to the delivery room in their beds in time to prepare them properly for delivery. Primigravidas are moved when the presenting part begins to distend the perineum, and multiparas are moved when they are 8 to 9 cm dilated.

The recent action to make the atmosphere of the hospital obstetric unit more homelike has led to the development of beds that can be used both during labor and for delivery. Such beds eliminate the need to transfer the patient to the delivery room and to a delivery table (Chapter 1).

As the presenting part descends deep into the pelvis during the second stage and begins to exert pressure on the pelvic floor, the patient will feel as though she needs to evacuate her rectum and will ask for a bedpan. Soon after this she will begin to hold her breath, tense her abdominal muscles, and strain or *bear down* in an attempt to expel the baby each time the uterus contracts. As this occurs, the relatively high-pitched cry at the time of the contraction changes to a sustained grunt, which can be recognized as indicating the second stage whenever it is heard. Bearing down during the first stage serves no useful purpose and should not be permitted because it will only tire the patient. The bloody vaginal discharge usually increases as cervical dilatation is completed, and the pressure of the presenting part may force small amounts of fecal material from the rectum.

NORMAL DELIVERY

Everyone in the delivery room should wear a cap that covers the hair completely and a face mask that covers both the nose and the mouth, and those participating directly in the delivery should wear sterile surgical gowns and gloves. Others wear clean surgical dresses or suits, and no one is admitted in street clothes.

An undelivered patient should never be left alone in the delivery room. She needs attention and support during the expulsive stage; in addition, she may deliver while the attendants are out of the room.

Fetal heart monitoring, either electronic or auscultatory, should be continued in the delivery room, which should have the capability of electronic recording. If the heart is being checked by stethoscope, the rate should be counted during and after almost every contraction.

When the patient is ready to deliver, she is placed in a suitable position. For spontaneous delivery, particularly of multiparas, the *dorsal recumbent position* is satisfactory. There is less stretch on the

perineum than in lithotomy position; hence perineal lacerations occur less often. Episiotomy can be performed, if necessary, but it is difficult to repair adequately in this position. Forceps delivery cannot be performed properly in dorsal recumbent position.

The *lithotomy position* is less comfortable for patients, but it provides better exposure of the perineum, making delivery easier with less likelihood of contamination. The lithotomy position is essential for any operative delivery and for adequate repair of more than a shallow episiotomy. A significant advantage is that the entire birth canal can be examined for injury after the placenta has been delivered; this is not possible in the recumbent position.

The vulva and anus, the upper portions of the thighs, and the skin over the pubis and lower abdomen are cleansed with an antiseptic solution, preferably one containing iodine, wiping from anterior to posterior and discarding the cotton sponge after each stroke. No attempt is made to cleanse the vagina; the constant discharge of amniotic fluid serves to keep it clean. Sterile leggings are placed over the feet and legs, and the abdomen is covered with a sterile sheet. In many hospitals a sterile sheet is also placed posteriorly covering the anus, but this is usually promptly saturated with blood and amniotic fluid and contaminated by fecal material expressed from the rectum. It is seldom necessary to catheterize the patient before spontaneous delivery because the bladder has been pulled up entirely out of the pelvis. The bladder should be emptied before forceps extraction.

Episiotomy, when necessary, is performed after the perineum has been flattened out well by the crowning head, and it should be deep enough to sever the fascia covering the lower surface of the levator muscles.

With each contraction, the head will extend, and more of the scalp will be visible through the dilated introitus. Delivery of the head can be controlled by *Ritgen's maneuver* (Fig. 31-19), with which upward pressure is applied through a sterile towel with the thumb and forefinger of the pronated right hand, or the first and second fingers with the hand supinated, first to the supraorbital ridges and later to the chin through the distended perineal body. The upward pressure, which increases extension and prevents the head from slipping back between contractions, is counteracted by downward pressure on the occiput with the fingertips of the other hand; this tends to prevent extension. With this maneuver, the delivery of the head can be readily controlled, and its rapid expulsion, which causes perineal tearing, can be prevented. As the head descends further, the perineum is pushed backward over the face and chin (Fig. 31-20).

As soon as the head is delivered, the physician feels for a loop of cord around the neck. If a long, loose loop is present, it can be slipped over the head; a shorter, tighter one can be slipped over the advancing shoulder. If there are several tight loops, it may be impossible to slip them either way, in which event the cord is doubly clamped, cut, and unwound.

After the head is delivered, the anterior shoulder descends and rotates to a position beneath the pubic arch. At this point the shoulder is said to be *impinged* beneath the pubis, but actually it can be considered to be delivered, since it and the upper humerus are visible. Impingement of the anterior shoulder can be aided by downward traction on the head (Fig. 31-21); little force should be applied to accomplish this because the brachial plexus may

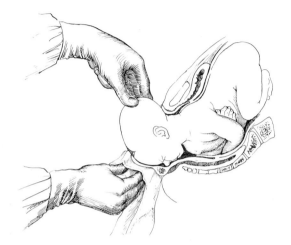

Fig. 31-19. Modified Ritgen's maneuver. (From Willson, J.R.: Atlas of obstetric technic, ed. 2, St. Louis, 1969, The C.V. Mosby Co.)

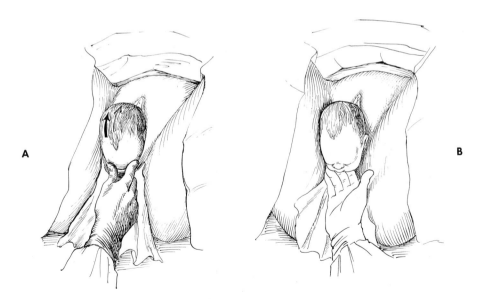

Fig. 31-20. Completion of delivery of head. **A,** Forehead is supported to maintain extension. **B,** Face is freed from perineum. (From Willson, J.R.: Atlas of obstetric technic, ed. 2, St. Louis, 1969, The C.V. Mosby Co.)

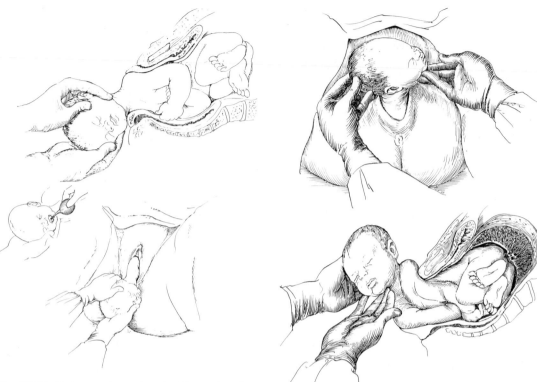

Fig. 31-21. Delivery of anterior shoulder and aspiration of nasopharynx. (From Willson, J.R.: Atlas of obstetric technic, ed. 2, St. Louis, 1969, The C.V. Mosby Co.)

Fig. 31-22. Delivery of posterior shoulder. (From Willson, J.R.: Atlas of obstetric technic, ed. 2, St. Louis, 1969, The C.V. Mosby Co.)

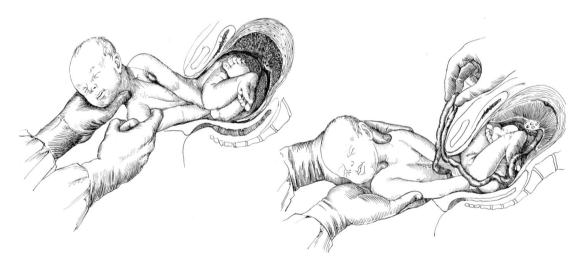

Fig. 31-23. Delivery of body. (From Willson, J.R.: Atlas of obstetric technic, ed. 2, St. Louis, The C.V. Mosby Co.)

be stretched and injured by the maneuvers. After the shoulder is visible, the physician waits for about 30 seconds to permit the muscle fibers in the fundus to retract and reduce the size of the uterine cavity, from which part of the baby has been delivered. During the wait mucus is aspirated from the nasopharynx. The head is then elevated toward the ceiling, and traction is applied to deliver the posterior shoulder over the perineum (Fig. 31-22). After another 30-second wait the remainder of the body is slowly extracted by traction on the shoulders (Fig. 31-23).

Some delay in clamping and cutting the umbilical cord probably is beneficial to the infant. If the newborn infant is held below the level of the introitus, blood will be infused from the placental vessels to the baby. The amount is determined by the time interval between delivery and cord clamping, but as much as a 75 to 100 ml increase in blood volume can be anticipated. Conversely, there is no transfer of blood if the infant is held above the level of the mother's abdomen.

The infant is placed in a heated crib with its head slightly lower than its body. The head-down position should not be too deep, neither should the infant be held upside down for any period of time because the pressure of the abdominal viscera against the diaphragm interferes with normal respiratory efforts.

PREMATURE LABOR AND DELIVERY

The term *premature delivery* indicates the termination of pregnancy before the end of the thirty-sixth week. In the past a diagnosis of premature or term delivery was made on the basis of the birth weight of the infant. If the baby weighed less than 2500 g (the average for white infants at the end of the thirty-sixth completed week), a diagnosis of prematurity was made automatically. The terms *low-birth-weight infant, small for gestational age,* or *growth retardation* may be more accurate because many infants weighing less than 2500 g actually are not premature by date; their low weight is the result of some other factor.

The fact that an infant weighs more than 2500 g at birth is no guarantee of maturity. The babies of mothers with diabetes are excellent examples; some may weigh 3500 to 4000 g at 35 or 36 weeks, but their development is comparable to that of infants of similar gestational age.

About 7% of all pregnancies terminate in the delivery of low-birth-weight infants; this occurs in from 3% to 5% of private and in about 15% of clinic patients. Low-weight infants are born more often to black than to white women.

It is not always possible to distinguish true premature delivery, in which pregnancy terminates before the thirty-seventh week, from delivery of growth-retarded infants, whose weight is less than that anticipated at any given week of pregnancy. This is particularly true in women who are first examined during the last weeks of pregnancy. If a patient is seen early and if uterine and fetal growth conform to the normal pattern, one can logically make a diagnosis of premature labor after the delivery of a small infant whose development is appropriate for the stage of gestation. Conversely, one can suspect growth retardation if fetal and uterine growth are behind those anticipated at specific periods of pregnancy and if the development of the infant at delivery corresponds to the dates, even though the baby weighs less than anticipated.

Etiologic factors. The reasons for premature labor are not completely understood, but it may occur in women with *placenta previa, abruptio placentae, multifetal pregnancy,* and *hypertensive cardiovascular disease.* It may also be necessary to induce labor prematurely in the treatment of these as well as other conditions, notably preeclampsia. The *membranes often rupture prematurely,* after which labor begins.

Bacterial contamination may play an important role in initiating premature labor. Bobitt and Ledger have demonstrated high bacterial counts in the amniotic fluid of women in premature labor. In the genital tract bacteria that often are cultured from amniotic fluid, Bejar and associates found an enzyme that releases prostaglandins. Naeye has found microscopic evidence of infection in the placenta and fetal membranes after the spontaneous onset of premature labor.

The infants of *women who smoke excessively* and

those addicted to heroin and other drugs weigh less at birth than the babies of nonusers. Low-birth-weight infants are born more often to *women at extremes of the reproductive years,* that is, to the young teenager and the woman over age 35, than to those between the ages of 18 and 30. The part played by *anemia, malnutrition, infection, general poor health,* and *inadequate medical supervision,* all so characteristic of women of the *lowest socio-economic levels* who have the highest rates of low-birth-weight delivery, has not been completely assessed. Many of these are examples of growth retardation rather than premature labor.

Premature delivery, with its consequently increased perinatal mortality, can also occur because of inappropriate early *elective induction of labor* or *elective repeat cesarean section.* These can be prevented by carefully documenting the relationships between presumed duration of pregnancy, uterine size, and fetal development during the prenatal period and by proving fetal maturity before elective delivery.

Prevention. Since the causes of premature labor are not always obvious, and since labor may begin early without warning, it is not always possible to prevent it. Under certain circumstances, however, the birth of premature infants can be prevented.

Delivery can usually be delayed until the fetus is mature when there is a minor degree of placenta previa with slight bleeding, with stabilized maternal hypertension, with well-controlled maternal diabetes, and with other medical problems. The delivery of premature infants after elective induction of labor or elective repeat cesarean section can be prevented by confirming fetal maturity before setting a date for delivery.

Ritodrine hydrochloride, a beta-mimetic agent, has a more potent inhibitory effect on uterine activity than does either *alcohol* or *isoxsuprine,* an ephedrine-like beta-adrenergic agonist. When given in early labor, ritodrine may prevent labor from progressing. The actions of this drug are not limited to the myometrium; there usually is an increase in maternal heart rate and an increase in systolic and a decrease in diastolic blood pressure. Tachycardia occurs in the fetus and in the mother. Metabolic effects include an increase in maternal glucose

and insulin levels and a drop in serum potassium. If these effects adversely influence the medical status of the mother, the use of the drug is contraindicated.

It may also be possible to stop uterine contractions with *alcohol,* which presumably suppresses pituitary oxytocin secretion. Fuchs and co-workers administered 9.5% alcohol in 5% dextrose in water intravenously to women 21 to 36 weeks pregnant who were having regular contractions. Uterine activity was inhibited in all; delivery was postponed in two thirds of those with intact membranes but in none whose membranes had ruptured. In a comparative study, however, significantly better clinical results were obtained with ritodrine than with alcohol. The principal dangers associated with the use of ethanol are vomiting, aspiration, and upper gastrointestinal bleeding.

Another agent that may reduce uterine activity is *magnesium sulfate* given intravenously. This drug is widely used during labor and is safe when the patient can be carefully monitored. Its major disadvantage is that it is less effective than is ritodrine. However, if ritodrine is contraindicated, magnesium sulfate may be an acceptable alternative.

Aspirin and *indomethacin* appear to decrease the intensity of uterine contractions and delay the onset of labor. The action presumably is from interference with prostaglandin synthesis. Prostaglandin inhibitors may produce premature closure of the ductus arteriosis in some animals, but not in the human.

The only reason to consider stopping premature labor is in the interest of the fetus. *Attempts to arrest premature labor are contraindicated* if (1) the pregnancy is of at least 37 weeks' duration, (2) the membranes are ruptured, (3) the cervix is 4 or 5 cm dilated, (4) the infant is abnormal, or (5) there is maternal disease such as hypertension, abruptio placentae, or another serious condition for which delivery is indicated.

Management. If premature labor cannot be prevented, one must do everything possible to protect the infant during labor and delivery.

Sedative and analgesic drugs should be administered in small amounts and only when there is no other alternative for pain relief. They depress fetal cerebral function, and if the infant is born during the period of depression, it may be unable to establish its vital functions. Morphine and meperidine often are given in an attempt to stop premature labor, but they should not be used because they have little effect on uterine contractions.

The fetus that weighs less than 1500 g does not tolerate the stress of labor well. For this reason, electronic monitoring is indicated during every premature labor. *Cesarean section* should be performed if persistent late decelerations or moderate-to-severe variable decelerations are recognized. As a general rule, cesarean section is preferred over vaginal delivery for stressed infants without obvious anomalies if their estimated weight is at least 800 g and if the labor is being conducted in a prenatal center with an intensive care neonatal nursery. Poor development of the lower uterine segment at this stage of pregnancy may preclude the use of a low transverse uterine incision; a vertical incision usually is preferred.

FETAL GROWTH RETARDATION

Fetal growth retardation is most likely to occur when the fetus develops abnormally because of congenital anomalies, intrauterine infection, or maternal disease or when there are abnormalities of placental development or function. The latter is probably the most common cause. For example, growth retardation, which is characteristic of severe chronic cardiovascular renal disease, probably begins because the placenta is usually smaller in women with vascular disorders than in normal women. Placental function is further compromised by infarction and by diminished uterine blood flow. The end result is that the reduced functional area of placenta is unable to meet all the requirements of the fetus and its growth is delayed. The fetus grows to the maximum size the placenta can support at any stage of pregnancy. Cessation of placental growth is followed by cessation of fetal growth and death if the fetus is not delivered. Although growth is delayed, development occurs at a reasonably normal rate.

Growth retardation can be anticipated in any high-risk pregnancy, particularly when the mother is very young, over age 40, malnourished, or chronically ill or has chronic vascular or renal disease. *Sonographic measurement* of the biparietal diameter of the fetal skull at 20 to 22 weeks provides baseline information to which growth of the head during the last weeks of pregnancy can be related.

If growth retardation is suspected, measurements of the biparietal diameter and abdominal circumference at 2-week intervals will indicate the rate at which the head and body are growing. As long as the biparietal diameter, abdominal circumference, and total intrauterine volume increase progressively, one can be reasonably certain that placental function is adequate. Conversely, if growth ceases, one can suspect that maximal functional capacity of the placenta has been reached and that the fetus is in jeopardy.

Growth retardation is of two types: *symmetric* if the fetal head and body grow at the same rate and *asymmetric* if there is a disparity between growth of the head and that of the body. In the latter the head often is spared; abdominal circumference and total volume are below those anticipated from the biparietal diameter. Differentiation of a symmetrically growth-retarded fetus from one that is normal but smaller than the average may be difficult.

Additional information concerning the status of the fetus can be obtained by *serial estriol assays* and *biophysical evaluation*. If estriol production increases progressively, even though it is lower than is expected for the stage of pregnancy, and if the fetal activity and heart rate tests are normal, the fetus probably has not reached the functional capacity of the placenta. If the fetus ceases to grow, estriol production levels off or decreases, and the biophysical tests become abnormal, prompt delivery is necessary to prevent fetal death.

One of the best indicators of the duration of pregnancy is accurate dating of the day of the onset of the last normal menstrual period. When this is combined with early examinations that substantiate the information provided by the menstrual history, there should be little confusion about the date of delivery (Chapter 20). If such information is available, one should not revise the anticipated delivery date solely because the fetus seems too small. Rather, one should assume that its growth is retarded and initiate the studies that will determine its status. When growth retardation is suspected but the dates are uncertain, the preceding suggested studies should be obtained.

As a general rule, the growth-retarded fetus should be delivered whenever there is evidence that it has outgrown the capacity of the placenta or when maturity can be established, even though there is no clear evidence of fetal deterioration. Ultrasonic evidence of a diminution or absence of amniotic fluid is an indication that the fetus is in jeopardy; it usually should be delivered promptly. Cesarean section often is the most appropriate method for delivery.

PROLONGED PREGNANCY

Sometimes pregnancy is prolonged for several weeks past the due date, during which time the fetus may die. This is most often observed in primigravidas, and according to some authorities, it is more frequently a cause of perinatal mortality with the first pregnancy than is prematurity. After excluding women with preeclampsia-eclampsia and antepartum hemorrhage the perinatal mortality is doubled at 42 weeks and tripled at 43.

The causes of true prolongation of pregnancy have not been established, but the fetus may play an important part in determining when labor begins. Pregnancy is prolonged by several weeks in certain animals if the fetal pituitary gland is absent or abnormal, and prolongation is associated with adrenal hypoplasia. This also occurs in humans, for example, with anencephaly without hydramnios.

After the forty-second week of gestation the amount of amniotic fluid decreases and vernix disappears; in affected infants the skin appears dry and cracked. Meconium, passed because of hypoxia, stains the placental surface, the umbilical cord, and the remaining vernix yellow-green. In more advanced cases the fingernails and toenails of the infant are also stained. The babies weigh less than the usual term infant and appear to have lost weight.

The cause of the abnormality in the infant is chronic hypoxia from placental dysfunction. The placenta can maintain the requirements of the infant only until it reaches a certain size, which is determined by the amount of functioning chorionic tissue. If the placenta is small or a portion of it has been destroyed, as occurs with chronic hypertensive disease, the baby will be smaller than usual; it often dies in utero before term and shows the same changes as the so-called postmature infant. *Placental deficiency syndrome* is therefore a better term than postmaturity.

Because of the danger to the infants in pregnancies

that have gone beyond the calculated due date, induction of labor or even cesarean section has been advised at the forty-second week. These recommendations should not be accepted without reservation; in most instances of presumed post-term pregnancy the baby is normal, and the due date probably was miscalculated. Thus is particularly true in multiparas.

However, if the dating of the pregnancy is accurate, the cervix favorable, and the fetus mature, an attempt can be made to induce labor at 42 weeks. If the induction fails or if the biophysical tests suggest that the fetus is compromised, cesarean section may be indicated.

If there is a question as to the actual duration of pregnancy, the management is determined by the maturity and condition of the fetus. If pregnancy extends past what is presumed to be 40 weeks, one should begin *biophysical testing*. If the biophysical tests indicate that the fetus is normal, nothing need be done. If placental function is normal, the fetus will continue to grow, but growth will stop when the maximum capacity of the placenta to support the fetus is reached.

Cesarean section is not often necessary in prolonged pregnancy, but it should be performed without hesitation when one establishes the need for delivery and when induction is unsuccessful or contraindicated.

PREGNANCY AND LABOR IN YOUNG PRIMIGRAVIDAS

Labor usually is normal in girls less than 16 years of age, and vaginal delivery can almost always be anticipated; but rates for maternal complications, low-birth-weight infants, and perinatal mortality are all increased.

The reported incidence of *preeclampsia-eclampsia* varies from 4.3% to 23.5%. Semmens, studying 12,857 pregnancies in teenagers, found a toxemia rate of 5.9% for the entire group but 17.7% in those less than 15 years of age. *Infections,* particularly *gonorrhea* and *syphilis; anemia,* and *malnutrition* are common. The figures collected by the Collaborative Perinatal Study indicate an increased rate of low-birth-weight infants born to teenagers. The rates for white girls and women are as follows: ages 10 to 15 years, 97.4; ages 16 to 17 years, 79.29; ages 18 to 19 years, 66.35; and ages 20 to 24 years, 67.04. Comparable figures for black girls and women are 172.92, 157.47, 149.53, and 130.47. The rates for children neurologically abnormal at 1 year of age delivered of white teenagers and women are as follows: ages 10 to 15 years, 35.40; ages 16 to 17 years, 19.7; ages

18 to 19 years, 10.97; and ages 20 to 24 years, 14.92. Comparable figures for black teenagers and women are 9.76, 13.86, 14.62, and 16.67.

Labor generally is of normal duration and terminates in spontaneous or low forceps vaginal delivery. In Semmens' study, labor was prolonged in 8%, and only 1.4% were delivered by cesarean section.

The fact that normal labor and delivery can be anticipated for almost all pregnant teenagers does not justify a complacent attitude. Pregnancy in a teenage girl is a high-risk pregnancy, and patients should be treated accordingly. Many are unmarried and of lower socioeconomic classes, and all need social counseling, in addition to medical care. If the number of pregnant teenagers justifies a special session, a "teenage clinic" should be established. Such a clinic is appropriately staffed by physicians, nurses, social workers, and psychiatrists who are familiar with the problems of teenage pregnancy. A major educational objective of such a clinic is to help patients develop the motivation necessary to prevent recurring pregnancies.

PREGNANCY AND LABOR IN ELDERLY PRIMIGRAVIDAS

A woman more than 35 years of age and pregnant for the first time is called an "elderly primigravida." Almost all will deliver without difficulty, but cesarean section is necessary more often than in younger patients. The incidence of essential hypertension, preeclampsia-eclampsia, heart disease, uterine fibroids, and other conditions that appear during the fourth decade is higher than in younger women. *Perinatal mortality* was increased two to three times, but recent studies show better results. The incidence of chromosomal abnormalities, particularly trisomies, increases after age 35. Genetic amniocentesis should be offered each patient (Chapter 2).

LABOR IN MULTIPARAS

Physicians tend to direct less attention toward multiparous women, particularly those who have had several children. This attitude cannot be justified, because both maternal and perinatal mortalities are increased. Disproportion, prolonged and obstructed labor, and ruptured uterus and fetal death may occur because babies tend to become progressively larger with each succeeding pregnancy and the uterine mechanism becomes less effective.

The impaired uterine mechanism also is responsible for a high incidence of postpartum hemorrhage. Hypertension and degenerative vascular disease are most common in multiparas because they are often in the older age groups.

PRECIPITATE LABOR AND DELIVERY

Precipitate labors, those lasting less than 3 hours, occur in only about 10% of all deliveries and are encountered more often in multiparas than in primigravidas. The baby may be injured during rapid, uncontrolled labor.

Patients who have delivered rapidly in previous pregnancies should enter the hospital at once if the membranes rupture or when contractions begin. Elective induction is indicated for those who live some distance from the hospital.

The physician should remain with the patient during her labor. It usually is wise to move her to the delivery room when she is about half dilated. If labor progresses so rapidly that it seems unlikely that she can be moved, it is safer to deliver her in bed than to risk the trip to the delivery room. Under no circumstances should the head be restrained forcibly or an anesthetic administered in an attempt to prevent delivery.

INDUCTION OF LABOR

Labor may be induced artificially by amniotomy or by the administration of oxytocic drugs. In some patients, particularly those with conditions that might be aggravated by continuing pregnancy, induction serves an important purpose; but it is contraindicated if the pregnancy is normal.

Selection of patients. It is difficult to induce labor safely unless it is about to begin spontaneously. Many complications associated with induction occur because it is attempted in women who actually are not yet ready to start. In most instances the condition of the cervix is the best indication of whether attempted induction is likely to be successful. If the cervix is firm, uneffaced, and occupies a position in the posterior part of the vagina, attempts at induction are likely to be unsuccessful. If immediate delivery is necessary, cesarean section should be considered. On the other hand, it usually is possible to initiate labor when the cervix is soft, effaced, partially dilated, and situated in the middle of the vagina. (Table 31-1).

Indications. Most indicated inductions are performed for preeclampsia-eclampsia or chronic hypertension, bleeding complications, and premature rupture of membranes.

PREECLAMPSIA-ECLAMPSIA OR CHRONIC HYPERTENSION. If advance in the severity of preeclampsia-eclampsia or chronic hypertension cannot be controlled by medical treatment, delivery is necessary. Most patients can be delivered vaginally after labor has been induced.

BLEEDING COMPLICATIONS. It may become necessary to deliver women with placenta previa or abruptio placentae to control bleeding. If this can be accomplished safely from below, it is preferable to cesarean section.

PREMATURE RUPTURE OF THE MEMBRANES. Premature rupture of membranes (that is, spontaneous rupture before labor begins) occurs in about 10% to 12% of all pregnant women. The principal complication associated with premature rupture of the membranes is infection, causing fetal and neonatal death.

The *latent period* is the interval between rupture and the onset of labor. The latent period usually is short when the membranes rupture near term, but the less advanced the pregnancy, the longer the latent period.

The principal clinical concern when the membranes rupture prematurely is for intrauterine infection and its consequences for both the fetus and the mother. The amniotic cavity may already have been invaded by bacteria when the membranes rupture; if not, the infection may develop afterward. The decision as to when to terminate the pregnancy is based on weighing the possibility of serious fetal and maternal infection against the risks of prematurity. The latter may be a greater hazard than is infection, particularly if neonatal intensive care is not available.

The patient should be examined to confirm rupture of the membranes and to determine fetal position and the degree of cervical effacement and dilatation. Occasionally, the sudden discharge of urine or of thin vaginal or cervical secretions may simulate the gush of fluid that occurs when the membranes rupture. If the cervix is exposed with a sterile speculum, one can determine the character of the fluid in the vagina. If *vernix caseosa* can be seen, the membranes clearly have ruptured. Amniotic fluid that is uncontaminated with blood, me-

conium, or vaginal secretions will produce a *fern pattern* when allowed to dry on a glass slide. The *pH of amniotic fluid* is alkaline. The identification of *orange-colored fetal cells* in a specimen stained with Nile blue confirms that it is amniotic fluid. Because of the possibility of introducing bacteria, no more examinations should be performed after rupture of the membranes has been confirmed.

Premature rupture of the membranes is usually an indication for delivery if the pregnancy is of at least 36 weeks' duration and the fetus is mature. The longer the membranes have been ruptured before the infant is delivered, the greater is the possibility of chorioamnionitis and fetal infection. Bacteria enter the fetus either by aspiration of infected amniotic fluid and exudates or through the fetal bloodstream from foci of infection in the placenta. However, some recent studies have had good newborn outcomes.

The decisions concerning the best time to deliver premature infants are difficult to make. Even though at least 50% of those weighing between 800 and 1000 g will survive if treatment in an intensive neonatal intensive care unit is started immediately after delivery, it is preferable to maintain them in a normal intrauterine environment rather than in a nursery. If neonatal intensive care is not available, patients with premature rupture of the membranes should be transferred to a perinatal center for delivery.

To help determine whether prompt delivery is necessary, samples of amniotic fluid can be obtained by transabdominal aspiration from isolated pockets identified by ultrasound. If the fluid is not infected, the risk for the fetus is low, and pregnancy can be allowed to continue. Conversely, if the amniotic cavity already is heavily contaminated, the pregnancy should usually be terminated, particularly if the infant is mature enough to have a good chance of surviving and of developing normally. There is no reason to delay in the hope that survival will be better if the fetus is stressed; evidence that this is effective is not available. One recent study showed a correlation between low amniotic fluid volume in these patients and an increased risk of infection. In the past, these high-risk patients could not be evaluated by amniocentesis.

The pregnancy should also be terminated if the mother

becomes febrile or begins labor. *Chorioamnionitis* can be diagnosed when the temperature rises and the uterus becomes tender. Cefoxitin or cefotetan should be administered, and electronic fetal monitoring started. If labor has already begun, it should be allowed to continue. There are no arbitrary time limits within which the fetus must be delivered, but labor should be terminated promptly if the fetus becomes distressed. If labor has not already started when chorioamnionitis is diagnosed, an oxytocin induction is appropriate.

Cesarean section is often necessary if labor does not progress or if fetal distress is recognized. Cesarean section is also appropriate if breech or another abnormal position is diagnosed or if any other abnormality such as prolapsed cord is detected.

Other indications. Other indications for induction include certain patients with *diabetes mellitus, prediabetes, Rh sensitization, recurrent pyelonephritis,* and *repeated intrauterine fetal death.*

ELECTIVE INDUCTION. The elective induction of labor is contraindicated for normal women.

Technique. Labor can be induced by *artificial rupture of the membranes,* by the infusion of 1:1000 *oxytocin solution* intravenously, by a combination of both, or with *prostaglandins.*

Labor will usually begin promptly after *amniotomy* if the head is well engaged and the cervix is soft, effaced, partially dilated, and in an anterior position (Fig. 31-24). Oxytocin supplementation is appropriate if labor has not yet begun within 6 hours after amniotomy.

The principal dangers from amniotomy to induce labor are prolapse of the cord, which may occur even though the head is well fixed in the pelvis, and failure. Unless contractions can be stimulated with oxytocin if amniotomy alone does not induce them, risks from infection are increased. Amniotomy should not often be performed unless the head is engaged.

Oxytocin must be administered with great caution, since the physician cannot determine in advance how responsive the uterus will be. An excessive dose may produce tumultous contractions, which may injure the baby or even rupture the uterus of a multiparous patient. An intravenous infusion of 5% dextrose is started, and the needle is secured in the vein. The needle from a second 1 L bottle of 5% dextrose to which 1 ml (10 U) of oxytocin has been added is connected through an infusion pump to the tubing of the first intravenous infusion set. The flow from the bottle of plain 5% dextrose solution is adjusted to about 5 drops/min, just enough to maintain a constant flow.

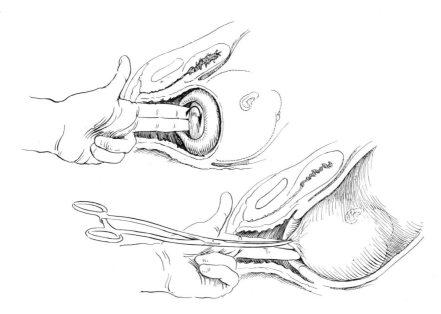

Fig. 31-24. Amniotomy to induce labor. Membranes are separated from cervix and lower segment, and bag of waters is torn with dressing forceps. (From Willson, J.R.: Atlas of obstetric technic, ed. 2, St. Louis, 1969, The C.V. Mosby Co.)

The dosage of oxytocin is calculated in milliunits (mU). If 1 ml of oxytocin (10 IU or 10,000 mU) is added to 1000 ml of 5% dextrose, each milliliter of the resultant solution contains 10 mU of oxytocin. The dosage necessary to stimulate contractions varies, but it may be as low as 0.5 mU/min; consequently, the constant infusion pump is set to deliver this dosage. If the uterus fails to respond within 20 to 30 minutes, the dosage can be increased to 1 mU/min. The dosage is gradually increased by 1 mU increments at 20- to 30-minute intervals until the contractions are similar to those of normal labor.

It is important that someone remain with the patient during an induction, recording the duration of each contraction and checking the patient's pulse and blood pressure frequently. During the early phase of the induction the uterine contractions and the fetal heart rate can be recorded from external monitors. As soon as is possible, these should be replaced by an intrauterine pressure recording system and a fetal scalp monitor. If the contractions become tetanic, recur too frequently, or last too long, the infusion rate must be reduced.

The total dosage of oxytocin in any uninterrupted period should be limited. Large dosages of oxytocin administered in electrolyte-free fluids over long periods of time are contraindicated because oxytocin may have an antidiuretic effect. This combination may produce edema or even water intoxication and convulsions. Abdul-Karim and Assali found the threshold dosage that produced antidiuresis in pregnant human subjects to be 15 mU/min and that a maximal response occurred at a rate of 45 mU/min. Munsick's study indicates that the antidiuretic effect occurs because of increased tubular reabsorption of water rather than altered glomerular filtration or renal blood flow.

Uterine contractions can also be initiated by the intravenous, intraamniotic, vaginal, or extraovular administration of *prostaglandin E_2 or $F_2\alpha$.* Although these substances appear to be as effective as oxytocin in inducing labor, much more study is necessary before they can be used clinically. They seem to be particularly effective in ripening the cervix before induction.

Contraindications. Any condition that makes labor hazardous for the mother or the fetus is a contraindication to induction. These include *abnormal fetal positions and presentations, obvious fetopelvic disproportion, uterine scars from previous cesarean sections, or uterine operations.* Oxytocin should be used with caution in *women of high parity*

because of the increased risk of uterine rupture. *Elective induction* is contraindicated.

REFERENCES

Abdul-Karim, R., and Assali, N.S.: Renal function in human pregnancy. V. Effects on renal hemodynamics and water and electrolyte excretion, J. Lab. Clin. Med. **57**:522, 1961.

Anderson, A.B.M., Laurence, K.M., Davies, K., Campbell, H., and Turnbull, A.C.: Fetal adrenal weight and the cause of premature delivery in human pregnancy, J. Obstet. Gynaecol. Br. Commonw. **78**:481, 1971.

Anderson, G.A.: Postmaturity: a review, Obstet. Gynecol. Surv. **27**:65, 1972.

Bejar, R., Curbelo, V., Davis, C., and Gluck, L.: Premature labor. II. Bacterial sources of phospholipase, Obstet. Gynecol. **57**:479, 1981.

Bishop, E.H.: Pelvic scoring for elective induction, Obstet. Gynecol. **24**:266, 1964.

Bobitt, J.R., and Ledger, W.J.: Amniotic fluid analysis: its role in maternal and neonatal infection, Obstet. Gynecol. **51**:56, 1978.

Caldeyro-Barcia, R., Noriega-Guerra, L., Cibils, L.A., Alvarez, H., Poseiro, J.J., Pose, S.V., Sica-Blanco, Y., Mendez-Bauer, C., Fielitz, C., and Gonzalez-Panizza, V.H.: Effect of position changes on the intensity and frequency of uterine contractions during labor, Am. J. Obstet. Gynecol. **80**:284, 1960.

Caldeyro-Barcia, R., and Poseiro, J.J.: Oxytocin and contractility of the pregnant human uterus, Ann. N.Y. Acad. Sci. **75**:813, 1959.

Calkins, L.A.: The second stage of labor: the descent phase, Am. J. Obstet. Gynecol. **48**:798, 1944.

Cibils, L.A., and Hendricks, C.H.: Normal labor in vertex presentation, Am. J. Obstet. Gynecol. **91**:385, 1965.

Danforth, D.N.: The fibrous nature of the human cervix, and its relation to the isthmic segment in gravid and nongravid uteri, Am. J. Obstet. Gynecol. **53**:541, 1947.

Danforth, D.N., Graham, R.J., and Ivy, A.C.: Functional anatomy of labor as revealed by frozen sagittal sections in Macacus rhesus monkeys, Surg. Gynecol. Obstet. **74**:188, 1942.

Danforth, D.N., and Ivy, A.C.: The lower uterine segment: its derivation and physiologic behavior, Am. J. Obstet. Gynecol. **57**:188, 1942.

Dawood, M.Y., Wang, C.F., Gupta, R., et al.: Fetal contribution to oxytocin in human labor, Obstet. Gynecol. **52**:205, 1973.

Friedman, E.A.: Labor in multiparas, Obstet. Gynecol. **8**:691, 1956.

Friedman, E.A.: Primigravid labor: a graphicostatistical analysis, Obstet. Gynecol. **6**:567, 1955.

Fuchs, A.R., et al.: Oxytocin receptors and human parturition: a dual role for oxytocin in the initiation of labor, Science **215**:1386, 1982.

Fuchs, F., Fuchs, A.R., Poblete, V.F., and Risk, A.: Effect of alcohol on threatened premature labor, Am. J. Obstet. Gynecol. **99:**627, 1967.

Gillespie, E.C.: Principles of uterine growth in pregnancy, Am. J. Obstet. Gynecol. **59:**949, 1950.

Hellman, L.M., and Prystowsky, H.: The duration of the second stage of labor, Am. J. Obstet. Gynecol. **63:**1223, 1952.

Husslein, P., Fuchs, A.R., and Fuchs, F.: Oxytocin and the initiation of human parturition, Am. J. Obstet. Gynecol. **141:**688, 1981.

Koh, K.S., Chan, F.H., Monfared, A.H., Ledger, W.J., and Paul, R.H.: The changing perinatal and maternal outcome in chorioamnionitis, Obstet. Gynecol. **53:**730, 1979.

Ledger, W.J.: Monitoring of labor by graphs, Obstet. Gynecol. **34:**174, 1969.

Ledger, W.J., and Wilting, W.C.: The use of a cervical dilatation graph in the management of primigravidae in labour, J. Obstet. Gynaecol. Br. Commonw. **79:**710, 1972.

Munsick, R.A.: Renal hemodynamic effects of oxytocin in antepartal and postpartal women, Am. J. Obstet. Gynecol. **108:**729, 1970.

Naeye, R.L.: Causes of perinatal mortality in the U.S. Collaborative Perinatal Project, J.A.M.A. **238:**228, 1977.

Niebyl, J.R., Blake, D.A., Johnson, J.W.C., and King, T.M.: The pharmacologic inhibition of premature labor, Obstet. Gynecol. Surv. **33:**507, 1978.

Reynolds, S.R.M.: Physiology of the uterus with clinical correlations, New York, 1949, Paul B. Hoeber, Inc., Medical Book Department, Harper & Brothers.

Schulman, H., and Ledger, W.J.: Practical applications of the graphic protrayal of labor, Obstet. Gynecol. **23:**442, 1964.

Seitchik, J., and Castillo, M.: Oxytocin augmentation of dysfunctional labor, Am. J. Obstet. Gynecol. **144:**289, 1982.

Semmens, J.P.: Implications of teenage pregnancy, Obstet. Gynecol. **26:**77, 1965.

Vintzikos, A.M., et al.: Degree of oligohydramnios and pregnancy outcome in patients with premature rupture of the membranes, Obstet. Gynecol. **66:**162, 1985.

Zuspan, F.R., Barden, T.P., Bieniarz, J., Cibils, L.A., Fuchs, F., Landesman, R., Mercer, J.P., Moawad, A.H., and Pauerstein, C.J.: Premature labor: its management and therapy, J. Reprod. Med. **9:**93, 1972.

32

J. Robert Willson

Obstetric analgesia and anesthesia

In 1847 the Scottish obstetrician James Y. Simpson reported to the Edinburgh Medical-Chirurgical Society that he had been able to abolish pain of delivery with chloroform and thereby initiated a new era in obstetrics. Among those most bitterly opposed to the use of anesthesia were some of the members of the clergy. They argued that according to the Bible women were meant to bring forth their children in "sorrow." Simpson countered with the point that anesthesia must be acceptable to God because He himself had put Adam to sleep to remove the rib from which Eve was created. Despite the controversy, chloroform was readily accepted by women in labor who were not particularly impressed by the theoretical arguments of the clergymen. The opposition was substantially reduced by Queen Victoria's acceptance of chloroform for the delivery of her eighth child in 1853.

Many drugs have been given to make labor and delivery less painful, but unfortunately all have disadvantages that limit their usefulness. The "perfect" agent must provide relief from pain while it neither interferes with the progress of labor nor adds to the maternal or fetal risk. Such an agent has not yet been discovered.

An important concept to remember is that anesthesia for delivery often is emergency anesthesia. There may be no time to prepare patients as there is before a planned surgical procedure. They may have eaten recently or have acute respiratory infections or other disorders that increase the anesthetic hazards.

CONTROL OF PAIN DURING LABOR

Our concept of a *normal childbirth* is one in which labor progresses at a regular rate and terminates in the birth of a healthy infant. This does not preclude the use of analgesia during labor and anesthetic for delivery, as long as neither increases the risk for the mother or the fetus.

Painless labors do occur, but, even in primitive societies, they are the exception rather than the rule. The amount of pain experienced is determined, in part, by the patient's attitude toward pregnancy, delivery, and motherhood in general, but other factors may be equally important. Gintzler observed a gradual increase in the pain threshold of rats throughout pregnancy with an abrupt rise just before parturition. He was able to abolish the increase by administering the narcotic antagonist naltrexone. His suggestion that the enhanced pain tolerance may be from increased secretion of endorphins in response to pain during labor is supported by studies in human beings. Hoffman and co-workers found that beta-endorphin concentrations in peripheral plasma were fairly stable during pregnancy, but increased from 49 ± 2.7 pg/ml during the third trimester to 202 ± 32 during early labor and to 398 ± 78 during late labor. The levels fell to 177 ± 22 within the first hour after delivery. Furthermore, plasma endorphins decreased from 189 ± 31 to 97.6 ± 12 after induction of epidural analgesia. Riss and Bieglmayer detected similar changes but also noted that, when meperidine (Demerol) was administered, the endorphin levels were higher than in women who had had no analgesia. This may be because meperidine occupies many of the opiate receptors, leaving more free endorphin in plasma. Facchinetti and associates found beta-endorphin and beta-lipotrophin concentrations to be lower in women who were delivered by cesarean section without having been in labor than in those who had had normal labor. In addition, the levels were even higher in women delivered by cesarean section after labor began than at similar stages of normal labor.

Oyama and colleagues found that the intrathecal injection of human beta endorphin in women abolished the pain associated with uterine contractions and delivery without affecting the course of labor or the fetus.

Fetal endorphins are less affected by labor than are maternal concentrations, except that, after the fetus has been stressed in utero, they are increased. The difference suggests that fetal endorphin secretion is unrelated to maternal changes.

As a general rule, women who approach delivery with a maximum of understanding and a minimum of apprehension require the least medication. A normal woman can achieve this state with the help of childbirth education classes designed to provide an understanding of labor as a normal and emotionally satisfying experience and of empathetic attendants who are willing to devote time and thought to meeting individual needs for prenatal education. The results of a similar program in women who are emotionally less well oriented toward pregnancy and motherhood often are unsatisfactory.

Women who have attended predelivery educational courses such as those in which the Lamaze and similar methods are taught often can proceed through labor and delivery with a minimum of discomfort. In many instances the labor progresses more rapidly than is anticipated.

It is essential that attendants understand that their principal role is supportive and that there is no need to interfere as long as labor is progressing normally and the mother is reasonably comfortable. However, it is equally important that the patient and her attendant reach an understanding of the goals before labor begins. The attendant must never force the patient to take an analgesic drug or anesthetic; neither must the patient think that she cannot have one simply because she has chosen one of the psychoprophylactic methods. On the other hand, they must agree that should the labor not progress normally, the physician automatically has the prerogative of ordering whatever medication is necessary for the procedure required to correct the abnormality.

The understanding, participation, and support of the attendant, the nursing staff, and the father are essential factors in a successful outcome.

There are many methods for providing analgesia during labor, no one of which is suitable for every individual. No "routine" method is possible because some women neither want nor need medication, and in others it may be contraindicated. Each dose should be ordered individually after the attendant is satisfied that it will benefit the patient.

Since no single method can be applied to all women, it is necessary that the attendant be familiar with more than one type. The techniques, however, must be ones that are safe in a particular environment. Certain methods that are permissible in large, well-staffed maternity hospitals may be too dangerous to use in smaller institutions or at home.

Systemic analgesia

The ability to reduce pain during labor with meperidine, morphine, and other narcotics is limited by their effects on the newly born infant. Since these drugs cross the placenta, they exert a cerebral depressant effect on the fetus as well as on the mother. This is not particularly important while the fetus is in the uterus, as long as the exchange of respiratory gases across the placenta is maintained at the usual rate. At birth the infant must breathe for itself; the onset of respiration may be delayed many minutes if the infant's respiratory center is depressed by the drugs administered to the mother. The effects of oversedation may last for several days.

Systemic analgesics should be used to reduce the discomfort to a tolerable level and to relax the patient enough to permit her to rest during the pain-free interval between contractions rather than to eliminate pain completely. This can be accomplished without increasing the risk for the infant.

Drugs used to provide systemic analgesia should be injected intravenously or intramuscularly because gastric motility and emptying time are considerably reduced during labor, thus making absorption of oral medications uncertain.

The most important factors to be considered when one prescribes a systemic analgesic are the *amount of the drug and the stage of labor at which it is administered.* Most women do not need analgesia during early labor when the contractions are relatively far apart and of short duration. An ataractic drug, such as promethazine (Phenergan), 50 mg, will usually relax them enough to permit them to rest, or even sleep, until labor is well established. For primigravidas the first injection of analgesic drugs should usually be delayed until the contractions are recurring at 2- to 3-minute intervals and the cervix is 4 to 5 cm dilated. Conversely, if the medication is given too late, the infant will be born during the period of its maximal effect and may well be depressed. Sedation should usually not be administered within 3 hours of delivery.

Meperidine. Meperidine relieves pain as well as morphine, and the usual doses do not alter the course of labor significantly. It does cross the placenta, and if too much is given or if it is administered too late in labor, the newborn infant may be depressed.

A combination of promethazine, 25 to 50 mg, and meperidine, 50 to 100 mg, injected intramuscularly provides excellent analgesia and relaxation without untoward effect on the infant. A maximal analgesic effect is reached in about 45 minutes. Subsequent doses of meperidine when necessary vary between 25 and 50 mg. A second injection of the phenothiazine can be given in 4 to 6 hours if the patient is restless or uncomfortable.

The drugs can be administered intravenously when a more rapid effect is desired. The usual initial dose by this route is no more than 50 mg meperidine and 25 mg promethazine.

Morphine sulfate. Morphine is an excellent analgesic for use during labor, but it may produce fetal bradycardia. It can be combined with a phenothiazine derivative. The initial intramuscular dose of morphine sulfate is 6 to 10 mg, given with 50 mg of promethazine. The morphine can be repeated if necessary.

Barbituric acid derivatives. These have no analgesic properties and therefore are not used for pain relief during labor. They exert a more profound depressant effect on the fetal respiratory center than do the narcotics, and they may produce considerable excitement in certain individuals.

Complications. The most important complication accompanying the use of systemic analgesics is *depression of the infant's respiratory center* and subsequent apnea neonatorum, which is particularly likely to occur if general anesthesia is also administered. This can be prevented by using small doses of the drugs and by attempting to time the last injection to precede delivery by at least 3 hours.

If the infant is narcotized by meperidine, morphine, or similar substances, the effect of the drugs can be neutralized by injecting naloxone (Narcan), 10 µg/kg, into an umbilical vein. Unlike nalorphine (Nalline), which is antagonistic only to morphinelike drugs and may increase the depression produced by barbiturates and inhalation anesthetics, naloxone has no other obvious pharmacologic effect.

The *heavily medicated patient cannot cooperate during the second stage;* thus the number of required operative deliveries is increased by excessive sedation.

Inhalation analgesia

Almost all the volatile anesthetic agents have been used to relieve pain during labor, but none is entirely satisfactory. The most often used is a mixture of *nitrous oxide (50%) and oxygen (50%),* which, when inhaled during each uterine contraction, will reduce the discomfort considerably. Somewhat higher concentrations of nitrous oxide can be used if necessary, but if the concentration of oxygen is reduced much below 30%, the fetus may become hypoxic.

This method is most valuable at the end of the first stage in multiparas and during the second stage in both multiparas and primigravidas. The gas can be inhaled intermittently for some time without interfering with uterine contractions or compromising the infant.

Regional analgesia

The transmission of pain impulses can be controlled by nerve block. With this type of analgesia the mother is awake and comfortable, and the baby rarely is depressed. Major nerve block techniques require an experienced individual to administer the anesthetic and supervise the patient during the rest of her labor and delivery; as a consequence, some of these forms of analgesia are usually available only in large institutions.

Pain sensations from the uterus, the cervix, and the upper vagina are transmitted to Frankenhauser's ganglions, which lie just lateral to the cervix; then through the inferior and superior hypogastric plexuses, and by way of the lumbar and lower thoracic sympathetic chains, to the spinal cord through nerves arising from T 10, 11, and 12 and L 1.

The major pain sensations from the lower vagina and posterior vulva and perineum, which are the principal sources of discomfort as the presenting part distends the lower vagina and delivers, are transmitted through the pudendal nerves, which are derived from the ventral branches of S 2, 3, and 4.

Paracervical (uterosacral) block (Fig. 32-1). The pain during the first stage of labor arises from the dilating cervix and upper vagina and generally can be controlled by blocking the sensory and autonomic nerves that supply these areas. To accomplish this an anesthetic agent is injected at about the junction of the uterosacral ligaments, through which the nerve fibers pass, and the cervix. The block usually is administered when painful contractions are recurring regularly and the cervix is dilated 5 to 6 cm in primigravidas and slightly earlier in multiparas.

A hollow metal guide, such as an Iowa trumpet, is inserted along the fingers into the vagina until its tip rests against the lateral fornix at about the 4 o'clock position. A 15 cm, 20-gauge needle is passed through the guide until its point punctures the vaginal epithelium. The tip of the needle is inserted to a depth of about 0.5 cm, and,

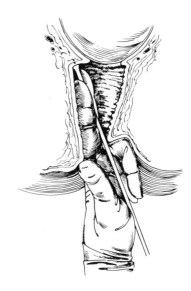

Fig. 32-1. Paracervical block. Needle is introduced through guide until it penetrates vaginal mucosa. Anesthetic agent is injected at 4 and 8 o'clock positions. (From Willson, J.R.: Atlas of obstetric technic, ed. 2, St. Louis, 1969, The C.V. Mosby Co.)

after aspiration to make certain that it has not punctured a blood vessel, 5 or 10 ml of 0.5% lidocaine (Xylocaine) is injected into the tissue. The procedure is repeated on the opposite side at the 8 o'clock position. The anesthetic agent must be injected superficially to avoid introducing it into a blood vessel, the uterus or even directly into the fetus.

Paracervical block provides prompt and effective pain relief in at least 75% of patients. The duration of action varies, but it often lasts an hour or more; the injection can be repeated if pain recurs and the cervix is still incompletely dilated.

In some patients, *uterine contractions stop* for a short time after the injection; however, when the contractions begin again, labor progresses normally. *Fetal bradycardia,* which has been observed frequently, is probably caused by absorption of the anesthetic agent into the fetal circulation or because of hypoxia resulting from spasm of the arteries in uterine muscle. If the concentration of the drug in fetal tissues is high enough, the infant may be depressed at birth or even die. Paracervical block should not be used if there is any suggestion of placental insufficiency or when uterine blood flow is reduced by hypertension.

The incidence of fetal bradycardia can be substantially

reduced by decreasing the dose of the drug used and by injecting it superficially in the vaginal wall rather than deep. If the needle is inserted too far, the anesthetic may be injected into the myometrium or into one of the large blood vessels in the broad ligament, thereby increasing the possibility that a large amount will reach the fetus.

This technique does not anesthetize the lower vagina or the perineal structures; consequently, pudendal block or local infiltration is necessary for delivery.

Epidural (peridural) block. The injection of an anesthetic drug into the extradural space controls pain by blocking the transmission of painful stimuli without interfering with the muscular activity of the uterus. Control of the voluntary muscles in the legs is maintained, but the pelvic muscles are relaxed, making delivery easier for both the mother and her infant. Because peridural block does not alter oxygenation unless the maternal blood pressure falls, it is particularly valuable during premature labor and in women with heart disease, diabetes, and pulmonary diseases.

The block is established by injecting an anesthetic agent into the peridural space between two lumbar vertebrae *(epidural block)* or through the sacral hiatus *(caudal block)*. The injection is made after labor is well established and is progressing normally and when the patient is uncomfortable enough to desire relief. Since the duration of pain relief from an injection is limited, *continuous caudal and epidural techniques* have generally replaced single injections. A polyethylene catheter is threaded through the needle and is left in place as the needle is withdrawn over it. Subsequent injections are made as needed to keep the patient comfortable until the infant is delivered.

Epidural anesthesia is *contraindicated* in patients with a skin infection near the proposed puncture site, in those with any disease of the spine or central nervous system, in those who are bleeding or in shock, and in those with hypertension. It is far more suitable for the delivery of primigravidas than of multiparas, particularly those who have had rapid easy labors in the past. Epidural block should not be attempted unless an experienced individual can supervise the insertion of the needle and catheter and the injections of the anesthetic agent throughout the labor.

The *complications,* some of which are potentially lethal, can be kept at a minimum by strict observation of the necessary precautions. The most serious complications are *massive spinal anesthesia* following the inadvertent injection of the agent into the subarachnoid space, *meningitis, epidural abscess, intravenous injection,* and

breakage of the needle or catheter. Less serious complications are *hypotension,* which is minimal in normal women, and *anesthetic failure.*

Although there may be a temporary depression of uterine activity after the injection, epidural block does not usually affect cervical dilatation. The second stage may be prolonged because the loss of pain sensation in the vagina and on the perineum eliminates involuntary expulsive efforts and interferes with voluntary attempts to use the secondary forces to expel the baby.

ANESTHESIA FOR DELIVERY

Relief of pain during the actual delivery of the infant plays an important part in modern obstetrics. Pain relief is not an important enough reason to justify an increase in maternal or fetal morbidity or mortality, but such an increase is not necessary if the physician selects the anesthetic most suitable for each patient and provides for its safe administration.

Inhalation anesthetic

Apprehensive women may demand inhalation anesthesia to obliterate all consciousness of what is happening during delivery. Although this can be accomplished with relative safety by the proper selection and administration of the agent, certain hazards accompany the use of inhalation anesthesia. *Vomiting* and *aspiration* are serious complications and a major cause of maternal deaths. Patients should be cautioned against eating after the contractions begin and not allowed anything by mouth during labor. Regional anesthesia should be used for women who have eaten recently, or if this is not available, the stomach should be emptied, and the patient should be given 30 ml of milk of magnesia or an antacid shortly before delivery to neutralize the remaining stomach contents. If she vomits and aspirates, there will be less pulmonary damage if acidity of the vomitus is reduced.

Prolonged deep anesthesia may *interfere with uterine contractions,* thereby increasing the incidence of bleeding during the third stage. Since the inhalation anesthetic agents cross the placenta, *the infant may be anesthetized and apneic at birth* if deep anesthesia has been induced. This need not occur during normal delivery, but prolonged anesthesia is a distinct hazard when the uterus must be relaxed with inhalation anesthesia.

This method generally is preferred over spinal or epidural anesthesia for women with hypotension from bleeding or other causes, for those with disorders of the spine or nervous system, or for emergency cesarean section when it is important to deliver the baby rapidly. Inhalation anesthesia is essential whenever it is necessary to abolish uterine contractions and relax the uterine muscle to complete delivery.

Inhalation techniques are being used less often for normal or forceps delivery as more obstetricians and their patients become aware of the advantages of conduction anesthesia. Many women want to be awake during the birth of their babies, and obstetricians are concerned over the potential dangers that are inherent with inhalation anesthesia. Fortunately, the variety of available conduction techniques permits the selection of one that is suitable under almost any circumstance. When conduction anesthesia is inappropriate, one of the following inhalation anesthetics can be used.

Nitrous oxide–oxygen. Nitrous oxide–oxygen mixtures are easy to administer, but they are not particularly potent anesthetic agents. They are most useful for the control of pain during the terminal phases of labor and for spontaneous delivery of multiparas.

Halothane. Anesthesia can be induced rapidly with halothane, which has a remarkable inhibitory action on uterine muscle activity. The inhibitory action, which causes excessive bleeding following delivery, makes it unsuitable as a general obstetric anesthetic agent. Its principal use is to produce complete uterine relaxation for total breech extraction and version and extraction. Since these operations are rarely performed, halothane has a limited use in obstetrics.

Conduction anesthesia

Some form of nerve block anesthesia usually is preferable to inhalation types because it permits the mother to be awake and it relieves pain without disturbing fetal oxygenation. Some methods, however, have a high potential mortality, but all must be administered with the greatest caution. The two principal types of regional anesthetic agents are those that produce loss of pain sensation by blocking the nerve roots and those that block the nerves peripherally (Fig. 32-2).

Nerve root block. For the most part these techniques relieve pain completely but do not interfere with the uterine contractions. There is an associated vasodilatation below the anesthetic level that may be responsible for a fall in blood pressure. These anesthetic technics do not depress the respiratory center and therefore are ben-

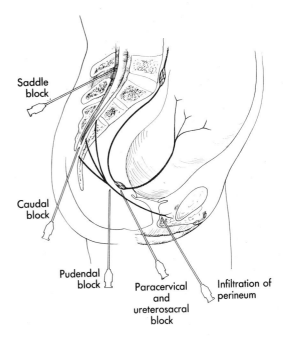

Fig. 32-2. Types of conduction anesthesia for delivery. (From Willson, J.R.: Atlas of obstetric technic, ed. 2, St. Louis, 1969, The C.V. Mosby Co.)

eficial to the fetus unless the maternal blood pressure falls enough to interfere with uterine blood flow, thus decreasing the amount of oxygen available to the fetus. Relaxation of the voluntary pelvic and perineal muscles decreases the pressure on the fetal head, but this loss of resistance may interfere with the normal mechanism of labor, particularly rotation. The relaxation makes forceps delivery easier and less traumatic, but the fact that uterine contractions are not altered makes nerve root block unsuitable for intrauterine manipulation.

Epidural anesthetic may be used for analgesia during labor and anesthesia for delivery and is particularly advantageous for women in whom the usual methods for relieving pain during labor and delivery are contraindicated. It can be administered only by trained and experienced individuals.

Epidural anesthesia may be unsatisfactory when given only for delivery when labor is progressing rapidly. It may take 20 to 30 minutes to insert the catheter and to obtain an adequate anesthetic level. If one starts too late, the patient may deliver before the anesthetic has become effective. This is particularly true in multiparas.

Spinal anesthesia has rightly been considered a dangerous method for producing anesthesia because the mortality is high if it is improperly used. The dangers that are inherent with this technique can be obviated by being aware of them and attempting to avoid them. The vasomotor system is unstable in gravid women, and shock may follow ordinary doses of medication given intraspinally.

Spinal anesthesia is of greatest value in primigravidas, to whom it is administered when the head is bulging the perineum. If given to multiparas too early, descent of the head often is prevented, even though uterine contractions continue, because the patient no longer has an urge to bear down. It should usually be administered to multiparas when the cervix is 8 to 9 cm dilated and the heat well below the ischial spines. It is only to be used in carefully selected patients in hospitals where there is sufficient help to treat the fall in blood pressure and other complications that may be associated with its administration.

Low spinal or *saddle block,* the type of spinal anesthesia most often used for delivery, is given with the patient sitting up. It is better used as a terminal anesthetic for delivery than to provide analgesia during labor. The agent used is *tetracaine (Pontocaine),* 3 to 5 mg, in 10% dextrose.

Headache often follows the administration of spinal or saddle block anesthesia for delivery. Bumgardner and Burns reduced the incidence substantially by the use of a 26-gauge needle rather than the standard larger sizes. The loss of spinal fluid through the dural defect, which is thought to be a major factor in the production of headache, is minimized when the small needle is used. Other more important complications of spinal anesthesia include *arachnoiditis, nerve root injury* from chemical

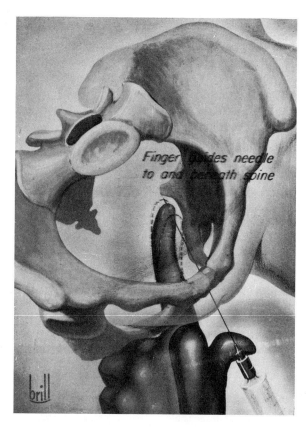

Fig. 32-3. Pudendal nerve block. Needle point is directed behind inferior tip of ischial spine by fingertip. (From Klink, E.W.: Obstet. Gynecol. 1:137, 1953.)

or direct trauma, and an *overdose of the drug*—any one of which may result in disability or death. Complications can be kept at a minimum by exercising every possible precaution during the preparation of the solution and its administration.

Peripheral nerve block. Local injection of anesthetic agents to block the peripheral nerve endings affords the same advantages to the fetus that nerve root blocks do, but they are less effective in relieving pain and providing muscle relaxation. They do not require unusual equipment or the presence of an anesthesiologist.

Simple infiltration of the perineum or injection along the line of the proposed episiotomy with 0.5% to 1% procaine or lidocaine is often sufficient for normal delivery but is usually inadequate for forceps delivery.

Pudendal nerve block by injection of 10 ml of 0.5% to 1% lidocaine around each perineal nerve trunk as it passes behind the ischial spine provides excellent pelvic

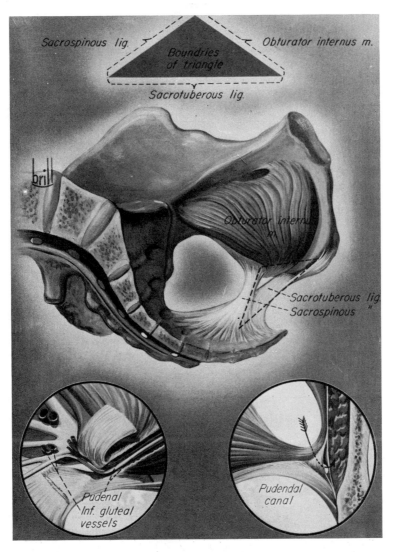

Fig. 32-4. Pudendal nerve block. Localizing landmarks in region of ischial spine and relationship of pudendal nerve to pudendal and inferior gluteal vessels. (From Klink, E.W.: Obstet. Gynecol. **1:**137, 1953.)

anesthesia for normal or low forceps delivery and for episiotomy and repair. It provides inadequate anesthesia for most manual or forceps rotations. It is safe, easy to learn, and requires no anesthesiologist or expensive equipment. This procedure should be suitable for almost all normal deliveries (Figs. 32-3 to 32-5).

A hollow metal guide such as an Iowa trumpet is passed along the palmar surface of the index or second finger toward the ischial spine. The tip of the guide is directed to a position just beneath the tip of the spine and is held firmly in place. A 15 cm, 20-gauge needle attached to a syringe containing lidocaine is inserted through the guide until its tip reaches the vaginal wall. With further pressure, the needle is pushed through the triangle formed by the sacrospinous and sacrotuberous ligaments and the obturator internus muscles until the

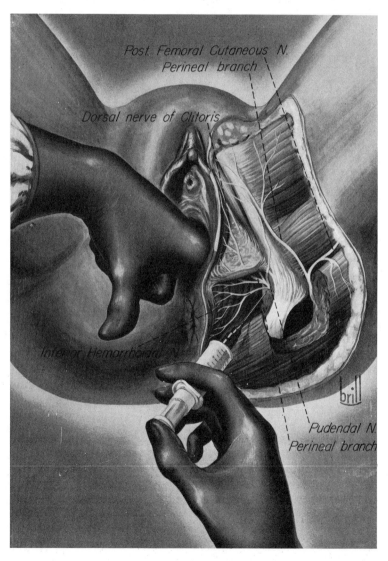

Fig. 32-5. Pudendal nerve block. Injection near main nerve trunk anesthetizes areas supplied by hemorrhoidal, perineal, and dorsal clitoral branches. Needle is usually inserted through vagina rather than through perineum. (From Klink, E.W.: Obstet. Gynecol. **1**:137, 1953.)

tip is in Alcock's canal, through which the pudendal nerve trunk runs. If the needle is properly placed, it can be moved back and forth without resistance. Blood can be aspirated if the pudendal artery or vein has been punctured; in this event the needle should be withdrawn slightly before the anesthetic agent is injected.

A 10 ml deposit of the lidocaine solution is made in the pudendal canal behind each ischial spine, where it is in direct contact with the pudendal nerve trunk. The anesthetic effect will be evident within 2 to 3 minutes. Muscular relaxation as well as anesthesia is effected and will last as long as an hour.

SPECIAL PROCEDURES

The judicious use of analgesics and anesthetics does not affect the outcome of normal labor adversely, but when complications are present, the choice of an inappropriate agent or method can add significantly to the risk for the mother or her baby. For instance, a combination of systemic analgesics and inhalation anesthesia for the *delivery of a premature infant* is generally contraindicated. A small infant is likely to be seriously depressed by these agents, whereas they have less effect on a mature fetus. Epidural or spinal anesthesia is generally contraindicated in women with *hypertension*, particularly when the blood pressure is labile, and for those who are bleeding from *placenta previa* or *abruptio placentae*. Conversely, conduction anesthesia is preferable for patients with *heart disease, pulmonary disease, diabetes (if the blood pressure is normal), and conditions that predispose to uterine relaxation and bleeding following delivery.* These are discussed elsewhere in the text with consideration of the specific complications.

REFERENCES

Arnolds, C.W., Anderson, C.J., and Sherline, D.M.: Prepared childbirth, Clin. Obstet. Gynecol. **24**:575, 1981.

Bumgardner, H.D., and Burns, F.D.: Effect of needle size on the incidence of postspinal headache, Am. J. Obstet. Gynecol. **69**:135, 1955.

Clark, R.B.: Conduction anesthesia, Clin. Obstet. Gynecol. **24**:601, 1981.

Cohen, S.E.: The aspiration syndrome, Clin. Obstet. Gynecol. **9**:235, 1982.

Evans, T.N., Morley, G.W., and Helder, L.: Caudal anesthesia in obstetrics, Obstet. Gynecol. **20**:726, 1962.

Facchinetti, F., et al.: Fetomaternal opioid levels and parturition, Obstet. Gynecol. **62**:764, 1983.

Gintzler, A.R.: Endorphine-mediated increases in pain threshold during pregnancy, Science **210**:193, 1980.

Hoffman, D.I., et al.: Plasma β-endorphine concentrations prior to and during pregnancy, in labor, and after delivery, Am. J. Obstet. Gynecol. **150**:492, 1984.

King, J.C., and Sherline, D.M.: Paracervical and pudendal block, Clin. Obstet. Gynecol. **24**:587, 1981.

Klink, E.W.: Perineal nerve block: an anatomic and clinical study in the female, Obstet. Gynecol. **1**:137, 1953.

Maduska, A.L.: Inhalation analgesia and general anesthesia, Clin. Obstet. Gynecol. **24**:619, 1981.

Oyama, T., Matsuki, A., Taneichi, T., Ling, N., and Guillemin, R.: Beta-endorphine in obstetric analgesia, Am. J. Obstet. Gynecol. **137**:613, 1980.

Riss, P.A., and Bieglmayer, C.: Obstetric analgesia and immunoreactive endorphin peptides in maternal plasma during labor, Gynecol. Obstet. Invest. **17**:127, 1984.

Scanlon, J.: Effects of obstetric anesthesia and analgesia on the newborn: a select and annotated bibliography for the clinician, Clin. Obstet. Gynecol. **24**:649, 1981.

Shnider, S.M., and Levinson, G.: Anesthesia for obstetrics, Baltimore, 1979, The Williams & Wilkins Co.

33

J. Robert Willson

Third stage of labor and postpartum hemorrhage

The third stage, the interval between the delivery of the infant and the delivery of the placenta, is the most dangerous part of the entire labor. Abnormalities of placental separation and expulsion are often accompanied by profuse bleeding that may end in death. At least 15% of maternal deaths result from postpartum hemorrhage, but most can be prevented if the attendant recognizes that blood loss is excessive, determines the cause, controls the bleeding, and replaces the lost blood promptly. Few postpartum hemorrhages occur so rapidly that there is no time for appropriate treatment. In most instances death occurs several hours after delivery when the patient has been exsanguinated by a steady trickle of blood rather than by a sudden overwhelming hemorrhage.

The total mortality from postpartum hemorrhage is not always obvious. Excessive bleeding may cause death by reducing the patient's ability to compensate for other complications such as infection. Douglas and Davis noticed an increase both in the incidence of infections and in their severity in women who had lost abnormal amounts of blood at delivery.

Blood loss during the third stage varies considerably. Newton reported the average measured blood loss during the first 24 hours after vaginal delivery to be about 650 ml. Pritchard and colleagues reported a similar figure and also observed

that 5% of women who delivered vaginally lost more than 1000 ml of blood. Ueland measured a blood volume loss of 610 ml 60 minutes after vaginal delivery. The highest measurements of blood loss are those of Quinlivan and Brock, who calculated the decrease in blood volume after delivery to be 1115 and 1023 ml by the two methods used. This corresponded to their measured loss of 1106 ml.

It has been customary to diagnose *postpartum hemorrhage* when the total blood loss with delivery and during the first 24 hours after delivery is *estimated* to exceed 500 ml. it is obvious from the studies in which blood loss was measured accurately, rather than estimated, that 500 ml is far too low a figure to accept as the upper limit of normal. A more logical maximum is 1000 ml.

NORMAL THIRD STAGE

Placental separation. Under normal circumstances the placenta is relatively noncontractile and has only limited ability to alter its size and shape to compensate for changes in the area of the uterine wall over which it is attached. As the uterus becomes smaller as the infant is expelled from the birth canal, the surface area of its cavity must of necessity diminish. As the area of the placental site is reduced, the placenta thickens, and its diameter decreases. Since placental size cannot be altered enough to equal the change in the muscular uterine wall beneath it, the placenta is at least partially sheared off as the uterus contracts during the expulsion of the fetus. The completeness with which the placenta is separated is determined by how much the subplacental area of the uterine wall is reduced (Fig. 33-1).

The separation occurs in the spongy portion of the decidua basalis; a thin layer of decidua remains on the uterine wall, and the remainder covers the cotyledons of the maternal surface of the placenta.

After the birth of the baby the uterus continues to contract regularly. At this stage the uterine muscle may be even more active than it was during late labor. The uterus is discoid, being wide transversely but relatively flattened in its anteroposterior diameter, and lies in the midline with its superior surface below the level of the umbilicus. The placenta has already been partially or completely separated during the expulsion of the baby, but it still is in the upper part of the cavity. The continuing uterine contractions complete the separation of the placenta and force it downward into the flaccid, distended lower segment.

As the placenta is expelled from the upper segment, this portion of the uterus becomes globular, its cavity is almost obliterated, and the thickness of the wall increases to as much as 5 cm. The bulky placenta distending the relaxed lower segment forces the globular fundus upward and to the right; the superior surface of the uterus can often be felt above the level of the umbilicus (Fig. 33-2).

The placenta ultimately is forced from the lower segment and vagina by voluntary bearing-down efforts of the mother or, as is more often the case, is expressed by the attendant.

The duration of the third stage will be from 15 to 30 minutes or even longer if the physician waits for the mother to expel the placenta herself. When the placental phase of labor is managed actively by the medical attendant, its duration can be less than 5 minutes in almost every instance.

Control of bleeding. The branches of the uterine arteries wind between the interlacing smooth-muscle bundles as they traverse the uterine wall, and they eventually open into the large sinuses in the decidua basalis at the placental site. *The source of the blood loss after delivery, except that caused by soft-tissue injury, is the sinuses that are left open by separation of the placenta.* Excess bleeding is prevented by firm contraction of the uterine muscle bundles, which kink and compress the vessels pass-

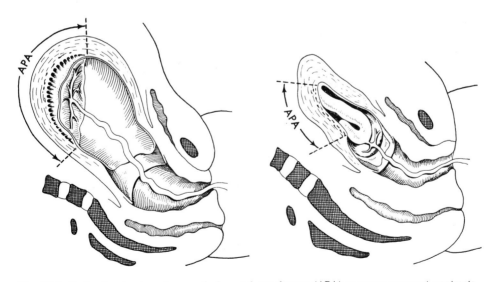

Fig. 33-1. Reduction in size of area of placental attachment *(APA)* as upper segment contracts, separates placenta, and expels it into lower uterine segment.

ing between them. This is followed by clot formation and retraction in the sinuses, the usual method by which bleeding from open vessels is controlled.

Placental expulsion. The so-called signs of separation of the placenta are more accurately evidences of its expulsion from the firmly contracted uterine fundus into the lower segment and vagina and indicate that it can be delivered. The signs consist of the following:

1. A *show of blood* appears as the uterus contracts and the placenta is forced downward. If the placenta is separated completely as the infant is delivered, it usually folds on itself like an inverted umbrella with the fetal surface preceding the periphery through the cervix. With this type of expulsion, the *Schultze mechanism,* the placenta occludes the cervical opening; and there is little obvious bleeding until it is expelled, at which time the blood retained within the uterus gushes out (Fig. 33-2). With the less common *Duncan mechanism,* there is a constant trickle of blood because an edge of the placenta, rather than an inverted surface, appears in the cervical opening and the blood can leave the uterus freely.

2. *The cord advances.* The length of cord visible outside the introitus is increased as the placenta descends into the lower segment and vagina.

3. *The fundus rises* and is deviated toward the right as the placenta, distending the lower segment, elevates the contracted upper portion.

4. *The shape of the uterus changes.* The uterus becomes globular rather than wide and flat after the placenta has been expelled into the lower segment.

5. *Nontransmission of impulse occurs.* As slight traction is made on the cord while the uterus is pushed downward by pressure on the fundus, the amount of cord outside the vagina increases. If the placenta is still in the upper segment, the cord is withdrawn into the vagina when the suprapubic pressure is released and the uterus is allowed to rise. If the placenta is detached and in the lower segment, the cord retracts very little when the uterus rises.

Management. During the second stage the physician should attempt to empty the uterus slowly, thereby permitting the muscle fibers to retract and decrease the size of the cavity gradually as the infant is being delivered. This encourages prompt

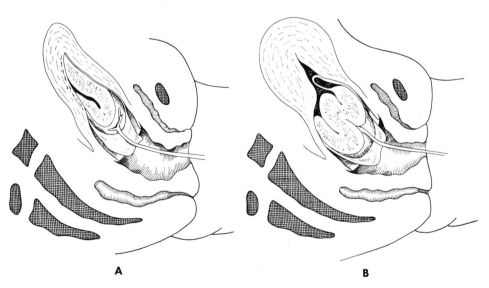

A   **B**

Fig. 33-2. **A,** While placenta is still in upper segment, uterus is discoid and flattened in anteroposterior diameter. **B,** Uterus becomes globular when placenta is expelled into lower segment.

and forceful contraction and more complete placental separation.

After the head has been born, the anterior shoulder is delivered beneath the pubic arch, where it is allowed to remain for 30 to 60 seconds. The head is then elevated, and traction is exerted until the posterior shoulder has cleared the perineum. After another 30- to 60-second wait to permit further readjustment of the uterine muscle fibers, the rest of the body is slowly and deliberately extracted. The physician should not try to restrain delivery if the spontaneous uterine contractions are forcing the baby through the birth canal, but the mother should be urged not to bear down lest the baby be expelled so rapidly that the soft tissues are torn.

After the cord has been clamped and cut, the uterus is gently palpated through the sterile drapes while the cord is held taut but without undue traction. The uterus should not be massaged and manipulated, and no attempt should be made to express the placenta until the uterus contracts. As the fundus becomes firm and globular, placental expulsion can be aided by downward pressure over the superior surface of the uterus with the palmar surfaces of the fingers; it should not be squeezed (Fig. 33-3). Downward pressure is no longer necessary after the placenta enters the lower segment; therefore, at the moment placental descent can be detected, the pressure is transferred from the fundus to the suprapubic area directly over the lower segment. As the contracted uterine fundus is pushed *upward* away from the placenta by firm pressure with the fingertips, the afterbirth, which by now should be visible at the introitus, can be delivered by applying slight traction on the cord (Fig. 33-4).

After the placenta has been delivered, the contracted fundus is kept from dropping back into the pelvis by maintaining upward pressure on it through the abdominal wall; this will promote muscular contraction and reduce bleeding. While a nurse or an assistant applies the pressure necessary to hold the uterus up, the physician examines the placenta to make certain it is intact and that none of its cotyledons has been left in the uterine cavity.

An oxytocic drug is usually given at this time to stimulate uterine muscle contraction.

Uterotonic (oxytocic) drugs stimulate firm uterine contraction and when properly used will reduce the blood loss accompanying placental separation and delivery. Some authorities recommend that an oxytocic drug be administered as soon as the anterior shoulder has been delivered, and others that it be given at the end of the second stage. Unless uterotonic drugs are used with great caution, the placental stage may be prolonged rather than shortened, and blood loss may be excessive. If a firm and sustained uterine contraction occurs while part or all of the placenta is still in the upper segment, its delivery may be delayed until the uterus relaxes as the effect of the drug diminishes. It generally is preferable to withhold uterotonic drugs until the placenta has been delivered.

The oxytocic activity of ergot has long been known, and it has been used extensively in obstetric practice. The purified ergot derivative *ergonovine maleate (Ergotrate),* when administered intravenously or intramuscularly in 0.5 to 1 ml (0.1 to 0.2 mg) doses, produces a sustained tetanic contraction of the uterine muscles that reduces the blood loss from the vessels at the placental site. Ordinarily, it is given intravenously as soon as the placenta has been delivered. *Methylergonovine maleate (Methergine),* a synthetic preparation, is equally effective in the same doses.

Ergonovine maleate, and to a lesser degree methylergonovine maleate, may produce vasoconstriction and an alarming rise in blood pressure in susceptible women. Neither should be given to women with hypertension or to those with labile blood pressures.

Oxytocin from which almost all the vasopressor factor has been removed can be administered instead of ergot preparations as an aid in managing the third stage. It is preferred over either ergonovine maleate or methylergonovine maleate for women with hypertensive disorders because it is less likely to produce alarming blood pressure elevations. The dosage is 0.1 to 0.2 ml (1 to 2 U) intravenously, 0.5 ml (5 U) intramuscularly, or 2 ml (20 U) dissolved in 1000 ml of 5% dextrose solution as an intravenous drip. The latter method is preferred if an intravenous infusion already is running.

Two potentially serious side effects of oxytocin are its cardiovascular and its antidiuretic actions. Hendricks and Brenner observed consistent and occasionally profound decreases in blood pressure after the rapid intravenous injection of a bolus of 0.5 ml (5 U) of oxytocin. This is less likely to occur with the small amounts ad-

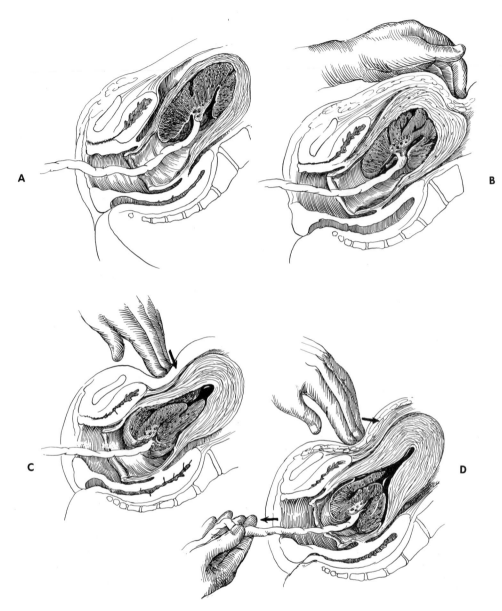

Fig. 33-3. **A,** Uterus before placenta is expelled. **B,** Manual pressure on fundus as uterus begins to contract aids expulsion of placenta into lower segment, **C,** from where it can be expressed by upward pressure on contracted fundus and tension on cord, **D.**

ministered in dilute solution and with intramuscular in-jection.

The most serious consequence of the antidiuretic effect is water intoxication, which may occur with the infusion of 20 mU or more of oxytocin per minute with a large volume of fluid. Since the effects of intravenously ad-

ministered oxytocin are brief, intoxication should occur much less often when it is used for a short time to control postpartum bleeding than when it is given for many hours during induction and augmentation of labor.

Manual removal of the placenta. Some obstetricians sep-arate and remove the placenta and explore the interior

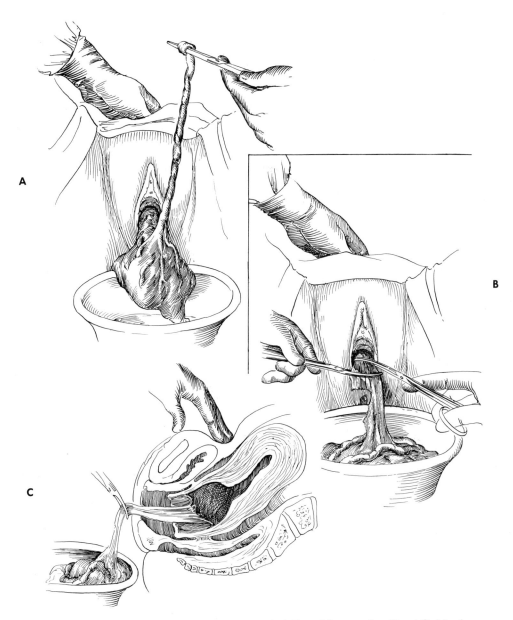

Fig. 33-4. A, Fundus is pushed upward as placenta is delivered from vagina. **B** and **C,** Membranes are peeled off lower segment. (From Willson, J.R.: Atlas of obstetric technic, ed. 2, St. Louis, 1969, The C.V. Mosby Co.)

of the uterus as a routine procedure. Although the risk is not great, it is an unnecessary procedure during which bacteria are inevitably introduced directly into the uterine cavity. Conversely, manual removal is indicated when the placenta fails to separate within a reasonable time

and as part of the treatment of postpartum hemorrhage.

Fetomaternal transfusion. A small amount of fetal blood probably enters the maternal circulation during almost every delivery. This accounts for some instances of Rh isoimmunization. The danger of immunization can be reduced by using a method of placental delivery that minimizes fetomaternal transfusion.

Simple expression of the placenta after spontaneous separation probably provides the smallest infusion of fetal blood from the placenta into the maternal blood in the choriodecidual spaces. Infusion may be increased by the injudicious use of oxytocic agents before the completion of the third stage and by manual removal of the placenta. Draining the placenta of fetal blood before it is delivered may reduce the incidence of massive transfusion.

POSTPARTUM HEMORRHAGE

Postpartum hemorrhage should occur in less than 5% of all deliveries. In almost every instance, excessive bleeding can be controlled, and the blood can be replaced so rapidly that no woman should die as a result of postpartum bleeding.

Etiologic factors. The most important causes of excessive bleeding at delivery or during the early puerperium are *uterine atony* and *soft-tissue injury*. Of these, the first is by far the more common.

The source of the bleeding is either the sinuses of the placental site that remain open after the placenta has separated because the uterus fails to contract properly or blood vessels of the birth canal that are torn during delivery. In either event the amount of bleeding is determined by the size of the involved vessels and the length of time before the blood loss is checked.

Predisposing factors. Certain factors increase the possibility that excessive bleeding will occur after delivery. Most of these interfere with the normal mechanism for controlling bleeding.

OVERDISTENTION OF THE UTERUS. If the uterus has been overdistended by twins, a large infant, or hydramnios, the muscle fibers have been stretched to a point from which they may not be able to retract rapidly enough and contract firmly enough to occlude the open vessels promptly after delivery. Delayed contraction also is likely to occur if the uterus is emptied rapidly.

ANESTHESIA. Deep inhalation anesthesia reduces the force of uterine muscle contraction and may inhibit uterine activity completely. Deep anesthesia therefore can eliminate the normal mechanism by which bleeding after delivery is controlled.

DYSFUNCTIONAL OR PROLONGED LABOR. Ineffective uterine contractions often continue into the third stage.

IMPROPER MANAGEMENT OF THE THIRD STAGE. Manipulation and massage in an attempt to express the placenta before it has separated completely may interfere with the normal mechanism and increase bleeding.

INJURY. A considerable amount of blood may be lost from vaginal lacerations, uterine rupture, or even the episiotomy. Odell and Seski state that the average blood loss from a mediolateral episiotomy is about 250 ml.

RETAINED PLACENTA. Excessive bleeding occurs if the uterus cannot expel a partially separated placenta or if a large fragment of placenta, for example, a succenturiate lobe, is retained.

HISTORY. Postpartum hemorrhage can be anticipated in multiparous women who have had excessive bleeding after other deliveries. The cause may not be obvious.

Clinical course. Deaths from postpartum bleeding are rarely caused by sudden overwhelming hemorrhage. None of the patients reported by Beecham died in less than 1½ hours, and only 11.5% died within 2 hours. The average time between delivery and death was more than 5 hours.

Excessive bleeding may occur while the placenta is still within the uterus or after it has been delivered. Excessive blood loss is usually the result of a prolonged trickle of blood rather than a single massive hemorrhage, but unless the flow is checked the end result is the same. Pregnant women, because of the expanded blood volume, withstand hemorrhage better than do nonpregnant women, but the amount any individual woman will tolerate cannot be determined in advance. *Those with anemia or chronic debilitating disease and those whose blood volume is decreased because of prolonged labor and dehydration or severe preeclampsia-eclampsia may go into shock with relatively minimal bleeding.*

Prevention. Most postpartum hemorrhages can be prevented, but since some cannot, all pregnant women should be considered potential candidates for excessive bleeding. Predisposing causes should be eliminated, and anemia and nutritional inadequacies should be corrected whenever possible.

Abnormal labor should be shortened by recognizing inadequate contractions early and instituting measures that will be helpful in preventing prolonged labor. Attempts to shorten either normal or abnormal labor by extracting the fetus before the presenting part has descended enough to make delivery safe or before the cervix is completely dilated only increases the possibility of severe injury and blood loss. Regional anesthetic should be used whenever possible, and the second as well as the third stage should be managed in a manner calculated to encourage retraction and firm contraction of uterine muscle fibers.

Treatment. The most important factors in preventing deaths from postpartum hemorrhage are to recognize abnormal bleeding before the blood loss has been excessive, to determine the source of the bleeding, to control it as rapidly as possible, and to replace lost blood promptly.

Before the delivery of women with conditions that predispose to excessive bleeding, an intravenous infusion of saline solution should be started through a 15-gauge needle. Blood should be administered to all in whom clinical evidence of blood loss can be detected, even though the amount of bleeding does not seem excessive.

Severe bleeding after the birth of the baby is more often the result of inadequate uterine muscle contraction than of injury. The first step in determining the cause therefore is to palpate the uterine fundus rather than to search for lacerations in the birth canal. If the uterus is soft and boggy, it is almost always the source of bleeding; this is particularly true if the placenta has not yet been delivered.

AT END OF SECOND STAGE. The placenta is expressed if possible or removed manually, and the uterus is pushed upward out of the pelvis and massaged between one hand inserted in the vagina and the other palpating through the abdominal wall to stimulate contraction. Oxytocin is added to the infusion fluid, or 1 or 2 U can be given intravenously while the uterus is being stimulated. If the uterus does not contract under the influence of oxytocin, methylergonovine, 0.5 ml (0.1 mg), can be given intravenously unless there is a contraindication to using it. If the uterus remains relaxed despite these measures, manual exploration to search for an injury or retained placental tissue should be performed promptly.

A *prostaglandin $F_2\alpha$ analogue, (15S)-15-methyl prostaglandin $F_2\alpha$ tromethamine,* has been used with some success in treating postpartum hemorrhage when the uterus fails to contract after the administration of oxytocin and ergot compounds. Hayashi, Costillo, and Noah were able to control bleeding in 86% of 51 patients after other methods had failed. The drug, in an initial dose of 0.25 mg, is injected intramuscularly or directly into the uterine wall. The latter site is appropriate during cesarean delivery or in hypovolemic patients in whom there might be a delay in transporting the material from the injection site to the uterus. A second injection can be given in an hour if necessary. The drug may produce acute hypertension; hence it probably is contraindicated in women with preeclampsia or chronic hypertension. Other side effects are nausea, vomiting and diarrhea, and temperature elevations. Prostaglandin preparations have not yet been approved for use in managing postpartum hemorrhage.

If bleeding continues, the physician must consider the possibility of a clotting defect and test for it.

Hysterectomy may be indicated if all other methods have failed to control bleeding. It should not be delayed until the patient is dying.

AT END OF THIRD STAGE. If abnormal bleeding begins after the placenta has been delivered, the physician should explore the uterus to make certain that it is intact and empty and then stimulate it by manual massage and oxytocics as described previously.

Postpartum hemorrhage from injury. Unless the vagina is extensively lacerated or there are deep cervical tears extending upward into the lower segment, bleeding from injury is less severe than that from atony. The usual cervical lacerations seldom bleed profusely. *Injury should be suspected and sought whenever vaginal bleeding continues despite a firmly contracted fundus.*

Bleeding from vaginal lacerations can usually be controlled with sutures, which must be placed precisely to make certain that they approximate the entire length of the injured area. An assistant to expose the laceration is essential if bleeding is excessive or if the upper vagina is involved. Continued oozing after the placement of sutures can usually be checked with pressure from a tight vaginal pack.

Cervical lacerations should be repaired regardless of whether they are bleeding. Deep lacerations that extend upward into the lower uterine segment will often bleed profusely; unless the upper end of the laceration can be identified and sutured, a laparotomy is necessary for adequate repair. Hysterectomy is usually necessary to control hemorrhage from ruptured uterus.

Delayed hemorrhage. Hemorrhage may occur at any time during the first 24 hours after delivery *(early delayed hemorrhage)* or several days later *(late delayed hemorrhage)*.

EARLY. Hemorrhage during the first 24 hours is most often the result of atony, retained placental fragments, or relaxation of the uterus, but it may be from the episiotomy or a laceration.

If the uterus is soft and distended with blood, it will contract with manual stimulation and the administration of an oxytocic. If the distention is a result of simple atony, it will usually stay contracted after these simple measures have been used.

If atony and bleeding recur, one must consider the possibilty of retained placental fragments or of bleeding from a vaginal or cervical injury. If the patient is lying in bed, blood from a vaginal tear can flow upward into the uterus, distending it and giving the appearance of atony.

If bleeding and relaxation recur after an oxytocic has been given, the vagina and uterine cavity must be explored.

LATE. Bleeding that begins or becomes profuse several days after delivery is most often caused by retained portions of placenta, although occasionally an injury may be responsible. In most instances the uterovaginal canal should be explored promptly. Placental tissue can be removed with a large curet.

Another form of late postpartum hemorrhage is that designated *placental site bleeding.* This usually begins suddenly between the twelfth and twenty-first days and may be profuse. It is presumably the result of separation of the crust of organized fibrin and hyalinized vessels covering the placental site and can usually be controlled by curettage. Blood transfusion may be necessary.

RETAINED PLACENTA

Occasionally, the third stage is prolonged because the placenta fails to separate or because the uterus cannot expel the placenta even though it is partially or completely detached. If the placenta is still completely attached, there can be no bleeding, but if it is partially separated the blood loss from the open placental site sinuses can be profuse. This is a common cause of excessive third-stage bleeding.

Failure of placental separation may be mechanical or

a result of abnormal penetration of the trophoblast into the uterine wall *(abnormally adherent placenta).* With a mechanical failure the uterine muscle at the placental site may be relaxed and boggy even though that of the rest of the upper segment is fairly firmly contracted. Because of failure of the muscle at the placental site to contract, the usual mechanism for placental separation does not come into play.

With abnormally adherent placenta all or part of the

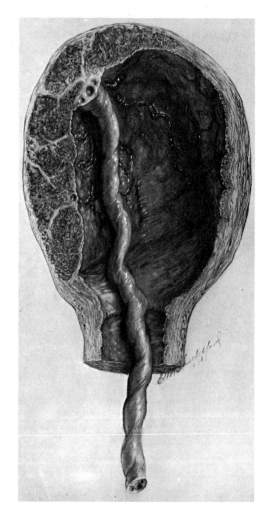

Fig. 33-5. Placenta increta. Abnormal fusion between placenta and uterine wall with deep invasion of uterine muscle by placental tissue. (From Willson, J.R.: Management of obstetric difficulties, ed. 6, St. Louis, 1961, The C.V. Mosby Co.)

decidua basalis is absent, and the chorionic tissue grows directly into the muscle, thereby eliminating the normal cleavage plane. The term *placenta accreta* indicates a relatively superficial penetration of the muscle. Deeper penetration is called *placenta increta* (Fig. 33-5); and *placenta percreta* indicates that the trophoblast has grown to or completely through the serosa.

Placenta accreta occurs more often in women of high than of low parity, in those who have been delivered by cesarean section, after the uterus has been curetted, and in association with placenta previa. In these patients the placenta implants over a scar or in an area is which the decidua is so poorly formed that the trophoblast invades the myometrium directly.

Placenta accreta can be *partial,* if only a portion of the placenta is abnormally adherent, or *complete;* with the partial type, bleeding can be profuse when the normal portion of the placenta separates because the uterus cannot complete the separation of the placenta and expel it. Bleeding cannot occur with complete placenta accreta because none of the placenta can separate from its abnormal attachment in the uterine muscle.

Management. If bleeding is active and the placenta cannot be expressed in the usual manner, it must be removed immediately by inserting the hand into the uterus, completing the separation, and extracting it (Fig. 33-6).

In the absence of bleeding it is safe to wait longer for spontaneous separation and expulsion, but there is no reason to delay more than 5 to 10 minutes.

Hysterectomy usually is necessary for placenta accreta unless the abnormally adherent portion of the placenta involves only a small area. The uterus may be perforated, or profuse bleeding may be produced by attempts to dig the cotyledons out of the uterine wall.

INVERSION OF THE UTERUS

Inversion of the uterus occurs rarely; but when it does, the mortality is high unless it is recognized and treated promptly. The inversion may be *partial* or *complete;* those discovered at delivery are *acute,* and those not detected until days or weeks later are *chronic.*

In most instances the uterine muscles near the placental site, which frequently is in the fundus, are relaxed, permitting the upper part of the uterus to prolapse through the dilated cervix. Vigorous attempts to deliver the pla-

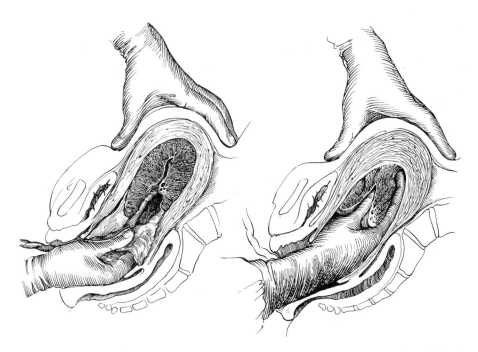

Fig. 33-6. Technique of manual removal of retained placenta. (From Willson, J.R.: Atlas of obstetric technic, ed. 2, St. Louis, 1969, The C.V. Mosby Co.)

centa by suprapubic pressure or by cord traction are probably important factors in inverting the fundus.

In most instances, shock develops promptly when the inversion occurs. The diagnosis can be suspected if the fundus is indented (incomplete inversion) or cannot be felt above the pubis (complete inversion). It can be confirmed by palpating the inverted fundus within the lower uterine segment or in the vagina.

The uterus can usually be replaced without difficulty if the diagnosis is made promptly, but if the inversion is not recognized at once, the constricting collar of muscle may contract and incarcerate the inverted uterus. The entire hand is inserted into the vagina, with the fingertips exerting equal pressure around the collar of uterus just within the cervical opening and the fundus resting on the palmar surface of the hand. The fundus is gradually replaced, and oxytocin or a prostaglandin $F_2\alpha$ analog is administered. The uterus can usually be replaced with minimal anesthetic if the inversion is recognized immediately. If there is a delay and the uterus is firmly contracted, it must be relaxed with deep inhalation anesthetic before replacement is attempted.

It is usually necessary to perform an operative procedure to correct chronic inversion.

POSTPARTUM PITUITARY NECROSIS

Partial or complete necrosis of the anterior pituitary gland may follow excessive bleeding during pregnancy. This condition, *Sheehan's syndrome,* usually cannot be detected in women who die soon after delivery because necrotic changes have not had time to develop. The entire anterior lobe or portions of it may be destroyed.

In the typical patient with severe damage the breasts remain flaccid, and no milk is secreted. Pubic and axillary hair may fall out. The genital organs atrophy, and the menses do not return. The endocrine glands that are under the control of the anterior pituitary cease to function. Complete pituitary necrosis is rarely seen, but the less severe states may be encountered occasionally. There may be enough tissue to carry on normal function, the deficiency only becoming obvious when the gland is subjected to unusual stress, such as another pregnancy, a surgical operation, or a serious infection.

Although the exact cause of pituitary necrosis is not known, prevention of excessive bleeding and the prompt replacement of blood may reduce the severity of pituitary damage.

AMNIOTIC FLUID INFUSION

The possibility that intravenous infusion of amniotic fluid could cause death was first suggested by Steiner and Lushbaugh. Reid, Weiner, and Roby suggested that amniotic fluid contains a thromboplastin-like substance that produces intravascular clotting and subsequent defibrination of blood and hemorrhage from the resultant clotting defect.

Amniotic fluid can enter the bloodstream through the vessels at the placental site or those opened by injury. The membranes must be ruptured to permit the escape of amniotic fluid, and the intrauterine pressure must be increased. Rupture of the membranes and the administration of an oxytocic to induce labor increases the possibility of amniotic fluid infusion, as does placenta previa.

Amniotic infusion is most likely to occur in women in labor at or near term, and many patients have been given oxytocin to induce or stimulate labor. Parous women are more often affected than are primigravidas. The symptoms occur suddenly, and the first evidence of the abnormality may be dyspnea and cyanosis or sudden shock. Death may occur promptly or be delayed for several hours. If a coagulation defect occurs, vaginal bleeding usually is evident.

The pathophysiologic changes, which result from sudden obstruction of the pulmonary capillaries by the particulate matter in the infused amniotic fluid, include acute cor pulmonale, decreased left atrial pressure, decreased cardiac output, and peripheral vascular collapse.

Treatment consists of cardiopulmonary resuscitation; insertion of a Swan-Ganz catheter; phlebotomy if central venous pressure is elevated; papaverine hydrochloride, 50 to 100 mg intravenously, to reduce bronchiole arteriospasm; atropine, 0.4 mg intravenously, to relax vagus-induced coronary and pulmonary arteriolar vasoconstriction; and vasopressors. Blood must be administered if the patient is bleeding excessively, and the coagulation defect corrected by appropriate treatment.

Amniotic fluid infusion can only be diagnosed with certainty by demonstrating the presence of fetal epithelial cells and amniotic debris in the lung capillaries. It can be suspected, however, in a patient in whom a state of collapse develops late in labor or immediately after delivery, and it is essential that treatment be instituted promptly.

REFERENCES

Beecham, C.T.: An analysis of deaths from postpartum hemorrhage, Am. J. Obstet. Gynecol. **53**:422, 1947.

Breen, J.L., Neubecker, R., Gregori, C.A., et al.: Placenta accreta, increta and percreta, Obstet. Gynecol. **49**:43, 1977.

Douglas, R.G., and Davis, I.F.: Puerperal infection: etiologic, prophylactic, and therapeutic considerations, Am. J. Obstet. Gynecol. **51**:352, 1946.

Fox, H.: Placenta accreta, 1945-1969, Obstet. Gynecol. Surv. **27**:475, 1972.

Hayashi, R.H., Costillo, M.S., and Noah, M.L.: Management of severe postpartum hemorrhage with a prostaglandin F_2-alpha analogue, Obstet. Gynecol. **63**:806, 1984.

Hendricks, C.H., and Brenner, W.E.: Cardiovascular effects of oxytocic drugs used post partum, Am. J. Obstet. Gynecol. **108**:751, 1970.

Hendricks, C.H., Eskes, T.K.A.B., and Saameli, K.: Uterine contractility at delivery and in the puerperium, Am. J. Obstet. Gynecol. **83**:890, 1962.

Magil, B.: PGF_2-alpha for postpartum hemorrhage—how well does it work? Contemp. Obstet. Gynecol. p. 111, 1984.

Newton, M.: Postpartum hemorrhage, Am. J. Obstet. Gynecol. **94**:711, 1966.

Odell, L.D., and Seski, A.: Episiotomy blood loss, Am. J. Obstet. Gynecol. **54**:51, 1947.

Price, T.M., Baker, V.V., and Cefalo, R.C.: Amniotic fluid embolism. Three case reports with a revies of the literature, Obstet. Gynecol. Surv. **40**:462, 1985.

Prichard, J.A., Baldwin, R.M., Dickey, J.C., and Wiggins, K.M.: Blood volume changes in pregnancy and the puerperium. II. Red blood cell loss and changes during and following vaginal delivery, cesarean section and cesarean section plus total hysterectomy, Am. J. Obstet. Gynecol. **84**:1271, 1962.

Quinlivan, W.L., and Brock, J.A.: Blood volume changes and blood loss associated with labor, Am. J. Obstet. Gynecol. **106**:843, 1970.

Read, J.A., Cotton, D.B., and Miller, F.C.: Placenta accreta: changing clinical aspects and outcome, Obstet. Gynecol. **56**:31, 1980.

Reid, D.E., Weiner, A.E., and Roby, C.C.: Intravascular clotting and afibrinogenemia, the presumptive lethal factors in the syndrome of amniotic fluid embolism, Am. J. Obstet. Gynecol. **66**:465, 1953.

Schneeberg, N.G., Perloff, W.H., and Israel, S.L.: Incidence of unsuspected "Sheehan's syndrome": hypopituitarism after postpartum hemorrhage and/or shock: clinical and laboratory study, J.A.M.A. **172**:20, 1960.

Secher, N.J., Arnsbo, P., and Wallin, L.: Haemodynamic effects of oxytocin (Syntocinon) and methylergometrine (Methergin) on the systemic and pulmonary circulations of pregnant anaesthetized women, Acta Obstet. Gynecol. Scand. **57**:97, 1978.

Sheehan, H.L.: Simmonds' disease due to postpartum necrosis of the anterior pituitary, J. Obstet. Gynaecol. Br. Commonw. **50**:27, 1943.

Steiner, P.E., and Lushbaugh, C.C.: Maternal pulmonary embolism by amniotic fluid as cause of obstetric shock and unexpected death in obstetrics, J.A.M.A. **117**:1245, 1941.

Ueland, K.: Maternal cardiovascular dynamics. VII. Intrapartum blood volume changes, Am. J. Obstet. Gynecol. **126**:671, 1976.

van Vugt, P.J.H., et al.: Inversio uteri puerperalis, Acta Obstet. Gynecol. Scand. **60**:353, 1981.

34

Russell K. Laros, Jr.

Care of the infant during pregnancy and labor and after delivery

During its intrauterine life the fetus is completely dependent on the transfer of respiratory gases and the materials essential for its growth from the maternal bloodstream. At birth, however, it must assume responsibility for maintaining all its functions. The highest mortality occurs during the first 24 hours of life while the infant is attempting to make this change.

The fetus in utero swallows amniotic fluid, which is absorbed from the intestinal tract and ultimately is excreted by the kidneys and returned to the amniotic sac. There is little peristaltic activity in the intestine of the normal infant until birth; the passage of meconium by the unborn infant usually indicates intrauterine hypoxia. Respiratory efforts that move amniotic fluid in and out of the nasopharynx and trachea and into the alveoli have been demonstrated in human fetuses and in experimental animals. The infant responds to tactile and auditory stimuli while it is still in the uterus. It is important that all the necessary functions be developed and in operation by the time the infant is born. Abnormally formed infants may be unable to survive outside the uterus. Those born before 26 weeks' gestation usually cannot cope with an independent existence, even though they are otherwise normal.

To survive, the infant must have developed normally and be born alive and uninjured. The hazards of labor and delivery are increased for the pre-mature infant whose delicate structures may be injured easily and for the excessively large infant who may be damaged during attempts to deliver it.

The goals of antepartum care, as far as the fetus is concerned, are the prevention of intrauterine death and the delivery of a healthy infant at term. This requires that the obstetrician recognize potential risk factors and treat them properly. There is a tendency to equate the effectiveness of antepartum care only with improved infant survival, but this is too limited a view. Four fetal deaths occur between the twentieth week of pregnancy and the onset of labor for every intrapartum death. Furthermore, the leading cause of neonatal death is prematurity. Thus any interventions that reduce fetal deaths and/or premature labor will have a significant effect on perinatal mortality.

Antepartum evaluation of the fetus is difficult because it must be done indirectly. We cannot ask it, "How do you feel today?" The methods by which we can evaluate the condition of the fetus in utero will be discussed in this chapter.

PRENATAL INFLUENCES ON THE FETUS

From time immemorial people have assumed that the growth of the fetus could be altered by maternal emotional experiences. We know now that most specific episodes cannot be correlated with congenital defects because they rarely occur at a time when the involved structure is developing, but we are learning more and more about the influence of drugs, chemicals, nutrition, infection, hypoxia, endocrine imbalance, and physical and even emotional stimuli on fetal growth and development.

The periods during which organs and tissues develop vary in length and occur at different stages of pregnancy. For each there exists an early stage during which the primordial tissue begins to differentiate; this is followed by a period of cellular growth and beginning development of the structure, and finally the period during which development is completed. Subsequent change is almost entirely one of growth. To produce an anomaly, a stimulus must be applied before development is completed; it will have little effect except to interfere with growth if it is applied after differentiation is completed. Almost all important organ systems are developed by the end of the twelfth week, but some take longer.

Most pregnant women are regularly exposed to stimuli of one kind or another that may alter fetal development. Fortunately, these stimuli are generally either too slight to affect the tissue, or they occur after the structure already has been formed. Physicians prescribe many medications for their pregnant patients, often with too little thought of their potential effect on the fetus. Most of these drugs have been thoroughly tested on experimental animals, but, unfortunately (thalidomide is an outstanding example), they may be toxic only to human fetal tissue. No animal model currently available accurately predicts damage to the human fetus.

Physicians and their patients are now aware of the possibilities of disturbing embryonic development and are becoming more reasonable about drug therapy during pregnancy—the physician about prescribing it and the patient about demanding it. *As a general rule no medication, no matter how innocuous it is presumed to be, should be prescribed during pregnancy unless there is a specific indication for its use and unless the patient may be harmed if it is not used.*

Hormones. Some of the *progestogens,* particularly the *19-norsteroids,* can cause maldevelopment of the genitals of the female fetus if they are administered during the first half of pregnancy. Since these medications are used almost exclusively in women who have aborted in previous pregnancies or are now threatening abortion, they are almost always administered when they might interfere with genital development. Fortunately, the major anomalies are clitoral hypertrophy and labial fusion, which can be corrected easily; the ultimate differentiation and function of the rest of the genital organs are usually normal. Since estrogens and progestogens are of no value in the treatment of threatened abortions, there is no reason to prescribe them.

Although the majority of current evidence suggests that pure progestogens are not teratogenic, as long as any doubt remains they should not be used as a test for pregnancy.

More than 400 clear cell adenocarcinomas of the vagina and numerous instances of adenosis, cervical lesions, transverse vaginal septa, and uterine and tubal anomalies have been diagnosed in women whose mothers were treated with *diethylstilbestrol* during the pregnancies that terminated in their births. Genital tract anomalies and infertility can also be produced in males. The development of these lesions, which are discussed in detail in Chapter 3, is not related to drug dosage or duration of treatment.

Antimicrobial agents. The *tetracyclines* are deposited in the actively growing epiphyses of fetal bones and may cause abnormal bone growth. They also are deposited in the enamel of teeth, producing permanent fluorescent mottling. Since limb buds appear at about the fifth week and tooth formation begins at about the twelfth week, these drugs should rarely be used during pregnancy.

Sulfonamides may displace bilirubin from its binding sites on serum albumin, and deposition of the free bilirubin in the basal ganglia may cause kernicterus. This does not occur while the fetus is in utero because the bilirubin is excreted across the placenta into the maternal blood. Sulfonamide therapy during late pregnancy, particularly with long-acting preparations, should not be used in women who are likely to deliver prematurely.

Chloramphenicol in large doses given to newborn premature infants may cause the gray syndrome and death. It has no obvious effect on the fetus.

All aminoglycosides may cause nerve deafness, as in adults.

Nitrofurantoin may cause anemia in infants with glucose-6-phosphate deficiency.

Chemotherapeutic agents. Antifolic acid agents such as *aminopterin* and *methotrexate* produce serious fetal deformities and even death; they should not be administered to pregnant women. *Chlorambucil* may have the same effect. No anomalies have been reported with the use of other agents. The wider use of a variety of chemotherapeutic agents in pregnant women with cancer should increase our information about the impact on the fetus.

Tranquilizers and sedatives. The information concerning these substances is not entirely clear, but *phenobarbital* in excess may cause bleeding in newborn infants. The *phenothiazines* may cause hyperbilirubinemia, and *meprobamate,* mental retardation.

Babies whose mothers receive large amounts of *medication during labor* are less attentive on second- and fourth-day testing than those whose mothers were less heavily sedated.

An increased incidence of chromosome breakage, the most common being chromatid and isochromatid breaks, has been found in *LSD users.* The same defect has been seen in children whose mothers used LSD during pregnancy. The significance of these findings is not yet obvious and may relate to the effects of total drug abuse and contaminants rather than to LSD specifically. Chromosome breaks have not been found when pure LSD is administered. Similar chromosome breaks have been reported when *marijuana* has been used. *Maternal alcohol abuse* is associated with the fetal alcohol syndrome characterized by intrauterine growth retardation, mental retardation, and craniofacial abnormalities.

X-radiation. During the early days of embryonic development the cells are chemically and structurally similar, but they soon begin to differentiate. Before differentiation the entire mass of cells is either destroyed or completely unaffected by x-radiation. Later, damage and interference with the growth of specific groups of cells may produce anomalies. X-ray film examinations, particularly of the abdomen and pelvis, should never be performed until the possibility of an unsuspected pregnancy has been eliminated by an accurate menstrual history and pregnancy test if it is indicated.

Narcotic addiction. The incidence of narcotic addiction, usually to heroin or methadone, in pregnant women is increasing. Many addicted women must resort to prostitution to purchase the drugs; consequently, *sexually transmitted diseases* occur frequently. Many addicted women are *malnourished* and *anemic,* and few obtain adequate prenatal care.

Labor and delivery usually are normal, but the *infant may be addicted.* The objective evidences of addiction in the newborn infant are irritability, tremors, vomiting, a high-pitched cry, sneezing, hypertonicity, hyperactivity, and convulsions. Neonatal morbidity and mortality are significantly increased.

Women taking small amounts of heroin can stop completely without affecting the pregnancy. Those taking larger amounts can be switched to methadone. Withdrawal symptoms in the infants of methadone addicts may be more severe than in those whose mothers are taking heroin, which may be related to the purity of the latter drug.

Miscellaneous. *Dicumarol* and related substances may be teratogenic when given during the first 12 weeks. They also may cause retroplacental hemorrhage and fetal death. *Heparin* does not cross the placenta; therefore it has no effect on the fetus. *Antithyroid substances,* such as propylthiouracil and potassium iodide, may cause goiter in the fetus. The babies of mothers who *smoke in excess* may be smaller than those born to nonsmoking mothers, and perinatal mortality is higher.

A specific series of fetal facial abnormalities have been reported in the newborns of mothers who received *phenytoin (Dilantin)* during pregnancy.

Valproic acid, an otherwise excellent anticonvulsant, and retinoic acid, used in the treatment of severe acne, also produces severe anomalies and must not be used during pregnancy.

Aspirin has a number of actions that may have an unfavorable impact on pregnancy. It is an effective antiprostaglandin agent, and its regular use has been associated with prolonged pregnancies and postterm delivery. In addition, it influences the ability of platelets to adhere to each other, and this action may last for up to 7 days. Prolonged maternal use has been associated with intracranial hemorrhage in newborns, particularly in those born prematurely.

A direct correlation exists between *older mothers and an increasing incidence of Down's syndrome* in the newborn. Affected fetuses can be detected by genetic amniocentesis or chorionic villus sampling (Chapter 1).

Asymptomatic bacteriuria has been associated with an unfavorable pregnancy outcome. A number of studies have indicated that infants of women with asymptomatic bacteriuria are smaller than those born to normal control subjects. The significance of this observation is still under study. At least one prospective study showed no increase in infant weights when asymptomatic bacteriuria was eliminated with antibiotic therapy.

TORCH (*t*oxoplasmosis, *o*ther, *r*ubella, *c*ytomegalovirus, and *h*erpes) refers to a series of maternal infections that have little impact on the mother, but that have a disastrous outcome for the fetus or the newborn. Monif has suggested that the German word for stork, *Storch,* with the *S* for syphilis, is an appropriate designation for these diseases. Syphilis and herpes are discussed in Chapter 26, and the other infections, in Chapter 21.

ERYTHROBLASTOSIS FETALIS RESULTING FROM Rh INCOMPATIBILITY

If the fetus' blood group is different from that of its mother, and if the mother has been sensitized to an antigen in the fetal blood cells, her blood will contain an antibody that can cross the placenta and hemolyze fetal red blood cells. Erythroblastosis is most often a result of Rh incompatibility, but differences in the ABO and other blood factors can also cause the disorder.

The fetus is more seriously affected by Rh incompatibilities than by most of the other types. The characteristic fetal manifestations, each of which is related to the hemolytic process, are (1) anemia; (2) erythroblastic hyperplasia of bone marrow; (3) extramedullary centers of erythropoiesis in the liver, spleen, kidneys, and other tissues; (4) erythroblastemia; (5) jaundice, particularly hemolytic but also hepatocellular, appearing soon after birth and with possible resulting kernicterus; (6) tissue damage from anoxia; (7) edema from cardiac failure and hypoproteinemia; and (8) purpura from complete bone marrow suppression.

Etiologic factors. The blood of about 85% of white people contains the Rh antigen; these are Rh_0 (D)–positive. The blood of the remaining 15% does not contain the factor, and these are Rh_0 (D)–negative. Individuals whose parents are both Rh_0 (D)–positive are *homozygous,* and those who had only one Rh_0 (D)–positive parent are *heterozygous;* half the sperm or ova of the heterozygous individuals will contain the Rh factor, and half will not.

When an Rh_0 (D)–negative woman is impregnated by a homozygous Rh_0 (D)–positive man, the fetus will be Rh_0 (D)–positive. Half the fetuses of heterozygous Rh_0 (D)–positive fathers will be Rh_0 (D)–positive and half Rh_0 (D)–negative.

If Rh_0 (D)–positive fetal red blood cells enter the maternal circulation, an antibody against them may be formed. Fetal blood cells may mix with the mother's blood in the intervillous spaces if placental blood vessels are torn during abortion or delivery, intact cells may cross the undamaged placenta by pinocytosis, or the products of disintegrated cells containing the antigen may enter the maternal circulation. Probably the most common method by which fetal red blood cells enter the maternal circulation is by disruption of the fetal placental vessels during the third stage of labor. Maternal antibodies of an IgG group will also be produced in response to blood transfusion with Rh_0 (D)–positive donor blood.

The Rh_0 (D) factor is the one most often responsible for sensitization, but others that may have the same effect are hr' (c), rh' (C), rh" (E), and hr" (e).

The maternal antibody crosses the placenta and enters the fetal circulation without difficulty; it hemolyzes fetal blood cells and produces the changes characteristic of erythroblastosis.

Although the potential for the development of erythroblastosis fetalis with an Rh_0 (D)–negative mother and Rh_0 (D)–positive father occurs in about 10% of all pregnancies, the actual incidence is about one in 250 births, or one in 20 in which Rh incompatibility exists. There are several reasons for this:

1. Unless women have been sensitized by blood transfusion or by an early abortion, they usually produce no antibodies during the first pregnancy, and the infant is unaffected.

2. Some women never become sensitized because Rh_0 (D)–positive fetal red blood cells never invade the maternal circulation, or, if they do, the number is so small that they stimulate only a weak response.

3. The father may be heterozygous Rh_0 (D)–positive so that some of the children will be Rh_0 (D)–negative.

4. The chances of erythroblastosis on an Rh basis are reduced with ABO incompatibilities (if the fetus has A or B antigens and the mother lacks them).

Although the first infant born of an Rh_0 (D)–negative mother and Rh_0 (D)–positive father almost always is normal, the second or subsequent ones may be affected. After a woman has borne one infant with erythroblastosis, the rest of her children are almost certain to have a similar condition if the father is homozygous Rh_0 (D)–positive. If he is heterozygous, half the spermatozoa will contain Rh factor, and half will contain none. As a general rule the disease in the first affected infant is mild, but one cannot predict what will happen during subsequent pregnancies. In some all the babies are only slightly affected, whereas in others the second and all subsequent fetuses develop hydrops or die in utero because of the severity of the hemolytic process.

The two principal types of Rh antibodies are *complete antibodies,* which can be detected in saline suspensions of Rh_0 (D)–positive red cells, and *incomplete antibodies,* which are detected by the indirect Coombs test. The latter ones enter the fetal circulation and react with Rh-sensitized red blood cells.

Management. An antibody screen should be performed on the serum of a pregnant woman during the first trimester. If the antibody screen is negative and the woman is Rh-positive, the antibody screen should be repeated at 28 weeks of pregnancy. This repeat screen is to detect sensitization to one of the antigens other than Rh_0 (D). If the woman is Rh-negative, the antibody screen should be repeated at 16 to 18 weeks and every 4 to 6 weeks thereafter. If the initial antibody screen is positive, the exact antibody must be identified, and a determination made as to whether it is of the IgG or IgM type.

Unfortunately, changes in antibody titer may not accurately reflect the condition. Fetal hydrops and intrauterine death have been observed with relatively low titers, and slightly affected or even Rh-negative babies have occurred when the titer had risen to astronomically high levels. As a consequence one cannot base treatment on Rh antibody titer alone.

A much more accurate evaluation of fetal conditions can be made by *spectrophotometric analysis of amniotic fluid.* The spectral absorption curves for amniotic fluid are determined for visible light-spectrum wavelengths between 350 and 700 nm. Optical density is then plotted as the ordinate, and wavelength as the abscissa. A normal curve will be fairly smooth, but the bilirubin in the amniotic fluid of fetuses affected by erythroblastosis alters the optical density and produces a deviation at about 450 nm.

The exact peak of this deviation from linearity is expressed as the difference between expected and actual optical density at 450 nm as measured from a tangent line drawn between 365 and 550 nm, using semilogarithmic graph paper. This difference indicates the severity of the disease.

Liley has established three zones for the purpose of evaluating the degree of fetal involvement. Fetuses in the *lower zone* (normal curve or a slight rise) are generally in no difficulty and often need no special treatment. Those in the *middle zone* (a higher peak) are more seriously involved and should be delivered early. Most of these will need exchange transfusions. Those in the *upper zone* (an even higher peak) are seriously involved and are likely to die in utero unless treated by intrauterine transfusion or delivery.

Treatment is based on spectrophotometric analysis, but a decision cannot be made on the basis of examining a single specimen unless the peak is already so high that there is little doubt that the fetus is seriously affected. The first study is made at about the twenty-fourth or twenty-sixth week of pregnancy, or even sooner if early fetal death has occurred in previous pregnancies; and subsequent ones are planned according to the result. If the peak is low, the next amniocentesis may be done at the thirty-second week; if it is higher, the next study may be made at the thirtieth week; if it is even higher, immediate treatment may be indicated.

Amniotic fluid should be examined only if the antibody titer is positive, because there is a risk of introducing fetal cells into the maternal circulation during needle amniocentesis. Before amniocentesis is performed, the *position of the placenta* should be determined with ultrasonography so that one can avoid passing the needle through it.

The babies of mothers who have experienced previous fetal death before the thirty-fifth week of pregnancy or those with a spectrophotometric study in the upper zone during the early part of the third trimester may be saved by *intrauterine intraperitoneal transfusion* with Rh_0 (D) donor cells. The largest experience with intrauterine transfusions (IUTs) has been reported by Bowman and Manning. They have performed over 1000 IUTs; the overall survival rate in recent years has been 92%.

Treatment of the infant. Whenever a patient who probably has an erythroblastotic baby is in labor or her delivery is planned, preparations should be made to examine and treat the baby as soon as it is born. A pediatrician experienced with exchange transfusion should be present at the delivery. A specimen of cord blood is obtained for blood typing, hematocrit, reticulocyte count, bilirubin, and a direct Coombs test. Exchange transfusion should be performed promptly if the baby has erythroblastosis and the hematocrit is low. Kernicterus, a major cause of death and disability in premature infants with erythroblastosis, can be almost completely prevented by exchange transfusions.

Prevention. Our present management of erythroblastosis is crude and ineffective when compared with what could be achieved by prevention. Rh_0 (D) hyperimmune human gamma globulin (RhIG) when injected intramuscularly into unsensitized Rh_0 (D)–negative individuals will prevent the development of an antigen against Rh_0 (D)–positive red blood cells. Ascari and co-workers, reporting on a cooperative study, found that only one of 1081 unsensitized Rh_0 (D)–negative women who were treated with this material after the delivery or an Rh_0 (D)–positive infant became sensitized, whereas 51 of 726 control women developed antibodies.

We now give RhIG to all unsensitized Rh_0 (Du)–negative women during the first 72 hours after they have delivered an Rh_0 (D)–positive infant. Those selected for treatment must be Rh_0 (Du)–negative without identifiable antibodies, and the baby must be Rh_0 (D)–positive with a negative direct antiglobulin (Coombs) test on cord blood. Because fetal cells pass into the maternal circulation during the course of pregnancy, approximately 2% of sensitizations occur before delivery. This sensitization can be largely prevented by the administration of RhIG at 28 weeks' gestation to all Rh-negative mothers with Rh-positive partners.

An Rh_0 (D)–negative patient who has aborted a pregnancy more than 8 weeks after the onset of the last menstrual period should also be treated if her husband is positive, even though the blood type of the embryo cannot be determined. An antibody study should be obtained 6 weeks after delivery and twice during subsequent pregnancies. Unsensitized women should be treated after each delivery. In addition, all Rh-negative unsensitized women requiring amniocentesis should be given RhIG after the amniocentesis has been performed.

ERYTHROBLASTOSIS FETALIS RESULTING FROM ABO INCOMPATIBILITY

A fetus of blood group A, AB, or B may develop hemolytic disease from maternal antibodies against any of the antigens not already present in the mother's blood. For example, if the mother is blood type O, she may become sensitized to either A or

B, or if she is A and her fetus is B or AB, she may become sensitized to B.

This situation is similar to Rh sensitization in several ways, but there are differences. Rh sensitization always occurs because of a transfusion of Rh_0 (D)–positive red blood cells into the maternal blood; ABO sensitization may develop in this manner, but there are naturally occurring antibodies that may already be present when the patient becomes pregnant for the first time. The antigen responsible for ABO sensitization is secreted in body fluids, as well as being contained in red blood cells. Thus a mother can become sensitized by the antigen "secreted" by the fetus into amniotic fluid from which it is absorbed into the maternal circulation.

There is no reliable way to prognosticate the development of ABO incompatibility during the prenatal period as there is with Rh erythroblastosis fetalis, but it can be anticipated by comparing the blood group of the mother with that of the child's father. If the mother's blood group is O and the father's A, B, or AB, the infant is a candidate for ABO incompatibility, and a direct antiglobulin (Coombs) test should be performed on cord blood. Fortunately, the process is almost never as severe as that caused by Rh sensitization and does not cause intrauterine fetal death. The treatment is exchange transfusion.

EVALUATION OF FETAL CONDITION DURING PREGNANCY

In the past, one could only assume that the fetus was healthy if it continued to grow and was active, since the only valid assessment of fetal well-being was the heart rate. There are now several reasonably accurate ways to assess fetal maturity (Chapter 20) and to determine the condition of the fetus before labor begins and while the membranes are still intact. The information gained by these tests frequently is helpful in making a decision as to the most appropriate time to terminate pregnancy.

These tests are of greatest value when *intrauterine growth retardation* on the basis of small or abnormal placenta is suspected, for example, in women with chronic hypertensive cardiovascular disease and cyanotic heart disease, or when the possibility of postmaturity exists. The tests also may be of value in patients with *diabetes* and other metabolic disorders that may affect the development of the fetus and whenever the *expected date of confinement cannot be determined accurately.*

Sonography. It is possible to measure the biparietal diameter of the fetal skull and femoral length with reasonable accuracy during pregnancy. If the size of the uterus at 16 and 20 weeks does not correspond to the date of the onset of the last menstrual period, an initial study should be obtained without delay. If the patient is not examined until late in the second trimester and the uterus is smaller than anticipated, ultrasonic fetal measurements should be obtained promptly.

Between the thirtieth and the fortieth weeks of pregnancy the biparietal diameter increases at a rate of about 2 mm/wk. The biparietal diameter will be greater than 8.7 cm in almost 100% of infants after the thirty-sixth week of pregnancy.

Sonographic measurement of the biparietal diameter and body size should be obtained at biweekly intervals whenever growth retardation is suspected. These studies will identify both symmetrical and asymmetrical growth retardation.

A steady normal increase in the various measurements provides good evidence that the placenta is capable of supplying the metabolic needs of the fetus and that the baby is growing at the usual rate. A less than normal increase or failure to increase at all is indicative of growth retardation and suggests that the fetus has outgrown the ability of the placenta to meet its needs.

Estriol excretion. Normal estrogen metabolism in the fetoplacental unit is dependent on a healthy fetus, an intact normal placenta, and a healthy mother. Estriol production increases as the fetus grows and decreases when growth ceases.

Serial maternal urinary estriol or serum unconjugated estriol determinations are only useful in two clinical conditions: (1) in identifying the fetus affected by the postmaturity syndrome, and (2) occasionally, are helpful in assessing fetal well-being in diabetes. In the former condition they must be done two times per week, and in the latter, daily.

The fetus probably is healthy, and placental function is normal if the first examination is within the normal range for the stage of pregnancy and if estriol production increases at the usual rate. Conversely, if the first estriol level is lower than anticipated, the fetus *may* be healthy, but younger than expected (inaccurate dates), or its growth may be retarded. The discrepancy can be clarified by repeated examinations; a progressive increase suggests a normal fetus, whereas stable or falling levels suggest an abnormality.

Counting of fetal movements. Fetal movements can be quantified by the mother. She is instructed to recline comfortably after a meal and then to count the number of "kicks" occurring during a 10-minute period. "Kick counts" for 10 minutes range between 5 and 20 in a healthy fetus. Generally, fetal movements decline rapidly over a day or two and are then absent for another 1 to 2 days before intrauterine death occurs.

Biophysical evaluation. New noninvasive techniques for recording fetal heart rate and uterine contractions and refined ultrasonic equipment have expanded our capabilities for evaluating the status of the fetus in utero. These techniques are almost 100% accurate in predicting a healthy fetus—that is, a normal test connotes a normal fetus—but they are less accurate in predicting an unhealthy fetus. There are many more abnormal tests than abnormal

newborns. Because of this, a need exists for more than one test when an abnormal biophysical evaluation occurs.

The *nonstress test* (NST) is designed to evaluate the reactivity of the fetus during the antepartum period. It is called nonstress because the mother is not given oxytocin to induce contractions. The great advantage of the test is that it is easy to do and requires no drug administration to the mother. Nonstress tests are most appropriate for women suspected of having placental dysfunction or insufficiency; for example, those with chronic hypertension or diabetes or with fetuses suspected of growth retardation or postmaturity.

A continuous record of fetal heart rate is made with Doppler or electrocardiographic equipment while the mother is resting in a lateral supine position. She is asked to report each fetal movement that she feels, and the effect of fetal movement on the heart rate is determined. A normal reaction to fetal movement is an acceleration in fetal heart rate of 15 beats/min or more above the baseline for 15 seconds or more (Fig. 34-1). If at least four such accelerations are seen in a 20-minute interval, the test is reactive, and the fetus is presumed to be healthy.

If only one or no accelerations occur during a

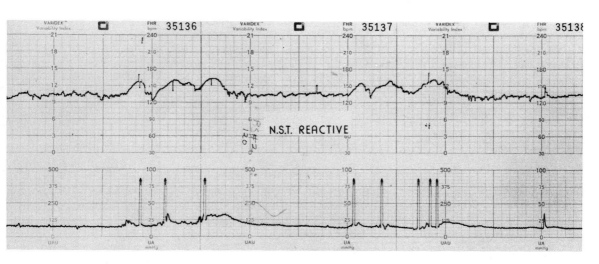

Fig. 34-1. Reactive nonstress test *(NST)*. Arrows on lower panel document timing of fetal movement. Strip has 12 minutes of observation, and accelerations are clearly evident.

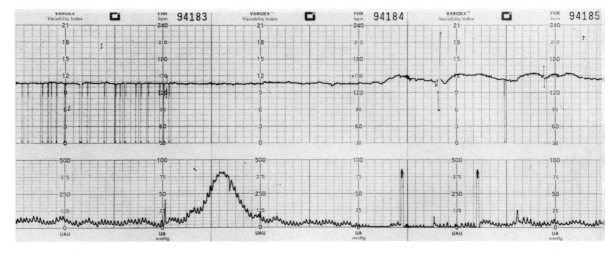

Fig. 34-2. Reactive nonstress test *(NST)* involving prolonged bradycardia, that is, more than 5 minutes. Patient who was beyond term was immediately transferred to labor and delivery area, where a carefully monitored induction was performed. Another prolonged bradycardia occurred, emergency cesarean section was performed, and infant with tight nuchal cord and thick meconium was delivered. Infant was resuscitated at birth and had uncomplicated course after birth.

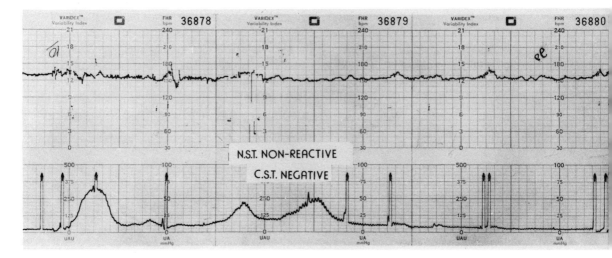

Fig. 34-3. Normal contraction stress test *(CST)*. No decelerations are seen.

20-minute period, the fetus may be unhealthy or simply resting. It is important to recognize the resting state because there are many more nonreactive tests than there are unhealthy fetuses. If no accelerations occur during an additional 20-minute observation period, a *contraction stress test* (CST) should be performed promptly.

The most ominous sign in nonstress testing is prolonged bradycardia, lasting for more than a minute (Fig. 34-2), which indicates incipient intrauterine fetal death. When bradycardia is recognized, fetal heart rate monitoring should be continued while the mother is moved to the labor and delivery area. Delivery by carefully monitored induction or by cesarean section is indicated if the bradycardia recurs. Fortunately, these serious pat-

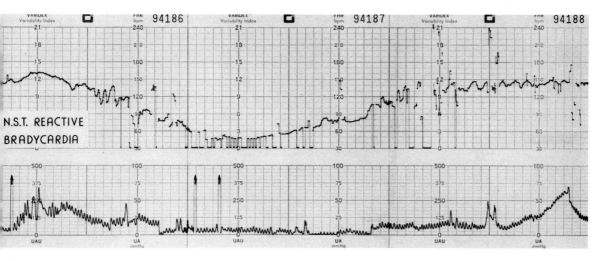

Fig. 34-2, cont'd. For legend see opposite page.

terns are rarely seen. The more usual problem is dealing with the patient with a nonreactive test.

The *CST, oxytocin challenge test, or nipple stimulation test* is designed to stress the fetoplacental unit and test the reserve of the fetus. Oxytocin is administered intravenously in a dosage that will produce three contractions in 10-minute intervals, and the effect of the contractions on heart rate is observed (Schifrin's "10-minute window"). Similarly, nipple stimulation can be used to cause uterine contractions. If late decelerations are seen with each contraction, the test is positive, and the patient should usually be delivered. If no decelerations occur during the 10-minute period, the test is normal (Fig. 34-3). This categorization is particularly important because it sharply reduces the number of equivocal tests, in which a late deceleration is occasionally seen.

A decision as to whether the patient should be delivered by cesarean section or vaginally cannot always be made on the basis of the test alone. The actual force of the uterine contractions cannot be measured by external recordings. Nearly half of women with a positive contraction stress test will go through labor without late decelerations.

Biophysical profile. Some authors have advocated use of a biophysical scoring system. The fetus is evaluated sonographically for fetal breathing move-ments, gross body movements, muscle tone, and the quantity of amniotic fluid and an NST is performed. The fetus is given a score of "2" or "0" for each of these five parameters. Fetuses having a score of "8" or more are at low risk for chronic asphyxia. Those scoring "0" or "2" are strongly suspected of being chronically asphyxiated; and the remainder form an intermediate, "suspicious" group.

FETAL HYPOXIA DURING LABOR

The fetus in utero is entirely dependent on the mother for its supply of oxygen, which it obtains from the maternal blood in the placental sinuses. Circulation of the blood through the sinuses is regulated by the mother's arterial blood pressure and by the activity of the uterine muscle. Maternal blood is injected into the sinuses in spurts from the open ends of spiral arterioles that are scattered, with corresponding venous channels, in the uterine wall beneath the placenta. Some of the blood is forced laterally into the marginal lakes, from which it is returned to the general circulation. Most of it, however, gravitates downward through the branching villi and leaves the intervillous space by way of the venous openings at the base.

The pressure within the intervillous space is about the same as or slightly higher than the amniotic fluid pressure, being about 5 to 10 mm Hg when the uterus is at rest and 55 mm Hg or more at the peak of a contraction. The intervillous pressure rises during a contraction because the veins are kinked and compressed by the uterine muscle fibers before the caliber of the more resistant arterioles is affected. Thus blood continues to flow into the spaces for some time after its means of egress are closed.

Under normal circumstances, during a uterine contraction the pressure within the intervillous space is lower than the capillary pressure in the placental villi, which is maintained by changes in fetal blood pressure. This prevents the villi from collapsing and impeding the flow of blood through the fetal vessels and permits the exchange of materials back and forth between the fetal and the maternal circulations even during a contraction.

The fetal oxygen supply can be reduced by any of the following:

1. *Reduction in blood flow through the maternal vessels.* The caliber of the arteries may be reduced by spasm in women with hypertensive complications of pregnancy, thus limiting blood flow. It is estimated that arterial blood flow can be reduced by as much as 50% in women with hypertensive disease.

The flow of blood will also be impaired whenever the maternal systolic blood pressure is lower than the amniotic fluid pressure. Fetal hypoxia is likely to develop when maternal blood pressure levels fall below 60 mm Hg.

2. *Reduction in blood flow through the uterine sinuses.* Blood flow through the intervillous space will be reduced if the veins or arterioles are compressed over long periods of time by forceful, rapidly recurring or prolonged tetanic uterine contractions. A reduction in maternal blood pressure will have the same result.

3. *Reduction of the oxygen content of maternal blood.* The available circulating maternal hemoglobin can be reduced by profound chronic anemia or hemorrhage, thereby reducing the total oxygen capacity.

4. *Alterations in fetal circulation.* The circulation of blood through the vessels of the infant's

body and placenta is maintained by the fetal heart. Anything that alters normal cardiac function will impair the circulation, as will compression of the umbilical cord. Placental infarction or separation will decrease the total area available for oxygen transfer from the maternal blood, and if a considerable portion of placenta is involved, the infant cannot survive.

Although a minority of predelivery intrauterine deaths occur during labor, that short time segment, usually less than 24 hours, makes it the most important portion of pregnancy for continuous observation of the fetus for evidence of stress associated with uterine activity.

Accurate assessment of fetal well-being during labor depends on an understanding of the physiology of the fetal heart rate tracing, so that proper interpretation can be made. Periodic changes in fetal heart rate during labor have been classified according to their relationship to uterine contractions. In *early decelerations* the onset of the decrease in rate begins with the onset of the contraction, and normal rate resumes as the uterus relaxes; in *variable decelerations* there is no constant relationship of the deceleration to contractions; and *late decelerations* begin after the contraction starts, and recovery is prolonged (Fig. 34-4). These periodic changes provide the physician with information concerning the types of stress to which the fetus is being subjected and the physiologic mechanisms involved.

Early decelerations are reflex, are related to pressure on the fetal head, and are mediated by the vagus. They are not associated with a poor outcome. *Variable decelerations* are caused by cord compression. They are reflex changes characterized by a sudden drop in the fetal heart rate and a rapid return to normal. Whether this will cause a problem for the fetus depends on the length of time the circulation is disturbed and the reserve of the fetus. *Late decelerations* are a sign of uteroplacental insufficiency.

The periodic changes in heart rate give the physician an understanding of the mechanisms of the stress to the fetus, but the most important point in the evaluation of the health of the intrauterine pas-

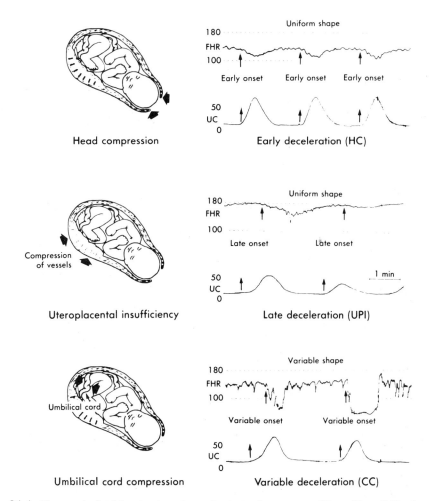

Fig. 34-4. Changes in fetal heart rate patterns due to various causes. (From Hon, E.H.: An atlas of fetal heart rate patterns, New Haven, Conn., 1968, Harty Press, Inc.)

senger is the presence or absence of significant *fetal distress*. This can be ascertained by the *beat-to-beat variability of the fetal heart rate* (Fig. 34-5). Good beat-to-beat variability indicates good fetal reserve. Poor beat-to-beat variability indicates either "distress" and little reserve or changes caused by exogenous medications such as meperidine given to the mother during labor. To differentiate these two conditions, *fetal scalp blood sampling* can be performed. Because fetal scalp PO_2 is technically difficult to measure and fluctuates rapidly, we generally use pH, PCO_2, and base excess to

assess the fetal acid-base status. A low pH is evidence of anaerobic tissue metabolism. The normal pH of fetal scalp blood is above 7.25; values between 7.25 and 7.20 suggest that hypoxia may be developing. Hypoxia can be diagnosed if the pH is less than 7.20 in the absence of maternal acidosis.

Since timing of uterine activity is important in the assessment of periodic changes and beat-to-beat variability accurately reflects fetal health, it is important for the physician to understand the limitations of instrumentation in current labor monitoring technology. Judg-

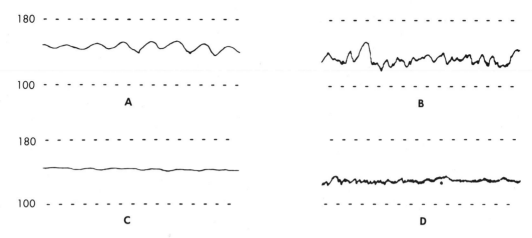

Fig. 34-5. Variability differences observed with fetal scalp electrode. **A,** Long-term variability only. **B,** Both long- and short-term variability. **C,** Neither long- nor short-term variability. **D,** Short-term variability only. (From Zanani, B., Paul, R.H., and Huey, J.R.: Am. J. Obstet. Gynecol. **136:**43, 1980.)

ments concerning the well-being of the fetus during labor should be made on the basis of the most complete data base. The *external tocodynamometer* provides incomplete information about uterine activity. This system usually assesses the frequency of uterine activity accurately but provides no information about resting uterine tone or the force of individual contractions. The accuracy of the tocodynamometer recording depends to a great extent on the ability of the patients to lie still and the frequency with which the labor floor staff will adjust the equipment. If there are problems in timing fetal heart rate accelerations, or when oxytocin is being administered, an *internal pressure catheter* to measure the force of uterine contractions and a *fetal scalp electrode* to record fetal heart rate should be introduced and connected to a transducer.

The major advantage of a fetal scalp electrode is that it provides an accurate fetal electrocardiographic signal. The R wave from this signal is used to count the heart rate, and the beat-to-beat variability is recorded on the monitor strip. None of the external systems can provide as accurate information about variability. The triggering signal from Doppler external monitoring is less clean, and the recorded result shows more variability than is seen with the internal system. Poor beat-to-beat variability on the external system means poor variability, but good variability on the external system may be recorded as poor by an internal electrode (Fig. 34-6).

The health of every fetus should be accurately evaluated during almost every labor. Although one study indicated that frequent evaluation by nurse midwives could give equivalent newborn survival when compared with electronic monitoring, the vast majority of reports have shown a decrease in newborn morbidity and mortality with complete use of electronic monitoring. All patients admitted to the labor-delivery unit, except those who are about to deliver, should have an external monitor applied. If decelerations are observed, an internal electrode should be applied to the fetal scalp to determine the nature of the decelerations and the amount of beat-to-beat variability. If variable decelerations occur, a vaginal examination should be performed to check for cord prolapse. If the cord cannot be felt, the patient should be positioned first on one side and then the other to determine if a change in maternal position will change the location of the cord and diminish cord compression during labor. So long as the variable decelerations do not get more severe and beat-to-beat variability persists, the labor can be allowed to continue. If late decelerations are seen, the patient should be positioned on her left side and given oxygen. If the late decelerations are mild and normal beat-to-

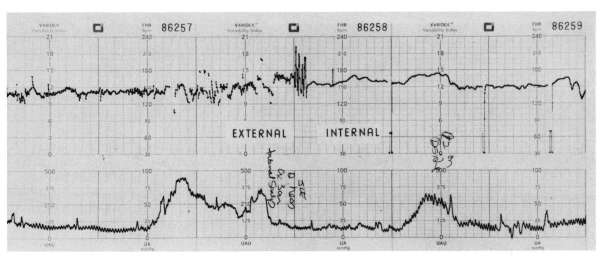

Fig. 34-6. Left side of upper portion of tracing shows good beat-to-beat variability with external monitor system. Immediately after internal electrode was applied, and much flatter fetal heart rate with decreased variability occurred.

beat variability is preserved, the labor can be allowed to continue. If variability is decreased, fetal scalp sampling is indicated. Labor may be allowed to continue if the pH is normal, but periodic scalp sampling will be necessary. If the fetus is acidotic, further labor is contraindicated, and cesarean section for fetal distress should be performed. If the capacity for fetal scalp sampling is not available, a cesarean section for fetal distress should be done if there are persistent late decelerations or severe variable decelerations, accompanied by loss of beat-to-beat variability.

Prolapsed umbilical cord. If a loop of the umbilical cord has prolapsed past the presenting part, it will be compressed against the pelvic wall with every uterine contraction. Each time this occurs, the blood flow through the umbilical vessels ceases, cardiac output is decreased, and the fetal blood pressure falls. The resultant hypoxia is indicated by a fall in the fetal heart rate and a variable deceleration pattern. Although prolapsed cord has no effect on the mother or the course of labor, the infant may die before delivery unless the obstruction to the fetal circulation is relieved.

The incidence of prolapse is about 0.5%; it oc-

curs less frequently when the presenting part fits the pelvis snugly, as it does with normal vertex or frank breech positions, than with certain abnormalities. The principal etiologic factors are those that prevent the presenting part from occluding the pelvic inlet. These include (1) complete and footling breech positions; (2) transverse lies, particularly those in which the back lies superiorly; (3) low-lying placenta with marginal insertion of the cord; (4) a long cord; (5) hydramnios; (6) premature rupture of the membranes; and (7) upward displacement of the presenting part during examinations or operations for delivery. The cord can only prolapse after the membranes rupture.

Cord pressure can be suspected whenever the heart rate during a contraction decreases more than 20 beats/min. The diagnosis can usually be made by vaginal examination. If the membranes have not yet ruptured, the cord may be felt in the intact forebag below the presenting part. This is called a *forelying cord* (Fig. 34-7) and is somewhat less serious than a complete prolapse. The forewaters provide a cushion that may impede descent of the infant and thereby reduce the pressure on the umbilical vessels. With *complete prolapse* (Fig. 34-

8), the cord falls through the cervix and descends into the vagina or even through the introitus. It can be seen or felt without difficulty.

An *occult prolapse* (Fig. 34-9) is one in which a loop of cord lies alongside the presenting part. The altered heart rate with each contraction is obvious, but the cord is so high that it may be impossible to feel it. Additional information can sometimes be obtained by manipulating the presenting part in the inlet. It is pushed against each lateral pelvic wall, the pubis anteriorly and the sacrum posteriorly, while the heart rate is counted. A significant decrease in rate when the head is pushed against a specific area of the bony pelvis suggests that it may be compressing a loop of cord.

Treatment of prolapsed cord is unsatisfactory, and infant mortality is high because the cord often is extruded early in labor before the patient has even entered the hospital. By the time the diagnosis is made, the infant has already died.

If a forelying cord is diagnosed during early labor, cesarean section is almost always indicated. Labor may be allowed to continue if cervical dilatation is almost complete, the presenting part is low in the pelvis, and the baby can be delivered promptly and easily when the

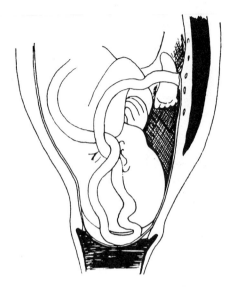

Fig. 34-7. Forelying umbilical cord.

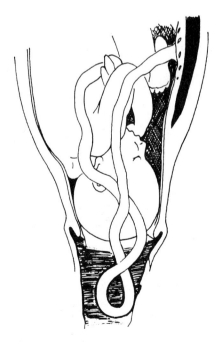

Fig. 34-8. Complete prolapse of umbilical cord.

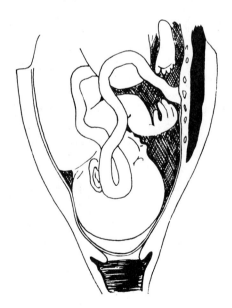

Fig. 34-9. Occult prolapse of umbilical cord.

membranes rupture. The patient should be transported to the delivery room, and the physician should scrub and be prepared to interfere at once if the cord prolapses.

When an actual prolapse is diagnosed during the first stage of labor, cesarean section should be performed if the fetus is alive and is likely to survive. While preparations for the operation are being made, the mother should be placed in the Trendelenburg position and given oxygen while the attendant holds the presenting part out of the pelvis with a sterile gloved hand in the vagina to present interruption of the fetal circulation. If the heart tones are absent, any form of operative interference is unwarranted.

If the cord prolapses during the second stage, it usually is possible to complete delivery by forceps or breech extraction.

Cord entanglement. If a long cord is looped several times around the neck, body, or extremities of the infant, it may be compressed as the loops are drawn tight during descent. The fetal heart rate decreases during each contraction, but no evidence of prolapse can be detected.

The patient suspected of having this condition is evaluated as are others exhibiting signs of hypoxia. Cesarean section should be performed if the variable deceleration pattern, which is characteristic of cord compression, increases and if beat-to-beat variability is lost. If variability and pH remain normal, the labor may be allowed to continue, even though the decelerations recur. One should be prepared to deliver the infant at any time if its condition deteriorates.

Head pressure. Occasionally, a marked depression in fetal heart rate will be detected late in the second stage when the head is distending the perineum. The decision concerning the need for prompt delivery can be made on the basis of beat-to-beat variability. If present, the labor can be allowed to continue.

CARE OF THE NEWBORN INFANT

Most infants make the change from intrauterine to extrauterine existence without difficulty, but some need the help of the physician and all should be observed closely during the immediate postnatal period. The normal infant cries and begins to breathe well within 1 minute of its birth without artificial stimulation. Mucus and blood should be aspirated from the mouth and nasopharynx after the head is born or soon after completion of the delivery. To minimize evaporative heat loss and subsequent cold stress, the infant should be dried and placed under a radiant heat source.

A standardized method for the assessment of the newborn was proposed by Apgar. It evaluates the condition of the infant at 1 and 5 minutes after birth on the basis of five objective signs. Each is scored as 0, 1, or 2 (Table 34-1). The highest possible score is 10; most normal infants score between 7 and 10. The lower scores indicate increasing degrees of severity of asphyxia and depression. Infants who are moderately affected usually have scores between 4 and 7. The muscle tone is somewhat reduced, and the infant is cyanotic; the heart beats at a rate of 100 beats/min or more. They respond to stimulation and can be resuscitated without difficulty.

Those with scores below 4 are severely depressed and must be treated promptly if they are to survive intact.

TABLE 34-1 Signs for determining condition of newborn infant

Sign	0	1	2
Heart rate	Absent	Below 100	Over 100
Respiratory effort	Absent	Slow, irregular	Good, crying
Response to catheter in nostril	None	Grimace	Cough or sneeze
Muscle tone	Limp	Some flexion of extremities	Active motion
Color	Blue, pale	Body pink, extremities blue	Completely pink

Modified from Apgar, V.: The role of the anesthesiologist in reducing neonatal mortality, N.Y. State J. Med. **55:**2365, 1955.

Asphyxia neonatorum

Asphyxia is the result of intrauterine hypoxia suffered by the fetus, most commonly during labor or delivery or both. Any interference with the supply of oxygenated blood to the fetus may be a reason for asphyxia. The most frequent causes are maternal hypotension, placental abnormalities, abruptio placentae, and cord complications. Among the factors making up the Apgar scores, the heart rate is the most sensitive indicator of the infant's oxygenation. A sustained rate of over 100 beats/min is the objective of any resuscitative effort.

Apnea

Infants may fail to breath initially. In addition to intrauterine hypoxia, this may be caused by narcosis from drugs administered to the mother, especially anesthetic agents. Birth injuries or malformations such as pneumothorax and diaphragmatic hernia may also cause immediate respiratory difficulties.

Resuscitation

The important steps in resuscitating asphyxiated infants are the establishment of an airway, the delivery of oxygen, and the establishment of ventilation. Thus initial aspiration of the nasopharynx and, if necessary, the trachea is followed by artificial ventilation. Although the most efficient means of artificial ventilation for newborn infants is the bag-to-endotracheal tube method, bag-to-mask ventilation is often useful while preparations for intubation progress rapidly. Artificial ventilation should not be used until the airway has been cleared. This is particularly important if the respiratory passages contain thick meconium; it will be forced into the lungs where it causes an intense reaction.

Aspiration of particulate meconium causes a chemical pneumonitis that, in turn, is the leading cause of death in full-term infants. Treatment of meconium aspiration is prevention that must be carried out in the delivery room. When thick meconium is present, the infant's mouth and nose should be suctioned as the head is delivered and before delivery of the thorax. After delivery, endotracheal intubation is performed, and the trachea suctioned. Ideally this should be performed before the first breath.

The infant should be positioned with a slightly dorsiflexed head. A laryngoscope with a newborn-sized blade is introduced at the right angle of the mouth, displacing the tongue to the left side. When the epiglottis is seen, the tip of the blade will be located between the tongue, and the epiglottis and must be lifted forward. This will make the vocal cords visible. Any foreign material encountered should be suctioned before an endotracheal tube is inserted. The internal diameter of the tube should be 3.5 mm for term infants and 3.0 mm for premature infants.

A self-inflating bag is connected to the tube and compressed at a rate of 30 to 40 times a minute. Continued bradycardia and failure to initiate spontaneous breathing will necessitate further procedures such as cardiac massage and administration of sodium bicarbonate through the umbilical vein.

All resuscitative maneuvers should be performed gently; there is no place for rough and potentially traumatic procedures such as holding the baby upside down and slapping it.

Stimulant drugs are not indicated in the resuscitation of the newborn. If the infant's depression is caused by administration of morphine or other narcotics to the mother, naloxone (Narcan), 0.01 mg/kg, should be injected into the umbilical vein.

Ligation of the cord

The blood in the fetal circulation is distributed between vessels in the infant's body and those in the placenta. At the end of the second trimester about half of the total blood is in the placenta; as the baby grows larger, relatively more is contained within the infant itself. Blood volume of the newborn is only 250 to 300 ml. Consequently, blood loss from the umbilical cord must be avoided. The ultimate amount of blood retained in the infant will depend on the relative position of the placenta, blood pressure, cord obstructions, and the timing of the cord clamping.

The cord should be ligated with a tie or clamp placed about 2 cm from the skin edge. Subsequently, an antiseptic preparation such as triple dye should be applied to curtail colonization by pathogens, especially staphylococci.

The *absence of one umbilical artery* is associated with congenital malformations of the infant, which usually are severe and obvious. Infants with single umbilical arteries who are normal on examination need no further investigation, but the fact should be recorded because one should be alert for the increased chance of urinary tract anomalies.

The cord mummifies and drops off on about the fifth day of life, leaving a small area at the umbilicus that heals rapidly. Occasionally, the stump of the cord becomes infected and serves as a source of sepsis.

Treatment of the eyes

Credé in 1884 suggested that silver nitrate solution be instilled in the eyes of the newborn infant as an aid in preventing gonorrheal ophthalmia. This has eliminated one of the major causes of acquired blindness. A drop of 1% silver nitrate solution is instilled into each conjunctival sac. Individual doses in wax ampules especially prepared for newborn infants should be used. Some infants develop a mild chemical conjunctivitis. The silver nitrate prophylaxis is required by law in almost all states, and it is not usually left to the physician's discretion to omit it or to use other agents such as antibiotics. Because of the concern over the possibility of chlamydial eye infections, some physicians are also using erythromycin or tetracycline eye ointments.

REFERENCES

Apgar, V.: Drugs in pregnancy, J.A.M.A. **190**:840, 1964.

Ascari, W.Q., Allen, A.E., Baker, W.J., and Pollack, W.: Rh₀ (D) immune globulin (human): evaluation in women at risk of Rh immunization, J.A.M.A. **205**:1, 1968.

Bowman, J.M., and Manning, F.A.: Intrauterine fetal transfusion: Winnipeg 1982, Obstet. Gynecol. **61**:203, 1983.

Carson, B.S., Losey, R.W., Bowes, W.A., Jr., and Simmons, M.A.: Combined obstetric and pediatric approach to prevent meconium aspiration syndrome, Am. J. Obstet. Gynecol. **126**:712, 1976.

Druzin, M.L., Gratacós, J., Keegan, K.A., and Paul, R.H.: Antepartum fetal heart rate testing. VII. The significance of fetal bradycardia, Am. J. Obstet. Gynecol. **139**:194, 1981.

Duenhoelter, J.H., and Pritchard, J.A.: Human fetal respiration, Obstet. Gynecol. **42**:746, 1973.

Evertson, L.R., Gauthier, R.J., Schifrin, B.S., and Paul, R.H.: Antepartum fetal heart rate testing, I. Evolution of the non-stress test, Am. J. Obstet. Gynecol. **133**:29, 1974.

Feingold, M., Fine, R.N., and Ingall, D.: Intravenous pyelography in infants with single umbilical artery, N. Engl. J. Med. **270**:1178, 1964.

Freeman, R.K.: The use of the oxytocin challenge test for antepartum clinical evaluation of uteroplacental respiratory function, Am. J. Obstet. Gynecol. **121**:481, 1975.

Haverkamp, A.D., Orleans, M., Langendoerfer, S., McFee, J., Murphy, J., and Thompson, H.E.: A controlled trial of the differential effects of intrapartum fetal monitoring, Am. J. Obstet. Gynecol. **134**:399, 1979.

Herbst, A.L., Kurman, R.J., Scully, R.E., and Postkanzer, D.C.: Clear-cell adenocarcinoma of the genital tract in young females, N. Engl. J. Med. **287**:1259, 1972.

Howard, F.M., and Hill, J.M.: Drugs in pregnancy, Obstet. Gynecol. **34**:643, 1979.

Liley, A.W.: Liquor amnii analysis in the management of pregnancy complicated by rhesus sensitization, Am. J. Obstet. Gynecol. **82**:1359, 1961.

MacDonald, D., Grant, A., Sheridan-Pereira, M.S., Boyalan, P., and Chalmers, I.: The Dublin randomized controlled trial of fetal heart rate monitoring, Am. J. Obstet. Gynecol. **152**:524, 1985.

Manning, F.A., Morrison, I., Lange I.R., Harman, C.R., and Chamberlain, P.F.: Fetal assessment based on fetal biophysical profile scoring: experience in 12,620 referred high-risk pregnancies, Am. J. Obstet. Gynecol. **151**:343, 1985.

Monif, G.: Personal communication.

Mulvihill, J.J., Klimas, J.T., Slokes, D.C., and Risemberg, H.M.: Fetal alcohol syndrome: seven new cases, Am. J. Obstet. Gynecol. **125**:937, 1976.

Neutra, R.R.: Effect of fetal monitoring on neonatal death rates, N. Engl. J. Med. **299**:324, 1978.

Rodriguez, S.U., Leikin, S.L., and Hiller, M.C.: Neonatal thrombocytopenia associated with antepartum administration of thiazide drugs, N. Engl. J. Med. **270**:881, 1964.

Schifrin, B.S., and Dame, L.: Fetal heart rate patterns: prediction of Apgar score, J.A.M.A. **219**:1332, 1972.

Stagno, S., and Whitley, R.J.: Herpes infections of pregnancy, N. Engl. J. Med. **313**:1270 and 1327, 1985.

Weinstein, L.: Irregular antibodies causing hemolytic disease of the newborn, Obstet. Gynecol. Surv. **31**:581, 1976.

Zanani, B., Paul, R.H., and Huey, J.R.: Intrapartum fetal heart rate: correlation with scalp pH in the preterm fetus, Am. J. Obstet. Gynecol. **136**:43, 1980.

Zelson, C., Lee, S.J., and Casalino, M.: Neonatal narcotic addiction: comparative effects of maternal intake of heroin and methadone, N. Engl. J. Med. **289**:1216, 1973.

35

William J. Ledger

Dystocia and prolonged labor

The maximal duration of normal labor has been set arbitrarily at 24 hours; labor that extends beyond this period is termed *prolonged*. Some classify multiparous labors of more than 18 hours' duration as prolonged. Long or difficult labors, to which the term *dystocia* is applied, can be caused by ineffective uterine contractions, by abnormalities in the size or position of the fetus, and by alterations in the structure of the birth canal.

DYSTOCIA FROM UTERINE DYSFUNCTION

At the onset of normal labor the uterine contractions often occur irregularly and last only a few seconds. Within 2 to 3 hours, however, they assume a more regular pattern and increase in frequency and intensity. The effect of normal uterine contractions is progressive cervical dilatation and expulsion of the infant.

Uterine dysfunction can be suspected if the contractions of early labor do not assume a normal pattern within a few hours. Although the contractions of dysfunctional labor may cause almost as much discomfort as those of normal labor, they are far less effective in dilating the cervix.

The gradient of force exerted by the uterine contractions during normal labor is from the fundus to the cervix, and, as labor advances, the upper segment progressively becomes shorter and its walls thicker as the individual muscle fibers retract. The

rising inferior border of the upper segment exerts traction on the lower segment and the effaced cervix, which are pulled upward around the presenting part as the latter is pushed through the gradually enlarging opening. This orderly sequence of events does not occur with uterine dysfunction; either the force of the contractions or the gradient of activity from the fundus downward toward the cervix is altered.

Although the type of uterine dysfunction cannot be determined precisely without special recording instruments, an abnormal latent or active phase of cervical dilatation can be recognized by clinical observation. During normal labor the upper portion of the uterus contracts firmly, whereas the lower segment feels much more relaxed. At the height of a normal contraction the uterus becomes so hard that it cannot be indented with firm finger pressure. In contrast, with uterine dysfunction the duration of each contraction is less, and the uterus is less firm and can easily be indented with pressure of the fingertips. Low amplitudes of the irregular contractions can be seen if intrauterine pressures are recorded directly.

As a result of the incoordinate activity, the muscle fibers of the upper segment fail to retract, development of the lower segment is incomplete, the cervix remains thick and dilates slowly, or dilatation may cease. The cervix often hangs down ahead of the presenting part instead of being applied tightly against it as in normal labor, and the cervix may become progressively thicker and more edematous. Under these circumstances, failure of the cervix to dilate in the usual manner is a result of inadequate uterine action rather than of local abnormality in the cervical tissues.

Abnormal progress in the latent or the active phase can be recognized promptly when cervical dilatation is plotted on a normal labor curve.

Latent phase abnormality. Normal, well-coordinated uterine activity is essential for completing effacement of the cervix and subsequently for dilating it. The contractions of early dysfunctional labor are uncoordinated and do not accomplish this effectively. As a consequence, the time required to complete effacement and to enter the active phase is usually longer than during normal labor. This is called *prolonged latent phase* (Fig. 35-1).

A statistical analysis of the length of the latent phase yields a range of observations in which approximately 95% fall within the mean and two standard deviations. The abnormal latent phases will be very short or very long. The major concern is in evaluating the patient who exhibits a possible prolongation of the latent phase. The obstetrician must make one or more of the following clinical decisions: whether the patient is in labor, whether she requires sedation, whether amniotomy should be performed, and whether she should be given oxytocin. There is no absolute amount of time that can be identified as normal for the latent phase; this can vary from service to service (Fig. 31-17). *On most services a latent phase of more than 10 to 12 hours in primigravidas and more than 6 to 8 hours in multiparas is considered prolonged.*

Active phase dysfunction. There are three possible *active phase patterns:* (1) *normal,* with cervical dilatation progressing at the anticipated rate; (2) prolonged, with the cervix dilating steadily but at a rate less than normal *(prolonged active phase);* or (3) one in which the early active phase may appear to be normal or may be progressing slowly, but progress ceases before cervical dilatation is complete *(active phase arrest)* (Fig. 35-1).

Since the cervix should dilate progressively during the active phase, abnormalities of this part of labor can be recognized early. With the use of a statistical analysis of primigravid labors at the University of Michigan as a baseline, a *prolonged active phase* can be diagnosed whenever cervical dilatation progresses at a rate less than 0.7 cm/hr in primigravidas and less than 1.1 cm/hr in multiparas. An *active phase arrest* can be diagnosed if cervical dilatation in the active phase does not change during a 2-hour period. By studying the slope of the active phase curve, the physician does not have to wait until the normal mean duration is exceeded to diagnose abnormal labor (Fig. 35-1).

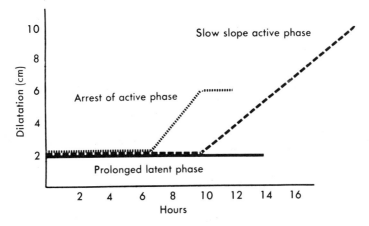

Fig. 35-1. Abnormal labor curves.

Etiologic factors. Uterine dysfunction is almost always encountered in *primigravidas* and is unusual during subsequent labors. This fact eliminates structural abnormalities of the uterus or faulty nerve supply as etiologic factors. It is frequently stated that a prolonged latent phase can be caused by the administration of *analgesic drugs* too early in labor, but this is doubtful. Women who are given drugs during the normal latent phase continue to progress at a regular rate, and the quality of the contractions during early normal labor often improves after the patient is relaxed by medication. Analgesics certainly can increase an abnormality already present, but they probably do not cause it. *Overdistention of the uterus* by hydroamnios or multiple pregnancy may decrease the efficiency of the uterine contractions, thus delaying progress. A prolonged *active phase,* during which the cervix dilates progressively but at a rate slower than anticipated, almost always occurs in primigravidas, and no specific cause can be found.

Active phase arrest, in which the cervix fails to dilate within 2 hours, is an ominous sign because it is a pattern that is encountered with cephalopelvic disproportion in primigravidas. Active phase arrest is less likely to occur with cephalopelvic disproportion in multiparas (Fig. 35-2).

Effect of uterine dysfunction. Prolongation of labor and the consequent multiple vaginal examinations increase the risk of *endomyometritis,* particularly if a cesarean section is required.

The defective uterine contractions usually continue into the third stage, thereby increasing the incidence of *postpartum hemorrhage.* This is far more serious if labor has been so long that the mother is exhausted and dehydrated and the intravascular space is concentrated. Blood loss may also be increased by injury from *operative delivery,* which is necessary more often than with normal labor.

Management of uterine dysfunction. Abnormal labor can usually be suspected within 6 to 8 hours after the labor begins because the contractions remain irregular and short and produce little change in the cervix or the station of the presenting part. The physician should not wait

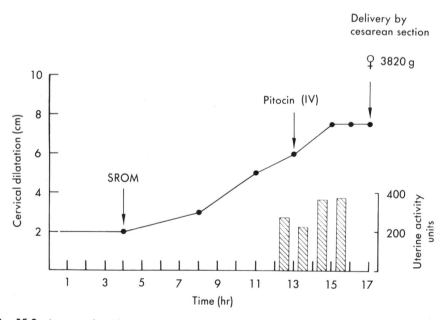

Fig. 35-2. Arrest active phase of cervical dilatation in 28-year-old gravida 3, para II. Uterine activity is noted in lower right portion of graph. Despite improvement in uterine activity with intravenous administration of oxytocin (Pitocin), cervical dilatation stopped at 7 cm, and cesarean section was performed. *SROM,* Spontaneous rupture of membrane.

until a prolonged latent or an abnormal active phase can be diagnosed on the basis of elapsed time before starting the study and treatment.

Certain principles are essential to the proper management of any prolonged labor regardless of the cause. These include evaluation, protection against infection, sedation, and hydration.

EVALUATION. A sterile vaginal examination should be performed as soon as abnormal labor is suspected. Unanticipated abnormalities in fetal position or cephalopelvic disproportion may be diagnosed, and the consistency and dilatation of the cervix can be determined.

PROTECTION AGAINST INFECTION. Vaginal examinations should be limited because bacteria are carried directly through the cervix on the fingers. Prophylactic antibiotics should not be necessary. There can be no need to treat infection if it is prevented by early recognition and proper management of abnormal labor.

SEDATION. Analgesic drugs administered as during normal labor will occasionally decrease both the force and the frequency of uterine contractions, but this is usually a short-term response. A phenothiazine preparation such as promethazine (Phenergan), 50 mg, will relax the patient and ease her tension without altering the contraction mechanism. If normal uterine activity can be achieved with oxytocics, any of the methods used to control pain during normal labor are applicable.

HYDRATION. Patients with prolonged labor should be kept well hydrated, particularly during the hot, humid summer months when loss through the skin is excessive. From 2 to 3 L of fluid are necessary every 24 hours. Since absorption from the stomach is reduced during labor, the fluid should be given intravenously.

PROLONGED LATENT PHASE. The frequency with which the diagnosis of latent phase prolongation is made is in part determined by the obstetrician's decision as to when labor began. To use labor graphs effectively, one must make an arbitrary decision when the patient is admitted that labor began at the time she first felt painful uterine contractions. Some of these women will actually be in false labor and will be discharged, but initial decisions concerning the onset of labor permit early recognition of latent phase abnormalities. A latent phase that extends beyond normal on a labor graph should not be ignored.

An attempt should be made to correct the abnormality as soon as it becomes evident that contractions have not assumed a normal pattern, that there is no appreciable change in the cervix, and that labor is not progressing at a normal rate (Fig. 35-3). At the end of the sixth or eighth hour of latent phase labor a *sterile vaginal ex-*

amination is performed to determine fetal position and station and the condition of the cervix.

Amniotomy performed at the time of the vaginal examination may be followed by improved contractions and conversion to a normal pattern. Since amniotomy commits one to completing delivery within a reasonable time, the physician must be as certain as possible that the problem is a prolonged latent phase and not false labor before rupturing the membranes. One must also plan each step of the treatment in advance and be prepared to perform cesarean section while it is still safe if an effective contraction pattern cannot be established.

If normal progress has not been established within an hour after amniotomy, the uterus should be stimulated with *oxytocin*. The method by which this solution is administered is described in the discussion on induction of labor (Chapter 31). The dosage necessary to stimulate normal contractions is usually small, and at the beginning no more than 0.5 to 1 mU/min of oxytocin should be delivered. If this is not enough to induce a normal contraction pattern, the dosage can be increased gradually at 1 mU/min increments every 20 to 30 minutes. One study by Seitchik and Castillo demonstrated this to be more effective than methods with larger increments given more rapidly. If the uterus does not respond to a dosage of 10 to 15 mU/min, a further increase is not likely to be effective. Since it is difficult to evaluate the quality of uterine contractions by palpation, intrauterine pressure recordings should be made during oxytocin infusion.

Almost all patients will enter the active phase with

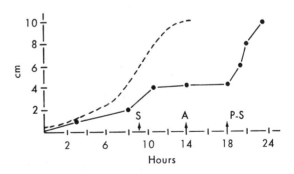

Fig. 35-3. Labor graph of primigravida with prolonged latent phase of labor. Sedative *(S)* was given at 9 hours, and amniotomy *(A)* performed at fourteenth hour. Latent phase persisted until oxytocin (Pitocin, *P*), was given. Position was right occipitoposterior; infant weighed 2405 g.

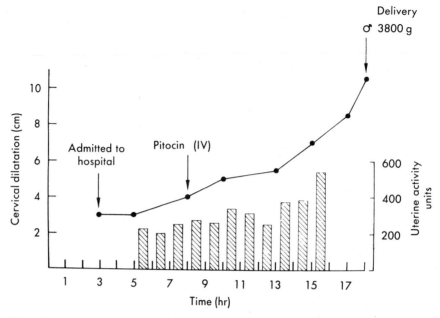

Fig. 35-4. Prolonged active phase in 20-year-old gravida 1, para 0. Progress of cervical dilatation was slow and steady despite intravenous administration of oxytocin (Pitocin).

amniotomy and oxytocin stimulation, and in some the labor will progress normally without continued stimulation, but many will develop active phase arrest if the oxytocin is stopped.

A *prolonged active phase* usually cannot be altered significantly by amniotomy or oxytocin. If cervical dilatation is progressing at a regular but reduced rate and if there is no concern over the adequacy of the pelvis, no active treatment is necessary. Oxytocin should be used if uterine contractions occur irregularly and if the recorded contractions are of low amplitude (Fig. 35-4).

ACTIVE PHASE ARREST (Fig. 35-5). Arrest during the active phase of labor is cause for concern, because it may be an indication of disproportion in primigravidas. If the contractions are irregular and progressive cervical dilatation ceases, vaginal examination is imperative. If absolute cephalopelvic disproportion is suspected, x-ray film pelvimetry should be ordered; this is rarely indicated in the 1980s. Treatment will depend on the degree.

Amniotomy, if the membranes are still intact, and *oxytocin stimulation* are both indicated if there is no disproportion or only a minor degree, which can probably be overcome with normal contractions. Amniotomy should be performed even though the presenting part is still high, particularly if the vertex is well applied to the cervix. It may be all that is needed to correct the abnormality and to eliminate the need for oxytocin and cesarean section. The possibility of cord prolapse is slight and is outweighed by potential risks of active phase arrest. Oxytocin should be started if the contractions do not improve within an hour after amniotomy. Oxytocin must be continued throughout the rest of the labor; if it is stopped, the abnormal contraction pattern will usually recur.

Cesarean section may become necessary if oxytocin-stimulated contractions fail to overcome what is considered to be minor disproportion or if normal progress in labor cannot be established. A decision can almost always be made during the first 4 to 6 hours of stimulation; although delivery may not occur within this time, the physician can determine whether it can logically be anticipated.

DELIVERY. The decision as to when a patient should be delivered is made on the basis of observed progress and an estimate of how long the total labor will be. If a *prolonged latent phase* is terminated and active phase abnormality does not develop, one can anticipate normal delivery. If the prolonged latent phase is not terminated by amniotomy and oxytocin, there is no choice but cesarean section.

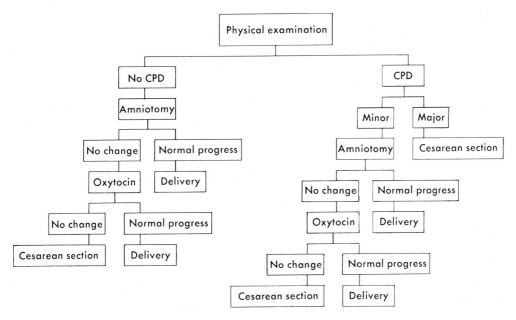

Fig. 35-5. Management of active phase arrest of cervical dilatation. *CPD*, Cephalopelvic disproportion.

In general, there is no need to interfere in *slow slope active phase* if measured uterine activity is normal and cervical dilatation and descent continue at a reasonable rate. Cesarean section may be justified if uterine activity is inadequate and continues after the administration of oxytocin and arrest occurs. Vaginal delivery usually occurs when *active phase arrest* can be corrected by oxytocin, and there is no disproportion.

Whether a patient can be delivered vaginally will be determined by the size of the pelvis; the position, station, and size of the infant; and the amount of difficulty anticipated. There is a natural tendency to terminate abnormal labor as soon as possible. This is reflected in the fact that 'poor progress in labor'' is one of the leading indications for cesarean section in the United States. Since the pelvis generally is normal, as is the mechanism of labor under the influence of oxytocin, there is little need for difficult midforceps delivery. If intervention is necessary, an atraumatic delivery should be the goal. A cesarean section is preferable to a difficult midforceps delivery.

Cesarean section should not be considered a last resort measure in the treatment of dysfunctional labor. With this attitude, perinatal morbidity and mortality can only increase. Cesarean section should be performed when

(1) uterine dysfunction cannot be corrected by amniotomy and oxytocin stimulation, (2) delivery becomes necessary because of fetal distress before the cervix is dilated, or (3) during the second stage unless easy forceps delivery is possible. On the other hand, cesarean section should not be used indiscriminately because abnormal labor usually occurs only in primigravidas and a uterine scar may complicate subsequent deliveries that are likely to be normal.

Since spinal or epidural anesthesia does not alter uterine tone but does relax voluntary muscle, it is more desirable than are inhalation methods.

The incidence of hemorrhage following delivery is increased because the abnormal contractions continue during the third stage and because injury occurs more frequently than with normal delivery.

CONSTRICTION RING DYSTOCIA

A constriction ring is a tetanic annular contraction of smooth muscle that may occur at any level in the uterine wall. The ring does not change position, and it may be applied so tightly around the infant's body that it prevents descent.

Constriction ring, although rare, should be suspected whenever the uterine contractions are irregular and uncoordinated and is particularly likely to develop with dysfunctional labor. The cervix and lower segment below the ring hang like a cuff ahead of the presenting part and are quiescent when the muscle in the fundus contracts. The infant may actually be pulled up rather than pushed down with each contraction. The diagnosis can only be made with accuracy by passing the hand upward into the uterine cavity until the band is felt.

It is usually impossible to relax a constriction ring except with deep inhalation anesthetic, which, of course, prevents further progress of labor. Cesarean section is almost always indicated.

PATHOLOGIC RETRACTION RING

A pathologic retraction ring (Bandl's ring) develops during obstructed but otherwise normal labor. The ring forms at the junction of the active upper and the relatively passive lower uterine segments and actually is the lower border of the unusually thick upper segment. Because descent and expulsion of the infant are impeded, the lower segment becomes excessively lengthened and thinned, and the upper segment shortened and thickened. Unless the obstruction is overcome, the uterus may rupture. In contrast to a constriction ring, a retraction ring itself does not prevent descent. It is a result rather than a cause of obstruction.

The ring can be felt and sometimes even seen as a ridge just below the umbilicus; it becomes more obvious as labor progresses. The treatment consists of delivery by the most expedient method; cesarean section is usually the preferred method because the basic reason for the ring is insurmountable disproportion.

DYSTOCIA OF FETAL ORIGIN

Dystocia of fetal origin may be the result of excessive size, abnormal development, or unusual positions in the birth canal.

Excessive development

The usual infant at term weighs slightly more than 3200 g (7 pounds) and is about 50 cm (19.5 inches) long. About 10% weigh at least 4000 g (9 pounds), but in no more than 1% or 2% is the birth weight over 4500 g (10 pounds).

The *birth weight often increases progressively in each pregnancy,* so the third or fourth infant may weigh much more than the first. Because of this the physician cannot assume that a multiparous woman will deliver without difficulty simply because she has before; the present infant may be too large to pass through the pelvis, although the measurements indicate that it is normal. Approximately 10% of primary cesarean sections in multiparas are performed because of disproportion. *Babies whose parents are large generally weigh more than those born to smaller individuals.* Fortunately, large women usually have large pelves that will permit the delivery of oversized infants without difficulty. *Maternal diabetes* is such an important factor that a glucose tolerance test should be performed in any woman who has been delivered of an infant weighing more than 4000 g. Fetal weight can be correlated with *maternal weight gain.* Women who gain more than 13.5 kg (30 pounds) during pregnancy are likely to have large babies.

Postmaturity has little to do with the development of large infants; in fact, the typical "postmature" baby is likely to be thin and undernourished because of placental insufficiency. Koff and Potter found that the gestational period for oversized infants averaged only 8 days more than for those of average weight.

The mortality for excessively large infants is increased, and many of them are injured during attempts at delivery. Sack's study of the outcome for 766 infants who weighed more than 4500 g (10 pounds) at birth illustrates the dangers for the fetus. The perinatal mortality was 7.2% (39 fetal and 16 neonatal deaths), and 16% of liveborn infants were severely depressed. A neurologic complication was diagnosed in 11.4% of 200 surviving infants who were followed up, and 4.5% died before the age of 7. Another interesting recent study showed increased morbidity related to the vaginal delivery of large infants by vacuum extraction.

The normal-sized pelvis should be adequate for the delivery of infants weighing 4000 to 4500 g if the uterine contractions are forceful enough. If the baby is too large, however, disproportion similar to that encountered with normal infants and contracted pelvis can occur; as a consequence, the infant may be injured during difficult extraction.

The physician must be on the lookout for large babies, particularly in women in whom there is a reason for their development. The size cannot always be determined accurately by palpation. *Sonographic measurements of the biparietal diameter and body circumference* are helpful in determining fetal size.

During labor the findings are similar to those in disproportion from contracted pelvis, except that the latter more often occurs in primigravidas. The head may fail to enter the pelvis, or descent may be slow despite what appear to be normal uterine contractions.

It is important to recognize fetopelvic disproportion

early in the course of labor. The uterus may rupture in multiparas with insurmountable disproportion because strong, forceful contractions continue despite the lack of descent. The primigravid uterus is more likely to respond by active phase arrest.

If disproportion is not too great, the head may descend and deliver, but the broad shoulders are not able to pass the inlet *(shoulder dystocia)* (Fig. 35-6). When this occurs, the chin will be pulled back tightly against the perineum as soon as the head is delivered through the

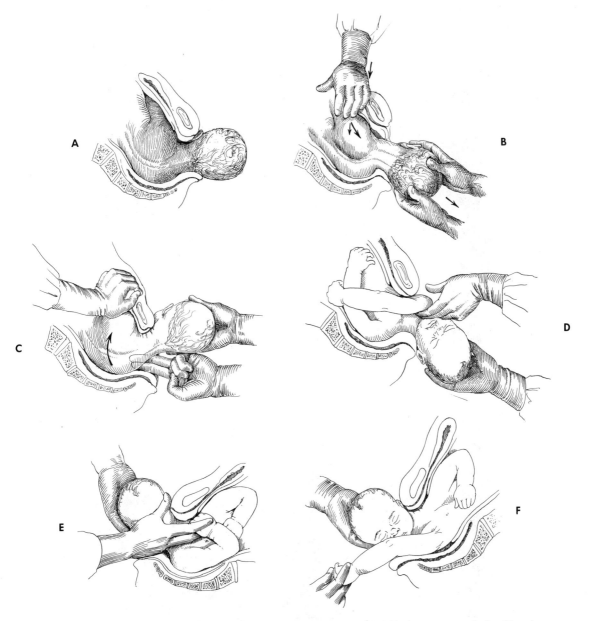

Fig. 35-6. Shoulder dystocia. **A,** Anterior shoulder cannot enter inlet. **B,** Attempt to push shoulder beneath pubis. **C** and **D,** Rotation of shoulders. **E** and **F,** Extraction of posterior arm. (From Willson, J.R.: Atlas of obstetric technic, ed. 2, St. Louis, 1969, The C.V. Mosby Co.)

introitus. Unless the infant is extracted promptly, it will die because its chest is compressed, preventing respiratory efforts, and the circulation through the cord is reduced.

The posterior shoulder usually has descended into the true pelvis below the promontory of the sacrum, but the bisacromial diameter is so long that the anterior shoulder, which lies above the pubis, cannot enter the pelvis. Under such circumstances forceful downward traction on the infant's head not only is ineffectual but may well stretch and injure the brachial plexus or even fracture the cervical spine. The physician should first attempt to push the anterior shoulder into the pelvis by direct pressure on it through the abdominal wall. If this cannot be accomplished, another maneuver must be tried at once. The hand is inserted into the vagina until the first and second fingers can be hooked in the posterior axilla. The posterior shoulder is rotated anteriorly and pulled down-

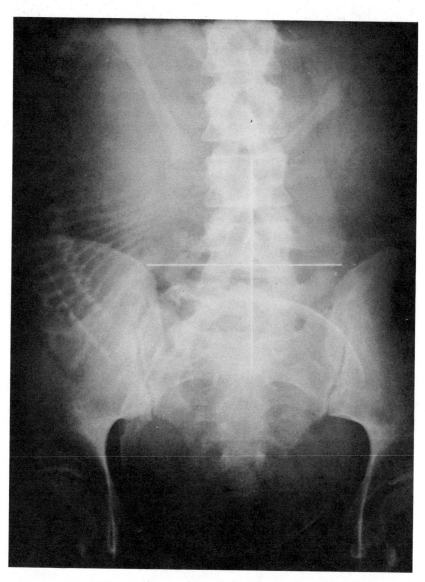

Fig. 35-7. Cephalopelvic disproportion from hydrocephalus.

ward simultaneously with a corkscrew motion. If this maneuver is successful, the anterior shoulder is rotated into the true pelvis below the sacral promontory while the posterior shoulder is delivered from underneath the symphysis anteriorly. From this point, delivery can be completed with little difficulty (Fig. 35-6, *A* to *D*).

If the shoulders are wedged into the inlet so tightly that they cannot be rotated, the hand is passed over the posterior shoulder and along the chest until the baby's hand can be seized and pulled downward over the chest and through the introitus. This releases the posterior shoulder and will permit its anterior rotation and delivery (Fig. 35-6, *E* and *F*).

All of these maneuvers to achieve vaginal delivery can result in soft tissue injury to the fetus. One new approach is to place the head back into the vagina and do an immediate cesarean section. The results seem to be good.

Developmental abnormalities

Developmental anomalies seldom cause dystocia, but in rare instances they may. This is particularly true of deformities such as hydrocephalus, enlargement of the body or abdomen, or conjoined twins.

With *hydrocephalus* (Fig. 35-7), labor is delayed because the head is too large to enter the inlet. The diagnosis can be suspected if a large mass is felt over the inlet. On vaginal palpation the presenting part is above the pelvic inlet; the sutures, if they can be reached, are wide; and the fontanels are huge. X-ray film or ultrasonographic examination will provide confirmatory evidence. With breech position, hydrocephalus is sometimes not diagnosed until it is impossible to extract the aftercoming head.

A hydrocephalic aftercoming head usually cannot be extracted unless it is decompressed. The fluid can be evacuated if the needle or trocar is inserted through the foramen magnum or the roof of the mouth. An alternative method is to aspirate the fluid after the needle has been inserted through the abdominal and uterine walls.

In recent years, cesarean section has been performed more frequently for the delivery of a hydrocephalic infant. Although preliminary results were encouraging, the long-term prognosis for a normal outcome after shunting in utero or after birth is small.

If a decision is made for vaginal delivery, there are techniques to withdraw fluid, collapse the head, and permit the normal progress of labor.

The fetal body may be enlarged by *tumors of the liver, abnormal development of the kidneys, urinary retention* from obstruction in the lower urinary tract, or other anomalies. In the past these abnormalities did not become apparent after the head had been delivered and the body did not follow. More widespread use of antepartum ultrasonography has increased the frequency of early diagnosis. In many cases intrauterine surgery to correct the obstruction has been performed. If not diagnosed in the antepartum period, their management is determined by the cause of the obstruction and whether it can be relieved by manipulation or operation through the maternal vagina.

DYSTOCIA FROM ABNORMALITIES IN POSITION AND PRESENTATION

Abnormalities in position and presentation frequently cause dystocia. If they are recognized promptly and are corrected, the results for both the mother and infant should be reasonably good.

Transverse lie

With transverse lie, the long axis of the infant lies at right angles to the longitudinal axis of the mother; its head lies in one flank, and its buttocks in the other. One of the shoulders lies over the inlet, the presenting part being the scapula or the achromial process. If the infant's back is directed toward the maternal spine, the presenting part will lie in the right or left posterior quadrant of the pelvis (right or left *scapuloposterior position*). If the back is directed anteriorly, the presenting part will lie in the right or left anterior quadrant (right or left *scapuloanterior position*) (Fig. 35-8). In an *oblique lie* the long axis of the fetus lies obliquely across the abdomen, with the head or the buttocks directed toward one or the other maternal iliac fossa.

Transverse lie occurs more often in multiparas than in primigravidas, but it complicates only about 0.25% to 0.5% of all pregnancies. If the placenta is implanted in the fundus or over the cervix, the infant may be forced to assume a transverse or an oblique position because the length of the uterine cavity is reduced. *In another third of all transverse lie, the placenta occupies the lower segment.* Transverse lie is more common in bicornuate or arcuate uteri than in those that have developed normally. It may occur because of hydramnios, which permits the fetus considerable freedom of motion.

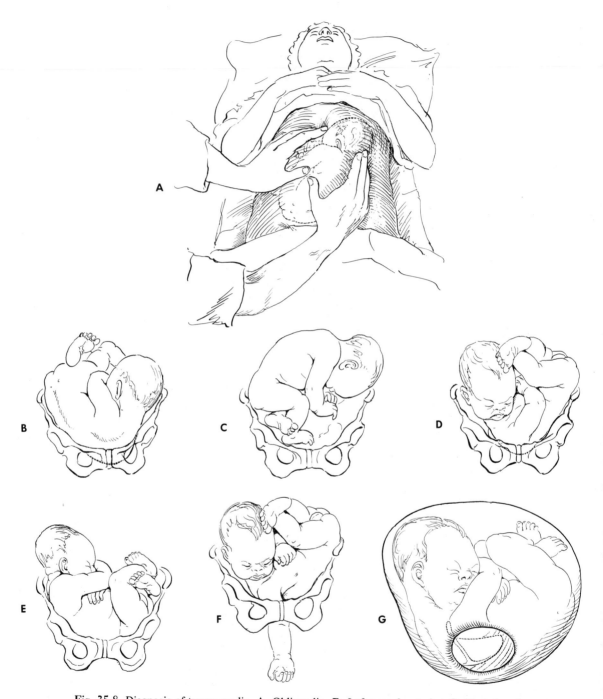

Fig. 35-8. Diagnosis of transverse lie. **A,** Oblique lie. **B,** Left scapuloanterior. **C,** Ventral surface of infant directed toward pelvic inlet and back toward fundus. **D,** Right scapuloposterior. **E,** Ventral surface of infant directed toward fundus and backlying over pelvic inlet. **F,** Right scapuloposterior with prolapsed arm. **G,** Transverse lie with back down. (A to H from Willson, J.R.: Atlas of obstetric technic, ed. 2, St. Louis, 1969, The C.V. Mosby Co.)   *Continued.*

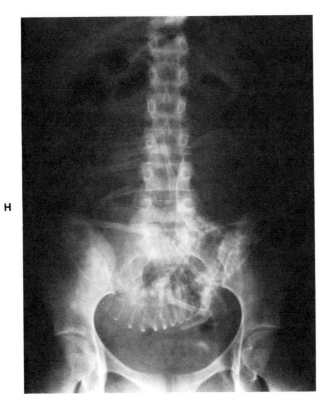

H

Fig. 35-8, cont'd. **H,** X-ray film examination.

Diagnosis. Transverse lie can be suspected if the abdomen looks wider than it does long. If the uterus is relaxed, the head can be felt on one side, and the breech on the other; there is no presenting part in the inlet. It may be possible to palpate the shoulder through the vagina, but if the membranes are intact, the presenting part is often so high that it cannot be reached. During labor, the membranes can be felt bulging through the partially dilated cervix with each contraction. Between contractions the scapula, the clavicle, the axilla, and the rib cage can be palpated. X-ray film study or sonography will confirm the findings (Fig. 35-8). The position of the placenta can be determined by *sonography.*

Vaginal or rectal examinations should not be performed in the physician's office on patients suspected of having transverse lies. If placenta previa is present, profuse bleeding can be precipitated.

Course of labor. Spontaneous delivery of a living normal-sized infant should not be anticipated with shoulder presentation. The cervix dilates around the forebag, and the shoulder is forced into the inlet, but it cannot descend. The membranes usually rupture early in the first stage, after which the hand and arm prolapse into the vagina. A small, macerated infant may sometimes be forced through the pelvis, but delivery must not be expected. More often descent is impossible, the lower segment becomes progressively thinner until it ruptures, or labor ceases with the uterus tetanically contracted. The infant is usually dead, and intrauterine infection has developed. This is termed *neglected transverse lie.*

Prognosis. If the abnormality is recognized early and treated properly, the maternal mortality should not be increased. Trauma to soft parts, particularly cervical laceration and rupture of the uterus, may occur as a result of attempts to complete delivery vaginally. Serious puerperal infection occurs less frequently now than in years past, but it still is a hazard, particularly when the abnormal position is not recognized and labor is prolonged.

Perinatal deaths are caused by anoxia from prolapsed cord, which occurs more often than with normal presentation; by infection; or by injury from prolonged labor or attempts at delivery. The perinatal mortality is as high as 30% to 50% with vaginal delivery, but most babies who are reasonably mature and in good condition should survive if delivered by cesarean section.

Management. If transverse or oblique lie is recognized during late pregnancy, *external version* to a breech or a vertex position should be attempted. If this is impossible, a sonographic examination for placental site should be obtained, and other possible causes of the abnormal lies sought. Many transverse presentations correct themselves spontaneously before labor begins.

During early labor, vaginal and x-ray film examinations should be performed, and external version attempted if it appears that vaginal delivery is possible with a more normal position. If the position cannot be corrected, cesarean section offers the best prognosis for the infant in either primigravidas or multiparas.

The patient with a neglected transverse lie is usually infected, dehydrated, and exhausted. Before anything else is done, she should be given antibiotics and intravenous fluid. Since the lower uterine segment is considerably thinned, any intrauterine manipulation may be enough to rupture the wall; consequently, cesarean section, with appropriate antibiotic therapy if the uterus is infected, usually is the preferred procedure.

Occipitoposterior position

In about a fourth of all vertex deliveries the occiput points toward one of the posterior quadrants during early labor. Almost all infants rotate to an anterior position spontaneously or deliver in the posterior position without difficulty; but, in a few patients, particularly those with abnormal pelves, the labor is prolonged and difficult.

One of the most important reasons for the occipitoposterior position (Fig. 35-9) is the shape of the bony pelvic inlet. If the transverse diameter of the inlet is narrowed and if the anteroposterior diameter is lengthened, as in an anthropoid pelvis, the head must descend with its long axis in an anteroposterior diameter. The occiput may be directed posteriorly or toward the pubis. If the anterior segment of the superior strait is narrow and of the android type, the head is also likely to descend in an oblique posterior position. The forehead fits the anterior segment of the inlet better than does the wider occipital area. In contrast, the infant's head is more likely to enter the gynecoid or the platypelloid pelvis in a transverse diameter, with its long axis in the longest axis of the inlet because it fits better; however, it can be in a posterior position if the pelvis is large.

Anterior rotation can be anticipated if the head is in an oblique occipitoposterior position and flexes as it descends, if the uterine contractions are effective, and if

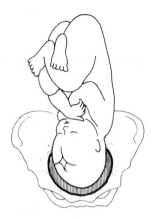

Fig. 35-9. Left occipitoposterior position.

the pelvic size and shape and the levator muscles are normal. In primigravidas the second stage may be slightly longer than usual, but in multiparas the head often descends to the pelvic floor in the posterior position and rotates and delivers with one or two contractions.

Failure to rotate may be the result of inadequate uterine contractions that do not provide enough force to push the baby downward or of relaxation and separation of the levator muscles, eliminating the inclined plane up which the occiput is forced, or it may be because the transverse diameter of the bony pelvis is so narrow that the head cannot turn within the birth canal.

The occiput also may fail to rotate anteriorly because the head is slightly deflexed, making some anterior portion rather than the occiput the presenting part. This area will naturally rotate anteriorly, thereby directing the occiput to the hollow of the sacrum, where it stays. This can occur when complete head flexion is not necessary because the head is small and the pelvis large.

If the head descends to the pelvic floor with the occiput in an oblique posterior position, the patient should be given an opportunity to rotate it herself. No interference is necessary as long as rotation is progressing, even though it is slow and the conditions of the mother and the baby are good. Conversely, delivery is indicated if the maternal or the fetal condition should change or if no progress is made during a period of an hour.

If the head descends in a direct occipitoposterior position (Figs. 35-10 and 35-11), anterior rotation is not likely to occur because the presenting part lies over the sacrum in the trough formed by the two levator muscles rather than on the inclined plane. If progress ceases, the

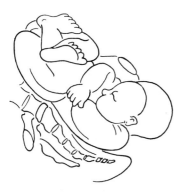

Fig. 35-10. Delivery of head in occipitoposterior position. Area of anterior fontanel stems beneath pubic arch.

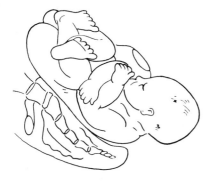

Fig. 35-11. Delivery of head in occipitoposterior position. Area at root of base stems beneath pubic arch. Longer diameters of head must come through introitus with this mechanism.

baby should be delivered. In many instances, particularly in multiparas with roomy pelves and relaxed soft tissues and in those with anthropoid pelves, spontaneous or low forceps delivery with the occiput in a posterior position is not only possible but is preferable to operative rotation. The longer diameters of the head may increase perineal injury slightly, but damage from rotation if the pelvis is abnormal may be even greater. Cesarean section is often indicated for an occipitoposterior position. On many services, this mode of delivery is considered to be the delivery of choice in place of a forceps rotation. The vacuum extractor has a theoretic advantage over forceps in rotation, but a poor fetal outcome caused by trauma to the baby has made this mode of delivery less popular in recent years.

Face position

When the head is completely deflexed, face position can be diagnosed (Fig. 35-12). The chin (mentum) is the presenting part, and relatively large diameters are presenting. Face positions occur in about 0.25% of all deliveries.

Complete deflexion may be primary, or it develops during descent of the head through the inlet; something holds the occiput up, thereby encouraging the anterior portion of the head to descend first. Deflexion increases as the head descends. Face positions may develop in women with *inlet contraction;* the bitemporal diameter is narrower than the biparietal and fits better in the inlet. The situation with a *large baby* is comparable. The *pendulous uterus in a multiparous woman* allows the infant to fall forward or to one side, thereby favoring abnormal positions. Flexion of the head may be prevented by *abnormalities of the neck or thorax* or by *loops of cord around the neck.* Almost all *anencephalic infants* present by the face.

Diagnosis. The fetal spine is extended, and the head is deflexed, with the occiput in contact with the back. On *abdominal examination* the smooth curve of the spine, which is characteristic of flexed attitudes, cannot be felt, but the extremities may be unusually prominent. The cephalic prominence can be felt on the side opposite the small parts. It often is difficult to make a diagnosis by abdominal palpation.

On *rectal examination* the face may feel like a breech, but if the cervix is partly dilated, the supraorbital ridges, nose, eyes, and mouth can be palpated *vaginally.* Great care must be taken not to injure the structures. The abnormal position can be visualized by x-ray film examination (Fig. 35-12).

Course of labor. The mechanism of labor (Fig. 35-13) for the face position is similar to that in the vertex position, but the chin rather than the occipital portion of the head is the presenting part. As the head descends, extension increases until the head is completely deflexed, with the occiput in contact with the infant's back. The chin is rotated because it is forced downward against the levator sling and the bony side walls of the lower pelvis; as labor continues it gradually rotates anteriorly until it lies beneath the pubic arch, with the occipital portion of the head directed toward the sacrum. The submandibular area stems beneath the pubis, while the occiput is forced upward over the perineum until it is free of the vagina. The head therefore is delivered by flexion. The delivery of the shoulders and body is like that in occiput positions.

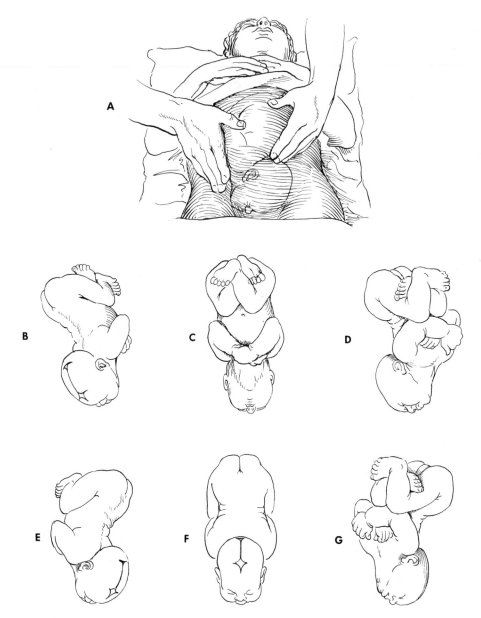

Fig. 35-12. Diagnosis of face positions. **A,** Right mentotransverse. **B,** Left mentoposterior. **C,** Mentoanterior. **D,** Left mentoanterior. **E,** Right mentoposterior. **F,** Mentoposterior. **G,** Right mentoanterior. (**A** to **I** from Willson, J.R.: Atlas of obstetric technic, ed. 2, St. Louis, 1969, The C.V. Mosby Co.)   *Continued.*

If anterior rotation of the chin fails to occur, *persistent mentoposterior position* can be diagnosed (Fig. 35-14). It is almost impossible for a normal-sized infant to deliver in a mentoposterior position because the chin, which lies in the hollow of the sacrum, can only be forced over the perineum by further extension of the head; this is impossible because it already is completely deflexed. Delay from mentoposterior position often occurs when the presenting part is relatively high in the pelvis. If the head descends with the chin pointed directly posteriorly, ro-

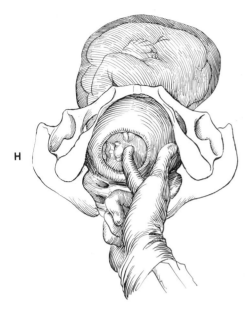

H

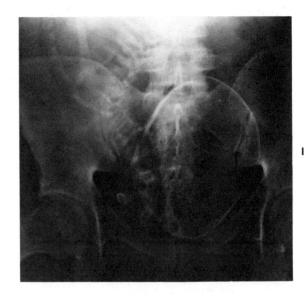

I

Fig. 35-12, cont'd. **H,** Vaginal palpation of right mentotransverse. **I,** X-ray film examination.

tation is not likely to occur. If it is directed obliquely posteriorly, rotation can be anticipated especially in multiparas, but it usually does not occur until the presenting part begins to bulge the perineum.

It is important to remember that when the face is presenting, the biparietal diameter does not pass the pelvic inlet until the chin reaches the pelvic floor; consequently, engagement occurs late in labor.

Management. The management of the face position depends on pelvic size, stage of labor, efficiency of the contractions, and parity. If an abnormal attitude is suspected by abdominal or rectal palpation, the patient should be examined vaginally. Unless delivery is imminent, x-ray film studies should usually be obtained because of the increased incidence of contracted pelvis with face position. If there is no obvious disproportion, and particularly if the chin is in an anterior or a transverse position, labor may be allowed to continue. If the chin is directed posteriorly and the head is wedged into the upper pelvis, the outlook for normal delivery is unfavorable. A short period of labor will usually indicate the outcome. In many instances, particularly in multiparas, face positions are not diagnosed until the patient is delivering.

If the chin does not rotate spontaneously to an anterior position during the second stage of labor, it may be possible to turn it manually, after which it can be extracted by forceps or allowed to deliver spontaneously.

Forceps extraction in the mentoposterior position cannot be performed on normal-sized infants without injuring them and the pelvic structures.

Cesarean section is indicated when progress ceases with the presenting part high in the pelvis or when mentoposterior positions cannot be corrected. It is more often necessary in primigravidas than in multiparas, many of whom deliver rapidly and spontaneously despite the abnormal position.

Brow position

Deflexed attitudes in which the brow is the presenting part occur about once in every 500 to 1000 deliveries and result from any of the factors that tend to prevent flexion and increase extension. Such causes are a large pelvis or a small infant, contracted pelvis, and abnormalities in the shape of the head.

Spontaneous delivery in the brow position will not always occur even if the pelvis is of normal size because the presenting diameter of the fetal head (occipitomental, 13.5 cm) is too large to come through the inlet without extensive molding (Fig. 35-15). However, the brow is frequently a transient position, and enough alteration in position may occur as labor progresses to permit pelvic delivery.

Diagnosis. The diagnosis of brow position is made by palpating the anterior fontanel in the middle of the cervical opening with the supraorbital ridges and the root

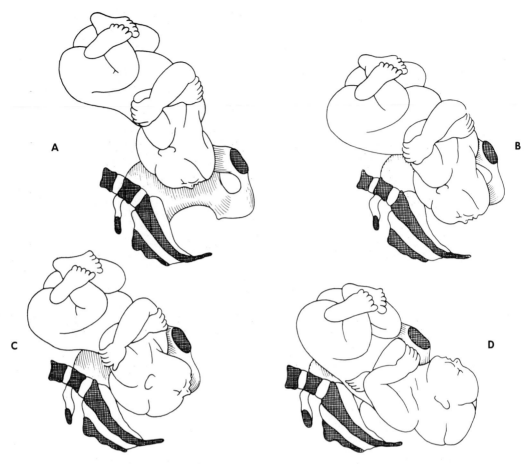

Fig. 35-13. Mechanism of labor in right mentoanterior positions. Head descends in left oblique diameter, **A,** until chin reaches levator sling. **B.** It then rotates anteriorly, **C,** until submandibular area lies beneath symphysis. **D,** Head is then delivered by flexion.

of the nose at one side. Ordinarily, the presenting part is well above the spines. On abdominal examination the deflexion may be suspected by the straight fetal spine with a cephalic prominence palpable on each side (Fig. 35-16). The findings can be confirmed by x-ray film examination, which will also help determine the preferred method for delivery.

Management. The management depends on the stage of labor, size of the infant, size of the pelvis, and findings on sterile vaginal and x-ray film examinations. Vaginal delivery can be anticipated if the infant is small and if the presenting part is below the spines at the time the abnormal position is recognized. Often the presenting part is unengaged and cannot be depressed into the pelvis. In this event, delivery without altering the position is not to be expected. Flexion of the head to an occiput position or extension to a face position might solve the problem, but neither of these is easy if the head is

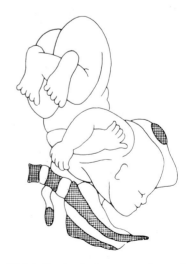

Fig. 35-14. Persistent mentoposterior position.

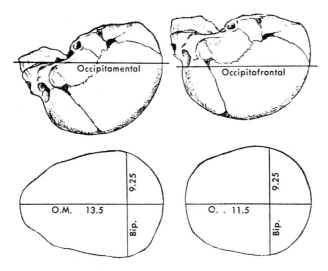

Fig. 35-15. With brow position, longest anteroposterior diameter of head (occipitomental) must pass through pelvis. (From Beck, A.C.: Obstetrical practice, Baltimore, 1955, The Williams & Wilkins Co.)

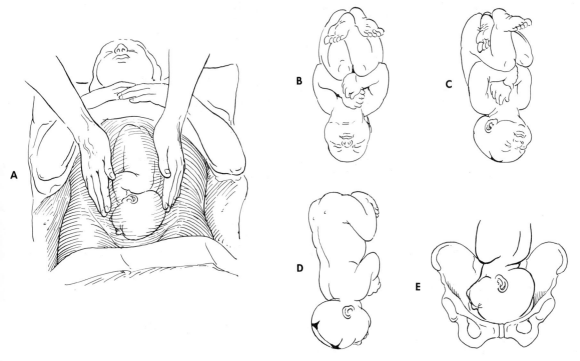

Fig. 35-16. Diagnosis of brow positions. **A,** Right frontotransverse. **B,** Frontoanterior. **C,** Left frontoanterior. **D,** Left frontoposterior. **E,** Right frontotransverse. (**A** to **J** from Willson, J.R.: Atlas of obstetric technic, ed. 2, St. Louis, 1969, The C.V. Mosby Co.) *Continued.*

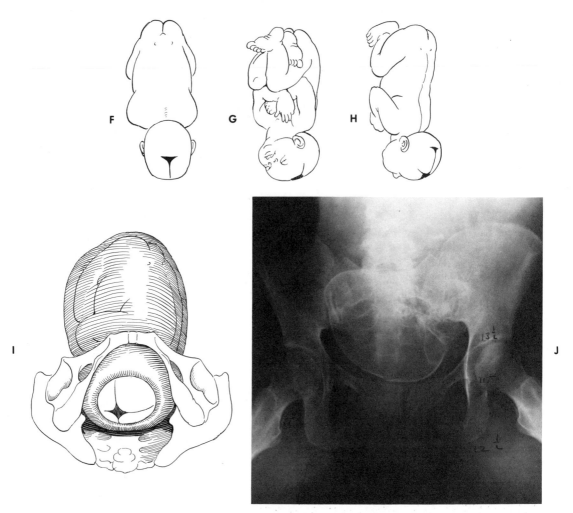

Fig. 35-16, cont'd. **F,** Frontoposterior. **G,** Right frontoanterior. **H,** Right frontoposterior. **I,** Right frontotransverse. **J,** X-ray film examination.

molded. Cesarean section frequently is the preferred method for delivery, particularly in the primigravida, when progress ceases with incomplete cervical dilatation or if the pelvis is contracted.

Compound presentation

Compound presentation can be diagnosed whenever one or more of an infant's extremities prolapse alongside the presenting head or breech. This occurs once in 700 to 1000 deliveries of viable infants. In most instances an upper rather than a lower extremity is involved. Com-

pound presentation occurs most often if the pelvic inlet is contracted or if the infant is premature and so small that it does not occlude the birth canal. It is encountered more often in multiparas than in primigravidas.

Labor usually progresses normally. Occasionally, however, the prolapsed extremity may be responsible for abnormal rotation of the presenting part, or, if large enough, it may even delay descent. Prolapsed cord occurs frequently with compound presentation, particularly if an extremity is prolapsed through the cervix.

No treatment for compound presentation is necessary

unless labor is delayed. A hand lying beside the infant's head, for example, will usually not prolapse completely because the increasing pressure against it as the head descends will hold it up. If an entire arm or leg has descended through the cervix, it may be necessary to disengage the head and replace the extremity within the uterine cavity. Neither cesarean section nor version and extraction is often warranted.

REFERENCES

Koff, A.K., and Potter, E.L.: The complications associated with excessive development of the fetus, Am. J. Obstet. Gynecol. **38:**412, 1939.

Sack, R.A.: The large infant, Am. J. Obstet. Gynecol. **104:**195, 1969.

Seitchik, J., and Castillo, M.: Oxytocin augmentation of dysfunctional labor, Am. J. Obstet. Gynecol. **144:**899, 1982.

36

William J. Ledger

Pelvimetry; dystocia from contracted pelvis

A clinical estimation of pelvic size is usually made at the initial prenatal visit because it is convenient to measure the pelvis at that time. Some physicians prefer to obtain the internal measurements later when the tissues are more supple and relaxed and when the patient is less tense. It makes little difference when the pelvis is measured as long as it is done before labor begins.

Most abnormal pelves can be at least suspected by clinical examination, but x-ray film study is necessary to obtain precise measurements and to determine pelvic shape accurately. There is much controversy about the importance of obtaining the additional information. Many obstetricians, weighing the benefits derived from x-ray film pelvimetry against the risks to the mother and the fetus, believe that it is indicated only under unusual circumstances.

NORMAL PELVIS

For obstetric purposes the pelvis is divided into the *false pelvis* and the *true pelvis,* or *pelvic cavity,* at the level of the sacral promontory; the linea terminalis on each side; and the upper border of the pubis anteriorly. The false pelvis serves no important purpose except to support the enlarging uterus and to direct the presenting part downward. The true pelvis—which is bounded by the sacrum posteriorly; the pelvic bones, muscles, and liga-

ments laterally; and the posterior surfaces of the rami of the pubis and the ischii anteriorly—is far more significant. Alteration in the size and shape of the pelvis may interfere with the mechanism of labor or even prevent normal delivery.

Pelvic inlet (Fig. 36-1). The pelvic inlet, or superior strait, the entrance to the true pelvis, is bounded by the promontory and alae of the sacrum, the lineae terminalis laterally, and the superior surface of the pubic bones anteriorly. It is oval in shape and its *angle of inclination,* the angle the plane of the inlet makes with the horizon with the patient standing, is about 55 degrees.

The *conjugata vera,* or *true conjugate,* extends from the midpoint of the sacral promontory to the superior surface of the symphysis and measures 10.5 to 11.5 cm. The *obstetric conjugate* extends from the promontory to the closest point on the convex posterior surface of the symphysis, which is about 0.5 to 1 cm below the upper margin. This measures about 0.5 cm less than the true conjugate. The *diagonal conjugate* extends from the promontory to the lower border of the symphysis and measures about 12.5 cm. This is the only anteroposterior measurement that can be obtained clinically (Fig. 36-1).

The *transverse diameter* of the inlet represents the greatest distance between each linea terminalis and usually forms a right angle with the true con-

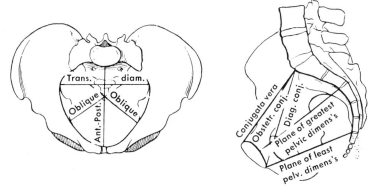

Fig. 36-1. Planes of pelvic inlet. (From Moloy, H.C.: Evaluation of the pelvis in obstetrics, Philadelphia, 1951, W.B. Saunders Co.)

jugate approximately 5 cm anterior to the promontory. It measures about 13.5 cm. The *oblique diameters* extend from each sacroiliac synchondrosis to the opposite iliopectineal eminence and measure about 12.5 cm. The right oblique diameter originates at the right sacroiliac synchondrosis and the left oblique diameter on the left side posteriorly (Fig. 36-1).

Pelvic cavity. The *plane of greatest pelvic dimensions,* the roomiest portion of the pelvic cavity, lies above the ischial spines at the level of a line that extends from the junction of the second and third sacral vertebrae to the middle of the posterior surface of the pubis. This measures about 12.75 cm (Fig. 36-2). The transverse diameter between the two iliac bones just above the superior surface of each acetabulum measures about 12.5 cm.

The *plane of least pelvic dimensions,* or the *midplane,* extends from the lower border of the pubis anteriorly to the lower sacrum at the level of the ischial spines and measures about 11.5 to 12 cm (Fig. 36-2). The transverse *bispinous diameter* is the smallest in the normal pelvic cavity, measuring about 10.5 cm.

Pelvic outlet. The pelvic outlet, or inferior strait, is even less a "plane" than is the inlet. Actually, it is made up of two triangles sharing a common base at a line joining the two ischial tuberosities. The apex of the anterior triangle is the lower border of the symphysis, and the sides are the descending

pubic rami and the ascending ischial rami. The apex of the posterior triangle is the tip of the sacrum, and the sides are the pelvic ligaments. The *bituberous* diameter measures 8 to 11 cm; and the *anteroposterior diameter,* or the distance between the lower border of the symphysis and the tip of the sacrum, is 11.5 cm (Fig. 36-2).

Many variations in the normal pelvis are produced by heredity, variations in hormone stimulation, pressure, and disease. Most pelves are adequate for childbearing, but in some the deviation may be sufficient to disturb the mechanism of labor.

Classification. Caldwell and Moloy have suggested a classification of normal pelves on the basis of the configuration of the inlet and the corresponding changes in the midpelvis and lower pelvis as demonstrated by x-ray film examination. This provides an accurate method for visualizing pelvic contour and for predicting the mechanism of labor and its outcome.

The pelvic inlet is divided into a *posterior segment,* behind the line representing the widest transverse diameter, and an *anterior segment* in front of it (Fig. 36-1). The information necessary to classify the inlet includes the length of the transverse diameter and the anteroposterior length of each segment.

The sacrosciatic notch can be visualized by a lateral film: a wide notch means that the sacrum is displaced posteriorly or that the curve is deep, thus

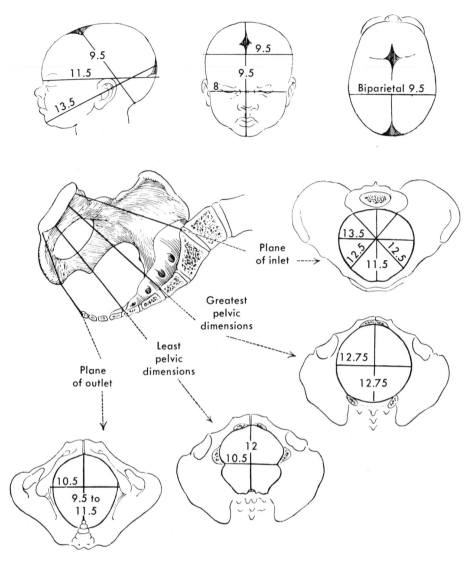

Fig. 36-2. Diameters in centimeters of various planes of pelvis and of fetal head that must pass through it.

increasing the anteroposterior diameter at the midpelvis. A narrow notch indicates a reduced anteroposterior diameter because the sacrum lies farther forward than usual.

Evaluation of the midpelvis and outlet includes measurement of the bispinous diameter and observation of the shape of the spinous processes and the length, width, and curve of the sacrum. The subpubic angle is estimated, and the contour of the

arch is noted. The degree of convergence or divergence of the lateral walls (splay) is also of importance; with considerable convergence toward the outlet, delay may be anticipated.

Female pelves are grouped into four pure and ten mixed types on the basis of morphology as determined by stereoscopic x-ray film study (Figs. 36-3 and 36-4).

GYNECOID PELVIS. Gynecoid pelvis occurs in

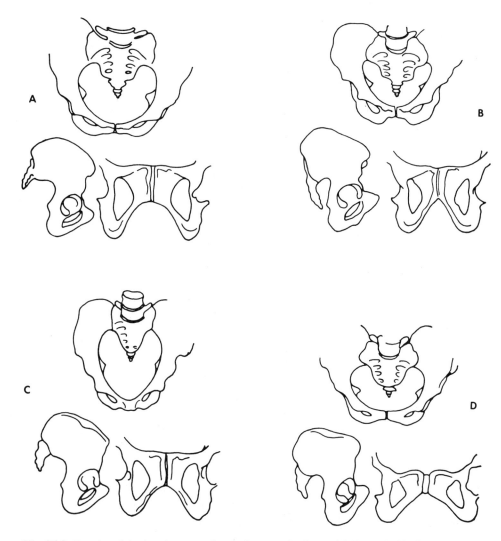

Fig. 36-3. Female pelvis showing normal growth types. **A,** Gynecoid. **B,** Android. **C,** Anthropoid. **D,** Platypelloid.

40% to 45% of women. The inlet of the typical female pelvis is rounded or slightly oval with both anterior and posterior segments rounded and spacious. The sacrum is well curved and of average length, and the sacrosciatic notch is of medium width. The subpubic angle is wide, and the sides of the arch are curved. The bispinous and bituberous diameters are wide, and the side walls are straight.

ANDROID PELVIS. Android pelvis, which occurs in 25% to 35% of white women and 10% to 15%

of black women, is a masculine type of pelvis with a wedge-shaped inlet. The posterior segment is wide and relatively flat, and the anterior segment is narrow with a narrow retropubic angle. The sacrum is straight and inclined forward, and the sacrosciatic notch is narrow. The subpubic angle is narrow, and the bones of the arch are straight. The side walls converge, reducing the bispinous and bituberous diameters. This is the typical *funnel pelvis.*

ANTHROPOID PELVIS. Anthropoid pelvis occurs

PURE TYPES MIXED TYPES MIXED TYPES

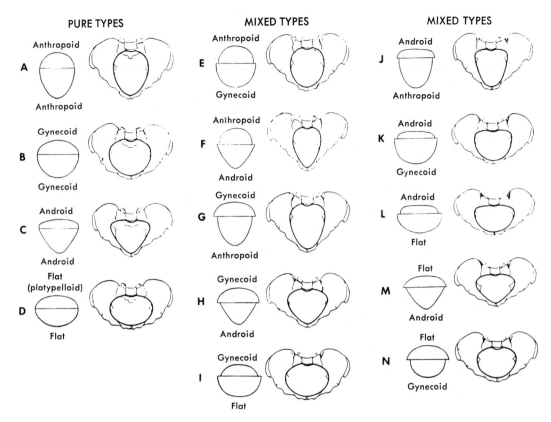

Fig. 36-4. Female pelvis showing pure and mixed types. (From Moloy, H.C.: Am. J. Obstet. Gynecol. **48:**149, 1944.)

in 20% to 30% of white women and 40% to 45% of black women. The transverse diameter of the inlet is reduced, making it a long narrow oval with an increase in the lengths of both the anterior and posterior segments. The sacrosciatic notch is wide and shallow, and the sacrum has an average curvature but is long and narrow. The subpubic arch is narrowed. The side walls of the pelvis are straight, but both the bispinous and the bituberous diameters are shortened.

PLATYPELLOID PELVIS. Platypelloid (flat) pelvis occurs in 2% to 5% of white women and only occasionally in black women. The transverse diameter of the inlet is lengthened, and the anteroposterior diameter is reduced. Both segments are rounded but flat, and the retropubic angle is rounded. The sacrum is normal, but the sacrosciatic notch is narrowed. The subpubic angle is wide.

The side walls are straight, but the bispinous and bituberous diameters are increased.

MIXED TYPES. Pelves in which the anterior and posterior segments are of different types are frequently encountered. They are named by mentioning first the shape of the posterior segment and then that of the anterior segment.

ESTIMATION OF PELVIC CAPACITY
Clinical pelvimetry

Clinical measurements are less accurate than those obtained by x-ray film examination, but they are adequate for almost all patients. In the past a ritual was made of measuring the external diameters, but these are of little clinical significance and give no information concerning the size of the cavity. Internal measurements can be made at any period of normal pregnancy and, if carefully per-

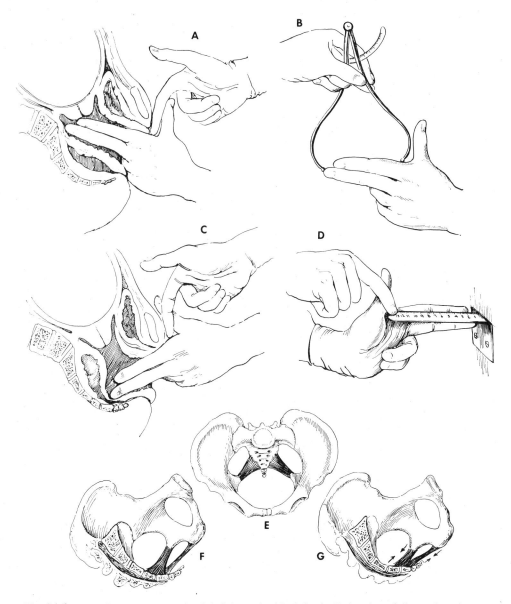

Fig. 36-5. Manual measurement of pelvic inlet and midpelvis. **A,** Estimation of diagonal conjugate diameter. **B** and **D,** Methods for measuring anteroposterior diameters. **C,** Estimation of anteroposterior diameter of outlet. **E** to **G,** Differences in length of sacrospinous and sacrotuberous ligaments estimated by sweeping examining finger along them. (From Willson, J.R.: Management of obstetric difficulties, ed. 6, St. Louis, 1961, The C.V. Mosby Co.)

formed, will provide a considerable amount of information concerning the pelvis.

Pelvic inlet. The only diameter of the inlet that can be measured with even reasonable accuracy is the *diagonal conjugate* (Fig. 36-5). From this mea-

surement the length of the conjugata vera can then be estimated.

With the patient in lithotomy position, legs abducted, and the buttocks slightly over the edge of the table, the examiner's index and second fingers are inserted through the introitus until the sacrum is reached. The elbow is depressed until it rests against the examiner's hip, with which firm pressure is exerted, pushing the palpating fingers upward along the sacrum toward the promontory as the flexed third and fourth fingers flatten the perineum. When the tip of the second finger touches the promontory or can be inserted no farther, the entire hand is pivoted forward until the radial surface of the index finger or its metacarpal presses against the apex of the pubic arch. The index finger of the opposite hand marks the point on the examining hand that touches the inferior border of the pubis, and the fingers are withdrawn from the vagina. The depth of insertion can be determined by measuring the distance between the tip of the second finger and the point at which the symphysis was contacted. If the promontory is touched, this represents the length of the diagonal conjugate (DC). If the promontory is not reached, the measurement should be recorded as the distance the fingers were inserted plus (DC = 10 cm plus), which will indicate that the greatest distance is greater than that noted.

The *conjugata vera* is estimated by subtracting 1.5 to 2 cm from the DC. If the pubic depth is short, 1.5 cm is subtracted; and if long, 2 cm. Physicians cannot even estimate the true conjugate if they fail to touch the promontory, but if the fingers can be inserted at least 11.5 cm, the anteroposterior diameter probably is normal.

The *transverse diameter* cannot be measured, but the width of the inlet can be estimated by attempting to palpate the linea terminalis. If the entire lateral border of the inlet can be touched on each side, the transverse diameter probably is shortened.

Midpelvis. The *bispinous diameter* cannot be measured clinically, but an impression as to the adequacy of the midpelvis can be obtained. The normal ischial spine projects only slightly into the cavity. If the spines are long, sharp, and heavy, the physician should suspect that the midpelvis is small. This is more likely to be true if the subpubic arch is narrow and if there is considerable resistance as the fingers are swept from one side of the pelvis to the other (Fig. 36-6).

If the sacral curvature is flattened, or if the sacrum is rotated farther anteriorly than usual, the anteroposterior diameter at the midpelvis and the outlet will be reduced. This is associated with shortening of the sacrospinous ligaments, which ordinarily are about 4 cm long. Posterior rotation of the sacrum increases both the anteroposterior diameter and the length of the sacrospinous ligaments (Fig. 36-5). The sacrum, the ischial spines, and the ligaments can be felt most accurately by rectal palpation.

Pelvic outlet. The *angle of the pubic arch* can be estimated by laying a thumb or forefinger along the inner aspect of each ramus with their tips meeting at the symphysis (Fig. 36-7). The normal subpubic angle is at least

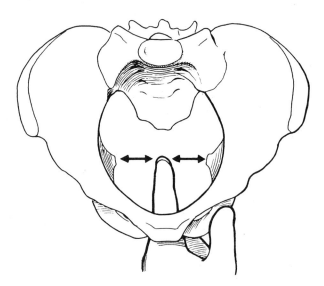

Fig. 36-6. Estimation of bispinous diameter. (From Moloy, H.C.: Evaluation of the pelvis in obstetrics, Philadelphia, 1951, W.B. Saunders Co.)

85 degrees. The angle probably is reduced if it is impossible to separate the index and second fingers placed side by side beneath the symphysis. The curvature of the pubic rami should also be studied.

The length of the *bituberous diameter* (Fig. 36-8) alone does not determine the adequacy of the outlet because the distance between the tuberosities varies with the depth of the pelvis and the subpubic angle. If the true pelvis is deep, the bituberous diameter may be of normal length even though the subpubic angle is considerably below normal (Fig. 36-9).

The bituberous diameter can be measured with a suitable pelvimeter, but the measurement is not particularly accurate. The amount of fat overlying the bone varies, and it may be difficult to determine exactly where the most widely separated points on the tuberosities are lo-

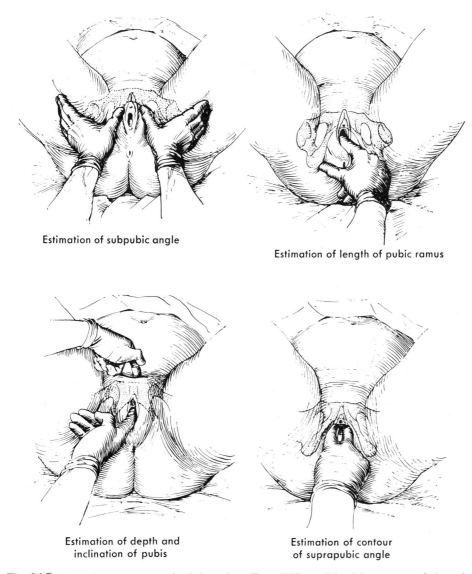

Estimation of subpubic angle

Estimation of length of pubic ramus

Estimation of depth and
inclination of pubis

Estimation of contour
of suprapubic angle

Fig. 36-7. Manual measurement of pelvic outlet. (From Willson, J.R.: Management of obstetric difficulties, ed. 6, St. Louis, 1961, The C.V. Mosby Co.)

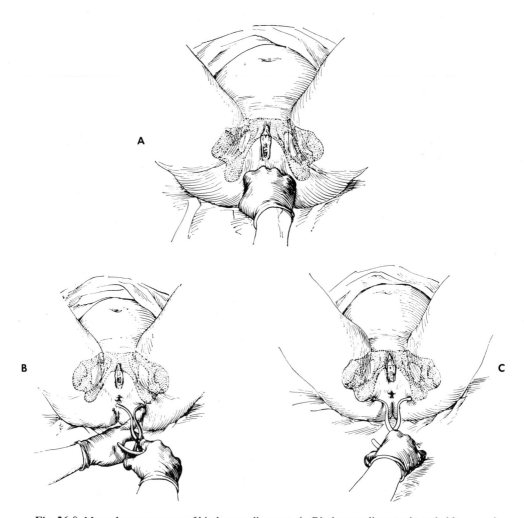

Fig. 36-8. Manual measurement of bituberous diameter. **A,** Bituberous diameter is probably normal if average-sized clenched fist can be inserted between tuberosities. **B** and **C,** Measurement with DeLee pelvimeter taken between inner surfaces of tuberosities as far posteriorly as possible. (From Willson, J.R.: Management of obstetric difficulties, ed. 6, St. Louis, 1961, The C.V. Mosby Co.)

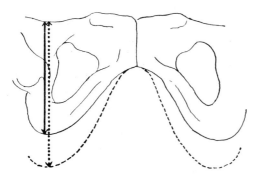

Fig. 36-9. Variations in width of bituberous diameter with differences in length of pubic rami. With deep pelvis, bituberous diameter may be normal even though angle is narrow. (From Caldwell, W.E., and Moloy, H.C.: Am. J. Obstet. Gynecol. **26:**479, 1933.)

cated. The measurement will be short if taken too far anteriorly. The physician can also estimate the adequacy of the outlet by attempting to insert a clenched fist between the tuberosities. If the average-sized male fist can be placed between the tuberosities, the outlet should be of ample size.

The *anteroposterior diameter* of the outlet is obtained in much the same manner as the diagonal conjugate. The fingers are inserted until the sacrococcygeal junction can be palpated, and the distance between the fingertip and the point at which the index finger contacted the lower border of the symphysis is measured.

Although each of these measurements is described individually and the pelvis is divided into the three main areas, variations rarely affect only one portion. For example, if the sacrum is straight and the bispinous diameter is reduced, the side walls usually converge, and the subpubic angle and the bituberous diameter are reduced.

CONTRACTED PELVIS

Any pelvis that is reduced in size or distorted enough to interfere with normal labor can be considered as contracted.

Classification. The classification of Caldwell and Moloy includes the normal growth types, as well as abnormalities caused by disease, injury, or congenital defects.

1. *Normal growth types:* Gynecoid, android, anthropoid, and platypelloid
2. *Abnormal growth types:* Infantile and dwarf
3. *Types caused by disease of the pelvic bones and joints:* Rachitic, congenital, inflammatory, atypical, and traumatic
4. *Types secondary to abnormalities of the spinal column:* Kyphotic, scoliotic, kyphoscoliotic, and spondylolisthetic
5. *Types secondary to abnormalities of the lower extremities:* Femoral luxation, atrophy, or loss of extremity

Other common terms used to describe abnormal pelves are *generally contracted,* which is equivalent to a gynecoid type; *funnel* or *masculine,* which is equivalent to the android type; and *simple flat,* which is equivalent to the platypelloid type. The configuration of each is like that of its normal parent growth type, but the measurements are reduced.

Effect on pregnancy. There usually is no change during pregnancy except in patients with pronounced contractions of the pelvic inlet. Because of the reduced measurements, the fetus is more likely to be carried high, and lightening is less likely to occur.

Effect on labor and delivery. Since lightening may not occur in women with inlet contraction, the head is likely to be unengaged or even above the pelvic brim when labor begins. Abnormal positions and presentations occur more frequently in women with contracted pelves; deflexed attitudes of the head, shoulder presentations, and compound presentations are encountered two to three times as often. The labor is likely to be prolonged and more difficult, and the incidence of cesarean delivery is increased.

Mechanism of labor. Significant alterations in the size or shape of the bony pelvis naturally affect the course of labor, but, since the shapes of many contracted pelves are like those of the normal growth types, the mechanism is often similar to that which occurs normally.

GYNECOID PELVIS. The mechanism in the small gynecoid pelvis is like that in the normal pelvis except that the head must flex at a higher level and mold more to descend through the inlet. Because all the diameters are reduced, resistance to descent is encountered at all levels of the birth canal.

PLATYPELLOID PELVIS. The main alteration in shape and size in the platypelloid pelvis involves the anteroposterior diameter of the inlet; consequently, delay occurs during the first and the early second stages of labor. The head must engage in the transverse diameter; therefore descent will be impeded if the anteroposterior measurement of the inlet is less than the biparietal diameter of the fetal skull (9.5 cm). The mechanism by which the head enters the small inlet is an exaggeration of the normal. The head assumes an attitude of exaggerated asynclitism, with the anterior parietal bone presenting over the inlet *(anterior parietal bone presentation)* and the sagittal structure in the transverse diameter just anterior to the promontory. With each contraction, the parietal bones are forced against the sacrum posteriorly and the pubis anteriorly, gradually causing their edges to approximate each other at the sagittal suture while the two parietal plates are elevated in relation to the frontal and occipital bones. This is called *molding* and serves to decrease the biparietal diameter. While the head is being molded, the anterior parietal bone is forced downward behind the pubis where it remains fixed, acting as a fulcrum on which lateral flexion takes place as the uterine contractions force the posterior parietal eminence past the promontory. As this occurs, the sagittal suture gradually approaches the anterior segment of the inlet. As soon as the biparietal diameter has passed the inlet, the head descends through the pelvis in the transverse diameter, usually not rotating until it reaches the pelvic floor.

The mechanism with *posterior parietal bone presentation,* which occurs somewhat less frequently, is the reverse of that just described.

If the parietal bosses ride above the promontory posteriorly and the pubis anteriorly with the sagittal suture near the center of the pelvis (synclitism), another mechanism may occur. Since the head cannot descend, it extends slightly with each contraction until the relatively short bitemporal diameter is forced into the inlet. This is one of the mechanisms by which deflexed attitudes are produced.

The primary effect of inlet contraction is on engagement, but it may also interfere with normal termination of labor. If much molding, elongation of the head, and caput formation occur, the lowest portion of the head can descend well down into the pelvis before the biparietal diameter passes through the inlet. The anteroposterior diameters are so short, and the head fits the inlet so tightly that it can neither rotate to an anterior position nor follow the curve of the sacrum anteriorly, so it remains wedged in the transverse position; consequently, descent ceases even though the capacity of the lower pelvis is ample. This is called *transverse arrest* of the head. *Deep* transverse arrest occurs with the lowest portion of the head below station 2, and *high* transverse arrest with the head near the spines.

ANDROID PELVIS. In the android pelvis the anterior segment of the inlet is wedge shaped, and the posterior segment is flattened; consequently, the head often descends in an oblique occipitoposterior position. In this position the relatively narrow frontal portion of the head fits better into the forepelvis than does the broad occipital area. The occiput usually descends to a point just below the ischial spines, but progress may cease at this level if convergence of the bony side walls is pronounced and if forward displacement of the sacrum considerably reduces the posterior sagittal diameter at the midpelvis. If the head can descend farther, the narrow lower pelvis may prevent anterior rotation of the occiput, but unless the diameters are too small, delivery in an occipito posterior position usually is possible.

ANTHROPOID PELVIS. In the anthropoid pelvis occipitoposterior positions are common; in fact, it may be impossible for the head to enter the pelvic inlet except in an occipitoposterior or occipitoanterior position. Because the transverse diameter is reduced along the entire length of the pelvis, the head usually descends and de-

livers without rotating. Occasionally, the head fails to enter the inlet, either because of extreme transverse narrowing or because it lies in a transverse or oblique position rather than an occipitoanterior or occipitoposterior position, which is more favorable in transversely contracted pelves.

Management of labor. For purposes of treatment, abnormal pelves can be divided into those in which the primary contraction is at the inlet and those in which the primary contraction involves the midpelvis and outlet.

Abnormal labor can be anticipated in women with reduced pelvic measurements or those in whom dystocia has occurred during previous labors. An unusual fetal position or a floating head at term should suggest the possibility of inlet disproportion, even though the measurements are normal.

A *sterile vaginal examination* with the patient in lithotomy position should be performed during early labor in any woman whose pelvic measurements are reduced or in whom there is any suggestion of disproportion. The biparietal diameter of the fetal head can be measured accurately by *sonography,* but this examination is of little help when disproportion is suspected.

INLET CONTRACTION. Inlet contraction can be diagnosed if the conjugata vera is 10 cm or less in length or if the diagonal conjugate measures 11.5 cm or less. The outcome of labor is in part dependent on the length of the true conjugate, but other important factors are pelvic configuration, size and position of the infant, and the effectiveness of the uterine contractions. Although it may not always be possible to prognosticate the eventual outcome, inlet contractions are usually relatively easy to manage as compared with the abnormalities involving the lower pelvis.

A reasonably accurate evaluation of whether the head will pass the inlet can be obtained at vaginal examination. Disproportion can be diagnosed if it is impossible to insert the first two fingers between the head in the inlet and the posterior surface of the pubis or if the head is overriding the pubis and cannot be forced into the inlet by downward pressure on the uterine fundus or on the suprapubic portion of the head. If the head can be pushed down to station minus 1 or 0, the size of the inlet probably is adequate. However, the inability to impress the head into the pelvis does not prove that there is significant disproportion. Reevaluation of cervical dilatation and descent after a period of electronically monitored active labor should provide the answer for the route of delivery.

Elective cesarean section. An elective cesarean section is usually indicated in women at least 38 weeks pregnant if the conjugata vera is 8.5 cm or less with vertex presentation. Any abnormality in pelvic shape and size justifies cesarean section for breech presentations.

Trial labor. Since most women with mild inlet contractions and some of those with more pronounced deformities will deliver vaginally if the uterine contractions are forceful enough, almost all should be allowed to undergo a trial labor. If the uterine contractions are of normal quality and recur every 3 to 5 minutes, the physician can ordinarily decide within 8 to 10 hours whether vaginal delivery is possible. If the inlet contraction can be overcome, the cervix will dilate, and the head will descend through the superior strait. If this occurs, labor can be permitted to continue with the expectation that it will terminate normally even though it may take longer than usual.

The physician must make certain that descent and engagement actually are occurring. In some instances the lower portion of the head descends into the pelvis, giving the appearance of steady progress in labor. In reality the apparent descent is a result of extreme molding and elongation of the skull and edema of the scalp (caput succedaneum) while the biparietal diameter remains stationary above the plane of the inlet. If there is any question concerning descent, a lateral x-ray film study should be done. If descent does not occur, cesarean section can be performed safely after an adequate trial labor.

The membranes usually rupture spontaneously during the course of labor, but, if they do not, they should be ruptured artificially. Intact membranes will sometimes prevent the head from descending, even though the pelvic capacity is perfectly adequate for delivery. The head often descends and delivers after amniotomy. There is some danger of the cord prolapsing if the amniotic sac is perforated while the presenting part is high. If this should occur, it is immediately obvious, and the infant can be delivered alive by cesarean section.

Unfortunately, a good trial labor is not always possible. Many women with contracted pelves also have abnormal labors with irregular, ineffective uterine con-

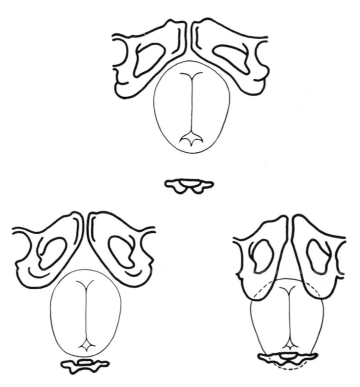

Fig. 36-10. Reduced bituberous diameter showing effect of length of posterior sagittal diameter on outcome. (From Willson, J.R.: Management of obstetric difficulties, ed. 6, St. Louis, 1961, The C.V. Mosby Co.)

tractions. Others will begin what appears to be a normal labor, cervical dilatation progressing to 6 to 7 cm after which the contractions become irregular and ineffective—an *active phase arrest*. This is a common response to cephalopelvic disproportion in primigravidas. Oxytocin stimulation is justified if the physician determines that the disproportion is minor. If it seems obvious that vaginal delivery will not occur, even with forceful uterine contractions, cesarean section should be performed. If the disproportion is insurmountable, the uterus can rupture.

Sedatives may be administered if the labor is normal. If the labor is abnormal, an intrauterine pressure catheter should be used, and the uterine activity improved with intravenous pitocin. The patient should be kept comfortable with sedation and/or an epidural anesthetic. Orificial examinations should be kept at a minimum to reduce the chance of infection; descent can be followed by palpating the anterior shoulder and measuring its distance above the pubis.

MIDPELVIC AND OUTLET CONTRACTION. There is no reliable method for evaluating the adequacy of the lower pelvis, and a trial labor is much less satisfactory than with inlet contractions. Sterile vaginal examination should be performed early in the course of labor; if the head has already reached the level of the spines and can be depressed farther, it probably will continue to descend and will deliver unless the outlet is too small. On the other hand, if the head is high, in a posterior position, and cannot be depressed past the long spines and the anteriorly projecting sacrum, the outlook is less favorable. Cesarean section is always preferable to a traumatic forceps extraction (Fig. 36-10).

If the head descends beyond station plus 2, vaginal delivery usually is possible. The head can be turned to an anterior position by manual or forceps rotation. If the attempt at delivery is unsuccessful or if it appears that extraction will be too traumatic, cesarean section should be performed.

Complications. Infant mortality and morbidity should not increase if the fetus is monitored electronically during labor and if a traumatic vaginal delivery is avoided. Injury to the brachial plexus may occur during attempts to overcome shoulder dystocia.

REFERENCES

Caldwell, W.E., and Moloy, H.C.: Anatomical variations in the female pelvis and their effect on labor with a suggested classification, Am. J. Obstet. Gynecol. **26:**479, 1933.

Caldwell, W.E., and Swenson, P.C.: The use of the roentgen ray in obstetrics. II. The mechanism of labor, Am. J. Roentgenol. **41:**719, 1939.

Javert, C.T., and Steele, K.B.: The transverse position and the mechanism of labor, Int. Abstr. Surg. **75:**507, 1942.

Kaltreider, D.F.: Pelvic shape and its relation to midplane prognosis, Am. J. Obstet. Gynecol. **63:**116, 1952.

Moloy, H.C.: Pelvic model manikins to show pelvic shape and to demonstrate labor mechanisms, Am. J. Obstet. Gynecol. **48:**149, 1944.

Steer, C.M.: Evaluation of the pelvis in obstetrics, Philadelphia, 1959, W.B. Saunders Co.

Tancer, M.L., and Vandenberg, W.: Disproportion in the multipara, Obstet. Gynecol. **14:**753, 1959.

37

J. Robert Willson

Multifetal pregnancy

Pregnancies in which more than one fetus is produced are associated with more complications than are single births.

Types. Twins are either *dizygotic* (double-ovum, or fraternal) or *monozygotic* (single-ovum, or identical). In *dizygotic twins,* two separate ova produced during the same period of ovulation are fertilized by two spermatozoa. The twins need not be of the same sex, and often they do not resemble each other any more than singly born siblings. There are two separate placentas with no communication between the two circulatory systems, although the placentas may be so completely fused that they look like a single structure. The infants are separated from each other by two layers of amnion and two of chorion (Fig. 37-1). About two thirds of all twin pregnancies are dizygotic.

Monozygotic twins occur in about a third of all twin pregnancies. Since both infants develop from a single fertilized ovum, they are always of the same sex and are either almost identical in appearance or are mirror images. In 25% to 30% of monozygotic twins the two daughter cells separate within 3 to 4 days after fertilization; as a consequence, each twin has its own complete placenta and membranes (Fig. 37-2). Occasionally, the separation into two distinct embryos occurs 7 to 13 days after fertilization but after the amniotic cavity has formed. In this type, *monoamniotic twins,* there

is a single placenta, and both infants develop in a common amniotic cavity. The *monochorionic-diamniotic placenta characteristic of 70% to 75% of monozygotic twin pregnancies* develops when separation occurs between these two extremes. The circulations of the two fetuses communicate with each other through the blood vessels in the shared placenta, and each fetus is enclosed in its own amniotic sac, but both sacs are surrounded by a single chorionic membrane. Thus, in contrast to dizygotic twins, monochorionic-diamniotic fetuses are separated from each other by only two layers of amnion.

Conjoined twins are formed when separation is incomplete. The degree of the deformity is determined by which area of the fetus failed to separate.

More than two fetuses develop by the same mechanisms as do twins, but there are more opportunities for variation in each pregnancy. For example, two of triplets may be monozygotic and the third from a second ovum, all may be fraternal if three ova were fertilized, or all may arise from one ovum. The same possibilities hold true for any number of fetuses.

Superfecundation is a term indicating that two ova produced at the same ovulation were fertilized after two separate acts of coitus. The pregnancies, of course, are always dizygotic. Superfecundation can be suspected if individuals of two or more races

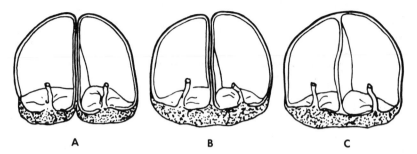

Fig. 37-1. Placenta and membranes in twin pregnancy. **A,** Dizygotic twins with two complete placentas and membranes. **B,** Dizygotic twins with double membranes and fused placenta. **C,** Monozygotic twins with double amniotic cavities enclosed within one chorion. (Modified from Eastman, N.J., and Hellman, L.M.: Obstetrics, New York, 1961, Appleton-Century-Crofts.)

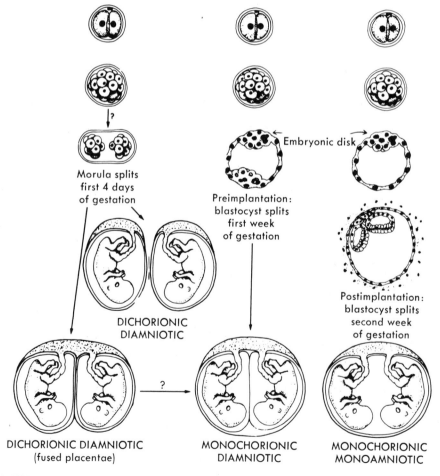

Fig. 37-2. Varieties of monozygotic twinning. (From Hafez, E.S.E.: J. Reprod. Med. **12:**88, 1974.)

are involved; each offspring will have the characteristics of its father superimposed on those of the mother. It can be proved by HLA testing of the children and the putative fathers. HLA haplotypes are so varied that it is unlikely that they are often duplicated by chance. Thus superfecundation can be substantiated if the haplotypes of each of two suspected fathers match those of each of two twins.

Incidence. Greulich reported the following incidences of spontaneous multifetal pregnancies in more than 21 million births: twins, 1:85; triplets, 1:7629; quadruplets, 1:670,734; and quintuplets, 1:41,600,000. These figures have been altered by a number of artificial etiologic factors.

Racial differences in the rate of twinning are interesting. According to Guttmacher spontaneous twinning occurs in ratios of 1:73.8 single births in black women and in 1:92.4 single births in white women. Comparable figures for triplets are 1:5631 and 1:9828. The lowest rate occurs in Orientals. The differences result from variations in the rates of dizygotic twinning; the rates of monozygotic twins are the same in all races.

Multifetal pregnancies occur much more often in some families than in others. *Genetic factors* influence only the rate of dizygotic (fraternal) twinning; monozygotic (identical) twins appear to develop by chance. The father has little influence on twinning. Women who themselves are dizygotic twins produce twins at a rate of 17.1/1000 deliveries, whereas the rate for wives of husbands who are dizygotic twins is only 7.9/1000 deliveries. Female siblings of dizygotic twins behave like female twins in this regard, but the male siblings behave like male twins.

The differences in dizygotic twinning probably are related to *differences in gonadotropin production*. The number of ovulations that can be stimulated in experimental animals is determined by the dosage of gonadotropin administered. It is well known that multiple ovulations can occur in women treated with clomiphene and human FSH. The hereditary factor in twinning may be that gonadotropin production is higher in women who produce dizygotic twins than in those who produce only singletons.

Martin and co-workers compared serum gonadotropins and estradiol concentrations during early and midfollicular phases of the menstrual cycle in seven women who had had two sets of dizygotic twins and one who had had one set with those of five who had had only singletons and one who had had monozygotic twins. During the early follicular phases both FSH and LH were higher, and during the midfollicular phases estradiol concentrations were higher in those who had had dizygotic twins than in the controls.

Maternal age and parity influence the rate of multifetal pregnancy. It occurs less often during the first pregnancy in young women than in multiparas past the age of 35.

Ron-El and colleagues reported an incidence of triplets of 1:1696 and of quadruplets of 1:5370 in their department between 1970 and 1978; 72% followed the use of *ovulation-inducing* agents.

Another minor factor is in vitro fertilization in which all fertilized ova are deposited in the uterus. As many as four have implanted and survived until delivery.

Rothman reported an increase in dizygotic twinning in women who conceived soon *after discontinuing the use of oral contraceptives*. Bracken confirmed this observation, but Harlap found an increased rate only in those who had used sequential preparations and in those taking oral contraceptives with high concentrations of estrogens. Any increase in oral contraceptive users may be related to age and fertility rather than to the drugs themselves.

The figures on incidence relate to deliveries rather than to conceptions. The actual number of multifetal gestations is unknown, because one or more embryos or small fetuses may die and be resorbed, leaving no trace of their existence. Occasionally, one of a set of double ovum twins may be aborted while the other continues to develop. This can also occur if pregnancies exist in both sides of a double uterus. The increasing use of ultrasound suggests that as many as 50% of women in whom two or more gestational sacs are identified early in pregnancy may deliver singleton babies. The exact incidence can only be determined by routine sonography during the first few weeks of pregnancy.

Sex ratios. The proportion of male to female fetuses in multifetal pregnancy is less than in single births. The discrepancy is exaggerated as the number of fetuses increases: 50.85% of twin fetuses are male as compared with only 46.48% of quadruplets.

FETAL DEVELOPMENT

Each twin at birth is usually smaller than a single infant of the same gestational age, but the combined weights of the babies are likely to be much more. More than 50% of individual twins weigh less than 2500 g.

Small differences in size are usually unimportant, but if one twin is much larger than the other, the physician should consider the possibility of *transfusion syndrome*. The larger twin is plethoric, edematous, and polycythemic and has cardiac and renal hypertrophy. There also is an accompanying hydramnios. The smaller twin is pale, anemic, and dehydrated and has less than the usual amount of amniotic fluid. The basic cause is an inequality in placental circulation resulting from anastomoses between the placental arteries of one twin and the placental veins of the other. The degree of change is determined by the number and size of anastomoses. With uncompensated arteriovenous anastomoses the recipient twin is constantly perfused by blood entering its circulation under high pressure from the donor twin's arteries. The recipient twin becomes plethoric, and the donor becomes hypovolemic and anemic.

In some instances one of the infants fails to develop and is deformed. One may die early and become compressed, whereas the other grows normally. This is called a *fetus papyraceus* (Fig. 37-3).

Malformations occur twice as often in twins as in singletons. More anomalies occur in monozygotic than in dizygotic twins. *Abortion* also occurs more often than when there is only one fetus.

CLINICAL COURSE

Nausea and vomiting may be more severe and persistent than in single-fetus pregnancies. Women with multifetal pregnancies are more uncomfortable because of the large uterus, and discomfort increases with each additional fetus. *Varicosities, backache, pelvic pressure, hemorrhoids, edema,* and *difficulty in breathing* occur frequently. The *volume of fluid in the combined amniotic sacs* is greater than with a single pregnancy, but the amount surrounding each infant is usually not abnormal, except with disorders such as the twin-to-twin transfusion syndrome or when other causes of hydramnios exist. The incidence of *pregnancy-induced hypertension* is increased, appears earlier, and is likely to be more severe. *Renal function* can be reduced significantly if the uterus is large enough to compress the ureters; kidney function returns to normal after delivery.

Labor usually begins before term, and the greater the number of fetuses the earlier it starts. Caspi and coworkers calculated the duration of pregnancy in 111 women in whom ovulation had been induced. Using a date 2 weeks before ovulation occurred as the beginning of pregnancy (comparable to the onset of the last menstruation in normal women) singletons delivered at 39 weeks, twins at 35 weeks, triplets at 33 weeks, and quadruplets at 29 weeks.

The *duration of labor* usually is normal. *Uterine dysfunction* may occur if the uterus is greatly overdistended. For the same reason *postpartum blood loss is often excessive.* Cephalopelvic disproportion is seldom encountered because each baby is relatively small.

The *position* of the infants is variable. Both heads may present, or one presentation may be a vertex and the other a breech. Occasionally, both present as breeches, or one may lie longitudinally and the other transversely.

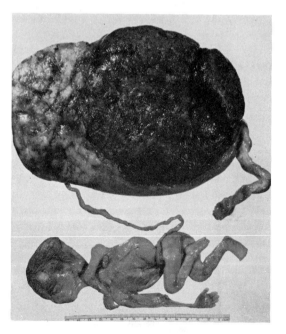

Fig. 37-3. Fetus papyraceus. Infarcted nonfunctioning placenta to which degenerated fetus is attached can be seen at left. Other infant was normal.

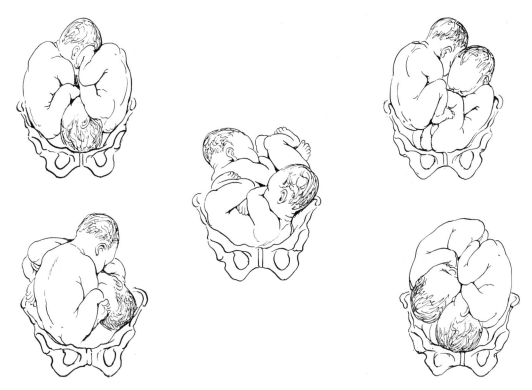

Fig. 37-4. Positions of twins in utero. (From Willson, J.R.: Atlas of obstetric technic, ed. 2, St. Louis, 1969, The C.V. Mosby Co.)

Abnormal position, particularly of the second twin, occurs more often than in single pregnancies (Fig. 37-4).

DIAGNOSIS

The diagnosis should be suspected if the uterus seems larger than it should for the calculated period of gestation, in the presence of an excessive amount of fluid, or if a profusion of small parts or more than one head or more than two fetal poles can be felt (Fig. 37-5). Unfortunately, multifetal pregnancy is often overlooked and, in as many as 50% of cases, is not diagnosed until late in pregnancy or after the first baby has been delivered.

The circumference of the abdomen at the umbilicus usually measures less than 100 cm in normal women at term; with multifetal pregnancy, it is usually larger. If two separate sets of fetal heart sounds that are widely separated and of different rates when counted simultaneously are heard, the diagnosis is certain.

Multifetal pregnancy can be diagnosed by *sonography* before the twelfth week if more than one gestational sac can be demonstrated and when the fetal skulls can be outlined. An ultrasound examination should be ordered whenever twin pregnancy is suspected and whenever pregnancy occurs after ovulation induction. It is preferable to x-ray film examination for confirming a clinical impression of multifetal pregnancy; unless the entire abdomen is scanned, however, the additional fetus(es) may be missed. *X-ray film examination* should generally be performed only late in pregnancy to determine the positions of fetuses if ultrasound examination is inconclusive.

This will permit the physician to anticipate problems that may arise during labor or delivery.

Concentrations of *chorionic gonadotropin, alpha-fetoprotein,* and *placental lactogen (chorionic somatomammotropin)* in maternal plasma are higher with twins than with a single fetus. These tests are not diagnostic of multifetal pregnancy.

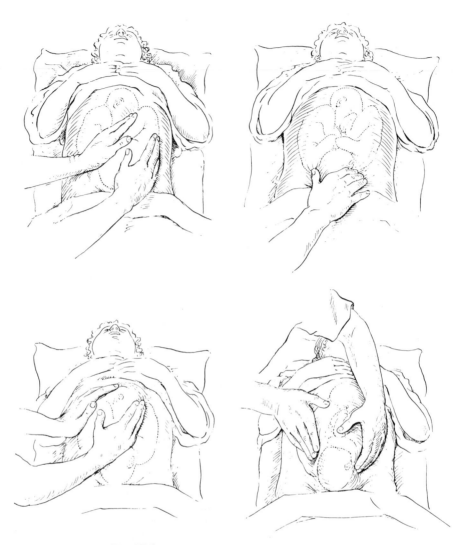

Fig. 37-5. Abdominal palpation of twin pregnancy.

Redford and Whitfield, however, have suggested that the level of alpha-fetoprotein may be a predictor of outcome in twin pregnancy. They measured maternal serum alpha-fetoprotein between 16 and 20 weeks in 145 twin pregnancies in which none of the fetuses had neural tube defects. When the serum concentration was less than two multiples of the mean for singletons, the outlook for pregnancy was good. Conversely, when the concentration was greater than four multiples of the mean for singletons, the outlook was poor. In the latter group perinatal mortality was 400/1000 as compared to 32.6/ 1000 in the others, mean duration of pregnancy was less, and mean birth weights were lower.

All the evidences of twin pregnancy are exaggerated when three or more infants develop. An exact count can be made only by x-ray film examination or sonography.

MANAGEMENT

Most women with multifetal pregnancy will be more comfortable with a maternity garment to support the large abdomen. Cervical effacement occurs earlier than with a single pregnancy, and, since labor usually begins before term, women with multifetal pregnancies should not travel during the last trimester.

The beneficial effect of prolonged bed rest, particularly as a way of preventing premature delivery, has not been proved conclusively. Persson and colleagues screened every pregnant woman in Malmö, Sweden, with ultrasound during the early second trimester; 86 of the total of 110 women with twin pregnancies agreed to participate in the study. They stopped work and rested at home until they were admitted to the hospital at the twenty-ninth week. The only treatment was bed rest. The outcome was compared with that of the remaining 24 women with twin pregnancies who were not in the study and with another group of 93 twins born in the same hospital 10 years before. Preterm delivery occurred in 20% of the study group and in 33% of the control subjects. Perinatal mortality in the study group was 0.6%, the same as for singletons, as compared with 10.5% in the 24 nonparticipants and 5.9% in those delivered 10 years before. This experience is confirmed by that of other investigators. Conversely, O'Connor and colleagues could detect no advantages of hospital bed rest for patients with twins as compared with those observed in a special "twins' clinic" and those managed by consultant obstetricians. The patients in the latter two groups were hospitalized only when complications arose or when progressive cervical dilatation was observed.

Although bed rest in the hospital during the early third trimester may be beneficial in prolonging pregnancy and in increasing fetal weight, it is costly. The average stay in the Malmö study was 55 days; one can plan on between 2 and 4 weeks. Bed rest is most effective if started early, at least by 30 weeks. There is no point in either starting after or in continuing after 36 weeks.

Cervical cerclage and *beta-sympathomimetic* agents have little effect on prolonging twin pregnancy and should be used only for indications other than multifetal pregnancy.

Labor and delivery. Compatible blood should be available to use if bleeding following delivery is excessive, and an intravenous infusion should be started through an 18-gauge needle when labor is well established. Twin pregnancy has little effect on the length of labor in either primigravidas or multiparas, but dysfunctional labor occurs more often than with single pregnancies. Artificial rupture of the presenting sac to reduce distention will generally improve labor.

If labor begins weeks before term, sedation must be used with caution; but when the pregnancy has pro-

gressed to 37 weeks or more, analgesic drugs ought not to harm the infants. However, *regional nerve block* is usually preferable.

The labor and delivery should be managed by an obstetrician who is experienced in the delivery of twins and who is capable of performing the operative maneuvers required for the delivery of both fetuses. If such a person is not available, most patients with twins should be transferred to a perinatal center for delivery, unless the fetuses are so immature that they have little chance of surviving. If there is no facility in the area, *cesarean section* is more appropriate than vaginal delivery if the fetuses are mature enough to survive.

Cesarean section should also be used more often for the delivery of premature twins, whenever breech or transverse presentations are diagnosed in one or both fetuses, when the second infant is considerably larger than the first, and for other complications such as premature rupture of the membranes when labor cannot be induced, dysfunctional labor that does not improve after amniotomy and the cautious administration of oxytocin, fetal distress during labor, prolapsed cord, and placenta previa or abruptio placentae or when delivery is necessary because of medical complications.

Vaginal delivery is appropriate when labor starts so early that the fetuses have little chance of surviving. It also may be selected for the delivery of mature infants when both are in vertex positions, if there are no contraindications to vaginal delivery, and if an experienced obstetrician, a capable anesthesiologist or anesthetist, and two attendants who are able to resuscitate depressed infants can be present at delivery.

The first child may be allowed to deliver spontaneously, or a low forceps delivery can be performed. The cord should be cut between two hemostats to prevent exsanguination of the second of monozygotic twins.

The position or even the lie of the second twin may change as the first baby leaves the uterus; consequently, the presenting part of the second infant should be identified soon after the first is delivered so that plans can be made for its delivery. This can be accomplished either by palpation or by ultrasound examination. As a general rule the membranes should be ruptured artificially, after which the vertex or breech usually descends into the upper pelvis. One must make sure that the cord did not prolapse after amniotomy. Uterine contractions usually recur when the membranes are ruptured; if they do, spontaneous delivery can be anticipated. If they do not, dilute oxytocin can be administered, or, depending on the conditions, a forceps extraction or breech extraction can be performed by an experienced obstetrician. As an alternative, cesarean section may be indicated for those who have had little experience in operative vaginal delivery. The fetal heart must be monitored constantly until the infant is delivered. The baby should be delivered immediately if bleeding suggesting placental separation occurs or for abnormal fetal heart rate patterns.

A prolonged wait after the delivery of the first fetus subjects the second to an undue hazard. The placenta may separate as the uterine muscle contracts, and cord prolapse is favored by the fact that the second presenting part is usually high or because the infant lies transversely. The results are best when the second twin is delivered within 10 to 15 minutes of the first.

If the second infant is lying transversely after the first delivers, a decision must be made promptly as to how it can be delivered with the least chance of injury. If the back is directed toward the fundus of the uterus, an experienced obstetrician can usually deliver it by bringing the legs through the cervix and extracting it as a breech *(version and extraction)*. The major problems are those encountered in any breech extraction. If the back lies over the cervix with the extremities in the fundus, version is difficult to perform, and the fetus is likely to be injured. Under these conditions cesarean delivery usually is preferred. Cesarean section may also be performed if the position of the second twin changes from vertex to breech or transverse during the delivery of the first infant and the operator has had little experience in delivering babies in these positions.

An alternative to cesarean section is to attempt external version on the second twin. Chervenak and co-workers were able to rotate 18 of 25 second twins from breech or transverse to vertex positions after the first had been delivered. Cesarean section was necessary after two successful versions, but the other 16 were delivered vaginally.

Regional anesthesia is preferable to inhalation anesthesia for vaginal twin delivery because pregnancy often terminates prematurely and because the distended uterus tends to contract poorly. Pudendal block alone or supplemented by nitrous oxide-oxygen during the delivery may be adequate. Intrauterine manipulation for delivery of the second twin usually cannot be performed with pudendal block or conduction anesthesia alone; hence deep inhalation anesthesia is necessary.

Occasionally, the placenta of the first infant will deliver while the second twin is still in the uterus, but more often both placentas are extruded simultaneously after both babies have been born. If the placenta cannot be expressed by the usual maneuvers, it must be removed manually. The placenta may separate partially after the first child is born. When this occurs, the second infant must be delivered or it will die of anoxia.

Most triplet and quadruplet pregnancies should be terminated by cesarean section in a perinatal center.

Complications. *Prolapsed cord* occurs more often than in single pregnancies and is more likely to complicate the delivery of the second infant than the first.

Collision between two fetal poles attempting to enter the inlet simultaneously may delay descent (Fig. 37-6). Cesarean section usually is preferable to trying to manipulate the fetuses into more favorable positions. If the first infant presents as a breech and the second as a vertex, *the heads may lock at the inlet* after the body of the presenting twin has been delivered (Fig. 37-7). According to Cohen, Kohl, and Rosenthal, locking occurs once in 817 twin deliveries and once in 87 with breech-vertex presentations. This is a grave complication, particularly for the first infant, who will usually die of anoxia during the manipulations necessary to free the heads. The problem can be prevented by early cesarean section.

An important way to reduce mortality is to recognize the *transfusion syndrome* promptly and treat the babies properly. The plethoric infant may develop cardiac failure; the dangers from this can be reduced by phlebotomy. The anemic baby needs blood and should be transfused. The blood withdrawn from the plethoric twin can be administered.

Prognosis. The perinatal mortality, 10% to 15%, is considerably higher than that for single births. The principal causes of death are the complications of prematurity, infection, prolapsed cord, anoxia during delivery of the aftercoming head, and injury. The mortality for monozygotic twins is two to three times that for dizygotic.

Many of the complications can be prevented if the labor and delivery are managed by an experienced obstetrician in a perinatal center. This is particularly true if vaginal delivery is planned. The mortality for the second twin is higher than that for the first because it may assume an abnormal position making vaginal delivery difficult; and because it may be larger than the first baby, the size may impede its delivery. The number of deaths can be reduced if the second infant is delivered promptly by forceps or breech extraction or by version and extraction, if the obstetrician has been trained to perform

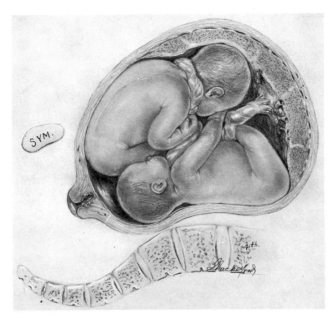

Fig. 37-6. Collision of twins at superior strait, preventing engagement of either. (From Willson, J.R.: Management of obstetric difficulties, ed. 6, St. Louis, 1961, The C.V. Mosby Co.)

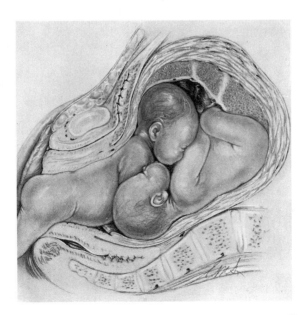

Fig. 37-7. Locking of twins. (From Willson, J.R.: Management of obstetric difficulties, ed. 6, St. Louis, 1961, The C.V. Mosby Co.)

these operations, or by cesarean section if that seems to be more appropriate.

The maternal risk is somewhat increased because of the relatively high incidence of postpartum hemorrhage.

REFERENCES

Benirschke, K., and Kim, C.K.: Multiple pregnancy, N. Engl. J. Med. **288:**1276, 1973.

Bracken, M.B.: Oral contraception and twinning: an epidemiologic study, Am. J. Obstet. Gynecol. **133:**432, 1979.

Caspi, E., et al.: The outcome of pregnancy after gonadotropin therapy, Br. J. Obstet. Gynaecol. **83:**967, 1976.

Chervenak, F.A., et al.: Intrapartum version of the second twin, Obstet. Gynecol. **62:**160, 1983.

Cohen, M., Kohl, S.G., and Rosenthal, A.H.: Fetal interlocking complicating twin gestation, Am. J. Obstet. Gynecol. **91:**407, 1965.

Greulich, W.W.: The incidence of human multiple births, Am. Natur. **64:**142, 1930.

Guttmacher, A.F.: The incidence of multiple births in man and some of the other unipara. Obstet. Gynecol. **2:**22, 1953.

Harlap, S.: Multiple births in former oral contraceptive users, Br. J. Obstet. Gynaecol. **86:**557, 1979.

Martin, N.G., et al.: Pituitary-ovarian function in mothers who have had two sets of dizygotic twins, Fertil. Steril. **41:**878, 1984.

Misenheimer, H.R., and Kaltreider, D.F.: Effects of decreased activity in patients with twin pregnancy, Obstet. Gynecol. **51:**692, 1978.

O'Connor, M.C., Arias, E., Royston, J.P., and Dalrymple, I.J.: The merits of special antenatal care for twin pregnancies, Br. J. Obstet. Gynaecol. **88:**222, 1981.

Olofsson, P., and Rydhstrom, H.: Twin delivery: how should the second twin be delivered?, Am. J. Obstet. Gynecol. **153:**479, 1985.

Persson, P.-H., Grennert, L., Gennser, G., and Kullander, S.: On improved outcome of twin pregnancies, Acta Obstet. Gynecol. Scand. **58:**3, 1979.

Redford, D.H.A., and Whitfield, C.R.: Maternal serum alpha-fetoprotein in twin pregnancies uncomplicated by neural tube defect, Am. J. Obstet. Gynecol. **152:**550, 1985.

Ron-El, R., Caspi, E., Schreyer, P., Weinraub, Z., Arieli, S., and Goldberg, M.D.: Triplet and quadruplet pregnancies and management, Obstet. Gynecol. **57:**458, 1981.

Rothman, K.J.: Fetal loss, twinning and birth weight after oral contraceptive use, N. Engl. J. Med. **297:**468, 1977.

Strandskov, H.H.: Plural birth frequencies in total, ''white'' and ''colored'' U.S. populations, Am. J. Phys. Anthropol. **3:**49, 1945.

Terasaki, P.I., Gjertson, D., Bernoco, D., Perdue, S., Mickey, M.R., and Bond, J.: Twins with two different fathers identified by HLA, N. Engl. J. Med. **299:**590, 1978.

White, C., and Wyshak, G.: Inheritance in human dizygotic twinning, N. Engl. J. Med. **271:**1003, 1964.

38

J. Robert Willson

Breech delivery

Breech positions, which occur in about 3.5% of all singleton deliveries of infants weighing more than 2500 g (5½ pounds), are longitudinal lies in which the buttocks alone or the buttocks and some portion of one or both lower extremities descend through the birth canal first. The sacrum is the guiding point; therefore the possible positions in the maternal pelvis are sacroanterior (SA), left and right sacroanterior (LSA-RSA), left and right sacrotransverse (LST-RST), left and right sacroposterior (LSP-RSP), and direct sacroposterior (SP) (Fig. 38-1).

VARIETIES OF FETAL ATTITUDE (Fig. 38-2)

In the *frank breech,* which is present in about two thirds of all breech deliveries of babies weighing more than 2500 g, the infant's hips are flexed on the abdomen, and the knees are extended so that the feet lie in front of the face or the head. In a *complete breech,* the attitude is one of complete flexion; both the hips and knees are flexed, and the feet present with the buttocks. With the less common *incomplete breech* attitudes, one foot *(single footling)* or both feet *(double footling)* descend through the cervix ahead of the buttocks because the hips and knees are partially extended. In the other type of incomplete breech, one or both *knees present* because of partial or complete extension of the hips, whereas the knees remain flexed.

ETIOLOGIC FACTORS

The capacity of the fundal area of the uterus is decreased when the placenta is implanted in one of the cornua. With cornual implantation the head may fit better in the fundus than will the larger mass of buttocks, feet, and legs. Fianu and Vaclavinkova, with ultrasound, found cornual placental implantations in 73% of women with breech presentations at or near term but in only 5% of those with cephalic presentations. When breech positions recur in successive pregnancies, congenital uterine anomalies such as bicornuate uterus may be a cause. Other factors include multiparity, hydramnios, multifetal pregnancy, fetal anomalies, and low implantation of the placenta.

Breech positions are common before the thirty-second week of pregnancy when the fetus can move freely within the uterus because the volume of amniotic fluid is relatively greater than it will be later in pregnancy. They can be diagnosed in almost a third of pregnancies between 25 and 28 weeks and in about 15% between 29 and 32 weeks.

Fetal motion plays an important part in decreasing the rate of occurrence of breech positions as pregnancy advances. When the knees are extended, the ability of the fetus to make crawling motions is eliminated, and conversion does not occur. Extension of the knees may account for the high percentage of frank breech positions in late pregnancy, most of those with flexed knees having converted to vertex. A small dead fetus, however, can be changed from breech to vertex position by uterine activity.

517

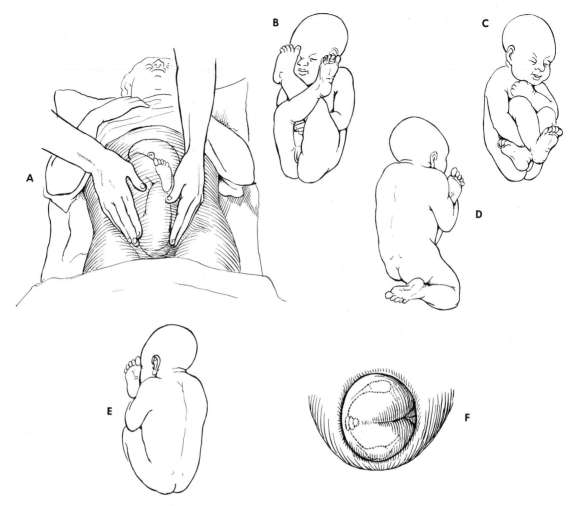

Fig. 38-1. Breech positions. **A,** Right sacrotransverse. **B,** Left sacroposterior. **C,** Right sacroposterior. **D,** Right sacroanterior. **E,** Left sacroanterior. **F,** Right sacrotransverse. (**A** to **H** from Willson, J.R.: Atlas of obstetric technic, ed. 2, St. Louis, 1969, The C. V. Mosby Co.)

PROGNOSIS

Breech presentations should not influence *maternal mortality,* but *morbidity* is likely to be increased. Cervical and vaginal lacerations and even uterine rupture may occur during vaginal delivery, particularly when breech extraction is performed. These, of course, increase blood loss and predispose to infection. *Hemorrhage* may also be caused by uterine atony from deep anesthesia required for breech extraction. Complications, particularly infection and those related to blood loss, are increased severalfold after *cesarean delivery.*

The gross uncorrected *perinatal mortality* may be as high as 20% to 30%, but for the normal fetus this should be reducible to a rate comparable to that for vertex presentation. The most important causes of perinatal mortality are associated with vaginal delivery and include the following:

1. *Anoxia* resulting from delay in delivery of the aftercoming head and from prolapsed cord,

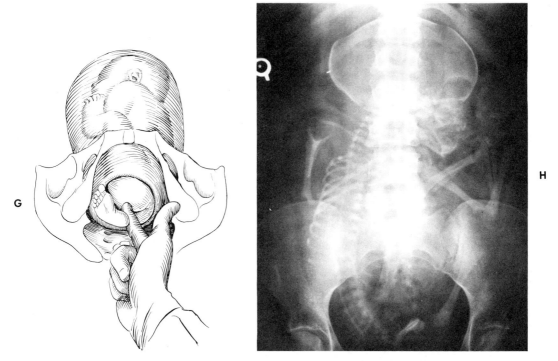

Fig. 38-1, cont'd. **G,** Vaginal palpation of left sacrotransverse. **H,** X-ray film examination.

which occurs about ten times more often than in vertex positions (Morley, studying 538 term breech deliveries conducted in the University of Michigan Hospital, found a 5% incidence of prolapsed cord with complete breech presentations, 15.7% with double footling, and 14.5% with single footling. No instance of prolapsed cord occurred in 345 patients with frank breech positions, presumably because the presenting part occluded the cervix as completely as does a well-applied head. Three of the babies with prolapsed cords died, and three others developed incapacitating neurologic deficiencies.)

2. *Injuries,* the most serious of which are those that cause intracranial hemorrhage, fractures of the spine associated with spinal cord injury, and rupture of the liver, spleen, and adrenals

3. *Complications of prematurity*

4. *Developmental anomalies,* which are present two to three times more often than with vertex presentations

DIAGNOSIS

The diagnosis of breech position can usually be made by abdominal examination alone (Fig. 38-1), but it may be necessary to perform other studies to confirm the impression obtained by palpation.

Abdominal examination. The firm, round, ballotable head can be felt in the fundus of the uterus and the irregular, softer breech over the pelvic inlet. A cephalic prominence cannot be palpated above the pubis. The fetal heart is usually best heard on the side of the abdomen toward which the back is directed and at or above the level of the umbilicus.

Vaginal examination. If the cervix is partly dilated, the physician can feel the triangular sacrum and coccyx with an ischial tuberosity on either side (Fig. 38-1). One or both feet can be palpated in

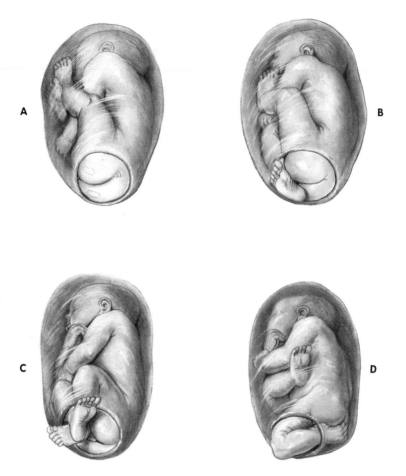

Fig. 38-2. Fetal attitudes in breech positions. **A,** Frank breech. **B,** Incomplete breech. **C,** Complete breech. **D,** Knee presentation. (From Willson, J.R.: Atlas of obstetric technic, ed. 2. St. Louis, 1969, The C. V. Mosby Co.)

the incomplete or complete breech attitudes. If the membranes are ruptured, fresh meconium may be present on the examining finger.

The most frequent error is mistaking the breech for a face or a shoulder. If the face is presenting, the bony orbits can be outlined, the sucking action of the mouth can be recognized, and there is no fresh meconium. With a shoulder presentation, the scapula and ribs can be identified.

X-ray examination. It is seldom necessary to resort to x-ray film examination only for diagnosis during the prenatal period (Fig. 38-1). An x-ray study is important at the onset of labor to identify factors

such as extension of the head or fetal positions that would make vaginal delivery hazardous if ultrasound is not available.

Ultrasound. Ultrasound is as accurate as is x-ray film for determining the exact position of the feet and legs and for identifying fetal anomalies.

MECHANISM OF LABOR (Fig. 38-3)

The cervix dilates at the usual rate in both primigravidas and multiparas if the uterine contractions are normal, but the presenting part may remain at or just above the level of the ischial spines until cervical dilatation is complete, after which it descends. The fact that the breech

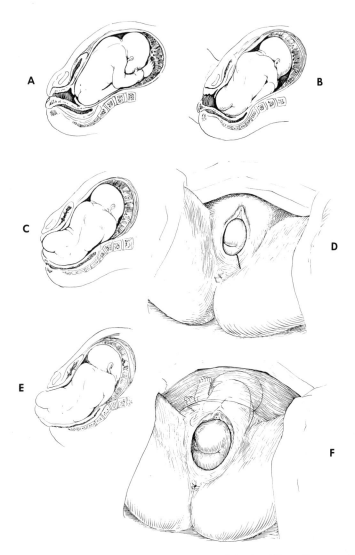

Fig. 38-3. Mechanism of breech labor. **A,** Breech enters inlet in oblique diameter. **B,** Rotation to sacrum left. **C** and **D,** Anterior hip appears in introitus. **E** and **F,** Both hips distending introitus. (From Willson, J.R.: Atlas of obstetric technic, ed. 2, St. Louis, 1969, The C. V. Mosby Co.)

remains high during the first stage does not indicate fetopelvic disproportion, as does failure of the presenting vertex to descend. The diameters of the breech are less than those of the head; consequently, size alone is usually not a factor in the presenting part's remaining high.

The presenting part usually enters the inlet with its widest diameter, the bitrochanteric, in the transverse or in one of the oblique diameters of the pelvis. It descends in this diameter until the anterior hip meets the resistance of the muscular pelvic floor and the bony pelvis. As descent continues, the increasing pressure of the anterior hip against the levator sling causes the hip to rotate 45 degrees anteriorly to a position beneath the pubic arch; the opposite hip is now directed toward the maternal sacrum, and the infant's spine is directed toward the lateral pelvic wall. With further descent, the anterior hip becomes visible in the introitus, at which time it impinges beneath the symphysis and remains relatively stationary while the posterior hip is forced upward and anteriorly over the perineum as the infant's spine bends laterally. After the posterior hip clears the perineum, it falls backward, permitting the expulsion of the anterior hip from the vagina.

With a few more contractions, the shoulders enter the inlet in the same oblique diameter that was occupied by the bitrochanteric diameter or in the transverse. They too descend until the anterior shoulder strikes the levator sling and rotates 45 degrees or more to a position beneath the pubic arch with the axilla visible; the posterior shoulder now lies in the hollow of the sacrum. The continuing uterine contractions force the posterior shoulder anteriorly over the perineum until it and the arm are delivered, after which it falls backward, permitting the anterior shoulder and arm to emerge from beneath the symphysis.

The head is usually incompletely flexed and enters the inlet with its long axis in either the transverse or in an oblique diameter, with the occiput directed obliquely anteriorly. The head descends, and the occiput is rotated anteriorly until the neck impinges beneath the pubis, after which the head becomes progressively more flexed as it descends; as a result the chin, nose, forehead, vertex, and occiput are forced over the perineum.

Variations. The previous description applies to most breech deliveries in women with normal pelves. Variations can be expected if the pelvis is small or with frank or incomplete varieties.

MANAGEMENT

Breech positions cannot be regarded lightly because, even though the deliveries are managed by experts, the perinatal mortality is greater than when the vertex presents. All breech deliveries should take place in a hospital. Family physicians and house staff should ask for consultation as soon as the position is recognized.

During pregnancy. If the breech can be converted to a vertex by *external version* (Fig. 38-4), the danger to the infant will be reduced. This maneuver should be attempted after the thirty-fourth week when most spontaneous versions will already have occurred, but it may also be possible to change the position at a later stage of pregnancy or even during early labor.

Ranney's experience with external version in 860 patients with breech presentations or transverse lies indicates that the procedure can reduce the incidence of breech presentations at term. Breech delivery occurred in only 0.6% of his patients. Fall and Nilsson reported a 70% success rate by giving a tocolytic agent before attempting version. Stine and co-workers were able to rotate 108 of 148 term fetuses from breech to vertex positions using terbutaline sulfate tocolysis. Fetal heart rate should be monitored during the manipulations. Phelan and associates recorded changes in fetal heart rate patterns in 39% of 141 fetuses after external version with beta-mimetic tocolysis. Most of these were bradycardias and/or decelerations, but in some tachycardia or sine-wave patterns were recorded. All the changes were transient, lasting 15 ± 12 minutes. The eventual outcome was unrelated to fetal heart changes.

External version should also be attempted during early labor if the breech is freely movable above the pelvic inlet and the membranes are intact. Ferguson and Dyson were able to rotate 11 of 15 breeches to vertex under ritodrine tocolysis during early labor.

The patient is placed in slight Trendelenburg position to allow the fetus to gravitate upward away from the pelvic inlet, and its exact position is determined. One hand manipulates the head toward the pelvis while the other attempts to mobilize the buttocks in the lower segment and push the breech toward the fundus of the uterus. The head is rotated in the direction that provides the shortest course to the pelvis. The fetal heart must be checked frequently during attempted version because cord entanglement or pressure or anything else interfering with fetal oxygen supply will be reflected in an alteration of cardiac rhythm. If the manipulations produce pain, the physician should desist.

The fetus will usually remain in the vertex position, but some will revert. This is likely to occur when the reason for the breech position is still present.

During labor. The principal responsibility of the obstetrician during late pregnancy and early in labor is to decided whether to deliver the patient vaginally or by cesarean section. The decision is made on the basis of parity, duration of pregnancy, estimated fetal size, pelvic capacity, condition of the cervix, quality of the uterine contractions, station, fetal attitude, and reaction of the patient to her pregnancy and delivery. One of the most

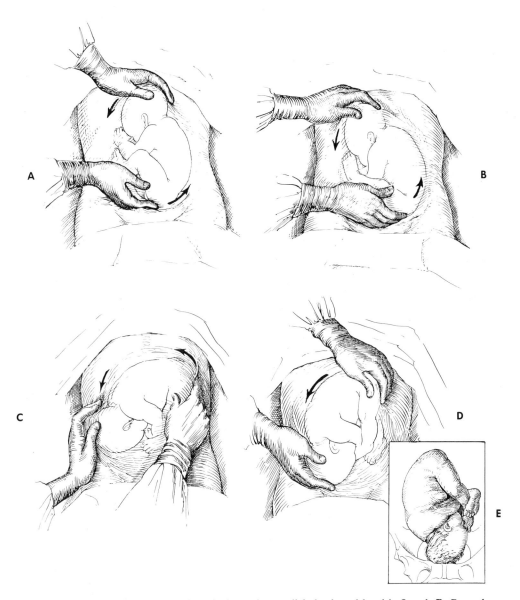

Fig. 38-4. External cephalic version. **A,** Buttocks are dislodged, and head is flexed. **B,** Buttocks are pushed upward and head downward until infant lies in transverse position. **C** and **D,** Version is completed by further manipulation. **E,** Position of fetus after completed version.

important factors in the decision is the experience of the physician who will conduct the delivery.

That cesarean section is not always necessary can be documented by several reports in which carefully selected patients have been allowed to deliver vaginally, Tatum delivered 174 patients at or near term with a corrected perinatal mortality of zero. Gimovsky, Petrie, and Todd compared the results of 130 vaginal breech deliveries in carefully selected and monitored patients with 78 who were not managed by their protocol, 130 vaginal vertex deliveries, and 130 patients who were delivered by elective cesarean sections for both vertex and breech presentations. There were no intrapartum or perinatal mortalities in the "protocol" group, the vaginal vertex deliveries, and the cesarean sections. In contrast, there was one intrapartum death and a neonatal mortality of 12.8% in the "non-protocol" group. Collea, Chein and Quilligan; Green and co-workers; and Watson and Benson have had equally good results.

An important factor in choosing between vaginal delivery and cesarean section is the experience of the obstetrician. Those who have trained since cesarean section has been used more liberally have had little opportunity to learn the technics for breech delivery. The possibility of disabling or lethal fetal injury is substantially increased when vaginal delivery is attempted by inexperienced operators. Sachs and associates studied neonatal mortality in 392,241 singleton births in Georgia between 1974 and 1978. The neonatal mortality rate for vaginal breech deliveries of infants weighing between 2501 and 4000 g was three times that for those delivered by cesarean section. The risk increased with decreasing size.

Vaginal delivery should be considered only if one anticipates a normal labor and delivery. The outlook is more favorable for multiparas who have delivered babies of at least normal size without difficulty than for those who have had problems with delivery in the past and for primigravidas. Vaginal delivery is also appropriate for women who are well advanced in labor when they arrive at the hospital, unless there is a reason for operative delivery. Hurried preparation for cesarean delivery may negate the positive effects of the operation.

Abdominal and vaginal examinations should be performed soon after labor begins to estimate fetal weight and to determine the amount of cervical effacement and dilatation, the status of the membranes, and the pelvic capacity. An ultrasound study to confirm fetal attitude and size is helpful in making the decision.

The *fetus should weigh between 2500 and 3500 g*. Vaginal delivery is less appropriate for premature infants and those with growth retardation than for those who are mature. The former are less able to compensate for even minor injuries and should be protected from trauma. Oversized babies are likely to be injured by the manipulations necessary for delivery. It is difficult to determine the weight of a fetus accurately, but a combination of palpation and ultrasound provides the best information on which to base the estimate.

The *pelvis should be of normal size and shape*. A trial of labor when the pelvis is thought to be small or misshapen is not appropriate when the breech is presenting. The body can descend through a pelvis too small to permit the passage of an unmolded aftercoming head. If the head is forcibly extracted, the baby will be injured. If it is allowed to mold and deliver gradually, the infant will die of anoxia.

Unfortunately, one of the most important bits of information needed to make the decision, a comparison of the size and shape of the fetal head with that of the pelvis, is not easy to obtain. Vaginal delivery should not be considered if there is any possibility that the head will not be able to pass through the birth canal easily.

The *most favorable fetal attitude* is the frank breech with a well-flexed head. The cord is less likely to prolapse if the cervical opening is plugged by the buttocks alone than it is with the footling varieties. The latter provide many chinks through which a loop of cord can slip. The fetal cervical spine and spinal cord is likely to be damaged during vaginal delivery if the head is extended.

Labor should have started spontaneously and should be progressing at a normal rate by the time the patient enters the hospital. We prefer not to try to induce labor when the breech is presenting.

An *obstetrician experienced in breech delivery* is essential to a favorable outcome. Cesarean delivery is almost always preferred when the fetus is mature enough to survive if the responsible physician has not had considerable experience with breech delivery.

Zatuchni and Andros have developed a scoring system on the basis of *parity, gestational age, estimated fetal weight, previous breech delivery, cervical dilatation*, and *station* to help in selecting patients for vaginal delivery (Table 38-1).

In patients with breech positions of normally developed single infants weighing more than 2500 g, the complications of labor and delivery occur with much greater frequency in those who score 3 or less. The duration of labor for low-score nulliparas was about 12 hours, and for those with high scores it was about 8½ hours. Comparable figures for multiparas were about 9 and 6 hours. Labor was abnormal in 23 of 30 low-score patients and in only 12 of the 109 patients with high scores. Six of the seven vaginal deliveries in low-score patients were complicated, whereas all but one of the 109 high-score patients were delivered without difficulty. The only infant death occured in a low-score patient, but five of the 29 surviving infants of mothers with low scores had nerve palsy, convulsions, or other complications. Bird and McElin confirmed the value of this scoring system in breech delivery.

The *membranes should not be ruptured artificially* in

TABLE 38-1 Zatuchni-Andros breech score*

Factor score	Parity	Gestational age	Estimated fetal weight (grams)	Previous breech delivery	Cervical dilatation	Station
0	Primigravida	>39 weeks	>3630	0	2 cm	Above −3
1	Multipara	38 weeks	3176 to 3629	1	3 cm	−2
2		37 weeks or less	<3176	2 or more	4 cm +	Below −1

Modified from Zatuchni, G.I., and Andros, G.J.: Am. J. Obstet. Gynecol. **98**:854, 1967.
*The breech score is the sum of the scores for each factor.

normal labors because this may permit the cord to prolapse past the irregular presenting part, which occludes the cervix less completely than does the firm, round head.

The fetal heart tones should be recorded constantly by an electronic monitor, since occult or complete prolapse of the cord occurs so frequently. The *passage of meconium* is of no significance during breech labors, but an attempt must be made to determine a cause for abnormal fetal heart tones whenever they are detected.

Delivery. The physician must be certain that the cervix is completely dilated before attempting breech delivery. The buttocks, the body, and even the shoulders can descend through a cervix that is not sufficiently dilated to permit passage of the head. This is particularly true with premature infants whose heads are larger than their shoulders. With a frank breech, the presenting part is smaller than the combined buttocks, feet, and legs of an infant in the complete breech attitude and will pass through a cervical opening much smaller than that required for the complete variety.

SPONTANEOUS DELIVERY. With spontaneous delivery the entire delivery is completed without manipulation by the attendant. This most often occurs with small, premature infants and in multiparas with large pelves and rapid labors.

PARTIAL BREECH EXTRACTION. Partial breech extraction, also known as *assisted breech delivery*, consists of spontaneous, controlled expulsion as far as the umbilicus, after which the shoulders and the head are extracted by the physician. When the breech begins to distend the introitus and about 8 to 10 cm of the presenting part is visible during a contraction, an episiotomy is performed if necessary. If this is done at the proper time, the next few contractions will force the buttocks and the abdomen

through the introitus, after which the rest of the body is extracted.

Downward traction is applied to the pelvic girdle with the thumbs placed parallel to each other over the sacrum or along the femurs, and the index fingers encircling the iliac crest (Fig. 38-5). Pressure and traction should be on bones rather than soft tissues, particularly the abdomen, to reduce the possibility of injury. Tank and associates described a number of soft-tissue injuries, including adrenal hemorrhage, attributable to trauma inflicted during breech delivery.

The body is gradually pulled downward, keeping the back directed anteriorly until the anterior axilla comes into view and the scapula emerges from beneath the pubic arch. Two fingers are introduced beneath the arch to a position along the humerus, and the arm is wiped down over the infant's chest and delivered (Fig. 38-6). The body is then lifted upward, and the posterior arm is delivered in the same manner (Fig. 38-7).

The head can usually be delivered by manual manipulation alone with the Celsus-Wigand-Martin maneuver (Fig. 38-8), by which it can be brought through the inlet in the transverse or oblique diameter and then rotated to the anteroposterior diameter of the lower pelvis and delivered over the perineum by flexion. The head can also be delivered by forceps after it has descended to the pelvic floor and has rotated to an anteroposterior position (Fig. 38-9). This is comparable to low forceps extraction of a presenting head. Forceps should never be used to try to bring the head through the pelvic inlet or through an incompletely dilated cervix.

If the pelvis is small, if the cervix is incompletely dilated, or if the fetus is extracted too rapidly, the arms may be swept upward beside the head *(extended arms)*. From there they can be rotated to a position behind the

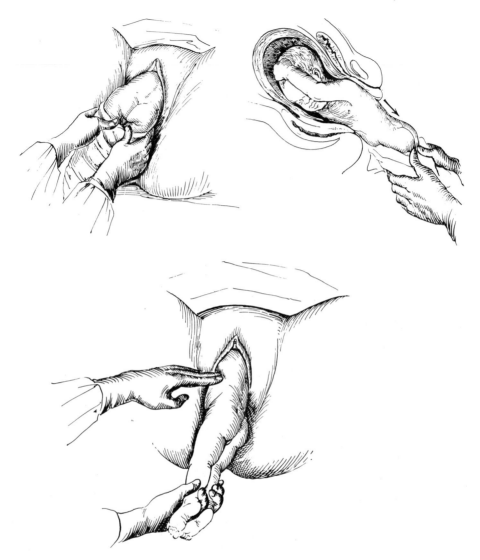

Fig. 38-5. Partial breech extraction. Traction is downward until anterior axilla appears beneath pubic arch. (From Willson, J.R.: Atlas of obstetric technic, ed. 2, 1969, The C. V. Mosby Co.)

fetal neck *(nuchal arms)* as the body is turned. This complication can usually be prevented by slow deliberate extraction of the body. Both can be corrected by freeing the arms and manipulating them downward across the fetal chest.

At this stage of the delivery the umbilical cord is compressed against the bony pelvis, and the blood flow is cut off. The fetus will become anoxic if it cannot begin to breathe. It is not necessary to deliver the entire head at this time; only the mouth must be exposed. Collea, Chein, and Quilligan have suggested that the fetus is not likely to suffer if the "umbilicus-to-mouth" delivery time is less than 4 minutes. More problems are caused by undue haste and forceful attempts at extraction than by deliberate performance of the required maneuvers.

COMPLETE BREECH EXTRACTION. In complete breech extraction the entire infant is extracted from the birth

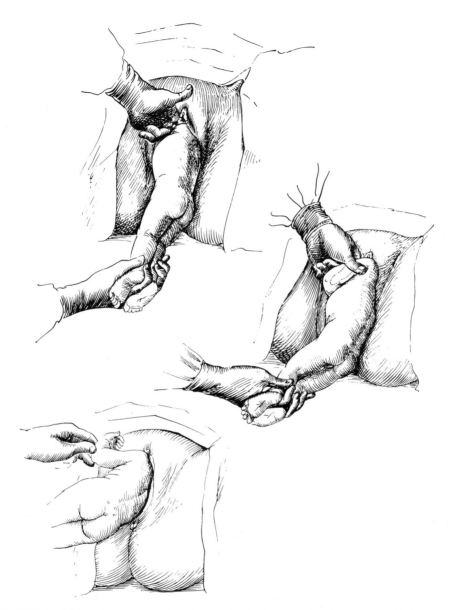

Fig. 38-6. Partial breech extraction. Anterior arm is wiped across chest by pressure with index and second fingers. (From Willson, J.R.: Atlas of obstetric technic, ed. 2, 1969, The C. V. Mosby Co.)

canal. This is one of the most difficult and potentially traumatic of all the obstetric operations and even when performed by experts results in unacceptably high perinatal morbidity and mortality. Cesarean section is preferable in almost every instance.

CESAREAN DELIVERY. Obstetricians have been loath to perform cesarean deliveries in a large percentage of breech presentations, even though the perinatal mortality is several times that for the vertex presentations, and serious physical and neu-

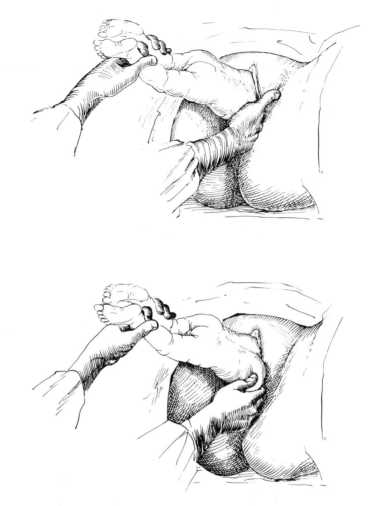

Fig. 38-7. Partial breech extraction. Delivery of posterior arm. (From Willson, J.R.: Atlas of obstetric technic, ed. 2, 1969, The C. V. Mosby Co.)

rologic sequelae in surviving infants delivered vaginally occur frequently. This attitude is changing because it is evident that the outcome for the infants is improved if cesarean delivery is selected for any breech presentation in which easy, uncomplicated vaginal delivery cannot be anticipated.

Between 1950 and 1964, the cesarean delivery rates for breech presentation in the University of Michigan Women's Hospital were 7.9% for primigravidas and 3.3% for multiparas. During this time eight term infants died (1.48%) as a result of vaginal breech delivery, and six more suffered se-

rious neurologic impairment, which was evident before they left the hospital. No deaths or neurologic damage are known to have occurred in the term babies after cesarean delivery.

During the next 7 years (1966 to 1972) the cesarean delivery rate for primigravidas with breech presentations increased to 75%, and that for multiparas to 38%. None of the infants delivered by cesarean section died, and none is known to have suffered neurologic impairment. Of those who were delivered vaginally, 0.4% died, and 0.9% had neurologic injuries recognized in the hospital. Cesarean

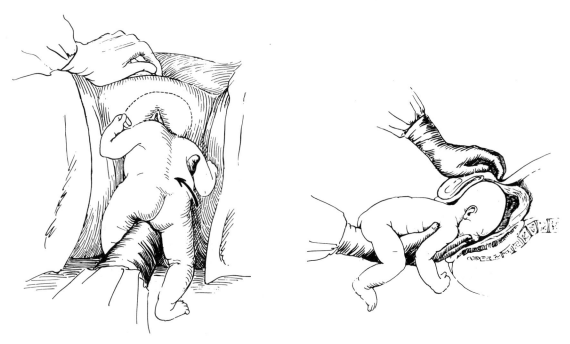

Fig. 38-8. Partial breech extraction. Delivery of head by Celsus-Wigand-Martin maneuver. (From *Atlas of obstetric technic*, ed. 2, 1969, The C. V. Mosby Co.)

rates for breech delivery in this institution have remained high, between 75% and 80% for primigravidas and 60% to 65% for multiparas, and the fetal outcome appears to justify the policy. The perinatal death rate for infants delivered vaginally now approximates that for those delivered by cesarean section. This suggests an appropriate selection of patients for both groups.

The availability of an excellent neonatal intensive care unit should encourage one to choose cesarean delivery even for small premature infants who have a reasonable chance of surviving, but there is a limit as to how far this concept can be extended. The survival of infants weighing between 1000 to 1500 g is now so good that babies in this weight range should usually be delivered by cesarean section. Vaginal breech delivery offers an unacceptable risk to infants of this size and should be chosen only under unusual circumstances.

Although the survival rates for those weighing between 700 and 1000 g are also improved by cesarean section and intensive neonatal care, the percentage of small babies with serious handicaps increases with decreasing size. Subjecting the mother to the risks of cesarean delivery can rarely be justified for infants weighing less than 700 g or when the pregnancy is much less than 28 weeks' duration. Kitchen and co-workers, studying 172 survivors of 326 babies of 24 to 28 weeks' gestational age, detected no significant improvement in neonatal mortality in those delivered by cesarean section. Moreover, the method of delivery did not influence the incidence of handicaps in 111 who were followed for 2 years.

Perinatal mortality alone does not provide all the information needed to justify cesarean section for premature breech delivery. Long-term follow-up of the survivors will indicate how many develop normally and how many are handicapped. A high percentage of defective children would suggest that cesarean delivery is inappropriate. The opposite appears to be true, at least in the larger premature

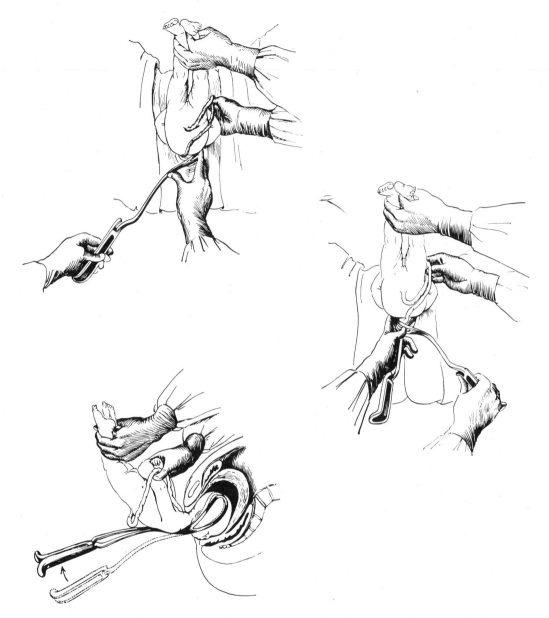

Fig. 38-9. Partial breech extraction. Forceps extraction of head. (From Willson, J.R.: Atlas of obstetric technic, ed. 2, 1969, The C. V. Mosby Co.)

infants. Ingemarsson, Westgren, and Svenningsen compared the development of 42 premature infants delivered by cesarean section with that of 48 who were delivered vaginally. All were between 28 to 36 weeks' gestational age. Perinatal mortality was 14.6% for those delivered through the vagina and 4.8% for those delivered by cesarean section. At 12 months of age, 10 of 41 survivors after vaginal delivery (24%) had significant neurologic disabilities as compared with one (2.5%) of those delivered by cesarean section.

One must make decisions concerning cesarean

or vaginal deliveries of tiny babies on the quality of the neonatal care available. One cannot justify a high cesarean rate if most of the small babies die or if a high percentage of those who survive are handicapped. If intensive neonatal care is not available, vaginal delivery may be appropriate for most breech presentations when pregnancy is terminated before 30 weeks. A preferable alternative, when possible, is to transfer the patient to a perinatal center for care.

Following are the *indications for cesarean section for breech presentation*:

1. *An estimated fetal weight between 1000 and 2500 g or more than 3500 g.*

2. *Suspected fetopelvic disproportion.* The time at which the fetus is most likely to be injured is during the delivery of the aftercoming head. It may die of anoxia if the head cannot be delivered relatively promptly. Conversely, forceful attempts to extract the head through a small pelvis may cause intracranial hemorrhage or injury to the spinal cord and nerve roots or to abdominal viscera.

3. *Footling breech presentations.* These presentations are acommpanied by a high incidence of prolapsed cord. Cesarean delivery usually is safer for both primigravidas and multiparas. Vaginal delivery should not usually be selected unless labor is well advanced when the patient arrives at the hospital.

4. *Hyperextension of the fetal head.* The manipulations necessary for vaginal delivery are responsible for a high incidence of spinal cord injury when the head is extended.

5. *Dysfunctional labor.* Dysfunctional labor can often be improved with oxytocin, but, as when the vertex presents, an operative extraction may be necessary if normal contractions cannot be induced. Breech extraction is accompanied by a risk of injury that can be eliminated by cesarean section. The same holds true *when descent is delayed during the second stage of labor.*

6. *Medical conditions and ruptured membranes.* Cesarean section is appropriate when early delivery of women with medical conditions, such as diabetes or hypertension, is indicated or when the membranes rupture while the cervix is still firm and uneffaced.

7. *History of abnormal labors or a perinatal death.* Cesarean should usually be selected over vaginal delivery whenever there is a history of abnormal labors or when an infant has died during or after delivery.

8. *Primigravidas.* Most primigravidas with breech presentations should be delivered by cesarean section.

Cesarean section does not guarantee an atraumatic delivery. The obstetrician can encounter the same difficulty in delivering an infant through an abdominal incision as through the vagina. Under these circumstances the advantages of cesarean delivery for the fetus are negated. In most instances a vertical incision in the lower uterine segment is preferable to a transverse. With the former the buttocks of the fetus usually appear in the incision, but they may be several centimeters above a transverse opening. Extraction is much easier through a vertical incision. In addition, the lengths of the uterine and the abdominal incisions are important. If the incision is too short the aftercoming head will be trapped, and the fetus may be injured during attempts to extract it. A long transverse muscle-cutting abdominal incision (Maylard) is preferable to a Pfannenstiel incision; the latter is far more likely to impede delivery.

The outcome for breech delivery should be comparable to the outcome for vertex presentations when the deliveries are conducted in a perinatal center, when most women with breech presentations are delivered by cesarean section, and when vaginal delivery is limited to those who are well advanced in normal labor and to those women who have no foreseeable complications, if they can be delivered by an obstetrician experienced in breech delivery.

REFERENCES

Bird, C.C., and McElin, T.W.: A six-year prospective study of term breech deliveries utilizing the Zatuchni-Andros prognostic scoring index, Am. J. Obstet. Gynecol. **121**:551, 1975.

Brenner, W.E., Bruce, R.D., and Hendricks, C.H.: The characteristics and perils of breech presentation, Am. J. Obstet. Gynecol. **118**:700, 1974.

Collea, J.V., Chein, C., and Quilligan, E.J.: The randomized management of term frank breech presentation: a study of 208 cases, Am. J. Obstet. Gynecol. **137**:235, 1980.

Fall, O., and Nilsson, B.A.: External cephalic version in breech presentation under tocolysis, Obstet. Gynecol **53**:712, 1979.

Ferguson J.E., II, and Dyson, D.C.: Intrapartum external cephalic version, Am. J. Obstet. Gynecol. **152**:297, 1985.

Fianu, S., and Vaclavinkova, V.: The site of placental attachment as a factor in the aetiology of breech presentation, Acta Obstet. Gynecol. Scand. **57**:371, 1978.

Gimovsky, M.L., Petrie, R.H., and Todd, W.D.: Neonatal performance of the selected term vaginal breech delivery, Obstet. Gynecol **56:**687, 1980.

Green, J.E., et al.: Has an increased cesarean section rate for term breech delivery reduced the incidence of birth asphyxia, trauma, and death? Am. J. Obstet. Gynecol. **142:**643, 1982.

Ingemarsson, I., Westgren, M., and Svenningsen, N.W.: Long-term follow-up of preterm infants in breech presentation delivered by caesarean section, Lancet **2:**172, 1978.

Kitchen, W., et al.: Cesarean section or vaginal delivery at 24 to 28 weeks' gestation: comparison of survival and neonatal and two-year morbidity, Obstet. Gynecol. **66:**149, 1985.

Morley, G.W.: Breech presentation: a 15-year review, Obstet. Gynecol. **30:**745, 1967.

Phelan, J.P. et al.: Observations of fetal heart rate characteristics related to external cephalic version and tocolysis, Am. J. Obstet. Gynecol. **149:**658, 1984.

Ranney, B.: The gentle art of external cephalic version, Am. J. Obstet. Gynecol. **116:**239, 1973.

Rovinsky, J.J., Miller, J.A., and Kaplan, S.: Management of breech presentation at term, Am. J. Obstet. Gynecol. **115:**497, 1973.

Sachs, B.P., et al.: Cesarean section: risks and benefits for mother and fetus, J.A.M.A. **250:**2157, 1983.

Stine, L.E., et al.: Update on external cephalic version performed at term, Obstet. Gynecol. **65:**642, 1985.

Tank, E.S., Davis, R., Holt, J.F., and Morley, G.W.: Mechanisms of trauma during breech delivery, Obstet. Gynecol. **38:**761, 1971.

Tatum, R.K.: Vaginal breech delivery of selected infants weighing more than 2000 grams, Am. J. Obstet. Gynecol. **152:**145, 1985.

Watson, W.J., and Benson, W.L.: Vaginal delivery for the selected frank breech infant at term, Obstet. Gynecol. **64:**638, 1984.

Zatuchni, G.I., and Andros, G.J.: Prognostic index for vaginal delivery in breech presentation at term, Am. J. Obstet. Gynecol. **98:**854, 1967.

39

J. Robert Willson

Forceps delivery

Obstetric forceps are instruments designed to *extract* the infant from the birth canal or to *rotate* its head within the vagina. They are never used to compress the head or to aid in dilating the cervix. Forceps are applied only to the head of the infant and never to any other part of its body.

More than 600 types of forceps have been designed, many of them for a specific purpose such as extraction of the aftercoming head in breech delivery or for rotation of the head from certain abnormal positions. All forceps are alike in that they consist of two blades that articulate at the point where the shafts cross and lead into the handles. The blades have a *cephalic curve,* which conforms to the contours of the infant's head, and most forceps have a *pelvic curve,* which approximates the curve of the pelvic canal. The blades may be fenestrated or solid. The left blade is the one that is inserted into the left half of the pelvis, the handle being held in the operator's left hand. This blade articulates with the right one by means of a flanged lock on the shafts of the instrument (Fig. 39-1).

TYPES OF FORCEPS APPLICATION

Forceps operations are classified according to the station and position of the presenting part at the time the forceps are applied (Fig. 39-2).

Low forceps application. The term *low forceps* indicates that the skull has reached the pelvic floor, the position is direct occipitoanterior, and the scalp can be seen in the introitus during each contraction. After the patient has been anesthetized for delivery, particularly with spinal or pudendal block anesthetic which eliminates perineal sensation and the urge to bear down, the head may retract slightly in the birth canal. One would still classify the extraction as low forceps if the criteria had been met before the anesthetic was administered.

Midforceps application. The term *midforceps* indicates that the head is engaged but the criteria for low forceps have not yet been met. The presenting part must have passed the level of the ischial spines but has not yet reached the pelvic floor, and the biparietal diameter must have passed through the plane of the inlet. The sagittal suture usually is in the transverse or in one of the oblique diameters of the pelvis.

High forceps application. The presenting part lies between the plane of the inlet and that of the ischial spines.

It is not sufficient merely to name the type of forceps delivery because some midforceps extractions are easy and atraumatic, whereas others are most difficult. Much more information is made available if an exact description of the station and

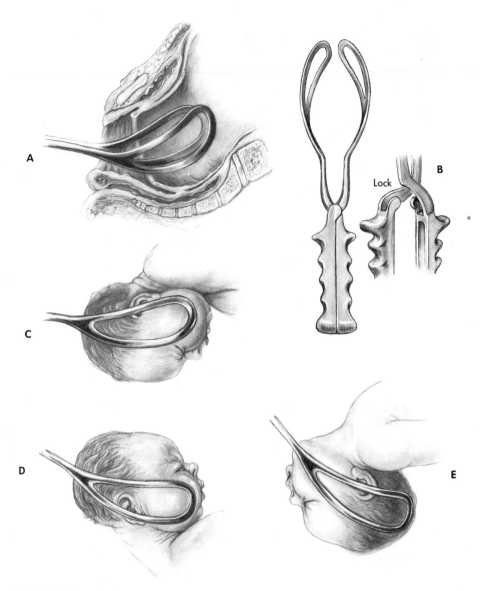

Fig. 39-1. Obstetric forceps. **A,** Forceps in transverse position with pelvic curve corresponding to curve of birth canal. **B,** Cephalic curve of blades and lock. **C** to **E,** Cephalic application. **C,** Occipitoanterior (ideal application). **D,** Occipitoposterior. **E,** Application to aftercoming head in breech presentation. (From Willson, J.R.: Atlas of obstetric technic, ed. 2, St. Louis, 1969, The C. V. Mosby Co.)

position of the head and the difficulties encountered during the application of the forceps and the delivery of the infant are recorded in the hospital record.

The *position* of the forceps in the pelvis is determined by the pelvic diameter that passes at a right angle through the center of the fenestra. If each blade is applied to the lateral pelvic wall with its pelvic curve directed anteri-

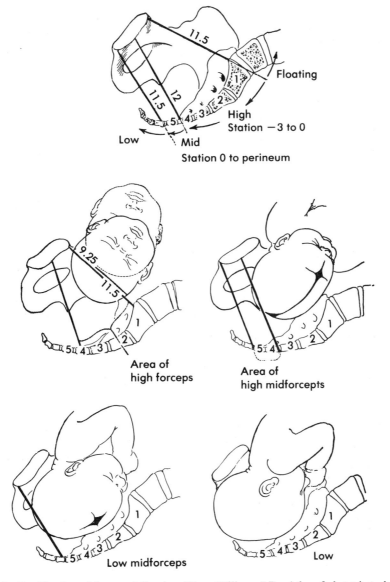

Fig. 39-2. Classification of forceps deliveries. (From Willson, J.R., Atlas of obstetric technic, ed. 2, St Louis, 1969, The C. V. Mosby Co.)

orly, the forceps are in the transverse diameter of the pelvis. If the blades are then rotated 45 degrees, they lie in an oblique diameter. If they are rotated another 45 degrees, the pelvic curve is directed toward the lateral pelvic wall with one blade overlying the sacrum and the other beneath the pubic arch; they are now in the anteroposterior diameter.

The blades are said to be in the *cephalic* or *ideal application* if they have been applied to the head in the occipitomental diameter and equidistant from the sagittal suture (Fig. 39-1). If the blades are applied to the sides of the pelvis with the front of the forceps directed anteriorly without regard to the position of the fetal head, they are in *pelvic application*.

INDICATIONS

The use of forceps is indicated whenever it is necessary to terminate labor in the interest of either the mother or the infant and when forceps extraction is the easiest and safest method for delivering the baby.

The principal indication for forceps delivery is *cessation of progress during the second stage of labor*. This may result from ineffective uterine contractions that do not improve with oxytocin stimulation, from an abnormal fetal position that can be corrected by manual or forceps manipulation, or from minor degrees of cephalopelvic disproportion that can be overcome easily by adding traction to the expulsive force of the uterine contractions. Forceps may also be used to *shorten a prolonged perineal phase of labor* or to eliminate it completely when bearing-down efforts are contraindicated, as they may be in patients with significant cardiac or pulmonary disease.

Forceps extraction is usually preferable to cesarean delivery when fetal distress is diagnosed late in the second stage of labor and when there are no contraindications to the use of forceps.

Elective low forceps. The elective low forceps operation is generally combined with episiotomy to eliminate the last 15 to 30 minutes of labor. Although this usually is not a definite indication for forceps delivery, it has many advantages. Normal vaginal support can be maintained if an adequate episiotomy is performed before the supporting structures have been injured by the advancing head and if they are carefully reconstructed after delivery. Extraction, which requires mainly extension of the fetal head as it is gently pulled through the introitus, reduces the risk of intracranial injury caused by prolonged pressure on the head as it distends the intact perineum.

REQUIREMENTS

Although a true indication for forceps delivery may be present, such an operation may be dangerous both to mother and baby unless the following requirements or conditions are met.

The operator must be familiar with the normal mechanism of labor and trained in the application and use of forceps. The physician who has not had special training in operative obstetrics should usually not perform forceps extractions. Consultation should be sought for all such problems.

The cervix must be completely dilated. No one can forcibly extract an infant through an undilated cervix without producing a laceration that may extend into the lower uterine segment.

There can be no marked disproportion between the size of the baby and the size of the pelvis.

The head must be engaged. The lower the head in the pelvis, the safer and easier will be the delivery. The physician must ascertain by pelvic and, if there is a question, by x-ray film examination that the head actually is engaged before attempting forceps extraction from a midpelvic location. If a huge caput has formed or if the head is molded and greatly elongated, its most dependent part may be deep in the vagina while the biparietal diameter is still above the plane of the inlet.

Forceps extraction from a high station, particularly in primigravidas, often results in deep soft-tissue lacerations as the head is drawn through the unprepared vagina.

The vertex or the face must be presenting in a position that will permit delivery, and the head must be large enough to be grasped by the blades.

Anesthetic must be adequate for the procedure. Pudendal block is satisfactory for most low forceps deliveries but inadequate for more difficult procedures, particularly when the head must be rotated. Spinal, epidural, caudal, or inhalation anesthesia will provide the muscle relaxation and pain relief required for these deliveries.

The membranes must be ruptured.

Contraindications. The use of forceps is contraindicated in certain *abnormal positions* such as impacted mentoposterior and brow, which cannot usually be corrected and delivered safely through the vagina, or for breech delivery, except to extract the aftercoming head. Forceps application also is contraindicated when progress is delayed by *significant cephalopelvic disproportion, before the presenting part has descended well below the level of the ischial spines,* and *when the cervix is incompletely dilated.* Cesarean delivery is almost always preferred under these circumstances.

SELECTION OF PATIENTS

The best results from forceps delivery are obtained when the operations are performed by expert obstetricians, but technique is not the only factor that influences the outcome. The operator must know when to interfere and when to allow labor to continue. Patient observation or oxytocin stimulation often permits spontaneous delivery or at least makes a potentially difficult operation easy if the head descends deeper into the pelvis. A reduction in unindicated and traumatic forceps extractions will improve both fetal and maternal outcomes.

Low forceps extraction. Low forceps extraction, when properly executed, does not add to the risk for the mother or the infant. This operation may be performed electively, or it may become necessary if the patient is unable to use her secondary powers to aid in the expulsion of the infant or if the uterine contractions become ineffectual late in the second stage. Under such circumstances, forceps delivery may be preferable to oxytocin stimulation.

TECHNIQUE. The patient, in lithotomy position and properly anesthetized, is examined to determine the exact position of the fetal head. Episiotomy usually is performed at this time. Laufe and Leslie measured the forceps traction force necessary to extract the head before and after episiotomy. Peak traction force was reduced 23% for primigravidas and 28% for para 1 women after episiotomy. The left blade of the forceps is introduced between the head and the guiding fingers of the physician's right hand until it lies in proper cephalic and pelvic application. The right blade is then introduced into the right side of the pelvis (Fig. 39-3). The forceps are locked after any necessary adjustments in their position have been made. If the forceps cannot be locked easily, the physician should suspect that the blades are not properly applied.

After a final examination to ascertain that the application is correct, the head is extracted (Fig. 39-4). Traction at first is directed toward the floor to pull the head through the proper axis of the birth canal. As soon as the occiput appears beneath the pubic arch, the handles of the forceps are elevated each time traction is applied. This tends to extend the head as it descends, a duplication of the sequence of events during normal labor. The forceps are removed in the reverse order of their application, the right one first and then the left (Fig. 39-5).

Midforceps extraction. Midforceps extraction is generally contraindicated unless there is a clear-cut reason to

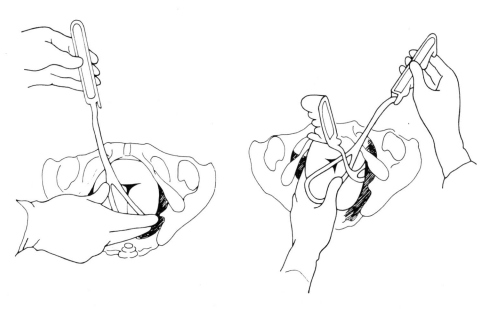

Fig. 39-3. Low forceps extraction showing application of blades.

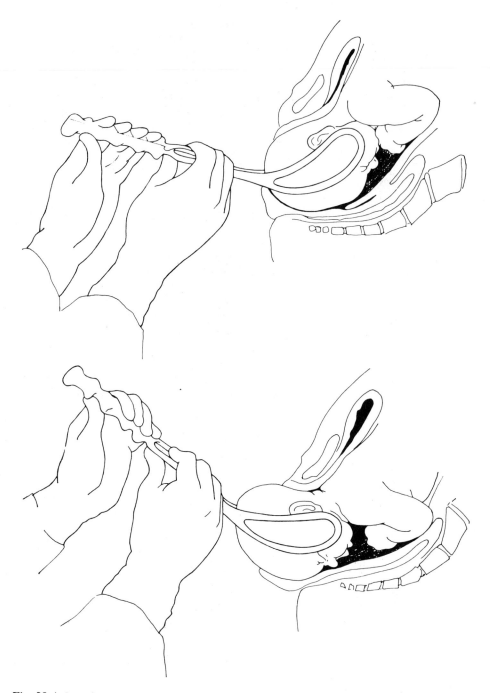

Fig. 39-4. Low forceps extraction of head. Traction force is downward as well as outward until occiput appears beneath pubic arch. Handles are then raised as traction is applied to extend head over perineum.

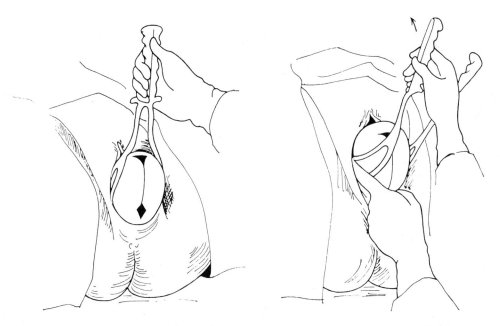

Fig. 39-5. Low forceps extraction showing completion of delivery of head and removal of forceps.

terminate labor. Most midforceps deliveries are performed because the orderly progress of the second stage of labor ceases. Forceps delivery should be considered whenever progress in descent and rotation ceases during a 1-hour period in the second stage if the uterine contractions are normal and if there is no significant disproportion, or when progress is so slow that a second stage of much more than 2 hours can be anticipated. Under such circumstances an unfavorable fetal position combined with mild disproportion often are the factors that interfere with labor and make the operation necessary. However, when the delay in labor is a result of ineffective contractions, a trial of oxytocin stimultion usually is preferable to immediate forceps extraction. If effective uterine activity can be restored, the labor may terminate spontaneously or at least progress until an easy low forceps extraction is possible.

When midforceps delivery becomes necessary, the head has usually not yet rotated to an anterior position. Although a transverse or even a posterior position does not contraindicate forceps delivery, it makes the application of the blades and the subsequent extraction more difficult. The head can be rotated to a more favorable position by manual manipulation. This can also be accomplished with forceps, and many obstetricians prefer this to manual rotation. In any event the physician must be completely familiar with the normal mechanism of labor and attempt to duplicate it during the manipulations for delivery.

Cesarean section is preferable to a traumatic mid-forceps delivery. This is particularly true if the presenting part has not descended below station plus 2, if it cannot be rotated to a favorable position for extraction, or if there is a definite cephalopelvic disproportion. On the other hand, if the presenting part is below station plus 2 and if there is no significant disproportion, atraumatic forceps extraction may well be possible.

High forceps extraction. High forceps deliveries can rarely be justified. Cesarean section is almost always preferable when the need for delivery arises before the head is engaged.

Trial forceps application. On rare occasions the physician may be able to apply forceps with ease but may not be able to extract the head because of insurmountable disproportion in the lower pelvis. When this occurs, cesarean section should be performed immediately. Bacteria are inevitably introduced during the manipulations necessary to apply forceps, and cesarean section after several hours is much more hazardous.

RESULTS

The mortality and morbidity for both mother and infant should be reduced if forceps are properly used. Low forceps extraction, when properly performed, does not increase morbidity, but the more difficult the procedure, the more dangerous it is. Mortality and morbidity will be increased if forceps deliveries are carelessly done or performed in the face of contraindications or failure to meet the requirements. Steer reported that the infant mortality attributed to midforceps extractions was 4%, whereas that caused by spontaneous expulsion was zero, and that by cesarean section, 0.1%. The only maternal death in 1295 patients studied occurred after midforceps extraction. Most of the patients who were delivered by difficult midforceps extraction in this series would now be delivered by cesarean section.

The main immediate danger to the mother is from hemorrhage from lacerations, which may also become infected. If the pelvic supporting structures are injured, cystocele, rectocele, and even uterine prolapse may develop later. Traumatic lesions in the infants from forceps delivery include skull fracture, intracranial hemorrhage, cephalohematomas, seventh nerve palsy, and soft-tissue laceration.

VACUUM EXTRACTION

The vacuum extractor is basically a suction cup attached to a traction handle. The cup is placed against the fetal scalp, and a vacuum of 0.6 to 0.8 kg/sq cm is produced. This permits the operator to exert traction on the fetal head and even to rotate it within the birth canal. Although the purpose of the extractor presumably is to reduce the damage produced by forceps manipulation, it is far from safe when it is used carelessly. The principal dangers for the infant are subaponeurotic hemorrhage, scalp abrasions and lacerations, and cephalohematomas. Plauche, in a literature review of 14,276 vacuum extractions, reported 18 subaponeurotic hemorrhages. In addition, scalp lacerations or abrasions occurred in 12.6%, cephalohematomas in 6%, and intracranial hemorrhages in 0.35%. There are fewer injuries with the silastic cup than there were with the original metal Malmström cup.

REFERENCES

Das, K.: The obstetric forceps: its history and evaluation. St. Louis, 1929, The C. V. Mosby Co.

Dennen, E.H.: Forceps deliveries. Philadelphia, 1955. F.A. Davis Co.

Dill, L.Y.: The obstetrical forceps. Springfield, Ill., 1953, Charles C Thomas, Publisher.

Laufe, L.E., and Leslie, D.C.: The timing of episiotomy, Am. J. Obstet. Gynecol. 114:773, 1972.

Maryniak, G.M., and Frank, J.B.: Clinical assessment of the Kobayashi vacuum extractor, Obst. Gynecol. 64:431, 1984.

Plauche, W.C.: Fetal cranial injuries related to delivery with the Malmström vacuum extractor, Obstet. Gynecol. 53:750, 1979.

Richardson, D.A., Evans, M.I., and Cibils, L.A.: Midforceps delivery: a critical review, Am. J. Obstet. Gynecol. 145:621, 1983.

Steer, C.M.: The effect of type of delivery on future childbearing, Am. J. Obstet. Gynecol. 60:395, 1950.

Willson, J.R.: Atlas of obstetric technic, ed. 2, St. Louis, 1969, The C. V. Mosby Co.

40

J. Robert Willson

Cesarean section

Cesarean section is an operative procedure by which the infant is delivered through incisions in the abdominal and uterine walls. This term should not be applied to the removal of an extrauterine abdominal pregnancy.

INCIDENCE

According to the National Institutes of Health Task Force on Cesarean Childbirth (Rosen), the cesarean birthrate in the United States increased from 5.5% in 1970 (195,000 operations) to 15.2% in 1978 (510,000 operations) and is still rising. In part the change has resulted from the increasing safety with which cesarean delivery can be performed: infection can be prevented or controlled, anesthetic techniques have been improved, and more labors that end in cesarean delivery are managed by trained obstetrician-gynecologists in sophisticated perinatal units. The improvements in neonatal care for the infant have permitted the extension of indications for the operation to include the delivery of infants of low birth weight and those who might be injured by prolonged labor or traumatic operative vaginal delivery.

The factors that have contributed most to the rising incidence of cesarean delivery are *dystocia* (30% increase), *repeat operations* (25% to 30% increase), *breech presentation* (10% to 15% increase), and *fetal distress* (10% to 15% increase).

INDICATIONS

The major indications for cesarean delivery, which are discussed in detail in the chapters concerned with specific complications, are reviewed briefly here.

Mechanical dystocia. Fetopelvic disproportion can result from abnormalities in the bony pelvis, excessive fetal size, or adnexal or uterine tumors that block the birth canal. Most decisions for cesarean section because of disproportion between pelvic and fetal size are made during labor, when it becomes evident that the fetus cannot be delivered safely through the vagina. Ovarian tumors that are recognized and removed during early pregnancy obviously cannot interfere with labor, but myomas located low in the posterior uterine wall may because they cannot be removed during pregnancy.

Unverified disproportion. Certain patients with unverified disproportion may be delivered by cesarean section. These include women with small pelves in whom the fetal membranes rupture prematurely when it may be difficult to induce labor because the cervix is still firm and uneffaced and those with serious cardiac lesions or other medical complications that might make a long trial of labor followed by cesarean section too dangerous to consider.

Dysfunctional labor. An increasing number of cesarean operations are performed because of "failure to progress''. Many of these are considered to be caused by fetopelvic disproportion, but in a substantial number the lack of progress is caused by dysfunctional labor. Cesarean delivery will certainly improve the outcome for the fetus if normal progress cannot be established by oxytocin stimulation.

Placenta previa. Almost all patients with complete placenta previa and most of those with incomplete varieties can be delivered more safely by cesarean section than through the vagina.

Abruptio placentae. Cesarean section may be performed to control profuse bleeding associated with complete placental separation when the conditions are not appropriate for induction of labor and vaginal delivery or for partial placental separation if one cannot anticipate early vaginal delivery and there is no indication that the fetus is seriously compromised.

Malposition of fetus. Cesarean section is indicated for most stable transverse lies, unless the baby already is dead or is so small that it is unlikely to survive; for abnormal vertex positions that cannot be corrected and delivered vaginally; and for most breech presentations.

Hypertensive diseases. Cesarean section is an appropriate method for delivering women with advancing severe preeclampsia, temporarily controlled preeclampsia or eclampsia, or serious chronic hypertensive cardiovascular renal disease when labor cannot be induced expeditiously.

Previous cesarean section. Until about 1980 elective repeat cesarean sections were performed almost routinely, even though the indication for the first operation was no longer present. Experience with large numbers of women indicates that many can deliver vaginally if the proper safeguards are available.

Uterine operations. Pregnancies that occur after plastic reconstruction of uterine anomalies and tubal transplantation through the uterine wall should be terminated by elective cesarean section because of the possibility of rupture through the scar during labor. Cesarean section should also be considered for patients on whom myomectomy has been performed if a large incision extended through the wall into the uterine cavity. Cesarean section

is not necessary after the removal of superficial myomas.

Fetal indications. The increasing safety with which cesarean section can be performed permits an extension of its use for terminating pregnancy in the interests of the fetus. Fetal indications for cesarean section include *prolapsed cord* when the cervix is incompletely dilated and the fetal condition is good, *intrauterine fetal distress, immature or growth-retarded fetuses* who may be injured during vaginal delivery, those *who must be delivered early before labor can be induced,* and many instances of *multifetal pregnancy.*

Elderly primigravida. The primigravida over 35 years of age need not be delivered by cesarean section simply because of her age, but the operation is used somewhat more liberally for the management of complications, particularly dysfunctional labor, disproportion, and abnormal positions.

CHOICE OF OPERATION

Classic section. In classic cesarean section the uterine incision is made through the upper contractile portion of the fundus above the dome of the bladder (Fig. 40-1). It is easy to perform but has certain disadvantages that make it undesirable. The incision in the thick, active upper segment bleeds more and may not heal as well as the low segment incision. It also cannot be peritonized; thus there is more chance for the development of adhesions and for infected uterine contents to seep into the peritoneal cavity, producing infection and ileus and distention. The risk of infection is high after this operation if the membranes have been ruptured or if the patient has been in labor. Rupture of the uterine scar in subsequent pregnancies occurs more often after the classic than the lower segment operations.

Classic cesarean section may be preferable to the lower segment operations if the bladder is firmly adherent to the uterus, for transverse lie, when the fetal back is directed toward the pelvic inlet, for anterior wall placenta previa, and when it is necessary to empty the uterus rapidly.

Classic cesarean section is contraindicated if the membranes have been ruptured for many hours or if there is evidence of chorioamnionitis.

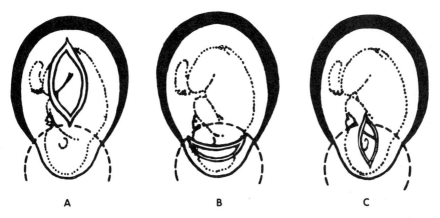

Fig. 40-1. Cesarean section showing position of uterine incision. Dotted line indicates approximate position of bladder. **A,** Classic incision. **B,** Low segment transverse incision. **C,** Low segment longitudinal incision. (Modified from Tenny, B., and Little, B.: Clinical obstetrics, Philadelphia, 1961, W.B. Saunders Co.)

Low segment section. In low segment cesarean section the uterine incision is made in the thin lower segment after the vesicouterine peritoneum has been cut and the bladder separated and pushed downward from its attachment to the anterior uterine wall. One advantage is that the incision is behind the bladder and can be completely covered by peritoneum; thus the seepage from the uterus is reduced and postpartum peritoneal infection is less likely to occur than with the classic method. The low segment section can be used more safely after the membranes have been ruptured or labor has been in progress for some hours.

A transverse incision in the lower segment is preferable to a vertical one because it requires less mobilization of the bladder and because the incidence of rupture in subsequent pregnancies is lower. Its major disadvantages are that it can extend into the huge uterine veins and that the manipulations necessary to deliver a fetus presenting as a frank breech or transversely are more difficult through a transverse opening. A vertical incision can extend either downward through the cervix or upward into the upper segment of the uterus and is more likely to separate during subsequent labors. Involvement of the contractile portion of the uterus, by deliberate incision or by traumatic extension, explains the increased possibility of rupture during a later pregnancy.

Extraperitoneal section. In extraperitoneal cesarean section the uterine incision is made in the lower segment behind the bladder after the peritoneum has been dissected off the dome of the bladder without entering the peritoneal cavity. The bladder is then pushed downward to expose the uterine wall. The extraperitoneal section is more difficult to perform, requiring a skilled operator, and bladder and ureteral injuries are more common than with the other operations. It does not solve the problem when infection has extended through the uterine wall, and it is not necessary in the potentially infected patient; therefore its value is limited.

Cesarean hysterectomy. Cesarean section followed by removal of the uterus is indicated if there is a definite reason for hysterectomy, for example, multiple fibroid tumors or uterine rupture. Its value in the infected patient is greatest if the uterine wall is deeply and heavily infected and contains multiple small abscesses that may produce a constant source of infected emboli.

Cesarean hysterectomy should not usually be considered as an alternative to cesarean section and tubal sterilization. The morbidity and potential mortality associated with hysterectomy is far greater than with tubal ligation.

ANESTHESIA

There should be no increase in maternal or fetal mortality from the anesthetic. The same factors that influence the administration of medication and anesthetic in vaginal delivery hold true with cesarean section. The fetus is narcotized or anesthetized by all the medication given the mother. Conduction anesthesia, except when contraindicated, is usually preferable to inhalation technics.

Conduction anesthesia provides excellent pain relief with limited effects on the fetus, unless the blood pressure falls to a level too low to maintain uterine perfusion. *Inhalation anesthesia* is preferable in patients who are bleeding and when rapid delivery is essential. The effects of the inhaled agent on the fetus can be minimized if the abdomen is prepared and draped and the surgical team is ready to start the operation as soon as an adequate anesthetic level has been reached. If the infant is delivered within 6 or 8 minutes, it will be little affected by the anesthetic.

An important cause of maternal morbidity and mortality is aspiration of vomitus as anesthesia is being induced or as the patient is reacting after inhalation technics. The effects of aspiration can be reduced by giving the mother 30 ml of an antacid solution preoperatively.

REPEAT CESAREAN SECTION

If a patient has been delivered by cesarean section in one or more previous pregnancies, there is always a question as to whether she should be delivered by elective cesarean section or whether she should be permitted to go into labor and deliver vaginally. The most important factor in arriving at a logical decision is the integrity of the uterine scar. If it is strong and well healed, labor will undoubtedly terminate uneventfully; but if it is weak, it may rupture late in pregnancy or after contractions begin. Unfortunately, there is no accurate method for evaluating the strength of the scar during pregnancy.

The scar of a classical section separates late in pregnancy, as the uterus becomes more active or during labor. The fetus is usually expelled into the peritoneal cavity where it dies. The separation of a lower segment incision is less dramatic. The rupture does not often extend into the peritoneal cavity because the old incision lies beneath the bladder. The defect in a transverse lower segment incision may be localized to a small area, or it may involve the entire scar. Most of these go unnoticed unless the defect is discovered at the time of cesarean section or when the uterus is explored after vaginal delivery. Separation of a vertical lower segment scar is more likely to be associated with profuse bleeding, because it may extend into the thick, vascular contractile portion of the uterus.

Since there is no way to evaluate the integrity of the uterine scar during pregnancy, many obstetricians advise *elective repeat cesarean section* sometime after the thirty-eighth week for almost all women who have been delivered by cesarean section. This practice prevents most of the catastrophic uterine ruptures of classic scars and those that extend upward from the lower segment. The increased use of transverse lower segment incisions, the good results of permitting vaginal delivery in carefully selected patients, and the inevitable increase in morbidity and mortality associated with cesarean delivery have prompted obstetricians to question the validity of the time-honored concept "once a cesarean, always a cesarean." The advantages of vaginal delivery over repeat cesarean section are a more rapid recovery, fewer complications, less discomfort and reduced cost.

Gibbs permitted 1192 (76%) of 1558 women who had had one previous lower segment transverse cesarean section and who had no contraindications to vaginal delivery to go into labor; 63% delivered uneventfully. Uterine rupture occurred three times in the 746 women who delivered vaginally, three times in the 446 who were delivered by cesarean section after a failed trial of labor, and three times in the 366 who were delivered by elective repeat cesarean section. There was no difference in the perinatal mortality. Febrile morbidity occurred in 1% of those delivered vaginally, in 17% of those delivered by elective repeat cesarean section, and in 27% of those delivered by cesarean section after a trial of labor.

Paul, Phelan, and Yeh permitted trials of labor in 751 of 1209 women who had been delivered previously by cesarean section; 614 (82%) delivered vaginally. There were no maternal or perinatal deaths attributable to the trials of labor, but there were 29 uterine ruptures. The incidence of dehiscence was similar in those delivered vaginally and those delivered by cesarean section. Meier and Porreco permitted trials of labor in 207 women who had been delivered previously by transverse lower segment cesarean section; 175 (84.5%) delivered successfully and without scar dehiscence. One scar separated in the 31 in whom the trial failed.

Women who are selected for trial labor should have been delivered through a transverse lower segment incision, should have no contraindications to vaginal delivery, should be delivered in a perinatal unit in which any type of maternal and infant complication can be managed expertly, and must be interested enough in normal delivery to accept the slight risk involved. *Trial labor is contraindicated* when the indication for the first cesarean section is still present (for example, a major contracted pelvis), if the original incision was vertical in either the body of the uterus or the lower segment, if there is more than one fetus, if the fetal position is abnormal, if there is a reason for delivery before labor starts spontaneously, or if the requirements for the prompt management of potential complications cannot be met.

The labor must be conducted by an experienced obstetrician; uterine activity and fetal condition should be monitored electronically; compatible blood should be available; and an operating room, an anesthesiologist, and a surgical team should be immediately available in case an emergency cesarean section is required. After delivery the interior of the uterus should be explored to ensure that the scar is still intact.

Cesarean section is performed promptly during trial labor if fetal distress is suspected, if there is a question concerning the integrity of the scar, or if significant fetopelvic disproportion is encountered.

Oxytocin stimulation of dysfunctional labor can be used cautiously. Before starting oxytocin, however, one must make certain that there are no abnormalities in fetal position and no significant fetopelvic disproportion. A previous cesarean section for "failure to progress" or for a minor degree of disproportion does not necessarily contraindicate trial labor.

Patients for whom repeat cesarean delivery is planned are admitted to the hospital sometime after the thirty-eighth week of pregnancy. The exact time is selected on the basis of the date of the last menstrual period, a comparison between the size of the uterus and the history at the first and subsequent examinations, confirmation of dates by ultrasound examination before the twentieth week, the dates at which fetal motion was first felt and the fetal heart was first heard, appropriate growth, the estimated size of the infant, and the condition of the cervix.

Although all deaths from the complications of prematurity cannot be eliminated, the number can be reduced. For example, almost every baby born by elective repeat cesarean section should survive, but too many do not. Jones reported that in 13 of 59 premature infants who died following delivery by cesarean section there was a discrepancy between the birth weight and the presumed duration of pregnancy. Each of these infants weighed less than 2500 g. Such deaths can be prevented by proving that the fetus is mature before scheduling a patient for elective cesarean section. When dates are uncertain, the operation should be delayed until amniotic fluid examination indicates that pulmonary maturity has been established.

STERILIZATION

The fact that a woman must be delivered by cesarean section does not necessarily limit her reproductive career, but repeated abdominal operations are more dangerous than an equal number of vaginal deliveries. A tubal ligation may be performed in conjunction with cesarean section if the patient requests it, but there is no reason to insist on the operation simply because of previous cesarean deliveries.

COMPLICATIONS

The mortality associated with cesarean section even under the most favorable conditions is greater than for normal delivery. The deaths are not all direct results of the operation itself; many are caused by the complication that made the cesarean delivery necessary.

There were 97 maternal deaths in 120,684 cesarean sections performed in Professional Activity Study (PAS) hospitals between 1967 and 1974, a rate of 80/100,000 operations. In contrast, the death rate for all 2,196,684 deliveries, including cesarean sections, in the same hospitals was 27/100,000. Jones reported two maternal deaths in 2563 cesarean operations: both occurred during the first 338 operations and were followed by 2225 consecutive procedures without a maternal death.

These figures and those from other reports suggest that between 80 and 100 of each 100,000 women who are delivered by cesarean section will die. Many of these deaths can be prevented by appropriate treatment of the complications that made the operation necessary and by paying meticulous attention to the details of the operation itself and to postoperative care. Support for this statement is that more than 10,000 consecutive cesarean sections were performed in the Boston Women's Hospital between 1968 and 1979 without a maternal death.

Infection. Infection, one of the most common of the complications of cesarean section, occurs more often after emergency operations performed during labor than after planned elective procedures. The number of serious infections can be reduced significantly by early decision to deliver patients in abnormal labor, by meticulous surgical technique, and by the judicious use of prophylactic antibiotics. (Chapter 42.)

Bleeding. Cesarean section is not a blood-conserving procedure; the blood loss averages at least 1 L, and many patients lose much more. The usual patient on whom cesarean section is performed need not be transfused, but replacement is desirable if the initial blood count is low or if blood loss is excessive.

Anesthetic. Unless the anesthetic is carefully controlled, it may contribute substantially to the mortality. Many of the deaths associated with aspiration of gastric contents can be prevented if the mother is given 30 ml of an antacid solution orally just before the anesthetic is administered. This neutralizes gastric acid and reduces lung damage if she aspirates vomitus.

Perinatal mortality. Cesarean delivery does not guarantee infant survival; in fact, the perinatal mortality associated with the operation is higher than that for delivery in general. Many deaths occur because of the complications that make delivery necessary.

One of the most important reasons for the increasing incidence of cesarean delivery is that infants who are born alive and undamaged have a better chance of developing normally than do those born after a difficult or traumatic vaginal delivery. Sachs and colleagues studied neonatal mortality in 392,241 singleton births in Georgia between 1974 and 1978. The neonatal mortality rate for vaginal breech deliveries of infants weighing between 2501 and 4000 was three times that for those delivered by cesarean section. The risk increased with decreasing weight. There was no significant advantage of delivering vertex presentations by cesarean section unless there was a serious maternal complication such as hypertension, bleeding, or infection. The best results for babies weighing between 1000 to 1500 g when delivery was made necessary by a maternal complication was by cesarean section in a tertiary care center.

Although cesarean section can now be used more liberally for small babies who are delivered in hospitals that provide excellent perinatal intensive care, there is a limit beyond which it offers no advantage. Barrett, Boehm, and Vaughan analyzed the outcome for 109 singleton neonates weighing between 501 and 1000 g. They could detect no advantage of cesarean section over vaginal delivery. They did note that the frequency of neonatal death was decreased in those who had not been in labor when the cesarean section was performed. Olshan and colleagues found no advantage of cesarean section for 345 infants weighing between 700 and 1500 g, even for breech presentations. Kitchen and co-workers, studying 172 survivors of 326 babies of 24 to 28 weeks' gestational age, also detected no significant improvement in neonatal mortality in those delivered by cesarean section. Moreover, the method of delivery did not influence the incidence of handicaps in 111 who were followed for 2 years.

Not everyone agrees that the increased incidence of cesarean section is necessary to maintain low perinatal mortality rates. O'Driscoll and Foley noted a decrease in perinatal mortality in 76,547 births from 42.1 in 1970 to 16.8 in 1980 at the National Maternity Hospital, Dublin. During this same period the cesarean section rate increased from 4.2% to only 4.8%. They accomplished this by being more aggressive in their management of dysfunctional labor, by encouraging vaginal breech delivery, and by reducing the number of repeat cesarean sections.

The figures in most reports relate only to mortality. One of the advantages of the increasing rate of cesarean section is decreased perinatal morbidity and mortality, for breech presentation, transverse lie, cephalopelvic disproportion, placenta previa, and other complications. In the past many babies were damaged during the vaginal management of these complications. Such babies are now much more likely to be born without injury.

REFERENCES

Barrett, J.M., Boehm, F.H., and Vaughan, W.K.: The effect of type of delivery on neonatal outcome in singleton infants of birth weight of 1000 g or less, J.A.M.A. **250**:625, 1983.

Chestnut, D.H., Eden, R.D., Gall, S.A., and Parker, R.T.: Postpartum hysterectomy: a review of cesarean and postpartum hysterectomy, Obstet. Gynecol. **65:**365, 1985.

Gibbs, C.E.: Planned vaginal delivery following cesarean section, Clin. Obstet. Gynecol. **23:**507, 1980.

Jones, O.H.: Cesarean section in present day obstetrics. Am. J. Obstet. Gynecol. **126:**521, 1976.

Kitchen W., et al.: Cesarean section or vaginal delivery at 24 to 28 weeks' gestation: comparison of survival and neonatal and two-year morbidity, Obstet. Gynecol. **66:**149, 1985.

Lowe, J.A., Klassen, D.F., and Loup, R.J.: Cesarean sections in U.S. PAS hospitals, PAS Reporter **14:**1, 1976.

Meier, P.R., and Porreco, R.P.: Trial of labor following cesarean section: a two-year experience, Am. J. Obstet. Gynecol. **144:**671, 1982.

O'Driscoll, K., and Foley, M.: Correlation of decrease in perinatal mortality and increase in cesarean section rates, Obstet. Gynecol. **61:**1, 1983.

Olshan, A.F. et al.: Cesarean birth and neonatal mortality in very low-birth-weight infants, Am. J. Obstet. Gynecol. **64:**267, 1984.

Paul, R.H., Phelan, J.P., and Yeh, S.: Trial of labor in the patient with a prior cesarean birth, Am. J. Obstet. Gynecol. **151:**297, 1985.

Rosen, M.G.: NIH consensus development statement on cesarean childbirth, Obstet. Gynecol. **57:**537, 1981.

Sachs, B.P., et al.: Cesarean section: risks and benefits for mother and fetus: JAMA **250:**2157, 1983.

Saldana, L.R., Schulman, H., and Reuss, L.: Management of pregnancy after cesarean section, Am. J. Obstet. Gynecol. **135:**555, 1979.

41

J. Robert Willson

Immediate and remote effects of childbirth injury; uterine retrodisplacement

Some damage to the soft-tissue structures of the birth canal and adjacent organs occurs during every delivery. It usually is more pronounced in primigravidas, whose relatively firm tissues offer more resistance to the descent of the baby than do those of multiparas. Damage to the pelvic supports, particularly those supporting the posterior vaginal wall, is usually caused by an injury that is obvious at delivery, but in some instances the skin and vaginal epithelium remain intact even though there are numerous small tears in the underlying fascia and muscle. In some women, notably blacks, the soft tissues are so readily distensible that they stretch without tearing to permit expulsion of the infant. Thus the supports remain intact even after several pregnancies. In contrast, extensive damage may occur in others, even though every effort is made to preserve the structures; these women may also develop varicose veins and diastasis recti, suggesting that they may have a generalized supporting-tissue deficiency that is basically responsible for the failure to heal properly.

The cervix, vagina, and perineum should be inspected after each hospital delivery, and obvious injuries should be repaired immediately unless there is a good reason for delay. Approximation of the injured tissues will permit them to heal faster and will limit the extent of the residual damage. Repair also reduces the possibility of infection.

The primary support of the uterus and the upper vagina is offered by the *cardinal ligaments* (Mackenrodt's ligaments), which are connective tissue condensations that extend laterally and posteriorly from the endopelvic fascia surrounding the cervix and upper vagina to fuse with the fascia overlying the obturator and levator muscles. The round ligaments and the broad ligaments have relatively little supporting function (Fig. 41-1).

The muscles making up each levator ani sweep downward from their attachments along the iliopectineal line and form the pelvic diaphragm, the superior surface of which is covered by a strong layer of endopelvic fascia (Fig. 41-2). The pubococcygeus portion of the levator surrounds the rectum and is intimately connected to the lateral walls of the urethra and vagina. The levator bundles are held together between the rectum and the vagina by the fascia, which, with the tissues in the lower portion of the rectovaginal septum, make up the perineal body (Fig. 41-3). The bladder and the rectum are supported by the muscle in the wall of each of the organs and the extensions of the endopelvic fascia in the rectovaginal and vesicovaginal septa.

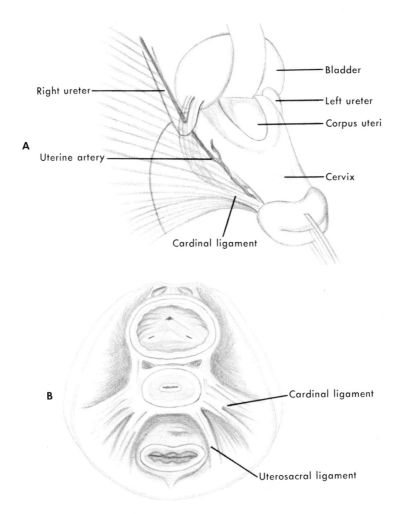

Fig. 41-1. Cardinal ligaments. **A,** Relationships of cardinal ligament as seen during vaginal hysterectomy. **B,** Cardinal and uterosacral ligaments and paracervical fascia at level just above internal cervical os.

PERINEAL LACERATIONS

Perineal lacerations are divided into four types, depending on their depth. In a *first-degree laceration* the tear extends through the skin and the superficial structures above the muscles. In a *second-degree laceration* the tear extends through the muscles of the perineal body but does not involve the sphincter ani. A *third-degree laceration* severs the sphincter, and with a *fouth-degree laceration* the anterior rectal wall is also torn. Perineal in-

juries usually occur as the structures at the vaginal outlet are overdistended during delivery of the head.

At least the lower vagina is involved whenever the perineum is injured. The vaginal portion of the tear often extends up one or both lateral sulci rather than up the midline; the depth depends on the extent of the perineal injury. The levator fascia is injured in all but the most superficial perineal lacerations (Fig. 41-4, *A*).

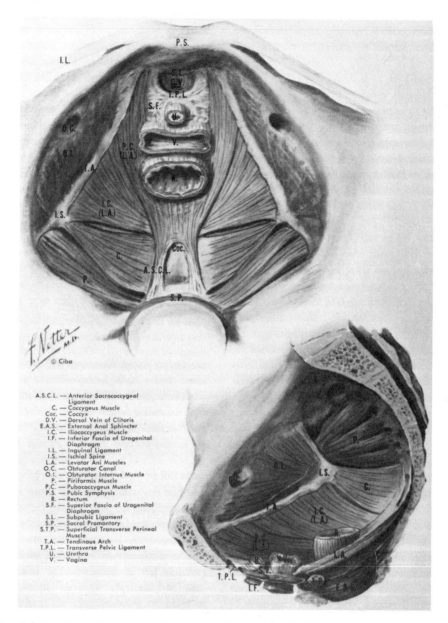

A.S.C.L. — Anterior Sacrococcygeal
　　　　　Ligament
　　C. — Coccygeus Muscle
　Coc. — Coccyx
　D.V. — Dorsal Vein of Clitoris
E.A.S. — External Anal Sphincter
　I.C. — Iliococcygeus Muscle
　I.F. — Inferior Fascia of Urogenital
　　　　　Diaphragm
　I.L. — Inguinal Ligament
　I.S. — Ischial Spine
　L.A. — Levator Ani Muscles
　O.C. — Obturator Canal
　O.I. — Obturator Internus Muscle
　　P. — Piriformis Muscle
　P.C. — Pubococcygeus Muscle
　P.S. — Pubic Symphysis
　　R. — Rectum
　S.F. — Superior Fascia of Urogenital
　　　　　Diaphragm
　S.L. — Subpubic Ligament
　S.P. — Sacral Promontory
S.T.P. — Superficial Transverse Perineal
　　　　　Muscle
　T.A. — Tendinous Arch
T.P.L. — Transverse Pelvic Ligament
　　U. — Urethra
　　V. — Vagina

Fig. 41-2. Muscles within pelvic cavity. (© Copyright 1954, 1965, CIBA Pharmaceutical Company, Division of CIBA-GEIGY Corporation. Reprinted with permission from The CIBA Collection of Medical Illustrations illustrated by Frank H. Netter, M.D. All rights reserved.)

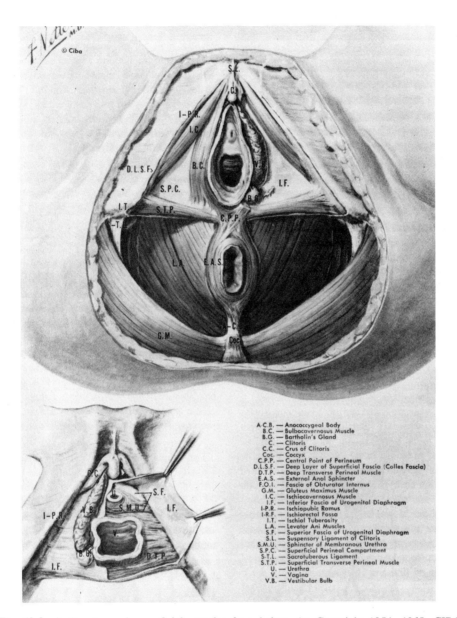

Fig. 41-3. A, Levator and superficial muscles from below. (© Copyright 1954, 1965, CIBA Pharmaceutical Company, Division of CIBA-GEIGY Corporation. Reprinted with permission of The CIBA Collection of Medical Illustrations illustrated by Frank H. Netter, M.D. All rights reserved.)   *Continued.*

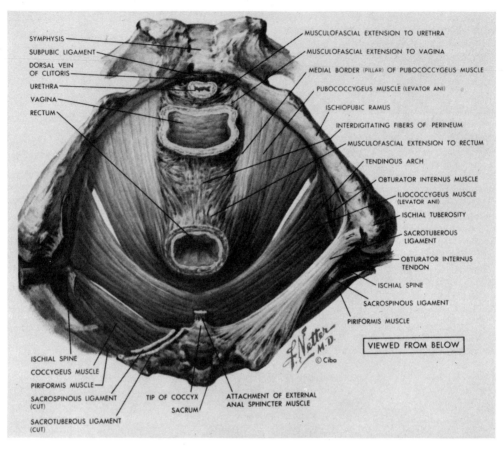

Fig. 41-3, cont'd. B, Levator muscles from below; superficial muscles removed. (© Copyright 1954, 1965, CIBA Pharmaceutical Company, Division of CIBA-GEIGY Corporation. Reprinted with permission of The CIBA Collection of Medical Illustrations illustrated by Frank H. Netter, M.D. All rights reserved.)

Treatment

Perineal lacerations should be repaired immediately with chromic no. 3-0 or 4-0 catgut or polyglycolic sutures. The most superficial ones can be closed with one layer of interrupted sutures, but two or more layers may be necessary for the more extensive injuries. It often is advantageous to use no. 4-0 sutures on an atraumatic needle to close the wounds near the clitoris, since the small needle and suture will provoke less bleeding. It is particularly important to repair third- and fourth-degree lacerations so that the patient can retain fecal continence (Fig. 41-4).

The rectal defect is closed by inverting the torn edges with two layers of interrupted catgut sutures carefully placed in the submucosal tissues but not through the mucosa itself. The cut ends of the sphincter muscle are located and approximated with two or three interrupted catgut sutures. The separated levator bundles and the more superficial muscles, which are also involved in the injury, are next approximated to complete the repair. No special postpartum care is required, but it usually is wise

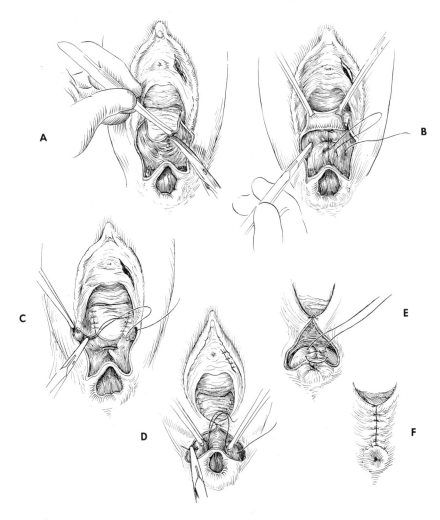

Fig. 41-4. Perineal lacerations. **A,** Bilateral sulcus tears, periurethral tear, and separation of anal sphincter. **B,** Exposure and approximation of levator structures. **C,** Approximation of torn bulbocavernosus muscle. **D** and **E,** Approximation of ends of anal sphincter. **F,** Complete repair. (From Willson, J.R.: Atlas of obstetric technic, ed. 2, St. Louis, 1969, The C.V. Mosby Co.)

to keep the stools soft for several days. It is not necessary to prescribe antimicrobial drugs.

Late results

Perineal injuries that do not involve the levator ani usually produce no permanent disability even though they are not repaired. If the severed ends of the superficial perineal muscles, particularly the bulbocavernosus, are not approximated, the vaginal introitus may gape.

If a sphincter tear is overlooked, the patient will probably be incontinent of feces unless the puborectalis portion of the levator ani muscle is strong enough to compensate for the torn sphincter. Since the levators and the sphincter are both involved in the injury, this usually does not occur.

If a third-degree laceration has been overlooked, and if the patient plans to have more children, the defect can be repaired satisfactorily at the next delivery. If she is past the childbearing age or desires no more children, the lesion can be corrected at her convenience by an experienced gynecologic surgeon.

VAGINAL LACERATIONS

Perineal injuries usually extend up the vaginal sulci and, if deep enough, will separate the levator ani from its attachments to the lateral vaginal and rectal walls. The vaginal wall may also be injured at the level of the ischial spines or in the vault. The tears in the vault are often circular and may be the result of forceps rotation, particularly if there is some degree of cephalopelvic disproportion.

Vaginal lacerations may bleed profusely, and, as a consequence, it is difficult to expose and repair them, particularly if the physician does not have adequate assistance.

INJURIES TO THE LEVATOR SLING

Perineal and vaginal lacerations may be relatively superficial, leaving the important deep supporting structures intact, or they may extend more deeply and interrupt the integrity of the levator sling and the endopelvic fascia. The extent of the visible laceration is usually obvious, but extensive damage to the deep supporting structures can occur even though there is no visible injury involving the skin or the vaginal wall.

As the presenting part descends through the birth canal and distends the lower vagina, the levator bundles are separated, and the levator fascia is stretched. If the fascial layer is unusually resilient, it can stretch enough to permit the birth of the baby and then return to normal, but more often it tears, permitting the levator muscles to separate and retract laterally.

The accompanying perineal and vaginal lacerations disrupt the fascial layer in the rectovaginal septum, destroying the support of the rectum anteriorly. The levator pillars may also be detached from the lateral walls of the rectum, further reducing its support. The lacerations usually are irregular, and the involved tissue is often badly bruised.

Serious lacerations can occur because labor terminates so forcibly and rapidly that the structures are torn apart rather than stretched slowly or because there is disproportion between the size of the infant and that of the pelvis. Another common cause is a narrow pubic arch. As the head is delivering, it cannot fit snugly beneath the symphysis but is forced backward toward the posterior pelvis, putting undue strain on the soft tissues as it passes through the introitus. Other less frequent causes are edema, extensive perineal scarring from past deliveries, and unskillful attempts at operative delivery.

Treatment

Immediate approximation of the torn levator structures and of the vaginal and perineal injuries will permit the tissues to heal and will reduce subsequent deformity. However, there may be a considerable amount of permanent relaxation of the repaired structures because they usually have been rather seriously injured by the extreme distention that preceded their final bursting.

Prevention

Even though the physician makes every possible effort to eliminate traumatic deliveries, the supporting structures will be injured unless special precautions are taken. *The most important measure for preventing serious posterior wall injury is episiotomy, or incision of the perineum and the underlying supporting structures.* Episiotomy should be performed on almost every primigravida and on most multiparas with intact pelvic supports.

If episiotomy is to offer maximum protection, the perineum must be incised before the tissues have already been stretched and injured by the advancing presenting part. The incision, which must be long enough to cut all the tissues holding the levator bundles together in the midline, is made when the perineum is flattened and bulging and when the vaginal opening is dilated about 6 cm during a contraction. A mediolateral or a median episiotomy (Figs. 41-5 to 41-7) will produce equally good results if the incision is made properly and at the

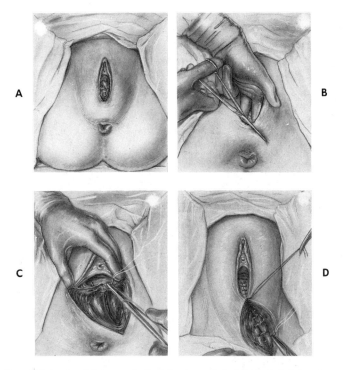

Fig. 41-5. Left mediolateral episiotomy. **A,** Incision is made before perineal structures are damaged. **B,** Incision from midline toward ischial tuberosity. **C,** Repair of vaginal wall. Sutures must include muscle layer, as well as epithelium. **D,** Approximation of levator bundles. (From Willson, J.R.: Atlas of obstetric technic, ed. 2, St. Louis, 1969, The C.V. Mosby Co.)

right time and if it is carefully repaired. With an adequate mediolateral incision, the fat in the ischiorectal fossa usually is visible in the lower angle, and a median incision usually exposes the sphincter ani.

Regional or general anesthesia is essential for the performance of an adequate episiotomy because it must be made before the tissues have been injured. The practice of making a small incision without anesthesia in the overstretched and blanched perineum offers no protection to the deep fascia and muscle; they already have been stretched to their maximum and have retracted so that only the superficial structures are cut.

The entire episiotomy is repaired meticulously with chromic no. 3-0 or 4-0 catgut or polyglycolic sutures, which produce relatively little local reaction. It is not necessary to take great sweeping bites of tissue with each stitch; neither must the physician tie the sutures tightly except when it is necessary to control bleeding. The repair should not be started until the placenta has been delivered and the uterus is well contracted. It is difficult to explore the uterus after the wound is closed unless the sutures are removed.

Late results

If injuries are left unrepaired, permanent defects in support may result. Occasionally, however, the same lesions develop in women whose injuries have been carefully repaired, in those in whom an attempt has been made to prevent lacerations, and even in those who have never been pregnant.

Rectocele (Fig. 41-8). Unrepaired posterior lacerations disrupt the fascial support of the rectal wall, permit the levator bundles to retract laterally, and destroy the perineal body, thereby eliminating the normal support of the lower vagina. One of the functions of the perineal body is to deflect stool posteriorly toward the anal canal, through which it is evacuated. Loss of the midline support in the

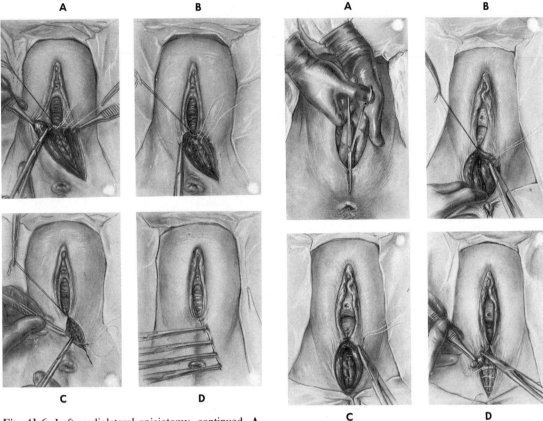

A   **B**

C   **D**

Fig. 41-6. Left mediolateral episiotomy, continued. **A,** Repair of bulbocavernosus muscle. **B,** Reconstruction of urogenital diaphragm. **C** and **D,** Skin closure. (From Willson, J.R.: Atlas of obstetric technic, ed. 2, St. Louis, 1969, The C.V. Mosby Co.)

A   **B**

C   **D**

Fig. 41-7. Median episiotomy. **A,** Incision to anal sphincter. **B,** Approximation of levator bundles. Vaginal incision has already been closed. **C,** Reconstruction of urogenital diaphragm. **D,** Skin closure. (From Willson, J.R.: Atlas of obstetric technic, ed. 2, St. Louis, 1969, The C.V. Mosby Co.)

lower vagina and introitus permits the rectum and the posterior vaginal wall to sag anteriorly. When the patient is on her feet, the weight of the abdominal contents produces an increase in descent of the rectal wall. Each time she strains in an attempt to evacuate her rectum, the fecal mass is forced downward against the relatively thin rectovaginal wall, stretching it a little more. The rectum gradually protrudes more and more into the vagina until eventually a large pouch may be visible through the relaxed introitus. This lesion, which is called a *rectocele,* is the most common late result of childbirth injury. Most rectoceles are small and produce few symptoms, but some are huge and bulge out-

side the vaginal canal whenever the patient stands up.

The rectocele often remains relatively small and produces a few symptoms until after the patient has gone through the menopause. When tissue atrophy develops because of withdrawal of the estrogenic hormones, the size of the rectocele increases rapidly.

SYMPTOMS. The symptoms produced by a rectocele are related to the loss of muscular and fascial support and the consequent disturbance of bowel function. If the lesion is large, most women will experience "bearing down" and a sensation of lack

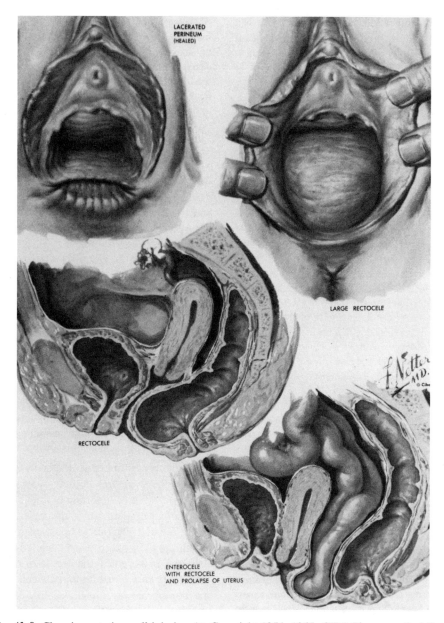

Fig. 41-8. Chronic posterior wall injuries. (© Copyright 1954, 1965, CIBA Pharmaceutical Company, Division of CIBA-GEIGY Corporation. Reprinted with permission from The CIBA Collection of Medical Illustrations illustrated by Frank H. Netter, M.D. All rights reserved.)

of support when on their feet. They feel as though all the pelvic organs are going to fall out through the introitus. They may also complain of the protrusion of a mass. Those with large rectoceles find it difficult to evacuate the rectum because the fecal material is pushed into the rectal pouch instead of being deflected toward the anal opening by the structures of the perineal body and the levator support of the lower rectum, which have been destroyed. If questioned, these women will usually state that they must hold the mass up with the fingers in the vagina to permit evacuation of fecal material. The fingers substitute for the intact vaginal wall and perineal body and divert the fecal mass downward into the anal canal rather than toward the vagina. The symptoms disappear when these women lie down.

DIAGNOSIS. The diagnosis is made by observing the mass protruding from the vagina and identifying it as a rectocele by performing rectal and vaginal examinations. The relaxed posterior vaginal wall can be inverted through the introitus by the rectal finger.

TREATMENT. Symptom-producing rectoceles can only be corrected by an operative procedure by which the separated levator muscles and their fascia and the structures of the perineal body are approximated in the midline between the anterior rectal and the posterior vaginal walls, thereby restoring the continuity of the supports. This procedure is performed with a vaginal approach and is called *perineorrhaphy* if the repair involves only the structures of the perineal body and lower rectum, *posterior colpoplasty* if the repair is more extensive, or more simply *posterior vaginal repair*.

Enterocele (Fig. 41-8). Enterocele, also called *posterior vaginal hernia* or *cul-de-sac hernia*, consists of herniation of the peritoneum of the posterior cul-de-sac downward between the uterosacral ligaments into the rectovaginal septum. The cul-de-sac in women who develop this defect probably is deeper than usual, and when its support is disrupted by childbirth injury, the weight of the intestine and omentum when the patient is on her feet gradually enlarges the sac and forces it downward between the rectum and the vagina. This lesion occurs frequently in association with prolapse of the uterus and after vaginal hysterectomy, particularly when it is performed as part of the treatment of vaginal relaxation.

SYMPTOMS. Enterocele produces few symptoms except pressure and a bearing-down sensation, which may be caused primarily by the relaxation of the other structures. It may protrude through the introitus.

DIAGNOSIS. On superficial inspection, an enterocele may resemble a rectocele, and in fact both lesions often are present in the same patient. Unless it is recognized and repaired, the first indication of its presence may be a persistent posterior wall bulge after rectocele repair or a herniation of the vaginal vault after vaginal hysterectomy.

The herniation can usually be recognized by performing a rectovaginal examination and feeling the increased thickness of the rectovaginal wall above the thin rectocele and by asking the patient to cough while palpating the bulge. If an enterocele is present, the increased intraabdominal pressure will be transmitted to the fingertip as through the usual type of hernia. In many patients the sac is discovered during an operation for vaginal repair.

TREATMENT. The hernia is usually treated by vaginal operation because rectocele and uterine prolapse are almost always present. The sac is opened, its contents are reduced, the peritoneal opening is closed, and the cul-de-sac defect is obliterated by approximating the uterosacral ligaments and the levator bundles in the midline. An abdominal operation that accomplishes the same thing can also be performed but is not usually necessary.

INJURIES TO THE ANTERIOR VAGINAL WALL

In nulliparous women the bladder is supported by the integrity of the vesical and vaginal walls and by an extension of the endopelvic fascia between the inferior vesical wall and the anterior vaginal wall. During labor the bladder, which is attached to the anterior surface of the uterus, is pulled up out of the pelvis as the lower uterine segment elongates. As a consequence, only the urethra, the vesical neck, and a portion of the bladder floor are vulnerable to injury.

As the presenting part descends and dilates the vagina, the structures in the vesicovaginal septum are stretched or even torn in multiple areas beneath the vaginal epithelium. If the infant is unusually large, the delivery precipitious, or the bony pelvis small, more damage occurs than from the usual delivery. If there is some degree of disproportion, there may be so little room between the head and the bony walls of the pelvis that the soft-tissue structures are pushed down ahead of the presenting part while the bladder is pulled upward each time the uterus contracts. The combination of counterforces may damage the supporting structures of the upper uretha, the vesical neck, and the bladder itself. The same effect is produced if the soft tissues are relatively rigid and do not dilate properly as labor progresses.

If the muscular structures of the posterior vaginal

wall are strong and heavy, the presenting part is forced anteriorly during the expulsive phase of delivery where it compresses the bladder neck and urethra against the pubis; descent also is delayed because it takes longer to overcome the soft-tissue resistance. The combination of prolongation of the expulsive phase and increased pressure against the bladder neck and urethra increases the chance of injuring these structures.

Treatment

The vaginal epithelium covering the anterior wall is seldom torn during delivery; consequently, there is little obvious soft-tissue damage and nothing can be repaired at the time of delivery. Tears in the lateral or posterior vagina and those in the vault do not affect the bladder.

Prevention

Injuries to the anterior wall can be minimized by a few simple procedures. The physician should not allow the bladder to become distended during labor. If the patient cannot void, she must be catheterized. The performance of episiotomy will eliminate the resistance offered by the muscle and fascia posteriorly and will permit the head to descend through the posterior portion of the outlet, thereby decreasing pressure on the urethra and vesical neck. Low forceps extraction combined with episiotomy, if the delivery of the head is delayed, will also reduce anterior soft-tissue trauma, but difficult forceps operations may increase it.

Late results

Relaxation of bladder and urethral supports can develop as a result of pregnancy even though there was no obvious soft-tissue damage at the time of delivery.

Cystocele (Fig. 41-9). A cystocele, the protrusion of the bladder downward into the vaginal canal, develops because the supporting structures in the vesicovaginal septum have lost their integrity. As with rectocele, anterior wall relaxation is not present immediately after delivery but develops over time and often after the patient has had several babies. The weakened anterior vaginal wall descends because of the force of gravity and the weight of the abdominal organs when the patient is on her feet. Repeated stresses, for example, increases in intraabdominal pressure from lifting, straining, and coughing and the weight of accumulated urine in the bladder gradually stretch the vesicovaginal septum until the bladder bulges into the vagina. With time cystocele enlarges until it may protrude through the introitus. A rectocele is usually present in women with relaxation of the anterior wall, and the bladder descends when the uterus prolapses.

The urethra may also be involved in anterior wall relaxation, since it, too, can be injured during the expulsion of the baby. *Urethrocele* rarely develops unless the bladder also is injured. The combined lesion is a *cystourethrocele* (Fig. 41-9).

SYMPTOMS. Small cystoceles, and even some huge ones, produce few symptoms. Some women complain only of bearing-down sensations in the pelvis and the protrusion of a mass through the introitus when they are on their feet. The pressure and the mass disappear when they lie down. Urinary control is maintained unless urethral and vesical neck function is disturbed. In fact, many women with large cystoceles find it difficult to initiate voiding unless they push the sagging bladder upward with their fingers. The bladder usually empties itself reasonably well, and in most instances there is little residual urine.

DIAGNOSIS. The diagnosis of cystocele is made by identifying the vaginal bulge as involving the anterior wall. Unless there is an associated urethral injury, the urethra and bladder neck may be well supported behind the pubis even when the patient strains and the cystocele is pushed downward. The size of the pouch and the degree of protrusion can often be better appreciated by examining the patient while she stands upright.

TREATMENT. The bulge of the cystocele is obliterated by plicating the bladder wall with interrupted sutures after the cystocele has been exposed by deflecting the vaginal mucosa off it. This can be accomplished only by a vaginal approach because the involved area cannot be reached through an abdominal incision. The fact that a cystocele is present does not mean that treatment is

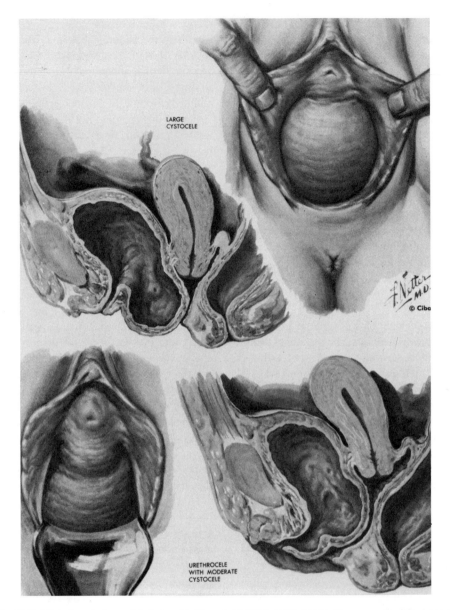

LARGE
CYSTOCELE

URETHROCELE
WITH MODERATE
CYSTOCELE

Fig. 41-9. Chronic anterior wall injuries. (© Copyright 1954, 1965, CIBA Pharmaceutical Company, Division of CIBA-GEIGY Corporation. Reprinted with permission from The CIBA Collection of Medical Illustrations illustrated by Frank H. Netter, M.D. All rights reserved.)

necessary; only those that produce symptoms should be operated on.

Urinary incontinence. Many women experience uncontrollable leakage of urine, which in most instances is the result of an injury sustained during childbirth. However, other causes must also be considered. Five major categories of conditions can disturb urinary control:

1. *Stress urinary (anatomic) incontinence.* The loss of urine occurs with sudden increases in intraabdominal pressure such as that generated by

sneezing or from sudden jarring movements. The loss is caused by structural injuries to the urethra and bladder neck.

2. *Detrusor dyssynergia.* The incontinence results from involuntary detrusor activity, which is triggered by a variety of stimuli.

3. *Urge incontinence.* Urge incontinence is characterized by the inability to keep from urinating when the urge to void occurs suddenly. Urge incontinence usually is caused by intrinsic disorders of the bladder and urethra, the most common being urethritis and urethral stricture, trigonitis, and cystitis.

4. *Neuropathies.* Neurologic disorders such as multiple sclerosis, diabetic neuritis, and diseases of or injuries to the spinal cord, disturb the nerve control of bladder function. Such disorders usually cause overflow or uninhibited detrusor incontinence.

5. *Congenital and acquired urinary tract abnormalities.* Urinary tract abnormalities include congenital defects such as ectopic ureter, abnormal muscular development of the vesical neck, neurologic disorders, and acquired lesions such as urinary fistulas (p. 570) and destruction of all or part of the urethra. The incontinence is usually constant and unrelated to voiding, to activity, or to position.

Continence of urine is dependent on normal urethrovesical support, normal anatomic configuration, innervation and function of the structures involved in voiding, and normal urethrovesical pressure relationships. In women who are continent the intraurethral pressure is always greater than the intravesical pressure except during voiding. When intravesical pressure is in the normal range, the differential is maintained principally by the primary urethral sphincter, an extension of the smooth muscle layers of the bladder wall that makes up the proximal 3 cm of the urethra. The tension provided by the voluntary muscle, fascia, and blood vessels that surround the urethra adds to the effect of the sphincter. Muscles in the lower urethra have little to do with urinary control; the entire distal third can be amputated without disturbing function.

When intravesical pressure is increased, for example, with coughing or straining, additional urethral pressure is supplied by voluntary contraction of the pubococcygeus muscle, which compresses the upper urethra and pulls it upward behind the pubis. The upper urethra and the urethrovesical junction lie within the abdominal cavity above the levator plate; hence increases in intraabdominal pressure are transmitted equally to the bladder and to the proximal urethra. Therefore changes in intraabdominal pressure do not affect the urethrovesical pressure relationships.

Voiding is initiated by relaxation of the voluntary muscles and the urethral sphincter and by contraction of the detrusor muscles. As a consequence, the urethral lumen is widened and shortened as its relaxed proximal wall is drawn up and funneled by the contracting longitudinal muscle fibers in the bladder wall. The short, relaxed urethra offers little resistance to the flow of urine from the contracting bladder.

STRESS URINARY INCONTINENCE. Stress incontinence is the involuntary loss of urine precipitated by coughing, sneezing, laughing, or lifting and by walking, running, or sudden jarring changes in position. Many multiparous women have slight stress incontinence during menstruation but maintain good control at other times. If the dysfunction is more pronounced, incontinence is present throughout the month. In the most severe cases the patient loses urine with the slightest provocation and must wear protective pads constantly.

Some women develop mild incontinence after the birth of their first babies; in others it does not appear until they have had several. Many women first become incontinent after the menopause, and in most the symptoms become more annoying as the effects of estrogen deprivation on the tissues and blood vessels in the bladder neck, the urethra, and the surrounding structures increase.

Stress incontinence, also called anatomic incontinence, usually results from changes in the structure and function of the urethra and the urethrovesical junction caused by injury during childbirth. The extent of the dysfunction is determined by how much the tissues were disrupted during delivery and how completely they recovered. The basic problem is that the mechanism for increasing intraurethral pressure is disturbed, and it cannot respond rapidly and completely enough to compensate for sudden rises in intravesical pressure such as those that occur with coughing or sneezing. When intraabdominal pressure and, simultaneously, intravesical pressure is increased suddenly, urine spurts from the incompetent urethra. The principal anatomic defects associated with stress incontinence are *changes in the posterior urethrovesical angle* and *changes in the relationship of the urethra to the pubis (urethral axis.)* The net result is that support of the vesical neck and the proximal urethra is altered and function is disturbed.

In the normal bladder the posterior wall of the urethra and the flat base of the bladder form a 90- to 100-degree angle with each other. In women with stress incontinence the angle is lost, and the bladder neck is funneled and lies at the most dependent portion of the bladder (Fig. 41-10). Since these changes are like those that occur in continent women when micturition is initiated, patients with stress urinary incontinence are always in the preliminary voiding phase. Any increase in the intravesical pressure forces urine through the urethra.

The urethral axis, the angle of inclination of the upper urethra to the perpendicular while in the upright position, is another important factor in urinary control. In normal women the angle is no more than 30 degrees. In incontinent women it is increased, often to more than 90 degrees, because the urethra is displaced backward and downward (Fig. 41-10). The degree to which the posterior urethrovesical angle is lost and the urethra is displaced is an indication of how much the urethral support was altered by the injuries sustained during delivery.

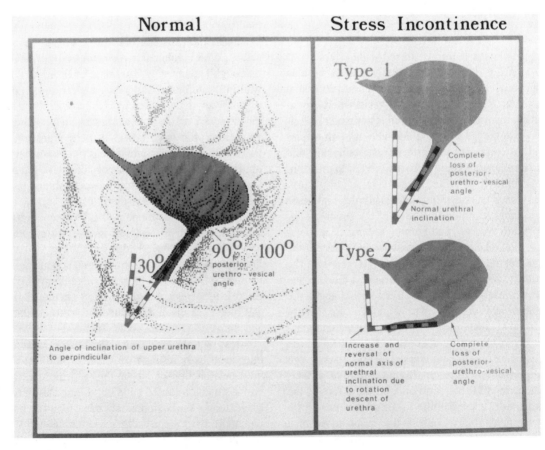

Fig. 41-10. Anatomic changes associated with incontinence. (From Incontinence in the female, A.C.O.G. Tech. Bull. no. 36, Feb. 19, 1976.)

An additional factor that may affect urinary control when urethral support has been disrupted is related to the transmission of intraabdominal pressure changes to the structures. The normally supported upper urethra lies above the intact levator plate and within the abdominal cavity. Increases in intraabdominal pressure are transmitted equally to the bladder and to the upper urethra; hence there is no unusual pressure differential and leakage of urine when intraabdominal pressure is increased suddenly. If the vesical neck is displaced downward because the levator plate is weakened, it may lie outside the abdominal cavity. Increases in intraabdominal pressure are then transmitted to the bladder but not to the urethra. The difference between the elevated intravesical pressure and the unchanged intraurethral pressure is followed by a spurt of urine.

Diagnosis. The diagnosis of stress incontinence is made on the basis of an accurate history, physical examination, and a variety of testing procedures. It is essential that stress incontinence be differentiated from other causes of incontinence because the treatment of each varies.

The typical patient with stress incontinence is multiparous, and many are already postmenopausal. The incontinence has gradually become more troublesome, and in some patients it may be so severe that they are wet much of the time. Characteristically, urine spurts from the urethra immediately whenever the intraabdominal pressure is increased by laughing, sneezing, or coughing or when they walk, run, or even step off curbs. The loss of urine can usually be stopped by voluntary muscle contraction. It does not occur at night, it usually does not occur with simple changes in position, and there is no discomfort associated with voiding.

Relaxation of the structures that support the urethra and bladder neck can be demonstrated by asking the patient to bear down. The axis of the normally supported urethra in the lithotomy position is usually horizontal; if the supports are weakened, the bladder and the urethra will rotate backward and downward when intraabdominal pressure is increased.

The degree of change can be measured by the *Q-tip test*. One inserts a lubricated cotton swab into the urethra to the level of the vesical neck and observes its change in relationship to the horizontal as the patient bears down. When the relaxed anterior vaginal wall and vesical neck descend as intraabdominal pressure is increased, the handle of the Q-tip rotates upward around the lower border of the pubis. If the structures are relaxed the handle of the swab will rotate through an arc of at least 30 degrees. There is little motion if the vesical neck is well supported.

The integrity of the sphincter mechanism can be tested by having the patient cough vigorously or by having her hold her breath and bear down. Urine will spurt from the urethra if muscle control is defective. Of course, this test is uninformative when the bladder is empty. If the patient has voided shortly before examination, enough water should be instilled into the bladder to produce an urge to void. If she does not lose urine in the lithotomy position, the test should be repeated with the patient standing.

The *cystometrogram* in stress incontinence is normal, in contrast to that in detrusor dyssynergia, uninhibited neurogenic bladder, or irritable bladder. *Urethral closure pressure profiles* measure pressure at various levels of the urethra. The pressure, particularly in the upper urethra, is reduced in women with stress urinary incontinence. Defective bladder neck function can be seen by *urethroscopy,* and bladder lesions with *cystoscopy; urograms* usually are not necessary.

Treatment. In some women, particularly those with relatively little descent of the bladder and urethra, stress incontinence can be corrected by *systematic muscle exercise.* The patient is taught how to contract the pubococcygeus muscles that pull the bladder neck upward and angulate it to constrict the distal urethra. If the patient contracts the muscles 80 to 100 times a day and attempts to check the flow of urine suddenly while she is voiding, the pubococcygeus may become strong enough to prevent leakage. The administration of *estrogen* may improve urinary control in postmenopausal women with a good bit of local atrophic change but little obvious tissue relaxation. In addition to estrogen an alpha-receptor stimulating drug (phenylpropanolamine) may increase baseline urethral tone.

Another simple treatment, which often is effective, is to insert a *Smith-Hodge vaginal pessary.* The retropubic portion of the ring elevates the vesical neck, lengthens the urethra, and may improve urinary control. This is particularly suited for elderly women who are unsuitable candidates for operation. This also may be used to indicate which patients will benefit from surgical repair.

Surgical treatment should be selected for patients with true stress incontinence that is not improved by muscle exercises and those who have large structural defects. Operation will make incontinence caused by neurogenic problems worse.

Most surgical procedures are directed toward restoring the integrity of the lost supports and particularly toward improving the function of the sphincter mechanism. If there is a large cystocele, this can usually be accomplished by plicating the bladder and urethra and restoring vesical neck support through a vaginal incision. This elevates the bladder neck, reestablishes the urethrovesical angle, and narrows the urethral orifice. For some women, particularly those whose angles of inclination approach 90 degrees but with little additional anterior wall relaxation, an abdominal approach is preferred. In the Marshall-Marchetti-Krantz, or retropubic vesical neck suspension, operation, the urethra and bladder neck are sutured to the posterior border of the pubis and the rectus fascia; this restores the urethrovesical angle and prevents the bladder neck from descending. More complicated procedures in which slings of rectus fascia or of plastic strips are used to support the bladder neck are seldom necessary.

DETRUSOR DYSSYNERGIA. Detrusor dyssynergia or unstable bladder is the responsible factor of incontinence in at least 10% of affected women. It can be suspected from the history and physical examination, but it can be diagnosed precisely only by urethrocystometry. The loss of urine occurs because of involuntary detrusor activity. The urine flow cannot be controlled voluntarily.

Diagnosis. Detrusor dyssynergia must be differentiated from both urge and stress incontinence, with which it shares some symptoms. The treatment for each varies.

The only symptom of mild detrusor dyssynergia may be frequency and urgency of micturition with occasional urge incontinence. The patient is unable to hold her urine long enough to get to the toilet after she first feels the urge to void. Incontinence is more troublesome in advanced cases.

Although there may be a component of stress incontinence in many women with detrusor dyssynergia, it differs from urine leakage caused by structural defects of the urethra and vesical neck. In the latter, a brief spurt of urine is induced immediately by the increase in intraabdominal pressure. In contrast, the flow of urine in women with detrusor dyssynergia may start 10 to 20 seconds *after* the stress and continues for 5 to 10 seconds. A large amount of urine is lost, and the stream cannot be stopped voluntarily. Incontinence may be triggered by running, walking, or a change in position, but it does not characteristically follow coughing and sneezing. Some women lose urine when they hear water running. Incontinence caused by detrusor dyssynergia usually does not occur during the night, but the patient may lose urine as soon as she arises from bed in the morning. There is no associated discomfort.

Bladder and urethral support usually is normal, and the patient generally cannot demonstrate incontinence by coughing and straining, even though the bladder is full. Neurologic examination is normal. Abnormal detrusor activity can be detected by measuring the urethral and bladder pressures simultaneously or, if instrumentation for this procedure is not available, by cystometry alone. Urethral pressures usually are normal because the defect is in the bladder. The volume of urine that stimulates detrusor activity measures the functional capacity of the bladder. Normal women experience a strong urge to void when the bladder contains 400 to 500 ml of urine. Voiding is voluntary and can be prevented. In contrast, in the patient with an unstable bladder, detrusor activity is usually stimulated at a lower volume of urine, and voiding cannot be inhibited. Uninhibited contractions can often be induced during the test if the patient changes position, walks in place, or bounces up and down on her heels.

Treatment. The treatment of detrusor dyssynergia is medical; the incontinence is usually made worse by surgical procedures. The patient should be reassured that there are no structural or neurologic abnormalities, and she should be urged to try to gradually prolong the intervals between voiding.

Anticholinergic drugs, which decrease excessive spontaneous bladder activity and uninhibited contractions, will usually relieve, or at least lessen, the symptoms.

OTHER CAUSES OF INCONTINENCE. Other than stress incontinence and detrusor dyssynergia, the major cause of incontinence in adult women is *urge incontinence* associated with urethral and bladder disorders. These include chronic urethrocystitis, the urethral syndrome, which may be caused by *Chlamydia* infection, urethral strictures, and other intrinsic bladder disorders. Urge incontinence must be differentiated from detrusor dyssynergia. Dysuria is not often a symptom of unstable bladder, but it often is present in women with urge incontinence because of the local disorder. The diagnosis is made by urethroscopy, cystoscopy, and urine culture. The incontinence can usually be corrected by treating the local condition appropriately. Other causes of incontinence can be diagnosed by urologic examination.

INJURIES TO THE UTERUS
Cervical lacerations

The cervix is usually torn during delivery, but most lacerations are shallow and bleed little; consequently, they rarely constitute a major cause of postpartum hemorrhage and need no repair. More extensive lacerations that extend upward and particularly those that involve the lower segment may produce serious bleeding. These are most often caused by precipitous delivery or by ill-advised attempts to "dilate" the cervix artificially or to extract the infant before dilatation is complete.

The cervix may also be injured if the anterior lip is caught and incarcerated between the descending head and the pubic bone (Fig. 41-11). This occurs most often with some degree of cephalopelvic disproportion. Since the trapped cervix cannot be retracted upward around the presenting part when the uterus contracts, the lower segment above it becomes excessively thinned and may even rupture. The anterior lip of the cervix becomes edematous and diffused with blood and may be almost

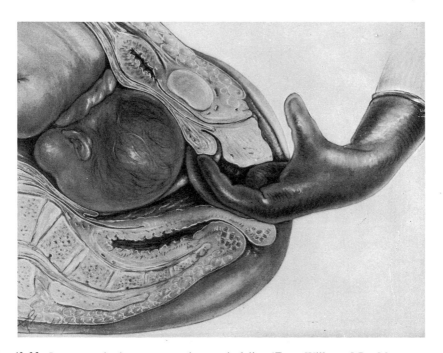

Fig. 41-11. Incarcerated edematous anterior cervical lip. (From Willson, J.R.: Management of obstetric difficulties, ed. 6, St. Louis, 1961, The C.V. Mosby Co.)

black. Unless it is freed by disengaging the head slightly and pushing the anterior lip upward with the fingers, the entire cervix may be torn loose, a so-called *annular amputation*.

The cervix should be exposed and inspected after each hospital delivery. If a laceration other than a shallow nick is found, the defect should be closed with interrupted chromic no. 3-0 catgut sutures (Fig. 41-12).

Rupture of the uterus

Rupture of the uterus is the most serious of the childbirth injuries, but fortunately it occurs only once in 1500 to 2000 deliveries. The uterus may rupture during pregnancy, but usually the wall gives way during labor.

Etiologic factors. During pregnancy the most frequent cause of rupture of the upper segment is *separation of a scar* from previous cesarean section. Rupture of the normal uterus except by direct trauma seldom occurs. The ruptures that occur during labor also may involve a scar, but an intact uterus also can rupture. Injuries to the lower segment are frequently the result of *obstructed labor* from cephalopelvic disproportion or malposition. The presenting part cannot descend through the pelvis, and the continuing contraction and retraction of the muscle fibers in the upper segment stretch and thin the lower segment to a point at which separation occurs. Uterine rupture occurs more often in multiparas than in primigravidas. In the latter the response to fetopelvic disproportion is usually active phase arrest. The multiparous uterus continues to contract until it ruptures.

Other traumatic causes are the *administration of oxytocin* in doses that are too large or to a patient in whom stimulation is contraindicated (for example, obstructed labor, abnormal positions) and *operative deliveries* such as version and breech extraction. Rupture is particularly likely to occur when operative delivery is attempted after labor

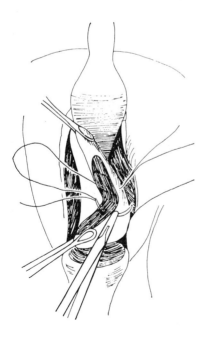
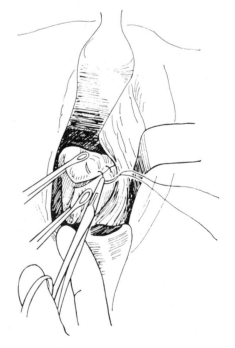

Fig. 41-12. Exposure and repair of cervical laceration. Interrupted sutures are placed through entire thickness of cervix.

has been prolonged and the lower segment is over-stretched or as a result of failure to relax the uterus and abolish its contractions by adequate anesthetic before such procedures are attempted. The uterus almost never ruptures during dysfunctional labor because the ineffective contractions do not stretch and thin the lower segment to a point at which the muscle fibers separate.

Pathologic anatomy. Traumatic ruptures during labor and delivery usually occur in the thin lower segment, but they may extend upward and involve the upper segment or downward into the cervix. They usually run transversely or obliquely unless they are extensions of a deep cervical laceration, in which event the tear is usually a longitudinal one in the lateral wall.

A *complete rupture* is one that extends through the entire uterine wall into the peritoneal cavity or the broad ligament; with an *incomplete rupture* the visceral peritoneum remains intact. With either type, hemorrhage is severe. The blood is lost directly into the peritoneal cavity, if the rupture is complete, or into the broad ligament with a lateral wall defect. The blood may dissect upward retroperitoneally sometimes as far as the diaphragm. There may be some external bleeding, but the major hemorrhage is often concealed within the broad ligament or the abdominal cavity unless the cervix as well as the uterine wall is involved.

Diagnosis. The diagnosis should be suspected when a pregnant woman or one in labor has sudden abdominal pain followed by clinical evidence of blood loss. If these symptoms occur during a labor that has been abnormally long or obstructed, or if a pathologic retraction ring has been detected, the diagnosis is more likely. When the uterus ruptures under such circumstances, the patient usually experiences a sharp agonizing pain, uterine contractions cease, and evidences of bleeding develop rapidly. If the baby has been extruded into the peritoneal cavity, it may be possible to palpate it outside the uterus, and the presenting part can no longer be felt through the cervix.

Rupture of a low-segment cesarean section scar may produce no symptoms. The separation occurs gradually as the lower segment elongates during late pregnancy and early labor. The fetus is usually not extruded from the uterus, because the opening is covered by bladder. Most injuries of this type bleed less than do those that involve the upper segment, and they may be found at the time of repeat cesarean section or when the interior of the uterus is explored after the patient has been allowed to deliver vaginally.

Treatment. The possibility that the uterus may rupture during abnormal labor should always be considered, and necessary precautions should be taken to prevent its occurrence. Since about two thirds of the ruptures of cesarean section scars occur after the thirty-eighth week of pregnancy or during labor, *elective repeat cesarean section* in those whose scars are most likely to separate will reduce the incidence of ruptures at this time (Chapter 40). Recognition of the cause and proper management of *prolonged labor,* adequate *anesthesia* for operative deliveries, and the judicious use of *oxytocic drugs* will also serve as preventive measures.

Expectant management of a ruptured uterus is almost never warranted. Prompt transfusion with whole blood and laparotomy are usually indicated; it is necessary to perform hysterectomy unless the laceration is small, in which event it may be possible to repair it and leave the uterus intact.

If the rupture occurs when the patient is ready for delivery, the infant should usually be extracted. This procedure may save its life and will permit the uterus to contract, thereby helping to control bleeding until the abdomen can be opened. If the infant lies in the peritoneal cavity, no attempt should be made to extract it through the vagina.

Prognosis. The *perinatal mortality* is almost 100% if the fetus is extruded from the uterus into the peritoneal cavity. If labor is well advanced and the presenting part is deep in the pelvis at the time of the rupture, the infant may remain within the birth canal, and prompt delivery can save its life. The *maternal mortality* is primarily from hemorrhage and can be kept at a minimum by prompt and adequate treatment, but it may be as high as 20% to 50%. Rupture of lower segment cesarean section scars are less lethal for both mother and fetus than are the ruptures that involve the upper segment. The former, which are discussed in Chapter 40, usually occur in a relatively avascular area and often produce no symptoms.

INJURIES INVOLVING UTERINE SUPPORT

The major support for the uterus and the upper vagina is provided by the thickenings of the endopelvic fascia known as the cardinal or Mackenrodt's ligaments. They extend from about the level of the internal os and vagina laterally to blend with the fascia covering the obturator internus muscle (Fig. 41-1). The round ligaments, broad ligaments, and uterosacral ligaments are more concerned with maintaining uterine position than with supporting it. The uterosacral ligaments are attached to the cervix posteriorly and below the level of the internal os. They pull the cervix upward and backward, thus rotating the fundus anteriorly. The round ligaments tense when the fundus rotates posteriorly and help return the uterus to an anteverted position.

Tearing of the cardinal ligaments during labor and delivery is rare, but they can be unduly stretched if descent is delayed by cephalopelvic disproportion, because of prolonged bearing-down efforts before the cervix is dilated or if attempts are made to complete delivery forcibly before the cervix is fully dilated.

Late results

If the ligaments are injured or stretched during labor and do not return to normal, they can no longer support the uterus, and it will sag backward and downward into the vagina. The axis of the uterus ordinarily forms an acute angle with the axis of the vagina, which in itself tends to prevent prolapse. Descent of the uterus can occur only when the other supporting structures such as the uterosacral ligaments and the cardinal ligaments relax, thereby altering the relationship of the uterus to the vaginal axis. This relaxation permits the cervix to sag downward into the vagina while the body of the uterus rotates posteriorly until its long axis lies in the axis of the vagina. If vaginal wall support also is compromised, the pressure of the abdominal organs on the uterus will gradually force downward through the vaginal tube. The latter is inverted, carrying the bladder and rectum with it as the uterus descends toward the introitus.

Descensus, or *prolapse*, of the uterus may occur in infants, nulliparous women, and multiparas (Fig. 41-13). Defects in innervation and in the basic integrity of the supporting structures account for descensus in the first two groups and childbirth trauma for the latter. The uterus often prolapses in children with spina bifida and with congenital extrophy of the bladder.

The uterus seldom descends immediately after delivery, but the defect develops gradually. The enlarging cystocele and rectocele that almost always accompany prolapse pull down on the uterus and cervix. The supravaginal portion of the cervix elongates because the weight of the sagging vaginal tissues pulls it downward, whereas the attached but weak cardinal ligaments tend to support it. As the cystocele enlarges and the cervix elongates, the ligaments become weaker until they can no longer hold the uterus in place. The more advanced stages of uterine prolapse are most often encountered in women past the menopause. Atrophy of the tissues eliminates whatever support was left.

A *first-degree prolapse* is one in which the cervix lies between the level of the ischial spines and the vaginal introitus. In *second-degree prolapse* the cervix protudes through the introitus, while the corpus remains within the vagina. In *third-degree,* or *complete, prolapse* both cervix and the body of the uterus have passed through the introitus, and the entire vaginal canal is inverted.

Symptoms. The symptoms of prolapse are primarily those related to the weight of the descending organs and their protrusion through the introitus. If the prolapsed cervix becomes ulcerated, it may bleed.

Diagnosis. The diagnosis is made by pelvic examination. The prolapse may reduce itself spontaneously when the patient lies down. Consequently, to determine the extent of the lesion it often is necessary to have the patient strain and push the cervix down, to exert traction on it with a tenaculum, and to examine her in an upright position. Prolapse must be differentiated from simple hypertrophy and elongation of the cervix that does not involve loss of uterine support.

Treatment. In general, the treatment of prolapse is operative, but, in certain poor-risk patients or those who are very old, a pessary may be inserted to hold the uterus in place. The physician should be certain that the patient actually is a poor operative risk before advising pessary support. Advanced age alone does not necessarily contraindicate surgical treatment.

Operative correction of prolapse rarely requires an abdominal operation. The faulty supporting structures

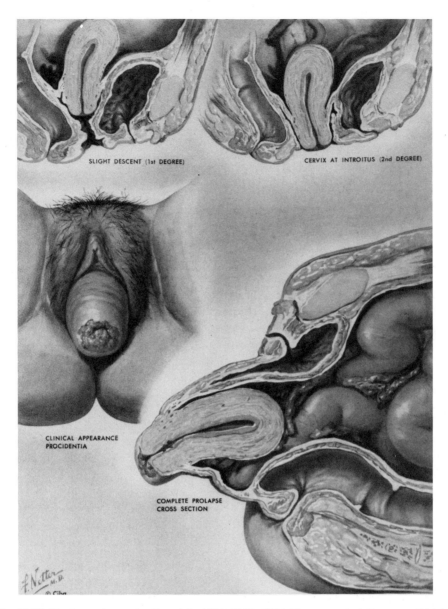

SLIGHT DESCENT (1st DEGREE)

CERVIX AT INTROITUS (2nd DEGREE)

CLINICAL APPEARANCE
PROCIDENTIA

COMPLETE PROLAPSE
CROSS SECTION

Fig. 41-13. Uterine prolapse. (© Copyright 1954, 1965, CIBA Pharmaceutical Company, Division of CIBA-GEIGY Corporation. Reprinted with permission from The CIBA Collection of Medical Illustrations illustrated by Frank H. Netter, M.D. All rights reserved.)

can only be approached vaginally; hence procedures such as abdominal suspension of the uterus often fail because they do not correct the fundamental pathologic change. An adequate, effective operative procedure must correct the cystocele and rectocele, return the uterus to a forward, position, shorten the elongated cervix, and shorten the cardinal ligaments. An alternate method is to remove the uterus. The following operative procedures will accomplish these aims: *Manchester-Fothergill operation* (cervical amputation and shortening of the cardinal ligaments and vaginal plastic repair), *vaginal hysterectomy* and vaginal repair, and *colpocleisis* (obliteration of the vagina by denuding and approximating the anterior and posterior vaginal walls).

GENITAL FISTULAS

Fistulous openings between the bladder and the genital tract (vesicovaginal, vesicocervical, or vesicouterine), between the ureter and the vagina (ureterovaginal), and between the rectum and the vagina (rectovaginal) are caused by radiation, operative trauma, or injuries during labor and delivery.

Urinary tract fistulas

The most common urinary tract fistula is that which forms in the anterior vaginal wall, a *vesicovaginal fistula*. In past years almost all such fistulas were caused by necrosis of the vesicovaginal septum from pressure during delayed labor, but today the majority follow hysterectomy. These may result from necrosis at the site of a suture in the bladder wall, from operative injury, or from interference with blood supply. They most often follow total or radical hysterectomy.

As a result of the abnormal opening, the patient is partially or completely incontinent of urine, and the constant flow of urine from the vagina excoriates the vulva and thighs. If the defect is large, all the urine will be passed through the vagina, but if it is small, the patient may void normally even though some of the urine seeps through the fistulous opening.

The diagnosis of vesicovaginal fistula is confirmed by demonstrating the opening between the bladder and the vagina and cystoscopic examination. If a small pack is placed in the vagina and methylene blue is instilled into the bladder, the dye will seep through the opening and discolor the pack.

Ureterovaginal fistulas usually develop because of devascularization or direct injury during radical operations for uterine cancer. The defect in the ureter develops near the ureterovesical junction, and the seepage of urine is usually first observed during the third week after the operation.

Ureterovaginal fistula can be suspected when the physician attempts to pass ureteral catheters. It often is impossible to insert the catheter beyond the constricted site of the fistula. Indigo carmine, when injected intrave-nously, will be excreted in the urine, and, if there is a ureterovaginal fistula, some of the dye will enter the vagina and stain a pack. Since this will also occur with a vesicovaginal fistula, one more test is necessary to differentiate the two lesions: methylene blue instilled into the bladder will enter the vagina through a vesicovaginal fistula, but this will not occur if the defect is in the ureter. These tests combined with cystoscopy and pyelography should localize any urinary tract fistula accurately.

Treatment. Most vesicovaginal fistulas can be closed satisfactorily by an experienced gynecologist through a vaginal approach. The treatment of a ureterovaginal fistula is determined by its location. For those near the ureterovesical junction, the ureter can be severed above the defect and implanted into the bladder *(ureteroneo-cystostomy)*. If the fistulous opening is several centimeters away from the bladder, the severed ends can usually be anastomosed, or a connecting tube of bladder wall can be constructed. Occasionally, it is necessary to remove the kidney on the involved side.

Rectovaginal fistulas

Rectovaginal fistulas are caused by infection in an episiotomy, a suture placed through the rectal wall during repair, or an unrecognized rectal injury incurred during delivery or vaginal repair. They may also be caused by extension of cervical cancer or from radiation necrosis after its treatment. Most of the traumatic lesions are found near the vaginal opening, whereas those caused by radium and cancer are higher. All result in fecal incontinence and passage of fecal material from the vagina. These lesions can be differentiated from incontinence caused by complete perineal laceration by the fact that with a fistula the sphincter ani is intact.

Treatment. Rectovaginal fistulas can almost always be corrected by a surgical procedure, but, since the operative field is infected, the repair may break down. The bowel should be prepared for several days preoperatively by reducing the diet to liquids for a day or two before operation, giving enemas, and prescribing antibiotics. Colostomy may be necessary before surgery for complicated rectovaginal fistulas.

INJURIES TO THE PELVIC JOINTS

The *symphysis pubis* always separates to some extent during delivery, but, if the baby is forcibly extracted or unusually large, a serious injury can be produced. When the patient attempts to move or stand on her feet after delivery, she experiences severe pain in the region of the symphysis and in the sacroiliac joints. The symphyseal area is tender, and the ends of the pubic bones are widely separated. The bone ends are unusually mobile and can be felt to shift several centimeters when the patient shifts her weight from one foot to the other. The bladder neck and the urethra may be injured, and as a result the urine may be bloody.

Treatment of separation of the symphysis consists of immobilization of the pelvic girdle by a tight binder or adhesive strapping until the pubis heals. The symptoms diminish rapidly.

If the *coccyx is dislocated,* the patient may complain of pain localized to the area and radiating down both legs. The dislocated coccyx can be felt overriding the end of the sacrum and can often be reduced by digital manipulation. Soreness and tenderness may persist for several weeks.

HEMATOMA FORMATION

A hematoma may form in the rectovaginal septum, in the episiotomy (Fig. 41-14), or in the base of the broad ligament after delivery. A large amount of blood can accumulate in the loose subcutaneous tissue of the labium without any evidence of external bleeding. The hematoma can also extend upward retroperitoneally, sometimes as high as the diaphragm. Evidence of shock may be one of the first signs of blood loss.

An enlarging hematoma causes pelvic pain and rectal pressure soon after delivery. Unfortunately, this is frequently attributed to the episiotomy and is treated symptomatically without examination. Inspection of the perineum generally reveals it to be distended and ecchymotic, and, when rectal examination is performed, it is easy to feel the tender mass. Women who have been delivered under epidural or saddle block anesthesia will usually be unable to appreciate perineal pain for several hours after delivery; consequently, a large hematoma may form without their being aware of the symptoms.

A hematoma in the episiotomy, unless it is small and stable, must be evacuated. If the bleeding vessel can be demonstrated, it should be ligated. Occasionally, it is necessary to pack the cavity to check diffuse oozing, but the bleeding can almost always be controlled by resu-

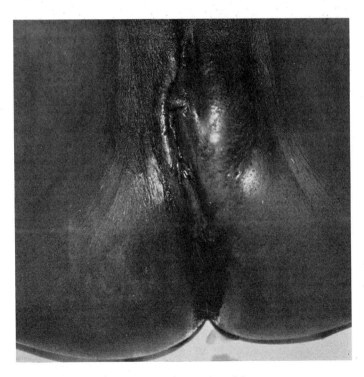

Fig. 41-14. Hematoma in episiotomy.

turing the episiotomy. Small hematomas in the vaginal wall generally need no treatment.

RETRODISPLACEMENT OF THE UTERUS
(Fig. 41-15)

The term *retrodisplacement* includes several situations in which the body of the uterus is displaced from its usual location overlying the bladder and occupies a position in the posterior pelvis. With *retroflexion* the fundus lies posteriorly, while the cervix retains its usual position in the vagina; the uterus is flexed in the region of the isthmus, the axis of the body forming an angle with the cervix. In *retroversion* the fundus rotates posteriorly and the cervix anteriorly around an axis at the level of the internal os. *Retrocession* indicates that the entire uterus has sagged backward into the posterior pelvis.

Retrodisplacement, which can be detected in 20% to 30% of all women, is caused by an alteration in the supporting structures of the pelvis. The uterus rotates in an anterioposterior plane around an axis situated approximately at the level of the internal os. Therefore anterior traction on the corpus or posterior and upward traction on the cervix will tend to rotate the uterus into an anterior position, with the fundus overlying the pubis and the cervix pointing toward the rectum, the long axis of the uterus forming an acute angle with the axis of the vagina. The anterior position of the uterus is maintained by a number of forces: the *uterosacral ligaments* pull the cervix backward and upward, and the *round ligaments* help return the fundus to an anterior position if for some reason it is rotated posteriorly.

When a woman assumes an erect posture, the *intraabdominal pressure* and the loops of *intestine* pressing on the posterior surface of the uterus force the fundus toward the pubis, thereby rotating the cervix backward and upward until it lies above the level of the corpus. With the patient lying on her back, the fundus is directed toward the ceiling and

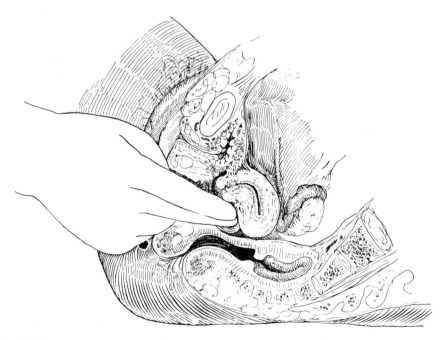

Fig. 41-15. Retrodisplacement of uterus. Cervix points in axis of vaginal canal, and corpus can be felt in posterior cul-de-sac. (From Titus, P.: Atlas of obstetric technic, ed. 2, St. Louis, 1949, The C.V. Mosby Co.)

may fall anteriorly or posteriorly; thus its position may vary from one examination to the next. If the bladder is distended, the fundus will be pushed posteriorly.

In some women the uterus is congenitally displaced and can be found lying posteriorly throughout their entire lives. In others, retrodisplacement develops after childbirth when the supporting structures are injured.

Symptoms. A retrodisplaced uterus may produce symptoms, but, when groups of women with retrodisplacements are compared with those whose uteri are in an anterior position, the same symptoms occur in about the same ratio in each group.

If the body of the retrodisplaced uterus is enlarged, boggy, heavy, and tender, it may cause pelvic pressure, low backache, and dyspareunia; and it may even interfere with evacuation of the rectum. The uterus can be bound down in the pos-

terior pelvis by the adhesions of endometriosis or those of the residua of pelvic infection, in which event symptoms are more often caused by the disease process itself than by the position of the uterus. A normal-sized, freely movable, retrodisplaced uterus rarely produces symptoms.

Diagnosis. The diagnosis of retrodisplacement is made by bimanual examination and by rectovaginal palpation. Either the axis of the cervix lies parallel with the axis of the vagina, or the tip of the cervix may point anteriorly toward the bladder. The body of the uterus can be felt lying in the posterior cul-de-sac by palpating behind the cervix through the posterior fornix (Fig. 41-15).

It sometimes is difficult to differentiate a retrodisplaced uterus from one in normal position with a fibroid arising from the posterior wall and occupying cul-de-sac or from an ovarian tumor prolapsed behind the uterus. If a sound is inserted into

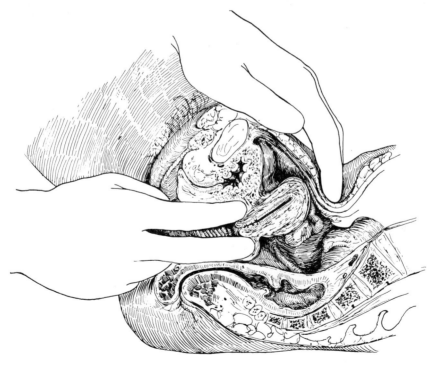

Fig. 41-16. Retrodisplacement of uterus. Corpus is pushed anteriorly by fingers in vagina until it can be held forward by fingers pressing abdominal wall inward. (From Titus, P.: Atlas of obstetric technic, ed. 2, St. Louis, 1949, The C.V. Mosby Co.)

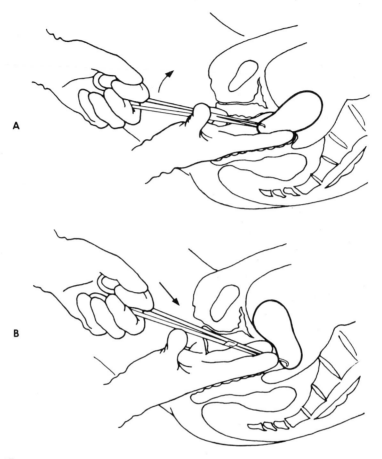

Fig. 41-17. Replacement of uterus with tenaculum. **A,** Cervix is grasped with tenaculum and pulled downward in axis of vagina until it is straight. Two fingers in vagina push upward on corpus. **B,** Cervix is pushed posteriorly between two fingers. Uterus can be held anteriorly by pressure against cervix while tenaculum is removed and pessary is inserted. (Modified from Tauber, R.: Gynecologic diagnosis, New York, 1949, Thomas Nelson & Sons.)

the uterine cavity, the physician can usually tell which way the fundus points.

Treatment. There is no need to suggest treatment for a retrodisplacement unless the patient has symptoms such as pelvic pain, dysmenorrhea, pressure, or infertility that could possibly be related to the position of the uterus. If the symptom is relieved after the uterus has been replaced and held in an anterior position by a proper pessary and recurs when it is permitted to fall posteriorly, the physician can suspect a relationship between the position of the uterus and the symptom. If, on the other hand, the symptom is still present after the retrodisplacement has been corrected, no such relationship can be assumed.

The initial therapeutic step in studying a patient with a retrodisplaced uterus and a pelvic symptom is actually diagnostic. The uterus is elevated by combined vaginal and abdominal manipulation, and a suitable pessary is inserted into the vagina to maintain the anterior position (Figs. 41-16 to 41-18). The manipulations can usually be performed with the patient in lithotomy position, but they sometimes are easier in the knee-chest position. The pessary is left in place for 2 to 3 months.

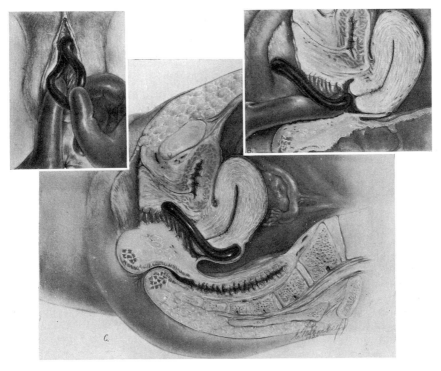

Fig. 41-18. Pessary support for retrodisplacement of uterus. **A,** Insertion while introitus is enlarged by downward traction on vaginal floor. **B,** Transverse bar of pessary is pressed downward and backward behind cervix. **C,** Some degree of descensus of uterus is always found in acquired retrodisplacements; anteflexion is maintained primarily by pressure of pessary on uterosacral ligament, drawing cervix backward. (From Willson, J.R.: Management of obstetric difficulties, ed. 6, St. Louis, 1961, The C.V. Mosby Co.)

If the symptoms are not eliminated by elevating the uterus, they obviously are not caused by its posterior position. If they are relieved while the pessary is in place and recur when the uterus falls backward after it is removed, it can be assumed that the symptoms are caused by the retrodisplacement, and surgical correction can be considered. Operation to correct retrodisplaced but otherwise normal uteri should rarely be necessary. In many instances the uterus falls back without the support of the pessary, but the symptoms do not recur. In such patients no further treatment is necessary. Long-continued pessary treatment is generally unwarranted.

Uteri that are fixed in the cul-de-sac by endometriosis or chronic tuboovarian infection are not suitable for pessary treatment because the uterus usually is so firmly bound down that it cannot be moved without an operation.

REFERENCES

American College of Obstetricians and Gynecologists: Urinary incontinence in the female, A.C.O.G. Tech. Bull. no. 36, Feb. 19, 1976.

Bhatia, N.N. and Ostergard, D.R.: Urodynamics in women with stress urinary incontinence, Obstet. Gynecol. **60:**552, 1982.

Bhatia, N.N., Bergman, A., and Gunning, J.E.: Urodynamic effects of a vaginal pessary in women with stress urinary incontinence, Am. J. Obstet. Gynecol. **147:**876, 1983.

Fothergill, W.: Anterior colporrhaphy and amputation of the cervix combined as a single operation for use in the treatment of genital prolapse, Am. J. Surg. **29:**161, 1915.

Gainey, H.L.: Postpartum observation of tissue damage, Am. J. Obstet. Gynecol. **70:**800, 1955.

Golan, A., Sandbank, O., and Rubin, A.: Rupture of the pregnant uterus, Obstet. Gynecol. **56:**549, 1980.

Green, T.H., Jr.: Urinary stress incontinence: differential diagnosis, pathophysiology, and management. Am. H. Obstet. Gynecol. **122**:368, 1975.

Hajj, S.N.: Female urinary incontinence: a dynamic evaluation, J. Reprod. Med. **23**:33, 1979.

Kegel, A.: Progressive resistance exercise in functional restoration of perineal muscles, Am. J. Obstet. Gynecol. **56**:238, 1948.

Langmade, C.F., and Oliver, J.A., Jr.: Simplifying the management of stress incontinence, Am. J. Obstet. Gynecol. **149**:24, 1984.

Mengert, W.F.: Mechanics of uterine support and position, Am. J. Obstet. Gynecol. **31**:755, 1936.

Ostergard, D.R., and McCarthy, T.A.: Diagnostic procedures in female urology, Am. J. Obstet. Gynecol. **137**:401, 1980.

Plauche, W.C., von Almen, W., and Muller, R.: Catastrophic uterine rupture, Obstet. Gynecol. **64**:792, 1984.

Ranney, B.: Enterocele, vaginal prolapse, pelvic hernia: recognition and treatment, Am. J. Obstet. Gynecol. **140**:53, 1981.

van Geelen, J.M., Lemmens, W.A.J.G., Esokes, T.K.A.B., and Martin, C.B., Jr.: The urethral pressure profiles in pregnancy and after delivery in healthy nulliparous women, Am. J. Obstet. Gynecol. **144**:636, 1982.

Zacharin, R.F.: Abdominal urethral suspension in the management of recurrent stress incontinence of urine—a 15-year experience, Obstet. Gynecol. **62**:644, 1983.

42

William J. Ledger

Obstetric and gynecologic infections

The most important of the many developments that have changed our concepts of infections in the female reproductive organs are (1) a better understanding of the bacteria involved; (2) a new classification of pelvic infections that differentiates low-risk from high-risk patients; and (3) a proliferation of new antibiotics, particularly cephalosporins and penicillins, imipenem, aztreonam, and quinolones, with broader spectrums of antibacterial activity.

In the past, every effort was made to identify a single "pathogenic" bacterial species, (for example, *N. gonorrhoeae*) to account for a specific infection. An antibiotic effective against that organism could then be prescribed. For the most part, only aerobic cultures were examined; hence anaerobic bacteria were not identified. As a consequence, cultures of pus from pelvic abscesses and similar infections, which almost always contain anaerobes, were usually reported to be "sterile." This is too simplified a concept; infections of the female pelvic organs are usually of multibacterial origin, and often three or more organisms can be isolated from the affected tissues. In addition, the importance of anaerobic bacteria, which can be recovered in about 70% of pelvic infections, is now appreciated. Few pelvic abscesses actually are "sterile"; anaerobes can be recovered in almost every instance, and a specific organism, *B. fragilis*, is isolated frequently. Anaerobic bacteria can also be cultured from the blood in 25% or more of women with pelvic infections and bacteremia.

Organisms other than anaerobic bacteria are important in the microbiology of pelvic infections. *Gram-negative aerobes* have been associated with serious infections, particularly in patients with septic shock. The gram-positive aerobe, *group B beta-hemolytic streptococcus,* has been implicated in both maternal and newborn infections. *Mycoplasma* species appear to be significant in some infections. Of greater clinical significance is *Chlamydia,* which is assuming an important role in the genesis of pelvic infections.

There are many pitfalls in the evaluation and treatment of women with pelvic infection. Definitive recommendations concerning proper treatment are not yet available because some of the end points of therapy have not been studied. For example, it is not known whether the results of hospital treatment of salpingo-oophoritis are better than those obtained by outpatient therapy. There is insufficient information to suggest that any one antibiotic regimen is superior to another. Of special significance is that we know little of one of the most important end points of therapy: the number of women whose tubes will function normally after antibiotic treatment is completed. It is easy to make a judgment about the patient's immediate response;

she becomes afebrile and asymptomatic, or she does not. If she fails to respond to the initial treatment, she may require different antibiotics, heparin for the treatment of septic pelvic thrombophlebitis, or some form of operative intervention to effect a cure.

The microbiologic identification of the bacteria at the site of infection before treatment is started and proof that the bacteria have been eliminated by the antibiotic regimen that results in clinical cure are important, but this is information that is impossible to obtain. The only access routes to the site of infection through which material for culture can be obtained are the vagina and the cervix. Both contain abundant aerobic and anaerobic bacterial flora that usually cannot be conclusively identified as either normal or pathogenic. The organisms listed in Table 42-1 have been recovered from pelvic sites of infection and can also be recovered from the lower genital tracts of asymptomatic women.

Because of the difficulties of clinical evaluation

TABLE 42-1   Organisms found in pelvic infections that can also be recovered from the lower genital tract of asymptomatic women

Gram-positive bacteria	Gram-negative bacteria
Aerobes	
Group B β-hemolytic streptococcus	*E. coli*
Enterococcus	*Klebsiella* species
Coagulase-positive staphylococcus	
Anaerobes	
Peptostreptococcus species	*Veillonella* species
Clostridium perfringens	*Bacteroides bivius*
	Bacteroides disiens
	B. fragilis
	Bacteroides melaninogenicus
	Fusobacterium species

in multibacterial pelvic infections, considerable effort has been exerted to develop an animal model applicable to human infections. The work of Weinstein and associates has had a profound impact on the antibacterial treatment of pelvic infections. In their experimental model, a gelatin capsule filled with rat feces is placed in the peritoneal cavity of rats. As the capsule dissolves, a biphasic response occurs to the heavy bacterial insult of the organisms in the rat feces. Peritonitis develops during the early onset phase. At this stage gram-negative *aerobic bacteria* can be isolated from the blood of the affected animals. Approximately 40% of the animals die as a result of the peritonitis. The survivors look fairly well for 2 to 3 days but then become sick as a result of the development of intraabdominal abscesses in which *anaerobic bacteria* predominate. Thus there is a biphasic response to a massive bacterial insult of mixed bacteria, an early onset phase with sepsis and death in which gram-negative aerobic bacteria are involved, and a late onset phase in which abscesses form and anaerobic bacteria predominate. This model is appealing because the end points of the bacterial insult and of the treatment are so clear. The presence of intraabdominal abscesses can be easily identified, and death is a specific end point.

After having demonstrated a predictable response to multibacterial insult, the investigators attempted to modify the course of the infections by administering antibiotics. They discovered that if the animals are pretreated with an aminoglycoside (gentamicin) before the bacterial insult, the early onset phase of the infection can be almost completely eliminated, but those which survive develop intraabdominal abscesses. With clindamycin, which is more effective against anaerobic bacteria than against aerobes, the early onset phase of infection is not influenced, but the survivors do not form abscesses. Finally, if a combination of drugs such as clindamycin and gentamicin is given, both phases of the infection can be almost completely eliminated.

Two questions must be answered before the results of animal experiments can be applied clinically: is the experimental infection like those that occur in humans, and can the regimen used in the animal model be applied to the treatment of mixed bacterial pelvic infections in women?

Many parallels exist between the model infections in animals and those that develop in humans. Early onset infections are often seen in clinical practice. The clinical course of a woman who developed an infection shortly after an uncomplicated labor and delivery is depicted in Fig. 42-1. The cause of the infection is obvious because of the temporal relationship between the event initiating the infection (that is, the delivery) and the onset of symptoms. In additon, gram-negative aerobes, usually *E. coli,* can often be isolated from the blood during the early stage of the infection. However,

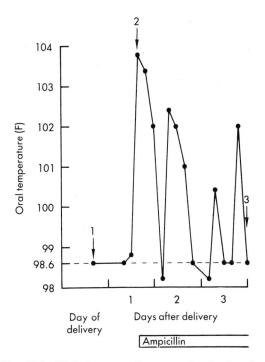

Fig. 42-1. Clinical course of woman who developed a pelvic infection. *1,* Patient delivered vaginally; *2,* blood cultures were obtained that subsequently yielded gram-negative aerobe; *3,* patient became afebrile and remained so throughout her hospitalization. (From Ledger, W.J.: In Wehrle, P.F., and Top, F.H., Sr., editors: Communicable and infectious diseases, ed. 9, St. Louis, 1981, The C.V. Mosby Co.)

other aspects of human experience are less like those in the animal model. Gram-positive aerobes such as the group B beta-hemolytic *Streptococcus* and anaerobic bacteria, both gram-positive and gram-negative, are often recovered from the bloodstream of patients who have a bacteremia associated with the early phase of a pelvic infection. Another difference from the animal model is that death from sepsis is now an unusual event in humans.

The late onset problems, however, are similar in human and experimental infections. In each, the abscesses develop relatively late after the initiating cause, and anaerobes are most often involved. Late infections may be difficult to recognize because of the long interval between the initiating procedure, the pelvic operation, and the development of the clinical signs of infection. Fig. 42-2 shows the clinical course of a patient who developed pelvic abscesses after vaginal hysterectomy.

The next question involves the reproducibility of the therapeutic results in the animal model as compared with human experience. The effectiveness of systemic antibiotics in experimental infections depends on the administration of the antibiotics before or at the time of the multibacterial insult. One of the realities of clinical experience is that the infection may already be well established when the physician first has an opportunity to treat it. There are important differences in the results of treating well-established infections as compared with those in which treatment can be started early in the clinical course of the disease. I studied a total of 501 patients who were treated for varying degrees of soft-tissue pelvic infections to evaluate this particular point. The patients were classified retrospectively as having had early infections if symptoms had been present for fewer than 5 days and if an indurated mass could not be felt when treatment was started. Patients with well-established infections had one of two clinical findings: symptoms for 5 days or more or an indurated pelvic mass that was considered to be a pelvic abscess. Table 42-2 shows the therapeutic result in these two groups of patients. Only one treatment other than the original antibiotic regimen is listed; this

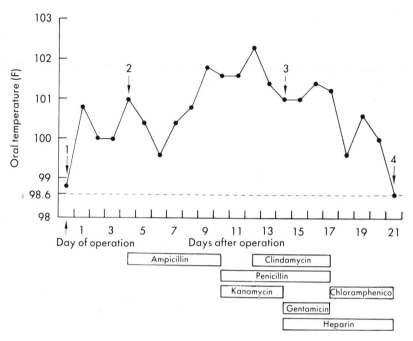

Fig. 42-2. Clinical record of woman who developed pelvic infection after vaginal hysterectomy. *1,* Vaginal hysterectomy was performed; *2,* respiratory infection was suspected, and ampicillin was begun; *3,* it was reported that prior blood culture was positive for *Bacteriodes fragilis; 4,* patient became afebrile and remained so throughout her hospitalization. (From Ledger, W.J.: Am. J. Obstet. Gynecol. **123:**111, 1975.)

TABLE 42-2 Treatment results in patients with early or well-established pelvic infections

	Early onset infection	Well-established infection
Number of patients	403	98
Cure*	337 (84%)	47 (48%)
Other antibiotics	38 (9%)	—
Heparin	2 (0.5%)	1 (1%)
Operation†	26 (6.4%)	50 (51%)

From Ledger, W.J.: Rev. Infect. Dis. **5**(Suppl.):98, 1983.
*Differences are statistically significant ($\chi^2 = 55.4$; $P < 0.001$).
†Differences are statistically significant ($\chi^2 = 120.1$; $P < 0.001$).

was judged to be the one needed to correct the most serious problem that required further care. For example, although almost every patient who eventually required an operation also was given additional antibiotics because of failure to respond to the initial treatment, only the operation was listed because this alternative therapy was thought to represent the most serious consequence of the poor response. The results are striking. There was a significantly higher number of responses to the initial treatment in women who were seen early in the clinical course of infection; more of the patients who were treated for a well-established infection required some form of operative intervention to effect a cure. This clinical classification is important for prognosticating the outcome of the treatment of soft-tissue pelvic infections. The prognosis for unsuccessful antibiotic therapy and the need for operative intervention are greater when treatment is delayed until the infection is well established.

An additional aspect of antibiotic therapy is the tremendous proliferation of new agents. There are now second- and third-generation cephalosporins and new penicillins that have a broader spectrum of activity against gram-negative bacteria than do the first-generation cephalosporins and that are effective against the gram-negative aerobic bacteria and the anaerobic bacteria that are most often responsible for obstetric and gynecologic infections. The great appeal of all of these agents is their low toxicity. In addition, imipenem has a broad spectrum of antibacterial activities. Some new antibiotics have appeal because of specific antibacterial actions. Aztreonam has great activity against gram-negative aerobes, whereas the quinolones show marked response against chlamydia.

There is justifiable concern regarding renal and eighth cranial nerve toxicity when aminoglycosides are prescribed and regarding toxicity associated with the use of clindamycin and chloramphenicol.

Categories of infection. The two broad categories of infection are those that are *community acquired*—that is, the patient already has the infection when she is admitted to the hospital—and those that are *hospital acquired,* or *nosocomial.* The second category includes infections that can be associated with the more resistant microorganisms.

COMMUNITY-ACQUIRED INFECTIONS
Infected abortion

A striking change has occurred in the medical problems related to infected abortion. The number of such infections has decreased, in part because of increased use of effective contraceptives and, probably of more significance, because of the ready availability of legal pregnancy termination services. Not only has there been an overall decrease in the number of patients with infected abortions, but the infections that occur are far less serious than were those encountered in the past. Fig. 42-3 is a visual presentation of the fever index, a quantitative evaluation of temperatures elevated above normal, in patients receiving antibiotic therapy for community-acquired infections. It is obvious that patients with infected abortions have a much better prognosis than do women with other types of community-acquired infection.

Clinical evaluation. The evaluation of each patient with an infected abortion includes assessment by physician examination, by accurate recording of the vital signs, and by appropriate laboratory tests. *Hypotension* or an *oral temperature above 39 C (102 F)* places the patient in a high-risk category because of the possibility of septic shock. *Generalized peritonitis,* an indication of extensive extrauterine involvement, also places the patient at higher risk. Uterine size is assessed, and the cervix is inspected for the presence of products of conception. Placental tissue can be removed from the cervical canal with ring forceps without causing significant discomfort. Perhaps the most important aspect of the pelvic examination is a careful assessment of the extent of the infection. More prolonged medical treatment is required when the infection has extended beyond the confines of the uterus than when it is localized.

Laboratory studies include a *complete blood count with a white blood cell count and differential.* Anemia and/or leukopenia identifies patients at higher risk. A low white blood cell count may be an early manifestation of septic shock. A number of *microbiologic samples* should be obtained before antibiotic therapy is started. The most important of these is a *blood culture,* which, when positive, identifies the most significant organisms involved with the infection. Anaerobic bacteria can often be identified in the bloodstream if appropriate culture techniques are used. This information will be particularly helpful if the patient fails to respond to the antibiotics that are administered first (Fig. 42-4). The results of one such study are given in Table 42-3.

There is little justification for relying on the results of anaerobic cultures obtained from the endocervical canal; the high frequency of surface anaerobic bacterial contamination invalidates the results. However, aerobic cultures should be obtained

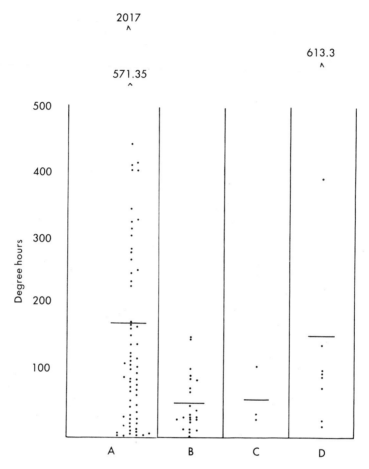

Fig. 42-3. Fever indices of patients admitted to inpatient gynecology service: those with, *A,* salpingo-oophoritis; *B,* infected abortions; *C,* postoperative infections, and *D,* postpartum infections. Bars represent mean values for each group. Lowest number of degree hours is noted in women with infected abortion. (From Ledger, W.J., Moore, D.E., Lowensohn, R.I., and Gee, C.L.: Obstet. Gynecol. **50:**523, 1977.)

from the cervix to ensure that serious pathogens are not present. The recovery of an aerobe such as *N. gonorrhoeae* or the group A beta-hemolytic streptococcus has great significance; these bacteria require strict isolation techniques for the patient and examination of the sexual partner.

X-ray film examination of the abdomen with the patient standing can be helpful. Free air beneath the diaphragm suggests that the uterus was perforated during an abortion attempt. Radiolucent foreign bodies that have been pushed through the wall

of the uterus into the peritoneal cavity can also be seen. Either of these indicates the need for an exploratory operation to estimate the extent of the infection and to remove the foreign body.

Treatment. The treatment of a patient with an infected abortion should be directed toward correcting the pathologic changes: infection that begins in the necrotic trophoblastic tissue within the uterine cavity and that can extend into or through the uterine wall.

Bacteria are introduced into the uterus during the

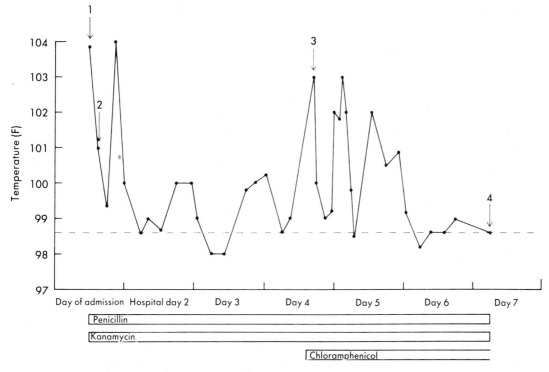

Fig. 42-4. Temperature response of patient with infected abortion. *1*, Blood cultures were obtained; *2*, curettage was performed; *3*, blood cultures were reported to have grown an enterococcus and *Bacteriodes fragilis*, and chloramphenicol was added; *4*, patient was discharged. (From Ledger, W.J.: Am. J. Obstet. Gynecol. **123**:111, 1975.)

manipulations necessary to disrupt the pregnancy. The risk is slight if the abortion is performed with sterile technique. The most serious infections follow abortion done by nonprofessional persons without concern for antisepsis. Such infections are infrequently seen in the United States since the liberalization of laws regulating termination of unwanted pregnancy. A fundamental right of women is control of the reproductive process. Attempts to eliminate this right will have serious medical consequences.

The point of entry for bacteria is through the placental site or through vaginal or uterine injuries. The bacteria advance by way of the veins (phlebitis) or the lymphatics (lymphangitis). The most common extrauterine infection is *parametrial cellulitis*, which may form *abscesses*. Pelvic and even generalized *peritonitis* also occurs with the most serious infections.

The use of *antibiotics* that usually are appropriate for the responsible organisms, primarily gramnegative aerobes and anaerobes, should be combined with curettage to remove the infected products of conception. Chow, Marshall, and Guze have shown that removal of the residual infected placental tissue is probably a more important factor in recovery than is antibiotic therapy. Although there is debate over the timing of curettage and concern about seeding the bloodstream with bacteria, it is usually safe to proceed whenever therapeutic levels of antibiotics have been achieved.

In most women with infected abortions one of the *second-generation cephalosporins* such as cefoxitin

TABLE 42-3 Bacteria isolated from the blood of 34 patients

Bacterium	Number of isolations
Strictly anaerobic	
Streptococcus	16
B. fragilis	9
Bacteroides funduliformis	4
B. melaninogenicus	3
Micrococcus	2
TOTAL	34
Microaerophilic (candle jar)	
Streptococcus	7
Haemophilus vaginalis	5
Actinomyces species	1
TOTAL	13
Aerobic	
E. coli	7
Group B *Streptococcus*	2
Group D *Streptococcus*	1
Pseudomonas aeruginosa	1
Diphtheroid	1
TOTAL	12

should be the first drug administered. If there is evidence of *septic shock*, a combination of clindamycin and gentamicin or metronidazole, penicillin, and gentamicin is more appropriate; these provide better coverage against *B. fragilis*. Either cefoxitin alone or the combinations with clindamycin or metronidazole provide good coverage for the important gram-negative aerobes and the anaerobes so frequently involved in extrauterine infection associated with abortion (Table 42-3).

Patients who are critically ill require more extensive therapy. Many such patients were more than 12 weeks pregnant when termination was attempted; the tissues are more likely injured during second-trimester abortions. These serious infections may occur in many ways. The infection may be caused by *Clostridium perfringens*, with widespread dissemination of its virulent exotoxins. This diagnosis should be considered in any patient with an infected abortion who has renal failure and evidence of intravascular hemolysis. It can be confirmed by x-ray film examination of the pelvis; the enlarged uterus has

an onionskin appearance because of gas formation in its wall. Additional supporting evidence is the presence of gram-positive bacilli with swollen ends in the endocervical smear. In addition to antibiotic therapy, hysterectomy should usually be performed promptly to remove the nidus of infection. This approach is not universally agreed on; British physicians are less aggressive, and the majority of women they treat are cured. This may be a result of differences in the interpretation of microbiologic results. *C. perfringens* can be recovered from the lower genital tract of normal, asymptomatic women; hence isolation of this organism in a culture from a patient with an infected abortion is not an indication for laparotomy unless serious infection is proved. Fortunately for the practitioner today, these infections are rare. This is in contrast to the more frequent problems with "gas gangrene" of the uterus when elective termination of pregnancy was not permitted.

Patients other than those with uterine infections may require operative intervention. Women with extensive uterine damage or infected pelvic hematomas may remain septic despite the use of appropriate antibiotics. In these patients laparotomy to drain or remove an abscess or the removal of pelvic organs will effect a cure.

PELVIC ABSCESS. In some patients, fever, pelvic pain, and signs of peritonitis persist despite antibiotic therapy and evacuation of the uterus. This suggests advancing parametritis and pelvic cellulitis, which may eventually end with pelvic abscess formation. Pelvic examination and sonogram should be frequently performed in such a patient in an attempt to detect the first evidence of fluctuation in the area of cellulitis. Most such abscesses eventually point into the vagina and can be drained by posterior colpotomy. Some, however, extend upward between the leaves of the broad ligament until they can be palpated above the pubis. These must be drained through an abdominal incision.

RENAL FAILURE. Soap or other toxic materials injected into the uterus in an attempt to produce abortion may enter the bloodstream, where they hemolyze red blood cells and damage renal tubular cells. Bacteria, especially *C. perfringens*, or their products may have the same effect on the kidney. This is a highly lethal complication with a high mortality. It must therefore be recognized early in its course. The treatment consists mainly of fluid restriction to an amount with which the patient will barely retain her weight, or even lose a little from day to day, and the maintenance of a reasonable electrolyte balance. The greatest danger is from hyperkalemia. Dialysis may be required if anuria persists and if the electrolyte levels are sufficiently altered to constitute a threat to life. Hysterectomy often is necessary.

RUPTURED UTERUS. Laparotomy should be performed if uterine perforation is diagnosed by x-ray film examination or is thought to be a possibility because of intraperitoneal bleeding or obvious local injury or if the uterus is perforated during surgical evacuation of the necrotic, infected contents. This concern applies to any lateral perforations of the uterus, and if the perforation occurs and a suction instrument has been turned on while outside of the uterus. With extensive lacerations it usually is necessary to remove the uterus. The bowel should be inspected because it often is lacerated if the uterus is ruptured.

THROMBOPHLEBITIS. Puerperal infection extends from its source in the uterine cavity through the wall and into the parametrium by progressive phlebitis and lymphangitis, as well as by direct tissue involvement. Thrombophlebitis eventually involves the veins on the lateral pelvic walls, the ovarian veins, and the vena cava. Septic emboli are transported to distant parts of the body where they set up secondary areas of infection, from which the patient may eventually die even though the pelvic lesion clears. When embolization continues despite antibiotic and anticoagulant therapy, ovarian and vena caval ligation may be lifesaving. With better knowledge of anaerobic organism involvement in infection and early use of antibiotics effective against anaeroba, this entity is rarer in the 1980s than it was in the 1960s.

SEPTIC SHOCK. Septic shock associated with an infected abortion is now an unusual clinical event. The successful treatment of the potentially lethal condition requires an understanding of the pathophysiologic changes and a marshaling of all available intensive care resources. Bacterial products, usually endotoxins from gram-negative aerobic bacteria, are disseminated from the site of infection and exert their deleterious effects on vital organ systems throughout the body. The toxin released from the lysed bacteria produces peripheral vasoconstriction, which is accompanied by reduced cardiac output, prolonged circulation time, hypotension, and tachycardia. The resultant reduced tissue perfusion becomes evident as urine secretion decreases or ceases completely. The hematocrit may be normal or elevated, even though blood loss has been excessive, because of the hypovolemia. The white blood cell count may be within the normal range even though it had been greatly elevated before signs of shock appeared.

The basic requirements for the successful treatment of septic shock include (1) the reduction of peripheral resistance, (2) the restoration of circulating blood volume, and (3) the treatment of infection. The response to the treatment program is monitored by determining the blood pressure, pulse rate, respiration rate, and urine output at 30-minute intervals and by measuring central venous pressure.

Serious therapeutic mistakes can be made in the care of these women if the physician focuses on symptoms while ignoring the underlying pathophysiologic conditions. A delay in performing a necessary operation while repeatedly administering fluid challenges to stimulate urine production, using vasopressors to restore blood pressure, or prescribing repeated steroid doses to combat the effects of endotoxic shock may cause the death of a patient who would have survived with proper care. *Septic shock in a patient with an infected abortion will be perpetuated as long as the nidus of infection exists. This requires curettage as the minimal operative procedure and hysterectomy if the infection is more extensive.* The steps in the management of a patient with septic shock following infected abortion are diagrammed in Fig. 42-5.

Salpingo-oophoritis

The criteria for the diagnosis of salpingo-oophoritis have changed remarkably in the last decade. Until the late 1970s, students were required to adhere to strict criteria for making a diagnosis of acute salpingo-oophoritis. Teachers believed that this was necessary to prevent physicians from ordering antibiotics indiscriminately when another form of treatment was indicated. A major concern was that inappropriate antibiotic therapy would delay operations for ectopic pregnancy. Following are the criteria formerly used for establishing a clinical diagnosis of salpingo-oophoritis:

1. Acute pelvic pain of a few days' duration
2. Temperature of 38 C (100.4 F) or higher
3. Tender adnexal swelling or mass
4. Increased erythrocyte sedimentation rate
5. Elevated white blood cell count

Recent studies in which laparoscopy was performed on patients admitted with a clinical diagnosis of salpingitis have revealed the shortcomings of this approach. Nearly half of women with laparoscopic evidence of acute salpingitis are afebrile

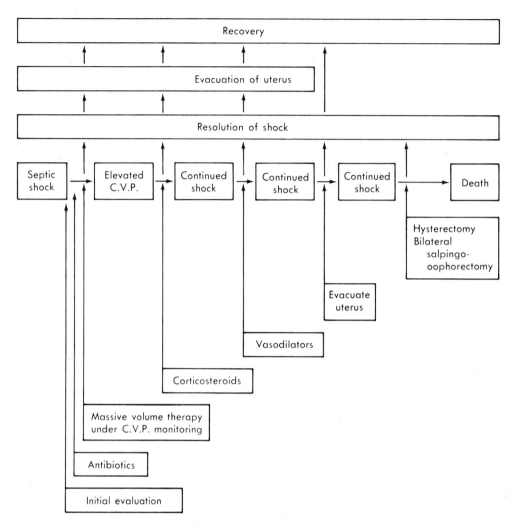

Fig. 42-5. Management of septic abortion with endotoxic shock. *C.V.P.,* Central venous pressure. (Courtesy R.K. Laros, Jr.)

at the time of admission, unilateral salpingitis is an accepted clinical entity, and elevated white blood cell counts or an increased sedimentation rate do not differentiate salpingitis from other noninfectious types of pelvic disorders. These facts indicate that the physician should consider pelvic infection in any woman with acute pelvic pain.

A wide variety of bacterial species has been implicated in the pathogenesis of salpingo-oophoritis, but a continuing emphasis on *N. gonorrhoeae* has

been maintained in the United States. Gonococci are often recovered from the endocervix of patients with salpingitis but less often from peritoneal fluid. The gonococcus was considered to be a bacterial trailblazer paving the way for subsequent colonization and infection of the endosalpinx with other bacteria. Recent studies by Sweet, Draper, and Hadley confirm the concept that salpingitis is a multibacterial infection and that the greatest variety of bacterial isolates can be recovered early in the course of the disease. Many gram-positive and gram-negative aerobes and anaerobes, in addition to *N. gonorrhoeae*, are involved in such multibacterial pelvic infections.

The role of other organisms is currently being evaluated. *Mycoplasma* species has been isolated occasionally from women with salpingo-oophoritis; its significance has not yet been established. Three observations suggest that *Chlamydia* species may play a significant role in pelvic infections. Chlamydiae were isolated in six of 20 biopsies of the fimbriae of fallopian tubes obtained at the time of laparoscopy in women with acute salpingitis. Chlamydiae also can be recovered from biopsies of pelvic adhesions in women with a past history of salpingitis. Women with blocked tubes as the cause of their infertility have a higher than expected incidence of *Chlamydia* antibodies in their blood. Confirmation of these findings will have an impact on future antibiotic strategies in women with salpingitis; chlamydiae are relatively susceptible to tetracycline, erythromycin, and clindamycin; but they are usually resistant to the cephalosporins and the newer penicillin.

Community-acquired infections caused by these organisms are also classified as *sexually transmitted diseases* because they are disseminated almost entirely by heterosexual or homosexual contact. *Gonorrhea* is the most common of the sexually transmitted diseases; the highest infection rates, in order of frequency, occur between the ages 20 and 24, 15 and 19, and 25 and 29.

The bacteria grow in the cervical crypts, producing an acute cervicitis, which may eventually become chronic and relatively asymptomatic. In less than half of cases the bacteria are carried upward through the uterus to the tubes. During the upward extension, which usually occurs during menstruation, a transient endometritis and then endosalpingitis develop. The tubal mucosa responds to the bacteria by producing a purulent exudate. The fimbriae become agglutinated in an attempt to prevent the infection from extending to the peritoneal cavity. The distended pus-filled tube is called a *pyosalpinx*. If there is an associated *peritonitis,* the bowel and omentum adhere to the involved tubes in an attempt to keep the infection confined in the pelvis. Both fallopian tubes usually are involved.

Variations from this clinical picture occur. Many patients obviously have had extensive endosalpingitis and even peritonitis because the tubes are closed, clubbed, and adherent, but they have no history of an acute infection. In others, particularly women who are using an intrauterine contraceptive device when they become infected, only one tube is involved.

Diagnosis. Because of these variations, the clinical diagnosis of acute salpingo-oophoritis may be difficult to establish. It should be suspected in all sexually active women who complain of lower abdominal discomfort or pain. Westrom has indicated that all women with laparoscopy-confirmed salpingitis have white blood cells in their vaginal fluid. In addition, *needle culdocentesis* is a helpful diagnostic technique in afebrile patients. The presence of bacteria in fluid obtained from the posterior cul-de-sac suggests intraperitoneal infection and indicates antibiotic therapy. A Gram stain should be made, and the fluid sent for aerobic and anaerobic culture. Two other examinations are important: one should try to determine whether there are inflammatory masses (an exact evaluation may be difficult because pronounced tenderness limits the accuracy of bimanual examination), and a sample of the cervical secretions should be sent for gonococcal culture and a gram-stained specimen examined for gonococci.

Treatment. Although guidelines for the antibiotic treatment of salpingitis are not yet based on properly designed prospective clinical studies, some observations influence therapeutic strategies. The recovery of *N. gonorrhoeae* from the endocervical canal of a patient with clinical evidence of salpingitis identifies a population with specific risk characteristics. These women usually respond rapidly to antibiotic therapy and subsequently have a lower rate of irreversible tubal damage. The sexual partners should also be treated before activity is resumed. In contrast to many stated beliefs, 20% to 40% of men from whom *N. gonorrhoeae* can be cultured are asymptomatic and can reinfect successfully treated women.

The results of treatment are also influenced by the status of the infection when the patient is first seen. Those with early infections are far more likely to respond successfully to antibiotic treatment than are those in whom the processes are well established (Table 42-2).

The clinical decisions concerning treatment of salpingo-oophoritis are made most logically on the basis of an overall view of the most effective antibiotic regimen. Following are the antimicrobial agents recommended by the Centers for Disease Control:

Outpatients

Either *cefoxitin*, 2.0 g intramuscularly; *ampicillin*, 3.5 g by mouth; *amoxicillin*, 3.0 g by mouth; or *aqueous procaine penicillin G (APPG)*, 4.8 million units intramuscularly at two sites

Each of these alternatives is given with probenecid, 1.0 g by mouth, followed by tetracycline, 500 mg by mouth, four times a day for 10 to 14 days, or doxycycline, 100 mg by mouth twice a day for 10 to 14 days.

Hospitalized patients

Doxycycline, 100 mg intravenously twice a day, plus *cefoxitin*, 2.0 g intravenously four times a day

Continue drugs intravenously for at least 4 days and at least 48 hours after patient defervesces.

Continue doxycycline, 100 mg by mouth twice a day after discharge from hospital to complete 10 to 14 days of therapy.

or

Clindamycin, 600 mg intravenously 4 times a day, plus *gentamicin* or *tobramycin*, 2.0 mg/kg intravenously, followed by 1.5 mg/kg intravenously three times a day in patients with normal renal function

Continue intravenous drugs for at least 4 days and at least 48 hours after patient defervesces.

Continue clindamycin, 450 mg by mouth four times a day after discharge from hospital to complete 10 to 14 days of therapy.

Unfortunately, these regimens are associated with a failure rate of 10% or more, particularly when ampicillin and tetracycline are prescribed. Second- and third-generation cephalosporins eradicate the infection at least 95% of the time. Therefore the most acceptable inpatient therapy for acute salpingitis is 2.0 g of cefoxitin intravenously every 8 hours, to be continued until the patient has been afebrile for 48 hours. Doxycycline, 100 mg taken orally twice a day, should be given for 10 days if outpatient therapy is deemed advisable. One therapeutic problem will be of increasing importance during the next few years. A new strain of *N. gonorrhoeae* that has absolute resistance to penicillin has emerged. Fortunately, these strains are susceptible to cefoxitin; this may be another reason to select this antibiotic.

More intensive antibiotic therapy is indicated for patients with indurated pelvic masses. Clindamycin, 600 mg intravenously every 6 hours, and gentamicin, 3 to 5 mg/kg/day in divided doses at 8-hour intervals, should be given. Because of the variations in serum levels achieved in patients receiving gentamicin, peak and trough blood concentrations of the antibiotics should be measured after 24 hours of therapy. The results will guide necessary dosage adjustment. *Ultrasonography* may be helpful in differentiating a tuboovarian complex from a tuboovarian abscess and in identifying patients who will most likely need an operation.

In recent years, the *operative care of women with salpingo-oophoritis* has been modified. There is general consensus on a number of therapeutic points. A ruptured *tuboovarian abscess* represents an operative emergency. Many women will die unless the infected pelvic structures are removed, the peritoneal cavity is lavaged, appropriate antibiotics are administered, and shock is treated. This diagnosis should be considered in every woman with diffuse peritonitis and a tachycardia out of proportion to the temperature elevation. The suspected diagnosis can be confirmed by a culdocentesis in which a free flow of purulent material is obtained. A *pelvic abscess* bulging into the vagina through a distended posterior cul-de-sac can be treated with transvaginal drainage. Operative evacuation of pelvic abscesses usually results in a clinical cure, and no further operative care is needed. It usually is necessary to remove the affected pelvic organs if the infection persists after it has been drained or if it recurs.

Other indications for surgery are more controversial. There is no standard definition of failure to respond to medical therapy. Although some gynecologists advocate laparotomy if there is no response after 48 hours of antibiotic therapy, most have been more conservative. The need for early operative intervention has decreased since more emphasis has been placed on the use of antibiotics such as clindamycin, metronidazole, or cefoxitin, which are effective against *B. fragilis,* and on longer periods of antibiotic therapy before deciding that the medical treatment has failed. A decrease in temperature after treatment has been started is an indication for continuing medical therapy.

Traditional teaching has stressed the bilaterality of pelvic infection and the need to remove both adnexa when an operation is necessary. This is not necessarily true. Unilateral tubal abscesses do occur, particularly in women who have used intrauterine contraceptive devices. In such patients only the involved adnexum need be removed. Some women respond initially to antibiotic therapy but have recurring bouts of pain. In the past, total abdominal hysterectomy and bilateral salpingo-oophorectomy was recommended to relieve the pain. This is still appropriate if repeated acute attacks have left the pelvic structures extensively damaged, but it is not always necessary. Lysis of adhesions to free the adherent tubes and ovaries, resection of structures that are most involved, and instillation of a high-molecular-weight dextran solution to help prevent reformation of adhesions may relieve the symptoms. The isolation of *Chlamydia* organisms from the adhesions is an indication for the use of a tetracycline.

POSTOPERATIVE INFECTIONS

Any patient who has undergone a pelvic operation may develop a *postoperative infection*. These infections are categorized as those of the operative site such as an infection in the abdominal incision or at the vault of the vagina after hysterectomy and those that are separate from the surgical field; for example, a postoperative respiratory tract infection.

Prevention. An important responsibility of surgeons who perform pelvic operations is to make every effort to prevent postoperative infection, but a number of time-honored hospital and operating room rituals may actually increase the infection rate. *The longer the preoperative stay, the greater the postoperative infection rate. Shaving the operative site* the evening before operation, the *use of cautery* rather than a sharp knife, *plastic adhesive drapes* instead of towels, or *wound drapes* all increase the number of abdominal wound infections.

Swartz and Tanaree have shown that closed-suction T-tube drainage of the space between the peritoneum and the vaginal cuff lowers the incidence of postoperative pelvic infections after hysterectomy. Several controllable procedures favorably influence the rate of *postoperative urinary tract infection*. Meticulous attention to maintaining a closed drainage system while an indwelling catheter is in place keeps urinary tract infections at a minimum. A correlation exists between the length of time a transuretheral catheter is in place and postoperative urinary tract infection. Indwelling catheters should be removed as soon as the patient is able to void. The number of infections can be reduced even more by the use of suprapubic bladder drainage instead of a transurethral catheter. These facts should be considered during the preoperative planning for the care of women scheduled for elective operations.

Systemic antibiotic prophylaxis has been used increasingly to lower the incidence of postoperative site infection. This represents a remarkable change in philosophy; prophylaxis had been condemned by many leaders in the field of infectious disease. The change made on the basis of a number of carefully controlled double-blind clinical studies that demonstrated the favorable impact of a short course of perioperative antibiotic prophylaxis on the postoperative infection rate. Fig. 42-6, a graphic representation of the cumulative quantities of elevated temperature in patients receiving either a placebo or a systemic antibiotic immediately before the operation, demonstrates clearly that systemic antibiotics decreased the postoperative infection rate. There is little disagreement that prophylactic antibiotics are effective in women undergoing vaginal hysterectomy. Although there has been less enthusiasm for prophylaxis with abdominal hysterectomy, most recent studies have shown that it does decrease postoperative infections after abdominal hysterectomies for benign disease and after radical operations for uterine cancer. The most commonly used antibiotics have been the cephalosporins, but penicillins have been equally effective. Although no carefully controlled studies have been done, antibiotic prophylaxis has also been used widely in women undergoing salpingolysis and elective tubal reconstruction. Since chlamydiae can sometimes be recovered from the pelvic adhesions that appear to be old and inactive, tetracycline would probably be a better choice than a penicillin or cephalosporin in these women.

Treatment. Despite preventive measures, postoperative infections still occur. Women with these infections should be studied systematically so that an appropriate treatment plan can be developed. A complete physical examination should be performed on every febrile postoperative patient in an attempt to determine the site of infection. This is important because the antibacterial agents selected for the treatment of a multibacterial pelvic infection differ from those that will eradicate a urinary tract infection caused by a single species of bacteria.

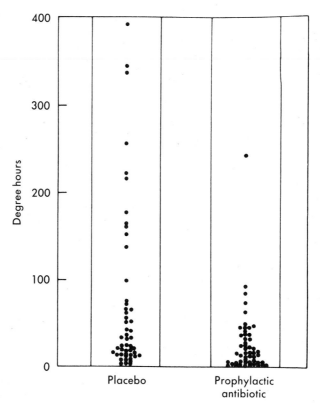

Fig. 42-6. Postoperative fever indices of patients undergoing vaginal hysterectomy who received either placebo or prophylactic antibiotic. (From Ledger, W.J., Gassner, C.B., and Gee, C.: J. Reprod. Med. **13**:128, 1974.)

In addition, a postoperative infection associated with a collection of infected material such as a vaginal cuff or an abdominal wound abscess is more effectively treated by drainage than by systemic antibiotics. Unless purulent material can be aspirated directly from the site of infection, culture for anaerobic bacteria is of little help; bacteria that grow may represent surface contaminants. *Blood cultures* for aerobic and anaerobic bacteria should be obtained before treatment is started.

If the infection is manifested only by induration and tenderness without fluctuation, good clinical results can usually be achieved with second-generation cephalosporins such as cefamandole and cefoxitin. Some patients who have been discharged from the hospital after what seems to have been an uneventful recovery will require readmission because they have developed clinical evidence of a postoperative infection. These patients' conditions usually respond best to a combination of genta-

micin and clindamycin. An operation to remove or drain an abscess or to remove the infected structure should be performed if the infection does not respond promptly to antibiotic therapy.

Abdominal wound infections, except small localized ones, are best treated by opening the entire wound. This ensures adequate drainage and permits the clinician to determine the integrity of the fascia. Systemic antibiotics are seldom needed unless there is spreading involvement of the wound edge. Rapidly spreading inflammation of the skin adjacent to the wound may herald the presence of a dangerous synergistic infection. If there is a possibility that this may be occurring, wide debridement may be lifesaving.

Most nonoperative site infections in the postoperative period involve the urinary tract. These problems usually are easily managed. Uncomplicated *urinary tract infections* usually respond promptly to sulfonamides or nitrofurantoins, which have limited antibacterial activity outside the urinary tract. However, any postoperative patient who develops acute pyelonephritis should be investigated for the possibility of ureteral injury related to the pelvic operation.

POSTPARTUM (PUERPERAL) INFECTIONS

In the tradition of Semmelweiss, obstetricians have maintained a consistent focus on maternal postpartum infections. In the past, statistics concerning obstetric infection rates were based on temperature recording. "Infectious morbidity" was defined as an oral temperature of 38 C (100.4 F) or more on any 2 of the first 10 postpartum days, excluding the first 24 hours. This standard is now much less useful than it was in the past. Few women remain in the hospital for 10 days after normal delivery; some are discharged within a few hours, and most have left by the fourth day. As a consequence, the first abnormal temperature elevation may occur after the patient has gone home. The day on which the temperature first rose in a series of women who developed puerperal infection is shown in Fig. 42-7. Unless the infection is a serious one, these patients are treated without readmitting them; thus they may not be included in hospital statistics as having developed postpartum infections. Another source of inaccuracy in compiling statistics on the basis of temperature morbidity is that systemic antibiotics are often prescribed for postpartum patients soon after the first temperature elevation and are continued for long periods. Many women receiving this treatment will not have postpartum infections that satisfy the definition based on temperature; hence reported infection rates may not reflect the reality of what is happening on a service. The postpartum infection rate should include the total number of patients who received systemic antibiotics, as well as those who met the temperature definition of infection.

Prevention. The prevention of postpartum infection requires a knowledge of the factors that increase risk. Women with a consistently high infection rate include those delivered by cesarean section, particularly those who have been in labor, and those from the lower socioeconomic populations.

One might suspect that factors such as prolonged labor, prolonged rupture of membranes, frequent internal examination during labor, or the use of invasive monitoring techniques would increase the risk of infection, but they do not do so consistently.

Cesarean section, particularly in patients who have been in labor, is followed by a high postpartum infection rate. The experience with prophylaxis with vaginal and abdominal hysterectomy suggests that systemic preventive antibiotics might be of value because the operative field is usually contaminated by the bacteria present in the amniotic cavity. Prospective, double-blind studies of *antibiotic prophylaxis for cesarean section* indicate that the infection rate usually is lower in patients who have been given systemic antibiotics, but questions about their use remain unanswered. One concern is that, even though the overall infection rate has been reduced, *serious* infections have not decreased significantly (Fig. 42-8). Of more importance is the concern about timing of antibiotic administration. Ideally for the mother, the antibiotics should be given before the operation is started, but this strategy results in a therapeutic level of antibiotics in the fetus, as well as in the mother. To prevent this problem, the first dose of the prophylactic is administered intravenously in the operating room as soon as the umbilical cord has been clamped. This approach is effective but not entirely without risk. Death from cardiovascular collapse has been reported in two patients after the intravenous injection of cephalothin in the operating room. The mechanism of action of this adverse effect is not known. Despite these concerns, the effectiveness of systemic antibiotics in reducing postpartum infections seems to mandate their use. Both the cephalosporins and penicillins are effective. A new development in preventive techniques may yield an alternative approach to the care of women with cesarean section. Lavage of the uterine wound, the peritoneal cavity, and the abdominal wound with a cefamandole solution has been accompanied by reduced incidence of postpartum infections. This approach prevents many of the potential problems possible with the use of systemic antibiotic prophylaxis. However, the results with this technique have not been universally successful.

Treatment. Despite these preventive techniques, postpartum infections still occur. Since effective treatment regimens must be established on the basis of the changes produced by the infection, an un-

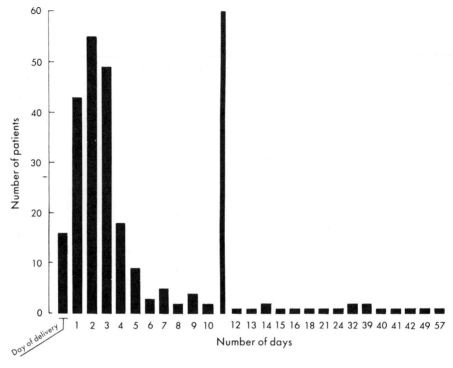

Fig. 42-7. Graph depicting first day of temperature elevation in postpartum patients with clinical diagnosis of bacterial infection. (From Ledger, W.J., Reite, A.M., and Headington, J.T.: Obstet. Gynecol. **37:**769, 1971.)

derstanding of the pathophysiology of puerperal infections is essential to their treatment.

Puerperal infection is for all practical purposes a wound infection. The point of entry for the bacteria from the uterine cavity is the placental site. From there they extend through the uterine wall by way of the veins (phlebitis), the lymphatics (lymphangitis), or direct extension through the muscle.

Endomyometritis, the most common type of puerperal infection, involves the endometrium and the superficial muscle layer of the uterine wall. Bacteria can be cultured from the uterine cavity in most women during prolonged or difficult labor and soon after normal delivery. Adherent bits of placenta in the area of the placental site, the shaggy decidua, and blood clots in the uterus serve as excellent media for the growth of bacteria, and as a consequence almost every recently delivered woman has a mild and inconsequential endometritis.

The clinically important infections are more obvious. With these infections, generally the temperature is slightly elevated from the day of delivery on, but by the third day it may be as high as 38.3 to 39 C (101 to 102 F). The patient has few symptoms other than malaise and perhaps slight abdominal tenderness. The lochia is usually profuse, purulent, and malodorous.

The clinical course of infections caused by group A or group B *beta-hemolytic streptococcus* is different from that of endomyometritis caused by other bacteria. The temperature rises abruptly to 39 to 40 C (102 to 104 F), frequently during the first 12 hours after delivery, and the patient looks and feels acutely ill. There may be little or no discharge from the uterus, and that present usually is not purulent.

Absence of the lochia is more often an evidence of *lochial block* than of beta-hemolytic streptococcal infection. This is produced by an obstruction

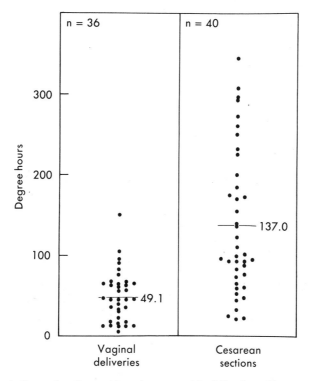

Fig. 42-8. Fever indices of patient with endomyometritis following either vaginal delivery or cesarean section. Less complicated infections were observed after vaginal delivery. (From Ledger, W.J., Kriewall, T.J., and Gee, C.: Obstet. Gynecol. **45**:603, 1975.)

to drainage of the uterine cavity by a sheet of retained membrane, a blood clot, or an abnormal position of the uterus. With this condition, the temperature rises abruptly when the drainage is impeded. It often is preceded by slight daily temperature rises.

The uterus in women with endomyometritis is usually boggy, larger, and less well contracted than it should be. It is tender, but the parametrial areas can be palpated without producing any great amount of discomfort. Unless the symptoms are caused by lochial block, there usually is a purulent discharge coming from the cervix.

In the more serious cases of endomyometritis the entire thickness of the uterine wall is involved and may even be the site of multiple small abscesses. This type of infection usually follows the early use of antibiotics ineffective against gram-negative anaerobes. All the symptoms and the findings that

characterize endomyometritis are exaggerated, and there usually is parametrial tenderness.

Further extension of the organisms along the blood vessels and lymphatics produces cellulitis within the peritoneal folds of one or occasionally both broad ligaments *(parametritis)*. The signs are similar to those with endomyometritis but are much more severe. The temperature may reach 39.5 to 40 C (103 to 104 F). The pulse is elevated, and the white blood cell count may be 30,000 or more. The uterus is boggy and tender, limited in mobility, and sometimes pushed to one side by tender induration filling half of the pelvis; the other side may be relatively normal.

An *abscess* may develop in the center of the area of cellulitis. As it enlarges, it may eventually dissect downward to point in the posterior cul-de-sac, or it may extend upward until it can be felt above the inguinal ligament. In either event, as an abscess develops, the evidences of pelvic infection become more pronounced.

Peritonitis almost always accompanies parametritis and pelvic cellulitis. It varies in severity from relatively mild involvement of the peritoneal covering of the broad ligaments to widespread generalized infection.

Since phlebitis in the pelvic and the ovarian veins occurs as part of every serious puerperal infection, *bacteremia* is common. A recent study of bacteremia from Texas indicated that those patients with an endomyometritis and a bacteremia were no more seriously ill than those without a bacteremia.

A general physical and pelvic examination should be performed before treatment is begun. Evaluation of the pelvis will provide information concerning the extent of the involvement of the pelvic structures will permit the clinician to remove membranes or placental tissue visible in the endocervical canal. In patients with *lochial block* the discharge of uterine secretions is reestablished and the temperature returns to normal after the obstructing tissue is removed with ring forceps.

Aerobic cultures from the lochia should be obtained in all febrile women suspected of having postpartum endomyometritis. There should be particular concern if the group A beta-hemolytic streptococcus is found because of its danger to the mother and its contagiousness. Attempts have been made to obtain anaerobic cultures uncontaminated by normal vaginal and cervical flora by using double-lumen aspirators to sample the endometrial cavity, transabdominal-transfundal aspiration, and needle culdocentesis to obtain peritoneal fluid. None of these ensures that contamination has been eliminated. It is difficult to interpret *standard blood studies* in evaluating postpartum patients. Normal women have a leukocytosis with a shift to the left.

There are rational guidelines for treating women with postpartum endomyometritis. The course of the infections that develop after vaginal delivery is much less complicated than that following cesarean section (Fig. 42-8). Because of this, a single antibiotic agent such as cefoxitin is often appropriate. Chlamydiae may be a factor in late postpartum endomyometritis following vaginal delivery; that

is, the patient has been discharged and, in a week to 10 days, is seen with an elevated temperature and a tender uterus.

For such infections one of the newer tetracyclines such as doxycycline is a logical choice.

Endomyometritis that follows cesarean section is more serious than that which develops after vaginal delivery. Traditionally, these patients have been treated with a combination of penicillin and an aminoglycoside, but recent studies have demonstrated the superiority of using clindamycin and either gentamicin or ampicillin as the first therapy. Better results have also been achieved with the newer cephalosporins and the newer penicillins. An abdominal wound infection should be suspected when patients fail to respond to systemic antibiotic therapy.

Many febrile postpartum patients will have *urinary tract infections*. This diagnosis can be suspected in a patient with no other clinical findings, the presence of bacteria on microscopic examination of an unspun catheterized urine sample, and a significant bacterial colony count. Women with these infections are best treated with nitrofurantoins whose activity is limited to the urinary tract. Any antibiotic given to the mother will appear in her breast milk.

THROMBOPHLEBITIS
Prenatal thrombophlebitis

Deep vein thrombophlebitis does not often occur during pregnancy. *Anticoagulant therapy* is indicated, but treatment is complicated by the pregnancy. *Warfarin (Coumadin)* crosses the placenta and may cause fetal death and hemorrhage in newborn infants. *Heparin* is preferable because it does not cross the placenta. In most instances the patient can learn to administer it. For serious infections, heparin should be continued throughout the entire pregnancy. It is discontinued when labor begins and restarted a few hours after delivery.

Puerperal thrombophlebitis

Although thrombophlebitis is an integral part of all puerperal infections, it is generally confined to the blood vessels in the uterine wall and is of little consequence. If the process extends laterally and involves the ovarian veins and the large vessels along the lateral pelvic wall, the prognosis becomes worse. *Pelvic thrombophlebitis* often is first suspected during the latter part of the first postpartum week, although in most instances the temperature has never been normal after delivery. The early use of antibiotics effective against gram-negative anaerobic bacteria had made this a much less frequent clinical entity than in the past.

The patient may complain of discomfort in the abdomen and pelvis, and tenderness may be elicited on deep pressure. There usually is no evidence of peritonitis. There is tenderness, often localized to one side of the pelvis, the uterus may be limited in mobility, and motion produces pain on the affected side. Occasionally, the involved veins may be palpated. The temperature remains elevated and in fact may become progressively higher.

Ovarian vein thrombosis is a distinct entity that should be suspected in any woman who develops unilateral lower abdominal pain, tenderness, and fever during the first few days after delivery. The pain is deep and constant and may radiate to the groin, the flank, or the costovertebral angle. Gastrointestinal symptoms usually are minimal, but ileus may be present. The abdomen is tender but soft, and a tender elongated mass can generally be felt on deep palpation. This differentiates it from pyelonephritis and the more common postpartum infections. Laparotomy often is necessary to confirm the diagnosis and to eliminate other lesions such as appendicitis.

The most serious involvement of the veins of the extremities is that of the *femoral vein,* which produces the process known as "milk leg." This usually appears at the end of the second week or later, and the patient experiences edema and pain in the affected leg and chills and fever. It seems likely that most postpartum involvements of the leg veins represent retrograde extensions from a pelvic thrombophlebitis.

Diagnosis. The diagnosis of pelvic thrombophlebitis is difficult, since involvement of the pelvic veins is difficult to discern. The physician should suspect the diagnosis in any postpartum patient with persistent unexplained fever, particularly if it is associated with a uterine infection and increasing pelvic pain and tenderness.

Heparin may be helpful in establishing the diagnosis. Puerperal pelvic thrombophlebitis can be diagnosed with reasonable accuracy when fever, which persists despite adequate antibiotic therapy, resolves within 48 hours after an appropriate dosage of heparin is added to the regimen.

Treatment. The treatment of postpartum thrombophlebitis is like that for nonpregnant women. Antibiotics will already have been prescribed for most women suspected of having puerperal thrombophlebitis; in fact, failure to respond to antibiotics is an important diagnostic feature of the condition. Since *Bacteroides* species are being recognized more and more often as the organisms responsible for thrombophlebitis, drugs to which they are susceptible should be added to the therapeutic regimen. *Anticoagulation* with heparin instituted early is essential in controlling the infection and in preventing serious vascular sequelae.

MASTITIS

Postpartum mastitis usually begins at least 2 weeks after delivery and is most common in women who are nursing or have attempted to nurse their infants. The bacteria are usually introduced through the nipples, and the incidence is not influenced by elaborate breast care. Infection is far more common in white than in black patients.

The patient may have pain in one quadrant of the breast, followed by fever, chills, and enlargement of the affected gland. The systemic reaction to a small area of infection may be pronounced. The breast is erythematous, indurated, and tender, and if the process is far enough advanced, fluctuation may be detected.

Treatment consists first of prevention, by prohibiting nursing by women whose nipples are inverted and abnormal, those in whom cracks and fissures do not heal promptly, those who have bleeding from the nipples, and those whose nipples are injured by the baby.

Curative treatment must be started early to be effective. Nursing is immediately stopped, the breast is immobilized with a tight binder, and ice is applied. Many breast infections are caused by penicillin-resistant staphylococci; consequently, an antibiotic preparation such as *oxacillin* is generally more appropriate than penicillin.

A Gram stain and culture of milk expressed during the examination may help determine appropriate treatment.

Such treatment usually aborts or cures the infection, but if the temperature remains elevated and fluctuation appears, incision and drainage become necessary. Extensive destruction of breast tissue may result from unrecognized abscess formation.

PELVIC TUBERCULOSIS

Tuberculosis of the pelvic organs usually is caused by tuberculous infection in some other part of the body, but frequently the primary source is quiescent at the time the pelvic involvement is discovered. The infection reaches the tube by hematogenous transmission or, less often, from an infection involving the peritoneum. It spreads downward along the tubal mucosa to the endometrium and then to the cervix and vagina. Since the extension is from above downward, the structures in the lower genital tract are not often involved. It is possible, however, that lesions on the external genitals, vagina, and cervix can come from an extrinsic source such as tuberculous epididymitis.

Tuberculous pelvic infection is encountered less frequently in the United States than in other parts of the world, where it is said to account for about 5% of all cases of salpingitis. Tuberculosis is found in from 5% to 10% of all women studied for infertility in Israel, Scotland, and some other countries, but much less often here. This picture may change. Refugees from the Caribbean and Southeast Asia have a high incidence of tuberculosis. We can expect an increase in the number of infertile women with unexpected pelvic tuberculosis.

The most characteristic lesions involve the tubes and the endometrium. There may be many small tubercles over the peritoneal surface, and the tube may be enlarged, thickened, and adherent. The lumen often contains cheesy, necrotic material, but, in contrast to the findings in other types of salpingo-oophoritis, the fimbriated end is open. Tubercles may be seen in any of the layers of the tubal wall. The ovarian involvement is usually superficial.

Endometrial tuberculosis is almost always a result of infection in the tubes and can usually be diagnosed microscopically without difficulty, particularly when the biopsy is obtained in the secretory phase of the cycle.

Diagnosis. The symptoms are variable and are determined by the structures involved. Extensive tubal tuberculosis with distortion and fixation generally causes dysmenorrhea and dyspareunia and may interfere with descent of the ovum. If the endometrium is involved, the menstrual cycle often is altered, but there is no characteristic change. The flow is increased and irregular at least as often as it is decreased. Most of the patients are infertile. Lesions of the vagina and cervix may resemble cancer and can be differentiated from it only by biopsy.

The diagnosis should be suspected in any person without a history of an acute pelvic infection who has pelvic pain and enlarged adherent adnexa. This is particularly true in virgins. In such a patient, *endometrial biopsy* or *curettage* may demonstrate the lesion. If the endometrium is involved, the tubes are almost certain to be infected also; but since the transmission is from above downward, tuberculous salpingitis can be present even though the endometrium is normal. Failure to demonstrate tubercles in the endometrium therefore does not eliminate the diagnosis. The lesion at this stage can sometimes be detected by *culture* of uterine discharge or from material obtained from aspiration of the endometrial cavity.

Treatment. Active and prolonged antibiotic treatment, often followed by total abdominal hysterectomy and bilateral salpingo-oophorectomy, is indicated for lesions that cause enlargement and distortion of the adnexal structures.

Medical treatment for minimal lesions is the same as that for more advanced disease, but operation is less important because the infection can usually be eradicated by the medications alone.

RARE INFECTIONS

Other forms of pelvic infection, such as those resulting from actinomycosis, should be considered if the symptoms do not fit the usual pattern or if treatment is ineffective, but they are too rare to consider here in detail.

REFERENCES

Berkeley, A.S., et al.: Imipenem/cilastatin in the treatment of obstetric and gynecologic infections, Am. J. Med. **78**:79, 1935.

Brown, T.K., and Munsick, R.A.: Puerperal ovarian vein thrombophlebitis: a syndrome, Am. J. Obstet. Gynecol. **109**:263, 1971.

Brunham, R.C., et al.: Chlamydia trachomatis infection in women with ectopic pregnancy, Obstet. Gynecol. **67**:722, 1986.

Chow, A.W., Marshall, J.R., and Guze, L.B.: A double blind comparison of clindamycin with penicillin plus chloramphenicol in treatment of septic abortion, J. Infect. Dis. **135**:535, 1977.

Curran, J.W., Rendtorff, R.C., Chandler, R.W., Wiser, W.L., and Robinson, H.: Female gonorrhea: its relation to abnormal bleeding, urinary tract symptoms, and cervicitis, Obstet. Gynecol. **45:**195, 1975.

Dodson, M.G., Faro, S., and Gentry, L.O.: Treatment of acute pelvic inflammatory disease with aztreonam, a new monocyclic β-lactam antibiotic, and clindamycin, Obstet. Gynecol. **67:**657, 1986.

Eschenbach, D.A., Buchanan, T.M., Pollock, H.M., Forsyth, P.S., Alexander, E.R., Lin, J.S., Wang, S.P., Wentworth, B.B., McCormack, W.M., and Holmes, K.K.: Polymicrobial etiology of acute pelvic inflammatory disease, N. Engl. J. Med. **293:**166, 1975.

Hawkins, D.F., Levitt, L.H., Fairbrother, P.F., et. al.: Management of septic chemical abortion with renal failure: Use of a conservative regimen, N. Engl. J. Med. **282:**722, 1975.

Henry-Suchet, J., Catalan, F., Loffredo, V. Serfaty, D., Siboulet, A., Perol, Y., Sanson, M.J., Debache, C., Pigeau, F., Coppin, R., de Brux, J., and Poynard, T.: Microbiology of specimens obtained by laparoscopy from controls and from patients with pelvic inflammatory disease or infertility with tubal obstruction: *Chlamydia trachomatis* and *Ureaplasma urealyticum,* Am. J. Obstet. Gynecol. **138:**1022, 1980.

Holmes, O.W.: Puerperal fever as a private pestilence, Boston, 1855, Tickner & Fields.

Ledger, W.J.: Anaerobic infections, Am. J. Obstet. Gynecol. **123:**111, 1975.

Ledger, W.J.: Anaerobic infections. In Wehrle, P.H., and Top, F.H., Sr., editors: Communicable and infectious diseases, ed. 9, St. Louis, 1981, The C.V. Mosby Co.

Ledger, W.J.: Selection of antimicrobial agents for treatment of infections of the female genital tract. Rev. Inf. Dis. **5:**98, 1983.

Ledger, W.J., and Peterson, E.P.: The use of heparin in the management of pelvic thrombophlebitis, Surg. Obstet. Gynecol. **131:**1115, 1970.

Ledger, W.J., and Headington, J.T.: Group A beta hemolytic streptococcus: an important cause of serious infections in obstetrics and gynecology, Obstet. Gynecol. **39:**474, 1972.

Ledger, W.J., Gassner, C.B., and Gee, C.: Operative care of infections in obstetrics-gynecology, J. Reprod. Med. **13:**128, 1974.

Ledger, W.J., Gee, C., and Lewis, W.P.: Guidelines for antibiotic prophylaxis in gynecology, Am. J. Obstet. Gynecol. **121:**1038, 1975.

Ledger, W.J., Kriewall, T.J., and Gee, C.: The fever index: a technic for evaluating the clinical response to bacteremia, Obstet. Gynecol. **45:**603, 1976.

Ledger, W.J., Moore, D.E., Lowensohn, R.I., and Gee, C.L.: A fever index evaluation of chloramphenicol or clindamycin in patients with serious pelvic infections, Obstet. Gynecol. **50:**523, 1977.

Ledger, W.J., Norman, M., Gee, C., and Lewis, W.: Bacteremia on an obstetric-gynecologic service, Am. J. Obstet. Gynecol. **121:**205, 1975.

Ledger, W.J., Reite, A.M., and Headington, J.T.: A system for infectious disease surveillance on an obstetric service, Obstet. Gynecol. **37:**769, 1971.

Mardh, P.A., Ripa, T., Svensson, L., and Westrom, L.: *Chlamydia trachomatis* infection in patients with acute salpingitis, N. Engl. J. Med. **296:**1377, 1977.

Nolan, G.H., and Osborne, N.: Gonococcal infections in the female, J.A.M.A. **42:**156, 1973.

Neuwirth, R.S., and Friedman, E.A.: Septic abortion, Am. J. Obstet. Gynecol. **85:**24, 1963.

Rotheram, E.B., and Schick, S.F.: Nonclostridial anaerobic bacteria in septic abortion, Am. J. Med. **46:**80, 1969.

Schachter, J.: Chlamydial infections (part I), N. Engl. J. Med. **298:**428, 1978.

Schachter, J.: Chlamydial infections (part II), N. Engl. J. Med. **298:**490, 1978.

Schaefer, G.: Antimicrobial treatment of tuberculous salpingitis, Am. J. Obstet. Gynecol. **77:**996, 1959.

Semmelweis, I.P.: The etiology, concept and prophylaxis of childbed fever, Baltimore, 1941, The Williams & Wilkins Co. (Translated by F.P. Murphy.)

Siegel, M.S., Thornsberry, C., Biddle, J.W., O'Mara, P.R., Perine, P.L., and Wiesner, P.J.: Penicillinase-producing *Neisseria gonorrhoeae:* results of surveillance in the United States, J. Infect. Dis. **137:**170, 1978.

Spruill, F.G., Minette, L.J., and Stumer, W.C.: Two surgical deaths associated with cephalothin, J.A.M.A. **229:**440, 1974.

Swartz, W.H., and Tanaree, P.: Suction drainage as an alternative to prophylactic antibiotics for hysterectomy, Obstet. Gynecol. **45:**305, 1975.

Sweet, R.L., and Ledger, W.J.: Puerperal infectious morbidity, Am. J. Obstet. Gynecol. **117:**1093, 1973.

Sweet, R.L., Draper, D.L., and Hadley, W.K.: Etiology of acute salpingitis: influence of episode number and duration of symptoms, Obstet. Gynecol. **58:**62, 1981.

Swenson, R.M., Michaelson, T.G., Daly, M.J., and Spaulding, E.H.: Anaerobic bacterial infections of the female genital tract, Obstet. Gynecol. **42:**538, 1973.

Weinstein, W.M., Onderdonk, A.B., Bartlett, J.G., et al.: Experimental intra-abdominal abscesses in rats: development of an experimental model, Infect. Immun. **10:**1250, 1974.

Westrom, L.: Incidence, prevalence, and trends of acute pelvic inflammatory disease and its consequences in industrialized countries, Am. J. Obstet. Gynecol. **138:**880, 1980.

White, C.: Treatise on the management of pregnant and lying-in women, London, 1973, E.C. Dilly.

Wong, R., Gee, C.L., and Ledger, W.J.: Prophylactic use of cefazolin in monitored obstetric patients undergoing cesarean section, Obstet. Gynecol. **51:**407, 1978.

J. Robert Willson

The puerperium

The puerperium is the period from 6 to 8 weeks after delivery during which the physical and physiologic changes produced by pregnancy regress.

NORMAL CHANGES

Uterus. The uterus, which at term weighs about 1000 g, returns to its nonpregnant weight of 60 to 80 g by a process known as *involution*. The uterus weighs about 500 g at the end of the first week and about 300 to 350 g at the end of the second week after delivery.

Normal pregnant women are in positive nitrogen balance during pregnancy, retaining an average of about 1.8 g daily. The retained nitrogen is used for the development of the fetus and placenta and for the growth of the uterus, the breasts, and other protein-containing structures. After delivery the excess protein in the uterine muscle cells is broken down by autolysis and excreted in the urine, or it is used, at least partially, if the patient is lactating. The increase in urinary nitrogen that is expected during involution is considerably reduced if the uterus is removed at or shortly after delivery. The number of muscle cells does not change during involution, but rather the size of each individual cell decreases by about 90%.

After the lower segment has regained its tone during the first few hours after delivery, the su-perior surface of the fundus can be felt below the umbilicus. The size of the uterus decreases rapidly, so that at the tenth to twelfth day it is at the level of the upper border of the pubis, and by the sixth week it usually has returned to normal size.

The more superficial layers of the decidua become necrotic and slough, but the bases of the glands that dip into the muscularis remain intact and active. The new endometrium, which eventually will line the entire cavity, regenerates from the remaining glandular epithelium.

The placental site is reduced to about half its predelivery size as the uterus contracts after expelling the placenta. It becomes progressively smaller, measuring only about 3 by 4 cm at the end of the second week. Immediate control of bleeding from the open choriodecidual sinuses is obtained by compression and kinking of the blood vessels leading to them. This is followed by clot formation in the open vessels. The remaining decidual and trophoblastic tissue at the placental site, the thrombosed choriodecidual sinuses and blood vessels, and a superficial layer of myometrium beneath the placental site are infiltrated with leukocytes; and tissue necrosis begins by the second day. Eventually the crust, composed of decidua, thrombosed vessels, endometrial glands, and myometrium, separates from the normal uterine wall beneath. This permits healing without significant scarring.

Regeneration of the endometrium from the remaining glandular tissue begins on the third day and progresses rapidly. The entire uterine cavity, except for the placental site, is covered by endometrium by the end of the third week. The placental site is reepithelized within another 2 to 3 weeks by endometrium growing in from the edges beneath the remaining crust.

The discharge from the uterus, which is made up of blood from the vessels of the placental site and debris from decidual necrosis, is called *lochia*. The discharge of pure blood from the open vessels soon changes to the *lochia rubra,* which is made up of necrotic decidua and blood. It gradually becomes less red as the vessels thrombose, but bloody discharge often persists for 4 to 5 weeks. The *serosanguineous lochia,* which is tan in color, contains less blood and finally changes to the serous *lochia alba*. Bloody discharge may persist if placental fragments remain in the uterus or if for some reason involution does not proceed at its usual rate.

The endometrial cavity is sterile from 6 to 24 hours after normal delivery but then becomes contaminated from the upward migration of vaginal bacteria. Bacterial growth in the shaggy necrotic decidua contributes to the discharge.

Cyclic ovarian function is suspended after conception, but the ovaries continue to secrete estrogen and progesterone throughout the pregnancy. According to Acar, MacNaughton, and Coutts, the corpus luteum produces progesterone but little estrogen; the latter is secreted by other ovarian tissues. Estrogen and progesterone are also elaborated by trophoblastic tissues.

The anterior pituitary–inhibiting effects of estrogen and progesterone are removed when the placenta is delivered and FSH and LH secretions gradually rise, but the levels are lower than those during menstrual cycles. The time required for return of normal ovarian function is governed by the rapidity with which both hypothalamic-pituitary activity and ovarian response are restored. This is determined principally by whether the mother is nursing her infant.

The studies of Bonnar and colleagues explain why ovarian function is inhibited in nursing mothers. Even though FSH and LH levels are well above those during the early puerperium, the high levels of prolactin inhibit the ovarian response to gonadotropin stimulation. The studies of Konner and Worthman on !Kung hunter-gatherers, who have an interval of about 44 months between births, supports this concept. !Kung mothers nurse their infants briefly, but frequently, several times an hour, until the children are 3 or more years old. Konner and Worthman compared the concentrations of prolactin, estrogen, and progesterone in 16 nursing mothers with those in eight who were menstruating. Estrogen and progesterone concentrations in the lactating mothers were comparable to those found in women with hyperprolactinemic amenorrhea.

Most women who do not nurse their babies will have a period of bleeding within 4 to 6 weeks of the baby's birth, whereas those who are lactating are often, but not invariably, amenorrheic as long as they nurse. Sharman reported the return of menstrual function in 91% of nonlactating multiparas and in a third of lactating primiparas within 3 months after delivery. Multiparas more often started to menstruate earlier, even though lactating. The first period of bleeding may be heavier than a normal menstrual period and often is anovulatory. By the third or fourth period, bleeding and ovulation should have returned to normal.

Sharman, studying postdelivery endometrial regeneration by biopsy, first found secretory endometrium, presumably resulting from ovulation, on the forty-fourth postpartum day. Kava and coworkers obtained secretory endometrium from 15 women between the thirty-third and forty-seventh postpartum days and on the ninety-third day in another patient.

Ovulation can occur in women who are lactating, even though menstruation has not been reestablished. Perez and associates reported that ovulation occurred in 14.1% of women who were on a full nursing schedule and in 28.8% of those nursing partially. The earliest ovulation occurred on day 36, and the latest on day 422. These figures indicate the need for contraception in all recently delivered women.

Cervix. Immediately after delivery the cervix is relaxed and flabby, but is regains its tone fairly rapidly. Within a few days the canal reforms as both the internal and the external os contract; by the end of 10 to 14 days the canal is well formed and narrow. Cervical lacerations heal by proliferation of fibroblasts.

Vagina. The vagina never returns completely to the pregravid state, and sometimes there may even be some relaxation after cesarean section. The tags of tissue that represent the hymenal ring are called *carunculae myrtiformes*. The vaginal epithelium looks thin and smooth like that of postmenopausal women until the ovaries again begin to function and produce estrogen.

Urinary tract. The bladder may be edematous and hyperemic, and there may even be areas of submucosal hemorrhage from the trauma of delivery. The hydronephrosis and hydroureter regress rapidly if the urinary tract is normal and within 2 to 3 weeks may have disappeared completely. Diagnostic urography should be delayed for at least 6 weeks to make certain that the gestational changes have regressed.

A marked diuresis begins within the first 12 hours after delivery in normal women; this is the mechanism by which the excess tissue fluid is eliminated. Naturally, the diuresis is more pronounced in women who have been edematous than in those with normal fluid retention.

Breasts. During pregnancy the glandular and ductal tissues of the breasts are stimulated by rising concentrations of estrogen, progesterone, human placental lactogen (hPL), prolactin, cortisol, and insulin. The concentrations of these hormones decrease promptly after delivery, and the time required for them to return to prepregnancy levels is determined in part by whether the mother nurses her infant. The complicated interactions of the various hormones and breast tissue are not yet clear, but prolactin appears to be essential for lactation. Prolactin concentrations rise abruptly, but temporarily, as a result of the stimulus of sucking. Women without anterior pituitary function do not lactate.

Colostrum, a thin, yellow, alkaline fluid is secreted by the glandular tissue of the breasts during late pregnancy and the first few days after delivery. Colostrum contains more protein but less fat and sugar than does milk. The concentration of globulin is greater than that of albumin.

On the third or fourth day after delivery the breasts become *engorged* and are distended, firm, tender, and warm, and milk can be expressed from the nipples. Engorgement may involve axillary breast tissue or even that in other accessory nipples along the milk line (Fig. 43-1). The breast distention is primarily from engorgement of blood vessels and lymphatics rather than from an accumulation of milk.

There is no large supply of ready-made milk; much of it is produced in response to the stimulus of nursing. The activity of the suckling infant stimulates prolactin secretion and initiates a stimulus from the nipple that releases oxytocin from the posterior lobe of the pituitary gland. Oxytocin stimulates the myoepithelial cells surrounding the mammary glands to contract and force the milk into the ducts and from the nipples. This is called milk ejection, or "letdown." In some instances the sight of the baby or even the thought of nursing will initiate the reflex.

Although prolactin stimulation is essential for milk production, there does not seem to be a direct quantitative relationship between prolactin and milk secretion. Howie and colleagues studied prolactin response to nursing during the first week of life. They found that suckling was followed by a prompt elevation in plasma prolactin, but they could not relate the concentration of the hormone to milk yield. Bunner, VanderLaan, and VanderLaan studied prolactin secretion in nursing mothers from 2 to 13 months after delivery. At 2 months, prolactin rose after nine of 18 nursing periods; at 6 months after five of 27 nursing periods; and, in the single patient who was studied at 13 months, after three of nine nursing periods. These studies suggest that a prolactin response is essential for the initiation of lactation but not for its continuation.

Both quality and quantity of milk can be altered by diet, activity, and emotional disturbances. The milk production can be halted almost overnight by

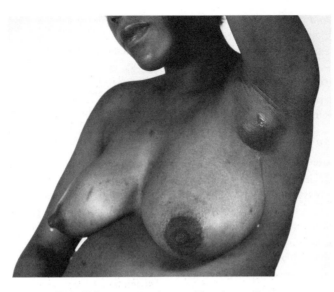

Fig. 43-1. Secretion from axillary breast tissue.

serious emotional shocks. A normal pregnancy diet supplemented with an additional pint of milk each day will usually replace the materials secreted in breast milk.

Vital signs. There should be no great change in *body temperature* during the puerperium. A rise usually indicates infection. The *pulse rate* often is low. A rapid pulse should suggest the possiblity of undue blood loss. *Blood pressure* should be altered only slightly in normal women.

Blood. The white blood cell count increases during labor and in the early puerperium. It may reach 20,000 to 30,000 if the labor has been prolonged. The rise is almost entirely the result of an increase in granulocytes. The count usually returns to normal within a few days.

As the plasma volume diminishes during the puerperium, the hemoglobin reading and the red blood cell count rise. The patient who has had an adequate iron intake during pregnancy and who has not bled excessively at delivery should not be anemic.

Body weight. An immediate weight loss of 4.8 to 5.8 kg (10 to 12 pounds) occurs at delivery. During the first few days of the puerperium the weight will decrease by 1.9 to 2.4 kg (4 or 5 pounds) more as the excess tissue fluid is eliminated. If the patient has been edematous, the loss will be greater. A further decrease will occur as the uterus involutes and plasma volume contracts.

Endocrine status. The major sources of hormone production during pregnancy are the placenta and the adrenal, thyroid, and anterior pituitary glands. Hormone secretion changes considerably after delivery.

The hormones that are produced by the trophoblastic cells are of necessity all reduced after placental delivery. Only a small amount of *chorionic gonadotropin* can be detected in the urine after the first day. *Estrogen* production is largely a function of the fetoplacental unit and ceases with delivery. The concentrations of estrone and estradiol reach the nonpregnant range within a week, but the estriol concentration decreases more slowly, this hormone being present for 2 to 3 weeks. *Progesterone* can no longer be detected after the first week.

Adrenal function is increased during pregnancy and returns to normal rather rapidly after delivery. *Aldosterone* production decreases promptly after delivery, and the excretion of *corticoids, 17-ketosteroids,* and *11-oxycorticosteroids* usually returns to normal levels during the first week.

The changes in *thyroid function* are reversed by delivery and slowly return to the normal level.

Pituitary function, except for the production of *prolactin* and *oxytocin,* which are increased by suckling, appears to be unchanged by delivery. The production of anterior pituitary gonadotropic hormones is gradually resumed.

CARE AFTER DELIVERY

The patient should remain in a recovery room for at least an hour after delivery. During this time her pulse and blood pressure should be checked every 15 minutes. The uterus should be palpated frequently to make certain that it remains well contracted, and the vulvar pad inspected for evidences of bleeding. The physician should not have to manipulate and massage the uterus to prevent relaxation; if this is necessary, something is wrong.

The patient may be returned to her room at the end of an hour if the pulse is below 100, the blood pressure is stable, the uterus remains contracted, there is no unusual bleeding, and she is awake. She must be checked frequently in her room for several hours.

Puerperal care is directed toward returning the patient to normal as rapidly as possible. In general, the patients are not ill and need not be treated like those who have undergone major surgical procedures.

Ambulation. The normal woman may be out of bed and become completely ambulatory as rapidly as she is able. Those who have had spinal or epidural anesthesia for delivery should not be allowed up until both sensation and voluntary muscle control have returned.

Diet. A general diet may be ordered as soon as the patient wants it. The diet is similar to that during pregnancy, but mothers who are nursing their babies should have at least an additional pint of milk to replace the protein, calcium, and other ingredients secreted in breast milk.

Lactation. Breast milk is clean, inexpensive, and readily available, and mothers should be encouraged to nurse their babies. It is well known that nursing infants develop passive immunity against certain infectious diseases from maternal antibodies that cross the placenta and that are present in colostrum and milk. Beer and Billingham have summarized the immunologic impli-

cations of breast-feeding. Maternal IgG antibodies are transferred to the fetus across the placenta before birth. The predominant immunoglobulin in human milk is secretory IgA, which provides protection within the infant's gastrointestinal tract. IgA contains antibodies against certain bacteria, for example, *E. coli,* to which the infant is regularly exposed and against which it has little or no immunity. The intestine also protects the infant against certain IgG antibodies such as those in immunized Rh-negative women. These antibodies, which are also present in breast milk, cross the placenta and affect the fetus but have no effect on newborn infants because they are not absorbed through the intestinal wall.

Many mothers notice painful contractions and an increase in vaginal discharge while the infant is at breast because nipple stimulation causes oxytocin release and uterine contraction.

The normal baby may be allowed to nurse before leaving the delivery room if the mother wishes. Babies and mothers, particularly primiparas, must be taught the techniques of nursing; consequently, the first attempts should be supervised by an experienced infant nurse. She can show the mother how to hold the infant and help it grasp the nipple.

At the first feedings the infant remains at the breast for only a few minutes, but nursing time is gradually increased to a 15- to 20-minute feeding period, which usually is adequate for an active baby. Suckling should not be limited too much because nursing success may depend on how frequently the infant nurses and is more likely if infants are fed on demand rather than by the clock.

If the nipples are flattened because of engorgement, they can be pulled out with a breast pump to permit the baby to grasp them. The intramuscular injection of 1 U of oxytocin or the use of a nasal spray of the same material just before the infant is put to breast will stimulate nipple erection and milk ejection.

The nipples should be washed with soap and water daily and cleansed with water before each nursing period. Antiseptics are unnecessary. The breasts are supported with a snugly fitting nursing brassiere that is changed at least daily.

If the nipples are sore or cracked, nursing on the affected side should be discontinued for 24 to 48 hours. During this time a bland ointment such as lanolin is applied, and the nipples are exposed to the air to help prevent maceration. When the tissues are healed, the baby may again nurse, starting with 1 to 2 minutes and gradually increasing. The baby should usually be taken from the breast if fissures cannot be healed or if they recur, if the nipples bleed, or if nursing causes severe pain. Inverted nipples are abnormal, and the epithelium often does not stand up under nursing.

Engorgement is temporary, the acute symptoms lasting only a day or two. The discomfort is mostly caused by lymphatic and venous engorgement rather than by distention with milk; pumping the breast may not be particularly helpful and may even increase the symptoms after relieving them temporarily. In most women the discomfort can be controlled with a tight, supporting binder, ice caps, and a simple analgesic.

Bromocriptine, 2.5 to 5 mg twice daily for 14 days, will usually prevent engorgement in women who choose not to nurse their infants. Some milk may be secreted while the patient is taking the drug, and engorgement may occur when she stops taking it.

Some drugs affect the quantity of milk produced, and others may affect the infant. Steroid hormones, notably *estrogen* and *oral contraceptives,* may reduce milk supply. *Atropine* decreases milk production and may poison the infant. *Cigarette smoking* may reduce milk volume, and nicotine intoxication of infants of lactating heavy smokers has been observed.

Most *antibiotics* are excreted in milk in low concentrations. They are not contraindicated, but the possible effects of large doses of antibiotics such as tetracycline and chloramphenicol must be considered when they are prescribed.

Radioactive iodine may be excreted in amounts sufficient to suppress the development of the infant's thyroid, and goiter might be produced by *thiouracil.*

Alcohol and *barbiturates* are excreted in breast milk, but the amount is small when they are ingested in moderate amounts. *Heroin* and *methadone* are excreted readily.

Other drugs that are excreted in milk and that may be toxic to the infant include *lead, mercury,* certain *fungicides* and *environmental intoxicants, ergot,* and certain *cathartics.*

Many drugs are excreted in amounts too small to have an adverse effect on the infant when prescribed in the usual doses. These include *morphine, codeine, salicylates, warfarin (Coumadin), heparin, antihistamines, phenobarbital, iodides,* and *reserpine.*

A good practice to follow is similar to that during pregnancy: the only drugs to be prescribed are those which are necessary and known to be innocuous to the infant.

Bladder care. The renal excretion of urine is increased during the early puerperium, but the patient may have difficulty in voiding because of perineal pain or local edema from trauma. The bladder may be atonic and can become remarkably distended without producing discomfort. If the patient voids spontaneously after delivery, no particular care is necessary except to check for the adequacy of urinary output and to palpate the abdomen frequently to make certain the bladder is not distended.

The patient who has not voided during the first 6 hours after delivery should be encouraged to try. If she is unsuccessful, the administration of codeine and aspirin orally or of a belladonna and opium suppository by rectum to relieve perineal pain may relax muscle spasm and aid in voiding. If she still is unable to void, she should be catheterized. This may be repeated every 2 to 4 hours, or more often if she is uncomfortable or if the distended bladder can be felt above the pubis, until she can urinate voluntarily. An indwelling catheter can be left in place for 24 to 48 hours if it is necessary to empty the bladder more than two or three times.

Bowel. Many women are constipated during the puerperium. Normal bowel function can be established by the use of stool softeners, suppositories, or mild laxatives such as milk of magnesia. Enemas are not often necessary.

Perineal care. If the patient must remain in bed, the vulva should be cleansed by the nurse two or three times daily and after each bowel movement. When she becomes ambulatory, she can cleanse the vulva herself after voiding and bowel movements with soft tissues and soap and water; no antiseptics are necessary. The perineum should be wiped from its anterior aspect toward the anus; the paper is discarded at the end of each stroke.

Tenderness in the episiotomy is usually caused by edema from too much suture material or sutures that have been tied too tightly. The discomfort can be relieved by the use of a heat lamp for 20 to 30 minutes three times daily or by the administration of aspirin and codeine or the insertion of a belladonna and opium rectal suppository three or four times daily. Hot sitz baths can be taken as soon as the patient can get into the tub.

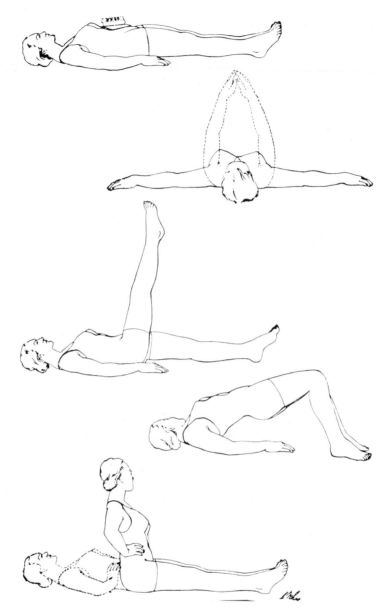

Fig. 43-2. Exercises to restore muscular tone after delivery. (From Willson, J.R.: Management of obstetric difficulties, ed. 6, St. Louis, 1961, The C.V. Mosby Co.)

Afterpains. Multiparas often are troubled by painful uterine contractions during the first 48 hours after delivery. These usually are stronger while the baby is nursing. The pain can be relieved with aspirin and codeine or a prostaglandin synthesis inhibitor. Primiparas rarely experience afterpains.

Exercises. Exercises such as leg or body raising to strengthen the abdominal muscles can be started any time the patient can perform them comfortably (Fig. 43-2).

The *pubococcygeus muscles* should be exercised systematically by contracting them slowly six to eight times in succession ten times daily. This will help prevent relaxation and urinary stress incontinence.

Blood count. The hematocrit should be determined before discharge. An iron preparation should be prescribed for all postpartum patients.

Bathing. Postpartum patients may shower whenever they are strong enough. Tub bathing may be resumed when the patient can get into and out of the tub comfortably.

Contraception. Most women will already have resumed intercourse before the first postpartum examination, and some of those who use no contraception will have conceived. Breast-feeding provides some protection against pregnancy because prolactin appears to reduce ovarian response to gonadotropins. However, the contraceptive effect of suckling cannot be relied on, particularly when the interval between nursings is increased to several hours. Ovulation may occur before the first period of uterine bleeding in both nursing and nonnursing mothers. Pregnancy spacing should be discussed with the patient before she leaves the hospital, and a suitable and reliable method of contraception should be prescribed.

Mothers who are nursing may use condoms, foam, or both until they return for postpartum examination. Oral contraceptives may be prescribed for those who are not nursing. Diaphragms cannot be fitted, and intrauterine devices inserted safely until the reproductive organs have involuted completely. Intercourse can be resumed when the episiotomy is healed and coitus is comfortable.

ROOMING-IN

The normal postpartum patient is perfectly able to assume increasing responsibility for her infant and should be encouraged to do so by having the baby with her in her room or an adjoining small nursery. An important advantage of the rooming-in plan is that it permits the mother to carry out, under supervision, all the details of infant care that were formerly the responsibility of the nurses, thereby making her transition from hospital to home far simpler than had the infant remained in the nursery except during the brief nursing periods.

Ideally, the baby should not be separated at all from its mother, but practically this is impossible. The most important time during which effective *bonding* is established seems to be the first hours of life; hence, whenever possible, the newborn infant should remain with its mother during this critical period. Skin stimulation, eye contact, and suckling appear to be important factors in establishing the relationship. The initial contact is expanded with rooming-in.

The infant may remain with the mother constantly, or the plan can be modified to include daytime care at the bedside, returning the baby to a central nursery or smaller peripheral nursery during the night. With the modified program, the baby is brought to the mother's bedside early each morning. During the day she assumes responsibility for its care under the supervision of the nurses, but before midnight the infant is returned to the nursery. The father should be encouraged to hold the baby and to change and feed it.

DISCHARGE FROM THE HOSPITAL

Most women who have had normal pregnancies and labors can be discharged by the third postpartum day; many will want to leave sooner.

Before the patient is discharged, the breasts, abdomen, perineum, and uterus should be inspected and palpated. The physician should be sure that she is voiding normally, that her blood pressure has stabilized, and that she is physically able to cope with her responsibilities at home. Each patient should be instructed specifically as to what she may and may not do after leaving the hospital. It is preferable that she limit her activity for a week or two after delivery, but this may be impossible if she has no help.

The increasing interest in *alternative methods of providing obstetric care* has led to some significant changes in hospital stay. Hospital delivery with a brief period of hospitalization is an acceptable alternative to home delivery with all its potential dangers. Patients may be offered all the advantages of hospital delivery and be discharged in 6 to 12 hours if the delivery is normal and the immediate puerperium is uncomplicated.

SUBSEQUENT EXAMINATIONS

Normal patients return to the office for examination when the infant is 6 to 8 weeks old. Those with abnormalities must, of course, be seen earlier. At the first visit the patient is weighed; her blood pressure is recorded; and the breasts, abdomen, and pelvis are examined. A clean-voided urine specimen should be examined, a urine culture should be ordered if she has had a urinary tract infection, and a blood count should be obtained if she was anemic when she left the hospital or has been bleeding. This is also a good time to obtain material for a cytologic examination.

If involution is complete, and if she appears normal physically, she should be instructed in some form of contraception if she wishes it and asked to return in 12 months. Any abnormalities present at this time should be corrected before the patient is discharged.

POSTPARTUM COMPLICATIONS

Bleeding. Abnormal bleeding can occur in any stage of the puerperium. Its management is discussed in Chapter 33.

Hemorrhoids. During labor and delivery, pressure from the presenting part impedes the flow of blood through the hemorrhoidal veins, and the resultant distention of the vessels may produce permanent injury to their walls. The hemorrhoids usually decrease in size rapidly and cause little discomfort, but some may produce severe pain, particularly if they thrombose.

The local application of witch hazel packs or ice reduces the distention and relieves discomfort. Belladonna and opium rectal suppositories provide relief for hemorrhoids that are more painful. The clot should be evacuated from those that thrombose, and prolapsed hemorrhoids should be replaced within the anorectal canal. Hot sitz baths may also be ordered.

Backache. Backache occurs frequently in puerperal women and is most often caused by the unusual activity necessary for the care of the new baby. A suitable support, rest, and heat will usually control it.

Pubic separation. The symphysis may be unusually mobile, and there may be considerable separation of the pubic bones. This causes severe pain when the patient attempts to walk. The area is tender to palpation, and the defect can be palpated readily. The only treatment necessary is adhesive strapping or a tight supporting garment to immobilize the pelvic girdle and rest in bed. Recovery usually is rapid.

Subinvolution. Involution of the uterus may be delayed by endometritis, inadequate uterine drainage, retention of placental fragments, uterine fibroids, and other less obvious causes. It occurs most often in multiparas.

With delayed involution, bloody discharge is more profuse and lasts longer than usual. The uterus is large, soft, boggy, and may be retrodisplaced. Generally, it is freely movable, and there is no evidence of infection.

Normal involution can be aided by promoting adequate uterine drainage during the early puerperium. This is best accomplished by ambulation and upright posture. The course of involution is influenced only slightly by oxytocic drugs, and they ordinarily need not be prescribed during the puerperium.

If the uterus has not yet reached normal size and if bloody discharge is still present 6 weeks after delivery, *subinvolution* can be diagnosed. Unless the delay in involution is a result of retained placental fragments or a far more serious but unusual complication such as choriocarcinoma, hot vaginal douches taken twice daily for a week or two will usually hasten the return to normal.

Amenorrhea. Return of menstruation may be delayed after delivery because of minor and easily correctable dysfunctions of the endocrine organs. Other disorders such as anterior pituitary necrosis (Sheehan's syndrome) are more difficult to treat. The *galacorrhea-amenorrhea syndrome,* which is characterized by amenorrhea and persistent lactation, is discussed in Chapter 9.

Uterine retrodisplacement. During the early puerperium the large, heavy uterus will often fall posteriorly, particularly when the patient lies on her back. As involution progresses, the uterus will assume its normal prepregnancy position unless the pelvic supports have been extensively damaged.

Most retrodisplaced uteri produce no symptoms and need no treatment, but if the uterus is large, boggy, subinvoluted, and retrodisplaced at the first postpartum visit, it can be replaced and held forward with a pessary. This may aid drainage and promote involution. When involution is complete, the pessary should be removed. If the uterus again assumes a retrodisplaced position, it can be managed as described in Chapter 41.

Cervicitis. The cervix is almost always injured during labor and delivery, and most multiparous women have some sort of cervical lesion, of which cervicitis is the most common.

An unepithelized area is often observed around the external os of recently delivered women, particularly if involution is not yet complete. If such a lesion is found at the first postpartum office visit, it can be treated with hot cautery or freezing if the pelvic organs have already returned to their normal nonpregnancy state. If the uterus is still enlarged and boggy, the cervical lesion may well heal spontaneously as involution progresses. Such patients should be advised to return for examination in 4 to 6 weeks. If the lesion is still present, it can be treated at that time; if it has healed, no therapy is necessary.

REFERENCES

Acar, B., MacNaughton, M.C., and Coutts, J.R.T.: Ovarian function in women immediately post partum, Obstet. Gynecol. **57:**468, 1981.

Anderson, W.R., and Davis, J.: Placental site involution, Am. J. Obstet. Gynecol. **102:**23, 1968.

Beer, A.E., and Billingham, R.E.: Immunology and the breast, Perinatology, p. 13, Jan.-Feb. 1981.

Bonnar, J., Franklin, M., Nott, P.N., et al.: Effect of breast-feeding on pituitary-ovarian function after childbirth, Br. Med. J. **4:**82, 1975.

Bunner, D.L., VanderLaan, E.P., and VanderLaan, W.P.: Prolactin levels in nursing mothers, Am. J. Obstet. Gyencol. **131:**250, 1978.

Delvoye, P., Demaegd, M., and Vwayitu-Nyampeta, R.C.: Serum prolactin, gonadotropins, and estradiol in menstruating and amenorrheic mothers during two years' lactation, Am. J. Obstet. Gynecol. **130**:635, 1978.

Howie, P.W., McNeilly, A.S., McArdle, T., Smart, L., and Houston, M.: The relationship between suckling-induced prolactin response and lactogenesis, J. Clin. Endocrinol. Metab. **50**:670, 1980.

Hull, V.J.: The effects of hormonal contraceptives on lactation, Stud. Fam. Plann. **12**:134, 1981.

Kava, H.W., Klinger, H.P., Molnar, J.J., and Romney, S.L.: Resumption of ovulation post partum, Am. J. Obstet. Gynecol. **102**:122, 1968.

Konner, M., and Worthman, C.: Nursing frequency, gonadal function, and birth spacing among !Kung hunter-gatherers, Science **207**:788, 1980.

Perez, A., Vela, P., Masnilk, G.S., and Potter, R.: First ovulation after childbirth, Am. J. Obstet. Gynecol. **114**:1041, 1972.

Sharman, A.: Postpartum regeneration of the human endometrium, J. Anat. **87**:1, 1953.

Sharman, A.: Menstruation after childbirth, J. Obstet. Gynaecol. Br. Commonw. **58**:440, 1951.

Simpson-Herbert, M., and Huffman, S.L.: The contraceptive effect of breast-feeding, Stud. Fam. Plann. **12**:125, 1981.

Williams, J.W.: Regeneration of the uterine mucosa after delivery with especial reference to the placental site, Am. J. Obstet. Gynecol. **22**:664, 1931.

Wilson, J.T.: Drugs in breast milk, New York, 1981, Adis Press.

44

J. Robert Willson

Diseases of the vulva

A great variety of developmental, trophic, inflammatory, and neoplastic disorders occur in the vulvar skin and its appendages. The following list includes some of the more common vulvar disorders:

1. *Epidermis and dermis:* the common dermatologic diseases, allergies, infections, nevi, dystrophies, and malignant neoplasms
2. *Skin appendages:* folliculitis, sebaceous cysts, hidradenomas, and Paget's disease
3. *Adjacent structures:* lipomas, hemangiomas, fibromas, and sarcomas
4. *Development:* vulvovaginal cysts and ectopic breast tissue
5. *Hormones:* atrophic changes occurring as a result of loss of estrogen stimulation after menopause

There often is a long delay in arriving at an accurate diagnosis of vulvar disease despite the facts that vulvar disorders occur frequently, that the lesions can be inspected and palpated without difficulty, that material can be obtained for culture directly from the lesions, and that biopsy is simple. *Too many physicians treat vulvar symptoms rather than vulvar disease, often without even a superficial examination.*

The *symptoms* most often produced by vulvar lesions are *pruritus* and *irritation.* Abscesses, other acute infections, and acute ulcerative lesions can cause *severe localized pain,* but most other lesions do not. *Bleeding,* except from ulcerated lesions of invasive cancer and that caused by trauma from injury or scratching, is unusual. An accurate *diagnosis* can usually be made by inspection, palpation, bacterial culture, and biopsy.

BENIGN CONDITIONS

The most common benign vulvar lesions are:

I. Inflammatory lesions
   A. Common skin infections
   B. Vulvitis associated with vaginal infections
      1. Trichomoniasis
      2. *Candida albicans*
      3. Atrophic vaginitis
   C. Sexually transmitted diseases
      1. Herpesvirus vulvitis
      2. Condylomata acuminata
      3. Molluscum contagiosum
      4. Chancroid
      5. Granuloma inguinale
      6. Lymphogranuloma venereum
      7. Syphilis
   D. Contact vulvitis
   E. Gland infections
      1. Bartholin glands
      2. Minor vestibular glands
II. Ulcers
   A. Simple acute ulcer
   B. Tuberculosis

III. Atrophy
IV. White lesions
  A. Pigment defects
    1. Leukoderma
    2. Vitiligo
  B. Hyperkeratotic lesions
    1. Intertrigo and other infections
    2. Dystrophies
      a. Lichen sclerosus
      b. Hyperplasia
        (1) Without atypia
        (2) With atypia
      c. Mixed (lichen sclerosus with foci of epithelial hyperplasia)
        (1) Without atypia
        (2) With atypia
V. Benign tumors
  A. Cystic tumors
    1. Sebaceous cysts
    2. Bartholin cysts
  B. Solid tumors
    1. Fibroma
    2. Lipoma
    3. Hemangioma
    4. Melanoma
    5. Hidradenoma (may be cystic)
    6. Papilloma

This classification obviously is incomplete, because the rare and unusual lesions have been omitted. Some of these lesions occur frequently, whereas others are less often encountered. All can be diagnosed without difficulty by using uncomplicated clinical techniques.

Inflammatory lesions

Common skin infections. The most common skin infections are *intertrigo* and *folliculitis*. They develop in the labial folds and inner surfaces of the thighs of obese women and often in women who wear pantyhose and tight slacks regularly. The basis for the infection is compression of the vulvar structures with decreased evaporation of normal vaginal and vulvar secretions followed by bacterial infection of the macerated skin and the hair follicles.

The basic treatment is to remove the cause by weight reduction in obese women and by substituting loose cotton undergarments and skirts for pantyhose and tight slacks, at least until the infection is eradicated. The vulva should be washed several times daily with bland soap. After it has dried completely, an unmedicated protective powder is applied. Antimicrobial ointments may be helpful in the initial stages of treatment. Itching, which may be intense until the condition improves, can usually be controlled by applying 0.5% to 1.0% hydrocortisone ointment three or four times daily.

PEDICULOSIS PUBIS, SCABIES, AND OTHER BITES. *Pediculosis pubis* is a common infection resulting from invasion of the hair-skin junction by the crab louse, *Pthirus pubis*. The outstanding symptom is pruritus; the skin may be excoriated from constant scratching. The eggs can be seen at the bases of the hairs with a magnifying glass. *Scabies* may involve the pubic hair and other hairy areas of the body. Both these conditions can be treated with topical medications that are designed to destroy the parasites. These include lindane shampoo (unless the patient is pregnant) and pyrethrins and piperonyl butoxide. *Insect, flea, bedbug,* and other bites are treated as they are in other parts of the body.

Vulvitis associated with vaginal infections. *Trichomoniasis, Candida vaginitis,* and *atrophic vaginitis* involve the vulva and the vagina secondarily (Fig. 44-1). The initial symptom is *pruritus,* which soon becomes intense and constant. *Vulvar irritation* is a result of changes in the vulvar skin, which is constantly bathed in the profuse discharge from the vagina.

Diagnosis and treatment are discussed in Chapter 45.

Sexually transmitted diseases

HERPESVIRUS INFECTIONS. Vulvar lesions resulting from infections with *herpes simplex viruses* are seen with great frequency. Herpes simplex virus vulvovaginitis is transmitted almost entirely by sexual contact. About 90% of the genital lesions are caused by herpesvirus type 2. These lesions may involve the vulva, the vagina, and the cervix. The remaining 10% result from herpesvirus type 1, the usual cause of herpetic lesions on the upper part of the body, particularly the lips (fever blisters).

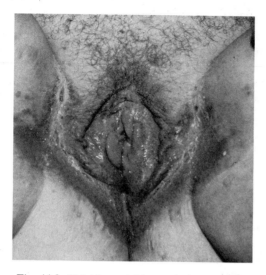

Fig. 44-1. Vulvitis caused by vaginal candidiasis.

Genital infections with this organism usually occur only on the vulva.

Herpesvirus type 2 genital tract infections are transmitted by sexual intercourse and involve the vulva, the vagina, and the cervix. Those resulting from herpesvirus type 1 are probably caused by orogenital contact, which may explain their localization primarily on the external structures.

The initial symptoms, intense vulvar pruritus, burning, and paresthesia, usually begin 6 to 10 days after the introduction of the virus. These symptoms are soon replaced by pain, which becomes progressively more intense as the infection advances. This, and the presence of the lesions, usually brings the patient to the physician.

At the onset there are many small papular and vesicular lesions scattered over the vulva, the vestibule, the perianal area, and even the inner surfaces of the thighs. The clear fluid in the vesicles soon becomes opaque, and the vesicles rupture, leaving painful ulcers. These may coalesce into large lesions. The vagina and the cervix may also be involved. In the most severe cases there may be so many lesions and so much reaction in the surrounding tissue that the patient cannot void. At this stage most patients feel ill and have low-grade temperature elevations. As the lesions regress, the pain

disappears. There is no residual scarring after the ulcers heal, but, with the first infection, resolution may take 2 to 4 weeks.

The lesions recur after the initial attack in at least 50% of patients. The lesions occur in the same places as did the first ones, but subsequent infections are usually less severe and of shorter duration than the first. The infections may continue to recur periodically for years.

The reason for the recurrences is that there is no effective treatment for herpes simplex virus infections, so the virus cannot be eradicated. The infection involves sensory nerves, and, as the tissues recover from the acute phase, the virus retreats to the sacral sensory nerve ganglia, where it remains dormant until a new attack is precipitated.

Antibodies against herpesvirus types 1 and 2 are produced as a result of an initial infection. These antibodies may offer some protection against subsequent infections. Patients who have developed antibodies against herpesvirus type 1 in childhood may have less severe herpesvirus type 2 infections than do those who have no antibodies against either type.

The clinical diagnosis is usually obvious, but it can be confirmed by culturing the virus from the lesions after rupturing the vesicles or removing the crusts and by demonstrating the presence of intranuclear inclusion bodies and multinucleated giant cells in exudate from the lesions.

Treatment is generally unsatisfactory because no specific systemic medication will eradicate the herpesvirus. *Acyclovir (Zovirax, 5%) ointment* applied directly to the lesions every 3 hours may decrease pain; healing time; and, when used during the *initial* attack, duration of viral shedding. It does not alter the course of recurrent attacks. Local anesthetic ointments may be prescribed during the painful stages of the infection. Oral acyclovir, in doses of 200 mg two to five times daily, reduces the recurrence rate significantly as compared to placebo-treated controls. Treatment for as long as 4 months does not appear to alter the frequency of recurrences after the drug is discontinued.

Herpes simplex virus infections during pregnancy are discussed in Chapter 26.

CONDYLOMATA ACUMINATA. Condylomata acuminata occur frequently as verrucous growths scattered over the vaginal introitus, the vulva, the perineum, and around the anus. There may be a few discrete lesions or confluent masses with a cauliflower appearance. Condylomata may also develop on the vaginal walls and the cervix.

The etiologic agent is the human *Papillomavirus,* one of several related viruses called the papovavirus group, all of which produce papillomas in a variety of animals. This virus may also cause the common warts so often found in other parts of the body. The virus is transmitted by direct contact, usually sexual, and it proliferates in the moist, warm genital tissues. The environment is even more supportive of viral growth if the genitals are constantly bathed by excessive vaginal secretions, particularly those accompanying a vaginitis. The virus also grows much more luxuriantly and spreads more rapidly in women who are pregnant, those with diabetes, and those with altered immunologic states. The lesions rarely spread to other parts of the body.

The verrucous pattern of the lesions and their characteristic distribution makes the diagnosis relatively easy. They must be differentiated from the raised, round or oval plaquelike lesions of secondary syphilis and from verrucous cancer. If there is any question as to the diagnosis, biopsy is imperative.

Treatment is often unsuccessful because it may be impossible to eliminate the underlying cause. Conversely, the lesions often disappear spontaneously, as do warts in other parts of the body. This suggests an altered immunologic state as a background.

Small, isolated condylomata can be destroyed by touching each one with *25% podophyllin* in tincture of benzoin, taking care to protect the surrounding skin from the medication. The vulva should be washed thoroughly after 6 hours. Podophyllin should not be used to treat large or numerous lesions in the vagina because the local and systemic reactions can be intense. Vaginal ulceration, polyneuritis, and paralysis have occurred after the medication has been applied to vaginal lesions. It also should be used during pregnancy.

Individual condylomata also can be destroyed with *liquid nitrogen, trichloroacetic acid, electrocautery, electrodesiccation,* or *cryocautery. Laser* therapy can also be used to destroy individual lesions. Ferenczy and co-workers biopsied the skin adjacent to condylomata after destroying the lesions with laser. In 45% papillomavirus was detected in the skin, and the lesions recurred in 67% of the patients with residual virus. In contrast, the lesions recurred in only 9% if the virus could not be detected in the skin edges. This suggests that a wide area of skin surrounding the lesion itself should be vaporized with the laser beam. Large masses of condylomata can be treated with laser or by excision.

MOLLUSCUM CONTAGIOSUM. This viral disease is thought to be transmitted by contact. The small, raised umbilicated lesions may occur anywhere on the vulva and the upper thighs. There is little inflammatory reaction, and most patients have few symptoms. The diagnosis can be confirmed by demonstrating the typical cytoplasmic inclusion bodies in excised lesions. Individual lesions are treated by expressing their contents and cauterizing the base of each with trichloroacetic acid.

Other sexually transmitted diseases. Other vulvar diseases that are transmitted by sexual intercourse include *chancroid, granuloma inguinale, lymphogranuloma venereum,* and *syphilis.*

CHANCROID. Also known as *ulcus molle* or *soft chancre,* chancroid is an infection disease that is presumed to be transmitted by sexual contact. The incubation period is 3 to 5 days. The infecting organism *Haemophilus ducreyi* can be identified by culture.

The lesion may occur at any point in the vestibule and, when first seen, usually is an irregular ulcer with a purulent base and little surrounding induration. Multiple lesions may occur because of several primary areas or by autoinoculation from the original lesions.

Inguinal adenitis appears about 1 week after the primary lesion is noted. The glands are tender and matted together and may suppurate.

The treatment is either erythromycin, 500 mg four times a day for 10 days, or trimethoprim/sulfamethoxazol, 160/800 mg twice a day for 10 days.

GRANULOMA INGUINALE. This disease may not appear

for several months after the contact. The initial lesion is a papule on the vulva or in the vagina. The lesions soon ulcerate; the ulcer has a red, granular base and a sharply defined margin.

The process spreads slowly by continuity and contiguity, forming superficial ulcers. The inguinal lymph nodes are involved by direct spread of the lesion, and a *pseudobubo,* which is actually a subcutaneous granuloma rather than an abscessed node, may develop in the inguinal area.

The primary lesions are painless at the onset, but the ulcers may be painful, since they are secondarily infected. Numerous small ulcers may coalesce into larger ulcerating areas, the bases of which are covered by granulation tissue that bleeds readily with manipulation. These ulcers usually do not heal spontaneously.

The organism that causes granuloma inguinale is a bacillus, *Calymmatobacterium granulomatis,* and the diagnosis is made by identifying *Calymmatobacterium* bodies or inclusions in the involved tissue.

The treatment is tetracycline, 500 mg four times daily for at least 14 days. The ulcers heal with appropriate treatment, but there is considerable residual scarring.

LYMPHOGRANULOMA VENEREUM. Lymphogranuloma venerum is a venereal disease that is prevalent in the southeastern states. After an incubation period of only a few days, a papule of pustule appears on the vulva, but it soon heals and almost always is overlooked. The infection spreads through the lymphatics and involves the inguinal lymph nodes. It may also extend along the lymph channels draining toward the rectum.

The involved inguinal nodes may coalesce and ulcerate. The ulcer is surrounded by an area of edema and fibrous induration.

Lymphatic drainage through the affected lymph channels is obstructed, and the vulvar tissues may be involved in a hyperplastic and hypertrophic lesion, accompanied by lymphostasis and lymphedema. The vulva and perineal area may be ulcerated. Eventually, scar tissue may contract and form vaginal and rectal strictures. Fistula formation is common.

Lymphogranuloma venereum is caused by organisms of the *Chlamydia trachomatis* group. The diagnosis is made by a specific complement-fixation test or by isolating *C. trachomatis* in cell cultures.

Treatment of acute lymphogranuloma is with tetracycline, 500 mg four times daily for 2 weeks, doxycycline, 100 mg twice a day for 16 days, or erythromycin, 500 mg four times a day for 14 days. It may be necessary to excise the enlarged vulvar structures, particularly if

ulcers do not heal. Colostomy may be necessary for tight rectal strictures.

Carcinoma of the vulva eventually may develop in the chronically infected scarred tissues. This adds an additional reason for removing persistent ulcerated areas.

SYPHILIS. The initial lesion of syphilis, a chancre, may occur on the vulva, but it usually is not recognized because it is transient and produces almost no symptoms.

A dark-field examination should be performed as part of the investigation of any vulvar ulcer in an attempt to identify spirochetes. This is the only way syphilis can be diagnosed in its earliest stages.

The raised, round or oval plaquelike lesions of secondary syphilis, *condylomata lata,* should not be confused with condylomata acuminata. The lesions may extend laterally and involve the upper thighs. There usually is a pronounced lymphadenopathy. Serologic test for syphilis generally is positive by the time the secondary lesions appear. Syphilis complicating pregnancy is discussed in Chapter 26.

Contact vulvitis. Contact vulvitis often represents a local reaction to undergarments made from synthetic materials, to detergents, and to medications. One type of preparation that produces a vulvar reaction is deodorant spray.

There is no evidence of vaginitis, and the vulvar skin and vestibule are red and edematous.

The acute symptoms can usually be relieved by oral antihistaminics, by local cortisone ointments, by wearing cotton panties rather than those made of synthetic fabrics or by wearing none at all, by washing underwear in bland soap and rinsing it well, and by discontinuing the use of any medication in the vagina or on the vulva.

Bartholin gland infections. The ducts of the Bartholin, or vulvovaginal, glands open on the medial surface of each labium minus at about the 4 and 8 o'clock positions just outside the hymen. An *acute bartholinitis* can develop in one or both glands. The responsible organisms are most often gonococci, streptococci, and *E. coli.*

The gland becomes swollen and red, and the tissues around it are edematous. If the duct is obstructed, a *Bartholin abscess* may form. An abscess will usually rupture spontaneously within about 3 days if it is not drained surgically.

The early stages of Bartholin gland infections

are usually not seen because patients are unlikely to seek help until the infection has been present for several days. Early acute Bartholin gland infections can be treated with hot soaks and an antimicrobial agent.

If the infection cannot be controlled and an abscess forms, or if the patient is first examined at this stage, the only logical treatment is surgical drainage. An incision is made over the medial bulging surface of the abscess, and the pus is evacuated. The infection usually subsides promptly.

If a wide opening persists, recurrent infections are not likely to occur, but they are common if the stoma closes.

Minor vestibular gland infections. Infections in the minor vestibular glands, which are located on the vestibular surface outside the hymen, have only recently been recognized as a source of vulvar symptoms. The gland openings, which can be seen best with a magnifying glass, are scattered over the vestibule with the major concentration being posterolaterally and posteriorly within the forchette.

The initial symptom is usually pruritus which is followed by burning, pain, and dyspareunia. The areas surrounding the gland ostia are reddened, and the erythematous areas may coalesce as more and more glands become involved. In advanced cases the entire vestibule is affected. Pressure on the red areas or brushing them with a cotton swab usually reproduces the symptoms.

The application of 3% acetic acid exposes numerous areas of white epithelium that are similar to flat condylomas on the cervix. Growdon and co-workers identified human papillomavirus in the lesions from 12 patients by the presence of koilocytotic epithelial cells and human papillomavirus capsid antigen. They also found similar penile lesions in the six consorts they were able to examine.

Woodruff and Parmley found that the symptoms could be relieved by surgical excision of the posterior hymeneal ring, the adjacent vestibule, and the skin over the perineal body. Growdon and associates obtained equally good results by applying 20% podophyllin in tincture of benzoin to individual lesions or to the entire vestibule. Carbon dioxide laser vaporization of individual lesions or of the vestibule to a depth of 2 mm can also be used; discomfort is greater, and healing may not be complete for several weeks.

Ulcers

The principal ulcerated vulvar lesions, other than those described previously in the discussion of sexually transmitted disease, are the simple acute ulcers. These may occur in the lower vagina or on the vulva. They often are situated on the medial surface of the labia majora. The ulcerated lesions may be moderately painful.

Atrophy

Atrophy occurs as a normal consequence of decreased estrogen secretion after the menopause. The labia become flatter, and the skin may hang loosely as a result of loss of subcutaneous fat (Fig. 44-2). The epithelium is pale, smooth, and thin. The introitus may become constricted. Atrophic changes cannot be reversed by estrogen, but in most instances they can be prevented when appropriate hormone therapy is started early.

White lesions

The white lesions of the vulva include a variety of conditions, some of which have little relationship to each other except for their color.

Pigment defects. The skin over the vulva may contain no pigment and appear perfectly white. The congenital absence of pigment is called *leukoderma,* and the secondary loss, *vitiligo.* Neither defect produces symptoms nor has any clinical significance.

Hyperplastic (hyperkeratotic) lesions. The hyperkeratotic lesions are characterized by a keratin layer thicker than that on normal vulvar epithelium. The hyperkeratotic lesions vary from benign lesions associated with chronic irritation (for example, intertrigo) to epithelial cancer.

Intertrigo is a hyperplastic lesion that occurs in the vulvar skin of obese women and women who wear pantyhose, tight synthetic fabric underwear, or tight slacks. All compress the vulvar structures and prevent evaporation of normal secretions. This

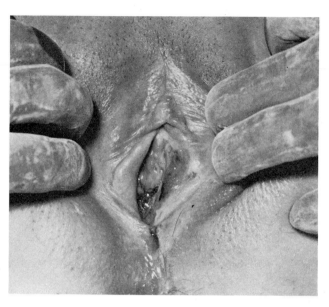

Fig. 44-2. Vulvar atrophy with almost complete effacement of labia minora and majora.

and localized infection produce continued irritation. The hyperkeratotic change in the skin will reverse if the irritation can be eliminated.

The outstanding symptom of *chronic vulvar dermatitis* is pruritus, which may be intractable. The itching is usually worse at night after the patient has gone to bed than during the day.

The vulva may appear normal except for mild irritation, or it may be pale and edematous. The skin may be thickened and white, and there may be linear excoriations on the surface or in the skin folds. If the itching has been severe, the skin may be excoriated and secondarily infected from constant scratching.

Any of the common skin infections can cause pruritus, scratching, and chronic vulvitis. Other causes include irritation from the discharge produced by long-standing vaginal and cervical infections such as trichomoniasis, candidiasis, atrophic vaginitis, or chronic cervicitis or from secondary infection of areas of contact vulvitis.

Intractable *pruritus vulvae* may occur in women with psychosexual problems and in those whose life situations create sexual frustrations.

A diagnosis of chronic vulvar dermatitis can be made on the basis of the history and clinical findings. Dysplasia and malignancy must be eliminated by biopsy of any suspicious areas before treatment is prescribed.

Chronic vulvar dermatitis cannot be treated successfully without eradicating the basic etiologic factor. The itching can usually be relieved by local application of 0.5% to 1.0% *hydrocortisone ointment* applied after the vulva is washed with a bland soap and patted dry. *Cool sitz baths* or *cold, wet compresses* also afford temporary relief. Vaginitis and cervicitis must be treated appropriately. *Topical antibiotic therapy* may be helpful if the vulva is secondarily infected. If there is a related emotional factor, the vulvitis will never be relieved until the conflict has been resolved.

Surgery rarely is necessary; in fact, the dermatitis will recur after operations unless the causative condition is eliminated.

Dystrophies

The vulvar dystrophies are disorders of epithelial growth characterized by a keratin layer that is thicker than the normal, changes in thickness of the epithelial layer, chronic subepithelial inflammatory infiltration, and changes in the subepithelial connective tissue. Almost all are benign, but abnormal hyperplasia does occur in some. The vulvar dystrophies include *lichen sclerosus* and *hyperplastic* and *mixed dystrophies*

Lichen sclerosus. Lichen sclerosus can occur at any age and in other areas of the body, but it is most often diagnosed in the vulvae of postmenopausal women.

In their earliest stages, the lesions are small, raised, bluish papules that eventually coalesce until they may involve the entire vulvar area and extend laterally to the thighs. In their late stages they are white. The affected skin looks thin, and frequently fissures and excoriations result from continued scratching. As atrophy advances, the tissues shrink, and the introitus may become smaller and smaller.

Lichen sclerosus is basically an atrophic lesion that is characterized by thin, atrophic epithelium covered by a keratin layer that varies in thickness. There is increased collagen formation in the subepithelial layer, and beneath this an infiltration of inflammatory cells.

The principal symptoms are pruritus and, as atrophy and shrinkage of the tissue progress, dyspareunia.

Lichen sclerosus is not a premalignant lesion unless abnormal hyperkeratosis also is present. Cancer develops in no more than 3% of women with the disorder; as a consequence, vulvectomy is not usually necessary. Before deciding on any treatment, however, multiple biopsies should be obtained to make certain that the condition actually is benign.

It is doubtful that lichen sclerosus can be prevented by estrogen therapy; although the condition is usually diagnosed in postmenopausal women, it can also occur in women with normal ovarian function and even in children.

Local treatment with *hydrocortisone ointment* will usually control the itching. Cortisone should be used only to provide temporary relief of symptoms. An ointment of 2% *testosterone proprionate in petrolatum* rubbed into the skin two or three times daily will usually eliminate the symptoms

and reverse many of the tissue changes. It may take several weeks to have an obvious effect and can be continued indefinitely.

Topical estrogen cream may be used in the vagina to eradicate atrophic vaginitis if it is present. The continuing irritation of the vulva by abnormal vaginal secretions may interfere with treatment of the vulvar disease.

Hyperplastic dystrophies. Epithelial hyperplasia, or the hyperplastic dystrophies, have no specific gross appearance: the lesions vary in color from dusky red when there is little hyperkeratosis to white when it is advanced; they may involve the labial and perineal structures diffusely, or they may be localized to small areas; and the borders may be poorly defined, or they may be distinct plaques that are raised above the surface of the surrounding skin (Fig. 44-3). The lesions often occur as a consequence of chronic irritation, but they may represent primary hyperplastic dysplasia; hence multiple biopsy is essential before treatment is started.

The microscopic changes in the hyperplastic lesions may show varying degrees of chronic dermatitis accompanying the epithelial hyperplasia, but there usually is no evidence of atypicality.

Atypia is classified as *mild, moderate,* and *severe,* each grade showing a progressive decrease in cellular maturation as dysplasia becomes more pronounced.

Mixed dystrophies. The mixed dystrophies are those that combine the gross and microscopic characteristics of both lichen sclerosus and a hyperplastic dystrophy. It is these in which cancer may develop.

The evaluation and treatment of the hyperplastic and mixed dystrophies are similar to those described for lichen sclerosus. Even though the symptoms are relieved and the lesions improve, one must be certain, by repeat biopsies, that the dysplastic change also has reversed.

Diagnosis of vulvar diseases. An accurate diagnosis is essential to successful treatment of vulvar lesions; this requires biopsy. Most vulvar lesions are benign, but, in some cases, premalignant and early malignant changes, which will not be obvious by gross inspection alone, can be diagnosed by histologic examination.

The areas selected for biopsy are thickened white plaques, pigmented lesions, fissures, any ulcerated area, and any other area that looks suspicious. Multiple biopsies are essential because carcinoma in situ of the vulva can be multifocal and the true diagnosis can only be made by sampling several areas. Adequate tissue can usually be obtained in the office, using local anesthesia and a 4 mm Keyes dermatologic punch with which a full thickness of skin can be removed. Excision biopsy of entire small lesions may be appropriate.

The use of *toluidine blue* to stain the vulvar tissues may be helpful in selecting biopsy sites. The entire vulva is painted with toluidine blue, which is a nuclear stain; after 3 minutes it is removed by dissolution with 1% acetic acid. The intact skin will be decolorized by the acetic acid, but a blue stain will be retained wherever there is a break in the epidermis. Toluidine blue is not a specific stain for cancer cells; rather it stains any cells that are exposed by injury or ulceration caused by infection or malignant lesions.

Benign tumors

Cystic tumors. The two most common benign cystic tumors of the vulva are *sebaceous cysts* and *Bartholin cysts.*

Sebaceous cysts of the vulvar skin occur frequently and are exactly like those that arise in other parts of the body. They can be excised if they produce symptoms or repeatedly become infected.

Bartholin cysts are more properly called *Bartholin duct cysts* because it is the duct rather than the gland itself that makes up the cyst wall. The main duct, or an accessory duct, is occluded. The gland continues its secretory activity, but the secretions cannot be discharged through the closed duct opening. The result is a retention cyst, which will continue to enlarge as secretions accumulate.

Bartholin cysts may follow obvious infections of the gland, but more often there is no specific antecedent cause.

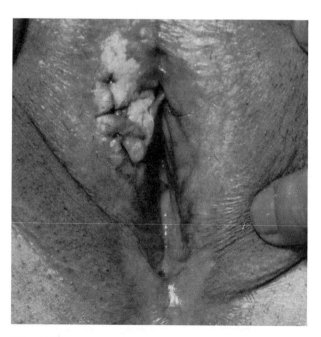

Fig. 44-3. Area of epithelial hyperkeratosis and early cancer.

Most Bartholin cysts produce no symptoms, and the patient is unaware of their presence. Generally, they are from 3 to 5 cm in diameter, but occasionally they may become much larger. Sometimes they become infected with a resultant abscess.

Asymptomatic Bartholin cysts need no treatment. Those that interfere with intercourse or are uncomfortable because of their size and those that repeatedly become infected should be treated surgically.

In most instances, *marsupialization* is preferable to excision of the cyst. In marsupialization a linear incision is made over the medial border of the cyst in the region of the occluded duct opening. The cyst lining is sutured to the vulvar skin and allowed to heal. If an incision of adequate length is made, the resultant opening will be widely patent, and the cyst will not often recur.

Solid tumors. The solid benign tumors of the vulva include a variety of *nevi, hemangiomas, fibromas, lipomas, papillomas,* and *hidradenomas.* Only the first three are common.

The importance of *nevi* is that the vulva is a frequent site for the development of *melanomas.* Suspicious nevi should be removed.

Hemangiomas occur frequently in infants and may be large enough to produce pronounced distortion of the vulvar structures.

The *hidradenoma* is a tumor arising in apocrine glands. It is a red, raised, often ulcerated, sessile tumor. The treatment is wide local excision.

MALIGNANT LESIONS

About 3% to 4% of primary malignancies of the reproductive organs occur in the vulva. The crude incidence for invasive cancer of the vulva is 1.9/100,000 women and for carcinoma in situ, 0.7/100,000. In contrast to carcinoma of the cervix and of the endometrium, there is little difference in incidence between black and white women, the age-adjusted rate being 1.7 in white women and 1.8 in black women.

Invasive carcinoma of the vulva (Fig. 44-4) can occur at any age, but it is basically a disease of older women and occurs most often after the age of 60 years. The delay period between the onset of symptoms and the first visit to a physician and from first visit to diagnosis is longer than for any other cancer of the genital organs. *The first symp-*

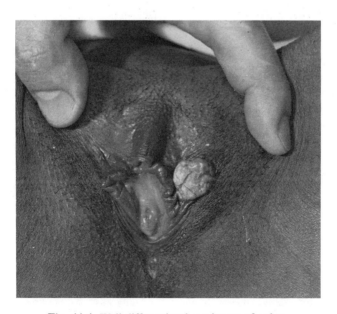

Fig. 44-4. Well-differentiated carcinoma of vulva.

tom, usually pruritus, is likely to be ignored by the patient and treated symptomatically by the physician, too often without adequate examination.

Carcinoma of the vulva is usually of squamous cell origin, but 10% to 15% may be a transitional cell type. Those beginning in *Bartholin's gland* may be squamous cell (from the duct orifice), transitional cell (from the duct itself), or adenocarcinoma (from the gland). Bartholin gland cancer is rare. *Basal cell cancer* also develops in vulvar skin.

Carcinoma of the vulva often is associated with carcinoma of the cervix or the vagina. Women who have been treated for carcinoma of the cervix may develop multiple foci of squamous cell cancer in the vagina and vulva. Conversely, women who have been treated for carcinoma of the vulva may develop cervical or vaginal neoplasms.

Carcinoma in situ of the vulva usually occurs in women who are much younger than those with invasive lesions, and it appears to be increasing in frequency. This may be related to the increasing incidence of papilloma virus infections.

The principal symptom of carcinoma in situ, like that of many other vulvar diseases, is pruritus. The lesions may be single or multiple papules, which may be discrete or coalesced. They often are darkly pigmented, but they may be white or red. The skin may be hyperkeratotic or scaly and eczematoid. Lesions of the bowenoid type appear as white keratotic islands on a red background.

The diagnosis is made by biopsy. Tissue should be obtained from obviously ulcerated and abnormal areas and from areas that retain toluidine blue stain. Since carcinoma in situ often is a multifocal lesion, multiple biopsies from all areas of the vulva are necessary for accurate evaluation.

If carcinoma in situ is localized to a single area or to several isolated areas and there are no premalignant changes elsewhere on the vulva, the lesion alone can be removed by wide local excision. Wide, superficial ("skinning") vulvectomy with skin graft may be appropriate for extensive lesions in young women. This operation preserves the normal vulvar contours. Total vulvectomy may be preferred for elderly women. Before closing the wounds the edges should be checked by fro-

zen section to make sure the tumor has been removed completely.

Surgical treatment for in situ vulvar cancer in young women should be restrained, because few cases become invasive.

Carcinoma in situ can be treated by the daily application of 5% fluorouracil cream for 10 weeks, but the results are equivocal. The lesions can also be eradicated with *laser therapy*, but too few patients have been treated to evaluate the results.

Paget's disease

Paget's disease of the vulva arises from apocrine glands. It is a malignant lesion that usually is intraepithelial, but it may be invasive. Grossly, the typical lesions are mutifocal, red with white patches and crusting. They may be located any place on the vulva and in the perianal region. The treatment of Paget's disease is wide vulvectomy. If invasion is found on the excised tissue, the inguinal and femoral lymph nodes should be removed.

All patients who have been treated for intraepithelial carcinoma of the vulva and Paget's disease must be examined at regular intervals. The lesions may recur in the vulvar skin at any time after the operation. Of even more importance is that women with in situ vulvar cancer have an increased incidence of malignancies in the vagina and cervix; Buscema and colleagues found cervical cancer in 27% of 106 patients with carcinoma in situ of the vulva. Only 4 of the 102 observed for 1 to 15 years developed invasive vulvar cancer.

Invasive cancer

The *first symptom* of invasive carcinoma of the vulva is persistent itching, which most patients treat with home remedies for several months. As the tumor grows, a lump may become obvious, and eventually the lesion becomes ulcerated. Exophytic lesions also are common. In contrast to in situ lesions, most invasive vulvar cancers are unifocal rather than multicentric. They also occur more often in elderly women than do the intraepithelial tumors.

Many women do not seek treatment until an ulcer or a fungating lesion several centimeters in diam-

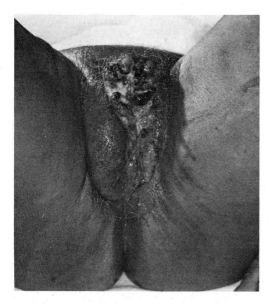

Fig. 44-5. Advanced carcinoma of vulva, involving entire vagina, urethra, and rectum. Total exenteration was necessary to remove growth.

eter is present. By this time the tumor often has metastasized to the regional lymph nodes (Fig. 44-5). The *diagnosis* is made by biopsy.

The *treatment* of invasive cancer of the vulva is radical vulvectomy and inguinal, femoral, and sometimes deep pelvic lymph node dissection.

All tissue from the anterior surface of the pubis, laterally well beyond the limits of the vulva and posteriorly to or around the anus, is removed. The dissection is carried downward to the fascia.

The inguinal and femoral lymph nodes are removed whenever there is more than a single area of minimal invasion. The value of deep pelvic lymph node resection has not yet been definitely proven. There may be a slight improvement in survival, particularly when the primary lesion is in the region of the clitoris, but the added surgical risk in elderly women may nullify the advantage.

Radiation therapy has almost no place as primary treatment for cancer of the vulva.

The potential for cure of cancer of the vulva is determined by the stage of the lesion when it is diagnosed and the quality of the treatment admin-

istered. Small, localized tumors can be eradicated completely; consequently, the cure rate can only be improved by early diagnosis. Early diagnosis is possible only if patients report symptoms at their onset and if physicians make accurate diagnoses rather than merely treat the symptoms produced by the vulvar disease.

Morley reported a 5-year survival rate of 66.8% among 374 patients treated for invasive cancer of the vulva in the University of Michigan Hospital. The corrected 5-year survival, eliminating those who died of intercurrent diseases unrelated to cancer, was 73.9%. The differences in survival for those in whom the tumor had extended to the lymph nodes is significant: 92.4% of those without metastases to inguinal lymph nodes and 38.7% of those with metastases survived at least 5 years.

Malignant melanoma

Malignant vulvar melanomas make up 3% to 5% of all melanomas in women, and they occur at all ages. The lesions are pigmented and may be either nodular or superficially spreading tumors. The edges usually are irregular, and they may ulcerate and bleed. A pigmented lesion that enlarges rapidly may be a melanoma. The treatment is wide local excision or vulvectomy, with lymph-node sampling or dissection, depending on the extent of the lesion. The prognosis is determined by the size of the tumor and the depth of invasion.

REFERENCES

Buscema, J., Woodruff, J.D., Parmley, T.H., and Genadry, R.: Carcinoma in situ of the vulva, Obstet. Gynecol. **55**:225, 1980.

Choo, Y.C., and Morley, G.E.: Multiple primary neoplasms of the anogenital region, Obstet. Gynecol. **56**:365, 1980.

Collins, C.G., Hansen, L.H., and Theriot, E.: A clinical stain for use if selecting biopsy sites in patients with vulvar disease, Obstet. Gynecol. **28**:158, 1966.

Douglas, J.M., et al.: A double-blind study of acyclovir for suppression of recurrences of genital herpes simplex virus infection, N. Engl. J. Med. **310**:1551, 1984.

Fenn, M.E., Morley, G.W., and Abell, M.R.: Paget's disease of vulva, Obstet. Gynecol. **38**:660, 1971.

Ferenczy, A., et al.: Latent papillomavirus and recurring genital warts, N. Engl. J. Med. **313:**784, 1985.

Friedrich, E.G., Jr.: Lichen sclerosus, J. Reprod. Med. **17:**147, 1976.

Friedrich, E.G., Jr.: The vulvar vestibule, J. Reprod. Med. **28:**773, 1983.

Friedrich, E.G., Jr.: Wilkinson, E.J., and Fu, Y.S.: Carcinoma in situ of the vulva: a continuing challenge, Am. J. Obstet. Gynecol. **136:**830, 1980.

Growdon, W.A., et al.: Pruritic vulvar squamous papillomatosis: evidence for human papillomavirus etiology, Obstet. Gynecol. **66:**564, 1985.

Jaramillo, B.A., et al.: Malignant melanoma of the vulva, Obstet. Gynecol. **66:**398, 1985.

Kaufman, R.H., and Woodruff, J.D.: Historical background in developmental stages of the new nomenclature, J. Reprod. Med. **17:**133, 1976.

Morley, G.W.: Infiltrative carcinoma of the vulva: results of surgical treatment, Am. J. Obstet. Gynecol. **124:**874, 1976.

Straus, S.E., et al.: Suppression of frequently recurring genital herpes: a placebo-controlled double-blind trial of oral acyclovir, N. Engl. J. Med. **310:**1545, 1984.

Wilkin, J.K.: Molluscum contagiosum venereum in a women's outpatient clinic: a venerally transmitted disease, Am. J. Obstet. Gynecol. **128:**531, 1977.

Woodruff, J.D., and Parmley, T.H.: Infection of the minor vestibular gland, Obstet. Gynecol. **62:**609, 1983.

45

William J. Ledger

Diseases of the vagina

Leukorrhea, a term applied to any nonbloody discharge from the vagina, may consist of physiologic secretions, or it may be produced in response to irritation or infection of the genital organs. A certain amount of vaginal discharge, made up of secretion of the cervical glands, endometrial debris, effusions from the vaginal mucosa, and exfoliated vaginal epithelium, is always present; but it is not obvious to most women. Normal secretions are nonirritating and usually are not profuse.

The adult vagina is lined by stratified squamous epithelium, the activity, thickness, and glycogen content of which are controlled primarily by variations in the level of estrogenic hormone. The pH of the vaginal secretions in the adult is between 3.5 and 4.5, the acidity being produced by the conversion of cellular glycogen to lactic acid by Döderlein's bacilli, which are normal vaginal inhabitants. Before the menarche and after the menopause, when estrogen production is low, the epithelium is inactive and only a few cell layers thick; the cells contain no glycogen, the Döderlein bacilli are absent, and the pH is between 6 and 7 (Table 45-1). The inactive unstimulated mucosa is especially susceptible to infection by an organism like *N. gonorrhaeae,* whereas the estrogen-stimulated vagina during the years of menstruation is rarely invaded by pathogenic bacteria.

The volume of secretions in the normal vagina varies throughout the menstrual cycle. In the immediate postmenstrual phase, when the estrogen level is low, the mucosa is thin and relatively inactive, and there is little secretion from the cervical cells. As estrogen production increases, the vaginal cells proliferate and exfoliate more rapidly, and the cervical cells secrete more and more mucus. At ovulation, when estrogen production is maximal, cervical mucus is profuse and watery, and vaginal desquamation reaches a peak. Some women are aware of discharge only at this time. The secretions then diminish until just before the onset of menstruation.

Secretions of the genital organs are also influenced by psychologic stimuli. Many women are aware of increased vaginal discharge during periods of emotional stress, and leukorrhea is a frequent complaint in women with pelvic congestion syndrome. The most powerful psychologic stimulant to genital tract secretion is sexual excitement. Before Masters' studies of coital physiology, vaginal lubrication before and during coitus was believed to come from an outpouring of secretions from cervical and Bartholin glands. Masters observed the formation of a smooth, shiny, lubricating covering for the vagina during sexual stimulation that started as a transudation of droplets of fluid from the vaginal wall during the excitement

TABLE 45-1 Changes in vaginal epithelium, flora, and secretions at various ages

	Newborn	Childhood	Premenarche	Adult midcycle	After menopause
Estrogen	High	Minimal	Increasing	High	Minimal
pH	3.5-5	6-8	4-5	3.5-4.5	6-7
Flora	Lactobacilli	Mixed	Mixed, lactobacilli	Lactobacilli	Mixed
Vaginal epithelium	Thick	Thin	Thickness increasing	Thick	Thin
Predominant cytology	Cornified squamous	Parabasal cells	Intermediate squamous	Cornified squamous	Parabasal cells
Glycogen	High	Absent	Increasing	High	Absent

phase and rapidly coalesced into a uniform coating.

Abnormal discharge is most often caused by infection of the vagina or the cervix; but it can be the result of chronic irritation, hyperemia, or endocrine disorders that are accompanied by excessive estrogen production. Diagnosis of a specific cause for a vaginal discharge cannot be made by gross inspection alone. The evaluation of these women requires a pH evaluation of the vaginal secretions and a microscopic examination of secretions in a saline and 10% potassium hydroxide solution.

TRICHOMONIASIS

Vaginitis caused by *Trichomonas vaginalis* is a common cause of leukorrhea in adults, but it is seldom encountered during the prepubertal period. A typical vaginitis can be produced by introducing pure cultures of the organisms into normal vaginas. The presence of trichomonads does not always indicate symptomatic infection because they can be demonstrated in the vaginal secretions of some women who have no symptoms.

The methods by which the infection is acquired are not always obvious, but since trichomoniasis can be produced by introducing organisms into normal women, it must be assumed that the organism is usually implanted in the vagina during sexual intercourse. Trichomonads have been found in the male urethra and prostate, and the highest inci-

dence of positive cultures occurs in women who have had frequent exposure to numerous sexual partners. Buxton, Weinman, and Johnson could not culture the organism from any of 157 female college students. Positive cultures were obtained in 6.9% of 575 women attending a private gynecologic clinic and in 15% of 715 inmates of a mental institution. In contrast, cultures were positive in 70% of 221 inmates of a women's prison.

The primary complaint of most women with trichomoniasis is of moderate to profuse discharge accompanied by intense itching and irritation of the vagina and vulva. They can have a vaginal burning sensation, and intercourse can be uncomfortable. The initial symptoms often begin during or immediately after a menstrual period; after the infection is established, both the discomfort and the discharge usually increase during the premenstrual phase of each cycle.

The vulva, vagina, and cervix are sometimes intensely inflamed, and punctate red ''strawberry spots'' can be seen scattered over the vaginal and cervical mucosa. The vagina contains a large amount of discharge that characteristically is foul smelling and thin, greenish yellow and bubbly in appearance. The vaginal pH is higher than 5.

The diagnosis is confirmed by identifying trichomonads in the secretion. A drop of the vaginal secretions is mixed with a small amount of warm saline solution in a test tube, and 2 or 3 drops of the suspension are placed on a clean glass slide and examined under the microscope at once without staining. Numerous motile trichomonads and pus cells can be seen. There are few epithelial cells.

Metronidazole (Flagyl), a trichomonacidal drug, is effective when taken orally and will kill the organisms in both men and women. The trichomonads can be eradicated with more certainty if partners also are treated because the infection often will recur unless foci in the male urethra and prostate are eliminated. A single dose of 2 g of the drug or 250 mg three times a day for 7 days will eradicate at least 90% of infections in women. If it does not, it can be repeated. If the infection persists after the second dose, a more detailed evaluation is in order. One must consider the possibility of reinfection rather than treatment failure and examine and treat infected sexual partners. If this is not the case, the possibility of more resistant trichomonads needs to be considered. A dosage of 3 g of metronidazole a day should be prescribed orally for 7 days. If the patient cannot tolerate this, he or she will have to be admitted for intravenous therapy. There have been no reports of anomalies in infants whose mothers were treated with metronidazole during pregnancy. Local therapy is preferable in the first trimester, but oral therapy can be prescribed after that.

Patients should not drink alcohol during treatment. Metronidazole enhances the systemic effects of alcohol and has an antabuse-like effect.

Transient relief from itching can be obtained with acid douches of vinegar (2 tablespoonfuls in 1 quart of warm water) once or twice daily. Although local agents are less effective than is metronidazole, iodine-containing products can rarely eradicate some infections. They may be used in women who cannot take metronidazole. Iodine-containing medications are contraindicated during pregnancy. Local treatment must be continued during menstruation because exacerbations usually occur at this time. Treatment should be continued for at least three menstrual cycles, even though the symptoms disappear and no organisms can be identified in the secretions. Patients should be advised to resume local therapy during each of the first three or four menstrual periods after daily treatment is stopped. The most important reasons for failure with these forms of treatment is that patients use the medications irregularly after the symptoms improve or they are reinfected by an asymptomatic male.

CANDIDIASIS

Candidiasis, which is also called *moniliasis* or *yeast infection,* occurs most frequently during pregnancy, in women using oral contraceptives or antibiotics, and in those who have diabetes. *C. albicans* is responsible for almost all vaginitis of this type. Thrush in infants may be contracted during delivery if vaginal contents containing the organisms enter the mouth.

The typical symptoms are watery discharge and intense itching of the vagina and vulva. The external genitals usually are edematous, intensely inflamed and irritated; and the vagina is fiery red and contains a considerable amount of thin, watery discharge as well as a thick, white cheesy exudate that may be adherent to the vaginal walls.

The diagnosis is confirmed by culture or by demonstrating mycelia and spores in a wet preparation. The addition of a drop or two of 10% potassium hydroxide to the wet preparation is of help in identifying yeastlike organisms. This chemical destroys most of the white blood and epithelial cells, leaving the mycelia clearly visible.

A simple and accurate culture method consists of the inoculation of a commercially prepared slant of Nickerson's medium with a specimen of discharge picked up on a dry sterile cotton applicator (Fig. 45-1). The cap is replaced, and the inoculated tube is kept at room temperature. If yeastlike organisms are present, they will appear as isolated brown or black colonies within 48 hours.

The most effective treatment for *Candida* vulvovaginitis is to instill *miconazole* (Monistat) or *clotrimazole* (Gyne-Lotrimin) *cream* into the vagina nightly for 3 to 7 days. Recently, a new preparation has been marketed, clotrimazole (Mycelex G) 500 mg, which is used for only one night. The cream can also be applied to the vulva several times a day during the first 2 or 3 days of treatment.

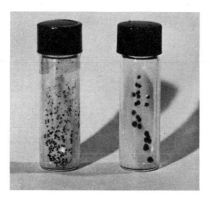

Fig. 45-1. Yeastlike organisms growing in Nickerson's medium.

Women who have regularly recurring infections, particularly those who are pregnant or using oral contraceptives, can usually keep them under control by instilling cream two or three times a week or by starting to use it as soon as the itching is felt. Before recommending this, one must be certain that the recurrences really are *Candida* infections. Antifungal treatment need not be prescribed prophylactically just because antibiotic therapy is necessary. However, it can be used if *Candida* vulvovaginitis recurs inevitably whenever antibiotics are used.

According to Miles, Olsen, and Rogers, recurrent vaginal candidiasis may come from a reservoir in the intestine. In studying young women with recurrent infections, they found that *Candida* organisms could always be recovered from feces when it was present in the vagina. Conversely, when the organisms were not present in the vagina, none could be found in feces. The obvious implication is that feces should be cultured in women with recurrent vaginal candidiasis.

There have been a number of new developments in the understanding of women with chronic or recurring episodes of *Candida* vaginitis. In some cases, men can be asymptomatic carriers of *Candida*. The ejaculate of the male sexual partner can be cultured for *Candida*. In addition, some women have a diminished lymphocyte response to *Candida*

that is reversible in some cases by the use of antiprostaglandins, such as ibuprofin.

The availability of an oral antifungal agent ketoconazole (Nizoral) has added another dimension to treatment. Two 200 mg tablets a day for 14 days can be prescribed. Rarely, liver toxicity has been noted, and liver function tests should be taken before treatment and at intervals if treatment is prolonged. This oral dose is helpful for the patient who carries yeast in her feces, has a chronic infection, needs long-term therapy because of an immunologic deficiency to yeast, or for the male who carries the organism.

Povidone-iodine gels and douches are often prescribed for women with *Candida* vulvovaginitis, but they are less effective than are other agents. In addition, they may have undesirable side effects. The iodine is absorbed readily, and serum concentrations of free and inorganic iodine are increased as much as fifteenfold from povidone-iodine preparations in the vagina. Thyroid hormonogenesis may be suppressed. *Povidone-iodine products should not be used during pregnancy; the absorbed iodine can induce goiter and hypothyroidism in the fetus.*

BACTERIAL VAGINOSIS OR NONSPECIFIC VAGINITIS

Bacterial vaginosis in the past was called nonspecific vaginitis because trichomonads, yeastlike organisms, and other common causes could not be identified.

The usual complaint of women with bacterial vaginosis is a discharge with a disagreeable odor. There is little, if any, evidence of vaginitis other than a gray exudate with a pH of 5 or more.

The diagnosis can be suspected by the symptoms and by the appearance of the vagina. It is confirmed by recognizing a *fishy odor* when a drop of 10% potassium hydroxide is added to fresh vaginal exudate on a glass slide and by identifying characteristic *"clue cells"* in a saline suspension of the vaginal secretion. Clue cells are vaginal epithelial cells with a stippled appearance and rather vague borders. The stippling is caused by many adherent short rods. Other bacteria can also adhere to epithelial cells, but most are gram positive in contrast to gram-negative *Gardnerella vaginalis*. The cause can also be suspected by the paucity of white blood cells, which usually cover the slide in trichomoniasis and candidiasis.

The infection responds to systemic therapy. There is controversy about the microbiologic cause of this disease. In the past, *G. vaginalis* was considered to be the cause, although many investigators now feel it is caused by an overgrowth of anaerobic bacteria. Metronidazole, 250 mg three times daily for 7 to 10 days, will usually eradicate it. Ampicillin, 500 mg four times daily for 5 days, also is effective, although with a lower cure rate.

Haemophilus vaginitis is a venereal infection; hence it may recur. Treatment of sexual partners whenever possible would seem appropriate, although it does not improve cure rates. As an alternative, the male can be counseled to use a condom.

ATROPHIC VAGINITIS

The pale, thin, smooth atrophic epithelium that lines the vagina in postmenopausal women is easily infected; even minor injuries may permit the entry of bacteria.

The patient usually complains of irritating vaginal discharge, pruritus, and, often, swelling and pain. The vagina is red and inflamed and may be covered with "strawberry spots" similar to those observed with trichomoniasis. The discharge is purulent and often profuse; in some women it is blood tinged. *If the patient has a bloody discharge, cancer must be suspected even though the physician can see a vaginal source for the bleeding.*

Estrogenic therapy will convert the atrophic epithelium to a thick, stratified squamous layer that is resistant to infection. Ordinarily, no other medication is necessary. Local treatment with an estrogenic vaginal cream nightly for 3 weeks will usually be effective, or oral estrogen can be used. Infection may recur as the epithelium returns to its pretreatment atrophic state, but it will respond to retreatment. Recurrences can usually be prevented by using the estrogenic material two or three times a week or by taking oral estrogen preparation daily for 25 days each month. There may be some systemic effect from vaginal applications of estrogen because estrogen is absorbed readily from the vagina.

If atrophic vaginitis is not treated, the vagina may become almost completely obliterated by atrophy and adhesions between denuded areas.

CHEMICAL AND ALLERGIC VAGINITIS

The vagina may become irritated in response to the introduction of certain chemicals. Some, such as creosote or potassium permanganate, which once were used as douches to induce abortion, can produce extensive tissue destruction. Chemical vaginitis can also be produced by medications being used to treat specific forms of vaginitis. Substances used in commercial douche powders, vulvar lotions, or aerosol sprays may cause allergic reactions in susceptible women. Recently, we have discovered some women who are allergic to the ejaculate of their male sexual partner.

This type of vaginitis should be suspected whenever the introduction of a substance into the vagina is followed by irritation that gradually subsides but recurs in response to reintroduction of the same material. The appearance of the vagina is determined by the tissue response to the irritant. Strong concentrations of creosote or potassium permanganate, for example, may produce deep ulcerations and bleeding. With allergic reactions the vagina is reddened and edematous, and secretions are usually thin and watery. They may become purulent if infection is superimposed.

Treatment of chemical vaginitis consists of recognizing the cause and discontinuing the use of the irritating preparation. Warm, plain water or saline solution douches may aid in relieving irritation. An antihistamine preparation, either taken orally or applied locally as ointment, may be helpful if the reaction is primarily an allergic one. Hydrocortisone ointment will relieve vulvar itching and irritation. If the allergy is to the male ejaculate, the use of a condom is helpful.

OTHER CAUSES OF LEUKORRHEA

Cervicitis, one of the most common causes of leukorrhea in adults, is discussed in Chapter 46, and herpesvirus infections in Chapter 44. Among the less common causes are foreign bodies (for example, tampons and pessaries); carcinoma of the cervix, endometrium, or tube; and certain rare infections of the genital organs.

TUMORS

Benign tumors. *Vaginal inclusion cysts* may develop at the site of injuries that occur with delivery. They frequently develop along the episiotomy scar. Inclusion cysts rarely cause symptoms and need not be treated.

Gärtner duct cysts are residual remnants of the paramesonephric ducts that do not atrophy. They usually are found in the lateral vaginal fornices or along the lateral walls of the upper third of the vagina. They rarely cause symptoms and, as a general rule, need no treatment.

Condylomata acuminata may involve the vagina as well as the vulvar structures. During pregnancy they may grow luxuriantly and actually fill the vagina. Extensive involvement may preclude vaginal delivery. The lesions often regress during the puerperium. Chemical cauterization of vaginal lesions is contraindicated, but some will regress when vaginitis is eradicated. One does not need to treat small scattered lesions that cause no symptoms. Those which are symptomatic can be destroyed by electrodesiccation, by cryocautery, or by laser (Chapter 44).

Vaginal adenosis may develop in young women who were exposed to diethylstilbestrol during embryonic and fetal life. A few may progress to clear cell adenocarcinoma. This lesion is discussed in Chapter 3.

Malignant tumors. *Primary squamous cell carcinoma* of the vagina is an unusual lesion. It may develop in the upper third of the vagina of women who have been treated for carcinoma of the cervix or of the vulva.

The diagnosis can be suspected by a report of an abnormal cytologic study, particularly in women who have been treated for cervical cancer or after hysterectomy.

The diagnosis is confirmed by biopsy of any obvious lesion or by multiple biopsies of the vagina if the cytology is abnormal but no lesion can be seen.

Vaginectomy is usually adequate treatment for carcinoma in situ of the vagina. The vagina can be reconstructed by vaginoplasty.

Invasive cancer is treated by radium application and external radiation. In some patients, particularly those in whom radiation has failed to eradicate the tumor, pelvic exenteration can be considered.

REFERENCES

Ansel, R., et al.: Nonspecific vaginitis. Diagnostic criteria and microbial and epidemiologic associations, Am. J. Med. **74**:14, 1983.

Buxton, C.L., Weinman, D., and Johnson, C.: Epidemiology of *Trichomonas vaginalis* vaginitis, Obstet. Gynecol. **12**:699, 1958.

Davis, M.E., and Pearl, S.A.: The biology of the human vagina in pregnancy, Am. J. Obstet. Gynecol. **35**:77, 1938.

Fleury, F.J.: Adult vaginitis, Clin. Obstet. Gynecol. **24**:407, 1981.

Masters, W.H.: The sexual response cycle of the human vagina; vaginal lubrication, Ann. N.Y. Acad. Sci. **83**:301, 1959.

Miles, M.R., Olsen, L., and Rogers, A.: Recurrent vaginal candidiasis, J.A.M.A. **238**:1836, 1977.

Muller, M., et al.: Three metronidazole-resistant strains of *Trichomonas vaginalis* from the United States, Am. J. Obstet. Gynecol. **138**:808, 1980.

Sobel, J.D.: Management of recurrent vulvovaginal candidiasis with intermittent ketoconazale prophylaxis, Obstet. Gynecol. **64**:435, 1985.

Vontver, L.A., and Eschenbach, D.A.: Role of *Gardnerella vaginalis* in nonspecific vaginitis, Clin. Obstet. Gynecol. **24**:439, 1981.

Vorherr, H., Vorherr, U.F., Mehta, P., Ulrich, J.A., and Messer, R.H.: Vaginal absorption of povidone-iodine, JAMA **244**:2628, 1980.

Witkin, S.S., Yu, I.R., and Ledger, W.J.: Inhibition of *Candida albicans*–induced lymphocyte proliferation by lymphocytes and sera from women with recurrent vaginitis, Am. J. Obstet. Gynecol. **1**:147:809, 1983.

46

J. Robert Willson

Benign and malignant diseases of the cervix

The relative ease with which the cervix can be exposed has permitted us to become familiar with the changes that occur normally throughout life. Its position also permits detailed study of pathologic conditions by direct inspection, colposcopy, biopsy, and chemical and microbiologic study of the secretions.

NORMAL CERVIX

The cervix, the most inferior part of the uterus, is derived from the fused caudal portions of the müllerian ducts. During reproductive life it protrudes into the vaginal canal at the apex of the vagina where the vaginal walls blend into the epithelial covering of its external surfaces. After the menopause the cervix atrophies as estrogen is gradually withdrawn until it is flush with the vaginal vault. The part of the cervix that lies above the level at which the vaginal wall is attached is the *supravaginal cervix,* and that below the attachment, the *portio vaginalis.* The supravaginal cervix is surrounded by pelvic fascia laterally and anteriorly and by the cul-de sac peritoneum posteriorly. The *cervical canal,* which is fusiform and 2 to 3 cm long, provides a passageway between the vagina and the uterine cavity.

The portio vaginalis of the normal cervix is covered by pink, smooth, stratified squamous epithelium much like that which lines the vagina. The cervical canal is lined by mucus-secreting columnar epithelium that is thrown into folds and grooves that form complex branching clefts and tunnels called *crypts.* The caudal end of the canal is constricted to form an opening into the vagina, the *external cervical os* (Fig. 46-1). The opening is round and centrally placed in nulliparous women. It is more likely to be represented by a transverse slit in those who have had children (Fig. 46-2). The upper end of the canal also is constricted at the opening into the uterine cavity called the *internal os.*

In contrast to the body of the uterus, which is principally a muscular organ, the cervical stroma is predominately collagenous connective tissue with some elastic fibers and a few smooth muscle cells. The change, which may be abrupt or gradual, occurs just above the internal os in an area known as the *isthmus.* The epithelium overlying the isthmus is more like that which lines the uterine cavity than that of the cervical canal.

The cervical epithelium responds to changes in ovarian hormone concentrations, but the responses of the stratified squamous epithelium on the portio are different from those of the columnar cells in the canal. The squamous cells proliferate under the stimulus of rising estrogen concentrations during the first half of the cycle and respond to progesterone after ovulation as do vaginal epithelial cells.

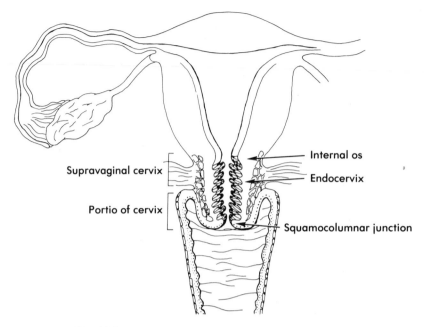

Fig. 46-1. Cervix and its relationship to vagina and uterus.

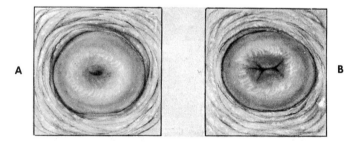

Fig. 46-2. Normal cervix. **A,** Nulliparous. **B,** Parous. (From Titus, P., and Wilson, J.R.: The management of obstetric difficulties, St. Louis, 1955, The C.V. Mosby Co.)

The columnar cells are also affected by changes in hormone concentrations, but the results are more obvious, because these cells secrete mucus. After a menstrual period the cervical mucus is thick and sticky, but it changes from day to day under the stimulus of increasing concentrations of estrogen. At about the time of ovulation the mucus is profuse, watery, and transparent and can be drawn out in strands 10 to 15 cm long *(spinnbarkheit).* After ovulation the mucus becomes thick and tenacious in response to progesterone. The pH at ovulation is 7 to 8 as compared with about 4.5 early and late in the cycle.

Arborization, or ferning, of cervical mucus is induced by the effect of estrogen and is inhibited by progesterone. Ferning is minimal during the postmenstrual phase, maximal at the time of ovulation, and then disappears as progesterone secretion increases (Chapter 2).

SQUAMOCOLUMNAR JUNCTION

The point at which the squamous epithelium that covers the portio joins the columnar epithelium of the cervical canal is the *squamocolumnar junction* (Fig. 46-3). The junction can be identified as the line of demarcation between the pale pink squa-

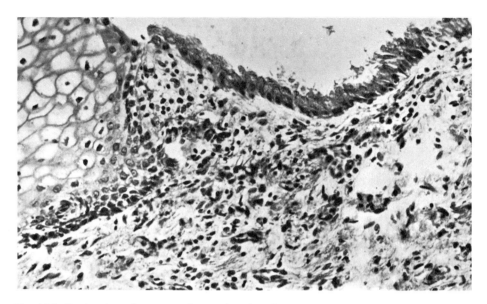

Fig. 46-3. Section through squamocolumnar junction. Squamous epithelium on left adjacent to tall columnar epithelium of endocervix. (×279.)

mous epithelium that covers the portio and the bright red columnar epithelium that lines the canal. The division may be at the external os, on the surface of the portio lateral to the opening, or within the cervical canal. The columnar epithelium often extends well beyond the external os in the diseased cervix and quite normally in newborn infants and during puberty and adolescence. In postmenopausal women the squamocolumnar junction may be high in the canal where it cannot be seen.

BENIGN DISEASES (Fig. 46-4)

Cervicitis. *Acute cervicitis* does not often occur as an isolated entity; rather, it accompanies an acute infection in some other part of the reproductive system. The acute infections that most often involve the cervix are those caused by *Trichomonas* vaginitis, *Haemophilus vaginalis* vaginitis, genital herpesvirus and *Chlamydia* infections, and gonorrhea. Acute cervicitis can also develop when foreign bodies such as menstrual tampons, are left in the vagina for long periods of time. Acute cervical infections occur regularly as part of puerperal and postabortal uterine infections.

The cervix is congested, edematous, and in-

flamed, and there usually is a profuse purulent exudate from the canal. The vagina may also be inflamed. The cervix is tender, and the parametrial areas may be indurated and tender when palpated.

The cause of the infection can be determined by bacterial culture of the exudate.

Chronic cervicitis occurs more often than does any other infection involving the female reproductive organs. Almost all women who have delivered babies or have had abortions have histologic evidence of chronic cervicitis. The vast majority of these infections cause no symptoms and are of no consequence. There is no known relationship between chronic cervicitis and cervical cancer.

The major involvement, *endocervicitis,* is in the cervical canal. Here the infection involves both the columnar epithelium lining the crypts and the underlying stroma. The secretion from the infected columnar epithelium is white, yellow, or green and thick and purulent in contrast to the normal clear mucus these cells usually secrete. In mild cases the portio may be completely covered by normal-appearing squamous epithelium, the only evidence of infection being the purulent secretion coming from the canal. In some instances the process extends outward from the canal, and one may see an irregular reddened area surrounding the external os. This may not be evident until the exudate is wiped away.

With the most severe infections the squamous epithelium that usually covers the portio is replaced by friable granulation tissue, and the cervix is edematous and hypertrophied. There may even be an associated parametritis as the process extends laterally through the lymphatic channels. These lesions often bleed after the slightest touch and can be differentiated from cancer only by biopsy.

Women with only histologic evidence of infection usually have no symptoms. Those with more extensive lesions may be annoyed by the discharge, which is present constantly but which usually increases at midcycle and premenstrually. Some have so much secretion that they must wear perineal pads to protect their clothing. Other symptoms such as lower abdominal pain, dyspareunia, and backache may accompany infections that extend beyond the cervix, but this is unusual.

Treatment. The treatment of *acute cervicitis* is determined by identifying the causative organism. Culture and sensitivity studies will indicate the appropriate medication.

Small areas of *chronic cervicitis* can be treated by *thermal cautery* or by *freezing (cryosurgery)*. The effect of both methods is to destroy the abnormal tissue; this is followed by healing and re-epithelization. The entire surface of the visible lesion and at least the lower 1 to 2 cm of the endocervical canal are treated. Nabothian cysts are usually destroyed in the process. The annoying discharge from the sloughing cervical tissue can be controlled with vinegar douches and the daily instillation of an antibiotic cream. This may be discontinued after 7 to 10 days.

Regeneration and healing may not be complete for 6 to 8 weeks; consequently, repeat treatment should be delayed at least that long. *Lesions that do not heal after adequate treatment should be biopsied to eliminate cancer as a cause of the failure.*

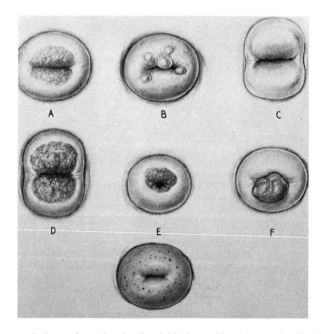

Fig. 46-4. Common lesions of cervix. **A,** Cervicitis in multiparous cervix. **B,** Nabothian cysts. **C,** Bilateral healed lacerations. **D,** Bilateral lacerations with eversion and endocervicitis. **E,** "Erosion" in nulliparous cervix, **F,** Cervical polyp. **G,** "Strawberry" spots with vaginal trichomoniasis. (From Kleegman, S.J.: Am. J. Surg. **48:**294, 1940.)

Local treatment of chronic cervicitis with douches and antibiotic creams or with chemical cautery (silver nitrate) almost always fails because the lesion is relatively deep seated in the tissue, and medications applied to the surface have no appreciable effect. Systemic antibiotics also are ineffective in the treatment of chronic cervicitis.

Large, cystic, infected cervices are best treated by *therapeutic conization*. The procedure is effective because the infected material is removed; at the same time, it provides the pathologist with an adequate block of tissue for study.

Erosion. An *erosion* is an extension of the columnar epithelium that lines the cervical canal outward across the vaginal face of the cervix. The squamocolumnar junction is at the periphery of the lesion rather than in the region of the external cervical os. Erosions are common at birth and in young girls. Linhartova found columnar epithelium on the portio in 42.7% of 103 autopsies on girls between the ages of 1 and 13. Erosions are seen frequently during adolescence, but most of them disappear as the reproductive organs and their functions mature.

The lesion is redder than the surrounding pink squamous epithelium and has a soft, velvety appearance. It does not usually bleed during manipulation. The secretion from the glandular epithelium covering the portio of the cervix is clear mucus like that produced by the glandular epithelium lining the cervical canal.

The term *erosion* is inaccurate because there is no actual loss of epithelium. Erosions heal as the medial border of squamous epithelium advances toward the external os by a process of metaplasia. The metaplastic epithelium is gradually transformed to a more mature squamous type. The stimulus for the replacement is unknown but may be estrogen, which increases before puberty or the resultant reduced pH. There may be patches of squamous epithelium intermixed with the columnar cells, and squamous cells may extend downward, displacing glandular epithelium. Areas of columnar cells may be trapped beneath the advancing squamous epithelium as the lesion heals (Fig. 46-5).

Erosions generally produce no symptoms, but some women may be aware of excessive, clear, nonirritating, mucoid secretion, which may be most obvious during the midcycle peak of estrogen stimulation.

Eversion. As one opens the speculum to expose

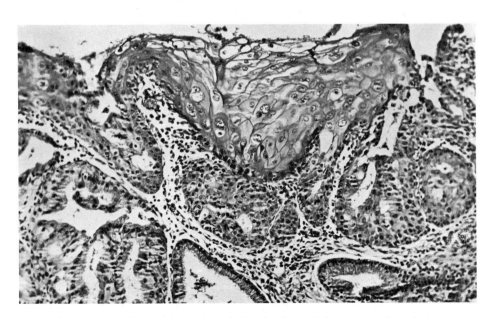

Fig. 46-5. Section showing squamous metaplasia of endocervical mucosa and contiguous crypts. (×164.)

the cervix, the anterior and posterior lips separate widely if the cervix has been deeply lacerated at the 3 and 9 o'clock positions during delivery. One looks directly at the cervical canal. The red endocervical tissue looks much like an erosion on the portio, but, as the speculum is withdrawn, the cervical lips fall together and the "lesion" disappears. This is a normal phenomenon unless there is an associated chronic endocervicitis.

Nabothian cysts. As squamous epithelium proliferates and replaces columnar epithelium that has extended onto the portio (for example, as an erosion heals), areas of columnar epithelium may become isolated beneath the advancing metaplastic squamous layer. The columnar cells continue to secrete mucus. Since there is no opening to the surface, the secretion accumulates, forming *nabothian cysts*. These structures are usually no larger than 1 to 2 cm in diameter. They are filled with normal-appearing cervical mucus, which does not become infected. Nabothian cysts cause no symptoms.

Diagnosis. Diagnostic procedures are relatively simple. Most benign lesions can be recognized with reasonable accuracy by gross inspection of the cervix, but one should use all available diagnostic aids if there is any question of the diagnosis. This is particularly true when a cervical lesion resembles cancer. Methods for diagnosing cervical lesions are discussed on pages 710 to 712.

POLYPS

Cervical polyps (Fig. 46-6) occur frequently. These small, pedunculated lesions arise in the endocervical canal and consist almost entirely of columnar epithelium with or without squamous metaplasia. They vary in size from a few millimeters up to 2 to 3 cm. They are soft, red, and friable. If cervical polyps are present, bleeding may be induced by the slightest trauma. Presumably, polyps have little to do with the development of malignancy in the cervix, and they rarely undergo carcinomatous change.

Cervical polyps are often responsible for episodes of slight vaginal bleeding. If the physician assumes that the polyp alone is responsible for the bleeding and does not perform an endometrial and endocervical curettage, a carcinoma may go undetected. This is particularly true in postmenopausal women.

Polyps can be removed in the office if there has been no abnormal bleeding. Although they rarely are malignant, they should be examined histologically.

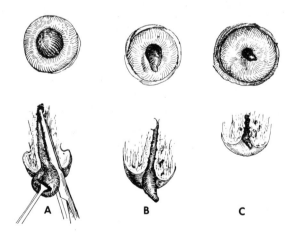

Fig. 46-6. Cervical polyps. **A,** Method for twisting a polyp off at its base. **B** and **C,** Usual appearance of endocervical polyps. (From Titus, P.: Atlas of obstetric technic, ed. 2, St. Louis, 1949, The C.V. Mosby Co.)

HYPERTROPHY

Both the diameter and the length of the cervix may increase severalfold. Usually the increase in diameter results from edema that accompanies a long-standing chronic infection. Vaginal relaxation and prolapse of the uterus, however, are frequently associated with a hypertrophy and lengthening of the supravaginal portion of the cervix. The weight of the cystocele and rectocele pulling on the cervix gradually stretches this portion of the uterus to several times it normal length. If the uterine supports remain reasonably intact, the cervix may elongate so that it protrudes far beyond the introitus, even though the uterus descends only slightly.

The treatment of hypertrophy alone depends a great deal on the accompanying pathologic findings and the age and physical condition of the patient. A high cervical amputation and a vaginal plastic operation may be all that is necessary if the uterus is normal and well supported. If the uterine supports are stretched, a vaginal hysterectomy and vaginal plastic repair are the procedures of choice.

STENOSIS

Stenosis of the cervical canal is caused by scar tissue contracting and by the agglutination of raw surfaces within the endocervix. Stenosis may follow cauterization, conization operations, cervical amputations, and intrauterine radium applications.

The major symptoms are related to menstruation. The flow may be scant, painful, and prolonged because of the stricture of the cervical canal. An acquired dysmenorrhea after cervical operations strongly suggests cervical stenosis. Obstruction may be complete in rare instances, with hematometra resulting. Severe cervical stenosis occasionally prevents cervical dilatation during labor, making cesarean section mandatory.

The uterus and cervix atrophy after the menopause. Contraction and stenosis may so completely close the endocervix that secretions from the atrophic endometrial cavity have no way to escape. The secretions and cellular debris accumulating within the body of the uterus may eventually become infected, and *pyometra* results. Pyometra may also occur with endometrial carcinoma or with

cancer of the cervix that obliterates the cervical canal.

Treatment consists of dilatation of the cervix and culture of the escaping purulent material. Appropriate antibiotics may be needed, although this is usually unnecessary. The cervix must be kept open by the passage of a 3 or 4 mm dilator once a week until the point of stricture remains open without force. This takes about four to six dilatations. In rare instances, patency cannot be maintained, and hysterectomy is indicated if the stenosis recurs. Diagnostic curettage is essential in women with pyometra because of its relationship to uterine cancer.

BENIGN NEW GROWTHS

In addition to the common polyp previously discussed, *myomas* often involve the cervix. These are considered in Chapter 47. Likewise, *endometriosis*, although infrequent in the cervix, does occur and is discussed in Chapter 11.

MALIGNANT DISEASES

Approximately 13% of all invasive cancers in women occur in the uterus, and, of these, about 40% arise in the cervix. It is estimated that 14,000 new invasive cancers of the cervix were diagnosed and that 6800 women died of the disease in 1986. The crude annual incidence of invasive carcinoma of the cervix is 17.3/100,000 women of all ages and 27/100,000 women over the age of 20 years. In addition to the invasive lesions, at least 45,000 noninvasive carcinomas of the cervix were also detected.

Although cancer of the cervix can occur at any age, invasive lesions are most often diagnosed in women between the ages of 35 and 65 years. Noninvasive lesions are diagnosed in women about 10 to 15 years younger.

EPIDEMIOLOGIC FACTORS

There are many similarities between carcinoma of the cervix and sexually transmitted diseases, sexual intercourse being an almost essential factor in the development of both.

Rotkin, studying 400 women with cervical cancer and an equal number of matched control subjects, found the most significant difference in the two groups to be the *age of first coitus.* Those with cancer started intercourse before the age of 20 years, many in their early teens. Related influences that appear to be important in the genesis of early cancer are: the number of sexual partners, the number of contacts of partners with other women, frequency of intercourse, and the number of marriages. Although most carcinomas of the cervix develop in parous women, the number of pregnancies seems to be less important than age at first coitus and the number and sexual habits of partners. Cervical cancer is unusual in nuns and virgins.

Carcinoma of the cervix occurs more often in *women of low socioeconomic status* than in those who are more affluent. *Cancer of the cervix also occurs more often in black than in white women.* The age-adjusted rate for invasive cervical cancer in black women is 33.6/100,000 as compared with 15/100,000 for whites. A similar ratio holds for carcinoma in situ: 62.6:32.5. The difference, which is at least partly caused by socioeconomic factors, may be eliminated as the age at which sexual activity is initiated decreases and as frequency of intercourse and number of partners in all races increase.

The incidence of cervical cancer is not increased in women whose first intercourse occurred after age 20. This is true even though other factors are similar to those for women who had intercourse early. One possible explanation is that an unidentified stimulus introduced during coitus induces anaplastic proliferation in the immature metaplastic epithelial cells of the transformation zone. Columnar epithelium, which often extends over the entire portio in young girls, undergoes a normal metaplastic change induced by the altered biochemical environment in the vagina after puberty. If the process continues without being disturbed, the metaplastic cells are converted to a mature squamous epithelium with the squamocolumnar junction near or just within the external cervical os. A mitogen introduced repeatedly before the conversion occurs and to which mature squamous epithelium is not particularly susceptible may induce an anaplastic reaction in the immature cells.

This is an attractive theory, but as yet an agent has not been identified. It was once thought that a substance in smegma might be responsible for inducing abnormal cell growth in the cervix and that smegma is more likely to be present in uncircumcised men. This theory, which has since been discarded, was used to explain the fact that *Jewish women do not often develop cervical cancer.* Jewish women have a protective mechanism, perhaps immunologic, because they do develop "premalignant" cellular changes. Czernobilsky and colleagues found cervicitis, reserve cell hyperplasia, squamous metaplasia, and dysplasia to be prevalent equally between Jewish and non-Jewish women.

There is evidence to suggest that *herpesvirus hominis type 2* could be a factor that induces abnormal cervical cell growth. Naib and co-workers observed 245 women with active herpesvirus genital infections for 5 or more years. Anaplastic cervical lesions developed in 58 (23%), including four with invasive cancer and 12 with carcinoma in situ. Anaplasia occurred in 1.6% with only one noninvasive and no invasive lesions in a matched control group without herpesvirus infection.

Catalano and Johnson identified herpesvirus hominis type 2 antibodies in 35.7% of women who subsequently developed carcinoma in situ of the cervix but in only 7.1% of matched control subjects who did not develop carcinoma in situ during the observation period. Antibodies were identified in 42% of patients with proved carcinoma in situ and in 17.7% of matched controls.

Another sexually-related infection that may play a role in the development of cervical cancer is that caused by *human papilloma viruses* 16, 18, 31, 33, and 35. Reid and colleagues were able to demonstrate papilloma virus in the cervix in 88% of uteri removed for cervical dysplasia and in 95% of those removed because of invasive cancer. Only 12.5% of control specimens were positive. Papilloma viruses have been identified in condylomata accuminata of the vulva and vagina and in warty growths in other parts of the body. Cervical condylomas are flat rather than sessile and are not usually visible on gross inspection. They are obvious, however, using the colposcope after 30% acetic acid has been applied to the cervix.

Although it has been assumed that there has been a recent increase in cervical condylomas that coincides with earlier onset of coitus and more frequent sexual activity in teenagers, this may not be true. Bernstein and co-workers reexamined 1264 cervical biopsy specimens that had been obtained in 1972 and found changes consistent with human papilloma virus in 36.5%; only 0.7% had been reported as positive on the initial examinations. Of 965 biopsies obtained in 1982, 34% showed viral changes. It seems likely, therefore, that the frequency of cervical condylomas has not changed much.

Further evidence that the viruses are sexually transmitted is that penile condylomas can often be identified in the sexual partners of women with cervical condylomata and cervical intraepithelial neoplasia.

Although papilloma virus has not been proved to be a direct cause of cervical cancer, there is no question that the two conditions are related.

The relationship between coitus and the development of cervical cancer and especially of the possibility of a male factor is strengthened by Kessler's study of 1087 second wives of men whose former partners had been treated for carcinoma of the cervix and 659 present wives of men whose former partners had not had the disease. Carcinoma in situ or invasive cancer has been detected in 29 (2.7%) of the study group and seven (1.1%) of the control subjects. Cervical cancer or an abnormal cytologic study has occurred in 14% of the study group and 8% of the controls.

Although it seems likely that male factors are responsible for inducing the cellular changes that precede invasive cervical cancer, they have not been precisely identified.

The *common benign lesions of the cervix* have long been suspected to be precursors of cancer, but the relationship has never been proven. Peyton and colleagues reported on the results of 38 years of ablation of abnormal cervical tissue by office cautery. Of the 6533 patients who were not cauterized, 81 developed in situ or invasive cancer: 27/1000. In contrast, the only malignancies diagnosed in the 6364 who underwent cauterization of the cervix were three carcinomas in situ: 0.5/1000.

TYPES

Most cervical carcinomas begin in the labile transformation zone. Subcylindrical (reserve) cells, which are found beneath the columnar epithelium at the squamocolumnar junction, form the metaplastic cells in the transformation zone. They proliferate, undermining and raising the columnar epithelium, as they advance across the portio. Metaplastic cells are usually transformed into mature epithelium, but in some instances they become atypical, a change that precedes dysplasia and cervical cancer.

About 90% of cancers of the cervix are of squamous cell origin, and about 10% arise in columnar epithelium. Rarely, sarcoma, mixed mesodermal tumors, or malignancies of the lymphoid series (for example, reticulum cell sarcoma or malignant lymphoma) may be primary in the cervix.

PATHOLOGIC FINDINGS

Basal cell hyperplasia is the earliest recognizable cellular alteration that *may* be a forerunner of invasive cancer. The arrangement of the undifferentiated basal cells is disorderly. They vary in size and shape, and many mitotic figures can be identified. The abnormal changes, which are called *dysplasia,* occur in single or multiple focal areas. In some, but not all, women the dysplasic change will become progressively more severe as the cells take on more of the characteristics of malignancy. Since it is impossible to tell in advance whether the lesion will progress or regress, dysplasia must be considered a step toward the development of cancer; hence the designation *cervical intraepithelial neoplasia (CIN).*

Since cervical intraepithelial neoplasia is usually associated with human papilloma virus infections, the cellular changes caused by the virus can often be identified in biopsy specimens. The most characteristic of these is the presence of *koilocytes,* which are squamous cells with dense, hyperchromatic, pyknotic nuclei surrounded by a clear cytoplasmic halo (Fig. 46-7).

With *mild dysplasia,* or *CIN I,* the undifferentiated cells are confined to the lower one third of the epithelial layer. The cells become progressively more differentiated toward the surface. In *moderate*

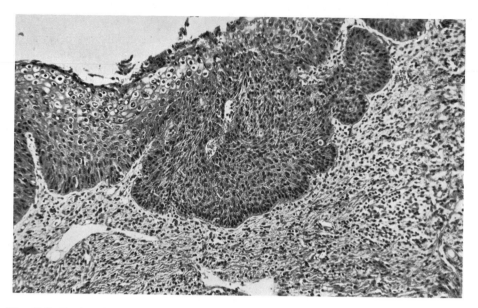

Fig. 46-7. Section showing dysplastic change. Prominent koilocytes in the superficial layers are characteristic of papilloma virus infection. (×255.)

dysplasia, or *CIN II* (Fig. 46-8), the lower 50% to 75% of the epithelial layer is replaced by undifferentiated cells, but the superficial layer is fairly well differentiated. It may be impossible to perceive the difference between *severe dysplasia* and *carcinoma in situ;* hence they are usually considered as a single entity, *CIN III.* The entire thickness of the epithelium is replaced by anaplastic cells, and there is no surface cornification (Figs. 46-9 and 46-10).

Dysplasia should be considered as a continuum, rather than a series of individual lesions. Any stage may regress to normal epithelium, but regression is more likely to occur with CIN I than with the more advanced lesions; the latter are likely to progress to invasive cancer.

Conversion of dysplasia to unmistakable carcinoma in situ takes about 4 years. The time interval between the *diagnosis* of dysplasia and of carcinoma in situ is determined by the severity of the dysplastic process when it is first recognized. It may take 5 or more years for mild dysplasia to become recognizable carcinoma in situ but only a few months for the more advanced lesions.

Most but not all carcinomas in situ continue to proliferate and eventually grow through the basement membrane and *invade the cervical stroma.* The exact period between the development of CIN and *invasive cancer* is not known but is probably between 10 and 15 years. One cannot rely on a specific time period, however, because more aggressively growing lesions may progress from dysplasia through carcinoma in situ to invasion within a 3- to 4-year period. Rarely, they may progress so rapidly that dysplasia and carcinoma in situ are not recognized.

Microinvasion, as the term suggests, is the earliest stage at which extension of the cancer beneath the basal epithelial layer can be recognized. Microinvasion is diagnosed when neoplastic cells invade the cervical stroma to a depth of no more than 3 mm below the base of the epithelium and when no obvious blood vessel or lymphatic invasion has occurred.

A band of carcinoma in situ and possibly another of dysplasia usually surround an area of invasive cancer. It is obvious that random punch biopsies may be inaccurate in assessing the extent of the

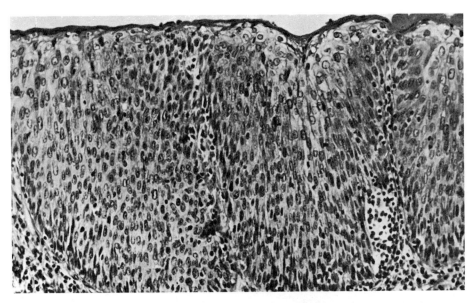

Fig. 46-8. Moderate to severe dysplasia. Cells are closely packed, and arrangement is fairly orderly. Upper half of epithelial surface shows maturation with some keratin production on surface. (×255.)

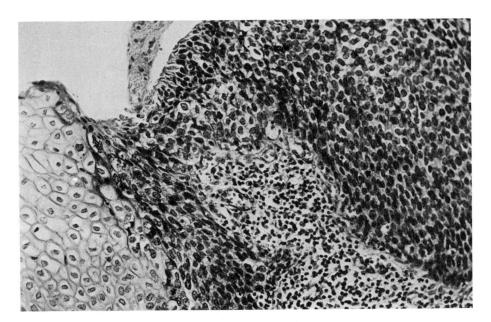

Fig. 46-9. Carcinoma in situ of cervix. Mature cells occur on left with abrupt change to complete loss of maturation on right, with intact basement membrane.

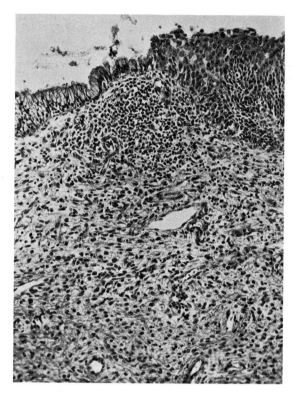

Fig. 46-10. Normal endocervical mucosa is seen on left with abrupt change on right where proliferation of reserve cells in transformation zone to incomplete maturation and carcinoma in situ is found. (×186.)

tumor because the tissue removed may not be representative of the entire lesion.

CLINICAL STAGES

The extent to which the cervix and surrounding structures are involved with cancer is referred to as the *clinical stage* of the disease. This factor definitely influences prognosis or cancer salvage. Small early lesions that are confined to the cervix have the best prognosis, whereas those that extend beyond the cervix have far less chance of a cure.

Carcinoma of the cervix spreads by direct extension and through the lymphatics. Since cervical cancer is disseminated through the lymphatics, the pelvic lymph nodes must, of necessity, be invaded as the tumor grows. Brunschwig and Daniel identified cancer in the pelvic lymph nodes in 13% of women with stage I lesions, 30% in stage II, 46% in stage III, and 53% in stage IV.

The *ureter* is particularly vulnerable in cervical malignancy because it passes through the parametrium just lateral to the cervix. Some degree of ureteral obstruction can be demonstrated in about two thirds of women with advanced invasive cancer of the cervix. The tumor grows laterally from the cervix and around the ureter, but the ureteral wall usually is not invaded. *Distant metastases* are uncommon, but they can occur in any part of the body.

The clinical stage or extent of the lesion, must be determined before treatment is started. Appropriate treatment differs, depending on the stage. Also, clinical staging permits a comparison of results of a variety of treatments.

The clinical stage of an individual tumor is determined by inspection, vaginal and rectal palpation, and biopsy. Obviously, clinical staging is not always accurate because involved lymph nodes and

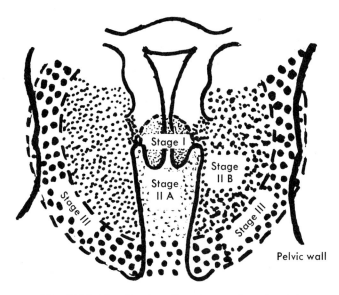

Fig. 46-11. Classification of carcinoma of cervix uteri.

other extensions of the disease cannot always be recognized.

The most widely accepted clinical staging classification of cervical cancer is that of the International Federation of Gynecology and Obstetrics (Fig. 46-11):

Stage	Description
0	Carcinoma in situ
I	Carcinoma confined to the cervix
IA	Microinvasion
IB	All other stage I lesions
II	Invasion of the vagina, except for the lower third, or infiltration of the parametrium, but no extension to the pelvic wall
IIA	Vaginal involvement, but no palpable parametrial extension
IIB	Parametrial infiltration
III	Involvement of the lower third of the vagina or extension to the pelvic wall and fixation
IIIA	Involvement of the lower third of the vagina
IIIB	Fixation to the pelvic wall
IV	Extension to the bladder or rectum or distant metastases

SYMPTOMS

There are no symptoms of early carcinoma of the cervix. An abnormality usually is first indicated by a *watery discharge* followed by *bleeding,* which characteristically is painless, bright red, intermenstrual or postmenopausal, and prone to follow trauma such as coitus or douching. Thus a tumor is not evident by palpation and gross inspection of the cervix until there is an ulcerative cervical lesion. With further growth, bleeding increases and may be constant and profuse.

Pain occurs only when the tumor has extended far enough to invade the pelvic nerves in the lateral pelvic wall and the nerve roots. Pain therefore indicates far advanced disease.

Since the bowel is not often involved until the tumor is in an advanced stage, most women with cervical cancer remain well nourished. *Weight loss* occurs only during the late stages of the disease.

DIAGNOSIS

Cervical carcinoma can be suspected if abnormal cells are found in a cytologic examination or by visual inspection, but it can only be diagnosed with certainty by biopsy.

Screening cytologic examination is an essential part of the periodic examination of presumably well women. It is usually performed at intervals of 12 to 18 months in women who have had several normal studies and are not likely candidates for cervical cancer. It should be performed more frequently in women who have been treated for dysplasia and in those who are at risk of developing cancer of the cervix.

Carcinoma of the cervix cannot be diagnosed with certainty by cytologic examination, but the presence of abnormal cells alerts the physician to the need for a more complete investigation.

One must be aware of the fact that cytology is not absolutely accurate in detecting either CIN lesions or invasive cancer. There is at least a 10% to 30% false-negative rate, which may be highest with invasive tumors. This suggests that lesions with the characteristics of cervical cancer should be biopsied, even though malignant cells are not detected by the cytologist.

Advanced invasive cancer can be suspected by visual inspection of the cervix, but benign conditions, particularly chronic cervicitis, can look almost exactly like malignant lesions, and a cervix containing an extensive invasive cancer may appear normal. An example of the former is *microglandular hyperplasia,* a benign lesion usually seen in women who are taking oral contraceptives. The gross appearance may be identical to that of invasive cancer, and its histologic appearance is much like that of adenocarcinoma.

The characteristic malignant lesion is either an *ulcer* or an *exophytic growth* (Fig. 46-12). In both instances the tissue is friable and usually bleeds readily when sponged with a cotton ball. A lesion that begins within the cervical canal may not be accompanied by bleeding and may not be visible. Such tumors often are far advanced when they are detected.

Abnormal epithelium can be identified by its failure to stain with iodine *(Schiller test).* The reaction is based on normal, glycogen-containing epithelial cells staining deep brown when Lugol's iodine solution is applied. Abnormal epithelial cells contain little or no glycogen and do not stain when iodine is applied. The absence of glycogen is not an infallible evidence of cancer; it only indicates an area of abnormal epithelium. Normal cervical and vaginal squamous cells in postmenopausal women contain little glycogen and may not stain.

Carcinoma of the cervix can only be diagnosed with certainty by *tissue biopsy.* This confirmatory examination is essential before treatment is started. Tissue can be obtained by *office punch biopsy* or *conization;* the choice depends on the location and extent of the lesion.

Multiple punch biopsy is an appropriate step if there is an obvious cervical lesion. Bits of tissue

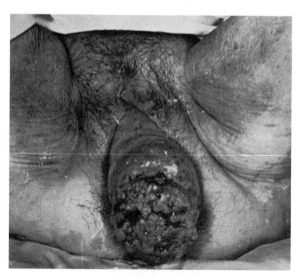

Fig. 46-12. Large carcinoma of cervix in patient with complete prolapse of uterus (rare).

are taken from several areas around the periphery of the lesion with punch biopsy forceps (Fig. 46-13). Samples from the squamocolumnar junction, if it can be identified, are important. If invasive cancer is found, one may proceed directly to treatment. If only CIN is diagnosed, more adequate biopsy is essential.

The accuracy of punch biopsy, particularly if the lesion is small or is not obvious, can be increased by the use of the *colposcope,* an instrument that provides a light source and binocular magnification of 10 to 40 times. Lesions on the portio and vagina can be studied easily, but those in the cervical canal can be more difficult to see. This is especially true when the external os is stenotic and the squamocolumnar junction lies within the canal.

Colposcopic examination is inconclusive unless the entire transformation zone, the squamocolumnar junction, and the entire cervical canal can be seen. Although experienced colposcopists can usually assess lesions accurately on the basis of their physical characteristics, the impression should be confirmed by *colposcopic-directed biopsy* before treatment is initiated. All abnormal areas should be sampled, and an endocervical curettage should be performed. The latter is particularly important if the upper edge of the lesion in the canal cannot be seen and biopsied.

Conization (cone biopsy) is an accurate method for studying the portio of the cervix and the entire cervical canal when invasive cancer is suspected because of abnormal cytology but colposcopy is not available, when colposcopic-directed biopsy does not confirm the diagnosis, or when the upper limits of endocervical CIN cannot be seen. The accuracy of conization is determined by how many sections of the specimen the pathologist examines.

Conization is mandatory when (1) the upper limit of the lesion in the cervical canal cannot be seen, (2) CIN is diagnosed in tissue removed by endocervical curettage, and (3) biopsy does not confirm invasive or microinvasive cancer suggested by colposcopy or cytologic examination.

TREATMENT

Dysplasia. The justification for treating cervical dysplasia vigorously is that it may be a precursor of cancer. Eradication of the areas of abnormal cell growth reduces the likelihood of this occurring.

The first step is to map the abnormal areas by colposcopic examination and biopsy and endocervical curettage.

Small lesions, which have been diagnosed as CIN I or II and which are confined to the portio of the cervix and the lower cervical canal, can be destroyed by *laser vaporization, cryocautery,* or *thermal cautery.* The tissue destruction must be deep enough to destroy lesions that involve the cervical clefts and tunnels and must include the entire involved area. More extensive lesions can be eliminated by *conization,* which should be wide and deep enough to remove any abnormal tissue on the portio and as much of the cervical canal as possible. The advantage of conization is that multiple sections can be made and the entire lesion studied. Severe dysplasia usually should be treated in the same manner as carcinoma in situ.

If the entire lesion is not removed or destroyed, the remaining abnormal tissue may continue to proliferate. Even though the lesion is completely removed, it may recur because abnormal stimuli responsible for its growth may continue. This suggests that women who have been treated for dysplasia must be observed closely with regular cytologic examinations for life even though the original lesion has been eradicated.

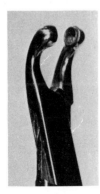

Fig. 46-13. One type of punch biopsy forceps that may provide adequate tissue to establish diagnosis of invasive carcinoma of cervix.

Carcinoma in situ. The justification for treating carcinoma in situ (CIN III) is that it is the immediate predecessor of invasive cancer. It is not a therapeutic emergency because there generally is an interval of months or years between its development and invasion. Even long delays before definitive treatment is applied can sometimes be justified.

Hysterectomy with conservation of the ovaries is usually the best treatment for carcinoma in situ of the cervix. This is a particularly appropriate operation in women who have had children and are no longer interested in childbearing. Hysterectomy does not completely eliminate the possibility of subsequent development of cancer. From 1% to 5% of women will develop another cancer in the vagina after hysterectomy. Since the new tumor may not appear for many years, patients who have been treated for carcinoma in situ must be followed up for life.

Cervical amputation, wide conization, laser vaporization, cauterization, and *cryosurgery* have all been recommended as an alternative to hysterectomy. Although they preserve menstrual and even childbearing functions, they provide less certain assurance of complete removal of the lesion than does hysterectomy.

Conization alone carries a significant risk of recurrence, even though the lesion is completely removed. The risk of cancer recurring after conization appears to be from 2% to 3%, but recurrence rates as high as 10% have been reported.

CIN III can be destroyed by *laser vaporization* with which lesions in the lower cervical canal, as well as those on the portio, can be eradicated. The failure rate may be as high as 10% with the first treatment, but this can be reduced to less than 5% by a second attempt.

Cryocautery appears to be less effective than laser in treating CIN III. Failure rates as high as 25% have been reported, probably because of failure to destroy the entire lesion on the portio, because the freeze in the canal does not penetrate deeply enough, or because the upper part of the lesion is not frozen. Furthermore, after cryocautery the squamocolumnar junction may retreat to a position within the cervical canal where it cannot be seen through the colposcope. This makes adequate follow-up difficult.

Extensive thermal cautery can also be used. This usually must be done under general anesthesia because cauterization necessary to destroy the lesion completely is too painful for most women to tolerate.

These forms of treatment are appropriate only for women who insist on retaining the reproductive function and who are willing to return at regular intervals for examination. All are more effective for small lesions on the portio or for those that extend only a short distance up the cervical canal than for those that are more extensive.

Occasionally, definitive treatment of carcinoma in situ can be delayed to permit pregnancy, but the extent of the lesion must be determined by colposcopy or diagnostic conization. This is particularly appropriate in childless women younger than 35 years of age. Cytologic studies and colposcopy are repeated at 3- to 6-month intervals while the patient is attempting to conceive. If studies suggest a shift toward invasive cancer, repeat conization should be advised.

It usually is easy to identify the transformation zone during pregnancy because the cervical canal is everted and is clearly visible. Colposcopic-directed biopsies can be taken even though bleeding is greater than in nonpregnant women. Conization during pregnancy carries a significant risk of hemorrhage and abortion and is not often indicated. The extent of the lesion can almost always be determined by colposcopy.

The patient in whom invasive cancer has been ruled out is observed closely throughout the prenatal period. Cytologic smears are obtained, and colposcopy is repeated every 2 months. Progressive changes constitute an indication for complete reassessment.

There is no evidence to suggest that vaginal delivery influences the course of carcinoma in situ adversely. Cesarean delivery is necessary only for obstetric indications. Elective cesarean hysterectomy can be considered for patients who want no more children.

Reevaluation of the lesion and definitive treatment can usually be delayed until involution is complete. Treatment may be delayed even longer if there is no evidence of residual tumor.

Invasive carcinoma. Invasive cancer of the cervix is most often treated by radiation therapy, but operation may be preferable for some. Patients with microinvasion, certain of those with stage I lesions, and those whose lesions either did not respond to radiation or recurred can be treated surgically.

Cancer of the female reproductive organs is best treated in centers that are equipped to provide all forms of cancer therapy. A therapeutic team made up of gynecologic oncologists and radiation therapists should be responsible for evaluating and directing the treatment of all women with invasive cancer. Survival figures for groups of patients treated in this manner are significantly better than for those who are treated by individual practitioners who have had limited experience in cancer therapy.

Pretreatment investigaton includes examination of the urinary tract by cystoscopy and intravenous pyelography to establish functional capacity and to detect any encroachment on the structures by the tumor. The bowel is studied by barium enema and sigmoidoscopy, and a chest x-ray film examination is obtained. Basic laboratory studies include hemoglobin and hematocrit, white blood cell count, blood urea nitrogen and serum creatinine concentrations, and urine examinations. Lymphangiograms or CT scans may be helpful in determining the extent of lymph node involvement (Fig. 46-14).

Radiation therapy. If radiation therapy is selected, the radiation therapist calculates the dose in rads to be delivered to the cervical tumor, the parametria, and the lateral pelvic wall where most of the lymph nodes are situated. Radiation is usually delivered from two sources:

radium or cesium, which is placed in the cervical canal and upper vagina (internal therapy), and supervoltage x-ray, telecobalt or linear accelerator, which is delivered to the pelvis through its walls (external therapy).

Radium or *cesium* is inserted into the cervical canal in tubes that are designed to filter out most of the alpha and beta rays while permitting the gamma rays to penetrate through the tumor. The effects of radiation from the cervical tandems are concentrated on the local lesion in the cervix, since its penetrating power is limited.

Additional sources are from ovoids placed lateral to the cervix in each lateral vaginal fornix. These are held in place by an applicator and tight vaginal packing. The effects of radiation from the vaginal containers is on the cervix medially, the parametrium adjacent to the cervix superiorly, and the vaginal wall and more distal parametrium laterally. One type of radium applicator with its ovoids for the vaginal sources and tandems for insertion into the cervical canal is shown in Fig. 46-15. An x-ray film of the radium in place is shown in Fig. 46-16.

The major effect of internal radiation is on the tumor in the cervix and in the nearby parametrium. An effective dose cannot be delivered to the lateral pelvic wall by radium alone.

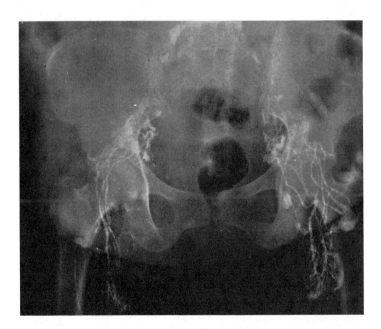

Fig. 46-14. Lymphoangiogram. Lymph nodes exhibit irregular defects. "Moth-eaten" appearance suggests extension of carcinoma to nodes.

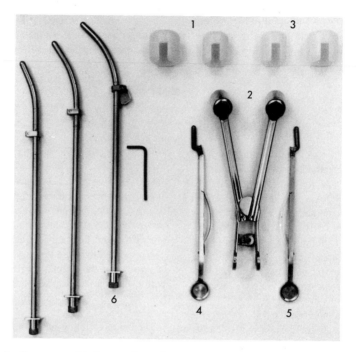

Fig. 46-15. Applicators used in intracavity radium therapy. *1* and *3*, Large and medium sleeves to fit over *2*, basic Fletcher applicator; *4* and *5*, steel tandems; *6*, plastic tandems.

External radiation is delivered to the pelvic structures through anterior portals over the lower abdomen and posterior portals over the lower back. The external radiation increases the dose delivered to the central portion of the lesion by the radium or cesium and also delivers a cancericidal dose to the lateral pelvis where the tumor may have spread.

The total dosage of radiation delivered by the two sources is planned to destroy the tumor whereever it is in the pelvis. Unfortunately, there is no accurate way to predict the response of individual tumors to radiation; some may respond to relatively small amounts, whereas others are much less easily affected. In most treatment plans a maximum of 10,000 rads is delivered to the central lesion by combined internal and external therapy and about 5000 rads to the lateral pelvic wall. The latter is almost entirely from the external source.

Since the beneficial effect of radiation is produced by tissue destruction and since there is no way to restrict the radiation to the tumor cells alone, normal tissue must inevitably be injured during radiation therapy. Fortunately, the *reactions* from well-planned and supervised treatment are usually not serious. Most women experi-

ence *diarrhea*, which starts after several days of treatment and is caused by irritation of the rectosigmoid. Generally, this is easily controlled with a low-fiber diet and antidiarrheal medication. Others may have some *bladder irritation* from the same source and, in addition, from urethrocystitis, which develops during radium implantation. This is treated with appropriate antimicrobial drugs.

Patients should be examined weekly while they are under treatment to evaluate the effects of the radiation.

Surgical therapy. The radical operation, which Wertheim introduced in 1898, now consists of removing the uterus and adnexa; the paracervical, parametrial, and upper paravaginal tissue; the upper vagina; and the pelvic lymph nodes. This procedure was used extensively until radiation therapy was improved enough to provide better results. Meigs revived radical hysterectomy and added regular complete and meticulous lymphadenectomy during the early 1940s. His total 5-year survival rate for women with stage I and II lesions was 78%; involvement of the lymph nodes reduced the rate to 26%, the same as for radiation in his clinic. Brunschwig and Daniel detected lymph node involvement of 13% in clinical

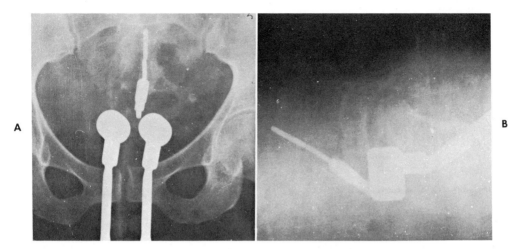

Fig. 46-16. Intracavity radium tandem in uterine canal and vaginal applicator with its two ovoids against lateral fornices. **A,** Anteroposterior view. **B,** Lateral view.

stage I patients, 30% in clinical stage II patients, and 46% in clinical stage III patients. Therefore it seems evident that well-designed radiation therapy is preferable to primary operation except for early lesions.

Operation is preferable for patients with *microinvasion,* in which there are focal areas of invasion that do not extend more than 3 mm into the stroma, and with which there is no evidence of lymphatic or vascular involvement. These women can be treated adequately with total abdominal hysterectomy without lymphadenectomy. Those with *small clinical stage I* lesions can be treated by radical hysterectomy and pelvic lymph node dissection, with results comparable to those with radiation. Since the ovaries can be preserved and the inevitable destructive effects of radiation on normal tissue avoided, operation is particularly appropriate for young women with limited lesions.

Radical surgical procedures are also appropriate when radiation therapy fails to halt tumor growth. Women who have undergone radiation therapy must be examined at monthly intervals for at least 6 months. If the cytologic analysis remains positive and tumor growth continues, an operation should be considered. Under these circumstances the operation may be a radical hysterectomy and node dissection (Fig. 46-17) or a far more radical procedure, depending on the extent of the lesion.

In a few patients, particularly those with recurrent disease, *pelvic exenteration operations* may be performed. With this operation, the uterus, vagina, pelvic lymph nodes, bladder, and rectum are removed. A co-

lostomy and ureteral diversion are essential. This is an extensive operation that is not often indicated. Morley and Lindenauer performed 70 exenterations with a surgical mortality of 2.8%. The 5-year survival rate in this group of patients, all of whom would otherwise have died of their tumors, was 61.8%; the 3-year survival rate was 63.6%.

Complications. Problems incident to surgery for carcinoma in situ are no different from those encountered with hysterectomy for other disease. Operative and postoperative complications resulting from radical hysterectomy and lymph node dissection for invasive cervical cancer occur frequently and may be lethal as well as annoying. Hemorrhage, infection, and urinary fistula formation are the most common problems encountered.

Radiation therapy also is attended by complications. For the most part, these affect the skin, large and small bowel, urinary tract, and fistula formation. Complications, whether associated with surgery or radiation, occur least often when treatment is carried out in a well-equipped center, staffed by qualified, well-trained individuals.

FOLLOW-UP CARE. Women who have been irradiated or operated on for cervical cancer require medical observation for the remainder of their lives.

Patients should be examined at monthly intervals during the first 6 months after treatment to assess the initial

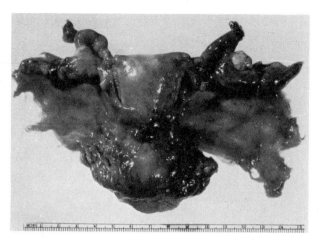

Fig. 46-17. Radical hysterectomy. Wide and deep dissection was necessary to remove parametrium and supporting structures.

effect of radiation on the tumor. If the cancer is resistant to radiation, *cytologic smears* will remain positive, and there will be palpable and perhaps visible evidence of continuing tumor growth. Induration in the paracervical areas, the uterosacral ligaments, and the base of the broad ligaments increases. Failure of response must be recognized early so that an attempt can be made to remove the tumor surgically before it becomes inoperable.

The majority of women treated for cervical cancer will, at the end of the first 6 months, show satisfactory response. Their cytologic smears will be normal and the cervix small, somewhat more mobile, and flush with the vaginal fornices. The supporting structures and paracervical and paravaginal areas will be smooth and fibrotic.

The time between follow-up appointments is then gradually lengthened, so that about 2 years from the completion of treatment, examinations are on a semiannual basis. Even though the initial response to therapy is satisfactory, the follow-up examiners must remain vigilant. Recurrence or regrowth may appear at any time.

The semiannual follow-up examination of a treated cancer patient should include an interval historic note and a reasonably complete physical examination. Taking a smear for cytologic evaluation is essential.

Of women being followed after treatment for one malignant growth, 5% to 8% develop another primary cancer. As many as five primary malignant

lesions have been seen in a woman treated for pelvic cancer.

Result of treatment. The most accurate method for evaluating and comparing the results of a treatment program for cervical cancer is the absolute survival rate, which makes no correction for the patients who die of conditions other than the cancer for which they were treated. Since most women who survive for at least 5 years after having been treated for cervical cancer will not have a recurrence of the original tumor, the basic figure generally used is the *5-year absolute survival rate.* The survival rate is determined by three principal factors: the extent of the lesion when treatment was started, the quality of the treatment, and the biologic response of the tumor.

According to the 1982 FIGO report the survival rates for 12,497 women treated for squamous cell cancer of the cervix in 82 institutions were:

	Radiotherapy only (percent)	Surgery alone or surgery combined with radiotherapy (percent)
Stage I	70.4	84.2
Stage II	52.4	68.6
Stage III	28.3	42.3
Stage IV	8.2	20

The survival for patients with adenocarcinoma was less for each stage.

Since these figures were derived from a number of different institutions in which there were variations in the quality of the treatment, they do not represent what can be achieved under the best of circumstances. Many clinics in the United States report higher survival rates, at least for the earlier stages of the disease.

PREGNANCY AND CERVICAL CANCER

Screening cytologic examination should be a part of each first prenatal examination, even though carcinoma of the cervix occurs only about once in every 2000 pregnant women. The procedure for further studies when the cytologist identifies abnormal cells is identical to that described for nonpregnant women: colposcopic-directed biopsies unless the lesion is obvious when direct biopsy may be appropriate. Conization is not often necessary and should be avoided if possible. Bleeding is profuse and difficult to control, and the membranes may be perforated during the operation or may rupture later, perhaps because of their proximity to the infected granulating cervix. The operation does not interfere with cervical dilatation during labor.

One may temporize in treating carcinoma in situ during pregnancy, but prompt treatment directed toward destroying the tumor is essential for invasive lesions.

Invasive cancer diagnosed during early pregnancy is treated much as though the patient were not pregnant and without regard for preserving the pregnancy. Lesions that are thought to be confined to the cervix can be treated by an appropriate surgical operation. Those that are more extensive are treated with radiation.

During approximately the first 20 to 22 weeks of gestation, external radiation is started despite the presence of the pregnancy. The fetus usually dies during the second or third week of treatment and is expelled from the uterus. External therapy is completed, and radium is applied after some involution has taken place.

If labor does not begin spontaneously, the uterus should be evacuated to permit proper radium application and because of the teratogenic effects of intensive radiotherapy.

If the pregnancy is so advanced that the infant has a reasonable chance of surviving, it should be delivered by cesarean section before radiation treatment is started.

This prevents fetal damage and also permits more adequate treatment of the tumor.

The results of treating carcinoma of the cervix during pregnancy are determined by the extent of the disease and the quality of the treatment rather than by the pregnancy. In most instances the outcome is the same or only slightly less successful than that in nongravid women.

CARE OF PATIENTS WITH ADVANCED DISEASE

Little can be done for patients in whom radiation or radical surgical procedures or both have failed to control the cancer. So far, no chemotherapeutic agent that will influence the growth of the tumor cells has been made available. As the disease advances, it invades the nerve roots, particularly the sciatic plexus, and constricts the ureters and possibly the rectosigmoid. Continued growth in the cervix itself produces a necrotic crater that may bleed with the slightest irritation. Death usually occurs from uremia caused by ureteral obstruction, infection, hemorrhage, or combinations of the three.

At this stage, one should prescribe whatever medications are needed to relieve pain and keep the patient reasonably comfortable. There is no place for heroic measures simply to prolong life.

PREVENTION

Invasive carcinoma of the cervix is a preventable disease. The proof of this statement is that the incidence of invasive cancer of the cervix decreased by 58% between the time of the second National Cancer Survey in 1947 and the third in 1970. There has been an even greater decrease in deaths. Bayes, Worth, and Anderson reported that in British Columbia the incidence of invasive cancer of the cervix in women over age 20 was reduced from 28.4/100,000 in 1955 to 7.6/100,000 in 1977, and that deaths declined from 11.4/100,000 to 3.8/100,000 during the same period.

The reduction has resulted principally from the increasing availability of screening cytologic analysis, which permits us to diagnose the disease in its earliest stages when it can almost certainly be cured.

The responsibility for early diagnosis rests with (1) *communities and public health services*, which must make screening facilities more readily available and acceptable, particularly to those women who are at greatest risk of developing the lesion; (2) *physicians,* who must provide the services for their patients; and (3) *patients* themselves, who must learn to assume more responsibility for their own health.

The controllable factors, in addition to periodic screening, include improved socioeconomic status, more concern for personal hygiene and cleanliness, and expanded sex education that should stress the relationship between coitus and cancer as well as between coitus and the other sexually transmitted diseases. Unless each individual assumes responsibility for minimizing the chances of developing cancer of the cervix and of detecting it in its earliest stages if it does develop, there will continue to be too many preventable deaths.

REFERENCES

Bayes, D.A., Worth, A.J., and Anderson, G.H.: Experience in cervical cancer screening in British Columbia, Gynecol. Oncol. **12:**143, 1981.

Bernstein, S.G., Voet, R.L., Guzick, D.S., et al.: Prevalence of papillomavirus infections in colposcopically directed biopsy specimens in 1972 and 1982, Am. J. Obstet. Gynecol. **151:**577, 1985.

Briggs, R.M.: Dysplasia and early neoplasia of the uterine cervix: a review, Obstet. Gynecol. Surv. **34:**70, 1979.

Brunschwig, A., and Daniel, W.W.: The surgical treatment of cancer of the cervix, Am. J. Obstet. Gynecol. **82:**60, 1961.

Burghardt, E., and Östör, A.G.: Site and origin of squamous cell cancer: a histomorphologic study, Obstet. Gynecol. **62:**117, 1983.

Catalano, L.W., and Johnson, L.D.: Herpesvirus antibody and carcinoma in situ of the cervix, J.A.M.A. **217:**447, 1971.

Czernobilsky, B., Zeituni, M., Lancet, M., et al.: The prevalence of cervicitis, reserve cell hyperplasia, squamous metaplasia, and cervical dysplasia in Jewish women, Obstet. Gynecol. **49:**587, 1977.

Dorman, S.A., Leigh, M.D., Wilson, D.J., et al.: Detection of chlamydial cervicitis by Papaniocolaou stained smears and cultures, Am. J. Clin. Pathol. **79:**421, 1983.

FIGO: annual report of the results of treatment in gynecologic cancer, vol. 18, Stockholm, 1982, Radiumhemmet.

Gallup, D.G., and Abell, M.R.: Invasive adenocarcinoma of the uterine cervix, Obstet. Gynecol. **49:**596, 1977.

Hacker, N.F., Berek, J.S., and Lagasse, L.D.: Carcinoma of the cervix associated with pregnancy, Obstet. Gynecol. **58:**735, 1982.

Jones, E.G., MacDonald, I., and Breslow, L.: A study of epidemiologic factors in carcinoma of the uterine cervix, Am. J. Obstet. Gynecol. **76:**1, 1958.

Kessler, I.I.: Venereal factors in cervical cancer, Cancer **39:**1912, 1977.

Kleger, B., Prier, J.E., Rosato, D.J., and McGinnis, A.E.: Herpes simplex infection of the female genital tract, I. Incidence of infection, Am. J. Obstet. Gynecol. **102:**745, 1968.

Linhartova, A.: Extent of columnar epithelium on the ectocervix between the ages of 1 and 13 years, Obstet. Gynecol. **52:**451, 1978.

Meigs, J.V.: Wertheim operation for carcinoma of the cervix, Am. J. Obstet. Gynecol. **49:**542, 1945.

Morley, G.W., and Lindenauer, S.M.: Pelvic exenterative therapy for gynecologic malignancy, Cancer **38:**581, 1976.

Naib, Z.M., Nahmais, A.J., Josey, W.E., and Kramer, J.H.: Genital herpetic infection: association with cervical dysplasia and carcinoma, Cancer **23:**940, 1969.

Nelson, J.H., Jr., Averette, H.E., and Richart, R.M.: Dysplasia, carcinoma in situ, and early invasive cervical carcinoma, CA **344:**306, 1984.

Papanicolaou, G.N., and Traut, N.F.: Diagnosis of uterine cancer by vaginal smears, New York, 1943, The Commonwealth Fund.

Peyton, F.W., Peyton, R.R., Anderson, V.L., and Pavnica, P.: The importance of cauterization to maintain a healthy cervix, Am. J. Obstet. Gynecol. **131:**374, 1978.

Reid, R., Stanhope, C.R., Herschman, B.R., et al.: Genital warts and cervical cancer. I. Evidence of an association between subclinical papilloma-viral infections and cervical malignancy, Cancer **50:**377, 1982.

Rome, R.M., Urcuyo, R., and Nelson, J.H., Jr.: Observations on the surface area of the abnormal transformation zone associated with intraepithelial and early invasive squamous cell lesions of the cervix, Am. J. Obstet. Gynecol. **129:**565, 1977.

Rotkin, I.D.: Epidemiology of cancer of the cervix. III. Sexual characteristics of a cervical cancer population, Am. J. Public Health **57:**815, 1967.

Roy, M., Morin, C., Casas-Cordero, M., and Meisels, A.: Human papillomavirus and cervical lesions, Clin. Obstet. Gynecol. **26:**949, 1983.

Sadeghi, S.B., Hseih, E.W., and Gunn, S.W.: Prevalence of cervical intraepithelial neoplasia in sexually active teenagers and young adults, Am. J. Obstet. Gynecol. **148:**726, 1984.

Shingleton, H.M., Gore, H., and Austin, J.M., Jr.: Outpatient evaluation of patients with atypical Papanicolaou smears: contribution of endocervical curettage, Am. J. Obstet. Gynecol. **126:**122, 1976.

Syrjänen, K.J.: Current concepts of human papillomavirus infections in the genital tract and their relationship to intraepithelial neoplasia and squamous cell carcinoma, Obstet. Gynecol. Surv. **39:**252, 1984.

J. Robert Willson

Benign and malignant diseases of the uterus

BENIGN DISEASES

The benign lesions that most often enlarge the uterus are multiple leiomyomas, symmetric hypertrophy of the muscular walls, and adenomyosis. Of these, leiomyomas are by far the most common.

LEIOMYOMAS

Benign uterine leiomyomas, also called *myomas, fibromyomas,* or, more commonly, *fibroids,* can be found in the uteri of 30% to 50% of all women past 30 years of age. They occur more often, appear at an earlier age, and grow more luxuriantly in black than in white women. Although they are often encountered in nulliparas, many women with fibroids are highly fertile.

Pathologic findings

The tumors probably develop from immature smooth-muscle cells of the uterine wall. The smallest ones are made up almost entirely of muscle, but strands of fibrous tissue appear between the bundles of unstriated muscle as the tumor enlarges. In some tumors the fibrous tissue predominates. Leiomyomas, although well circumscribed, have no true capsule; a layer of compressed uterine muscle surrounding each neoplasm forms a pseudocapsule.

The tumors may occur singly, but they more often are multiple. They vary in size from those that are visible only under the microscope to huge masses that almost fill the abdominal cavity. They may occupy any portion of the uterine wall. When sectioned, they are firm and white, and the whorled, trabeculated muscular bundles are characteristic.

The tumor types are designated according to their position in the uterine wall (Fig. 47-1). *Submucous* tumors lie beneath the endometrium and protrude into the uterine cavity. If there are many fibroids in this area or if they are large, the endometrial cavity may be tremendously enlarged and distorted. *Intramural* or *interstitial* tumors occupy the central portion of the uterine wall, whereas those of the *subserous* variety lie beneath the peritoneal covering and protrude into the abdominal cavity. If the tumors are predominantly intramural or subserous, they may grow to a remarkable size without altering the size and shape of the uterine cavity. However, intramural tumors that grow toward the center of the uterus rather than toward the peritoneal surface may enlarge and distort the endometrial cavity as much as do the subserous types. *Cervical* fibroids develop from the musculature of the cervical portion of the uterus (Fig. 47-2). Tumors that grow laterally between the leaves of the broad ligament are called *intraligamentous.*

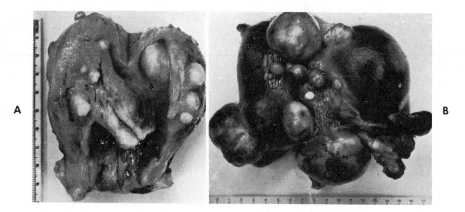

Fig. 47-1. Types of fibroid tumors. **A,** Large submucous tumor projecting into cavity of opened uterus and smaller one near left cornu. Several intramural tumors also are visible. **B,** Subserous fibroids of varying sizes on surface of unopened uterus that also contains large intramural tumors.

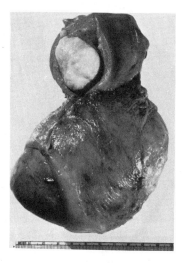

Fig. 47-2. Large cervical fibroid. Small opened uterus containing white submucous tumor can be seen at top of specimen. Large mass is cervical fibroid that can be seen protruding through dilated external os at left.

Submucous, subserous, and cervical myomas, particularly those located near the surface, can become *pedunculated* as they gradually grow away from the myometrium. Occasionally, a subserous growth loses its connection to the uterus completely and becomes a *wandering* or *parasitic* fibroid, deriving its blood supply from the omentum or some other extrapelvic source.

Degenerative changes. The blood supply, which comes through the pseudocapsule from the vessels in the uterine wall rather than by way of a single blood vessel, frequently becomes inadequate as the tumor enlarges; as a result degenerative changes are common. In *hyaline degeneration,* the type most often observed, the fibrous and muscle tissues are partially or completely replaced by hyaline tissue, which grossly is smooth, relatively soft, and lacks the usual whorl-like appearance. Under the microscope the hyalinized areas are homogeneously pink stained and may be completely acellular. *Cystic degeneration* or *liquefaction* occurs when the hyaline material breaks down from a further reduction in blood supply (Fig. 47-3). With *calcification,* which occurs most often after the menopause, the tumor may be stonelike because of a deposition of calcium; this type of tumor can often be detected by x-ray film examination (Fig. 47-4). *Fatty degeneration* is rare.

Necrosis of a tumor may occur if its blood supply is compromised. This is most often encountered when pedunculated tumors twist on their pedicles, completely occluding the vessels, but it may also happen in rapidly growing leiomyomas of other types. Necrotic submucous tumors often become secondarily *infected.*

Red, or *carneous, degeneration* occurs during pregnancy and affects at least half of all fibroids in gravid women. When sectioned, the tumor bulges out of its bed, and the characteristic dark red color produced by hemorrhage into the tissue is obvious (Fig. 47-5).

Sarcomatous degeneration occurs in about 1/1000 (0.1%) leiomyomas. The cut surface is pink and soft and

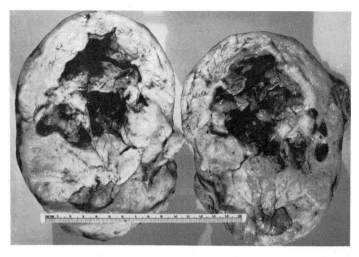

Fig. 47-3. Cystic degeneration in large pedunculated fibroid.

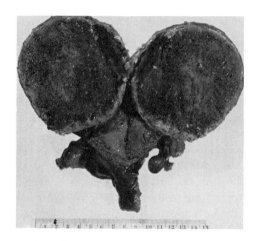

Fig. 47-4. Large, hard, calcified fibroid.

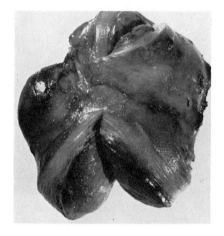

Fig. 47-5. Red degeneration in fibroids in postpartum uterus. Color is dark, and cut surface of tumor bulges out.

has been compared to the appearance of raw pork. Later the tissue may become friable with ragged cavitation in the center.

Etiologic factors

The cause of leiomyomas is unknown, but the growth of the tumor is in some way related to stimulation by estrogen. This theory is supported by the fact that the tumors do not often occur before the ovaries have functioned for several years and that growth usually ceases after the menopause. In addition, rapid enlargement of leiomyomas occurred in some women who were taking the early oral contraceptive pills, which contained relatively large amounts of estrogen. This rarely happens with the present low-dosage forms.

Farber and colleagues found that tissue from leiomyomas bound 20% more estradiol per milligram of cytoplasmic protein than did normal endometrium. Spellacy could detect no difference in plasma estradiol concentrations in women with leiomyomas as compared to those with normal uteri. Otubu and associates found significantly higher concentrations of estradiol in leiomyomas than in normal endometrium. Estrone concentrations were slightly higher in myometrium than in tumors, but progesterone concentrations were similar. Gabb and Stone could detect no differences in estradiol-to-estrone conversion in myomas as compared to myometrium. Pollow and associates, however, found conversion to be lower in tumor tissue than in myometrium. Deligdish and Loewenthal and Farrer-Brown, Beilby, and Tarbit reported that glandular hyperplasia can be found regularly in the endometrium adjacent to submucous myomas. This suggests locally increased concentrations of estrogen.

Wilson, Yang, and Rees found a significant increase in cytoplasmic estrogen receptors in leiomyomas as compared to myometrium from the same patients, but they did not relate the receptor concentrations to the stage of the menstrual cycle. Soules and McCarty found more estrogen receptors in tumor tissue than in myometrium during the first 18 days of normal menstrual cycles. Concentrations were similar in both tissues during the postovulatory phase.

Although none of these studies clarifies the exact cause of leiomyomas, they do support the relationship of their growth to estrogen.

Signs and symptoms

Symptoms vary with the size and location of the tumors. Some huge growths cause no discomfort or disturbance of the menstrual pattern, whereas much smaller ones may produce severe pain or exsanguinating hemorrhage.

Bleeding. An alteration in menstrual bleeding is the most frequent single symptom produced by uterine fibroids. *The characteristic bleeding pattern associated with leiomyomas is excessive or prolonged flow or both, with little if any change in the cycle.* As the tumors enlarge, the amount of bleeding increases, but the change may occur so gradually that the patient is not aware of the increasing flow.

Abnormal bleeding is almost always caused by submucous or intramural tumors that enlarge and distort the uterine cavity. Subserous tumors, even the largest ones, which do not alter the size and shape of the endometrial cavity, are ordinarily not accompanied by abnormal bleeding.

The source of the bleeding is the endometrium, and the mechanism is the same as that responsible for menstruation in the normal uterus. The endometrial glands and stroma respond to the changes in ovarian hormone levels in the same manner as in normal women. The excessive bleeding is at least in part caused by the increased endometrial surface in the uterus containing a number of large submucous tumors. Sehgal and Haskins found that the endometrial surface area may increase from about 15 cm^2 in normal uteri to as much as 200 cm^2 in those with myomas. An additional factor, described by Farrer-Brown, Beilby, and Tarbit, is an increase in the number and size of endometrial veins in association with submucous tumors. This may be a result of abnormal hormone stimulation or of pressure from the tumors.

Acyclic bleeding can occur in women with myomas as a result of infected or ulcerated submucous tumors, hormonal disturbances (dysfunctional bleeding), or cervical or endometrial cancer; however, *uncomplicated leiomyomas do not cause intermenstrual or postmenopausal bleeding.*

Pressure and pain. Many women experience increasing pressure on the bladder and frequency of urination as the tumors grow. Occasionally a large tumor in the anterior uterine wall will push the fundus posteriorly into the cul-de-sac and rotate the cervix anteriorly beneath the pubis where it compresses the vesicle neck. As the tumor grows it becomes progressively more difficult to initiate urination, and finally complete obstruction may occur. Large posterior wall tumors may fill the cul-de-sac, making it difficult to evacuate the rectum.

Pain may indicate that the tumor itself is degenerated, twisted, or infected or that it is pressing on another organ or on the pelvic nerve roots. Small tumors may cause more symptoms than large ones if they are located where they can exert pressure on sensitive areas.

Dysmenorrhea. Severe, cramping, laborlike pains may occur as the uterus attempts to expel a pedunculated submuous tumor. However, dysmenorrhea is not usually a characteristic symptom of fibroids.

Infertility. Many women with leiomyomas are infertile, but it is not always possible to relate the presence of the tumors to the failure to conceive, because other women with tumors of equal size or larger are normally fertile. Occasionally, growths in the cornual areas distort the fallopian tubes or disturb their function, but more often the lumina are patent. Some women experience long periods of infertility before small fibroids are first detected, making the presence of the tumors an unlikely etiologic factor.

Spontaneous abortion occurs more frequently in those who do conceive, perhaps because the implantation site is near or on a submucous myoma where the endometrium cannot respond appropriately. *Premature delivery* also occurs more often.

Diagnosis

The diagnosis is made by abdominal and bimanual palpation of the uterus, which is enlarged and nodular as a result of the presence of numerous leiomyomas. The tumors vary in size from some that are too small to be detected by physical examination to those that are 15 to 20 cm or more in diameter. Individual myomas are smooth, firm, and nontender, unless they have degenerated. The uterine mass may be fixed or freely movable, depending on the size and location of the neoplasms.

Differential diagnosis. Several pelvic lesions are at least superficially similar to uterine fibroids.

CANCER. Endometrial and cervical carcinomas cause irregular intermenstrual bleeding and develop in fibroid uteri as often as in those that are normal. Benign uterine tumors do not predispose to the development of cancer. Necrotic, bleeding, pedunculated, submucous tumors protruding through a normal but dilated external os may look much like cervical carcinoma. Malignancy should be excluded by cytologic examination, dilatation and curettage, and cervical biopsy in women with irregular or postmenopausal bleeding before they are treated for fibroids.

PREGNANCY. Large, soft leiomyomas, particularly large single tumors growing on the fundus of the uterus, may simulate pregnancy, and women with uterine fibroids may conceive. Most errors in diagnosis are made because the history of amenorrhea, and the softening of the cervix and the lower part of the uterus are ignored. Even a remote possibility of pregnancy should be eliminated by pregnancy test or sonography before the patient is operated on (Chapter 26).

OVARIAN NEOPLASMS. These tumors usually are separate from the uterus, but it my be difficult to differentiate a pedunculated fibroid from a solid ovarian neoplasm. The symptoms produced by either an ovarian neoplasm or a pedunculated leiomyoma twisting on its pedicle are similar, and degenerated or cystic fibroids situated in the lateral uterine wall or those that are pedunculated may simulate cystic ovarian tumors. Neoplasms of the ovary usually do not alter the menstrual cycle, whereas increased bleeding occurs frequently with uterine fibroids.

Treatment

There are several methods for treating women with uterine fibroids, and the one selected will be determined by the age, parity, and physical condition of the patient; the size of the tumors; and the symptoms they produce. Cancer must always be suspected if the bleeding is irregular, intermenstrual, or postmenopausal and can be excluded by dilatation and curettage and cervical biopsy. Anemia can be corrected by iron therapy or, if it is profound enough, by blood transfusion.

Observation. As a general rule, leiomyomas of almost any size need not be treated unless they are producing symptoms, because they do not predispose to malignancy, seldom undergo malignant degeneration, and do not interfere with the functions of other pelvic organs. Active treatment can be instituted at any time if symptoms develop or if the tumors begin to enlarge rapidly. In the majority of cases, active treatment never becomes necessary. If the enlarged uterus fills the pelvic cavity, it may exert pressure on the ureters. X-ray film pyelography should be ordered if large tumors are to be observed.

Observation is especially appropriate for women near the menopause because, after ovarian function ceases, bleeding will stop and the uterine mass will no longer grow and may become smaller. Fibroid tumors in postmenopausal women rarely need to be removed unless they continue to grow.

One need not change the schedule of periodic examinations after the menopause in women known to have uterine fibroids. No special examinations are necessary unless the tumors continue to grow or symptoms appear. Conversely, if a pelvic tumor is found in a postmenopausal woman whom one has never examined before, a more precise diagnosis must be made. It is impossible by physical examination alone to differentiate a benign uterine fibroid from an ovarian neoplasm. Sonography may be helpful; if not, a diagnostic laparoscopy will usually provide the necessary information.

Surgical removal. Large fibroids and those that produce symptoms should usually be removed.

Myomectomy, or the removal of individual tumors from the uterine wall, should be considered for young women in whom it is desirable to maintain both menstruation and reproductive function. This operation is of particular value in the management of pedunculated, subserous, and submucous tumors. Myomectomy occasionally corrects infertility, but it should be reserved for those in whom all other possible factors have been eliminated. Myomectomy should be considered for young women who have had no children and who do not plan to become pregnant for several years. If the tumors are not removed, they may grow enough to be a factor in infertility or to increase the risk of pregnancy complications.

The removal of the tumors alone, except the pedunculated submucous variety in an otherwise normal uterus, may not alter excessive bleeding. If bleeding occurs irregularly, and if endometrial biopsy a few days before an anticipated period of bleeding is productive of proliferative endometrium or of benign hyperplastic endometrium (dysfunctional bleeding), hysterectomy is a preferred procedure, because the bleeding is probably caused by an endocrine disorder rather than by the tumors.

Although most myomectomies are performed through abdominal incisions, small submucous tumors can sometimes be removed by *hysteroscopic resection*. Obviously, such operations should be attempted only by those with considerble experience in hysteroscopic surgical procedures.

Leiomyomas recur, or those that are overlooked grow, in about 15% of women after myomectomy. About 10% of these will require treatment, either repeat myomectomy or hysterectomy. Treatment usually is not necessary when myomectomy has been performed after ages 35 to 40. The remaining tumors grow slowly and they probably will not cause symptoms before the menopause occurs.

Hysterectomy, or removal of the uterus, is the operative procedure most often selected for the treatment of fibroid tumors. It is indicated for large and multiple tumors producing considerable distortion of the uterine cavity, for those that have grown rapidly, for those accompanied by profuse and irregular bleeding, and for those producing pressure symptoms. In young women, one or both ovaries should be left in place if they appear normal.

Special problems in treatment

Pedunculated submucous fibroids. Pedunculated submucous fibroids occasionally grow to a diameter of 10 to 12 cm, and they often undergo necrosis and become infected. The patient may experience severe, cramping, laborlike pains and profuse bleeding during the menses as the uterus attempts to expel the tumor. If the infected tumor protrudes through the dilated cervix, it should usually be removed vaginally after preliminary treatment with an antibiotic preparation and, when necessary, blood transfusion. If there are no other fibroids in the uterus, further treatment may not be necessary; but if hysterectomy is required, it usually should not be performed until the residual uterine infection has been eliminated.

Degeneration and infection. Degenerative changes and subsequent infection usually develop because of interference with the blood supply to the tumor. If the blood flow is obstructed, antibiotic preparations cannot reach the tumor. Consequently, removal is necessary before the surrounding intraabdominal structures become involved in the inflammatory process.

Sarcomatous degeneration. Malignant degeneration in a fibroid tumor seldom occurs, but it should be suspected whenever a rapid increase in size is detected. Prompt removal of rapidly growing tumors is indicated.

Contraception

Although estrogen appears to be the responsible factor in the growth of leiomyomas, their presence does not contraindicate the use of *oral contraceptives* with low estrogen content or those containing only progesterone.

HYPERTROPHY

Another type of uterine enlargement is that termed *diffuse symmetric hypertrophy* (Fig. 47-6); the uterus is smooth, heavy, enlarged, and frequently retrodisplaced. Menstruation is often excessive, and the patient may experience moderate-to-severe discomfort and pressure, particularly when the pelvic structures are congested before and during menses.

Because this syndrome is usually encountered in multiparous women, the uterine enlargement has been attributed to chronic subinvolution. That this is not always the case is indicated by the fact that the same change occasionally occurs in nulliparous women with chronic retrodisplacements. Taylor has termed this the congestion-fibrosis syndrome and believes that an emotional disturbance plays an important part in the genesis of the symptoms.

Dilatation and curettage usually is indicated to eliminate the possibility of carcinoma and small submucous fibroids, and the procedure may sometimes control the bleeding, at least temporarily. If the bleeding and dis-

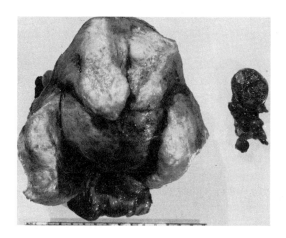

Fig. 47-6. Diffuse symmetric hypertrophy of uterus. Note thickness of walls and absence of fibroids. Uterus was removed because of persistent excessive bleeding.

comfort cannot be controlled by relatively simple means, hysterectomy may be considered.

ADENOMYOSIS

Adenomyosis, a benign uterine condition in which endometrial glands and stroma are found deep in the myometrium, is often considered to be a form of endometriosis, but they probably are not related disorders. The frequency with which adenomyosis is diagnosed depends largely on how many sections of uterine wall are studied. The reported incidence varies from about 10% of all hysterectomies to about 90%. It is diagnosed most often in women between the ages of 40 and 50.

The histogenesis is not entirely clear, but adenomyosis is related in some way to estrogen stimulation, particularly when the action of estrogen is unopposed by progesterone. The cells in the basal portions of the endometrial glands grow downward between the myometrial muscle bundles and may lose their connection to the uterine cavity. The lesions are usually diffuse with patches of endometrial tissue scattered throughout the entire thickness of the uterine wall. The process may be extensive enough to enlarge the uterus, but not often beyond a size comparable to a pregnancy of 8 to 10 weeks. Occasionally, the process may be more circumscribed with the formation of a distinct nodule, an *adenomyoma*, but this is much less common than is diffuse involvement. Adenomyosis is often associated with uterine fibroids.

The ectopic endometrial tissue responds to variations in ovarian estrogen concentration, but, like the epithelium in the bases of the glands from which it originates, it is less active than are the more superficial portions of the endometrial glands and stroma. It does not often undergo a progestational change.

The most frequently reported symptoms are *colicky secondary dysmenorrhea* and *abnormal bleeding,* but many women with adenomyosis have no symptoms. The pain is caused by first swelling and then hemorrhage in the uterine wall as the confined patches of endometrium grow under the stimulus of a rising estrogen concentration and then disintegrate and bleed as the stimulus is withdrawn. Excessive bleeding may reflect the expanding endometrial surface as the uterus enlarges. Increased and irregular bleeding may also occur because of ovulatory failure (dysfunctional bleeding).

The diagnosis is suspected in a woman over 40 who complains of increasingly severe dysmenorrhea and excessive bleeding if the uterus is enlarged and tender. Oral contraceptives relieve the pain of ordinary dysmenorrhea and that associated with endometriosis, but these preparations have little effect on the pain associated with adenomyosis.

The only uniformly successful treatment for adenomyosis is hysterectomy. However, operation will not be necessary if the menopause can be expected to occur soon and if the dysmenorrhea can be controlled. The symptoms will disappear after ovarian hormone secretion ceases. Replacement estrogen therapy is not contraindicated.

MALIGNANT DISEASES

The comparative incidences of cancers involving the female reproductive organs have changed considerably. Formerly, carcinoma of the cervix and carcinoma of the body of the uterus (endometrial carcinoma) were diagnosed in a ratio of at least 4:1. There now are more endometrial than cervical cancers. It is estimated that 37,000 new invasive cancers of the body of the uterus and 15,000 new invasive cancers of the cervix were diagnosed in 1985.

According to Walker and Jick, endometrial cancer rates for women between the ages of 50 and 59 peaked in 1975 at 133/100,000 women at risk per year. The rates then began to drop, reaching 72 in 1978, the same rate as in 1970. Rates for women between the ages of 60 and 69 and for those over 70 have continued to rise. This change has occurred in all parts of the United States.

Although carcinoma of the endometrium can occur at any age, it is most common in women past age 50 with the median age being about 61; 75% of women with corpus cancer are postmenopausal. This is in contrast to cervical cancer, which occurs in younger women. The incidence of carcinoma of the cervix is 14.5/100,000 women between the ages of 25 and 29 years, whereas that of endometrial cancer in the same age range is 1.1/100,000 and does not reach 14/100,000 women until ages 40 to 44 years.

Because endometrial cancer occurs in an older age group, it often is complicated by degenerative conditions such as hypertensive cardiovascular disease, obesity, and diabetes. These and other medical complications add immeasurably to the problem of establishing an adequate treatment program.

ETIOLOGIC FACTORS

The etiologic factors responsible for the development of endometrial carcinoma are different from those causing carcinoma of the cervix. In addition to the *age difference,* the ratio of black to white women who develop the disease is reversed. The age-adjusted incidence for corpus cancer in black women is 12.2/100,000 women and for white women, 21.6. Comparable figures for carcinoma of the cervix are 33.6 and 15/100,000 women.

Carcinoma of the cervix is a disease that affects poor women more often than those who are more affluent. Cancer of the endometrium occurs *predominantly in middle- and upper-class women. Jewish women* do not often develop cervical cancer, but they are not protected against endometrial carcinoma.

Estrogen is in some way implicated in the pathogenesis of carcinoma of the endometrium, but its exact role has not been clarified.

Endometrial cancer develops more often in women with *estrogen-secreting ovarian neoplasms* and in young women with *polycystic ovarian disease* than in women with normally functioning ovaries. In each of these conditions the effects of estrogen are unopposed by progesterone.

Until the 1960s estrogen was used extensively to control climacteric symptoms, but for limited periods of time. The dosage was usually decreased gradually after the flushes were brought under control; most women were able to stop using the drug after 2 to 3 years. The concept of "estrogen forever" was introduced because more women were living longer and were subject to the atrophic changes related to estrogen deficiency during the many years after they stopped menstruating. The coincidence of the remarkable increase in estrogen use by perimenopausal and postmenopausal women and a steady rise in the incidence of endometrial cancer prompted numerous investigators to seek a connection. Most reports indicated that estrogen does increase the risk of developing endometrial cancer at least three to four times and as much as tenfold. These studies also indicated that the cancer rate increased only after estrogen had been used for from 3 to 5 years. Before this the incidence was similar to that for nonusers of the same age. Both patients and doctors became concerned, and estrogen use decreased. This was followed by a nationwide fall in the incidence of endometrial cancer.

Other observations suggest that estrogen plays a role in the genesis of uterine cancer. There are reports of endometrial cancer developing in women with gonadal dysgenesis who have taken estrogenic substances for many years. Peterson, studying 32 women under age 40 with endometrial cancer, found that 26 were obese, 16 had never been pregnant, and 26 had grossly irregular or anovulatory bleeding. Many of these women must have had long exposures to excessive and unopposed estrogen stimulation.

The results of most studies suggest that the *major risk factor is long-term unopposed exposure to estrogen. Cancer is less likely to develop in those whose endometria are stimulated periodically by progesterone.*

Many studies of hormone excretion patterns have been made in women with endometrial hyperplasia and carcinoma of the endometrium. Hausknecht and Gusberg and MacDonald and Siiteri have studied extragonadal conversion of Δ 4-androstenedione to estrogen in postmenopausal women. Their findings indicate that the major conversion is to estrone and that the conversion rate is increased over the normal in women with benign postmenopausal bleeding. There is a further increase in women with endometrial cancer. Sall and Calanog reported that the excretion pattern of steroid metabolites is the same in women with benign postmenopausal bleeding and normal women of the same age. Conversely, the excretion of androsterone in women with endometrial hyperplasia and carcinoma is lower than that of normal women. This may represent extragonadal conversion of androgenic substances to estrogen and continued low-level stimulation of the endometrium by the latter hormone. Nisker and colleagues found a significant elevation in free serum estradiol in women with endometrial cancer as compared with that in control subjects. They attribute this to a decreased sex hormone–binding globulin capacity. Since only free estradiol is biologically

active, an increase in activity might be related to the induction of uterine cancer.

The fact that estrogen stimulates benign and adenomatous hyperplastic changes in normal-appearing endometrium is well known. These changes usually regress when the stimulus is withdrawn. Since similar hyperplastic changes precede frank endometrial cancer, it seems likely that estrogen can actually induce a malignant change if the endometrium is biologically prepared to respond to the stimulus. Estrogen is probably not the "cause" of endometrial cancer, but its long-term stimulation may well induce the lesion in certain susceptible women.

It had been said that the prototype woman who is most likely to develop endometrial cancer is obese, hypertensive, and diabetic. Recent studies suggest that this may not be true. Lucas and Yen could find no differences in carbohydrate metabolism between 16 thin women with endometrial cancer and control subjects. Although hypertension appears to be somewhat more prevalent in women with carcinoma of the endometrium than in those who are normal, its effect is not clear-cut. Hulka and colleagues, for example, found that nonobese, nonhypertensive women had the greatest risk of developing endometrial cancer after long-term estrogen therapy.

All studies implicate obesity as the principal metabolic disturbance in women with endometrial cancer. Since fat is a major site in which androgenic steroids are converted to estrogen, obese women are subjected to higher levels of estrogen than are those at or below normal weight. According to Hulka and associates, the addition of exogenous estrogen does not increase the risk of obese women developing uterine cancer.

One might then suspect that the woman most likely to develop carcinoma of the endometrium is postmenopausal and obese. She may have had a long history of ovarian dysfunction, as indicated by infertility and abnormal bleeding associated with anovulation. She may also have hypertension or diabetes, but these probably are coincidental. The greatest risk is from obesity.

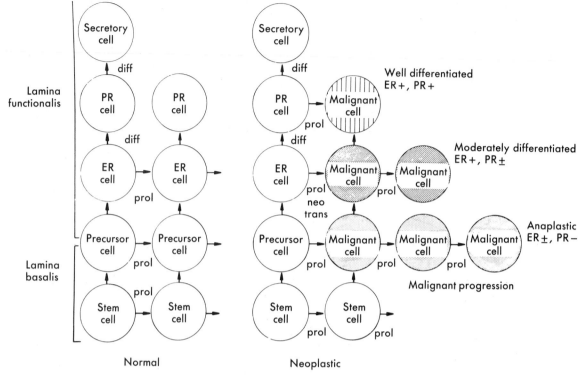

Fig. 47-7. Origin of endometrial cancer from abnormal stem cell differentiation. *PR,* Progesterone receptor; *ER,* estrogen receptor; *diff,* differentiation; *prol,* proliferation; *neo trans,* neoplastic transformation. (From Satyaswaroop, P.G., and Mortel, R.: Am. J. Obstet. Gynecol. **140:**620, 1981.)

Satyaswaroop and Mortel have proposed a model designed to explain the development of carcinoma of the endometrium (Fig. 47-7). It is based on the concentrations of estrogen and progesterone receptors in endometrial cells and on the effects of reproductive hormones during normal menstrual cycles. The regeneration of endometrium after a menstrual period begins by proliferation of estrogen-responsive precursor cells in the basalis. As these cells proliferate, estrogen and then progesterone receptors develop. These receptors permit the cells to respond to the reproductive hormones. Satyaswaroop and Mortel suggest that endometrial carcinoma begins by abnormal proliferation of either precursor cells or of those more highly differentiated. Tumors that originate in precursor cells are anaplastic and have no progesterone receptors. Those that are moderately differentiated come from cells that have well-developed estrogen receptors and some progesterone receptors. The well-differentiated tumors contain both. Although this is

an attractive theory, it still does not explain why cells develop abnormally.

PATHOLOGIC FINDINGS

Cancer of the endometrium, like malignant lesions in other anatomic areas, is preceded by abnormal cell changes, which are comparable to those observed in basal cells before the development of invasive cervical cancer.

Retrospective studies of endometrium obtained during bleeding episodes that preceded the development of endometrial carcinoma indicate a progression from normal-appearing proliferative endometrium through *cystic hyperplasia* to *adenomatous hyperplasia* (Fig. 47-8). With the latter lesion the gland cells are overactive, and the glands, which lie back to back, may be dilated or

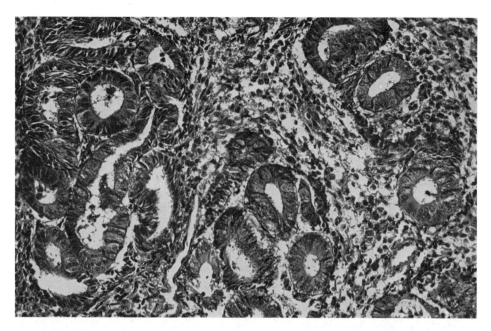

Fig. 47-8. Adenomatous hyperplasia of endometrium. Glands are dilated and in their characteristic back-to-back position.

irregularly shaped, with papillary projections into the lumina. The individual cells are fairly well oriented to each other, but the nuclei may be hyperchromatic, and mitoses may be present.

As the process advances, more cellular evidences of malignancy can be detected. At the stage of *atypical hyperplasia,* or *carcinoma in situ* (Fig. 47-9), the cells are larger and more disoriented, and the nuclei often are eccentrically placed and irregular in size and staining characteristics. The stromal cells are not affected. This change is followed by invasive cancer.

With few exceptions, malignancy of the uterine body is an *adenocarcinoma*. This lesion may be so anaplastic that there is complete loss of glandular pattern. Conversely, some are so well differentiated that it may be difficult to differentiate them from atypical hyperplasia.

Invasive endometrial carcinoma is of two types: circumscribed and diffuse (Fig. 47-10). In the more common *circumscribed adenocarcinoma*, malignancy starts as a small local growth and invades the myometrium faster than it spreads laterally across the endometrium.

In *diffuse adenocarcinoma,* the growth starts as a superficial and almost uniform condition and may penetrate the myometrium slowly. It often is almost entirely removed by diagnostic curettage. This type of cancer causes enlargement of the uterine body earlier than does circumscribed neoplasm.

Although most endometrial cancers are pure adenocarcinomas, an increasing number with a squamous component are being recognized. The squamous epithelium apparently develops as a metaplastic change in glandular basal cells. Adenosquamous tumors in which benign-appearing squamous epithelium is mixed with adenocarcinoma are called *adenoacanthomas*. Those in which both components are malignant are called *mixed* or *adenosquamous carcinomas*. Most reports suggest that mixed carcinomas are more aggressive and respond less well to treatment than do pure adenocarcinomas.

Secondary carcinoma of the corpus uteri may develop from metastases from carcinoma of the ovary, breast, or gastrointestinal tract. Women with carcinoma of the stomach may present no symptoms other than uterine bleeding from a metastatic lesion.

Sarcoma. Sarcoma of the uterus is rare and may arise either in fibroids or in otherwise normal muscle (Fig.

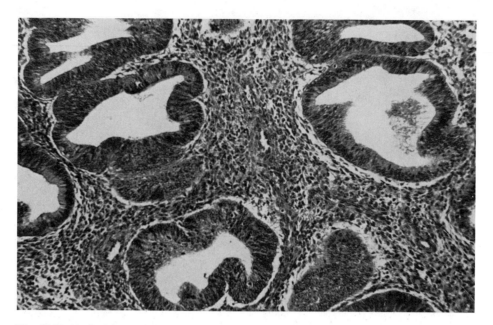

Fig. 47-9. Atypical hyperplasia, or carcinoma in situ, of endometrium. Glands are well formed, show no secretory activity, and have large cells, some cellular disorientation, and disparity in size.

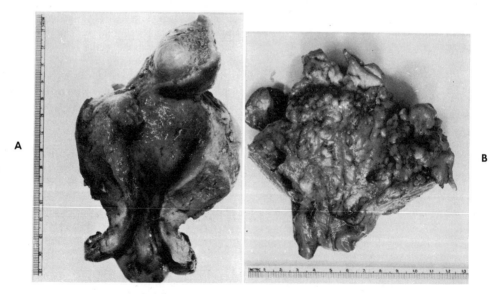

Fig. 47-10. Invasive carcinoma of corpus. **A,** Circumscribed adenocarcinoma; superficial raised area 2.5 cm in diameter is at right cornu. **B,** Diffuse, far-advanced carcinoma.

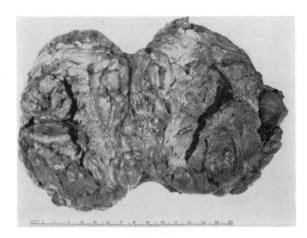

Fig. 47-11. Leiomyosarcoma of uterus.

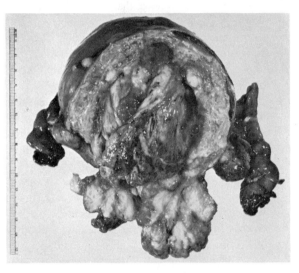

Fig. 47-12. Sarcoma botryoides, uterine tumor of mixed mesodermal origin.

47-11). No more than 0.1% of myomas undergo this type of malignant change.

Carcinosarcoma is a rare and highly malignant uterine tumor in which cells have the characteristics of sarcoma and carcinoma are found. Two distinct cell types from a carcinosarcoma have been grown in tissue culture. Metastatic lesions may show either carcinoma or sarcoma rather than the mixed pattern of the primary tumor.

Müllerian stroma is capable of giving rise to highly malignant tumors with a variety of histologic patterns. For this reason, it is often suggested that all these growths be grouped together and referred to as *tumors of mixed mesodermal origin*. Sarcoma botryoides (Fig. 47-12), a highly malignant polypoid growth usually found in infants, is of this type.

Stromatosis is a term to designate a rare, slow-growing tumor with a monotonous cellular pattern not unlike endometrial stroma. These growths should be regarded as sarcomatous, but they are much less aggressive than the usual *stromal sarcomas*.

CLINICAL STAGES

The clinical stages of endometrial cancer, like those of carcinoma of the cervix, are based on the pattern of extension of the lesion from its site of origin in the endometrium. The paths of extension are different from those of cervical lesions. *Lymphatic spread* is less predictable in that the tumor may invade the periaortic lymph nodes without involving those on the pelvic wall. The metastatic patterns of tumors that develop near the cervix may be more like those of primary cervical lesions. Tumor cells *invade the myometrium* directly and, in fact, may grow completely through to the serosal layer. *Hematogenous* and *peritoneal spread* occur frequently; and distant metastases, particularly to lung, pleura, and liver, are common.

Clinical stage can only be determined after the uterus has been removed and examined; consequently, staging is less helpful in planning therapy than is clinical staging of cancer of the cervix.

Clinical stages of carcinoma of the corpus uteri, adopted by the International Federation of Gynaecology and Obstetrics, are as follows:

Stage	Description
0	Carcinoma in situ; histologic findings suspicious of malignancy (Cases of stage 0 should not be included in any therapeutic statistics.)
I	Carcinoma confined to the corpus
IA	Length of the uterine cavity 8 cm or less
IB	Length of the uterine cavity more than 8 cm
	The stage I cases should be subgrouped with regard to the histologic type of the adenocarcinoma as follows:
	Group 1: Highly differentiated adenomatous carcinomas
	Group 2: Differentiated adenomatous carcinomas with partly solid areas
	Group 3: Predominantly solid or entirely undifferentiated carcinomas
II	Involvement of the corpus and the cervix
III	Extension outside the uterus but not outside the true pelvis
IV	Extension outside the true pelvis or obvious involvement of the mucosa of the bladder or rectum (A bullous edema as such does not permit allotment of a case to stage IV.)
IVA	Involvement of adjacent organs
IVB	Involvement of distant organs

SYMPTOMS

Endometrial cancer often produces early symptoms, the first of which usually is a *serous, malodorous discharge*. All too frequently it is not regarded seriously by the patient or her physician. It is not long before the watery leukorrhea is replaced by a *bloody discharge, intermittent spotting of blood,* or *steady bleeding.* If these symptoms are disregarded, the bleeding will ultimately become frank hemorrhage. The increasing blood loss indicates progressive growth of the cancer and enlargement of its area of ulceration.

DIFFERENTIAL DIAGNOSIS

The possibility of carcinoma of the corpus is immediately suggested when irregular uterine bleeding occurs near the menopause or when bleeding recurs in those who have already ceased menstruating.

Although only 20% of postmenopausal bleeding is caused by pelvic carcinoma, one cannot afford to disregard this important early sign of the lesion. It is unwise to assume that a cervical polyp, a fibroid, atrophic vaginitis, or any other benign lesion is the cause of abnormal bleeding. *The physician cannot make a definite diagnosis until a fractional curettage has been performed, and a biopsy of the cervix has been made.*

Exfoliative cytologic studies are less helpful in diagnosing endometrial cancer than cervical lesions. The cytologic examination reveals positive findings in no more than 50% of women with invasive endometrial cancer.

The diagnosis can be made by *outpatient endometrial biopsy* if malignant tissue is removed with the curet or by suction. *Dilatation and curettage* is essential, however, if the tissue is normal or if only hyperplasia, dysplasia, or carcinoma in situ is identified in the biopsy specimen. An area of invasive tumor may have been missed.

PREVENTION

It is obvious that deaths from endometrial cancer can be eliminated if its development can be prevented or if definitive treatment is instituted during its preinvasive phases.

The relationship between long periods of unopposed estrogen stimulation and endometrial abnormalities seems to be fairly well established. It is also likely that regular intervals of progesterone stimulation followed by endometrial shedding will reduce its incidence. The cyclic administration of progesterone to women with polycystic ovarian disease and anovulatory bleeding (Chapter 8) and during postmenopausal estrogen therapy (Chapter 50) reduces the incidence of uterine cancer.

If abnormal changes already have developed, they may not be reversible. Even though the administration of progesterone converts abnormal endometrium to a normal pattern, it may not be logical to continue hormone therapy for many years, for example, in women with endometrial dysplasia diagnosed near or after menopause. Under these circumstances hysterectomy is indicated. Conversely, progesterone therapy might be appropriate in young women if there is a reason to preserve the uterus temporarily. Women who have recurrent bleeding after dilatation and curettage during the climacteric or postmenopausal periods, particularly if there is an endometrial abnormality, are best treated by hysterectomy.

TREATMENT

It has been customary in most clinics to use radiation in one form or another as a preliminary step to hysterectomy for endometrial carcinoma. Whether the uterus is radiated by multiple radium or cesium sources from within the cavity or by external x-radiation or telecobalt radiation makes little difference in survival figures.

Surgery. Abdominal hysterectomy and bilateral salpingo-oophorectomy with pelvic and paraaortic node sampling is the operation most frequently indicated and is the most important part of the treatment of endometrial carcinoma. Vaginal hysterectomy often is preferrable to an abdominal operation in extremely obese women, but it may be difficult to evaluate the lymph nodes and to remove the tubes and ovaries if the structures are atrophic.

Primary hysterectomy is most appropriate for women with early endometrial cancer and minimal enlargement of the uterus from the tumor. Unfortunately, the size of the uterus does not always indicate the depth to which the tumor has penetrated. If there is deep myometrial penetration, the end results from primary hysterectomy are inferior to those in patients who have been treated with radium before surgery.

Radiation. Some women with endometrial carcinoma are poor candidates for any operation, and their entire treatment must be by radiation. A preliminary course of telecobalt therapy followed by intrauterine radium or cesium applied in Heyman's capsules gives the best result. The uterus is tightly packed by the multiple-radiation sources. The 5-year survival rate in patients treated with radiation alone is lower than that with surgery alone or when hysterectomy is combined with radiation.

Combined therapy. The combination of preoperative intrauterine radium or cesium therapy followed by hysterectomy has more advantages than either form of treatment alone. Preoperative radiation devitalizes tumor cells and reduces the total mass of bulky tumors, thus making the subsequent operation easier. Hysterectomy is performed a few days after radium implantation.

Another important beneficial effect of preoperative radiation is a decreased incidence of vaginal metastases. This complicaton occurs in as many as 10% to 12% of women who are operated on primarily and in less than 1% if they are treated before the operation is performed.

POSTOPERATIVE RADIATION. Far-advanced carcinoma of the endometrium may extend directly through the uterus at any point. Generally, this occurs near the lower uterine segment and involves the parametrial or broad ligament areas or both. This may preclude wide dissection; in fact, the gynecologist may be forced to cut across the tumor at some point. Other patients with advanced carcinomas may be free of direct extension but have one or more positive lymph nodes. Preoperative external radiation is preferred under these circumstances, but when it has not been given, postoperative treatment is appropriate.

Treatment of vaginal metastases. Vaginal metastases often occur because the tumor already has extended beyond the uterus by the time the operation is performed or because live tumor cells are disseminated during the operation. One of the major benefits of preoperative radiation is that the incidence of postoperative vaginal metastases is less than that after a primary surgical procedure.

Metastases are best treated by radium in a mold; occasionally, radium needles are preferred.

Treatment with progestogens. Kelley and Baker's report on the benefits of high dosages of progesterone in the treatment of metastatic endometrial carcinoma led to the use of 17-alpha-hydroxyprogesterone (Delalutin) and medroxyprogesterone acetate. The effect of progesterone in producing remission is most pronounced on pulmonary metastases, but control of local pelvic recurrence also has been observed. Well-differentiated tumors are more likely to respond favorably than are more anaplastic lesions. Response to progestins appears to be determined by the presence of cytoplasmic progesterone receptors. Well-differentiated tumors contain more progesterone receptors than do those that are anaplastic, which may explain the lack of response in the latter. Progesterone therapy must be considered as palliative rather than curative.

RESULTS OF TREATMENT

The prognosis is determined by the clinical stage of the disease when it is diagnosed, the size of the uterus and the depth of penetration of its wall, the histologic pattern and the degree of differentiation of the tumor, the quality of treatment, and the general health of the patient. The 5-year survival of women with stage I disease is about 90%. Treatment failures increase with more advanced lesions. Many failures reflect the conditions of the patients, as well as the disease and its treatment. Many women with endometrial cancer are poor risks for any form of treatment, and others have disease that is too extensive to eradicate.

REFERENCES

Bird, C.C., McElin, T.W., and Manalo-Estrella, P.: The elusive adenomyosis of the uterus—revisited, Am. J. Obstet. Gynecol. **112:**583, 1972.

Deligdish, L., and Loewenthal, M.: Endometrial changes associated with myomata of the uterus, J. Clin. Pathol. **23:**676, 1970.

Ehrlich, C.E., Cleary, R.E., and Young, P.C.M.: Which endometrial cancers respond to progestin therapy? Contemp. Obstet. Gynecol. **15:**139, 1980.

Farber, M., Conrad, S., Heinrichs, W.L., and Herrmann, W.L.: Estradiol binding by fibroid tumors and normal myometrium, Obstet. Gynecol. **40:**479, 1972.

Farrer-Brown, G., Beilby, J.O.W., and Tarbit, M.H.: Venous changes in the endometrium of myomatous uteri, Obstet. Gynecol. **38:**743, 1971.

Gabb. R.G., and Stone, G.M.: Uptake and metabolism of tritiated oestradiol and oestrone by human endometrial and myometrial tissue *in vitro*. J. Endocrinol. Great Britain **62:**615, 1974.

Gallup, D.G., and Stock, R.J.: Adenocarcinoma of the endometrium in women 40 years of age or younger, Obstet. Gynecol. **64:**417, 1984.

Gambrell, R.D., Jr., Bagnell, C.A., and Greenblatt, R.B.: Role of estrogens and progesterone in the etiology and prevention of endometrial cancer: review. Am. J. Obstet. Gynecol. **146:**696, 1983.

Gusberg, S.B.: The individual at high risk for endometrial carcinoma, Am. J. Obstet. Gynecol. **126:**535, 1976.

Hammond, C.B., Jelovsek, F.R., Lee, K.L., Creasman, W.T., and Parker, R.T.: Effects of long-term estrogen replacement therapy. II. Neoplasia, Am. J. Obstet. Gynecol. **133:**537, 1979.

Hart, W.R., and Yoonessi, M.: Endometrial stromatosis of the uterus, Obstet. Gynecol. **49:**393, 1977.

Hausknecht, R.U., and Gusberg, S.B.: Estrogen metabolism in patients at high risk for endometrial carcinoma. II. The role of androstenedione as an estrogen precursor in postmenopausal women with endometrial carcinoma, Am. J. Obstet. Gynecol. **116:**98, 1973.

Hausknecht, R.U., and Gusberg, S.B.: Estrogen metabolism in patients at high risk for endometrial carcinoma. I. Urinary metabolites of H3-estradiol in normal postmenopausal women and those with endometrial carcinoma, Am. J. Obstet. Gynecol. **105:**1161, 1969.

Henriksen, E.: The lymphatic dissemination in endometrial carcinoma, Am. J. Obstet. Gynecol. **123:**570, 1975.

Hulka, B.S., Fowler, W.C., Jr., Kaufman, D.G., Grimson, R.C., Greenberg, B.G., Hogue, C.J., Berger, G.S., and Pulliam, C.C.: Estrogen and endometrial cancer: cases and two control groups from North Carolina, Am. J. Obstet. Gynecol. **137**(1):92, 1980.

Jick, H., Watkins, R.N., Hunter, J.R., Dinan, B.J., Madsen, S., Rothman, K.J., and Walker, A.M.: Replacement estrogens and endometrial cancer, N. Engl. J. Med. **300:**218, 1979.

Kelley, R.M., and Baker, W.H.: Progestational agents on the treatment of carcinoma of the endometrium, N. Engl. J. Med. **264:**216, 1961.

Lucas, W.E., and Yen, S.S.C.: A study of endocrine and metabolic variables in postmenopausal women with endometrial carcinoma, Am. J. Obstet. Gynecol. **134:**180, 1979.

MacDonald, P.C., and Siiteri, P.K.: Relationship between extraglandular production of estrone and the occurrence of endometrial neoplasia, Gynecol. Oncol. **2:**259, 1974.

McDonald, T.W., Malkasian, G.D., and Gaffey, T.A.: Endometrial cancer associated with feminizing ovarian tumor and polycystic ovarian disease, Obstet. Gynecol. **49:**654, 1977.

Neuwirth, R.S.: Hysteroscopic management of symptomatic submucous myomas. Obstet. Gynecol. **62:**509, 1983.

Nisker, J.A., Hammond, G.L., Davidson, B.J., Frumar, A.M., Takaki, N.K., Judd, H.L., and Siiteri, P.K.: Serum sex hormone-binding globulin capacity and the percentage of free estradiol in postmenopausal women and without endometrial carcinoma, Am. J. Obstet. Gynecol. **138:**637, 1980.

Otubu, J.A., Buttram, V.C., Besch, N.F., and Besch, P.K.: Unconjugated steroids in leiomyomas and tumor-bearing myometrium, Am. J. Obstet. Gynecol. **143:**130, 1982.

Patanaphan, V., Salazar, O.M., and Chougule, P.: What can be expected when radiation therapy becomes the only curative alternative for endometrial cancer? Cancer **55:**1462, 1985.

Peters, W.A., III, Andersen, W.A., Thornton, W.N., Jr., and Morley, G.W.: The selective use of vaginal hysterectomy in the management of adenocarcinoma of the endometrium, Am. J. Obstet. Gynecol. **146:**285, 1983.

Peterson, E.P.: Endometrial carcinoma in young women, Obstet. Gynecol. **31:**702, 1968.

Pollow, K., et al.: *In vitro* conversion of estradiol-17-beta into estrone in normal human myometrium and leiomyoma, J. Clin. Chem. Clin. Biochem. **16:**493, 1978.

Salazar, O.M., DePapp, E.W., Bonfiglio, T.A., Feldstein, M.L., Rubin, P., and Rudolph, J.H.: Adenosquamous carcinoma of the endometrium, Cancer **40:**119, 1977.

Sall, S., and Calanog, A.: Steroid excretion patterns in post-menopausal women with benign and neoplastic endometrium, Am. J. Obstet. Gynecol. **114:**153, 1972.

Satyaswaroop, P.G., and Mortel, R.: Endometrial carcinoma: an aberration of endometrial cell differentiation, Am. J. Obstet. Gynecol. **140:**620, 1981.

Sehgal, N., and Haskins, A.L.: The mechanism of uterine bleeding in the presence of fibromyomas, Am.J. Surg. **26:**21, 1960.

Soules, M.R., and McCarty, K.S., Jr.: Leiomyomas: steroid receptor content. Variation within normal menstrual cycles. Am. J. Obstet. Gynecol. **143:**6,1982.

Spellacy, W.N.: Plasma growth hormone and estradiol levels in women with uterine myomas, Obstet. Gynecol. **40:**829, 1972.

Taylor, H.C., Jr.: Vascular congestion and hyperemia: their effect on structure and function of the female reproductive system, Am. J. Obstet. Gynecol. **57:**2, 1949.

Walker, A.M., and Jick, H.: Declining rates of endometrial cancer, Obstet. Gynecol. **56:**733, 1980.

Wilson, E.A., Yang, F., and Rees, E.D.: Estradiol and progesterone binding in uterine leiomyomata and in normal uterine tissues, Obstet. Gynecol. **55:**20, 1980.

48

J. Robert Willson

Ovarian neoplasms

The ovary has a greater potential for tumor growth than does any other structure in the body. A variety of neoplastic tumors arise from glandular and connective tissues and from embryonic remnants, which often are present within normal ovaries.

It is essential that physicians be familiar with the changes that occur in the ovary during a normal menstrual cycle. Those who do not understand the normal physiologic changes will be unable to differentiate the functional ovarian enlargements, which usually need no treatment, from neoplasms for which the proper treatment almost always is surgical removal.

NONNEOPLASTIC CYSTS

Normal ovaries of newborn infants contain one to two million primordial follicles. Many of these degenerate before the menarche. During active reproductive life many follicles begin to grow under the stimulus of FSH during the preovulatory phase of each menstrual cycle. One or occasionally two or more follicles mature and produce ova that are capable of being fertilized. The rest become atretic. Ovulation occurs about 14 days before menstruation begins, and a corpus luteum develops and persists until just before the next menstrual period. This cycle is repeated, except during pregnancy, until the climacteric phase of life.

A *follicular cyst* occurs with each normal menstrual cycle. The follicle reaches its maximum size just before ovulation when the ovary may be 4 to 5 cm in diameter. The cyst disappears with ovulation.

Occasionally, the follicle fails to rupture and may even continue to grow, sometimes reaching a diameter of 8 to 10 cm. Such *persistent follicular cysts* are thin walled and contain clear serous fluid. Granulosa and theca cells can be identified in the walls of the smaller tumors, but, as the cyst enlarges, these cells become flattened and look like those lining a serous cyst. These are frequently diagnosed histologically as *simple cysts*. The large, persistent follicular cysts usually have no hormone activity, but the fluid in the normal follicle contains a high concentration of estrogen.

The normal corpus luteum is a cystic structure and may enlarge the ovary slightly. Rarely, the corpus luteum may fail to involute. It continues to secrete progesterone, thus delaying the onset of menstruation, and may even grow. *Corpus luteum cysts* may produce pain as they expand or with intraperitoneal rupture, and the combination of a delayed period, pain, and bleeding may simulate ectopic pregnancy. Persistent corpus luteum cysts probably do not occur often in the absence of pregnancy. In fact, undiagnosed pregnancy may be the cause of almost all persistent corpora lutea.

Women are usually unaware of the presence of normal follicles and corpora lutea or even large follicular cysts because they produce no symptoms unless a complication develops.

Nonneoplastic functional cysts of the ovary occur frequently and usually need no treatment. They can be recognized by their relationship to the menstrual cycle; for example, enlargement caused by the development of a follicle occurs just before ovulation, and enlargement caused by the corpus luteum just before menstruation. In addition, 95% or more of tumors of the ovary that are less than 5 cm in diameter are nonneoplastic, whereas true neoplasms are almost all larger.

Whenever a small ovarian enlargement is discovered, the patient should be reexamined before definitive treatment is considered. The most appropriate time for reexamination is at the end of a menstrual period when ovarian activity is at a minimum. If the enlargement has disappeared, one can assume that it was a functional cyst. The patient should be examined again within 2 to 4 months.

If the enlargement is still present after menstruation and is less than 5 cm in diameter, the patient should be reexamined in 4 to 6 weeks. Operation may be indicated if the ovary is larger, or further observation if it is smaller or unchanged. One may also prescribe a cycle or two of *oral contraceptives* if the ovary is still slightly enlarged when the patient is reexamined after menstruation. Small, persistent follicular cysts may regress when pituitary gonadotropin secretion is inhibited.

The exception to observation of small ovarian enlargements is in postmenopausal women. After the menopause the ovaries become progressively smaller and cannot be felt. If one does feel an adnexal enlargement of any size, particularly if it has not been felt before, a neoplasm should be suspected. Laparoscopy or, in some instances, laparotomy is indicated.

A functional cyst that requires surgery because it grows or fails to regress under observation is usually single, thin walled, unilocular with a smooth lining, and filled with clear serous fluid. It usually should be resected. Oophorectomy is not often necessary.

Excessive production of chorionic gonadotropin overstimulates the theca-lutein cells, producing *theca-lutein cysts,* which are made up of many follicles of varying sizes surrounded by luteinized theca cells. These cysts characteristically develop in women with hydatidiform moles, but they may occur with multiple pregnancy and Rh sensitization. They also follow ovarian overstimulation by gonadotropins given to induce ovulation. Theca-lutein cysts are bilateral, and the involved ovary may be as large as 20 to 25 cm in diameter. They usually cause no symptoms unless they undergo torsion. These cysts regress when the stimulus is withdrawn at delivery.

Another tumor caused by gonadotropin stimulation is the *luteoma.* These tumors probably develop from hyperplastic overgrowth of luteinized theca cells. They occur during normal pregnancy and are less likely to be bilateral than are theca-lutein cysts. Although luteomas may be 15 to 20 cm in diameter, they usually produce no symptoms and are generally overlooked unless found at cesarean delivery.

About 25% of mothers with luteomas are virilized because of the large amounts of androgenic steroids produced by the luteinized cells. Female fetuses may be born with clitoromegaly and fused labia.

Theca-lutein cysts and luteomas regress after pregnancy is terminated. About the only indication for their removal is torsion.

Germinal inclusion cysts, which are caused by infolding of the germinal layer, are often seen on the surface of the ovaries in postmenopausal women. They have no clinical significance.

Polycystic ovarian disease, with which multiple small cysts develop, is discussed in Chapter 9.

Endometriomas, which are discussed in Chapter 11, should not be confused with endometrial ovarian neoplasms.

Ruptured functional cysts. Occasionally, during the course of follicular rupture, a blood vessel on the surface of the ovary is torn. The amount of intraperitoneal bleeding from *rupture of an ovarian follicle* is determined by the size of the blood vessel. The scant bleeding that occurs normally may produce no symptoms, but, if there is extensive intraperitoneal bleeding, the patient may develop the typical signs of hemorrhagic shock.

The clinical picture of extensive intraperitoneal bleeding from a ruptured follicle may be like that of ruptured ectopic pregnancy, but these situations often can be distinguished from each other by the history. The former occurs at midcycle after a normal menstrual period and is usually not accompanied by vaginal bleeding, although there may be slight spotting as a result of the sudden fall in estrogen level.

Intraperitoneal bleeding from a *ruptured corpus luteum* presents an identical clinical picture except that it occurs just before menstruation rather than at midcycle.

The *diagnosis* of either of these lesions is made by clinical history, pelvic examination, culdocentesis in an attempt to aspirate blood, and laparoscopy.

No *treatment* is necessary unless bleeding from the ovary does not stop spontaneously. Bleeding that continues can be controlled by resecting the follicle or the corpus luteum and repairing the defect in the ovary. Oophorectomy is rarely necessary.

NEOPLASMS

Ovarian neoplasms occur less often than do the functional cysts, but they are far more important. They may grow to a large size, secrete hormones that alter normal physiologic functions, and be malignant.

There are many classifications of ovarian neoplasms, but the one we have found most useful is that proposed by Abell:

I. Neoplasms of germ cell origin
   A. Germinoma
   B. Embryonal teratoma (embryonal carcinoma)
   C. Partially differentiated teratoma (malignant teratoma, solid teratoma)
   D. Mature teratoma (benign cystic teratoma)
   E. Mixed germ cell neoplasms (teratocarcinoma)
   F. Carcinoma or sarcoma arising in a mature teratoma

II. Neoplasms of coelomic (germinal) epithelium and its derivatives
   A. Serous (tubal cell) type
      1. Benign
         a. Cystadenoma
         b. Papilloma
         c. Cystadenofibroma
         d. Adenofibroma
      2. Malignant
         a. Papillary cystadenocarcinoma
   B. Mucinous (cervical cell) type
      1. Benign
         a. Cystadenoma
         b. Cystadenofibroma
         c. Adenofibroma
      2. Malignant
         a. Cystadenocarcinoma
   C. Endometroid (endometrial cell) type
      1. Benign
         a. Cystadenoma
      2. Malignant
         a. Cystadenocarcinoma
         b. Acanthoadenocarcinoma
   D. Brenner tumors
   E. Mixed and unclassified cell types

III. Neoplasms of specialized gonadal stroma (sex cords and mesenchymal)
   A. Granulosa-theca cell group
      1. Granulosa cell tumor
      2. Theca cell tumor
      3. Granulosa-theca cell tumor
   B. Sertoli-Leydig cell group
      1. Sertoli cell tumor
      2. Leydig cell tumor (hilus cell)
      3. Arrhenoblastoma
   C. Luteomas
   D. Gynadroblastoma

IV. Neoplasms of nonspecialized stroma and heterotopic elements
   A. Fibroma-fibrosarcoma
   B. Leiomyoma-leiomyosarcoma
   C. Angioma-angiosarcoma
   D. Adrenocortical adenoma-adrenocortical carcinoma
   E. Mesonephric cystadenoma-mesonephric carcinoma
   F. Lymphoblastoma

The histogenesis of ovarian neoplasms is illustrated in Fig. 48-1.

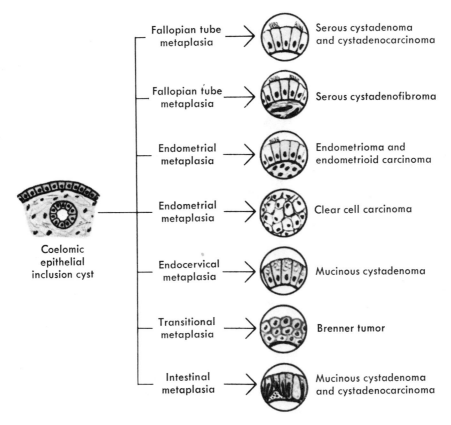

Fallopian tube metaplasia → Serous cystadenoma and cystadenocarcinoma

Fallopian tube metaplasia → Serous cystadenofibroma

Endometrial metaplasia → Endometrioma and endometrioid carcinoma

Endometrial metaplasia → Clear cell carcinoma

Endocervical metaplasia → Mucinous cystadenoma

Transitional metaplasia → Brenner tumor

Intestinal metaplasia → Mucinous cystadenoma and cystadenocarcinoma

Coelomic epithelial inclusion cyst

Fig. 48-1. Histogenesis of ovarian neoplasms. (From Fenoglio, C.M., and Richart, R.M.: Contemp. Obstet. Gynecol. **9:**64, 1977.)

Neoplasms of germ cell origin

A variety of ovarian neoplasms can arise from germ cells. For example, embryonal teratomas (Fig. 48-2) occur infrequently and are highly malignant. Others such as benign cystic teratomas are common and almost always benign. These tumors presumably arise from primordial germ cells; this concept is supported by the fact that almost all ovarian neoplasms in this group have a 46 XX chromosomal pattern.

Benign cystic teratomas. Benign cystic teratomas, or dermoid cysts, comprise about 15% to 20% of all ovarian neoplasms. They occur at any age but account for about 60% of benign ovarian neoplasms in girls under age 15. They are the second most common ovarian neoplasms in women of all age groups, being outnumbered only by serous cystadenomas.

Benign cystic teratomas usually are between 5 and 10 cm in diameter when they are diagnosed. Sometimes tiny tumors are discovered when the ovary is bisected, and occasionally a dermoid may be 15 cm or more in diameter (Fig. 48-3). About 10% are bilateral. These tumors are gray, glistening, smooth, and tense. They are cystic, usually with a single cavity filled with oily, sebaceous fluid and a mass of matted hair (Fig. 48-4). There usually is a solid prominence in the tumor wall adjacent to the ovary.

The most prominent tissue is of ectodermal origin, but endodermal and mesodermal structures can usually be identified. The tissues most often

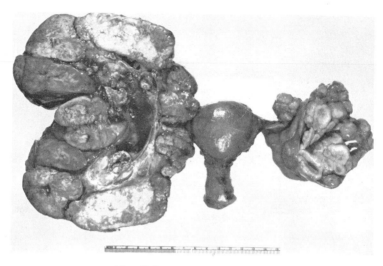

Fig. 48-2. Malignant teratoma.

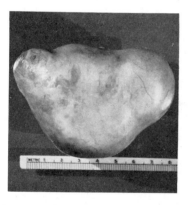

Fig. 48-3. Benign cystic teratoma with corpus luteum cyst on left.

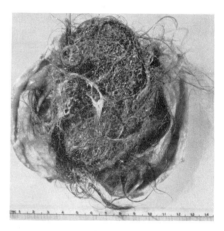

Fig. 48-4. Opened benign cystic teratoma, contents of which are mainly hair and sebaceous material.

recognized are skin and its appendages, cartilage, respiratory epithelium, and neural elements. All the tissues are mature. Fairly well-formed teeth often can be seen by x-ray film examination (Fig. 48-5). In the absence of calcification, a teratoma may still be suspected by x-ray film examination. Teratomas are more radiolucent than other ovarian neoplasms, and the capsule is usually clearly delineated. However, there is no need to obtain an x-ray film study if the tumor is large enough to require operation; a precise diagnosis will not influence treatment.

Occasionally, an area of *malignancy* may develop in an otherwise benign teratoma. This is almost always squamous cell carcinoma, but adenocarcinoma and even stromal malignancies can occur.

Struma ovarii is an unusual variation in which thyroid tissue dominates the tumor. Thyrotoxicosis can result.

Dysgerminomas. Dysgerminomas are malignant germ cell tumors, 80% of which are diagnosed during the early reproductive years, frequently in

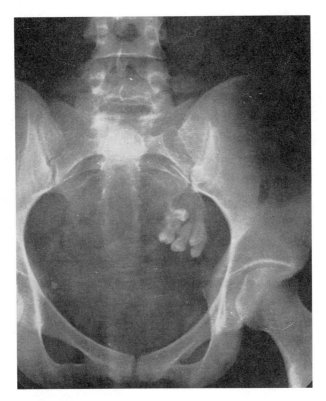

Fig. 48-5. Well-developed teeth within benign cystic teratoma demonstrated by x-ray film examination.

teenagers and occasionally before the menarche. The tumor is smooth, gray to yellow, and usually of a firm, rubbery consistency. The size varies from a small nodule to a mass that fills the entire abdomen.

There usually are no symptoms; the patient first becomes aware of the tumor because of progressive abdominal enlargement. Although dysgerminomas have no endocrine activity, they may occur in association with ambiguous sexual development.

Dysgerminomas are almost always unilateral, and they respond well to radiation. The *treatment* usually is to remove the tumor alone unless the other reproductive organs are invaded. Recurrent tumor often regresses completely when treated by external radiation.

Solid teratomas. The solid teratomas are composed of immature tissues and are highly malignant.

Neoplasms of coelomic (germinal) epithelium and its derivatives

The most common coelomic epithelial neoplasms are the serous and mucinous cystadenomas, which account for about 50% of all benign ovarian neoplasms.

Serous cystadenomas (Figs. 48-6 and 48-7). These tumors occur more frequently than do the mucinous types. They are diagnosed most often between the ages of 20 and 50 years, with a peak incidence during the fourth decade of life.

The surface of the tumor is usually pearly gray, glistening, and lobulated because of its multilocular interior (Fig. 48-6). The lining may be smooth or covered with papillary projections. Similar excrescences are often seen on the surface of the tumor. The fluid is thin and pale unless there has been hemorrhage into the cavity of the tumor. The exact

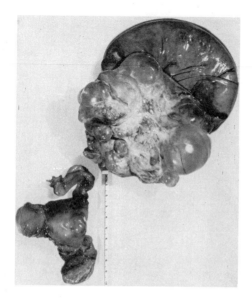

Fig. 48-6. Multilocular serous cystadenoma.

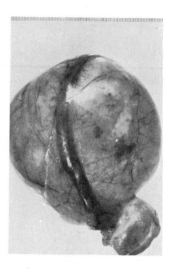

Fig. 48-7. Interligamentous serous cystadenoma; tube is stretched out over tumor.

incidence of bilateral serous cystadenomas has not been established, but both ovaries are involved in 20% to 25% of cases.

The cells lining the cyst cavities may resemble germinal epithelium, but more characteristically they are secretory and ciliated like those of the lumen of the normal fallopian tube. Small, calcified granules called *psammoma bodies (calcospheroids)* are sometimes present in the cyst wall. These represent degeneration and subsequent calcification of small papillae. Psammoma bodies serve to differentiate serous from mucinous cystadenomas; they do not occur in the latter. Psammoma bodies may also be seen in serous cystadenocarcinomas but not in malignancies of the mucinous type.

Mucinous cystadenomas. It may be impossible to differentiate these tumors from serous cystadenomas by gross inspection. Mucinous cystadenomas, however, are likely to be larger; cysts of this type weighing as much as 300 pounds have been reported (Fig. 48-8).

Mucinous cysts are usually multilocular and contain thick, straw-colored, viscid fluid. Papillary growths occur less often than in the serous cystadenomas. Only 5% to 7% of mucinous cystadenomas are bilateral.

The cells lining the cyst cavity are tall and columnar, with clear cytoplasm and dark nuclei located close to the basement membrane. Goblet cells are seen frequently. The cells resemble those normally found in the endocervix or colon.

Pseudomyxoma peritonei is an unusual condition characterized by the transformation of peritoneal mesothelium to mucus-secreting epithelium. Pseudomyxoma peritonei occurs in association with mucinous cystadenomas and appendiceal mucoceles. Huge amounts of mucinous material are secreted, and bowel obstruction and death can occur. There is no way to treat this condition successfully.

Other neoplasms from coelomic epithelium. Other less common neoplasms arise from germinal epithelium, including *papillomas, adenofibromas,* and *cystadenofibromas* (Fig. 48-9). These resemble serous cystadenomas more than the mucinous variety.

Brenner tumors. These are unusual solid tumors in which nests of epithelial cells grow in connective tissue stroma. They rarely become malignant and secrete no hormones. In about a third of these cases another tumor, often a mucinous cystadenoma, is present in the same or opposite ovary. The diagnosis is usually made only by histologic examination.

Malignancy in coelomic epithelial neoplasms. Both serous and mucinous cystadenomas can be malignant from their onset or undergo malignant change

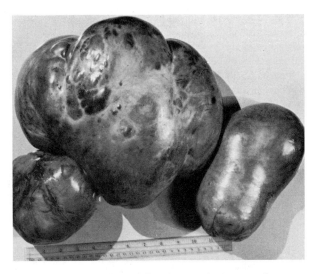

Fig. 48-8. Bilateral, multilocular mucinous cystadenoma.

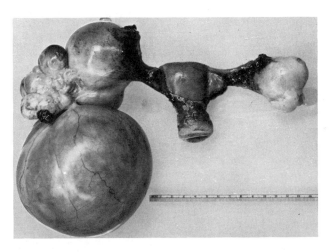

Fig. 48-9. Bilateral adenofibroma of ovary. Areas of cystic degeneration are visible.

after many years. These account for about two thirds of all malignant ovarian tumors. Almost all are carcinomas. If the entire tumor is made up of malignant cells, it is not possible to determine whether it was malignant from the onset or an extensive malignant change occurred in a benign neoplasm. If there is a small focus of malignancy in a large serous or mucinous cyst, one must accept the fact that it represents malignancy developing in a benign tumor.

From 30% to 45% of serous tumors are malignant *(serous cystadenocarcinoma)* in contrast to only 5% to 10% of those of the mucinous variety *(mucinous cystadenocarcinoma)*. About half of all ovarian adenocarcinomas are of the serous type, and about 15% are mucinous.

If the capsule is intact, these tumors look very much like benign cystadenomas. Serous cystadenocarcinomas are almost always bilateral, whereas mucinous cystadenocarcinomas are more likely to be unilateral. Not all bilateral cysts are malignant, neither are unilateral ones necessarily benign. There may be papillary growths on the surface of the tumor and on the surrounding peritoneal tissues. Often the amount of peritoneal fluid is increased, and tumor cells may be found in the fluid even though the wall of the tumor is smooth, intact, and not adherent to surrounding structures. This means, of course, that the possibility of widespread metastasis exists.

In advanced cases the pelvis may be completely filled with a mass of papillary tumor to which bowel and omentum are adherent. The omentum may be infiltrated with tumor, and there may be metastatic areas on the bowel and the parietal peritoneum. The tumor may invade the wall of the uterus, and cells shed into the peritoneal cavity may pass through the tubes and uterine cavity and be identified in cervical cytologic studies. The tumor also metastasizes through lymphatic channels.

Endometrioid carcinoma. These tumors probably develop in coelomic epithelial inclusions. They are far less common than the serous and mucinous types but much less lethal. They are of low-grade malignancy, and, although they do invade locally, they do not metastasize widely.

Ovarian cancer is usually diagnosed at a stage when it cannot be treated successfully because it is so far advanced.

Neoplasms of specialized gonadal stroma (sex cords and mesenchymal)

Neoplasms of specialized gonadal stroma are unusual neoplasms. Almost all secrete either estrogen or androgen, each of which produces its characteristic effect on the patient.

Granulosa-theca cell tumors (Fig. 48-10). These tumors may be made up predominately of granulosa cells, theca cells, or a combination of both. Most neoplasms in this group secrete estrogen; hence they are also called *feminizing tumors*. This is not strictly accurate because virilization may occur in some women with theca cell tumors.

Granulosa cell tumors are diagnosed most frequently during the climacteric and postmenopausal periods, although they may also develop in premenarchal girls. Only about 10% are bilateral.

The principal symptoms of feminizing tumors

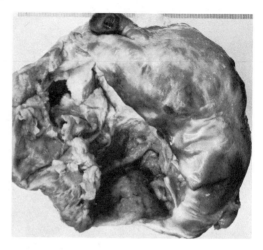

Fig. 48-10. Huge granulosa-theca cell tumor of ovary.

are those resulting from estrogen, which most of these tumors secrete. In young girls the estrogen stimulates breast and genital maturation and uterine bleeding (isosexual precocious puberty). Postmenopausal women with estrogen-secreting tumors may also experience uterine bleeding as a result of stimulation of the endometrium. The vaginal epithelium will become cornified, and the uterus may enlarge slightly. The breasts feel full and may be tender.

The *diagnosis* may be difficult because the ovarian tumor may be so small that it cannot be felt or seen by the usual methods of examination. The presence of an estrogen-secreting tumor should be suspected whenever bleeding recurs after the menopause. One should look for evidences of estrogen stimulation, which are usually not present when endometrial cancer occurs in elderly women. In young girls, estrogen-producing tumors must be differentiated from constitutional precocious puberty. This may be easy if ovulation is occurring, as it does with the latter condition. Estrogen production from tumors is likely to be more steady than is that during anovulatory ovarian cycles. In anovulatory cycles, bleeding occurs as estrogen production subsides periodically.

Dilatation and curettage and cervical biopsy are important diagnostic steps. The endometrium in women with granulosa cell tumor is usually hyperplastic, and there may be atypical areas. Endometrial adenocarcinoma also occurs more often in women with estrogen-secreting tumors. The diagnosis is confirmed by identifying the tumor in the ovary.

About 10% of granulosa cell tumors recur after they are removed. They grow slowly and may recur locally many years after the primary lesion was removed. Since the 5-year survival rate is at least 90%, only the involved structures need be removed in young women. The normal-appearing ovary should be inspected carefully and even bisected; about 10% of granulosa cell tumors are bilateral. The uterus and the other tube and ovary should be removed in women near or past the menopause.

Thecomas, which arise from stromal cells, are solid, benign, and almost always unilateral. They occur less often than do granulosa cell tumors, but they, too, secrete estrogen. Occasionally, thecomas may have a virilizing effect.

Sertoli-Leydig cell group. These rare gonadal stromal tumors usually have a virilizing effect.

The *arrhenoblastoma* is the most frequently diagnosed neoplasm in this group. Most arrhenoblastomas occur in women between the ages of 20 and 40 years. They are rare in children. The principal effect is defeminization followed by virilism. The first evidence is usually amenorrhea and decreased breast size. This is followed by increased hair growth with a male distribution, deepening of the voice, coarsening of the skin with an acneform eruption, and hypertrophy of the clitoris. Some arrhenoblastomas are hormonally inert.

The *diagnosis* is made by identifying an ovarian tumor, and *treatment* is its removal. Its malignant potential is similar to that of granulosa cell tumors; hence conservative surgical procedures are appropriate in young women.

Leydig (hilus) cell tumors are rare and usually cause virilization. The hilus cells from which these neoplasms arise are thought to be similar to Leydig cells in the testis. *Sertoli tumors* are composed of tissue that resembles fetal seminiferous tubules.

Gynandroblastomas are rare tumors with a mixture of tissues that resemble both arrhenoblastoma and granu-losa-theca cell tumors. They usually produce virilism and are likely to be malignant.

Neoplasms of nonspecialized stroma and heterotopic elements

The most important in this group of tumors is the *fibroma.* This neoplasm occurs most frequently during the fifth and sixth decades of life. Fibromas usually are unilateral, and they are not often malignant.

Meigs described an interesting association of ascites and hydrothorax with ovarian fibromas *(Meigs' syndrome).* Ascites and hydrothorax can also occur in the presence of other kinds of ovarian neoplasms. One should consider the possibility of an ovarian neoplasm in any woman with ascites and pleural effusion. It may not be possible to feel the tumor until after the fluid has been removed.

Metastatic carcinoma

Tumors that most often metastasize to the ovaries are those that originate in the breast, gastrointestinal tract, and endometrium.

Metastatic breast cancer is found in as many as 20% of ovaries removed prophylactically in treating the primary lesion. The ovary will be involved in about 5% of corpus carcinomas. Typical Krukenberg tumors may be a result of malignancy in the gastrointestinal tract (Fig. 48-11). Occasionally, the metastatic ovarian tumor is the first evidence of the primary disease.

Benign tumors

Symptoms. *Most ovarian neoplasms produce no symptoms and are found during examinations of women who do not suspect that anything is wrong.* As the tumor is growing, the patients may experience a *sense of pressure in the pelvis,* but even this may be absent if the tumor can move freely within the peritoneal cavity. Large tumors cause *enlargement of the abdomen.*

Fixed or incarcerated tumors may produce *painful micturition, painful defecation, rectal tenesmus,* or *pain during coitus. Menstrual disturbances* occur in only 10% to 15% of women with benign ovarian neoplasms.

Acute episodes of pain may occur if the *ovarian neoplasm twists on its pedicle (twisted ovarian neo-*

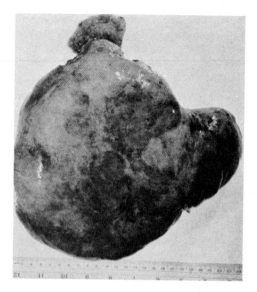

Fig. 48-11. Krukenberg tumor, metastatic from stomach.

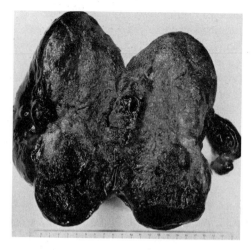

Fig. 48-12. Hemorrhage into ovarian tumor. Tumor has been opened. Long pedicle on right was completely occluded by 360-degree twist.

plasm). This obstructs the blood supply suddenly. Torsion occurs most often with tumors of moderate size, 8 to 12 cm in diameter. Larger ones are usually not mobile enough to rotate, and smaller ones are not heavy enough. In addition, smaller neoplasms can untwist easily because of their size.

The twist usually occurs suddenly and is accompanied by sharp pain in the pelvis. The pain subsides if the twist is reversed and circulation is restored, but it becomes progressively more severe if the obstruction is not relieved. Many patients have transitory recurrent attacks of mild pain before the final episode.

If the vascular obstruction persists, the tumor becomes necrotic and hemorrhagic (Fig. 48-12). It is exceedingly tender to palpation. Pain increases, and signs of pertoneal irritation appear. The treatment is prompt surgical removal.

Diagnosis. Ovarian neoplasms can usually be diagnosed by pelvic examination, except in their early stages when they are too small to feel. They are often found during periodic examinations of presumably well women. Neoplasms develop in retained ovaries after hysterectomy at the same rates that they do with the uterus in place; hence regular examinations are important after the uterus

has been removed. Ovarian tumors should also be suspected as a cause of vague pelvic discomfort and of mild gastrointestinal distress.

If one suspects that there is an enlarged ovary, the patient should be reexamined after a cleansing enema and at the end of a menstrual period when physiologic cysts are not likely to be present. If one is still uncertain, *diagnostic ultrasound* may be helpful. *Diagnostic laparoscopy* is justified if sonography is inconclusive.

It is particularly important that an exact diagnosis be made whenever one suspects the ovary to be enlarged in a postmenopausal woman. At this stage of life the normal ovary is too small to feel; hence an enlarged ovary is likely to be abnormal.

One must also be suspicious of an abnormality when an ovary that has previously been freely movable is felt to be larger and adherent in the cul-de-sac or to the posterior leaf of the broad ligament.

Treatment. Since a true ovarian neoplasm will continue to grow and may ultimately undergo malignant degeneration, the treatment is surgical removal. When the ovary is more than 5 cm in diameter, the enlargement is almost always caused by a true neoplasm, and operation is indicated. Although all ovarian neoplasms are at some time smaller than 5 cm in diameter, they are rarely discovered at this stage because of the total lack of symptoms.

Since at least 95% of ovarian enlargements under 5 cm are nonneoplastic, immediate removal of slightly enlarged ovaries is containdicated. Such an enlargement is usually a result of a normal follicle or corpus luteum, and at reexamination after menstruation it will have disappeared. Observation of these small cysts every 3 to 6 months is the only treatment required. Should they increase in size, a true neoplasm is to be suspected, and removal may then be considered. The low incidence of malignancy in these small tumors makes the risk from observation negligible.

Observation is contraindicated if an ovarian neoplasm is suspected in women past the menopause. It is impossible to feel tiny atrophic ovaries; hence any palpable and adnexal structure, particularly if it has not been felt before, may be a malignant neoplasm.

Unilateral *cystectomy* or *cystoophorectomy* is the treatment of choice for young women with single benign lesions, but in each instance the opposite ovary must be carefully inspected or even *bisected* in an effort to detect a small neoplasm that may grow later.

Benign cystic teratomas are usually easily resectable, and much normal ovarian tissue can be preserved. The almost total lack of malignant change makes conservative surgery a highly desirable practice for benign cystic teratomas in young women.

Benign serous cystadenomas are likely to develop bilaterally; hence bilateral cystoophorectomy often is necessary. In young women with a unilateral serous cystadenoma, the normal ovary and the uterus can be left in place. If the excised tumor proves to be malignant, hysterectomy with removal of the other ovary usually is appropriate.

Mucinous cystadenomas are likely to be unilateral, and the incidence of malignancy is far less than with the serous variety. It is usually possible therefore to remove the involved ovary and leave the normal-appearing one.

Bilateral salpingo-oophorectomy and hysterectomy usually are indicated in women over 40 years of age with ovarian neoplasms, particularly serous cystadenomas, because of the increased possibility of malignancy at that age.

Complete hysterectomy and bilateral removal of the adnexa are indicated for ovarian tumors diagnosed after the menopause.

Ovarian neoplasms with torsion of the pedicle must be considered an acute surgical emergency, and immediate operative removal is indicated.

As a general rule the ovaries can be removed at the time of hysterectomy in women who are approaching the menopause and certainly in those whose periods have ceased.

Malignant tumors

The incidence of carcinoma of the ovary is increasing steadily. It now accounts for about 4% of all cancers and for about 5% of all cancer deaths in women. It is estimated that 18,500 new cancers of the ovary were diagnosed in 1985 and that 11,600 women died of the disease. It is the fourth leading cause of cancer deaths in women, being surpassed only by cancer of the breast (36,483), lung (29,797), and colon and rectum (27,350). Cancer of the ovary is unusual before the age of 20, but it increases steadily thereafter. It occurs at a rate of about 6 or 7/100,000 women aged 20 to 44, 27/100,000 at ages 45 to 54, 70/100,000 at ages 65 to 74, and 140 to 150/100,000 for those over 75. The average age at which it is diagnosed is about 50. It occurs somewhat more often in white than in black women.

The lesions are often far advanced and impossible to cure when the patient first seeks treatment. She may have had mild gastrointestinal disturbance, which she attributed to "indigestion," and perhaps a slight increase in girth but no other symptoms. She often goes to a physician only after she feels a mass in the abdomen or has an attack of pain.

The only method for detecting ovarian cancer is periodic abdominal and pelvic examination. This is likely to fail. Small malignant tumors may be overlooked because they cannot be felt; by the time they grow enough to become palpable, the disease has spread throughout the peritoneal cavity. Ovaries that can be felt in postmenopausal women, particularly when previous examinations were considered to be normal, are suspect. Any ovary larger than 5 cm in diameter at any age may well contain a neoplasm and cannot be ignored.

Treatment. The results of treatment are in a large measure determined by the extent of the disease. The possibility of cure is greater if the tumor is confined to the ovary than if it has extended to the surrounding structures. It is not now possible to eradicate cancer of the ovary that has disseminated throughout the peritoneal cavity.

Cancer of the ovary is staged, as are carcinomas of the uterus, to permit the development of appropriate treatment plans and so that a physician may compare results with those of colleagues.

The following groups were established by the Cancer Committee of the International Federation of Gynaecology and Obstetrics:

Stage	Description
I	Growth limited to the ovaries
I A	Growth limited to one ovary
I B	Growth limited to both ovaries
I C	Growth limited to one or both ovaries with ascites showing malignant cells
II	Growth involving one or both ovaries with pelvic extension
II A	Extension and/or metastases to the uterus and/or tubes
II B	Extension to other pelvic tissues
III	Growth involving one or both ovaries with widespread intraperitoneal metastasis to upper half of abdomen (the omentum, the small intestine, and its mesentery)
IV	Growth involving one or both ovaries with distant metastasis outside the peritoneal cavity.

NOTE: The presence of ascites will not influence the staging for stages II, III, and IV.

The initial treatment of women with carcinoma of the ovary is *surgical*. The type of operation is determined by the extent of the disease and the nature of the lesion.

Whenever possible, a total hysterectomy, bilateral salpingo-oophorectomy, and omentectomy should be performed. Ascitic fluid or peritoneal washings should be collected for cytologic examination, and selected lymph nodes should be removed for histologic examination. Tumor nodules that involve the pelvic peritoneum should be removed.

If the tumor has metastasized widely, the bulky masses should be removed as completely as possible.

Occasionally, cancer will be diagnosed unexpectedly in a unilateral ovarian neoplasm. As a general rule, a second operation at which the uterus and the remaining tube and ovary are removed should be performed promptly unless the tumor is one that is almost always unilateral and there are reasons for preserving reproductive function.

The surgical treatment is supplemented by postoperative external radiation and/or chemotherapy, even though there was little chance that tumor was disseminated during the operation. A possible exception to this is selected patients with stage IA disease.

Five thousand rad are delivered to the pelvis from an external telecobalt source. In addition, if the lesion has obviously spread beyond the pelvis, the upper abdomen can also be treated. The dose to this area must be less than that to the pelvis because the organs in the upper abdomen tolerate radiation poorly.

If the tumor appears to be confined to the pelvis but there is a large quantity of ascitic fluid, tumor cells have certainly been disseminated into the upper abdomen. Under these circumstances or if there is gross evidence of widespread involvement, chemotherapeutic agents may be used alone or to supplement pelvic irradiation. The drugs do not often cure cancer of the ovary, but they may reduce fluid formation and maintain patients in a reasonable state of general health for many months.

Prognosis. As is true for all malignant tumors, the results of treating carcinoma of the ovary are determined by the type of tumor, the extent of its growth when diagnosed, and the quality of the treatment. Unfortunately, many ovarian cancers are beyond the hope of salvage by the time they are recognized.

The general 5-year survival rate for all types of ovarian cancer was 32% for both white and black women between 1900 and 1963. This had increased to 37% and 40%, respectively, between 1976 and 1981. Almost no patients with more advanced disease survive for 5 years.

REFERENCES

Abell, M.R.: The nature and classification of ovarian neoplasms, Can. Med. Assoc. J. **94:**1102, 1966.

Barber, H.R.K.: Ovarian cancer: diagnosis and management, Am. J. Obstet. Gynecol. **150:**910, 1984.

Demopoulos, R.I., et al.: Characterization and survival of patients with serous cystadenocarcinoma of the ovaries, Obstet. Gynecol. **64:**557, 1984.

Doss, N., Jr., Forney, J.P., Vellios, F., and Nalick, R.H.: Covert bilaterality of mature ovarian teratomas, Obstet. Gynecol. **50:**651, 1977.

Evans, A.T., III, Gaffey, T.A., Malkasian, G.D., and Annegers, J.F.: Clinopathologic review of 118 granulosa and 82 theca cell tumors, Obstet. Gynecol. **55:**231, 1980.

Fenoglio, C.M., and Richart, R.M.: Mucinous tumors of the ovary, Contemp. Obstet. Gynecol. **9:**64, 1977.

Garcia-Bunuel, R., Berek, J.S., and Woodruff, J.D.: Luteomas of pregnancy, Obstet. Gynecol. **45:**407, 1975.

Gordon, A., Lipton, and Woodruff, J.D.: Dysgerminoma: a review of 158 cases from the Emil Novak Ovarian Tumor Registry, Obstet. Gynecol. **58:**497, 1981.

Heintz, A.P., Hacker, N.F., and Lagasse, L.D.: Epidemiology and etiology of ovarian cancer: a review, Obstet. Gynecol. **66:**127, 1985.

Hallatt, J., Steele, C.H., Jr., and Snyder, M.: Ruptured corpus luteum with hemoperitoneum: a study of 173 surgical cases, Am. J. Obstet. Gynecol. **149:**5, 1984.

Hibbard, L.T.: Adnexal torsion, Am. J. Obstet. Gynecol. **152:**456, 1985.

Meigs, J.V.: Cancer of the ovary, Surg. Gynecol. Obstet. **71:**44, 1940.

Pantoja, E., Axtmayer, R.W., Colon, F.E., and Pelegrina, I.A.: Ovarian dermoids and their complications, Obstet. Gynecol. **30:**1, 1975.

Tazelaar, H.D., et al.: Conservative treatment of borderline ovarian tumors, Obstet. Gynecol. **66:**417, 1985.

49

J. Robert Willson

Aging

The biologic changes that accompany chronologic aging begin early in life, but most of those that occur before the ages of 40 to 45 are of little significance. The most obvious evidence of aging is cessation of menstruation, the menopause, which clearly marks the transition from the reproductive phase of life to senescence. Many other less evident changes are important determinants of physical and emotional health and well-being.

In most mammalian species the capacity to reproduce is maintained until late in life. The menopause and the atrophic changes that occur during the postmenopausal period are unique to humans and undoubtedly are attributable to increased longevity. Former generations of women were likely to have died at an early age from complications of repeated pregnancies or from infectious diseases, both of which can now effectively be prevented.

Aging women must cope with societal and socioeconomic, as well as physical problems, many of which occur because they live longer than men. In 1982 the average life expectancy at birth was 78.7 years for white women and 75.2 years for nonwhite women as compared to 71.4 years for white men and 66.5 years for nonwhite men. Life expectancy at age 65 is 18.5 years for white women, 14.2 years for white men, 16.5 years for black women, and 12.9 years for black men.

In 1982 about 34 million (28%) of the 119 million women in the United States were at least 50 years old; about 6 million were aged 50 to 54, about 12 million were 55 to 64, about 9 million were 65 to 74, and about 7 million were 75 or older. The fastest growing segment of the older population is that over age 85. It is anticipated that by 2010 about 4.5 million people will be older than 85, and, unless life expectancy of men increases dramatically, most of these will be women. One obvious consequence of the differences in death rates is that a greater proportion of elderly men than women are living with spouses; 7.5% of men aged 65 to 74 and 21.8% of those over 75 are widowed as compared to 38.3% and 68.5% of women at the same ages. This will not improve.

It has been customary to think of aging in women only in terms of the menopause, but this is too limited a concept. Aging is a continuing process that begins during embryonic life and ends with death. During the *climacteric* or *perimenopausal phase of life,* reproductive capacity is lost. The climacteric begins several years before the menopause and terminates when ovarian function ceases. The *menopause,* an episode in the climacteric period, indicates complete cessation of menstruation. The *postmenopausal phase of life* includes the late climacteric period and the subsequent years during which atrophic changes progress.

CLIMACTERIC

Sometime after the age of 40 the ovaries begin to lose their ability to respond to pituitary gonadotropin stimulation by the orderly sequence of follicle growth, maturation of the ovum, and ovulation, and by the secretion of normal amounts of estrogen and progesterone. This change is directly related to a significant decrease in the number of responsive ovarian follicles. The maximum number of primordial follicles, 8 to 10 million, can be found in the fetal ovary at about the twentieth gestational week. Most of these are lost or degenerate as pregnancy advances, so that at birth there are only about 1 to 2 million left. About 300,000 to 400,000 remain at menarche. During each menstrual cycle many follicles are "recruited" and begin to grow, but, in most instances, a single dominant follicle matures and ovulates; the rest become atretic. Since most normal women ovulate about 400 to 450 times during their reproductive lives, as many as 1000 follicles may begin to grow during each menstrual cycle.

After the age of 40 ovulation begins to occur less regularly than it had in the past. The relatively few remaining follicles are less likely to respond appropriately to gonadotropin stimulation. This may be because the estrogen peak necessary to release LH may not be reached or because the most responsive follicles have already been used. As a consequence, anovulatory cycles occur more and more frequently. Before the actual cessation of menstruation, bleeding may occur irregularly because of the erratic pattern of estrogen secretion. As the months go by, the diminishing number of remaining follicles produce less and less estrogen, and, finally, when there no longer are any that can respond, both estrogen secretion and bleeding cease.

As ovarian function declines, the concentrations of FSH and LH rise because there is no longer enough estrogen to inhibit their secretion. The reproductive hormone pattern during the early climacteric, therefore, is gradually declining estrogen, no progesterone after ovulation no longer occurs, and corresponding rises in FSH and LH. Later, when ovarian function ceases, FSH rises

tenfold to twentyfold and LH about threefold, reaching a maximum in 1 to 3 years (Fig. 49-1).

Menopause

The menopause, the complete cessation of menstruation and the most obvious evidence of termination of reproductive function, is the outstanding event of the climacteric phase of life. Menopause is the antithesis of menarche, an event during adolescence that marks the onset of reproductive capacity. Menopause can be diagnosed after a period of amenorrhea of 1 year.

The average age at which the menopause occurs is about 51. Some women stop menstruating as early as age 35, whereas others may continue until age 55 or even longer. Although both these limits may be normal, they are unusual.

In some women the periods continue to recur at regular intervals until they stop abruptly and permanently. More often the change is gradual. During the last 1 to 3 years of the climacteric, the amount of bleeding decreases, the interval between bleeding episodes lengthens, and periods of amenorrhea, which increase in duration, occur. The final periods may be represented by only slight spotting. The change in bleeding pattern occurs because of a progressive decline in ovarian estrogen secretion. Bleeding ceases permanently when too little estrogen is being produced to cause endometrial growth.

Some women have increased bleeding before the menopause. Periods of bleeding that may recur as often as every 2 to 3 weeks and that may be prolonged and profuse occur because of erratic increases and decreases in estrogen secretion. This is similar to dysfunctional bleeding in younger women. *Increased and irregular bleeding cannot be accepted as a consequence of declining ovarian function until uterine malignancy has been eliminated as a cause.*

Hormone secretion

The concentration of circulating estrogens decreases significantly after the menopause, and there is a reversal of estrogen fractions. Most of that which is available in postmenopausal women is estrone rather than estradiol. Neither the ovary nor

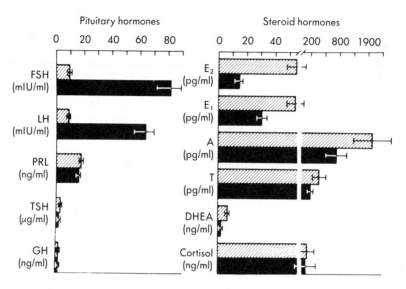

Fig. 49-1. Circulating concentrations of pituitary and steroid hormones in premenopausal women on days 2 to 4 of cycle *(lined bars)* and postmenopausal women *(black bars)*. *FSH,* Follicle-stimulating hormone; *LH,* luteinizing hormone; *PRL,* prolactin; *TSH,* thyroid-stimulating hormone; *GH,* growth hormone; E_2, estradiol; E_1, estrone; *A,* androstenedione; *T,* testosterone; *DHEA,* dehydroepiandrosterone. (From Yen, S.S.C.: J. Reprod. Med. **18:**287, 1977.)

the adrenal gland secretes significant amounts of estrogen during the postmenopausal period of life. The major source is peripheral conversion of androstenedione to estrone. Most of the androstenedione is derived from the adrenal cortex, but some comes from ovarian stroma. The ovary also produces testosterone, some of which may be converted to estradiol. The principal site of conversion is fat, although other tissues, especially the liver, do contribute. In some women enough estrone is produced by peripheral conversion to cause endometrial growth, even to the stage of hyperplasia, and bleeding. Since the prototypic candidate for endometrial cancer is obese, one can hypothesize that the exaggerated estrone production in adipose tissue may play a role in the genesis of the tumor.

Occasionally ovarian stromal and hilus cells will become hyperplastic, with a resultant increase in androgen secretion. Aromatization of these may produce enough estrone from androstenedione and estradiol from testosterone to cause endometrial hyperplasia and bleeding. These women may also be at risk of developing endometrial carcinoma.

The concentrations of pregnenolone, 17-hydroxy-pregnenolone, progesterone, and 17-hydroxyprogesterone are similar to those during the proliferative phase of a normal ovulatory cycle.

The menopause can be precipitated by removing the ovaries: *surgical menopause.* In contrast to the natural climacteric, during which ovarian function is reduced slowly, it is terminated abruptly and completely by oophorectomy. FSH and LH concentrations begin to rise almost immediately and remain elevated indefinitely.

PHYSIOLOGIC CHANGES ACCOMPANYING AGING

The changes that occur with aging affect all structures and functions of the body.

Changes in reproductive organs

The outstanding physical changes in the reproductive organs after the menopause are directly related to the withdrawal of the tissue-stimulating effects of estrogen. Labial fat is gradually reabsorbed, so the labia majora are flattened and, in elderly women, the skin may hang in folds. The labia minora may actually disappear.

The vagina gradually becomes smaller, the fornices become shallower, and the mucosa becomes progressively thinner. The vaginal smear reflects the change; as estrogen secretion diminishes, superficial cornified cells disappear, and eventually the cell type is predominantly parabasal and basal cells with a few of the intermediate type—a typical estrogen-deficient pattern.

Vaginal pH increases from the normal 3.5 to 4.5 in menstruating women to 5.0 or more after the menopause. The change is a result of decreased glycogen production in vaginal epithelial cells and the consequent decreased conversion of carbohydrate to lactic acid by Döderlein lactobacilli. There also is *less vaginal fluid,* which parallels the *decrease in vaginal blood flow.*

The supporting structures of the uterus, bladder, and rectum lose much of their tone and premenopausal strength because of atrophic changes in the tissues themselves accompanied by a significant decrease in vascularity that further reduces their integrity. These changes and the atrophy of the vaginal wall contribute to the development of cystocele, rectocele, and uterine prolapse. Stress urinary incontinence often increases or may begin after the menopause.

The cervix gradually decreases in size, but this may not be evident for some years; however, the secretory activity of the cervical glands decreases early in the climacteric. The mucus becomes scant and viscid, and the arborization phenomenon, which is a function of estrogen, is either absent or greatly reduced. Part of the atrophic change is a retreat of the squamocolumnar junction from its normal position on the portio or at the external os to a position well within the cervical canal (Fig. 49-2).

As a result of thinning of the myometrium, the uterus gradually becomes smaller until it resembles the uterus of the prepubertal girl. The endometrium as a rule becomes thin and atrophic, but various forms of retrogressive hyperplasia may occur in response to extragonadal estrogen stimulation (Figs. 49-3 and 49-4).

General body changes

A variety of changes in many physiologic functions occurs with aging. These physiologic changes include decreased thyroid function, decreased renal function, decreased insulin release in response to glucose challenge, hyperparathyroidism, impairments in thermoregulation, decreased tissue response to catecholamines, increased conversion of androstenedione to estrone, changes in fat distribution, and excessive hair growth. Neurologic changes include loss of memory, confusion, and impairments in balance control, which often result in falls.

Cardiovascular changes. There is conflicting and confusing information concerning the effect of the menopause on the occurrence of cardiovascular disease. The fact that the incidence of coronary artery disease, hypertension, and strokes is lower in premenopausal women than in men of similar ages led to the assumption that estrogen might have a beneficial effect. There is, however, no definite evidence to support the belief that estrogen protects against the development of atherosclerosis and myocardial infarction in women who experience natural menopause. The rate of cardiovascular disease in women increases in a linear manner, whereas there is an abrupt increase in men at about age 40. By the eighth or ninth decades of life the rates are similar in men and women.

In one study men who survived myocardial infarction and who were treated with estrogen had a higher incidence of reinfarction than did nontreated controls. The rate of recurrence was positively related to the amount of estrogen. The mortality from cardiovascular disease is increased in men with prostate carcinoma who are treated with estrogen. Klaiber and colleagues found that serum estradiol concentrations were significantly higher in men with acute myocardial infarction and in men with unstable angina as compared to men who were not hospitalized. There was a slight but insignificant rise in men who were hospitalized in a coronary care unit because a diagnosis of myocardial infarction was suspected but could not be made. Serum estrone concentrations were elevated in all patients.

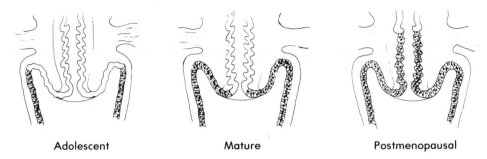

Adolescent   Mature   Postmenopausal

Fig. 49-2. Position of squamocolumnar junction at various life stages.

Conversely, Rosenberg and colleagues reported a sevenfold increase in myocardial infarctions after bilateral oophorectomy performed before age 35. A similar increase was not observed after hysterectomy with ovarian conservation. Others have suggested that early natural menopause increases the risk of cardiovascular disease, but this concept could not be confirmed by Lapidus, Bengtsson, and Lindquist.

Obviously there are differences in the responses of men and women to estrogen, and the exact role of each in the development of cardiovascular disease requires further study.

Bone changes. Bone loss begins at about age 30 and is progressive throughout adult life in both sexes. An abrupt acceleration occurs after the menopause, either natural or artificial, and the increasing length of life has compounded the associated problems. Postmenopausal women lose bone at an average rate of 1% to 2% a year. Those in their eighties may have lost half or more of their skeletons. *Osteoporosis* is accompanied by an increased risk of disability and death. Osteoporosis occurs more often in Caucasian and Asian than in black women, in thin than in fat women, and in smokers than in nonsmokers. It is more prevalent in those who have a family history of osteoporosis, in those receiving glucocorticoid therapy, and in those who, by choice or of necessity, are physically inactive. See box on page 686.

Bone loss appears to occur as a result of bone resorption, which is not balanced by reconstruction as it is in younger women. The precise mechanism

by which osteopenia and osteoporosis develop is not yet known. Available calcium may be reduced by inadequate dietary intake and by decreased intestinal absorption, both of which may occur in elderly women. Bone in elderly persons may become increasingly sensitive to the effects of parathyroid hormone. A calcitonin deficiency has been suspected, but Tiegs and colleagues found basal immunoreactive calcitonin in high concentrations and normal calcitonin reserves in women with osteoporosis.

One of the most important factors appears to be decreasing concentrations of estrogen. Richelson and colleagues, studying women whose ovaries had been removed early in life and women who were well past the menopause, none of whom was taking estrogen, found bone mineral densities at the midradius, the femoral neck, the intertrochanteric area, and the lumbar spine to be significantly reduced as compared to normal perimenopausal women who were still secreting estrogen. They concluded that estrogen deficiency is a more significant factor in the development of osteoporosis than is age alone. The exact mechanism for the protective effect of estrogen is not known.

Lindsay found that mestranol, 2.5 mg taken daily, prevented bone loss after bilateral oophorectomy. In contrast, control subjects who received no hormone lost bone at a rate of 1% a year. One group maintained bone density during 4 years of estrogen replacement but lost bone at a rate of 2.5% a year when the drug was stopped. Others have substantiated these findings. Another observation

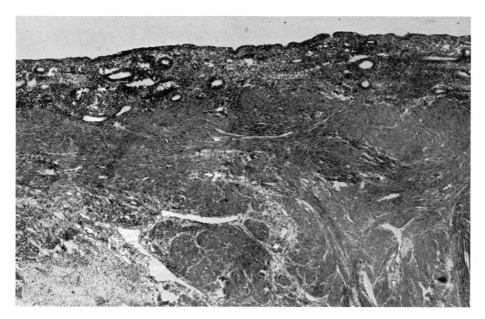

Fig. 49-3. Atrophic endometrium. Endometrium is thin, stroma is compact, and glands are few in number, narrow, and straight. (×60.)

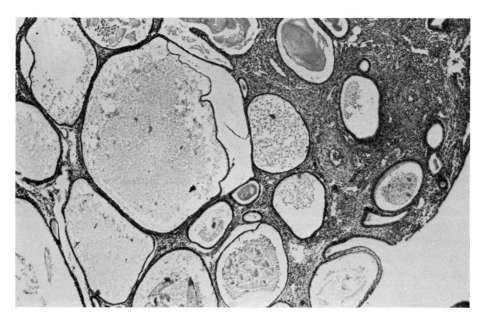

Fig. 49-4. Retrograde hyperplasia. Senile cystic endometrium resembles Swiss cheese hyperplasia. Stroma in this condition is more fibrous, and lining cells of glands are low cuboidal or flattened. (×60.)

RISK FACTORS FOR OSTEOPOROSIS
Hereditary
Female gender
Ovarian agenesis
Positive family history
Small bone mass
Caucasian or Oriental
Endocrine
Amenorrhea
Diabetes mellitus
Menopause
Thyrotoxicosis
Nulliparity
Adrenal steroid therapy
Nutritional
High alcohol intake
High caffeine intake
High animal protein intake
High sodium intake
High vitamin D intake
Low calcium intake
Life-style
Cigarette smoking
Inactivity
   Bedridden
   Inadequate exercise
   Weightlessness

suggesting that estrogen is important in maintaining normal bone metabolism is that hypogonadal women are likely to develop severe osteoporosis.

Bone loss begins first in trabecular bone and somewhat later in cortical bone. Demineralization of trabecular bone in the dorsal and lumbar vertebrae is followed by compression fractures that may first appear soon after the menopause. About 60% of women over 60 who are not taking estrogen will develop vertebral compression fractures. The only evidence may be gradual loss of height and the development of kyphosis. Pain occurs when nerves are compressed. Fractures through cortical bone occur somewhat later. Women have more long-bone fractures than do men of comparable ages. More than 40% of women will have had a fracture by age 75. At least 80% of women who develop hip fractures after age 40 are at least 75 years old. Most hip fractures are intertrochanteric and in osteoporotic bone. The cost of caring for patients with hip fractures may be as much as $2 billion a year, and as many as 26,000 women in the United States may die each year from the complications of hip fractures.

Symptoms

The most distressing symptoms in aging women begin to appear before the menopause and continue after the periods cease. Few of the symptoms are directly related to changes in hormone secretion. Many of the same symptoms occur in men. In both sexes they result from the general physical and emotional changes that accompany aging.

Vasomotor symptoms (hot flush). The most characteristic symptom of the menopause is the *hot flush*. The typical hot flush appears suddenly, with the first symptom being a sensation of heat in the chest, neck, and head that increases rapidly and lasts 3 or 4 minutes. The flush is followed by chilling and diaphoresis, which may be profuse enough to saturate the clothing. Hot flushes occur at night and during the day, and they are often accompanied by vertigo, palpitation, and a feeling of faintness.

The frequency and duration of the flushes vary. Some women have no vasomotor symptoms, but at least 75% experience flushes. In the majority the flushes are mild and may occur several times a day, but interfere little with usual activities. In the minority they recur many times during the day and at night and are so severe that they are disabling.

The flush follows rapid and localized vasodilatation, which often is evident because the face and neck become bright red. Core body temperature decreases slightly, but temperature in the fingers and toes rises because of vasodilatation and increased blood flow. Blood pressure is unchanged. Each flush coincides with a pulsatile release of LH, but FSH does not change. No significant changes take place in plasma dopamine, epinephrine, or norepinephrine.

The frequency with which flushes occur and their intensity usually begin to decrease in a few months. Most women are comfortable by 24 to 30 months, except during periods of emotional stress, when flushes usually are more troublesome.

The flushes are related to the decreasing secretion of estrogen as ovarian function declines. They do not occur in preadolescent girls or in women with primary hypogonadism before they are treated with estrogen. However, young women with gonadal dysgenesis who have been treated with exogenous estrogen will develop typical flushes if the medication is stopped. Women receiving clomiphene citrate (an antiestrogen) and danazol (which suppresses gonadotropin release) often experience flushes. It seems likely that a period of estrogen stimulation followed by withdrawal is an essential factor in the development of hot flushes.

The possibility that hot flushes are caused by high levels of gonadotropins has been considered, but it seems unlikely. Many women do not experience flushes despite the normal increase in gonadotropin concentration after the menopause. Untreated women with gonadal dysgenesis, who have elevated levels of gonadotropins, do not have hot flushes. Flushes can be eliminated by amounts of estrogen too small to suppress gonadotropin production to preclimacteric levels.

Obviously, factors other than estrogen and gonadotropins are responsible for the vasomotor symptoms. Emotional responses to the changing hormone pattern, the alterations in general physiologic processes, and the life situation in general may serve as accessory factors in the genesis of vasomotor symptoms. Flushes are usually more severe in anxious, neurotic women and usually are intensified in normal women whenever they are subjected to unusual stresses.

Nervous and psychologic symptoms. Headache, insomnia, vertigo, depression, and feelings of hopelessness, worthlessness, and self-condemnation are often experienced during the climacteric. These symptoms are of emotional origin and are not a direct result of estrogen deficiency. The basic personality is an important factor in determining the severity of psychologic symptoms. There is no evidence to suggest that psychoses are precipitated by menopause.

Few women understand the physiologic changes that occur during the climacteric and that are responsible for the menopause. Many have bizarre ideas of what to expect. Their fears include obesity, excessive hair growth, and other changes in their bodies that will make them less attractive; loss of sexual appetite; the development of psychoses; and, of course, the undeniable fact that they are getting old.

Many women who have been busy caring for their families find that their children no longer need them and their husbands are preoccupied with their jobs. These women now have less and less to do, and too few know how to make use of the many free hours available to them. Those who are working may realize that there is no hope of advancing to more interesting or responsible positions.

Many women become more sexually active when the fear of pregnancy is removed. Others lose libido completely when menstruation ceases. Sexuality and sexual activity have little relationship to estrogen secretion.

Genital symptoms. Most of the genital tract symptoms in postmenopausal women are caused by the atrophic changes that develop as a result of estrogen deprivation. The principal one is *atrophic vaginitis* (Chapter 45). *Dyspareunia* may occur because of decreased precoital lubrication, vaginitis, or constriction of the vagina or introitus. *Pruritus vulvae* also occurs frequently after the menopause.

The severity of symptoms associated with cystocele, rectocele, and uterine prolapse is determined by the extent of the changes in the supporting structures. Stress urinary incontinence is common in postmenopausal women.

Skeletal symptoms. Pain and stiffness in the joints is a common complaint in climacteric women and is often called *menopausal arthralgia*. Physical and x-ray examinations do not disclose any arthritic changes. The discomfort may be caused by an obscure change in the soft tissues surrounding the joints, or it may arise in muscles and tendons that are not exercised enough.

Osteoporosis involves most of the bone mass. It is particularly noticeable in the spine, with the formation of "dowager's hump" (dorsal kyphosis). Pain occurs only with fractures.

Differential diagnosis

Women who have periods of amenorrhea during the climacteric often fear that they may be pregnant. This can be ruled out by pelvic examination, demonstration of arborization in cervical mucus, and a pregnancy test when other examinations are inconclusive.

Not infrequently, the physician sees women in their forties who are still menstruating regularly but who complain of headache, dizziness, insomnia, fatigue, and some degree of depression. The temptation to blame these symptoms on the menopause is strong. Most often the patient is suffering from a condition that is totally unrelated to estrogen deprivation. The physician should hesitate to make a diagnosis of "menopausal syndrome" in patients who are still menstruating regularly, especially if vasomotor phenomena are not prominent features of the illness.

Treatment of the climacteric patient

Many women see no physician other than their gynecologists regularly. Therefore it is essential that obstetrician-gynecologists acquire more understanding of aging and provide appropriate examinations for their elderly patients. It is equally important that internists and family physicians who are responsible for the total care of elderly women be aware of the general physiologic changes of aging in addition to the gynecologic problems that may develop.

Since many of the changes attributed to aging are much like those that occur with prolonged periods of reduced physical activity, disuse may play an important role in the aging process. The most important changes that occur with inactivity are decreases in oxygen consumption, cardiac output and stroke volume, and body fluid. There is an increase in urinary nitrogen, in total cholesterol and triglycerides, and in the risk of thromboembolism. Bone loss is increased significantly by inactivity. Blood pressure, which may be elevated in elderly people, is often decreased by exercise. It seems essential that aging women be encouraged to remain active and that they be instructed in exercise programs that are within their limits of tolerance.

The best exercises, particularly to decrease the risk of osteoporosis, are those that stress bone; walking and aerobic exercises are excellent.

Dietary instruction is important. Many elderly women are undernourished because they cannot afford nutritious food, because they have no interest in preparing meals if they live alone, because they are edentulous or have poor dentures and cannot chew solid food, or because they are unaware of their nutritional needs. The diet should be adequate in protein and vitamins, particularly vitamin D, but a particularly important ingredient is calcium. An intake of 1500 mg of calcium is recommended to prevent postmenopausal bone loss. This can be reduced to 1000 mg in women who are taking estrogen. Most women will need additional calcium to supplement that taken in their diets; this can be given as calcium carbonate.

Periodic examinations are even more important for women during the climacteric and after the menopause than in younger women. The incidence of many malignancies increases as do degenerative changes in other organ systems. Emotional problems that may have caused little discomfort while a woman was busy caring for her family may become far more serious and even disabling as physical discomfort increases and responsibilities decrease. The symptoms may be magnified by her children leaving home and by the death of her husband.

The examination should be designed to detect the disorders that first appear or that are more prevalent in older than in younger women. For example, pregnancy, genital herpes, and gonorrhea rarely occur during the climacteric period, but cancer, both genital and extragenital, hypertension, obesity, degenerative diseases, diabetes, nutritional deficiencies, and anemia are common. Young women have little concern for death and aging, but these are of great importance after the menopause.

An *appropriate periodic examination* for the presumably well elderly woman includes a history update, complete physical examination including tonometry, breast, pelvic and rectal examinations, with a check for occult fecal blood. Basic laboratory studies should include a Pap test, hemoglobin and hematocrit studies, and urine examination. Other laboratory studies are ordered as indicated. A yearly mammogram will help to detect early breast abnormalities. There are no tests comparable to cervical cytology to detect early uterine or ovarian cancer, but if one is able to palpate an ovary in a postmenopausal woman an abnormality should be suspected and investigated. The normal ovary is so small that it cannot often be felt (Chapter 48).

Since osteoporosis is one of the most important consequences of the menopause it should, if possible, be recognized before fractures occur. Standard x-ray film evidence of bone loss suggests that the process is well advanced. *Single photon densitometry* involves assessment of bone thickness in the radius. Midshaft determinations reflect principally cortical bone, whereas those near the wrist reflect trabecular bone. *Dual photon densitometry* is used primarily to assess the femoral head and spine. These studies are costly and not generally available and need not be used for patients at low risk of developing osteoporosis. This is particularly true of those who are taking estrogen-progestogen. They should be considered as part of the assessment of high-risk women.

Depression is almost universal in elderly people, and physicians often do not recognize the less obvious forms. Loss of memory and episodes of mental confusion also may occur. As physical and mental functions deteriorate, day-to-day living becomes more difficult. Physicians must be prepared to recognize these changes and to help patients cope with them.

Psychotherapy. An unhurried discussion of the meaning and manifestation of the menopause is the first and perhaps most important step in therapy for the climacteric patient. This provides authoritative guidance and reassurance to the middle-aged woman who at this time finds herself in need of both. No woman can blithely disregard the change in her appearance and the prospect of progressive aging.

A well-adjusted, emotionally secure woman can be encouraged to draw psychologic strength from her past successes and to turn her resources and energies to new pursuits. Reeducation, reassur-ance, and mild manipulation of the patient's environment constitute the methods of superficial psychotherapy that are available to all interested physicians. Such measures will be sufficient for the vast majority of climacteric women. The patient with profound changes in personality or one who becomes extremely depressed should be referred to a psychiatrist for more specialized treatment.

Hormone therapy. Since the symptoms and physiologic alterations that accompany the menopause occur in women whose ovarian function is failing, it seems logical to assume that ovarian hormone replacement therapy should be beneficial. This assumption is true. Although psychotherapy and other measures are appropriate and may be helpful, they do not often eliminate the symptoms caused by estrogen deficiency.

ESTROGENS. The principal reasons for prescribing estrogen therapy are *to eliminate hot flushes, to prevent or delay atrophy of the genital structures,* and *to prevent osteoporosis.*

There are many effective estrogen preparations that differ in their derivation, potency, duration of action, and cost. The dosage is regulated by the degree to which hot flushes are relieved, insomnia corrected, and a feeling of well-being produced. The amount required to accomplish this usually also prevents genital atrophy and unusual bone loss.

The preparations most often used are sodium estrone sulfate, in daily dosages of 0.625 to 1.25 mg, and ethinyl estradiol, 0.05 to 0.2 mg. There is rarely a reason for giving estrogen parenterally.

Unopposed estrogen stimulation appears to be an important factor in the genesis of endometrial cancer, but the risk can be reduced substantially if a progestogen is added during the last 10 to 14 days of the treatment cycle. Gambrell reported the incidence of endometrial cancer to be 242.2/100,000 population in postmenopausal women who were taking no hormone, 434.4/100,000 in women taking estrogen alone and 70.8/100,000 in women taking estrogen-progestogen combinations (Table 49-1).

The initial dose of estrogen should be the lowest one might expect to control symptoms while still

TABLE 49-1 Endometrial cancer and hormonal therapy*

Therapy	Patient years observation	Incidence/100,000
None	2477	242.2
Estrogen	2303	434.4
Estrogen-progestogen	7063	70.8
Estrogen vaginal cream	1318	75.9

*From Gambrell, R.D., Jr.: The menopause, Fertil. Steril. **37:**457, 1982.

preventing atrophic changes in the reproductive organs and bone loss. In most women *0.625 mg of sodium estrone sulfate daily during the first 25 days of each month* will accomplish these aims. The frequency and severity of flushes are either decreased significantly or eliminated. If the symptoms persist, 1.25 mg can be prescribed. It is unusual that a dose larger than this is needed.

The prescription of *10 mg of medroxyprogesterone acetate* (Provera) daily starting on the sixteenth day of the treatment cycle will reduce the risk of abnormal endometrial hyperplasia. Unfortunately, the combination of estrogen and progesterone often stimulates withdrawal bleeding, whereas estrogen alone may not. This, together with the possibility that the combination will produce symptoms like those during the premenstrual phase of the normal cycle, makes many women reluctant to continue the regimen. Since withdrawal bleeding usually decreases and stops within a few years, they should be encouraged to persist.

An alternative method, which reduces the likelihood of significant bleeding while still offering the protective effect of a progestogen, is to prescribe combined treatment to be taken continuously. Staland has treated 265 women with 17 beta-estradiol, estrone, and norethisterone acetate continuously with good relief of flushes and minimal bleeding. By the end of 4 months endometrial biopsy revealed the endometrium to be atrophic in 92% and incompletely atrophic in 6%. Such a regimen reduces the incidence of annoying bleeding and, since it prevents hyperplasia, should provide excellent protection against malignancy.

In the past it was thought necessary to limit the duration of estrogen use. The dosage schedule was determined by the fact that untreated women became free from symptoms after about 24 to 30 months. The initial dose that controlled the symptoms was continued for 12 to 18 months, then gradually reduced and eventually withdrawn completely. Gradual reduction was necessary to acclimatize the patient to a progressively lower dosage. If estrogen is stopped abruptly, flushes almost always return.

The risk of death and disability from the complications of osteoporosis are far greater than that of developing endometrial cancer, particularly in women who are taking an estrogen-progestogen combination. Although there is not yet enough experience to determine whether the protective effect of estrogen therapy on bone loss will continue indefinitely, serious consideration should be given to continuing estrogen therapy indefinitely if there is no contraindication to its use. It should certainly be continued in women who are at risk of developing osteoporosis. These include thin white or Asian women, smokers, those with family histories of osteoporosis, those who are receiving glucocorticoid therapy, and those who are bedridden or inactive. They, too, can be treated with estrogen-medroxyprogesterone or estrogen-methyltestosterone combinations. They should also be given supplemental calcium and encouraged to exercise vigorously.

One of the important indications for estrogen therapy is *atrophic vaginitis*. This is better managed by estrogenic cream applied to the vagina than by oral estrogen. The vaginal cells are stimulated to proliferate and cornify, which permits them to overcome the infection without the use of other agents. Estrogen is absorbed from the vagina and may produce systemic effects. Atrophic vaginitis is discussed in detail in Chapter 45.

Estrogen may also be helpful in controlling *stress urinary incontinence* that begins after the menopause. The atrophy of the tissues and the loss of vascularity in the structures surrounding the vesicle neck may permit them to relax enough to interfere with urinary control. The symptoms may be relieved by estrogen therapy. Estrogen will have no effect in premenopausal women, nor can it be expected to correct incontinence that is associated with extensive vaginal relaxation nor that caused by unstable bladders. Pubococcygeus exercises should also be recommended (Chapter 41).

There is little evidence to support the concern that estrogen plays a role in the genesis of cancers of the cervix or ovary or of malignancies in other parts of the body, particularly when it is administered with a progestogen. The major concern is for breast lesions. Gambrell reported an incidence of breast cancer of 500/100,000 population in women taking no medication, 137.3/100,000 in women taking unopposed estrogen, 135.3/100,000 in women taking estrogen-androgen combinations and 95.6/100,000 in women taking estrogen and progestogen (Table 49-2).

Treatment of asymptomatic women. Postmenopausal women who have no flushes obviously need no medication to control them. Since these women appear to be able to aromatize enough androgens to provide the estrogen necessary to prevent flushes, they may develop endometrial hyperplasia. Gambrell has suggested that such women be given 10 mg of medroxyprogesterone acetate daily for 10 days (Progestogen Challenge Test): if they have no withdrawal bleeding, they are not secreting enough estrogen to stimulate the endometrium. Conversely, if they do bleed after estrogen withdrawal, monthly courses of a progestogen should be recommended to prevent hyperplastic changes. The progestin can be discontinued when it no longer stimulates withdrawal bleeding. These women should be given the same advice concerning diet and exercise as those who are taking estrogen.

Uterine bleeding. Most women who take estrogen-progestogen preparations have withdrawal bleeding, which may continue in decreasing amounts until about age 60. After that it decreases, but in some bleeding will continue as long as progestogen is administered. Most authorities believe

TABLE 49-2 Breast cancer and hormonal therapy*

Therapy	Patient years observation	Incidence/100,000
None	3799	500.0
Estrogen	10,928	137.3
Estrogen-progestogen	7322	95.6
Estrogen vaginal cream	1811	55.2

*From Gambrell, R.D., Jr.: The menopause, Fertil. Steril. **37:**457, 1982.

that no investigation is necessary if the bleeding occurs only after progestogen withdrawal. Conversely, if it occurs at any other phase of the cycle, endometrial biopsy or curettage is essential to determine the cause.

Women who are taking estrogen alone should be given a Progestogen Challenge Test of 10 mg medroxyprogesterone acetate from time to time. If bleeding occurs the endometrium may be overstimulated and regular courses of progestogen should be recommended. If there is no bleeding, there probably is so little endometrial stimulation that it cannot respond to progestogen. It probably is safe for these women to continue taking estrogen alone.

CONTRAINDICATIONS. Estrogens are contraindicated in women with *acute liver disease* or *whose liver function is significantly reduced,* those who have had severe *thrombophlebitis* or *thromboembolism,* those with *estrogen-dependent malignant neoplasms,* or those with *abnormal vaginal bleeding for which the cause has not yet been determined.*

Progesterone. Medroxyprogesterone acetate may be used to control hot flushes when estrogen is contraindicated. It may be given orally as Provera, 20 mg daily, or by injection as Depo-Provera, 150 to 200 mg monthly. Although progesterone may eliminate flushes, it is not a complete substitute for estrogen. Progesterone may have a depressive effect on some women.

Nonhormonal treatment. There are alternative methods of treating climacteric symptoms in women who do not want to take estrogen or those in whom it is contraindicated. Mild symptoms can often be ameliorated by superficial psychotherapy and the prescription of small doses of phenobarbital or tranquilizers. These drugs have a limited effect on women who are disabled by the flushes. The antihypertensive agent clonidine may reduce the severity of the flushes.

REFERENCES

Bartuska, D.G.: Physiology of aging: metabolic changes during the climacteric and menopausal periods, Clin. Obstet. Gynecol. **20**:105, 1977.

Bush, T.L., and Barrett-Connor, E.: Noncontraceptive use and cardiovascular disease, Epidemiol. Rev. **7**:80, 1985.

Bortz, W.M., II: Disuse and aging, J.A.M.A. **248**:1203, 1982.

Chang, R.J., and Judd, H.L.: The ovary after menopause, Clin. Obstet. Gynecol. **24**:181, 1981.

Gambrell, R.D.: The menopause: benefits and risks of estrogen-progestogen replacement therapy, Fertil. Steril. **37**:457, 1982.

Gambrell, R.D.: Sex steroid hormones and cancer, Curr. Probl. Obstet. Gynecol. **7**:1, 1984.

Hammond, C.B., and Maxson, W.S.: Current status of estrogen therapy for the menopause, Fertil. Steril. **37**:5, 1982.

Judd, H.L., Cleary, R.E., Creasman, W.T., Figge, D.C., Kase, N., Rosenwaks, Z., and Tagatz, G.E.: Estrogen replacement therapy, Obstet. Gynecol. **58**:267, 1981.

Klaiber, E.L., et al.: Serum estrogen levels in men with acute myocardial infarction, Am. J. Med. **73**:872, 1982.

Lapidus, L., Bengtsson, C., and Lindquist, O.: Menopausal age and risk of cardiovascular disease and death, Acta Obstet. Gynecol. Scand. (Suppl.) **130**:37, 1985.

Lindsay, R., Hart, D.M., and Clark, D.M.: The minimum effective dose of estrogen for prevention of postmenopausal bone loss, Obstet. Gynecol. **63**:759, 1984.

Lindsay, R., Hart, D.M., MacLean, A., Clark, A.C., Kraszewski, A., and Garwood, J.: Bone response to termination of oestrogen treatment, Lancet **1**:1325, 1978.

Lobo, R.A., et al.: Depo-medroxyprogesterone acetate compared with conjugated estrogens for the treatment of postmenopausal women, Obstet. Gynecol. **63**:1, 1984.

Monroe, S.E., and Menon, K.M.J.: Changes in reproductive hormone secretion during the climacteric and postmenopausal periods, Clin. Obstet. Gynecol. **20**:113, 1977.

Natl. Inst Health Consensus Conference Statement: Osteoporosis, Bethesda, 1984, National Institute of Arthritis, Diabetes, and Digestive and Kidney Diseases.

Persson, I.: The risk of endometrial and breast cancer after estrogen treatment: a review of epidemiologic studies, Acta Obstet. Gynecol. Scand. (Suppl) **130**:59, 1985.

Richelson, L.S., et al.: Relative contributions of aging and estrogen deficiency to postmenopausal bone loss, N. Engl. J. Med. **311**:1273, 1984.

Rigg, L.A., Hermann, H., and Yen, S.S.C.: Absorption of estrogens from vaginal creams, N. Engl. J. Med. **298**:195, 1978.

Rosenberg, L., Hennekens, C.H., Rosner, B., Belanger, C., Rothman, K.J., and Speizer, F.E.: Early menopause and the risk of myocardial infarction, Am. J. Obstet. Gynecol. **139**:47, 1981.

Schiff, I., Tulchinsky, D., Cramer, D., and Ryan, K.J.: Oral medroxyprogesterone in the treatment of postmenopausal symptoms, J.A.M.A. **244**:1443, 1980.

Semmens, J.P.: Estrogen deprivation and vaginal function in postmenopausal women, J.A.M.A. **248**:445, 1982.

Staland, B.: Continuous treatment with a combination of estrogen and gestagen—a way of avoiding endometrial stimulation, Acta Obstet. Gynecol. (Suppl.) **130**:29, 1985.

Tiegs, R.D., et al.: Calcitonin secretion in postmenopausal osteoporosis, N. Engl. J. Med. **312**:1097, 1985.

Tulandi, T., and Lal, S.: Menopausal hot flush, Obstet. Gynecol. Surv. **40**:553, 1985.

Worley, R.J.: Age, estrogen, and bone density, Clin. Obstet. Gynecol. **24**:203, 1981.

Yen, S.S.C.: The biology of menopause, J. Reprod. Med. **18**:287, 1977.

Index

A

Abdominal examination, 14
  fetal position and, 394-396
  during labor, 419
  during pregnancy, 290, 394-396
Abdominal wall, pregnancy and, 255-256
Abdominal hysterectomy, hydatidiform mole and, 244
Abdominal hysterotomy for abortion, 207
Abdominal pregnancy, 227, 231
Abdomen
  ovarian neoplasms and, 675
  wound infection and, 590
Abell classification of ovarian neoplasms, 668
Abnormal uterine bleeding, 88-96; *see also* Uterine bleeding
ABO incompatibility, 152, 461-462
ABO status of rape victim, 73
Abortion, 10, 210-224; *see also* Fetal death
  amniocentesis and, 34
  appendicitis and, 332
  bleeding and, 89
  breast cancer and, 140-141
  care of patient after, 208
  complete, 214, 218
  complications of, 206-207
  diabetes mellitus and, 306
  elective, 206
  glomerulonephritis and, 340, 341
  habitual, 214-215, 218, 219
    treatment of, 218, 220-221
  heart disease and, 317, 319
    kyphoscoliotic, 310
  hypertension and, 376
  illegal, 210, 222-223
  incomplete, 213-214, 216-218
  indications for, 205-206
  induced, 221-223
  inevitable, 213, 216
  infected, 211, 219-220, 222-223, 581-585

Abortion—cont'd
  intrauterine device and, 198
  legal, 6, 205-208, 210
  leiomyomas and, 653
  missed, 214, 218
  multifetal pregnancy and, 510
  physician responsibility and, 206
  placenta previa and, 386
  radioreceptor assay for, 29
  rape and, 74
  rubella during pregnancy and, 293
  septic, 210, 222
  spontaneous, 10, 210-218
  surgery during pregnancy and, 331
  technique of, 207-208
  threatened, 213-216, 235
  thyroid disorders and, 308
  tubal, 228, 229, 231
  tuberculosis and, 314
Abrasion, scalp, 540
Abruptio placentae, 376, 386-391
  anesthesia and analgesia and, 443
  cesarean section and, 542
  differential diagnosis of, 332, 389-390
  enema during labor and, 419
  fibrin degradation product and, 387
  hypertension and, 378
  neonatal death and, 11
  premature labor and, 425
Abscess
  endomyometritis and, 593
  epidural, 438
  infected abortion and, 583
  pelvic, 584, 588
  periareolar, 135
  tuboovarian, 588
Acceleration phase of labor, 417
Accessory nipples, 135

Acetate, 159
Acetic acid, 613
Acid phosphatase screening test, 73
Acid-base balance, 270; *see also* Acidosis
    parathyroid disorders and, 309
Acidosis
    diabetes mellitus and, 298, 299, 304
    nausea and vomiting during pregnancy and, 327, 328
Acrodysesthesia, 359
Acromegaly, 106
Acrosomal reaction, 146
ACTH; *see* Adrenocorticotropic hormone
Actinomyces, 584
Actinomycin D, 248-249
Actinomycosis
    breast lesion and, 136
    intrauterine device and, 198
    pelvic infection and, 596
Active phase of labor, 417
    arrest of
        contracted pelvis and, 506
        dystocia and, 475, 476
        uterine dysfunction and, 478-479
Active transfer by placenta, 154
Actomyosin, 408
Acute fatty liver of pregnancy, 329-330
Acute tubular necrosis, 387
Acyclovir, 610
Addiction, infant and, 458
Addison's disease, 109, 310
Adenoacanthomas, 659
Adenocarcinoma
    clear cell, 42-43
    diethylstilbestrol and, 42
    endometrial cancer and, 659, 660
    endometriosis and, 127
    teratoma and, 670
Adenofibromas, 672
Adenoma, 658-659
    oral contraception and, 202
    parathyroid, 310
Adenomatous carcinomas, uterine, 662
Adenomatous hyperplasia, 658-659
Adenomyoma, 310, 655
Adenomyosis, 126, 131, 655-656
    abnormal uterine bleeding and, 89
    definition of, 122
Adenosine triphosphate, 408
Adenosis
    breast and, 137
    vaginal, 41-43
Adenosquamous carcinomas, 659
ADH; *see* Antidiuretic hormone
Adhesions
    amenorrhea and, 101

Adhesions—cont'd
    endometriosis and, 123
    peritubal, 226
Adnexal mass, 16
Adolescence, 56-57
    abnormal uterine bleeding and, 91-93
    amenorrhea and, 98
    contraception and, 193
    and diet in pregnancy, 284-285
    gynecologic problems in, 49-50
    pregnancy and, 6-7
Adrenal atrophy, 310-311
Adrenal corticosteroids
    placenta and, 161
    thrombocytopenic purpura and, 324
Adrenal crisis, 310
Adrenal gland
    amenorrhea and, 109, 112
    diseases of, 45-46, 310-311; *see also* Adrenal hyperplasia
        insufficiency in, 310, 341, 428
    eclampsia and, 374
    infarction of, 310
    pregnancy and, 267
        prolonged, 428
    tumor of, 47, 49
Adrenal hyperfunction, 311
Adrenal hyperplasia, 45-46, 311; *see also* Congenital adrenal
        hyperplasia
    amniotic fluid and, 164
    heterosexual precocity and, 49
    hormone assay and, 18
Adrenal hypoplasia, 428
Adrenal insufficiency, 310
    immunosuppressives and, 341
Adrenal medullary hyperfunction, 311
Adrenal tumor, 47, 49
Adrenalectomy, 140
Adrenocortical extracts, 310
Adrenocortical failure, acute, 310
Adrenocorticotropic hormone
    adrenal atrophy and, 310
    congenital adrenal hyperplasia and, 45
    placenta and, 161
Aerobic bacteria, 578
Aerosol foam contraception, 196
Afterpain, 604
Agammaglobulinemia, 149
Age; *see also* Aging
    carcinoma and, 656
    gestational, 524
    maternal, Down's syndrome and, 459
    menstruation onset, 85
Agenesis, vaginal, 40
Agglutination inhibition principle, 28
Aging, 682-692; *see also* Age; Menopause

Aging—cont'd
  climacteric and; *see* Climacteric
  multifetal pregnancy and, 509
  nervous symptoms and, 687
  physiologic changes in, 682-686
  symptoms in, 686-688
  treatment of, 688-692
AID; *see* Artificial insemination
AIH; *see* Artificial insemination
Alanine amninotransferase, 329
Albright's syndrome, 49
Albumin, plasma, 329
Albumin-globulin ratio, 258-259
Alcock's canal, 443
Alcohol
  breast-feeding and, 603
  maternal abuse of, 212, 458
  megaloblastic anemia and, 322
  pregnancy and, 212, 288-289
  premature labor prevention and, 426
  sex therapy and, 68
  trichomoniasis and, 623
Alcohol/drug screening, rape and, 74
Aldohexose, 153
Aldosterone
  placenta and, 161
  pregnancy and, 263, 264, 267
  puerperial changes and, 601
Alkaline pH of saliva, 264
Alkaline phosphatase, 161-162, 329
Alkalosis, 309
Allergic vaginitis, 625
Alpha thalassemia, 323
Alpha-fetoprotein
  diabetes mellitus and, 301, 303
  pregnancy and, 259
    multifetal, 511, 512
  serum, 301
17-Alpha-hydroxyprogesterone
  endometrial cancer and, 663
  habitual abortion and, 221
  inevitable abortion and, 213
5-Alpha-reductase, 103-104
ALT; *see* Alanine aminotransferase
Alternative birth center, 4-5
Aluminum hydroxide
  hiatus hernia and, 329
  hypoparathyroidism and, 309
Amastia, 135
Ambulation after delivery, 602
Ameboid mass, 150
Amenorrhea, 56, 97-114
  adolescence and, 98
  diagnosis in, 109-111
  etiologic factors and, 97-109

Amenorrhea—cont'd
  anatomic, 99-101
    gonadal, 101-108
    physiologic, 99-100
  exercise and, 108
  hormone assay in, 18
  oral contraception and, 201, 203
  postpartum, 606
  pregnancy and, 276
  primary, 50, 85, 97
  psychogenic, 108
  secondary, 97
  thyroid disorders and, 308
  treatment for, 111-113
Amenorrhea-galactorrhea, 106, 606
American Board of Obstetrics and Gynecology, 1
American Cancer Society, 133, 135
American Fertility Society, 124
Amethopterin, 248-249
Amino acids, 263
Aminoglycosides, 578, 584, 588, 590
  endomyometritis and, 594
  side effects in infant and, 458
  subacute bacterial endocarditis and, 318
Aminopterin, 458
Amniocentesis, 34-35, 164
  complications of, 34-35
  diabetes mellitus and, 302
  diagnosis and, 34-35, 149
  genetics and, 276
  indications for, 34
  Rh incompatibility and, 461
Amniography, hydramnios and, 170
Amnion, 147, 150
  abnormality of, 169-170
  ultrastructure of, 163-164
Amnionitis, 168
Amnioscopy, 35
Amniotic fluid, 163-166; *see also* Amniocentesis
  fetal age and, 283
  fetal cells from, 165, 166
  multifetal pregnancy and, 510
  pH of, 430
  spectrophotometric analysis of, 460
  volume abnormality of, 33
Amniotic fluid infusion, 454
Amniotomy
  contracted pelvis and, 505
  hydramnios and, 170
  labor and, 431
  uterine dysfunction and, 477, 478-479
Amobarbital
  eclampsia and, 373
  vomiting and, 328
Amoxicillin, 588

Amoxicillin—cont'd
    rape and, 74
Ampicillin, 579, 588
    bacterial vaginosis and, 625
    endomyometritis and, 594
    pyelonephritis and, 338
    rape and, 74
    urinary tract infection and, 337
Amylase, 330
Amytal; *see* Amobarbital
Anaerobe, 578
Anal phase, 55-56
Anal sphincter, separation of, 553
Analgesia; *see also* Anesthesia
    hypoadrenalism and, 310
    inevitable abortion and, 216
    obstetric, 434-438
    premature labor and, 426
Anatomic incontinence, 560, 561-564; *see also* Stress urinary
    incontinence
Androgens
    amenorrhea and, 103
    fetus and, 61-62
    luteomas and, 666
    male external genitals and, 45
    tests for, 23
Androgyny, 54
Android pelvis, 497, 498, 504
Androstenedione, 23
    aging and, 682
    placenta and, 159
Anemia
    infected abortion and, 581
    iron-deficiency, 321-322
    macrocytic, 322
    megaloblastic, 322
    narcotic addiction and, 458
    pernicious, 322
    postpartum hemorrhage and, 450
    pregnancy and, 256-257
    premature labor and, 426
    sickle cell, 322-324
    young primigravidas and, 428
Anencephaly, 149
    face position and, 487
    placenta and, 158
Anesthesia; *see also* Analgesia
    cesarean section and, 546
    diabetes mellitus and, 304
    episiotomy and, 555
    forceps delivery and, 536
    heart disease and, 318, 319
    hypoadrenalism and, 310
    infant and, 438

Anesthesia—cont'd
    inhalation, 544
    obstetric, 434-435, 438-443
    postpartum hemorrhage and, 450
    spontaneous abortion and, 212
    surgery during pregnancy and, 331
    vaginal twin delivery and, 514
Aneuploidy, 148
Aneurysm, cerebral, 358
Angiotensin and angiotensinogen, 264
Angle of inclination, 494
Ankylosis, sacrococcygeal, 362
Annular amputation, 566
Anorexia, pregnancy and, 329
Anorexia nervosa, 56, 108
Anovulatory cycle, 25
Anoxia
    breech delivery and, 520
    fetal death and, 10
    placenta previa and, 386
Antacid, 546
Antepartum care, 456
Antepartum fetus evaluation, 456
Anterior displacement of uterus, 350
Anterior fontanel, 171
Anterior parietal bone presentation, 410, 411
    platypelloid pelvis and, 503
Anterior pituitary gland, 76, 77, 78
Anterior rotation, 486
Anterior segment, 495
Anteroposterior diameter, 491, 495, 496, 499, 500,
    503
Anthropoid pelvis, 497-498, 504
Antibiotics
    abortion and, 581, 582
    breast-feeding and, 603
    cervicitis and, 630
    cesarean section and, 591
    fetus and, 457
    pelvic masses and, 588
    postoperative infection and, 589, 590
    pyelonephritis and, 338
    surgery during pregnancy and, 331
    vulvular dermatitis and, 614
Antibody
    antisperm, 190
    herpesvirus and, 610
    pregnancy and, 275
    Rh incompatibility and, 460
Anticholinergic, 565
Anticholinesterases, 357, 358
Anticoagulants
    disseminated intravascular coagulation and, 324
    thrombophlebitis and, 594-595

Antidiuretic hormone
  diabetes insipidus and, 306
  pregnancy and, 263
Antiestrogen
  breast cancer and, 140
  hot flush and, 687
Antiglobulin test, 461, 462
Antihistamines
  breast-feeding and, 603
  herpes gestationis and, 360
  vulvitis and, 612
Antihypertensives, 377
Antimicrobial agent; *see* Antibiotics
Antiplatelets, 324
Antipyrine, 268
Antispasmodics, 333
Antisperm antibody, 190
Antithyroid drugs, 309, 458
Anuria
  abruptio placentae and, 391
  eclampsia and, 368
Anus, vaginal ectopic, 41
Aorta
  coarctation of, 319
  compression on, 316
Apgar score, 471
Apnea, infant, 436, 438, 472
Appendicitis
  blood count and, 17
  infertility and, 179
  pregnancy and, 331-332
    ectopic, 235
Appendix, pregnancy and, 265, 332; *see also* Appendicitis
APPG; *see* Aqueous procaine penicillin G
Apresoline; *see* Hydralazine
Aqueous procaine penicillin G, 588
Arachnoiditis, 440
Arborization, 20, 628
  menstruation and, 84-85
Areola
  pregnancy and, 256
  secondary, 277
Arm, partial breech extraction and, 525
Arrhenoblastoma, 675
  amenorrhea and, 103, 105-106
Arterial blood pressure, 260
Arterial oxygen saturation, 173
Arteriolar spasm, 366
Arteriovenous oxygen difference, 261
Arteriovenous shunt, 169
Arthralgia, 687
Artificial insemination, 188-189
Ascites, 675
Ascorbic acid, 322, 328
Asherman's syndrome, 101

Asian influenza, 314
Aspartate aminotransferase test, 329
Aspermia, 178
Asphyxia neonatorum, 472
  diabetes mellitus and, 300
Aspiration
  inhalation anesthesia and, 438
  of mucus, eclampsia and, 373
  of particulate meconium, 472
  vabra, 23
Aspiration biopsy of breast, 134-135, 138
Aspirin
  fetus and, 459
  premature labor prevention and, 426
  urination after delivery and, 603
Assault, sexual, 70-75
Assisted breech delivery, 525-526, 527, 528, 529, 530
AST; *see* Aspartate aminotransferase test
Asthma, 314
Asymmetric retardation, 427
Asymmetrical breasts, 135
Asymptomatic bacteriuria
  fetus and, 459
  pregnancy and, 336, 337
  pyelonephritis and, 338
Asynclitism, 410, 411
Atony, uterine, 452
Atresia
  of cervix, 100
  of vagina, 39, 99, 100
Atrial fibrillation, 316, 317, 318
Atrophic vaginitis, 609, 610, 625, 687, 690
  dyspareunia and, 64
Atrophy
  endometrial, 683, 685
  vulva and, 613, 614
Atropine
  amniotic fluid infusion and, 454
  breast-feeding and, 603
  ptyalism and, 326
Attitude
  fetal, 393
  sexual response and, 62-63
Atypia, 615
Atypical hyperplasia of endometrium, 659, 660
Auscultation of fetal heart, 396
  during labor, 419
Autoimmunity
  endometriosis and, 127
  habitual abortion and, 218
Autosomal deletion, 148
Azoospermia, 178
Azotemia, 339
Aztreonam, 577, 581

B

Baby boom, 5
Bacilli, Döderlein's, 621
Backache
    multifetal pregnancy and, 510
    postpartum, 606
Bacteremia, 168, 594
Bacteria
    in blood, 594
    culture of, 17
    infected abortion and, 584
    placental transfer and, 154
    premature labor and, 425
    rape and, 74
    in urine; *see* Bacteriuria, asymptomatic
Bacterial endocarditis, 318, 319
Bacterial vaginosis, 74, 624-625
Bacteriuria, asymptomatic
    fetus and, 459
    pregnancy and, 336, 337
    pyelonephritis and, 338
Bacteroides bivius, 578
Bacteroides fragilis, 577, 578, 588
    infected abortion and, 583, 584
    pelvic thrombophlebitis and, 595
Bacteroides disiens, 578
Bacteroides funduliformis, 584
Bacteroides melaninogenicus, 578, 584
Bag-to-endotracheal tube resuscitation, 472
Bag-to-mask ventilation resuscitation, 472
Ballottement, 277-278
Bandl's ring, 480
Barbiturates, 603
Barbituric acid derivative, 436
Barr body, 143-144, 145
Bartholin gland, 14
    abscess of, 612
    cyst of, 616-617
    infection of, 612-613
        pregnancy and, 343, 344
    vulvar carcinoma and, 618
    young girls and, 36
Basal body temperature, 25-27
    natural family planning and, 195, 196
    ovulation and, 186
    pregnancy testing and, 29
    progesterone and, 23, 80
Basal cell, 18-20
Basal cell cancer
    vulva and, 618
    cervical, 635
Basal metabolic rate, 266
Basalis layer of endometrium, 84

Bathing
    after delivery, 605
    pregnancy and, 288
Battledore placenta, 168
Bearing down
    cystocele and, 559
    in delivery, 422
    labor and, 408
Beat-to-beat variability of fetal heart rate, 467, 468
Bed rest
    multifetal pregnancy and, 513
    preeclampsia and, 371
    threatened abortion and, 215
Bedbug bite, 609
Behavior therapy for sexual dysfunction, 67-68
Belladonna, tincture of, 326
Belladonna and opium suppository, 603
Bell's palsy, 359
Bendectin, 328
Benign conditions
    of cervix, 629-632
    of ovary, 675-677
    of uterus, 649-656
    of vagina, 626
    of vulva, 608-609, 616-617
Benign cystic teratomas, 669-670, 677
Benign intracranial hypertension, 358
Benign serous cystadenomas, 677
Benzathine penicillin, 345
Beta cell hyperplasia, 301
Beta subunit of human chorionic gonadotropin, 29, 216
Beta-adrenergic drugs, 331
Beta-endorphin, 434-435
17-Beta-estradiol, 690
Beta-blockers, hypertension and, 377
Beta-subunit radioimmunoassay, 29
Beta-sympathomimetic agent
    breech delivery and, 522
    dysmenorrhea and, 117
    multifetal pregnancy and, 513
Beta-thalassemia, 323
Bicarbonate value, plasma, 270
Bile acids, 329
Bilirubin, 339, 457
Bimanual examination, 15
    retrodisplacement of uterus and, 351
Biofeedback, 117
Biophysical evaluation
    diabetes mellitus and, 303
    fetal status in, 427, 465
        prolonged pregnancy and, 428
Biopsy
    cervical, 15, 30-31, 640
        endometrial cancer and, 662

Biopsy—cont'd
  endometrial, 22-23, 27
    pelvic tuberculosis and, 596
    suction curet, 93
  excision, 136, 137
  multiple punch, 640-641
  vulvar, 615-616, 619
Biparietal diameter, 396, 462; *see also* Fetal skull
Biphasic curve of body temperature chart, 25
Birth, 5-6
  illegitimate, 6
  nonlethal effects of, 12
  percentages of live, 7
  post-term, 400
Birth asphyxia, 472
  diabetes mellitus and, 300
Birth canal, stations of, 412
Birth center, 4-5
Birth weight
  dystocia and, 480
  maternal weight gain and, 284
Birthrate, 5-6, 7; *see also* Birth
Bisexuality, 63
Bishop score, 405, 406
Bispinous diameter, 495, 500
Bitemporal diameter, 396
Bites, vulva and, 609
Bituberous diameter, 495, 496, 501-503
  contracted pelvis and, 505, 506
Bladder
  labor and, 421
  postpartum care and, 603
  pregnancy and, 263-264, 276, 288
    bleeding in late, 391
  radiation therapy and, 644
Blastocyst, 147
Blastodermic vesicle, 147
Bleeding
  abnormal uterine, 88-96, 476; *see also* Uterine bleeding
    adolescent dysfunctional, 50
  abruptio placentae and, 387
  adenomyosis and, 655
  blood dyscrasia and, 92
  breakthrough, 89, 200-201, 203
  carcinoma of cervix and, 639
  cesarean section and, 546
  climacteric, 95
  colon cancer and, 96
  dysfunctional uterine, 89-90
    adenomyosis and, 655
  endometrial cancer and, 657, 662
  endometriosis and, 127
  estrogen withdrawal, 89
  implantation and, 148

Bleeding—cont'd
  induction of labor and, 430
  intraperitoneal, 16
  irregular, 681
  labor and, 419
  menstruation and, 82-84
  perimenopausal, 95-96
  placenta previa and, 380-382
  postmenopausal, 95, 625
  postpartum, 445, 606
    multifetal pregnancy and, 510
  pregnancy and, 260-261, 322, 380-392
    abruptio placentae and, 386-391
    early weeks of, 216
    ectopic, 231
    placenta previa and, 380-386
    one side of double uterus, 352-353
    second trimester of, 216
    third stage of labor and, 444
    threatened abortion in, 215
  progesterone breakthrough, 89
  uterine; *see* Uterine bleeding
  vulvar lesions and, 608
Block, nerve; *see* Nerve block
Blood; *see also* Bleeding
  changes in
    puerperium and, 601
    pregnancy and, 256-257
  examination of, 16-17
  fetal hypoxia and, 466
  placental expulsion and, 446
  in uterus, pregnancy and, 252
  vaginal, decrease in, 683
Blood count
  abnormal uterine bleeding and, 92
  after delivery, 605
  infected abortion and, 581
  rape and, 74
Blood culture
  infected abortion and, 581
  postoperative infection and, 590
Blood diseases, 320-324
  abnormal uterine bleeding and, 92
Blood glucose, 275-276, 300-301
Blood pressure
  contractions and, 316
  coronary artery disease and, 319
  eclampsia and, 368, 373
  fetal, 174
  labor and, 419, 420
  oxytocin and, 447-448
  preeclampsia treatment and, 371, 372
  pregnancy and, 260-261
  puerperium and, 601

Blood sampling
  fetal, 149-150
  postpartum infection and, 594
Blood serology, syphilis and, 344, 345
Blood sugar, 275-276, 300-301
Blood transfusion
  multifetal pregnancy and, 510, 514
  placental separation and, 390
  sickle cell trait and, 323
Blood type, 275
  preabortion testing of, 207
Blood urea nitrogen, 327
Blood volume
  fetal, 174
  intestinal obstruction and, 333
  pregnancy and, 256, 257, 320
Blutpunkt, 142
Body temperature, ovulation and, 186
Bonding, 58, 605
Bone and joint disorders
  aging and, 684, 686
  pregnancy and, 265-266, 356, 361-363
    coccygeal dislocation in, 362
    osteogenesis imperfecta in, 362-363
    sacrococcygeal ankylosis in, 362
    sacroiliac relaxation in, 362
    spinal fusion in, 362
    spondylolisthesis in, 362
    symphyseal separation in, 362
Bone marrow, pregnancy and, 257-258
Bones, pregnancy and, 265-266; *see also* Bone and joint dis-
    orders
Bowel
  pregnancy and, 264-265, 288
  puerperium and, 603
Bowel lesion
  bleeding during late pregnancy and, 391
  endometriosis and, 128
Bowel resection, 131
Brachialgia statica dysesthetica, 359
Brachystasis, 402
Bradycardia
  fetal, 464
    paracervical block during labor and, 437, 438
  infants of mothers with intrahepatic cholestasis and, 329
Bradykinin, 116
Brain
  eclampsia and, 374
  female, 55
  male, 55
Brassiere, maternity, 288
Braxton Hicks contraction, 253, 277, 402-403, 406
Breakthrough bleeding, 89, 200-201, 203,
Breast, 133-141
  adolescent and, 133

Breast—cont'd
  amenorrhea and, 98
  aspiration biopsy of, 134-135
  asymmetrical growth of, 135
  benign disorders of, 136-141
  cancer of, 137, 138, 675
    aging and, 691
    death rate of, 133
    metastatic, 675
    pregnancy and, 140-141
  care of, pregnancy and, 288
  changes in
    pregnancy and, 256, 276-277, 290
    puerperium and, 600
  development of, 133, 135
  disorders of, 135-136
  estrogen and atrophy of, 80
  examination of, 133-135
    pregnancy and, 290
  massive hypertrophy of, 135
  newborn, hypertrophy of, 133
  self-examination of, 134
  supernumerary, 135
Breast budding, 98
Breast-feeding; *see also* Lactation
  emotions and, 57-58
  environmental intoxicants and, 603
  epilepsy and, 356
  hyperthyroidism and, 309
Breech delivery, 517-532
  complete, 518, 526-527
  diagnosis of, 520
  fetal attitude variations and, 518-520
  management of, 522-531
  mechanism of labor and, 520-522
  morbidity and, 520
  neonatal death and, 11
  partial, 518, 525-530
  premature, 529-531
  prognosis and, 520
  Zatuchni and Andros score and previous, 524
Breech position, 399, 517, 518
  complete, 518
  frank, 518
  incomplete, 518
  placenta previa and, 382
Breech presentation, 393; *see also* Breech position
  cesarean section and, 541
Bregma, 396
Brenner tumor, 669, 672
Broad ligament pregnancy, 227-228
Bromocriptine
  amenorrhea and, 113
  breast engorgement and, 603
  hyperprolactinemia and, 106

Bromocriptine—cont'd
  premenstrual syndrome and, 120
Bronchial asthma, 314
Bronchial endometriosis, 128
Brow position, 398
  dystocia and, 489-492
Brown discharge, 215
BSP; *see* Sodium sulfobromophthalein
Bulbocavernosus muscle, torn, 553
Bulimia, 56, 108
Bullous edema, uterine, 662
Butaline sulfate tocolysis, 522
Bypass, jejunoileal, 334

C

Cachexia, 107
Caffeine, 120
Calcification
  leiomyoma and, 650, 651
  placenta and, 167-168
Calcitonin, 684
Calcium
  aging and, 688
  dysmenorrhea and, 117
  hyperparathyroidism and, 310
  hypoparathyroidism and, 309, 310
  pregnancy and, 266, 269-270
  premenstrual syndrome and, 119
Calcium antagonist, 117
Calcium carbonate, 688
Calcium gluconate, 310
Calcium lactate, 309
Calcospheroid, 672
Calculi
  biliary, 333
  renal, 310
  ureteral, 332
  urinary, 339-340
Caldwell and Moloy classification, 503
Calendar method of family planning, 195
Calories, fetalgrowth and, 284-285
Calymmatobacterium granulomatis, 612
Cancer
  breast
    aging and, 691
    death rate of, 133
    pregnancy and, 140-141
  cervical; *see* Cervical cancer
  chronic cervicitis and, 630
  colon, abnormal uterine bleeding and, 96
  endometrial, 30, 32, 656
  endometriosis and, 127
  invasive; *see* Invasive cancer

Cancer—cont'd
  leiomyomas and, 653
  lichen sclerosus and, 615
  lung, 2
  tests for, 29-32
  vaginal, 625
  vulvar, 618-619
Candida albicans, 347
  vaginitis and, 609, 610
  vulvitis and, 343
  vulvovaginitis and, 623-624
    preadolescent and, 38
Candidiasis; *see Candida albicans*
Capacitation, fertilization and, 146
Capillary permeability, 261
Capsule, Heyman's, 663
Carbohydrate intolerance, 298; *see also* Diabetes mellitus
Carbohydrates
  adrenal insufficiency and, 310
  pregnancy and, 269
  premenstrual syndrome and, 119
18-Carbon or 21-carbon compound, 80
Carbon dioxide laser vaporization, 613
Carcinoma
  abnormal uterine bleeding and, 89
  cervical; *see* Cervical cancer
  endometrial, 30-32, 656
    aging and, 689
    biopsy and, 31-32, 662
    estrogen and, 80
  endometrioid, 669, 674
  inflammatory, 138
  lobular, 137
  mammary; *see* Breast, cancer of
  metastatic, 675
  mixed, 659
  ovarian
    clinical stages of, 678
    endometriosis and, 128
    incidence of, 677
  papillary, 137
  rectal, 333
  scirrhous, 137
  secondary, 659
  squamous cell, 30
    cervical, 635
    teratoma and, 670
    vaginal, 626
  thyroid, 308
  of vulva, 617-618
Carcinoma in situ, 31
  cervical, 31, 639, 642
    diethylstilbestrol and, 42
    endometrial cancer and, 659, 660
    dysplasia and, 636, 637
    pregnancy and, 647

Carcinoma in situ—cont'd
  uterine, 662
  vulvar, 618
Carcinosarcoma, uterine, 661
Cardiac arrhythmias, 309
Cardiac catheterization, 315
Cardiac decompensation, 316, 317, 318, 319
Cardiac output, 315-316
  fetal, 174
  position of patient and, 316
  pregnancy and, 261
Cardinal ligament, 548, 549
  injury to, 567-570
Cardiomegaly, 301
Cardiomyopathy, 319
Cardiovascular changes
  aging and, 683-684
Cardiovascular disease, 315-320
  diabetes mellitus and, 301
  oral contraception and, 201
Carneous degeneration of leiomyoma, 650, 651
Carotid artery ischemia, 358; *see also* Cerebral hemorrhage
Carpal tunnel syndrome, 359
Carunculae myrtiformes, 600
Catechol estrogen, 80
Catecholamines, 77, 78
  adrenal hyperfunction and, 311
  urinary-free, 267
Cathartics in breast milk, 603
Catheter
  epidural block and breakage of, 438
  indwelling, infection and, 589
  radial artery, 318, 374
  Swan-Ganz, 318, 454
  urination after delivery and, 603
Caudal anesthesia, 438
  appendicitis and, 332
Cautery
  cervical, 635
    carcinoma in situ and, 642
  postoperative infection and, 589
  thermal
    chronic cervicitis and, 630
    dysplasia and, 641
  tubal, 204
Cefamandole, 590, 591
Cefotetan, 431
Cefoxitin, 584, 588
  chorioamnionitis and, 431
  infected abortion and, 583-584
  postoperative infection and, 590
Cellulitis
  parametrial, 583
  pelvic, 584, 594

Celsus-Wigand-Martin maneuver, 525, 529
Centers for Disease Control, 588
Central nervous system lesion, 48
Central venous pressure, placental separation and, 390
Cephalexin, 337
Cephalic application of forceps, 534, 535
Cephalic curve, 533
Cephalic prominence, 396
Cephalic version, external, 522, 523
Cephalohematomas, 540
Cephalopelvic disproportion
  forceps delivery and, 536
  uterine dysfunction and, 476
Cephalosporin
  endomyometritis and, 594
  infections and, 577
  pelvic infection and, 581
  postoperative infection and, 589
  salpingo-oophoritis and, 587
  second-generation
    infected abortion and, 583
Cephalothin, 591
Cerebral calcification, 295
Cerebral cortex, 77
Cerebral hemorrhage
  oral contraception and, 202
  pregnancy and, 376
Cerebral signs of preeclampsia, 370
Cerebrovascular accident; *see* Cerebral hemorrhage
Cervical amputation, 642
Cervical biopsy
  cancer and, 30-31
  feminizing tumor and, 674
Cervical canal, 627
Cervical cancer, 626, 633-648, 656
  advanced, 647
    visual inspection and, 640
  clear cell adenocarcinoma in, 41, 42-43, 669
  clinical stages of, 638-639
  diagnosis of, 639-641
  epidemiology of, 633-635
  normal cervix and, 627-628
  Paget's disease and, 618
  pathology of, 635-638
  polyps and, 632
  pregnancy and, 348, 647
  prevention of, 647-648
  squamocolumnar junction and, 628-629
  squamous cell, 30
  stenosis and, 633
  survival rate and, 646
  symptoms of, 639
  treatment of, 641-647
  types of, 635

Cervical cerclage
  habitual abortion and, 220
  multifetal pregnancy and, 513
Cervical collar in child, 42
Cervical dysplasia, diethylstilbestrol and, 42
Cervical ectopy, 41-43
Cervical ectropion, 42, 253
Cervical erosion, 630, 631
Cervical eversion, pregnancy and, 253, 631-632
  preadolescent and, 42
Cervical fibroid, 649, 650
Cervical fibromyoma, 100
Cervical gland in young girls, 36
Cervical incompetence
  habitual abortion and, 220, 221
  spontaneous abortion and, 219
Cervical intraepithelial neoplasia, 635-636, 637
Cervical laceration
  childbirth injury and, 565-566
  postpartum hemorrhage and, 451-452
  repair of, 566
  spontaneous abortion and, 211
Cervical lip, incarcerated edematous anterior, 565
Cervical microinvasion, 639
Cervical mucus, 24-25, 628
  changes in
    cyclic, 180, 181
    menstruation and, 84-85
  examination of, 20-22
    postcoital, infertility and, 187
  infertility and, 179, 187
  pH of, 146
  progesterone and, 23
  viscous, 188
Cervical polyp, 630, 632
  pregnancy and, 347-348
Cervical stromal invasion, 636
Cervicitis, 31, 626, 629-632
  postpartum, 606
Cervix, 24-25; *see also* Cervical entries
  atresia of, amenorrhea and, 100
  benign proliferative adenomatous growth on, 202
  biopsy of, 15, 30-31, 662
  carcinoma of; *see* Cervical cancer
  changes in
    pregnancy and, 253, 277
    puerperium and, 600
  consistency of, 15
  cockscomb, in pediatric patient, 42
  dilatation of
    forceps delivery and, 536
    preoperative, abortion and, 207
    stenosis of cervix and, 633
    Zatuchni and Andros breech score and, 524

Cervix—cont'd
  diseases of, 627-648
    abnormal uterine bleeding and, 93
    benign, 629-632
    bleeding during late pregnancy and, 391
    fibroids in, 649, 650
    fibromyoma in, 100
    hypertrophy and, 633
    malignant, 633-648; *see also* Cervical cancer
  effacement of, 404, 405
  hypertrophy of glands of, 255
  incomplete, 219, 220, 221
  induced labor and, 429
  infection of, spontaneous abortion and, 219-220
  infertility and, 180, 187
  lesions of, 630; *see also* Cervix, diseases of
  portio of, 628
  prepared, 405, 406
  ripe, 405, 406
  stenosis of, 633
  supravaginal, 627, 628
Cervix-corpus ratio, 36
Cesarean hysterectomy, 543
Cesarean section, 541-547
  anesthesia and, 543-544
  breech delivery and, 520, 523, 527-531
  choice of operation and, 542-543
  classic, 542
  complications of, 545-546
  congenital heart lesions and, 319-320
  contracted pelvis and, 504-505
  diabetes mellitus and, 304
  elective repeat
    prematurity and, 426
    risk of scar rupture and, 567
  endomyometritis and, 594
  face position and, 489
  heart disease and, 318
  hemoglobin C disease and, 323
  herpes and, 296
  hysterectomy and, 543
  immature fetus and, 542
  incidence of, 541
  indications for, 431, 541-542
  kidney transplant and, 342
  low segment, 543
  multifetal pregnancy and, 513
  ovarian neoplasms and, 350
  placenta previa and, 380
    complete, 386
    incomplete, 384
  postpartum infection and, 591
  premature labor and, 427
  rectal carcinoma and, 333

Cesarean section—cont'd
  repeat, 542, 544-545
    prematurity and, 426
    rupture of scar and, 567
  sickle cell disease and, 323
  sterilization and, 545
  thrombocytopenic purpura and, 324
  uterine dysfunction and, 478, 479
Cesarean section scar rupture, 567
Cesium
  cervical invasive carcinoma and, 643
  endometrial cancer and, 663
Chadwick's sign, 255, 277
Chancroid, 611
Chemical agent exposure, breast cancer and, 138
Chemical diabetes, 304
Chemical vaginitis, 625
Chemotherapy
  breast cancer and, 140
  fetus and, 458
  influenza and, 314
  ovarian cancer and, 678
  pyelonephritis and, 338
Chenodeoxycholic acid, 329
Chest x-ray film examination
  pregnancy and, 275
  tuberculosis and, 313
Chickenpox, 295
Childbearing period, 57-59
  abnormal uterine bleeding and, 93-95
Childbirth, definition of normal, 434; *see also* Delivery
Childbirth education, 418
  attitude to, 58
Childbirth injury, effects of, 548-572
  genital fistulas and, 570
  hematoma and, 571-572
  lacerations and
    perineal, 549, 552-554
    vaginal, 554
  levator sling and, 554-558
  pelvic joints and, 570-571
  uterine support and, 567-570
  uterus and, 565-567
  vaginal wall and, 558-565
Childhood, 55-56
Chlamydia, 577, 589, 629
  cervicitis and, 38
  infertility and, 180
  lymphogranuloma venereum and, 612
  preadolescent and, 38
  pregnancy and, 346
  rape and, 74
  salpingo-oophoritis and, 587
  urinary incontinence and, 565
Chloasma, 256

Chlorambucil, 458
Chloramphenicol
  breast-feeding and, 603
  infected abortion and, 583
  pelvic infection and, 581
  pregnancy and, 339
  premature infants and, 458
Chocolate cyst, 124
Cholecystitis or cholelithiasis
  oral contraception and, 202
  pregnancy and, 333
Cholestasis
  idiopathic, pruritus and, 360
  intrahepatic, 329
  oral contraception and, 202
Cholesterol, 329, 333
Cholestyramine, 329
Cholic acid, 329
Cholinesterase, plasma, 329
Chorea, Sydenham's, 357
Chorea gravidarum, 357
Chorioamnionitis
  cesarean section and, 542
  rupture of membranes and, 430, 431
Chorioangioma, 168
Choriocarcinoma, 247-250
Choriodecidual spaces, 152
Chorion, 147
Chorion frondosum, 150
Chorion laeve, 150
Chorionic gonadotropin, 23; *see also* Gonadotropin
  death of embryo and, 212
  hydatidiform mole and, 243, 244
  missed abortion and, 214
  placental hormones and, 155-156
  predicting abortion and, 216
  pregnancy and, 28, 211-212, 280
    ectopic, 232-233
    multifetal, 511
  puerperium and, 601
  radioreceptor assay for, 29
  thyroid disorders and, 308
Chorionic human placental lactogen, 269
Chorionic phospholipase A_2, 409
Chorionic somatomammotropin, 511
Chorionic villi, 147
  testing of, 35, 149
Chorioretinitis
  cytomegalovirus and, 295
  toxoplasmosis and, 296
Chromatin, 143, 144
Chromic catgut suture, 552, 555
Chromosomal aberration, 148-149; *see also* Chromosomes
  amniotic fluid and, 34, 164
  ectopic pregnancy and, 226-227

Chromosomal aberration—cont'd
  hydatidiform mole and, 240
  spontaneous abortion and, 219
Chromosomes; *see also* Chromosomal aberration
  female, 143, 144
  idiogram of, 145
  LSD and, 458
  male, 143, 144
  marijuana and, 458
  number variance in, 148
  nondisjunction of, fertilization and, 143
  sex, 143, 144
  Y, 44
Cigarettes
  abortion and, 212
  breast-feeding and, 603
CIN; *see* Cervical intraepithelial neoplasia
Circhoral, 78
Circulation
  changes at birth, 173-174
  fetal development and, 171-173
Circulatory system
  diseases of, 315-320
  pregnancy and, 256-261
Cirrhosis, 330
Classic estrogen, 80
Classic cesarean section, 542
Clean voided specimen, 16
Clear cell adenocarcinoma, 41, 42-43, 669
Cleft lip or palate, 149
Climacteric, 59-60, 680, 681-682; *see also* Aging
  abnormal uterine bleeding and, 95
Clindamycin, 578, 588
  endomyometritis and, 594
  infected abortion and, 584
  pelvic infection and, 581
  postoperative infection and, 590
  salpingo-oophoritis and, 587
Clomid; *see* Clomiphene citrate
Clomiphene citrate
  amenorrhea and, 112
  in amenorrheic women, 201
  hot flush and, 687
  infertility and, 189-190
  polycystic ovarian syndrome and, 105
Clonidine
  aging and, 692
  hypertension and, 377
Clostridial infection, 578, 584
  stained smear and, 17
Clot observation test
  abruptio placentae and, 389
  complete placental separation and, 390
Clothing, pregnancy and, 288
Clotrimazole, 623

Clotting disorder; *see also* Coagulopathy
  abnormal uterine bleeding and, 92
  abruptio placentae and, 387, 388
  amniotic fluid infusion and, 454
  complete placental separation and, 390
  oral contraceptives and, 202
Club foot, 149
Clue cells, 624
Coagulase-positive staphylococcus, 578
Coagulation of blood; *see* Clotting disorder; Coagulopathy
Coagulopathy; *see also* Clotting disorder
  abortion and, 218
  disseminated intravascular; *see* Disseminated intravascular coagulation
Coarctation of aorta, 319
Coccyx, dislocated, 362, 571
Cockscomb cervix, 42
Codeine, 603
Coelomic epithelium, ovarian neoplasms of, 671-674
Coital physiology, Masters' study of, 621
Coitus
  age of first, cervical cancer and, 634, 635
  hyperemesis and, 327
  sexual dysfunction and, 66
Coitus interruptus, 193-194
Colicky secondary dysmenorrhea, 655
Colitis, ulcerative, 331
Colloid carcinoma, 137
Colon cancer, 96
Colostrum, 600
  pregnancy and, 256, 277
Colpocleisis, 569
Colpoplasty, posterior, 558
Colposcopy, 31
  in cervical carcinoma, 641
    in situ, 642
    in pregnancy, 647
Colpotomy, posterior, 584
Columnar epithelium of cervix, 635
Combined oral contraception, 200
Comedocarcinoma, 137
Comedomastitis, 136
Commissurotomy, 317
Communication, sexual problems and, 65, 68
Community health service, cervical cancer and, 647
Community-acquired infection, 581-589
Compacta, endometrium and, 84
Compazine; *see* Prochlorperazine dimaleate
Complement-fixing antibody
  Rh incompatibility and, 460
  rubella in pregnancy and, 294
Complete abortion, 214, 218
Complete breech, 518, 526-527
Complete inversion of uterus, 453-454

Complete placenta accreta, 453
Complete placenta previa, 380, 386
Complete placental separation, 386, 390-391
Complete prolapse
    of umbilical cord, 469-470
    of uterus, 568
Compound presentation, dystocia and, 492-493
Compression, vena caval, 316
Compression fractures, 686
Conception rate, 177
Condom, 197
Conduction anesthesia, 544
Condylomata acuminata
    pregnancy and, 343, 344
    vagina and, 626
    vulva and, 611
Condylomata lata, 612
Cone biopsy, 31, 641
Confinement, date of expected, 282-283
Congenital adrenal hyperplasia
    amniotic fluid and, 164
    compensated, 45
    heterosexual precocity and, 49
    hormone assay and, 18
    masculinization of genitals and, 45
    sexual ambiguity of newborn and, 45-46
Congenital anomaly, 40-41
    anticonvulsants and, 356
    diabetes mellitus and, 300
    fetal death and, 10
    fusion, infertility and, 190
    genital tract during pregnancy and, 351-354
    immunosuppressives and, 341
Congenital goiter, 307, 308
    iodine and, 314
Congenital heart lesions, 319-320
Congenital polycystic kidney disease, 341
Congenital stricture of vagina, 353
Congestion-fibrosis syndrome, 655
Conization, cervical, 640, 641
    cervicitis and, 631
    pregnancy and, 647
    wide, 642
Conjoined twin, 507
Conjugata vera, 494, 499, 500
    cesarean section and, 505
    inlet contraction and, 504
Conjugate, 494
    diagonal, 494, 495
    true, 494
Conjugated estrogen; *see also* Estrogen
    abnormal bleeding and, 202, 203
    pregnancy interception and, 204
Conjunctivitis of newborn, inclusion, 346

Constipation, pregnancy and, 264-265, 288
Constriction ring dystocia, 479-480
Consumption coagulopathy, 387; *see also* Coagulopathy; Disseminated intravascular coagulopathy
Contact vulvitis, 612
Contraception, 193-205
    adolescents and, 63, 192-193
        pregnancy in, 6-7
    barrier, 196-197
    chemical, 196
    after delivery, 605
    effectiveness of, 193
    factors in selection of, 194
    hormonal, 199-204
    intrauterine device, 197-199
        infertility and, 179
    kidney transplant and, 341
    oral; *see* Oral contraception
    physiologic, 193-196
    record of, for pregnant patient, 275
    surgical, 204-205
    withdrawal, 193-194
Contracted pelvis, 503; *see also* Gynecoid pelvis
Contraction stress test, 464-465
    diabetes mellitus and, 302, 303
    preeclampsia and, 371
    previous fetal death and, 378
Contractions
    inlet, 487, 504
    labor and, 403-404, 420
        true, 416
    midpelvic, 506
    myometrial, 152
    outlet, 506
    small, 402
    stroke volume and, 316
    uterine
        abruptio placentae and, 389
        Braxton Hicks, 253, 277, 402-403, 406
        labor and, 403-404, 416, 420
        normal, 407
        pregnancy and, 277
Convulsion
    cytomegalovirus disease and, 295
    eclampsia and, 373
    hypoparathyroidism and, 310
    toxoplasmosis and, 296
Coombs' test, 460, 461, 462
Copper, intrauterine device and, 199
Cord; *see* Umbilical cord
Cornification, 18, 19, 20
Cornual placental implantation, 519
Cornual pregnancy, 228
Coronal suture, 171, 396

Coronary artery disease, 319
Coronary occlusion, 319
Corpus albicans, 81
Corpus luteum, 77, 78
  fertilization and, 142
  menstruation and, 81
  pregnancy and, 211-212
    surgery during, 331
Corpus luteum cyst, 666
  amenorrhea and, 103
  ectopic pregnancy and, 235
Corpus uteri, malignant lesions of, 662
Cortex, hyperplasia of, 267
Cortical necrosis, 374
Corticoids after delivery, 601
Corticosteroids
  asthma and, 314
  carbohydrate metabolism and, 269
  herpes gestationis and, 360
  infertility and, 190
  inflammatory bowel disease and, 331
  lupus erythematosus and, 361
  pregnancy and, 267
  thrombocytopenic purpura and, 324
  thrombotic thrombocytopenic purpura and, 324
Cortisol
  congenital adrenal hyperplasia and, 45
  placenta and, 161
  pregnancy and, 267
Cortisol-binding globulin, 80
Cortisone
  adrenal insufficiency and, 310, 311
  adrenal tumor and, 47
  congenital adrenal hyperplasia and, 45
  contact vulvitis and, 612
  placenta and, 161
  pregnancy and, 263
  subclinical diabetes and, 304, 306
Cortisone glucose tolerance test, 306
Corynebacterium, 346
Co-therapist, sex therapy and, 68
Cotyledon, 162
Coumadin; *see* Warfarin
Counseling
  abortion and, 206
  teenage pregnancy and, 7
Couvelaire uterus, 387
Coxsackievirus B, 314
Creatinine
  amniotic fluid and, 166
  fetal age and, 283
  preeclampsia treatment and, 371
  pregnancy and, 259, 263, 336
    renal function in, 263

Creosote, 625
Cretinism, 307, 308
Crohn's disease, 331
Crown-rump length of embryo, 283
Cryocautery; *see also* Cryosurgery
  condylomata acuminata and, 611
  dysplasia and, 641
Cryoprecipitate
  disseminated intravascular coagulation and, 324
  placental separation and, 390
Cryosurgery; *see also* Cryocautery
  cervical carcinoma in situ and, 642
  chronic cervicitis and, 630
Crypts, 627
Cryptomenorrhea, 99, 100
CST; *see* Contraction stress test
Cul-de-sac hernia, 557, 558
Culdocentesis, 668
  ectopic pregnancy and, 234
  salpingo-oophritis and, 587
Cultures, 17-18
  candidiasis and, 623
Curettage
  abnormal uterine bleeding and, 95
  abortion and, 207
    incomplete, 216-218
  ectopic pregnancy and, 235
  endometrium and, 27
    biopsy of, 31-32
    cancer of, 662
  feminizing tumor and, 674
  infected abortion and, 583, 585
  pelvic tuberculosis and, 596
Cushing's disease, 106
Cushing's syndrome, 311
  amenorrhea and, 109
  placenta and, 161
Cyclic dyschezia, 128
Cyclic hemoptysis, 128
Cyclic hormone therapy, 95, 96
Cyst
  androgen secreting, 103
  chocolate, 124
  corpus luteum
    amenorrhea and, 103
    ectopic pregnancy and, 235
  dermoid, 43-44
  epididymal, 42
  estrogen secreting, 103
  follicular, 103, 666
  neoplastic
    amenorrhea and, 103
    diagnosis of pregnancy and, 280
  nonneoplastic ovarian, 350, 666-668

Cyst—cont'd
  placental, 168
  sebaceous, 135, 616
  teratomas and, 669-670, 677
  theca-lutein, 241
  vaginal, in infant, 41
  vulvar tumor and, 616-617
Cystadenocarcinoma, 669
  mucinous, 673-674
Cystadenofibromas, 669, 672
Cystadenoma, benign serous, 671, 677
  mucinous, 669, 672, 673, 677
Cystectomy, ovarian, 350, 677
Cystic degeneration, 650, 651
Cystic fibrosis, 164
Cystic hyperplasia, 90, 658-659
Cystic ovarian neoplasm, pregnancy and, 280
Cystine-amino-peptidase, 161, 260
Cystinuria, 149
Cystocele, 559-560, 568, 569, 683
Cystometrogram, 563
Cystoophorectomy, 677
Cystoscopy
  hematuria and, 340
  pregnancy and, 336
  stress incontinence and, 563
  ureterovaginal fistula and, 570
Cystourethrocele, 559, 560
Cytology, 14
  for cancer, 30
    of cervix, 642, 646
    of endometrium, 662
  changes in, at various ages, 622
Cytomegalovirus
  fetus and, 459
  hepatitis and, 330
  pregnancy and, 295-296
Cytoplasmic estrogen receptor, 652
Cytotrophoblast
  human chorionic gonadotropin and, 155
  placenta and, 150

D

Dactinomycin, 248-249
Danazol
  endometriosis and, 130, 131
  hot flush and, 687
  mastodynia and, 136
  premenstrual syndrome and, 120
  side effects of, 130
DAO; *see* Diamine oxidase
Dark-field examination, 344
Dead fetus syndrome, 218

Death; *see also* Mortality
  abortion and, 207-208
  fetal, 6, 7, 9, 10
  hebdomadal, 9
  maternal, 3, 8
  neonatal, 6, 9, 10-11
  obstetric, 8
  perinatal, 9, 337
  postneonatal, teenage pregnancy and, 6
Decapeptide, 78
Deceleration phase of labor, 417, 466, 467
Decidua, 147, 148
  menstruation and, 82
  invasion of, by trophoblastic tissue, 327
Decidua basalis, 147, 148
Decidua capsularis, 147, 148
Decidua vera, 147
Decompensation, cardiac, 316, 317, 318, 319
Deflexion of head, 393, 394
Degeneration
  leiomyoma, 654
  red, 348, 349, 650, 651
  medical abortion and vascular, 206
Dehydration
  hepatitis and, 330
  hypoadrenalism and, 310
  nausea and vomiting during pregnancy and, 328
  postpartum hemorrhage and, 450
11-Dehydrocorticosterone, 161
Dehydroepiandrosterone, 23
  aging and, 682
  pregnancy and, 158, 159
  amenorrhea and, 103
Delalutin; *see* 17-Alpha-hydroxyprogesterone
Delayed menarche, 98
Delayed menstruation, 85
DeLee pelvimeter, 502
Delivery, 400-401, 422-433; *see also* Labor
  alternative birth centers and, 4-5
  of body, 424, 425
  breech; *see* Breech delivery
  cardiac valve disease and, 318-319
  care after, 602-605
  cesarean; *see* Cesarean section
  diabetes mellitus and, 304
  elderly primigravidas and, 429
  emotions during, 58
  fetal growth retardation and, 427-428
  forceps; *see* Forceps delivery
  of head, 422-423
  at home, 5
  hydramnios and, 169
  multifetal pregnancy and, 513-514
  normal, 422-425
  obstructed, malposition of uterus and, 353

Delivery—cont'd
  pain control during, 438-443
  precipitate, 429
  premature, 425-427; *see also* Premature labor and delivery
    acute glomerulonephritis and, 340
  prolonged pregnancy and, 428
  shoulder, 424, 425
  at term, 400
  tuberculosis and, 313-314
  uterine dysfunction and, 478-479
  vaginal
    breech delivery and, 524; *see also* Breech delivery
    multifetal pregnancy and, 513
  young primigravidas and, 428-429
Delivery room, transfer to, 421-422
Demerol; *see* Meperidine
Densitometry, single photon, 689
Dentalcare, pregnancy and, 288
Dentin, 270
Deoxycholic acid, 329
Depo-medroxyprogesterone, 131
Depo-Provera; *see* Medroxyprogesterone acetate
Depression
  abnormal uterine bleeding and, 95
  aging and, 689
  oral contraception and, 200
  sexual fulfillment and, 61
Dermatitis, papular, 360
Dermoid cyst, preadolescent and, 43-44
DES; *see* Diethylstilbestrol
Descensus of uterus, 568-570
  pregnancy and, 351
Descent in labor, 410,411
Desoxycorticosterone acetate, 310
Detrusor dyssynergia, 561, 564-565
Development
  fetal, 170-174; *see also* Fetus
  of placenta, 150-166; *see also* Placenta
Developmental abnormality, 148-150
  antenatal diagnosis of, 149-150
  breast, 135
  breech delivery and, 520
  of fetus, dystocia and, 483
  of uterus, abortion and, 211
Dexamethasone
  amenorrhea and, 112
  polycystic ovarian syndrome and, 105
DHEAS; *see* Dehydroepiandrosterone
Diabetes insipidus, 306-307
Diabetes mellitus, 298-304
  anesthesia and analgesia during delivery and, 443
  chemical, 304
  diagnosis of, 298
  dystocia and, 480
  eclampsia and, 375

Diabetes mellitus—cont'd
  endometrial cancer and, 657
  fetal development and, 462
  hydramnios and, 169, 170
  incidence of, 298
  induction of labor and, 431
  influence of, on pregnancy, 299-301
  influence of pregnancy on, 298-299
  latent, 304-306
  management of, 301-304
  medical abortion and, 206
  overt or clinical, 304
  polycystic ovarian syndrome and, 105
  prediabetes and, 304
  subclinical, 304, 304-306
Diabetogenic effect of oral contraception, 202
Diagnostic methods, 13-35
  amniocentesis and, 34-35
  cancer tests in, 29-32
  chorionic villus sampling and, 35
  fetoscopy and, 35
  history and, 13-14
  hormone assay and, 18-28
  hysteroscopy and, 34
  laboratory tests and, 16-18
  laparoscopy and, 33-34
  magnetic resonance imaging and, 33
  physical examination and, 14-16
  pregnancy tests and, 28-29
  ultrasound and, 33
  x-ray and, 32-33
Diagonal conjugate, 494, 495, 499
  inlet contraction and, 504
Diamine oxidase
  placental enzyme and, 161
  pregnancy and, 260
Diaphragm, contraception and, 196-197
Diarrhea, radiation and, 644
Diastasis recti, 256
Diazepam
  eclampsia and, 373
  status epilepticus and, 357
DIC; *see* Disseminated intravascular coagulation
Dicumarol, 458
Dieckmann salt test, 366, 367
Dieckmann signs and symptoms, preeclampsia and, 370
Diet
  aging and, 688
  after delivery, 602
  diabetes mellitus and, 302
  dysmenorrhea and, 117
  eclampsia and, 368-369
  gallbladder disease and, 333
  jejunoileal bypass and, 334
  nausea and vomiting and, 328

Diet—cont'd
　during pregnancy, 283-287
　premenstrual syndrome and, 120
　vegetarian, 284-285
Diethylstilbestrol
　abnormal uterine bleeding and, 92
　examination and management of women exposed to, 42-43
　fetus and, 457
　functional abnormality in exposed males and, 42
　infertility and, 178-179
　neoplasm and, 41
　pregnancy interception and, 204
　vaginal adenosis and, 626
Diffuse adenocarcinoma of endometrium, 659
Diffuse symmetric hypertrophy of uterus, 655
Digestive tract disorder in pregnancy, 326-334
　acute fatty liver in, 329-330
　gingivitis in, 326
　heartburn in, 328
　hiatus hernia in, 328-329
　inflammatory bowel disease in, 331
　jaundice in, 329
　nausea in, 326-328
　pancreatitis in, 330-331
　peptic ulcer in, 330
　ptyalism in, 326
　surgery and, 331-334
　teeth care and, 326
　viral hepatitis in, 330
　vomiting in, 326-328
Digitalis, 317, 318
Digoxin, 96
Dihydrotestosterone, 103-104
Dilantin; *see* Phenytoin
Dilatation
　cervical, 407
　　placental edge during stages of, 382
　and curettage
　　in abnormal uterine bleeding, 95
　　ectopic pregnancy and, 235
　　endometrial cancer and, 662
　　feminizing tumor and, 674
　renal pelvis, 262, 335
　ureteropelvic, 340
Dimple, skin, ectopic anus and, 41
Diphtheroid, 584
Direct obstetric death, 8
Discharge
　from hospital, 605
　serosanguineous, 38, 599
　serous, 662
　vaginal
　　brown, threatened abortion and, 215
　　diagnosis and, 13-14
　　endometrial cancer and, 662

Discharge—cont'd
　vaginal—cont'd
　　labor and, 416
Discoid lupus erythematosus, 361
Diseases
　Addison's, 310
　Crohn's, 331
　Cushing's, 106; *see also* Cushing's syndrome
　Hodgkin's, 324
　Hurler's, 149
　Mondor's, 136
　Paget's, 137, 618
　Tay-Sachs, 149
Dislocation, coccyx and, 362, 571
Displacement of uterus, anterior, 350
Disproportion
　cephalopelvic
　　forceps delivery and, 536
　　uterine dysfunction and, 476
　fetopelvic
　　cesarean section and, 531
　　induction of labor and, 432
　unverified, cesarean section and, 541
Disseminated intravascular coagulation, 324
　abortion and, 207
　abruptio placentae and, 387
　eclampsia and, 369
Distant metastases, 638, 639
Dizygotic twins, 507, 508
Döderlein bacilli, 621
Donovan body, 346, 347
Dopamine
　adrenocortical failure and, 310
　hot flush and, 686
　menstruation and, 78
　pseudocyesis and, 280-281
Doppler apparatus, fetal heart tones and, 278
Dorsal kyphosis, 687
Dorsal recumbent position for delivery, 422
Double footling, 518
Double-ovum twins, 507, 508
Douche
　candidiasis and, 624
　menstruation and, 86
　postcoital, contraception and, 196
　vinegar, cervicitis and, 630
Dowager's hump, 687
Down's syndrome, 148, 459
Doxycycline, 588
　lymphogranuloma venereum and, 612
　postpartum infection and, 594
Doxylamine succinate, 328
Drape, wound, 589
Droplet transfer, 154
Drug
　antithyroid, 309, 458

Drug—cont'd
  immunosuppressive, 341
  labor and, 458
  pregnancy and, 289, 457
    toxic effects of, 339
  premature labor and addiction to, 426
  sex therapy and, 68
  sexual dysfunction and, 66-67
  stage of labor and, 436
  transfer of, through placenta, 164
Drug overdose, spinal anesthesia and, 440
Dual photon densitometry, 689
Dual puncture technique, laparoscopy and, 128, 186
Duchenne's muscular dystrophy, 149
Ductus arteriosus, 173
Duncan mechanism, 446
Dyscrasia, blood, 92
Dysfunctional labor
  cesarean section and, 531, 541-542
  postpartum hemorrhage and, 450
Dysfunctional uterine bleeding, 89-90
  adenomyosis and, 655
Dysgenesis, gonadal
  amenorrhea and, 101-102, 111
  infertility and, 178, 180, 189
Dysgerminomas, 670-671
Dysjunction, fertilization and, 142
Dysmenorrhea, 50, 56, 115-118
  definition of, 86
  endometriosis and, 126
  leiomyomas and, 652-653
  pelvic tuberculosis and, 596
  primary, 115-116
  secondary, 115
Dyspareunia, 64-65
  aging and, 687
  endometriosis and, 126-127
  hyperemesis and, 327
  infertility and, 179
  pelvic tuberculosis and, 596
Dysplasia
  cervical cancer and, 635-636, 638
  cone biopsy and, 31
  conversion of, to carcinoma in situ, 636
  treatment of, 641
Dystocia
  anterior displacement of uterus and, 350
  cesarean section and, 541
  contracted pelvis and, 494, 503-506; *see also* Pelvis
  definition of, 474
  prolonged labor and, 474-493
    active phase in, 475, 476
    constriction ring dystocia and, 479-480
    fetal origin and, 480-483
    latent phase in, 475

Dystocia—cont'd
  prolonged labor and—cont'd
    pathologic retraction ring and, 480
    position and presentation in, 483-493
    uterine dysfunction and, 474-479
  shoulder, 481-483
Dystrophy
  Duchenne's muscular, 149
  vulva and, 614-615
Dysuria
  urethrocystitis and, 337
  urge incontinence and, 565

E

E_1; *see* Estrone
E_2; *see* Estradiol
E_3; *see* Estriol
Early abortion, 205-208
Early deceleration, 466, 467
Ecchymosis
  mammary necrosis and, 136
  rape in preadolescent and, 40
Eclampsia, 365-375; *see also* Preeclampsia
  diabetes mellitus and, 299
  hospital treatment of, 373-374
  hypertension and, 364, 375
  immunologic factors in, 369
Ectopic anus, preadolescent and, 41
Ectopic pregnancy, 225-238; *see also* Tubal pregnancy
  abnormal uterine bleeding and, 89
  course and termination of, 228-230
  diagnosis of, 233-235
    differential, 235
  etiology of, 226-227
  human chorionic gonadotropin and, 29
  implantation sites and, 225
  laboratory findings and, 232-233
  management of, 236
  monoclonal antibody test and, 28
  pathologic anatomy and, 227-228
  physical signs of, 231-232
  prognosis for, 237
  rates for, 225
  symptoms of, 230-231
  treatment of, 235-237
  ultrasound and, 33
Ectopic ureter, 40-41
Ectopy, cervical, 41-43
Ectropion, cervical
  preadolescent and, 42
  pregnancy and, 253
EDC; *see* Expected date of confinement

Edema
  definition of, 364
  gestational, 365
  low-sodium diet and, 287
  multifetal pregnancy and, 510
  preeclampsia-eclampsia and, 365
  pregnancy and, 366
  premenstrual syndrome and, 119
  pulmonary, 374
Edrophonium chloride, 358
Education
  pregnancy and, 274, 290
  sex, teenage pregnancy and, 6-7
Effacement, cervical, 404, 405
Eisenmenger's syndrome, 319
Ejaculation, premature, 66, 179
Elderly primigravida, 429
  cesarean section and, 542
Elective abortion, 206
Elective induction of labor, 431-432
Elective low forceps extraction, 536
Electrocardiography, fetal, 420-422, 463-465
Electrocautery, 611
Electrodesiccation, 611
Electrolyte concentration, 327
Electrode, fetal scalp, 468, 469
Electronic monitoring
  of fetal heart, 420-422, 463-465
    in diabetes mellitus, 302, 303
  of uterine contraction, 420
Embryo, development of, 170
Embryonal teratomas, 669, 670
Emotional factors
  abnormal uterine bleeding and, 90
  infertility and, 190
  patient care and, 52
  spontaneous abortion and, 212
Empty-sella syndrome, 107
Empyema
  pregnancy and, 333
Encephalitis, 296
Endocarditis, bacterial, 318, 319
Endocervical curettage, 641; *see also* Curettage
Endocervical metaplasia, 669
Endocervicitis, 629-630
Endocervix, 628
Endocrine disorders, 298-312; *see also* Endocrine gland
  adrenal gland diseases in, 310-311
  diabetes insipidus in, 306-307
  diabetes mellitus in, 298-304; *see also* Diabetes mellitus
  parathyroid gland diseases in, 309-310
  subclinical diabetes in, 304-306
  thyroid gland diseases in, 307-309
Endocrine gland
  amenorrhea and, 106-108

Endocrine gland—cont'd
  disorders of; *see* Endocrine disorders
  pregnancy and, 266-268
    nausea and vomiting during, 327
  placenta and, 154
  puerperium changes and, 601-602
  sexual response and, 61-62
  spontaneous abortion and, 211-212
Endocrine therapy
  breast cancer and, 139-140
  surgery during pregnancy and, 331
Endogenous opiate peptide
  menstruation and, 78
  premenstrual syndrome and, 119
Endometrial biopsy, 22-23, 27
  cancer and, 31-32, 662
  estrogen and, 22
  pelvic tuberculosis and, 596
  premenstrual, 23
  suction curet for, 22-23, 93
Endometrial carcinoma, 30, 31-32, 656
  aging and, 689
  estrogen and, 80
  malodorous discharge and, 662
Endometrial decidua, 80
Endometrial failure, 109
Endometrial gland, 147
Endometrial hyperplasia, 93
Endometrial infection, 219-220
Endometrial metaplasia, 669
Endometrial polyp, 89, 93
Endometrial tuberculosis, 596
Endometrial wash technique, 32
Endometrioid carcinoma, 669, 674
Endometriomas, 123, 666, 669
  ovarian, 124, 127, 131
Endometriosis, 122-132
  abnormal uterine bleeding and, 89
  adenomyosis and, 131
  amenorrhea and, 99
  bronchial, 128
  cervix and, 633
  classification of, 125
  differential diagnosis and, 128
  dyspareunia and, 64
  etiology of, 122-123
  external, 122
  infertility and, 179
  internal, 122, 126
  nodular cul-de-sac, 128
  pain and, 127
  pathology and, 123-126
  spontaneous abortion and, 211
  symptoms of, 126-128
    relief of, 131

Endometriosis—cont'd
 treatment for, 128-131
Endometritis, postoperative, 101
Endometrium, 77, 78
 abortion and infection of, 219-220
 abnormal uterine bleeding and, 89, 90, 93
 aging and, 683, 685
 amenorrhea and, 101, 109
 biopsy of; *see* Endometrial biopsy
 carcinoma of, 30, 31-32, 656
  aging and, 689
  estrogen and, 80
 late secretory, 23
 menstruation and, 76, 83
 metaplasia and, 669
 polyps of, 89, 93
 pregravid, fertilization and, 148
 prolactin and, 80
 proliferative phase and, 23
 retrograde hyperplasia of, 683, 685
 tuberculosis and, 596
Endomyometritis, 592-593
 cesarean section and, 594
 fever and, 593, 594
 uterine dysfunction and, 476
 vaginal delivery and, 594
Endorphins, fetal, 434, 435
Endosalpingiosis, 122
Endosalpingitis, 226
Endotoxins, 86
Endotracheal intubation, 373
Enema, labor and, 419
Engagement
 face position and, 489
 labor and, 412, 416
Engorgement, 600-601, 603
Enlargement, spleen, 301
Enterobacter, 336, 337
Enterocele, 557, 558
Enterococcus, 578, 583
Environmental intoxicants, breast-feeding and, 603
Enzymes
 menstruation and, 84
 placental, 161-162
 placental transfer and, 154
 serum, pregnancy and, 259-261
Eosinophils
 infant of diabetic mother and, 301
 pregnancy and, 321
Epidemic puerperal mastitis, 136
Epididymal cyst, 42
Epidural abscess, 438
Epidural anesthesia, 438
 contracted pelvis and, 506
 control of pain during delivery and, 439

Epidural anesthesia—cont'd
 delivery in women with appendicitis and, 332
 needle breakage and, 438
Epigastric pain, appendicitis and, 332
Epilepsy, 356
Epinephrine
 hot flush and, 686
 pregnancy and, 267
Episiotomy, 422, 554-555, 556
 elective low forceps delivery and, 536
 median, 554-555, 556
 mediolateral, 554-555, 556
Epithelial cilia, fertilization and, 144
Epithelial hyperkeratosis of vulva, 615, 616
Epithelium
 cervical, 627-628
 coelomic, ovarian neoplasms from, 671-674
 vaginal, 18-19
  menstruation and, 85
 vulvar, 614-616
Epstein-Barr virus, 330
ER; *see* Estrogen receptor
Ergonovine maleate
 heart disease and, 319
 placental expulsion and, 447
Ergot
 breast-feeding and, 603
 placental expulsion and, 447
Ergotrate; *see* Ergonovine maleate
Erosion, cervical, 630, 631
Erythroblastosis fetalis
 ABO incompatibility and, 461-462
 hydramnios and, 169
 Rh incompatibility and, 459-461
Erythrocytes, 258
 sheep, 28, 29
Erythrocyte protoporphyrin, 320
Erythromycin
 chancroid and, 611
 chlamydial vaginitis and, 38
 lymphogranuloma venereum and, 612
 newborn eye ointment and, 473
 rape and, 74
 salpingo-oophoritis and, 587
 syphilis and, 345
Erythropoiesis
 extramedullary, diabetes and, 301
 megaloblastic, 339
 pregnancy and, 256
Escherichia coli, 578, 579
 abortion and, 584
 Bartholin gland and, 612
 breast-feeding and, 602
 early stage of infections and, 579
 urinary tract infection and, 336, 337

Esterase-D, 73
Estradiol
  aging and, 682
  inevitable abortion and, 213
  leiomyomas and, 651-652
  menstruation and, 76, 78, 79
  ovaries and, 80
  placenta and, 159
  plasma concentration of, 23
  pseudocyesis and, 280
  radioimmunoassay for, 23
Estriol
  cessation of production of, 281
  diabetes mellitus and, 302, 303
    subclinical, 306
  fetal condition and, 462-463
  ovaries and, 80
  placental hormones and, 158
  radioimmunoassay for, 23
  urinary excretion of, 160, 303
Estriol/creatinine ratio, 302, 303
Estrogen
  abnormal uterine bleeding and, 90, 92
  adenomyosis and, 655
  age and, 622, 656, 689-691
  amenorrhea and, 112
  atrophic vaginitis and, 625
  breakthrough bleeding and, 203
  breast cancer and, 138
  breast changes during pregnancy and, 256
  breast-feeding and, 603
  classic, 80
  after coitus, pregnancy interception and, 204
  combined oral contraception and, 200
  congenital adrenal hyperplasia and, 45, 47
  conjugated
    abnormal uterine bleeding and, 92
    breakthrough bleeding and, 203
    pregnancy interception and, 204
  death of embryo and, 212
  endometrium and, 84
    cancer of, 656
  fat metabolism during pregnancy and, 269
  hypothyroidism and, 308
  immunologic assay for, 23
  infant and, 36
  jaundice during pregnancy and, 329
  labial agglutination and, 39
  lichen sclerosus and, 615
  menstruation and, 76, 77, 78, 79, 82-84, 85
  myocardial infarction and, 683, 684
  oral contraception and, 199, 202
  osteoporosis and, 684
  Papanicolaou technique and, 19, 20

Estrogen—cont'd
  placenta and, 156, 158
  postpartum blues and, 58
  pregnancy and, 211-212
  premenstrual syndrome and, 118
  pruritus gravidarum and, 329
  puerperium changes and, 601
  sexual desire and, 61
  stress incontinence and, 563
  teratogenesis and, 41
  tests for, 18-20
  thyroid function and, 266
  vaginal epithelial cells and, 19
  vaginitis and, 38
  vascular changes and, 320
Estrogen de novo, placental hormones and, 156, 158
Estrogen receptor
  breast cancer and, 139, 140
  endometrial cancer and, 658
Estrogen secreting cyst, 103
Estrogen withdrawal bleeding, 89
Estrogen-androgens, breast cancer and, 691
Estrogenic effect, 19
Estrogen-medroxyprogesterone, 690
Estrogen-methyltestosterone, 690
Estrogen-progesterone
  aging and, 689, 690
  amenorrhea and, 112
Estrogen-progestin, abnormal uterine bleeding and, 92, 95
Estrogen-progestogen, endometriosis and, 129, 130
Estrogen-secreting ovarian neoplasm, 656
Estrone
  aging and, 682, 690
  leiomyomas and, 652
  ovaries and, 80
  placenta and, 159
  plasma, 23
Ethambutol, 313
Ethinyl estradiol
  aging and, 689
  oral contraception and, 199
  pruritus gravidarum and, 329
Ethisterone, hazard of, 221
Ethylene oxide, 212
Euglycemia, 302
Eversion, cervical, 631-632
  preadolescent and, 42
  pregnancy and, 253
Examination
  abdominal, 14
    abruptio placentae and, 389
    breech delivery and, 520
    face position and, 487
    labor and, 420
    placenta previa and, 382

Examination—cont'd
  bimanual, 15
    retrodisplacement of uterus and, 572, 573-574
  breast and, 133-135
  digital, placenta previa and, 382-383
  gynecologic, 14-16
  laboratory, abruptio placentae and, 389
  pelvic, 14-16
  physical, 14-16
    sexual assault and, 71-74
  postpartum, 605
  pregnancy and initial, 274-276
  premarital, 273
  prepregnancy, 273
  rectal, 16
    face position and, 487, 488, 489
  rectovaginal, 16, 37
  vaginal
    abruptio placentae and, 389
    breech delivery and, 520
    contracted pelvis during labor and, 504
    diagnosis of fetal position and, 396
    labor and, 419, 420-421
    placenta previa and, 382
    uterine dysfunction and, 477
  x-ray film and; *see* X-ray examination
Exchange transfusion, 461-462
Excision biopsy, 136, 137
Excitement phase of sexual response, 62
Excretion of hormones, placenta and, 154
Exenteration, pelvic, 645
Exercise
  aging and, 688
  amenorrhea and, 108, 111
  after delivery, 604-605
  dysmenorrhea treatment and, 117
  premenstrual syndrome treatment and, 120
  prenatal care and, 287
  pubococcygeus muscle, 288, 604-605, 691
  stress incontinence and, 563
Exfoliative cytology; *see* Cytology
Exhibitionism, 63
Exophytic growth, cervical, 640
Expected date of confinement, 282-283
Expulsion, placental, 446-450
Exsanguination, placenta previa and, 386
Extended arm, partial breech extraction and, 525
Extension during labor, 414, 415
External cephalic version, 522, 523
External cervical os, 627
External endometriosis, 122
External radiation for cervical cancer, 643, 644, 647
External rotation during labor and, 415-416
External tocodynamometer, 468-469

External version
  breech delivery and, 522, 523
  dystocia and, 486
Extraction
  breech, 522-531
  delivery of second twin and, 514
  forceps; *see* Forceps delivery
  Malmström cup, 540
  vacuum, 540
Extragenital injury in rape, 70
Extramedullary erythropoiesis, 301
Extraperitoneal cesarean section, 543
Extrasystoles, 260
Extrauterine pregnancy; *see* Ectopic pregnancy
Eye infection, newborn, 473
  chlamydial vaginitis and, 38
Eyelids, ptosis of, 357

F

Face position, 398-399
  dystocia and, 487-489
  forceps delivery and, 536
Face presentation, 393
Facilitated diffusion in placenta, 154
Facilities for obstetric care, 2-3
Fallopian tube; *see also* Tubal entries
  infertility and, 179-180
    treatment for, 189-190
  metaplasia of, 669
  pregnancy and, 253
  sterilization and, 204
Fallot's tetralogy, 319
False labor, 416
False pelvis, 494
Family planning, 192-209
  abortion and, 205-208
  contraception and, 193-205
  teenagers and, 192-193
Fasting diabetes test, pregnancy and, 275-276, 299
Fats, pregnancy and, 269
Father, labor and, 419
Fatty acids
  carbohydrate metabolism and, 269
  diabetes mellitus and, 299
  nonsterified, 269
  plasma, 299
Fatty degeneration, 650
Fatty liver of pregnancy, 329-330
Febrile morbidity, 544
Fecundability, 177
Fellows of the American College of Obstetricians and Gyne-
  cologists, 1
Female brain, 55

Female zygote, 143, 144
Femininity, 54-55
Feminizing tumor, 44, 674
  ovarian, 48-49
Femoral hernia during pregnancy, 333
Femoral vein, thrombophlebitis and, 595
Ferning, 20, 628
  cervical mucus and, 24-25
  endometrial biopsy and, 22
  infertility and, 180
  rupture of membranes and, 430
Ferrous gluconate, 322
Ferrous sulfate, 322
Fertile period, 194
Fertility rate, 6, 177
Fertilization, 142-150
  basal body temperature and, 25, 26
  due date and, 282
  in vitro, 227, 509
Fetal blood sampling, 149-150
Fetal cell
  age determination and, 283
  membrane rupture and, 430
Fetal death, 9, 10
  cesarean section and, 545
  hypertension and, 378
  intrauterine
    acute glomerulonephritis and, 340
    appendicitis and, 332
    labor induction and, 431
    ultrasound and, 33
  teenage pregnancy and, 6
Fetal death ratio, 7
Fetal distress, 467
  cesarean section and, 541, 542
Fetal heart monitoring
  abruptio placentae and, 389
  beat-to-beat variability and, 467, 468
  delivery and, 422
  diabetes mellitus and, 302, 303
  due date determination and, 282
  fetal death and, 281
  labor and, 420-421
  position diagnosis and, 396
Fetal heart tone, 278
Fetal hemoglobin, 321, 322, 323
Fetal length calculation, 170
Fetal mortality, 9, 10
Fetal movement
  cessation of, 281
  counting of, 463
  diagnosis of pregnancy and, 278
Fetal pole, 279
Fetal position
  determination of, 393-399

Fetal position—cont'd
  labor induction and, 432
Fetal scalp blood sampling, 467
Fetal scalp electrode, 468, 469
Fetal skeleton, 279-280
Fetal skull
  biparietal diameter of, 33, 283
  bitemporal diameter of, 396
  landmarks of, 172
Fetal surveillance of diabetic pregnant woman, 302-304
Fetal weight, breech delivery and, 524, 531
Fetomaternal transfusion, 449-450
Fetopelvic disproportion
  cesarean section and, 531
  labor induction and, 432
Fetoplacental circulation, 171
α-Fetoprotein; *see* Alpha-fetoprotein
Fetoscopy, 35, 150
Fetus; *see also* Fetal entries
  abortion of; *see* Abortion
  antepartum evaluation of, 456
  ballottement of, 277-278
  development of, 170-174
    amniocentesis and, 34, 164
    dystocia and, 480-483
    multifetal pregnancy and, 510
  erythroblastosis fetalis and, 459-462
  evaluation of, during pregnancy, 462-465
  growth of
    chart of, 170
    ultrasound and, 33
    retardation of; *see* Growth retardation
  immature, 542
  palpation of, 277-278
  prenatal influences on, 456-459
  role of, in initiation of labor, 410
  signs of life or death of, 281
Fetus papyraceous, 510
FFA; *see* Free fatty acid
Fibrin, 167
Fibrin degradation products, 387
Fibrinogen
  complete placental separation and, 390
  pregnancy and, 259
Fibrinous layer of Nitabuch, 152
Fibroadenoma, 137
Fibrocystic disease, 134-135, 136-137
Fibroid
  pedunculated submucous, 654
  wandering, 650
Fibroma, 675
  vulva and, 617
Fibroid, 649-655
Fibromyoma; *see* Uterine leiomyoma

Filtration fraction, 263
Fimbria, 144-145
Fimbria ovarica, 144
First-degree laceration, 549
First-degree prolapse of uterus, 568
Fistulas, 570
Flagyl; *see* Metronidazole
Flat pelvis, 497, 498
Flea bites of vulva, 609
Flexion, 413
Flora, age and, 622
Flow, menstrual; *see* Menstruation
Flufenamic acid, 117
Fluid
    amniotic; *see* Amniotic fluid
    excessive storage of, in pregnancy, 284
    interstitial, 257
    preeclampsia treatment and, 371
    premenstrual syndrome and, 118-119
    pyelonephritis and, 338
Fluorescent treponemal antibody-absorption test, 344
Fluoroscopy, 184
Fluorouracil cream, 618
Foam, contraceptive, 196
Foaming tablets, contraceptive, 196
Folate levels, 322; *see also* Folic acid
Foley catheter, 101
Folic acid
    deficiency of, 322
    epilepsy and, 356
    pregnancy and, 270
Follicle
    fimbriae enclosing, 145
    preantral, 81
    rupture of, 146, 235, 667-668
Follicle-stimulating hormone, 23, 24
    aging and, 681, 682
Follicular cyst, 666
    amenorrhea and, 103
Follicular phase of menstruation, 76
Folliculitis, 609
Fontanel, 171, 172, 396
Food, labor and, 419, 421
Footling breech presentation, 518, 531
Foramen ovale, 173
Forceps delivery, 533-540
    low; *see* Low forceps extraction
    partial breech extraction and, 525, 530
    uterine dressing and, 22
Forces in labor, 406-408
Foreign body, vaginal, 626
    preadolescent and, 39
    radiolucent, 582
Forelying cord, 469, 470

Formiminoglutamic acid, 322
Fourth-degree laceration, 549
Fractional curettage, 662
Fractures, compression, 686
Frank breech, 518
Fraternal twins, 507, 508
Free fatty acids
    carbohydrate metabolism and, 269
    diabetes mellitus and, 299
Free thyroxine index, 308
Freestanding center, 4
Frigidity, 65
Frontal suture, 171
Frontanel, posterior, 171
Frontoanterior position, 491, 492
Frontoposterior position, 491, 492
Frontotransverse position, 491, 492
FSH; *see* Follicle-stimulating hormone
FTA-ABS; *see* Fluorescent treponemal antibody-absorption test
FTI; *see* Free thyroxine index
Fundal dominance, 407
Fundus, elevation of, 446
Funduscopic examination, 301
Fungal infection, vulvovaginal, 347
Fungicide, 603
Funnel pelvis, 497, 503
Fusion, spinal, 362
Fusobacterium, 578

G

Galactocele, 137
Galactorrhea, 135
Galactorrhea-amenorrhea syndrome, 106, 606
Galactosemia, 164
Gallbladder, 265, 333
Gallstones, 333
Gametogenesis, 143, 144
Gamma globulins, 294
Ganglionic blocker, 377
Gantrisin; *see* Sulfisoxazole
Gardnerella infection, 346, 625
Gärtner duct cyst, 626
Gas gangrene, 584
Gastric acidity, 264
Gastric motility, 264
Gastrointestinal tract, pregnancy and, 264-265
Gender identity, 55
Generative organs, 251-255
Genetics, 44
    amniotic fluid and, 164
    endometriosis and, 123

Genetics—cont'd
  multifetal pregnancies and, 509
Genital herpesvirus, 629
  pregnancy and, 345-346
  spontaneous abortion and, 211
Genital tract; *see also* Genitals
  aging and, 687
  estrogen and, 689
  fistula and, 570
  pregnancy and, 343-355
    congenital anomalies and, 351-354
    neoplasia and, 347-350
    uterus malposition and, 350-351
    vulvovaginal disorders and, 343-347
  spontaneous abortion and, 211
Genitals; *see also* Genital tract
  atrophy of, 80
  of child, 36
  pregnancy and, 277
  rape and, 70
Genotype, 143
Gentamicin, 584, 588
  endomyometritis and, 594
  postoperative infection and, 590
Germ cell
  maturation of, 142
  ovarian neoplasms and, 669-671
German measles, 293
German silver Graefenberg ring, 197
Germinal inclusion cyst, 666
Gestational age, 524
Gestational edema, 365
Gestational hypertension, 364
Gestational proteinuria, 365
Gestational sac, 232, 279
Gestational trophoblastic neoplasm, 239-250
  abnormal uterine bleeding and, 89
  choriocarcinoma and, 247-250
  hydatidiform mole and, 239-246
  invasive mole and, 247
Gingivitis, 264, 326
Girdle, maternity, 288
Glandular hyperplasia, 652
Glomerular endotheliosis, 374
Glomerular filtration, 262-263, 335
Glomerulonephritis, 340-341, 361
Glucagon, 299
Glucocorticoids, 684
Glucose, 269
  diabetes mellitus and, 298, 302
    subclinical, 306
  fasting levels of, 299
  premenstrual syndrome and, 118
  renal threshold for, 298
  in saline, 310

Glucose oxidase reagent strips, 302
Glucose oxidation, 174
Glucose screening, 306
Glucose tolerance test, 298, 306
Glucose-6-phosphate dehydrogenase deficiency, 339, 458
Glutamic oxaloacetic transaminase, 260, 329
Glutamic pyruvic transaminase, 260, 329
Glycogen, 18, 19
  age and, 622
  menstruation and, 82
Glycogen storage disease, 149, 164
Glycohemoglobin, 306
Glycosuria, 298
  pregnancy and, 263, 269
  subclinical diabetes mellitus and, 306
Glyoxalase I, 73
GnRH; *see* Gonadotropin-releasing hormone
Goblet cells, 672
Goiter
  congenital, 307, 308
    iodine and, 314
  hyperthyroidism and, 308
  povidone-iodine products and, 624
  simple colloid, 307
Gonadal dysgenesis
  amenorrhea and, 101-102, 111
  infertility and, 178, 180, 189
Gonadal sex, 44
Gonadal stroma, 674-675
Gonadectomy, 103
Gonadotrope, 78
Gonadotropin; *see also* Chorionic gonadotropin
  dizygotic twinning and, 509
  hot flush and, 687
  hydatidiform mole and, 243, 244
  luteoma and, 666
  tests for, 23
Gonadotropin-releasing hormone
  menstruation and, 76
  sexual precocity and, 48
Gonorrhea, 587, 629
  bacterial culture and, 17
  contraception and, 197
  infant and, 344
  preadolescent and, 38
  pregnancy and, 344
  rape and, 40, 74
  testing for, 73
  treatment for, 344-345
  young primigravidas and, 428
Goodell's sign, 277
Graafian follicle; *see* Follicle
Graefenberg ring, 197
Gram stain, 17, 577, 578

Gram stain—cont'd
  illegal abortion and, 222
  salpingo-oophritis and, 587
Gram-negative or gram-positive bacteria, 577, 578; *see also*
    Gram stain
Granulocytosis, 331
Granuloma inguinale, 611-612
  pregnancy and, 346
Granulosa cell tumor, 674
Granulosa-theca cell tumor, 674-675
  amenorrhea and, 103
Graves' disease, 109
Gravid uterus, 252
Gravida, term of, 400
Gray syndrome, 339
Group rape, 70
Growth
  adolescents and, 49-50
  exophytic, 640
  neoplastic, 347-350
  retardation of; *see* Growth retardation
  of uterus in pregnancy, 251
Growth hormone
  aging and, 682
  pregnancy and, 263
Growth retardation
  anticonvulsants and, 356
  cesarean section and, 542
  definition of, 425
  delivery and, 427-428
  diabetes mellitus and, 300
  hypertension and, 376
Guillain-Barré syndrome, 357
Gynandroblastomas, 675
Gynecoid pelvis, 496-497, 498, 503
Gynecologic examination, 14
Gynecology, pediatric, 36-51; *see also* Pediatric gynecology
Gyne-Lotrimin; *see* Clotrimazole

H

Haase's rule, 170
Habitual abortion, 214-215, 218, 219
  treatment of, 218, 220-221
Haemophilus vaginitis, 625, 629
  infected abortion and, 584
  pregnancy and, 346-347
Halban's syndrome, 89
Halothane, 439
hCG; *see* Chorionic gonadotropin
Head, fetal
  characteristics of, 171, 172
  delivery of, 422-423
  early decelerations and, 466, 467

Head, fetal—cont'd
  forceps delivery and, 536
  hyperextension of, 531
  labor and, 410-411
Head-down position, 425
Health, psychology and, 52
Health care team, 2
Heart; *see also* Heart disease
  fetal; *see* Fetal heart monitoring
  hypoparathyroidism and, 310
  oral contraception and, 201-202
  pregnancy and, 260-261
  rheumatic lesion of, 316
Heart disease, 315-318, 319
  delivery and, 443
  medical abortion and, 206
Heart failure, 316, 318, 319
Heart rate
  fetal; *see* Fetal heart monitoring
  pregnancy and, 315-316
Heart valve prostheses, 317-318
Heartburn, 328
Heat-stable alkaline phosphatase, 161-162
Hebdomadal death, 9
Hegar's sign, 277
HELLP syndrome, 369
Hemagglutination inhibition test, 28, 29
  rubella and, 294
Hemangiomas, 617
Hematochezia, 128
Hematocolpos, 99, 100, 101
Hematocrit, 16
  blood count, 258
  eclampsia and, 368
  iron-deficiency anemia and, 321
  labor and, 419
  pregnancy and, 275
  sickle cell trait and, 323
Hematogenous spread, 662
Hematoma, 571-572
Hematometra
  amenorrhea and, 99, 100
  diagnosis of pregnancy and, 280
Hematosalpinx, 99, 100
Hematuria
  endometriosis and, 128
  pregnancy and, 340
Hemoconcentration, 368
Hemodialysis, 341
Hemoglobin, 16, 258, 321, 322-324
  A, 306
  A_{1c}, 300, 306
  C, 323, 324
  electrophoresis of, 324
  labor and, 419

Hemoglobin—cont'd
  pregnancy and, 320
  S, 324
  total, 256
Hemoglobin C disease, 323, 324
Hemoglobinopathies, 322-324
Hemolytic anemia, 295
Hemolytic streptococcal vaginitis, 38
Hemophilia, 149
Hemorrhage; *see also* Bleeding
  abruptio placentae and, 387
  breech delivery and, 520
  cerebral, 376
  postpartum, 444, 450-454
    intrahepatic cholestasis and, 329
    placenta previa and, 386
    uterine dysfunction and, 476
  subaponeurotic, 540
  subarachnoid, 358
Hemorrhoidectomy, 333
Hemorrhoids
  multifetal pregnancy and, 510
  postpartum, 606
  pregnancy and, 333
Hemosiderin, 128
Heparin
  breast-feeding and, 603
  disseminated intravascular coagulation and, 324
  fetus and, 458
  pelvic infection and, 579
  thrombophlebitis and, 578, 594, 595
  valve disease and, 318
Hepatic splenomegaly, 296
Hepatitis, 330
Hepatomegaly, 301
Hepatosplenomegaly, 295
Heredity; *see* Genetics
Hermaphroditism, 48
Hernia
  cul-de-sac, 557, 558
  hiatal, 265, 328-329
  pregnancy and, 333-334
  vaginal, 557, 558
Herniorrhaphy, 334
Heroin
  breast-feeding and, 603
  fetus and, 458
  premature labor and, 426
Herpes gestationis, 360
Herpesvirus, 609-610, 626
  cervical cancer and, 634
  fetus and, 459
  pregnancy and, 296, 345-346
  rape and, 74
  spontaneous abortion and, 211

Herpesvirus—cont'd
  vulva and, 609-610
Heterologous insemination, 188-189
Heterosexual precocity, 48, 49
Heterotopic elements, neoplasms of, 675
Heterozygosity, 459
Heyman's capsule, 663
HI; *see* Hemagglutination-inhibition test
Hiatal hernia, 265, 328-329
Hidradenomas, 617
High forceps extraction, 533, 535, 539
High transverse arrest, 504
High-risk pregnancy, 290
  diagnosis of, 273-274
  neonatal death and, 11
Hilus cell tumor, 675
  masculinizing, 106
Hip dislocation, congenital, 149
Hirsutism, 18
Histaminase, 161
Histamine vasopressor test, 311
Histidine, 263
History
  diagnosis and, 13-14
  rape victim and, 71-74
  sexual response and, 63-64
Hodgkin's disease, 324
Home delivery, 5
Homologous insemination, 188-189
Homozygosity, 323, 459
Hormone assay, 18-28
  androgens and, 23
  estrogen and, 18-20
  gonadotropins and, 23
  ovulation and, 23-28
  progesterone and, 23
Hormone excretion curve, 154-155
Hormone therapy, 103, 112
  abnormal uterine bleeding and, 95
  aging and, 689-691
  endometriosis and, 129
  habitual abortion and, 220-221
Hormones
  aging and, 681-682
  menstruation and, 78-80
  nausea and vomiting during pregnancy and, 327
  placental, 154-161
  pregnancy and, 457
  spontaneous abortion and, 219
Hospital, 3-4
  discharge from, 605
  labor and, 419
Hospital-based birth center, 4
Hot flush, 686-687
  estrogen and, 689

Hot flush—cont'd
  phenobarbital and, 692
hPL; *see also* Human placental lactogen
hPr; *see* Human prolactin
HSAP; *see* Heat-stable alkaline phosphatase
Human anti-D gamma globulin, 207
Human chorionic gonadotropin; *see* Chorionic gonadotropin
Human leukocyte antigen testing, 509
Human menopausal gonadotropin, 112, 190
Human papilloma virus
  cervical cancer and, 634, 635
  rape and, 74
Human placental lactogen, 160-161
  diabetes mellitus and, 299
  pregnancy and, 256, 266
Human prolactin, 266
Hurler's disease, 149
Hyaline degeneration, 650
Hyaline membrane disease, 304
Hydatidiform mole, 239-246
  hormone assay and, 18
  invasive, 247
  nausea and vomiting during pregnancy and, 327
  ultrasound and, 33
Hydralazine
  eclampsia and, 373
  hypertension and, 377
  preeclampsia and, 372
Hydramnios, 168, 169-170
  diabetes mellitus and, 299, 306
Hydrocephaly
  cytomegalovirus disease and, 295
  dystocia and, 482, 483
  toxoplasmosis and, 296
Hydrocortisone
  adrenal insufficiency and, 310, 311
  lichen sclerosus and, 615
  vulvar
    dermatitis and, 614
    infection and, 609
Hydronephrosis, 262
Hydrothorax, 675
Hydroureter, 262
17-Hydroxycorticosteroids, 161
2-Hydroxyestrone, 80
4-Hydroxyestrone, 80
17-Hydroxypregnenolone
  aging and, 682
  placenta and, 159
17-Hydroxyprogesterone
  aging and, 682
  endometrial cancer and, 663
  habitual abortion and, 221
  placenta and, 159

17-α-Hydroxyprogesterone; *see* 17-Alpha-hydroxyprogesterone
Hygiene of menstruation, 86
Hymen
  dyspareunia and, 64
  imperforate
    amenorrhea and, 99, 100
    preadolescent and, 39, 40
  infertility and, 179
  rape and, 73
  young girls and, 36
Hyperbilirubinemia, 300, 304
Hypercalcemia, 310
Hypercortisolism, 106
Hyperemesis gravidarum, 327
Hyperglycemia, 304
Hyperglycemic hyperinsulinemia, 299
Hyperkalemia, 584
Hyperkeratosis of vulva, 613-614, 615
Hyperlipidemia, 105
Hypermenorrhea, 85, 88
Hyperparathyroidism, 310
Hyperplasia, 32
  diabetes mellitus and, 301
  endometrial
    abnormal uterine bleeding and, 90
    retrograde, 683, 685
  glandular, 652
  islet of Langerhans, 300
  microglandular, 640
  polycystic ovarian syndrome and, 104
Hyperplastic dystrophy, 615, 616
Hyperplastic lesion of vulva, 613-614
Hyperprolactinemia
  amenorrhea and, 106, 107
  correction of, 189
  diabetes mellitus and, 299
  infertility and, 180
  premenstrual syndrome and, 119
Hyperptyalism, 264
Hypersegmentation of neutrophils, 322
Hypertension; *see also* Hypertensive disorders
  abortion and, 206
  abruptio placentae and, 386-387
  adrenal hyperfunction and, 311
  anesthesia and analgesia and, 443
  benign intracranial, 358
  cesarean section and, 542
  definition of, 364
  diabetes mellitus and, 304
  endometrial cancer and, 657
  gestational, 364
  kidney transplants and, 341
  labor induction and, 430
  oral contraception and, 202

Hypertension—cont'd
  polycystic ovarian syndrome and, 105
  postpartum hemorrhage and, 451
  pregnancy and, 375-378
    hydatidiform mole and, 242
    multifetal, 510
  pulmonary, 316, 317, 318
  pyelonephritis and, 339
Hypertensive disorders, 364-379; *see also* Hypertension
  cardiovascular, premature labor and, 425
  chronic, 375-378
  classification and diagnosis of, 364-365
  diabetes mellitus and, 302
  incidence of, 365
  preeclampsia-eclampsia and; *see* Eclampsia; Preeclampsia
Hyperthecosis, 105
Hyperthyroidism, 307, 308-309
  hydatidiform mole and, 242
Hypertonic saline solution, 207
Hypertrophy
  of breast, 135
  of cervix, 633
  of uterus, 655
Hyperventilation
  pregnancy and, 261-262
  tetany and, 309
Hypoadrenalism, 310
Hypocalcemia
  diabetes mellitus and, 300, 304
  hypoparathyroidism and, 310
Hypoestrogenic state, 101
Hypoglycemia
  diabetes mellitus and, 300, 304
  fetal, 171
  hypoadrenalism and, 310
  newborn, 302, 306
  premenstrual syndrome and, 119
  shock and, 299
Hypogonadotropic hypogonadism, 108, 178
Hypomenorrhea, 85
Hypoparathyroidism, 309-310
  impetigo herpetiformis and, 360
Hypophosphatemia, 299
Hypophysectomy, 140
Hypopituitarism, 106
Hypoplastic testes, 42
Hypospadias, 179
Hypotension, 438, 581
Hypothalamic amenorrhea, 107-108
Hypothalamic-hypophyseal complex, 78
  amenorrhea and, 98
Hypothalamic-pituitary dysfunction, 189-190
Hypothalamic-pituitary-ovarian axis, 48, 76
Hypothalamus, 77, 78
  menarche and, 49

Hypothalamus—cont'd
  menstruation and, 76
Hypothyroidism, 307, 308
  abnormal uterine bleeding and, 93, 96
  amenorrhea and, 106, 109
  infertility and, 178
  neonatal, 309
  povidone-iodine products and, 624
  sexual precocity and, 49
Hypovolemic shock, 388
Hypoxia, fetal, 171
  appendicitis and, 332
  labor and, 465-471
  surgery during pregnancy and, 331
Hysterectomy
  abnormal uterine bleeding and, 95
  cervical carcinoma in situ and, 642
  endometrial cancer and, 663
  endometriosis and, 129, 131
  hydatidiform mole and, 244
  infections and, 584
    abortion and, 585
  leiomyomas and, 654
  ovarian neoplasms and, 677, 678
  radical, 644, 645, 646
  uterine fibromyoma and, 349
  uterine prolapse and, 569
Hysterogram
  abnormal uterine bleeding and, 94, 95
  ectopic pregnancy and, 235
Hysterosalpingography
  abnormal uterine bleeding and, 91
  infertility and, 184, 185, 186
  x-ray film and, 32
Hysteroscopy, 34
  abnormal uterine bleeding and, 91, 95
  amenorrhea and, 101
  resection and, 654
Hysterotomy, 207

I

[131]I; *see* Radioactive iodine
Ibuprofen, 117, 624
Icterus, 329
Identical twins, 507, 508
Idiopathic autoimmune thrombocytopenic purpura, 324
Idiopathic cardiomyopathy, 319
Idiopathic cholestasis, 360
Illegal abortion, 210
Illegitimate births, 6
Imaging, radionuclide, 341
Imipenem, 577, 581
Immune globulin preparation, 330

Immunization
  influenza, 314
  poliomyelitis and, 357
  during pregnancy, 296
Immunofluorescent staining, 38
Immunoglobulins, 602
Immunologic estrogen assay, 23
Immunology
  eclampsia and, 369
  infertility and, 181-182
  pregnancy testing and, 28
  spontaneous abortion and, 220
Immunosuppressive drugs, 341
Imperforate hymen
  amenorrhea and, 99, 100
  preadolescent and, 39, 40
Impetigo herpetiformis, 360
Implantation, 147
  ectopic pregnancy and, 227
Implantation bleeding, 148
Impotence, 65, 66
  infertility and, 179
In vitro fertilization
  ectopic pregnancy and, 227
  infertility and, 190
  multifetal pregnancy and, 509
Incarceration of gravid uterus, 351
Inclination, angle of, 494
Inclusion conjunctivitis, 346
Incompetent cervical os, 219, 220, 221
Incomplete abortion, 235
Incomplete antibody, 460
Incomplete breech, 518
Incomplete placenta previa, 380, 381
  treatment of, 384, 385
Incomplete placental separation, 386
  treatment of, 391
Incontinence, urinary, 560-564, 565
  menopause and, 683, 690-691
  stress, 683, 690-691
Indigo carmine, 570
Indirect obstetric death, 8
Indomethacin, 426
Induced abortion, 221-223
Induction of labor, 429-432
Infant; *see also* Newborn
  care of
    after delivery, 456, 471-473
    during labor, 456, 465-471
    during pregnancy, 456-465; *see also* Fetus
  diabetic mother and, 299-300, 305
  genital herpesvirus and, 345-346
  liveborn, 9
  low-birth-weight, 10-11, 170, 425

Infant—cont'd
  at term, 170-171
  urinary retention of, 483
  viable, 400
Infant mortality, 10
Infantilism, sexual, 102
Infarction
  adrenal gland, 310
  hypertension and, 376
  oral contraception and, 201-202
Infection, 293-297, 577-597; *see also* specific infection
  abdominal wound, 590
  abortion and, 222-223, 581-585
    spontaneous, 211, 219-220
  Bartholin gland, 343, 344
  breast and, 135-136
  cervical, 219-220
  cesarean section and, 545-546
  community-acquired, 581-589
  dyspareunia and, 64
  early onset, 579
  endometrial, 219-220
  eye, in newborn, 613
  fetal death and, 10
  herpesvirus; *see* Herpesvirus
  hospital acquired, 581
  infertility and, 178
  intrauterine, 430
  intrauterine device and, 198
  iron-deficiency and, 322
  late onset problems of, 579, 580
  leiomyomas and, 654
  mastitis, 595-596
  necrosis and, 650
  nosocomial, 581
  pelvic, 128, 596
    treatment for, 579-581
  placental, 168
  postoperative, 589-591
  postpartum, 591-594
  premature labor and, 426
  rare, 596
  respiratory, 314
  thrombophlebitis, 594-595
  Trichomonas, 347, 622, 629
    preadolescent and, 38
  urinary tract; *see* Urinary system, infections of
  uterine dysfunction and, 477
  vestibular gland, 613
  yeast, 623
  young primigravidas and, 428
Infectious disease, 293-297
Infectious morbidity, 591
Inferior strait, 495
Infertility, 177-191

Infertility—cont'd
  causes of, 178-182
  definition of, 177
  emotions and, 59
  endometrial cancer and, 657
  endometriosis and, 127, 130-131
  hormone assay and, 18
  infection and, 178
  investigation of, 182-187
  Kallmann's syndrome and, 178
  Klinefelter's syndrome and, 178
  leiomyomas and, 653
  male and female history and, 183
  primary, 177
  relative, 177
  reproduction factors and, 177-178
  secondary, 177
  treatment of, 187-191
Inflammatory carcinoma, 138
Inflammatory disease
  bowel, 331
  pelvic, 179
Inflammatory lesion of vulva, 609
Influenza, 314
  immunization and, 296
Infundibulopelvic ligament, 253, 255
Inguinal hernia, 333
Inhalation anesthesia, 544
Injury; *see also* Trauma
  breech delivery and, 520
  postpartum hemorrhage and, 450, 451-452
  uterine, childbirth and, 565-567
Inlet, pelvic, 494
  contracted pelvis and, 504
  face position and, 487
  occipitoposterior position and, 486
Insect bites of vulva, 609
Insemination, 188-189
Insulin
  diabetes mellitus and, 302, 304
  placental barrier to, 300
  placental degradation of, 299
  plasma, 306
  pregnancy and, 269, 299
Insulinase, 299
Intelligence, impaired, 295
Intercourse
  infertility treatment and, 188
  painful, 64-65
  pregnancy and, 288
Intermediate cell
  fetal, 165, 166
  menstrual, 85
Intermenstrual bleeding, 652
Internal cervical os, 627, 628

Internal endometriosis, 122, 126
Internal pressure catheter, 468-469
Internal radiation therapy, 643
Internal rotation, 413-415
International Federation of Gynecology and Obstetrics staging
  of corpus uteri carcinoma, 662
  of cervical cancer, 639
Intersexual state, 44
Interstitial fluid volume, 257
Interstitial tumor, 649, 650
Intertrigo, 613-614
  vulva and, 609
Intervillous pressure, 466
Intervillous space, 147
Intestinal metaplasia, 669
Intestinal obstruction, 332-333
Intraabdominal pressure, 572
Intraamniotic saline injection, 207
Intracranial hemorrhage, 459
Intracranial hypertension, 358
Intraductile carcinoma, 137
Intraepithelial neoplasia, cervical, 635-636, 637
Intragastric pressure, 328
Intrahepatic cholestasis, 329
Intraligamentous pregnancy, 227-228
Intraligamentous tumor, 649, 650
Intramural tumor, 649, 650
Intraperitoneal bleeding, 16
Intrauterine device, 199
  ectopic pregnancy and, 226
  infertility and, 179
Intrauterine growth retardation, 462
Intrauterine intraperitoneal transfusion, 461
Intrauterine pregnancy, 198
Intrauterine pressure, 403, 406
Intravascular coagulation, disseminated; *see* Disseminated intravascular coagulation
Intravenous fluid, 328
Intravenous injections, 38, 438
Intubation, endotracheal, 373
Inulin, 336
Invasive cancer
  cervical and, 633, 642-644
  endometrial, 659, 660
  pregnancy and, 647
  vulvar, 618-619
Invasive mole, 247
Involution, 598
Iodide, 603
  clearance of, 263
Iodine
  asthma and, 314
  radioactive, 266, 308, 603
  trichomoniasis and, 623

Iowa trumpet, 442
Iron
    abnormal uterine bleeding and, 93, 95
    iron-deficiency anemia and, 321, 322
23
    heart disease and, 317
    parenteral, 322
    pregnancy and, 270, 320
    serum, 320, 321
Iron-beta globulin complex, 320
Iron-binding capacity, 320, 321
Iron-deficiency anemia, 321-322
Irregular shedding, uterine, 90
Ischemic necrosis, 167
Islets of Langerhans, 300
    hyperplasia of, 299, 305
Isochromosome, 149
Isoniazid, 313
Isosexual precocity, 48, 674
Isoxsuprine, 426
Isthmus of uterus, 402, 403, 627
IUD; *see* Intrauterine device
IVF; *see* In vitro fertilization

J

Jarcho's classification of uterine malformations, 352-354
Jaundice
    cytomegalovirus and, 295
    hepatitis and, 330
    oral contraception and, 202
    pregnancy and, 329
    tetracyclines and, 339
    toxoplasmosis and, 296
Jejunoileal bypass, 334
Johnson, V.E., 68
Johnson Rape Kit, 73
Joints, 265-266
    disorders of, 356, 361-363; *see also* Bone and joint disorders

K

Kallmann's syndrome
    amenorrhea and, 108
    infertility and, 178
Karyotyping, 34
Keflex; *see* Cephalexin
Kernicterus
    erythroblastosis and, 461
    sulfonamides and, 339
Ketoacidosis, 302

Ketoconazole, 624
Ketohexose, 153
Ketoprofen, 117
6-Ketoprostaglandin $F_1\alpha$, 127
Ketosis, 334
17-Ketosteroids
    congenital adrenal hyperplasia and, 45
    placenta and, 161
    pregnancy and, 267
    puerperium and, 601
Keyes dermatologic punch, 32, 616
Kick count, 463
    diabetes mellitus and, 303
Kidney, 341
    dystocia and, 483
    eclampsia and, 374
    single, pregnancy and, 341
    transplant of, pregnancy and, 341-342
Klebsiella, 578
Klinefelter's syndrome, 45
    chromosomal aberration and, 148
    fertilization and, 144
    infertility and, 178
Knee presentation, 518-519
Koilocytes, 635, 636
Krukenberg tumor, 675, 676
Kyphoscoliotic heart disease, 320
Kyphosis, dorsal, 687

L

Labia majora, 682-683
Labia minora, 683
Labial agglutination, 39
Labor, 400-433
    abruptio placentae and, 387
    breech delivery and, 520-522
    cardiac valve disease and, 318-319
    care during, 419-422
    cause of, 408-410
    cessation of, during second stage, 536
    changes preceding, 401-406
    clinical course of, 416
    contracted pelvis and, 504-506
    diabetes mellitus and, 302-304
    duration of, 416-418
        multifetal pregnancy and, 510
    dysfunctional
        breech delivery and, 531
        cesarean section and, 541-542
        postpartum hemorrhage and, 450
    dystocia and; *see* Dystocia
    elderly primigravidas and, 429

Labor—cont'd
  emotions during, 58
  false, 416
  fetal growth retardation and, 427-428
  first stage of, 417, 418
  forces in, 406-408
  immature, 210
  induction of, 429-432
    early elective, 426
  mechanism of, 410-416
  multifetal pregnancy and, 513-514
  multiparas and, 429
  observations during, 419-421
  obstructed, 566
  onset and diagnosis of, 416
  pain control in, 434-438
  patient education and, 418-419
  postpartum hemorrhage and, 450
  precipitate, 429
  preeclampsia and, 373
  premature, 425-427; *see also* Premature labor and delivery
  preparation for, 418-419
  primigravida and, 417, 418
  prolonged; *see* Prolonged labor
  prolonged perineal phase of, 536
  prolonged pregnancy and, 428
  stages of, 416
  third stage of, 444-450
  trial, 505-506, 544
  tuberculosis and, 313-314
  young primigravidas and, 428-429
Labor curve, abnormal, 475
Labor graph, 419, 420-421
Laboratory study
  preeclampsia and, 370, 371
  pregnancy and, 275, 390
Laceration
  cervical; *see* Cervical laceration
  degrees of, 549
  perineal, 549, 552-554
  vaginal, 451, 554
Lactation, 602-603; *see also* Breast-feeding
  amenorrhea and, 99
Lactobacilli, 622
Lactose, 269
Lactotrope, 78
Lamaze method, 435
Lambdoid suture, 171, 396
Laminaria stick, 207
Landrey's ascending paralysis, 359
Langhans' cell, 150, 152
Laparoscopy, 33-34
  dysmenorrhea and, 117
  ectopic pregnancy and, 234
  endometriosis and, 128

Laparoscopy—cont'd
  hermaphroditism and, 48
  infertility and, 184, 186
  neoplasm and, 668
    ovarian, 676
Laparotomy
  ectopic pregnancy and, 234
  feminizing tumor of ovary and, 49
  true hermaphroditism and, 48
Laryngoscopy, 472
Laser therapy
  carcinoma in situ and
    cervical, 642
    vulvar, 618
  condylomata acuminata and, 611
  dysplasia and, 641
Lassar's paste, 38
Late deceleration, 466, 467
Latency phase, 56
Latent diabetes mellitus, 304-306
Latent period, 430
Latent phase abnormality, 475
Lateral umbilical ligament, 173
Latex particle, 28
Lead, 603
Lecithin/sphingomyelin ratio, 164, 166
  diabetes mellitus and, 302-303
  fetal age and, 283
Lee-White clotting time, 389
Left adnexum, 15-16
Left sacroanterior position, 517, 518
Left sacroposterior position, 517, 518
Legal abortion, 205-208, 210; *see also* Abortion
Legal considerations for sexual assault, 74-75
Leiomyoma
  abnormal uterine bleeding and, 89
  abortion and, 211, 220, 221
  diagnosis of pregnancy and, 280
  uterine, 649-655
Leiomyosarcoma, 661
Lesbians, 52
Lesion
  bladder, 391
  bowel, 128, 391
  cervical, 391, 630
  heart valve, 316
  malignant; *see also* Cancer; Carcinoma
    breast and, 137-141
    vulva and, 618-619
  organic, 89
  resection of, 129
  urinary tract, 128
  white, 613
Leukemia, 91, 324
Leukocytosis, 258, 331

Leukoderma, 613
Leukopenia, 581
Leukorrhea, 621
Levator muscle, 548, 551-552
Levator sling, 554-558
Leydig cell, 44
Leydig cell tumor, 675
LH; *see* Luteinizing hormone
LHRBI; *see* Luteinization inhibitor receptor–binding inhibitor
LH-releasing hormone; *see* Luteinizing hormone–releasing hormone
LI; *see* Luteinization inhibitor
Libido, 61
    oral contraception and, 200
Lichen sclerosus, 615
    preadolescent and, 39
Lidocaine
    paracervical block and, 437
    pudendal block and, 442
Lie, 393
    longitudinal, 393, 396-399
    transverse, 399
Life stages of women, 52-60
Ligament
    infundibulopelvic, 253, 255
    round, 253, 572
Ligamentum arteriosum, 173
Ligamentum teres hepatis, 173
Ligamentum venosum, 173
Ligation
    of cord, 472-473
    of fallopian tube
        cesarean section and, 545
        sickle cell hemoglobin C disease and, 325
        sterilization and, 204
Lightening, 503
Lindane shampoo, 609
Linea nigra, 256
Linear salpingostomy, 237
Lipids
    oral contraception and, 202
    serum, 259
Lipomas, 617
Lipoproteins, oral contraception and, 202
Liquefaction, 650, 651
Liquid nitrogen, 611
Liquor folliculi, 81
Lithium carbonate, 120
Lithotomy position, 422
Liveborn infant, 9
Liver
    disease of, 691
    eclampsia and, 374
    enlargement of, 301

Liver—cont'd
    fatty, 329-330, 339
    pregnancy and, 265
    tumors of, 483
Liver function test, 624
Lobular carcinoma, 137
Lochia, 599
    block of, 592, 594
Lochia alba, 599
Lochia rubra, 599
Locking of twins, 514, 515
Loestrin 1/20; *see* Norethindrone acetate
Longitudinal lie, 393, 396-399
Love, sexual response and, 63
Low forceps extraction, 533, 535
    appendicitis and, 332
    heart disease and, 318
    patient selection for, 537
Low segment cesarean section, 543
Low spinal block, 440
Low-birth-weight infant, 170
    definition of, 425
    perinatal death and, 10-11
Lower zone, 460
Low-sodium diet, 287
L/S ratio; *see* Lecithin/sphingomyelin ratio
LSD, 458
LUE; *see* Luteinized unruptured follicle syndrome
Lugol's iodine, 19, 29-30
    cervical cancer and, 640
    clear cell adenocarcinoma and, 43
Lung cancer, 2
Lupus anticoagulant factor, 361
Lupus erythematosus, 361
Lupus glomerulonephritis, 361
Luteal phase of menstruation, 76
    progesterone level in, 23
Luteal phase defect
    abnormal uterine bleeding and, 89
    abortion and, 219, 220
    infertility and, 186, 190
Luteinization inhibitor, 81
Luteinization inhibitor receptor–binding inhibitor, 81
Luteinized unruptured follicle syndrome
    endometriosis and, 127
    infertility and, 180
Luteinizing hormone, 23, 24
    aging and, 681, 682
    rapid, 27
Luteinizing hormone–releasing hormone, 78
Luteolysis, 81
Luteoma, 666
Lymphadenectomy, 644
Lymphadenopathy, 296
Lymphangitis, 583

Lymphatic spread, 661-662
  cervical cancer and, 638
Lymphedema, 102
Lymphoangiogram, 643
Lymphogranuloma venereum, 612
  pregnancy and, 346

M

Mackenrodt's ligament, 548, 549, 567
  injury to, 567-570
Macroadenoma, 106, 107
Macrocytic anemia, 322
Macrodantin; *see* Nitrofurantoin
Macrophage, 127
Macrosomia, 300, 302
Maculine pelvis, 503; *see also* Android pelvis
Magnesium, 372
Magnesium sulfate
  eclampsia and, 373
  preeclampsia and, 372
  premature labor and, 426
Magnesium trisilicate, 329
Magnetic resonance imaging, 33
Malaria, 296
Male brain, 55
Male chromosome, 143, 144
Male factor, cervical cancer and, 635
Male pseudohermaphroditism
  amenorrhea and, 103-104
  preadolescent and, 48
Male zygote, 143, 144
Malformation, multifetal pregnancy and, 510
Malignancy
  breast; *see* Breast, cancer of
  cervical, 633-648; *see also* Cervical cancer
  ovarian, 677-678
  stromal, 670
  uterine, 656-664
  vaginal, 626
  vulval, 617-619
Malignant melanoma, 361, 617, 619
Malignant teratoma, 670
Malmström cup, 540
Malnutrition
  narcotic addiction and, 458
  premature labor and, 426
  young primigravidas and, 428
Malposition, fetal, 542
Mammary carcinoma; *see* Breast, cancer of
Mammary duct ectasia, 136
Mammary glands; *see* Breast
Mammary necrosis, 136

Mammography, 134
  aging and, 689
  breast cancer and, 138
  fibrocystic disease and, 136
Mammoplasty, 135
Manchester-Fothergill operation, 568
Mannitol, 268
Marfan's syndrome, 319
Marginal lake, 152
Marginal sinus, 152
Marijuana, 458
Marital history, 14
Marshall-Marchetti-Krantz operation, 563-564
Marsupialization, 617
Masculinity, 54-55
Masculinizing hilus cell tumor, 106
Mask of pregnancy, 256
Mastectomy, 138-139, 140
Masters, W.H., 68, 621
Mastitis, 595-596
  plasma cell, 136
Mastodynia, 136-137
Masturbation, 56, 68
Maternal mortality, 8-9
  abruptio placentae and, 391
  breech delivery and, 520
  cesarean section and, 545
    scar rupture from, 567
  hospital size and, 3
  hypertension and, 378
  placenta previa and, 386
Maternal Mortality Review Committee, 9
Maternal obstetric paralysis, 359
Maternity units, 3
Maturation of germ cells, 142
Maturation index, 19
Maturity
  fetal, 164-166
  life stages of female and, 57
Mayer-Rokitansky-Kuster-Hauser syndrome, 99
Maylard incision, 531
McIndoe procedure
  amenorrhea and, 113
  vaginal agenesis and, 40
Mean corpuscular volume, 324
Measles, 293
Meconium, 525
Median eminence, 77, 78
Median episiotomy, 554-555, 556
Medication; *see* Drug
Mediolateral episiotomy, 554-555, 556
Medroxyprogesterone acetate
  abnormal uterine bleeding and, 89, 95, 96
  aging and, 690, 691

Medroxyprogesterone acetate—cont'd
  amenorrhea and, 112
  endometrial cancer and, 663
  endometriosis and, 131
  hazard of, 221
  mastodynia and, 136
  polycystic ovarian syndrome and, 105
  sexual precocity and, 48
Medullary hyperfunction, adrenal, 311
Mefenamic acid
  dysmenorrhea and, 117
  premenstrual syndrome and, 120
Megaloblastic anemia, 322
Megaloblastic erythropoiesis, 322, 339
Meigs' syndrome, 675
Meiosis, 142
Melanoma, 617, 619
  pregnancy and, 361
Membrane rupture, 419
  artificial, 431-432
    breech delivery and, 524-525, 531
    forceps delivery and, 536
  premature, 425, 430-432
Menarche, 49, 50; *see also* Menstruation
  delayed, 98
  preparation for, 67
Meningitis, 438
Menometrorrhagia, 104
Menopausal arthralgia, 687
Menopausal syndrome, 688
Menopause, 680, 681; *see also* Aging
  life stages of female and, 60
  nervous symptoms of, 687
  psychologic, 60
  surgical, 682
Menorrhagia, 88
Menotropin, 112, 190
Menstrual molimina, 86; *see also* Dysmenorrhea
Menstruation, 76-87
  adolescents and, 49
  age at onset, 85
  associated symptoms of, 86, 118-120
  attitudes toward, 53-54, 56
  cervical mucus and, 84-85
  clinical aspects of, 85-86
  delayed, 85
  duration of, 85
  dysmenorrhea and, 116
  endometriosis and, 122
  feedback response and, 78
  flow during, 86
  history of, 13
  hormones and, 77, 78-80
  hygiene and, 86
  menarche and; *see* Menarche

Menstruation—cont'd
  ovarian changes and, 81
  periodicity of, 85
  precocious, 85
  uterus and, 81-84
  uterine fibroids and, 652
  vaginal epithelium and, 85
Mental retardation, 296
Mentoposterior position, 488-489, 490
Meperidine
  fetal distress and, 467
  heart disease and, 318
  labor and, 435, 436
    premature, 426
Meprobamate, 458
Mercury, 603
Mesenchymal neoplasms, 674-675
Mesoblast, 150
Mesodermal tumor, 43-44
Mesonephric duct, 44-45
Mestranol
  bone loss and, 684
  oral contraception and, 199
Mesylate, 113
Metabolism during pregnancy, 268-270
Metanephrines, 311
Metaplasia, 122, 669
Metastatic carcinoma, 675
Methadone
  breast-feeding and, 603
  fetus and, 458
Methergine; *see* Methylergonovine maleate
Methotrexate
  fetus and, 458
  gestational trophoblastic neoplasm and, 248-249
15-Methyl prostaglandin $F_2\alpha$ tromethamine, 451
Methyldopa, 377
Methylene blue, 570
Methylergonovine, 451
Methylergonovine maleate, 447
Methylxanthine, 137
Metronidazole, 584, 588
  bacterial vaginosis and, 625
  Trichomonas and, 38, 347, 623
Metroplasty, 190
Metrorrhagia, 88
Miconazole, 623
Microcephaly
  cytomegalovirus and, 295
  toxoplasmosis and, 296
Micrococcus, 584
Microglandular hyperplasia, 640
Microinvasion, 636
  cervical, 639

Microinvasion—cont'd
surgery and, 645
Micturition, 564
Middle zone, 461
Midforceps extraction, 533, 535
selection of patients for, 537, 539
Midpelvic contraction, 506
Midplane of pelvic cavity, 495, 496
Midwife, 2
Milk ejection, 600
Milk line, 133
Minerals, 269-270
Minilaparotomy, 204
Minipill, 200
Missed abortion, 33
Mitral commissurotomy, 317
Mitral lesions, 316
Mixed carcinomas, 659, 675
MN; *see* Metanephrines
Molding, 503
Mole, hydatidiform; *see* Hydatidiform mole
Molimina, 86; *see also* Dysmenorrhea
Molluscum contagiosum, 347, 611
Mondor's disease, 136
Mongolism, 149
Monilia; *see Candida albicans*
Monistat; *see* Miconazole
Monoamniotic twins, 507
Monoclonal antibody test, 28, 216
Monophasic curve, 25, 26
Monozygotic twins, 507, 508
arteriovenous shunt and, 169
Montevideo unit, 253
Montgomery's tubercle, 256
Moos' Menstrual Distress questionnaire, 118
Morphine
breast-feeding and, 603
heart disease and, 318
labor and, 435, 436
premature, 426
Mortality; *see also* Death
eclampsia and, 374-375
fetal; *see* Fetal death
infant, 10
lupus erythematosus and, 361
maternal; *see* Maternal mortality
neonatal; *see* Neonatal mortality
perinatal; *see* Perinatal mortality
second twin and, 514
subarachnoid hemorrhage and, 358
Mortality conference, 10
Morula, 147
Mosaicism, 102, 148-149
Mother-infant bonding, 58, 605

Mouth gag, 373
Mucinous cystadenocarcinoma, 673-674
Mucinous cystadenoma, 669, 672, 673, 677
Mucoid secretion, 343
Mucopolysaccharidosis, 164
Mucous plug
passage of, 416
pregnancy and, 253
Mucus, cervical; *see* Cervical mucus
Müllerian duct, 44-45
Müllerian dysgenesis, 111
Müllerian-inhibiting substance, 45
Multifetal pregnancy, 507-516; *see also* Twins
cesarean section and, 542
premature labor and, 425
Multipara, 400, 429
Multiple birth, 112
Multiple punch biopsy, 640-641
Multiple sclerosis, 358
Mumps, 178, 295
Mumps-orchitis, 178
Murmur, systolic, 260
Muscles
bulbocavernosus, 553
levator, 548, 551-552
obturator, 548, 551-552
pelvic cavity, 548
pubococcygeus, 604-605
Muscular dystrophy, 149
Myasthenia gravis, 357-358
Mycelex G; *see* Clotrimazole
Mycoplasma, 577
infertility and, 180
salpingo-oophoritis and, 587
spontaneous abortion and, 211, 219
Mycotic vulvovaginitis, 347
Myocardial infarction
estrogen and, 683, 684
oral contraception and, 201-202
Myomas
cervical, 633
pedunculated, 94, 650
submucous, 180
uterine, 190, 348
Myomectomy
infertility and, 190
leiomyomas and, 654
pregnancy and, 349
Myometrium
contraction of, 152
invasion of, 662
pregnancy and, 251-252
Myotonia, 62
Myxedema, 308

N

Nabothian cyst, 630, 632
Nalline; *see* Nalorphine
Nalorphine, 436
Naloxone
  labor and, 436
  premenstrual syndrome and, 119
  resuscitation of newborn and, 472
Naproxen sodium
  dysmenorrhea and, 117
  premenstrual syndrome and, 120
Narcan; *see* Naloxone
Narcotic addiction, fetus and, 458
Nasopharynx, 425, 426
National Collaborative Diethylstilbestrol Adenosis Project, 42
National Institutes of Health Task Force on Cesarean Childbirth, 541
National Surgical Adjuvant Breast Project, 139
Natural family planning, 194-196
Nausea
  pregnancy and, 276, 326-328
    multifetal, 510
  surgical emergencies and, 331
Necrosis
  ischemic, 167
  mammary, 136
  postpartum pituitary, 454
  renal cortical, 376, 387
  tubular, 387, 391
  tumor, 650
Needle culdocentesis
  ectopic pregnancy and, 234
  salpingo-oophritis and, 587
NEFA; *see* Nonesterified fatty acid
Neglected transverse lie, 485
Neisseria gonorrhaeae, 577, 621
  infant and, 344
  infected abortion and, 582
  infertility and, 179
  new strain of, 588
  salpingo-oophoritis and, 586, 587
Neonatal hypoglycemia, 302
Neonatal hypoparathyroidism, 310
Neonatal mortality, 9-11; *see also* Newborn
  cesarean section and, 546
  diabetes mellitus and, 300
  teenage pregnancy and, 6
Neonatal osteogenesis imperfecta, 363
Neonatal tetany, 310
Neoplasms; *see also* Carcinoma; Tumor; specific neoplasms
  adrenal, 47, 49
  of genital tract, 347-350
  mesenchymal, 674-675

Neoplasms—cont'd
  ovarian; *see* Ovarian neoplasms
  pediatric, 41
Neoplastic cyst, ovarian, 103
Neoplastic tranformation, 658
Neostigmine, 358
Nephrectomy, 339
Nephritis, 340-341
Nephrotomography, 341
Nerve block, 439-441
  multifetal pregnancy and, 513
  paracervical, 437
    incomplete abortion and, 216-218
  peripheral, 441-443
  pudendal, 440, 441-443
    forceps delivery and, 536
Nerve root injury, 440
Nervous symptoms of menopause, 687
Nervous system disorders during pregnancy, 356-360
Neural tube defect, 164
Neurectomy, presacral
  dysmenorrhea and, 117
  endometriosis and, 130
Neuritis, 359
Neurogenic factors in labor initiation, 409-410
Neuropathy, 561
  peripheral, 358-360
Neutrophil hypersegmentation, 322
Nevi, 617
  spider, 256, 320, 329
New York Heart Association functional classification of heart disease, 315
Newborn; *see also* Infant
  apnea in, 438
  care of, 471-473
  hypoglycemia in, 302
  hypoparathyroidism and, 310
  mortality in; *see* Neonatal mortality
  osteogenesis imperfecta in, 363
  resuscitation of, 472
  sexual ambiguity of, 45-47
  tetany in, 310
Nickerson's medium, 17, 623, 624
Nifedipine, 117
Nipple
  accessory, 135
  engorgement and, 602
Nipple stimulation test, 465
Nitrofurantoin
  infants and, 458
  infertility and, 179
  pregnancy and, 339
  urinary tract infection and, 337, 590-591, 594
Nitrogen, 268

Nitrogen—cont'd
 blood urea, 327
  nausea during pregnancy and, 327
  puerperium and, 598
Nitrous oxide-oxygen, 436, 439
Nizoral; *see* Ketoconazole
Nocturia, 336
Node dissection, 645
Nodular cul-de-sac endometriosis, 128
Non-A–non-B hepatitis, 330
Nonesterified fatty acid, 269
Nonneoplastic ovarian cyst, 350, 666-668
Nonobstetric death, 8
Nonspecific vaginitis, 624-625
 preadolescent and, 38
Nonsteroidal antiinflammatory medication, 95
Nonstress test, 463-464
 diabetes mellitus and, 302, 303
 preeclampsia and, 371
 previous fetal death and, 378
Norepinephrine
 hot flush and, 686
 menstruation and, 78
 pregnancy and, 267
Norethindrone acetate, 200
 abnormal uterine bleeding and, 95
 hazard of, 221
 mastodynia and, 136
Norethisterone acetate, 690
Norgestrel, 200
Normal active phase uterine dysfunction, 475
19-Norsteroids
 fetus and, 457
 hazard of, 221
Nosebleeds, 320
Nosocomial infections, 581
NPH insulin, 302
NST; *see* Nonstress test
Nuchal arm, 526
Nucleated squamae fetal cell, 166
Nulligravida, 400
Nullipara, 400
Nutrition
 amenorrhea and, 111
 infertility and, 180-181
 placenta and, 154
 premenstrual syndrome and, 119
 spontaneous abortion and, 211
 total parenteral, 287

O

Obesity
 amenorrhea and, 108

Obesity—cont'd
 endometrial cancer and, 657
 pregnancy and, 285
 subclinical diabetes mellitus and, 306
Oblique diameter, 495
Oblique lie, 393
 dystocia and, 483
Obliterated hypogastric ligament, 173
Obstetric care, 2-3
 alternative methods of, 5, 605
Obstetric conjugate, 494
Obstetric death, 8
Obstetric forceps, 533, 534; *see also* Forceps delivery
Obstetric history, 14, 275
Obstetric nurse, 275
Obstetric paralysis, 359
Obstetric team, 274
Obstruction, intestinal, 332-333
Obturator muscle, 548, 551-552
Occipitomental diameter of head, 489, 491
Occipitoposterior forceps, 534
Occipitoposterior position, 486-487
Occiput position, 396-399
Occlusive cerebral arterial disease, 358
Occult prolapse of cord, 470
Office punch biopsy, 640
Oligohydramnios, 170
Oligomenorrhea, 85, 97
 polycystic ovarian syndrome and, 104
Oligoovulation, 93
Oligospermia, 178
 infertility and, 188
Oliguria, 119
Omentectomy, 678
OMI; *see* Oocyte maturation inhibitor
Oocyte maturation inhibitor, 81
Oophorectomy, 131
Operation; *see also* specific operation
 emotions during, 59
 endometriosis and, 129
 repeat cesarean section and, 541
Ophthalmia neonatorum, 38, 344
Opioid, 77, 78
Optical density, 460
Oral contraception, 199; *see also* Contraception
 abnormal uterine bleeding and, 92
 advantages of, 203
 amenorrhea and, 112
 biphasic preparations and, 203
 breast-feeding and, 603
 combined, 200
 contraindications for, 204
 cyst and, 666
 dysmenorrhea and, 117
 endometriosis and, 129, 130

Oral contraception—cont'd
  leiomyomas and, 655
  limitations and cautions for, 203
  multifetal pregnancy and, 509
  premenstrual syndrome and, 120
  progestin-dominant, 204
  selection of, 203-204
  triphasic preparations and, 203-204
Oral hypoglycemic agents, 306
Oral phase of life stages, 55
Organogenesis, 170
Orgasm, 62
  dysfunction in, 64, 65, 66, 327
  uterine contractions after, 288
Osteogenesis imperfecta, 362-363
Osteomalacia, 270
Osteopenia, 684
Osteoporosis, 684
  aging and, 689
  estrogen and, 80
  risk factors for, 686
Outlet contraction, 506
Out-of-wedlock pregnancy, 6
Ovarian agenesis XO, 45
Ovarian androgen excess, 180
Ovarian cancer; *see* Ovarian neoplasms
Ovarian cyst, 350
  nonneoplastic, 350, 666-668
Ovarian disease, polycystic; *see* Ovarian syndrome, polycystic
Ovarian dysfunction, 89-90
  endometrial cancer and, 657
Ovarian endometriomas, 124, 127, 131; *see also* Endometriomas
Ovarian endometriosis; *see* Endometriosis
Ovarian follicle; *see* Follicle
Ovarian function, 89-90
  amenorrhea and, 103
  endometrial biopsy and, 31-32
  endometrial cancer and, 657
  hormone assay and, 18
  infertility and, 180, 189
  nursing mothers and, 599
  puerperium and, 599
Ovarian neoplasms, 43-44, 666-679
  amenorrhea and, 105-106
  benign tumors and, 675-677
  clinical stages of, 678
  of coelomic epithelium, 671-674
  diagnosis of pregnancy and, 280
  endometriosis and, 128
  estrogen-producing, 96
  of germ cell origin, 669-671
  of germinal epithelium, 671-674
  hemorrhage into, 676

Ovarian neoplasms—cont'd
  histogenesis of, 669
  hormone-secreting, 18
  incidence of, 677
  leiomyomas and, 653
  malignant tumors and, 677-678
  metastatic carcinoma and, 675
  nonneoplastic cysts and, 666-668
  of nonspecialized stroma and heterotopic elements, 675
  preadolescent and, 43-44
  pregnancy and, 349-350
  of specialized gonadal stroma, 674-675
  twisted, 675-676
Ovarian syndrome, polycystic, 666
  amenorrhea and, 104-105
  endometrial cancer and, 656
  infertility and, 180, 190
Ovarian vein thrombosis, 595
Ovarian wedge resection
  amenorrhea and, 113
  infertility and, 190
Ovary
  carcinoma of; *see* Ovarian neoplasms
  endometriosis and, 123-124
  enlargement of
    cyst and, 666; *see also* Ovarian cyst; Ovarian syndrome, polycystic
    ultrasound and, 33
  feminizing tumor of, 48-49
  function of; *see* Ovarian function
  hormones and, 80
  menstruation and, 76, 81
  pregnancy and, 253-255
Overt diabetes, 304
Overweight women
  amenorrhea and, 108
  endometrial cancer and, 657
  pregnancy and, 285
  subclinical diabetes mellitus and, 306
Ovral
  abnormal uterine bleeding and, 92
  pregnancy interception and, 204
  rape and, 74
Ovulation, 76-79
  basal body temperature and, 25
  infertility and, 180, 186-187
  natural family planning and, 195-196
  tests for, 23-28
Ovulation-inducing agent, 509
Ovum
  blighted, 210-211
  ectopic pregnancy and, 226
  migration of, 144-146
Oxacillin, 595
11-Oxycorticosteroids, 601

Oxygen
    eclampsia and, 373
    fetal development and, 173-174
    fetal hypoxia and, 466
    heart disease and, 318
    labor and, 436
    pregnancy and, 261
Oxytocic drug, 447
    inevitable abortion and, 216
    subinvolution and, 606
Oxytocin
    artificial rupture of membranes and, 431-432
    blood pressure and, 447-448
    breast engorgement and, 602
    cesarean section scar and, 566, 567
    contracted pelvis and, 506
    diabetes insipidus and, 307
    heart disease and, 319
    nonstress test and, 463
    placental expulsion and, 447
    placental separation and, 390
    postpartum hemorrhage and, 451
    pregnancy and, 266
    previous cesarean section and, 545
    puerperium and, 602
    receptor for, 408, 409
    uterine dysfunction and, 477, 478-479
    uterine rupture and, 566, 567
    water intoxication and, 448
Oxytocin challenge test, 465
    diabetes mellitus and, 304
Oxytocinase, 161, 260

P

P₄; *see* Progesterone
Pacemaker, 406
Pagano-Levin medium, 17
Paget's disease, 137, 618
PAH; *see* Para-aminohippurate
Pain
    abdominal, 231
    cervical cancer and, 639
    coitus and, 675
    defecation and, 675
    delivery and, 438-443
    endometriosis and, 126
    labor and, 434-438
    leiomyomas and, 652
    micturition and, 675
    pelvic, 61
    suprapubic, 337
Palmar erythema, 256, 320, 329

Palpation
    bimanual, 15, 16
    of fetus, 277-278, 394-396
    perineal, 420
    rectovaginal, 570
Palsy, Bell's, 359; *see also* Paralysis
Pancreatic islet cells, 300, 301
    hyperplasia of, 299, 305
Pancreatitis
    pregnancy and, 330-331
    tetracycline and, 339
Papanicolaou smear, 19, 20
    abnormal uterine bleeding and, 93
    aging and, 688
    rape and, 73-74
Papaverine hydrochloride, 454
Papillary carcinoma, 137
Papilledema, 358
Papillomas, 617, 672
Papillomavirus, 635, 636
    condylomata acuminata and, 611
    vestibular gland infection and, 613
Papules, pruritic, 360-361
Para-aminohippurate, 262
Parabasal cells, 622
    estrogen and, 18-20
    fetal, 165, 166
    menstruation and, 85
Paracervical block, 437
    incomplete abortion and, 216-218
Paralysis
    Bell's, 359
    Landrey's ascending, 359
    maternal obstetric, 359
Paramesonephric duct, 44-45
Parametrial cellulitis, 583
Parametrial infiltration, cervical, 639
Parametritis, 584, 630
    endomyometritis and, 593
Parasitic fibroid, 650
Parathyroid adenoma, 310
Parathyroid gland disorders, 309-310
    pregnancy and, 266
Paraurethral gland, 36
Parenteral nutrition, 287
Parenteral medication, 38, 438
Parietal bone presentation, posterior
    labor and, 410, 411
    platypelloid pelvis and, 504
Parity, 400
    multifetal pregnancy and, 509
    Zatuchni and Andros breech score and, 524
Parlodel; *see* Bromocriptine
Paroxysmal tachycardia, 316

Partial breech extraction, 525-530
Partial inversion of uterus, 453-454
Partial placenta accreta, 453
Partial separation of placenta, 386, 391
Parturient, 400
Patency, tubal, 184-186
Pathologic retraction ring, 480
Pco_2, 300
PCO; *see* Polycystic ovarian syndrome
Pearl's formula, 193
Pediatric gynecology, 36-51
  abnormal sexual development and, 44-49
  adolescents and, 49-50
  cervical ectopy and, 41-43
  congenital anomalies and, 40-41
  mixed mesodermal tumors and, 43-44
  neoplasms and, 41
  preadolescents and, 38-40
  vaginal adenosis and, 41-43
Pediculosis pubis, 609
Pedunculated submucous fibroid, 654
Pedunculated submucous myomas, 94, 650
Pelvic abscess, 584, 588
Pelvic application of forceps, 535
Pelvic capacity, 498-503
Pelvic cavity, 494, 495, 548
Pelvic cellulitis, 584, 594
Pelvic congestion syndrome, 621
Pelvic curve, forceps and, 533
Pelvic examination, 14-16
  patient's reaction to, 54
  pediatric, 36
  pregnancy and, 275
  rape and, 73
  threatened abortion and, 215
Pelvic exenteration, 645
Pelvic infection
  endometriosis and, 128
  treatment results for, 579-581
Pelvic inflammatory disease, 179
Pelvic inlet, 494
  contracted, 504
  face position and, 487
  occipitoposterior position and, 486
Pelvic joint, childbirth injury to, 570-571
Pelvic organs, 37
Pelvic outlet, 495, 500-503
Pelvic pain, 61
Pelvic pressure
  multifetal pregnancy and, 510
  ovarian neoplasms and, 675
Pelvic thrombophlebitis, 595
  septic, 578
Pelvic tuberculosis, 596

Pelvimetry, 494-506
  bispinous diameter in, 495, 496, 500-503
  estimation of pelvic capacity in, 498-503
  normal pelvis in, 494-498
Pelvis
  android, 497, 498, 504
  anthropoid, 497-498, 504
  breech delivery and, 524
  contracted, 494, 503-506
  false, 494
  forceps delivery and, 536
  funnel, 497; *see also* Android pelvis
  gynecoid, 496-497, 498, 503
  normal, 494-498
  platypelloid, 497, 498, 503-504
  true, 494
Pemphigoid gestationis, 360
Pendulous uterus, 487
Penicillin, 577, 584, 588
  aqueous procaine, 588
  bacterial endocarditis and, 318
  endomyometritis and, 594
  parenteral, 38
  pelvic infections and, 581
  postoperative, 589
  rape in preadolescent and, 40
  salpingo-oophoritis and, 587
  syphilis and, 345
Penis envy, 56
Peptic ulcer, 330
Peptidase-A, 73
Peptostreptococcus, 578
Perforation of uterus, 198, 582
Pergonal; *see* Menotropin
Periareolar abscess, 135
Peridural block, 438
Perihepatitis, 38
Perimenopausal bleeding, 95-96
Perimenopausal phase of life, 680; *see also* Aging
Perinatal center, 3
Perinatal mortality, 9-12
  abruptio placentae and, 391
  breech delivery and, 520
  cesarean section and, 531, 546
    rupture of scar from, 567
  diabetes mellitus and, 301
  eclampsia and, 375
  elderly primigravidas and, 429
  glomerulonephritis and, 340
  low-birth-weight infant and, 10-11
  maternal heart disease and, 316
  multifetal pregnancy and, 514
  placenta previa and, 386
  reasons for, 10

Perinatal mortality—cont'd
  socioeconomic factors and, 11-12
  transverse lie and, 485
Perineal care, 603
Perineal laceration, 549, 552-554
Perineal palpation, 420
Perineorrhaphy, 558
Perineum, 419
Periodic fetal activity test, 378
Peripartum idiopathic cardiomyopathy, 319
Peripheral nerve block, 441-443
Peripheral neuropathy, 358-360
Perisalpingitis, 179
Peristalsis, 264-265, 335
  tubal, 144-145
Peritoneal spread, 662
Peritonitis
  appendicitis and, 332
  fetal death and, 332
  infected abortion and, 581
  parametritis and, 594
  salpingo-oophritis and, 587
Peritubal adhesion, 226
Periurethral tear, 553
Pernicious anemia, 322
Peroneal nerve, 359
Persistent follicular cyst, 666
Persistent mentoposterior position, 488-489, 490
Pessary
  uterine prolapse and, 569
  uterine retrodisplacement and, 351, 574-575, 606
Pfannenstiel incision, 531
PG; *see* Phosphatidylglycerol
PGI$_2$ infusion, 324
PgR; *see* Progesterone receptors, cancer and
PGSI; *see* Prostaglandin synthetase inhibitor
pH
  salivary, 264
  umbilical cord blood, 300
  vaginal
    aging and, 622, 683
    pregnancy and, 255
Phallic phase of life stages, 56
Phenergan; *see* Promethazine
Phenobarbital
  breast-feeding and, 603
  epilepsy and, 356
  fetus and, 458
  hot flushes and, 692
Phenolsulfonphthalein, 263, 336
Phenothiazines
  fetus and, 458
  heart disease and, 318
  labor and, 436
Phenotype, 143

Phentolamine tests, 311
Phenylpropanolamine, 563
Phenytoin, 356, 458
Pheochromocytoma, 311
Phlebitis, 583; *see also* Thrombophlebitis
Phosphatidylglycerol, 283
  amniotic fluid and, 166
  diabetes mellitus and, 302
Phosphoglucomutase, 73
Phosphorus
  hyperparathyroidism and, 310
  pregnancy and, 269-270
Photon densitometry, 689
Physical examination, 14-16; *see also* Pelvic examination
  sexual assault and, 71-74
Pica, 287
PIF; *see* Prolactin-inhibiting factor
Pigment defect of vulva, 613
Pill, contraceptive, 199; *see also* Oral contraception
Pinocytosis, 459
  placental transfer and, 154
Pinworms, 38
Piperonyl butoxide, 609
Pitocin; *see* Oxytocin
Pitressin; *see* Vasopressin
Pituitary adenoma, 106, 107
Pituitary gland
  adenoma of, 106, 107
  amenorrhea and, 106-108
  anterior, hormone assay and, 18
  menarche and, 49
  menstruation and, 76
  posterior, 77, 78
  pregnancy and, 266
  puerperium and, 602
    hemorrhage in, 454
Placenta, 150-170
  abnormally adherent, 452
  abnormally implanted, premature separation of; *see* Placenta previa
  battledore, 168
  calcification of, 167-168
  cysts of, 168
  development and physiology of, 150-166
    circulation in, 152
    enzymes in, 161-162
    hormones in, 154-161
    immunologic properties in, 150-152
    term placenta and, 162-166
    transfer mechanisms in, 152-154
  disorders of, 166-170
  expulsion of, 446-450
  fetal surface of, 164
  formation of, 147

Placenta—cont'd
  insertion variations of, 168-169
    spontaneous abortion and, 211
  insulin and, 299, 300
  low-lying, 380
  manual removal of, 448-449
  maternal surface of, 163
  normally implanted, premature separation of; *see* Abruptio
    placentae
  oxygen utilization by, 165, 166
  postpartum hemorrhage and, 452-453
  retained, 450, 453
    malposition of uterus and, 353
    postpartum hemorrhage and, 452-453
  selective activity of, 154
  separation of, 444-446
    complete, 386, 390-391
    partial, 386, 391
  term, 162-166
  true knots and, 168
  twin pregnancy and delivery of, 514
  vascular anomalies and, 169
  velamentous insertion of, 168-169
Placenta accreta, 453
Placenta bipartita, 166
Placenta circumvallata, 166, 167
Placenta increta, 452, 453
Placenta membranacea, 166-167
Placenta percreta, 453
Placenta previa, 380-386
  abruptio placentae and, 389-390
  anesthesia and analgesia during delivery and, 443
  cesarean section and, 542
  dystocia and, 483
  enema during labor and, 419
  neonatal death and, 11
  premature labor and, 425
Placenta succenturiata, 166
Placenta tripartita, 166
Placental barrier, 152-154
  lupus erythematosus factor and, 361
Placental deficiency syndrome, 428
Placental edge, cervical dilation and, 382
Placental enzymes, 161-162
Placental hormones, 154-161
Placental infarct, 167, 168
  working during pregnancy and, 287
Placental lactogen, pregnancy and, 266
  multifetal, 511
Placental localization, 33
  placenta previa and, 382, 383
Placental migration, 383
Placental separation, 444-446
  complete, 386, 390-391
  partial, 386, 391

Placental site, puerperium and, 598
  delayed hemorrhage and, 452
Placental transfer, 154; *see also* Placental barrier
Placental vessel, rupture of, 391
Plane of pelvic dimensions, 495, 496
Plaques, pruritic, 360-361
Plasma
  oral contraception and, 202
  thrombotic thrombocytopenic purpura and, 324
Plasma albumin, 329
Plasma bicarbonate, 270
Plasma cell mastitis, 136
Plasma cholinesterase, 329
Plasma epinephrine, 267
Plasma estriol, 302, 303
Plasma estrone, 23
Plasma free fatty acids, 299
Plasma progesterone, 23
Plasma proteins, 258-259
Plasma testosterone, 23
Plasma volume
  heart disease and, 315, 316
  preeclampsia-eclampsia and, 368
  pregnancy and, 257, 320, 321
Plastic adhesive drape, 589
Plateau phase of sexual response, 62
Platelet concentrates, 324
Platypelloid pelvis, 497, 498, 503-504
PMS; *see* Premenstrual syndrome
Pneumonectomies, 315
Pneumonia, 314, 315
  immunization against, during pregnancy, 296
  neonatal, 346
  placental transfer and, 154
  sickle cell trait and, 323
Podophyllin
  condylomata acuminata and, 343, 611
  vestibular gland infections and, 613
Polar body, 142
Poliomyelitis, 357
Polycystic kidney disease, 341
Polycystic ovarian disease, 666
  amenorrhea and, 104-105
  endometrial cancer and, 656
  infertility and, 180, 190
Polydipsia, 306
Polyglycolic suture, 552, 555
Polyhydramnios, 302
Polymenorrhea, 85, 88
Polymorphonuclear cell, 332
Polyneuritis, 357, 359-360
Polyps, cervical, 347-348, 630, 632
Polyradiculopathy, 357
Pontocaine; *see* Tetracaine

Portio of cervix, 628
Portio vaginalis, 627
Position; *see also* Lie; specific position
    dystocia and, 483-493
    forceps delivery and, 536
    labor and, 421
    mentoposterior, 488-489, 490
    multifetal pregnancy and, 510-511
Postcoital diethylstilbestrol, 204
Postcoital douches, 196
Posterior colpoplasty, 558
Posterior fontanel, 171
Posterior parietal bone presentation, 410, 411
    platypelloid pelvis and, 504
Posterior pituitary, 77, 78
Posterior sacculation of uterus, 351
Posterior vaginal hernia, 557, 558
Postmaturity, 480
Postmenopausal bleeding, 95
    leiomyomas and, 652
Postmenopausal phase of life, 680; *see also* Aging
    uterine bleeding in, 95, 652
    enlarged ovary and, 676
    neoplasms and, 666
Postneonatal death rate, 6
Postoperative infection, 589-591
Postoperative orgasmic dysfunction, 59
Postovulatory phase, 85
Postpartum blues, 58
Postpartum care, 319
Postpartum complications, 606
Postpartum hemorrhage, 444, 450-454; *see also* Hemorrhage,
        postpartum
Postpartum infection, 591-594
Postpartum pituitary necrosis, 454
Postpartum psychosis, 58-59
Postterm birth, 400
Potassium hydroxide, 624
Potassium iodide, 458
Potassium permanganate, 625
Povidone-iodine gel, 624
Prazosin, 377
Preadolescent gynecologic problems, 38-40
Preantral follicle, 81
Precipitate labor, 429
Precocious menstruation, 85
Precocious puberty, 48-49
    isosexual, feminizing tumors and, 674
    pseudoisosexual, 48-49
Precocity, sexual, 48-49
Prediabetes, 304, 431
Prednisone, 112
Predunculated tumor, 349
Preeclampsia, 284, 365-375; *see also* Eclampsia

Preeclampsia—cont'd
    acute, 376
    adrenocortical failure and, 310
    diabetes mellitus and, 299
    gallbladder disease and, 333
    hypertension and, 364
    labor induction and, 430
    laboratory signs of, 370
    low-sodium diet and, 287
    mild, 365
    postpartum hemorrhage and, 450
    severe, 368
    treatment of, 370-372
    vascular resistance and, 366
    young primigravidas and, 428
Pregnancy
    abdominal, 227, 231
    abdominal wall and, 255-256
    alcohol during, 212, 288-289, 458
    basal body temperature and, 29
    bathing and, 288
    bleeding in, 380-392; *see also* Bleeding
    blood pressure and, 260-261
    bones and joints in, 265-266; *see also* Bone and joint dis-
        orders
        disorders of, 356, 361-363
    breast cancer in, 140-141
    broad ligament and, 227-228
    cervical, 228
    cervical cancer and, 647
    changes in, 255-256
    circulatory system in, 256-261
    clothing and, 288
    contracted pelvis and, 503; *see also* Gynecoid pelvis
    cornual, 228
    diabetes mellitus and; *see* Diabetes mellitus
    diagnosis of, 274-281
    diet in, 286
    drug use in, 289, 339, 457
    duration of, 281-287
    ectopic, 225-238; *see also* Ectopic pregnancy
    elderly primigravida and, 429
    endocrine system in, 266-268
    endometriosis and, 129-130
    exercise in, 287
    extrauterine; *see* Ectopic pregnancy
    gastrointestinal tract in, 264-265
    generative organs in, 251-255
    genital tract disorder and, 343-355; *see also* Genital tract,
        pregnancy and
    high-risk, 290
        diagnosis of, 273-274
        neonatal death and, 11
    hypertensive disorders and, 364-379; *see also* Hypertensive
        disorders

Pregnancy—cont'd
  illegitimate, 6
  immunizations in, 296
  infectious diseases in, 293-297; *see also* Infection
  interception of, 240
  intercourse and, 288
  intraligamentous, 227-228
  intrauterine, 198
  leiomyomas and, 653
  life stages of female and, 57-59
  mask of, 256
  metabolism in, 268-270
  multifetal, 507-516; *see also* Multifetal pregnancy
  nausea and vomiting of, 276, 326-328
  nervous system disorders in, 356-360
  ovarian, 228
    intrauterine device and, 199
  prolonged, 428
  respiratory system in, 261-262
  skin disorders in, 356, 360-361
  teenage, 6-7
  termination of; *see also* Abortion
    eclampsia and, 374
    hypertension and, 377
    preeclampsia and, 372-373
  tests for, 28-29, 280
    fetal death and, 281
    rape and, 74
  thyroid function tests in, 309
  tobacco and, 289, 458
  travel and, 288
  tubal; *see* Tubal pregnancy
  urinary system in, 262-264
  weight gain in, 283-287
  work and, 287
  young primigravida and, 428-429
Pregnancy cell, 266
Pregnanediol, 156, 157
Pregnanetriol, 45
Pregnenolone, 158, 159
  aging and, 682
Premarin, 38
Premarital examination, 67, 273
Premature ejaculation, 66, 179
Premature labor and delivery, 425-427
  anesthestics and analgesics for, 443
  appendicitis and, 332
  breech, 529-531
  diethylstilbestrol and, 42
  glomerulonephritis and, 340
  leiomyomas and, 653
  placenta previa and, 386
Premature sexual activity, 6-7
Premenopause, 99

Premenstrual endometrial biopsy, 23
Premenstrual syndrome, 86, 118-120
Prenatal care, 287-291
  chronic hypertension and, 376-377
  diabetes and, 301-302
Prenatal influences on fetus, 456-459
Prenatal sex determination, 34, 164
Preovulatory interval, 85
Prepared cervix, 405, 406
Prepregnancy examination, 273
Presacral neurectomy
  dysmenorrhea and, 117
  endometriosis and, 130
Presentation, 393; *see also* Lie
  breech; *see* Breech presentation
  dystocia and, 483-493
  face, 393
  knee, 518-519
  parietal bone, 410, 411, 504
  shoulder, 481
Presenting part, 393
  ballottement of, 395
  floating, 413
  stations of, 412-413
Primary abdominal pregnancy, 227
Primary amenorrhea, 50, 85, 97
Primary dysmenorrhea, 115-116
Primary force in labor, 406-407
Primary hypothyroidism and amenorrhea, 109
Primary infertility, 177
Primary sexual dysfunction, 64
Primigravida, 400
  cesarean section for breech delivery and, 531
  elderly, 429
  uterine dysfunction and, 476
  young, 428-429
Primipara, 400
PRL; *see* Prolactin
Probenecid, 74, 588
Prochlorperazine dimaleate, 328
Progesterone
  abnormal uterine bleeding and, 90, 95
  aging and, 682, 691
  appendicitis and, 332
  assays for, 23
  basal body temperature and, 25
  breast changes in pregnancy and, 256
  embryonic death and, 212
  endometrial cancer and, 657, 662-663
  endometrial response to, 186-187
  inevitable abortion and, 213
  infertility and, 190
  labor and, 409
  leiomyomas and, 652

Progesterone—cont'd
  luteal phase deficiency and, 220-221
  menstruation and, 82-84, 85
  in oil, 190
  ovulation and, 78, 80, 186-187
  puerperium and, 601
  placenta and, 156, 159
  plasma, 23
  pregnancy and, 211-212
  premenstrual syndrome and, 118
  pseudocyesis and, 280
  sexual desire and, 61
  surgery during pregnancy and, 331
  tests for, 23
  threatened abortion and, 215
  urinary tract and, 335
  vaginal suppository for, 190
Progesterone breakthrough bleeding, 89
Progesterone receptors, cancer and
  breast, 139, 140
  endometrial, 658
Progestin
  abnormal uterine bleeding and, 96
  amenorrhea and, 109, 112
  intrauterine device with, 199
  masculinization of fetus and, 47
  oral contraception and, 92, 199, 200
Progestin-dominant oral contraceptive steroid, 92
Progestogen
  endometriosis and, 129, 130, 131
  fetus and, 457
Progestogen challenge test, 691
Prolactin
  aging and, 682
  amenorrhea and, 109
  menstruation and, 78, 79
  pregnancy and, 266
    breast changes in, 256
  pseudocyesis and, 280-281
  puerperium and, 602
  serum, 93
Prolactin-inhibiting factor, 106
Prolactinoma, 98
Prolapse
  ovarian, 64
  umbilical cord, 469-471
    cesarean section and, 542
    multifetal pregnancy and, 514
    neonatal death and, 11
  urethral, 39
  uterine, 351, 568-570, 683
Proliferation, endometrial cancer and, 658
Proliferative phase of menstruation, 76, 81-82
Prolonged active phase of labor, 475, 476

Prolonged labor, 450, 474-493
  constriction ring dystocia and, 479-480
  of fetal origin, 480-483
  pathologic retraction ring and, 480
  position and presentation abnormalities and, 483-493
  uterine dysfunction and, 474-479
Prolonged latent phase of labor, 475
Promazine, 29
Promethazine
  labor and, 436
  uterine dysfunction and, 477
Prophylaxis
  antibiotic, 589, 590
  sexual dysfunction and, 67
Propranolol, 309
Propylthiouracil, 309, 458
Prostaglandin E_2, 432
Prostaglandin $F_{2\alpha}$
  labor induction and, 432
  menstruation and, 84
Prostaglandin $F_{2\alpha}$ analogue, 451
Prostaglandin inhibitor, 120
Prostaglandin synthetase inhibitor, 117
Prostaglandins
  abnormal uterine bleeding and, 95
  abortion and, 207
  artificial rupture of membranes and, 314, 431-432
  dysmenorrhea and, 116
  labor and, 409
  preeclampsia-eclampsia and, 367
  thrombotic thrombocytopenic purpura and, 324
Prostanoids, 127
Prostheses, heart valve, 317-318
Prostigmine; *see* Neostigmine
Protein
  deficiency of
    fetal brain and, 285-286
    hydatidiform mole and, 240
  plasma, 258-259
  pregnancy and, 268, 284-285
  premenstrual syndrome and, 119, 120
  urinary excretion of, 371
Protein hydrolysate solution, 328
Proteinuria
  definition of, 364
  gestational, 365
  polycystic kidney disease and, 341
  preeclampsia-eclampsia and, 365, 367
Protoporphyrin
  iron-deficiency anemia and, 321
  pregnancy and, 320
Provera, 691
Pruritic folliculitis, 360

Pruritic urticarial papules and plaques of pregnancy, 360-361
Pruritus
  pregnancy and, 329, 360-361
  vulvar lesions and, 608, 609
    carcinoma in, 618
Pruritus gravidarum, 329, 360-361
Pruritus vulvae, 614, 687
  sexual fulfillment and, 61
Psammoma bodies, 672
Pseudobubo, 612
Pseudocyesis, 56, 130, 280-281
  amenorrhea and, 108
Pseudohermaphrodism, 46, 48, 103-104
Pseudoisosexual precocity, 48
Pseudomonas aeruginosa, 584
Pseudomyxoma peritonei, 672
Pseudopregnancy state; *see* Pseudocyesis
Pseudotumor cerebri, 358
PSP; *see* Phenolsulfonphthalein
Psychiatric condition abortion and, 206
Psychoanalysis, 67-68
Psychogenic amenorrhea, 108
Psychogenic polydipsia, 306
Psychogenic uterine bleeding, 90-91
Psychologic factors; *see also* Psychology
  aging and, 60, 687, 689
  amenorrhea and, 108
  dysmenorrhea and, 117
  habitual abortion and, 221
  infertility and, 181
  polydipsia and, 306
  postpartum illness and, 58-59
  sexual dysfunction and, 62, 65-68
  uterine bleeding and, 90-91
Psychologic menopause, 60
Psychology, 52-60; *see also* Psychologic factors
  femininity and masculinity and, 54-55
  woman and physician and, 53-54
Psychosexual dysfunction, 65-68
Psychosis, postpartum, 58-59
Psychosocial role, sexual response and, 62
Psychotherapy; *see also* Psychologic factors
  aging and, 689
  habitual abortion and, 221
  sexual dysfunction and, 67-68
Pthirus pubis, 609
Ptosis of eyelids, 357
Ptyalism, 326
Pubic arch, angle of, 500-501
Pubis, 570
  depth and inclination of, 500-501
  separation of, 265, 362
    postpartum, 606
  urethra and, 562

Pubococcygeus exercises, 288, 604-605, 691
Pudendal nerve block, 440, 441-443
  forceps delivery and, 536
Puerpera, 400
Puerperium, 598-607
  care after delivery and, 602-605
  changes in, 598-602
  complications and, 606
  hospital discharge and, 605
  infection in, 591-594
  rooming-in and, 605
  sterilization in, 204
  subsequent examinations and, 605
  thrombophlebitis and, 594-595
Pulmonary artery catheter, 318
Pulmonary disease
  delivery and, 443
  tuberculosis and, 313-314
Pulmonary edema, 374
Pulmonary function, 313, 315
Pulmonary hypertension, 316, 317, 318
Pulmonary maturation, fetal, 304
Pulmonary resection, 315
Pulmonary tuberculosis, 313-314
Pulmonary wedge pressure, 390
Pulse
  preeclampsia-eclampsia and, 366, 373
  pregnancy and, 260
  puerperium and, 601
Punch biopsy, 31
PUPPP; *see* Pruritic urticarial papules and plaques of pregnancy
Purpura, thrombocytopenic, 324
Pyelography, 570
Pyelonephritis
  diabetes mellitus and, 302
  labor induction and, 431
  pregnancy and, 338-339
  sickle cell trait and, 323
  single kidney during pregnancy and, 341
  urinary tract infection and, 336, 337
Pyometra, 633
Pyosalpinx, 587
Pyrethrin, 609
Pyrexia, 179
Pyridoxine, 119, 120, 328

Q

Q-tip test, 563
Quickening, 276, 282
Quinolone, 577, 581

R

Rabbit anti-human chorionic gonadotropin, 28
Radial artery catheter
  eclampsia and, 374
  heart disease and, 318
Radiation
  breast cancer and, 138, 139
  cervical invasive carcinoma and, 643
  endometrial cancer and, 663
  fetus and, 458
  internal, 643
  ovarian cancer and, 678
Radical hysterectomy, 644, 645, 646
Radical mastectomy, 138-139, 140
Radioactive iodine
  breast-feeding and, 603
  pregnancy and, 266
  thyroid disorders and, 308
Radioimmunoassay
  beta-subunit, 28
  estradiol and, 23
  estriol and, 23
  plasma estrone and, 23
  predicting abortion and, 216
  pregnancy testing and, 29
Radioisotope scan, 135
Radiolucent foreign body, 582
Radionuclide imaging, 341
Radioreceptor assay, 28, 29
Radium, 643, 644, 663
Rape, 70-75
  preadolescent and, 40
Rapid estradiol assay, 27
Rapid luteinizing hormone, 27
Recommended daily dietary allowances, 286
Rectal carcinoma, 333
Rectal defect, 552
Rectal examination, 16
Rectal operation, 333
Rectal tenesmus
  endometriosis and, 126-127
  ovarian neoplasms and, 675
Rectocele, 555-558, 568, 569, 683
Rectosigmoid tract, 124, 131
Rectovaginal examination, 16, 573
  pediatric, 37
Rectovaginal fistula, 570
Red blood cells, 256, 320, 321
Red degeneration, 650, 651
  uterine fibromyoma and, 348, 349
Reduction division, 142
Reduction mammoplasty, 135
REF; *see* Renal erythropoietic factor

Regional nerve block, 513
Registry of Clear Cell Adenocarcinoma of the Genital Tract
    in Young Females, 41
Regression, spontaneous, 230
Relative infertility, 177
Relaxin, 160-161, 265-266
Renal blood flow, 366
Renal cortical necrosis, 376
Renal disease; *see* Renal function
Renal erythropoietic factor, 256
Renal function, 262-264, 335-342
  abortion and, 584
  diabetes mellitus and, 301, 302
  eclampsia treatment and, 373
  medical abortion and, 206
  multifetal pregnancy and, 510
  polycystic kidney disease and, 341
  preeclampsia and, 368, 372
  pregnancy and, 262-264, 336
Renal insufficiency, 339
Renal pelvis dilatation, 262, 335
Renal plasma flow, 262, 335
Renal sign, 370
Renal threshold for glucose, 298
Renal transplantation, 310
Renal tuberculosis, 339
Renal vein thrombosis, 301
Renin, 264, 267
Renin substrate, 264
Reproduction
  aging and, 682-683
  essential factors for, 177-178
Resection
  bowel, 131
  pulmonary, 237, 315
Reserpine
  breast-feeding and, 603
  hypertension and, 377
Resistant ovary syndrome, 103
Resolution phase of sexual response, 62
RESOLVE, 190
Respirations; *see also* Respiratory system
  depression of infant's, 436
  eclampsia and, 373
  fetal development and, 171
  placenta and, 154
  vital capacity and, 261
Respiratory distress syndrome, 283
  diabetes mellitus and, 300
  perinatal death and, 386
Respiratory infections
  acute, 314
  chlamydial vaginitis and, 38
  heart failure and, 317

Respiratory system; *see also* Respirations
    diseases of, 313-315
    pregnancy and, 261-262
Restitution, labor and, 414, 415
Resuscitation, newborn, 472
Retained placenta, 450
    manual removal of, 453
Retardation
    fetal growth, 427-428
    mental, 296
Reticulocyte, 258
Retinal vessel, 371, 374
Retinoic acid, 459
Retinopathy, 301, 302
Retraction ring, 404, 405
    pathologic, 480
Retrocession of uterus, 572
Retrodisplacement of uterus, 351, 548, 572-575
Retroflexion of uterus, 572
Retrograde hyperplasia of endometrium, 683, 685
Retrograde tubal transmission, 122
Retroversion of uterus, 572
    dyspareunia and, 64
Reye's syndrome, 330
Rh antibody, 460
    initial examination and, 275
    preabortion, 207
Rh antigen, 459
Rh sensitization, 449-450, 459-461
    amniocentesis and, 34
    immunoglobulins for pregnant woman and, 207, 290, 461
    labor induction and, 431
    theca-lutein cyst and, 666
    transfer mechanism and, 152
Rh_O (D) factor, 459, 460
Rh_O hyperimmune human gamma globulin, 461
Rheumatic chorea, 357
Rheumatic heart lesions, 316
RhIG; *see* Rh_O hyperimmune human gamma globulin
RhoGAM; *see* Human anti-D gamma globulin
Rhythm, 194-196
Ridges of vagina or cervix, 42
Rifampin, 313
Right sacroanterior position, 517, 518
Right sacroposterior position, 517, 518
Right sacrotransverse position, 517, 518
Ring
    Bandl's, 480
    constriction, 479-480
    retraction, 404, 405
        pathologic, 480
Ripe cervix, 405, 406
Ritgen's maneuver, 422-423
Ritodrine, 426, 522

Rooming-in, 605
Rotation, labor and, 413-416
Round ligament
    pregnancy and, 253
    uterine retrodisplacement and, 572
Rubella
    fetus and, 459
    medical abortion and, 206
    pregnancy and, 275, 293
    vaccination for, 294-295
Rubella antibody study, 294
Rubella antibody titer, 275
Rubella-specific immunoglobulin M antibody response, 294
Rubeola, 293
Rubin test, 184
Rudimentary horn, 354
Rupture
    corpus luteum, 668
    functional cyst, 667-668
    tubal, 230
    uterine, 567

S

Sacculation, posterior, 351
Sack's study, 480
Sacroanterior position, 517, 518
Sacroposterior position, 517, 518
Sacrotransverse position, 517, 518
Sacrococcygeal joint ankylosis, 362
Sacroiliac relaxation, 362
Sacroiliac synchondroses, 265-266
Sacrosciatic notch, 495-496
Sacrospinous ligament, 499, 500
Sacrotuberous ligament, 499, 500
Saddle block, 440-441
Sadomasochism, 63
Safe period, 194-196
Sagittal suture, 171, 396
Salicylates, 603
Saline solution
    abortion and, 207
    postpartum hemorrhage and, 451
Saling fetal scalp blood examination, 174
Saliva, 264
Salk vaccine, 357
Salpingectomy, 237
Salpingitis, 38
    ectopic pregnancy and, 235
    infertility and, 179
Salpingo-oophorectomy
    bilateral endometriosis and, 129
    endometrial cancer and, 663

Salpingo-oophorectomy—cont'd
  ovarian neoplasms and, 677, 678
Salpingo-oophoritis, 582, 585-589
  abnormal uterine bleeding and, 89
  blood count and, 17
  dyspareunia and, 64
Salt intoxication, 207
Salt replacement, 710
Salt-losing syndrome, 45
Sarcoma
  stromal, 661
  uterine, 659, 660
Sarcoma botryoides, 43, 661
Sarcomatous degeneration, 650-651, 654
Scabies, 609
Scalp abrasion, 540
Scalp traction, 386
Scapuloanterior position, 483
Scapuloposterior position, 483
Scar tissue
  ectopic pregnancy and, 226
  uterine rupture and, 566, 567
Scarlet fever, 38, 295
Schifrin's 10-minute window, 465
Schiller's test for cancer, 29, 43, 640
Schultze mechanism, 446
Sciatic neuritis, 359
Scirrhous carcinoma, 137
Scopolamine, 318
Screening cytology
  cervical cancer and, 639
  prenatal examination and, 647
Scuba diving, 287
Sebaceous cyst
  breast infection and, 135
  vulva and, 616
Secondary abdominal pregnancy, 227
Secondary areola, 277
Secondary carcinoma, 659
Secondary dysmenorrhea, 115
Secondary force in labor, 407-408
Secondary sexual dysfunction, 64
Second-degree laceration, 549
Second-degree prolapse of uterus, 568
Secretion
  breast, 135
  vaginal, 17-18
Secretory phase of menstruation, 76, 82
Sedation
  excessive, 436
  fetus and, 458
  preeclampsia and, 372
  premature labor and, 426
  uterine dysfunction and, 477

Sedimentation rate, 331
Seizures, 356-357
Self-examination of breast, 134
Selye's fear andfight reaction, 58-59
Semen, 182-184
Semmens' study of labor in young primigravidas, 428-429
Senescence, 60
Sensate focus, 68
Sensitive end-organ response, 48
Septate uterus, 220
Septate vagina, 353
Septic abortion, 210, 223, 581, 584, 585, 586
Septic pelvic thrombophlebitis, 578
Septic shock
  abortion and, 223, 223, 581, 584, 585, 586
  pyelonephritis and, 338
Serial estriol assay, 427, 462
Serophene; *see* Clomiphene citrate
Serosal theory, 122
Serosanguineous discharge, 38, 599
Serous cystadenocarcinoma, 673
Serous cystadenofibroma, 669
Serous cystadenoma, 669, 671
Serous discharge, 662
Sertoli tumor, 675
Sertoli-Leydig cell group, 675
Serum alkaline phosphatase, 329
Serum alpha-fetoprotein, 301
Serum cystine aminopeptidase, 260
Serum enzymes, 259-261
Serum glutamic oxaloacetic transaminase, 260, 329
Serum glutamic pyruvic transaminase, 260, 329
Serum human chorionic gonadotropin; *see* Chorionic gonado-
    tropin
Serum iron, 320, 321
Serum lipids, 259
Serum prolactin, 93
Serum protein, 258-259
Serum theophylline, 314
Serum thyroid-stimulating hormone, 93
Serum thyroxine, 308, 309
Serum unconjugated estriol determinations, 462
Sex
  changing attitudes toward, 62-63
  determination of fetal, 34, 164
  genetic, 44
  gonadal, 44
  ratio of, in multifetal pregnancy, 510
Sex chromatin mass, 143-144, 145
Sex chromosome, 143, 144
Sex cord neoplasms, 674-675
Sex education, 6-7
Sex steroid-binding globulin, 80
Sex therapy, 67-68

Sexual ambiguity of newborn, 45-47
Sexual assault, 70-75
  chlamydial vaginitis and, 38
  medical record for, 71
  preadolescent and, 38
Sexual desire, inhibited, 64, 65-66
Sexual development
  abnormal, 44-49
    sexual precocity and, 48-49
  differentiation of genitals and, 44
Sexual dysfunction
  inhibitions and, 64, 65-66
  primary or secondary, 64
  treatment for, 67-68
Sexual education
  healthy attitude towards sex and, 67
Sexual excitement, inhibited, 64, 65-66
Sexual fantasy, 66
Sexual history, 14, 63-64
Sexual precocity, 48-49
Sexual problems, 64-69
  discussion of, with doctor, 59
Sexual response of women, 61-69
Sexually transmitted disease, 587
  narcotic addiction and, 458
  preadolescent and, 38
  rape and, 74
  vulva and, 609-613
SGOT; *see* Serum glutamic oxaloacetic transaminase
SGPT; *see* Serum glutamic pyruvic transaminase
Shaving, postoperative infection and, 589
Sheehan's syndrome, 107-108, 454, 606
Sheep erythrocytes, 28, 29
Shock
  hypoglycemic, 299
  postpartum hemorrhage and, 450
  septic; *see* Septic shock
Shoes, pregnancy and, 288
Shoulder dystocia, 481-483
Sickle-cell anemia, 322-324
Sickle-cell beta-thalassemia, 323
Sickle-cell hemoglobin C disease, 322-323
Sickle-cell hemoglobin F disease, 323
Sickle-cell trait, 322, 323
  urinary tract infection and, 336, 337
Silver nitrate
  cervicitis and, 631
  newborn eyes and, 473
Simple cyst of ovary, 666
Simple flat pelvis, 503
Sims-Huhner test, 187
Sinciput, 396
Single footling, 518
Single photon densitometry, 689

Single-gene disorder, 149
Single-ovum twins, 507, 508
Sitz bath
  chronic vulvar dermatitis and, 614
  vaginitis and, 38
Sinus, urogenital, 46
Skeletal symptoms, aging and, 687
Skeleton, fetal, 279-280
Skin
  pregnancy and, 256
    disorders in, 356, 360-361
  infections of vulva and, 609
  vaginal ectopic anus and, 41
Skin testing for tuberculosis, 275, 313
Skinning vulvectomy, 618
Skull, fetal, 279, 396
Slide test, 28, 29
Slow slope active phase, 479
Small for gestational age, 425
Small-for-date infant, 170
Smears, vaginal secretion, 17-20
Smith-Hodge vaginal pessary, 563-564
Smoking; *see also* Tobacco
  oral contraception and, 202
  perinatal mortality and, 289
  premature labor and, 425
  spontaneous abortion and, 212
Socioeconomic status, cancer and, 634, 656
Sodium; *see also* Saline solution
  preeclampsia-eclampsia and, 366
  pregnancy and, 263, 287, 335
Sodium estrone sulfate, 689, 690
Sodium sulfobromophthalein excretion, 329
Soft chancre, 611
Soft-tissue injury, postpartum, 445, 450
Solid teratomas, 671
Solid tumor, 617
Somatesthetic role in sexual response, 62
Sonography, 32, 33
  abruptio placentae and, 389
  bleeding in pregnancy and, 215-216
  breast and, 135
  breech delivery and, 520
  contracted pelvis during labor and, 504
  delivery date and, 283
  ectopic pregnancy and, 233
  fetal condition and, 462
  fetal diameters and, 378, 427
  fetal heart motion and, 279, 281
  gallbladder disease and, 333
  hematuria and, 340
  hydatidiform mole and, 243
  indurated pelvic masses and, 588
  large babies and, 480

Sonography—cont'd
    malformation diagnosis and, 149
    ovarian neoplasms and, 676
    ovulation and, 28
    placenta previa and, 383, 384
    pregnancy diagnosis and, 279, 280, 511
    transverse lie and, 485
Spectrophotometry of amniotic fluid, 460
Speculum, 14
Sperm, 146
    contraception and, 196-197
    infertility and, 178, 179
    rape and, 73
Sperm penetration assay, 179
Spermatogenesis, faulty, 178
Spermicidal jelly, 196-197
Spider nevi, 256, 320, 329
Spina bifida, 149
Spinal anesthesia, 438, 439
Spinal fusion, 362
Spinnbarkheit, 24, 628
    infertility and, 180
    menstruation and, 84
Spirochete, 154, 344
Spironolactone, 120
Spleen enlargement, 301
Splenectomy, 324
Splenomegaly, 301
Spondylolisthesis, 362
Sponge contraceptive, 196
Spongiosa, 84
Spontaneous abortion, 10, 210-218
Spontaneous regression, 230
Spotting, 662
Squamocolumnar junction, 628-629
    aging and, 683, 684
Squamous cell carcinoma, 30
    of cervix, 635
    teratoma and, 670
    of vagina, 626
Stages of life, female, 55-60
Stains, 17
    Gram, 17, 222, 577-578, 587
    immunofluorescent, 38
Staphylococcus aureus, 86
Stations of birth canal, 412
    Zatuchni and Andros breech score and, 524
Status epilepticus, 357
Stenosis of cervix, 633
Sterility, 177
Sterilization
    abortion and, 208
    abruptio placentae and, 378
    cesarean section and, 545
    ectopic pregnancy and, 226

Sterilization—cont'd
    elective, 204
    epileptic retarded women and, 357
    glomerulonephritis and, 341
    kidney transplants and, 342
    puerperal, 204
    tubal, 317, 319
Steroidogenesis, 76
Stillbirth, 10
    diabetes mellitus and, 300
Stomach tone, 264-265
Stones; *see* Calculi
Storch syndrome, 459
Strangulation of hernia, 334
Streptococcus, 577, 578, 579, 594
    abortion and, 582, 584
    endomyometritis and, 592
Stress
    physiologic function and, 59
    sex therapy and, 68
Stress test, contraction; *see* Contraction stress test
Stress urinary incontinence, 560, 561-564
    menopause and, 683, 690-691
Striae gravidarum, 256
Stroke, 358
Stroke volume, 316
Stroma, 82
    malignancy of, 661, 670
Stromatosis, 661
Struma ovarii, 670
Subacute bacterial endocarditis, 318, 319
Subaponeurotic hemorrhage, 540
Subarachnoid hemorrhage, 358
Subclinical diabetes, 304
Subinvolution, postpartum, 606
Submucous leiomyoma, 180, 220, 221
Submucous tumor, 180, 220, 221, 649, 650
Subnuclear vacuolization, 82, 83
Subserous tumor, 649, 650
Suction curettage; *see also* Curettage
    abortion and, 207
        incomplete, 216-218
    endometrial biopsy and, 31-32
Sulcus tear, 553
Sulfamethizole, 337
Sulfasalazine, 331
Sulfisoxazole, 337
Sulfonamides
    chlamydial vaginitis and, 38
    fetus and, 457
    pregnancy and, 339
    urinary tract infection and, 590
Sulfurylation, 159
Superfecundation, 507, 509
Superficial cell, 85

Superior strait, 494
Supernumerary breasts, 135
Supine hypotensive syndrome, 387
Suppositories, contraceptive, 196
Suprapubic pain, 337
Supravaginal cervix, 627, 628
Surgery; *see also* specific procedure
 endometrial cancer and, 663
 leiomyomas and, 654
 pregnancy and, 331-334
 stress incontinence and, 563-564
Surgical menopause, 682
Suspensions of vaginal secretions, 17-18
Swan-Ganz catheter, 318, 374, 454
Swimming, pregnancy and, 287
Swyer's syndrome
 amenorrhea and, 113
 gonadal dysgenesis and, 102
Sydenham's chorea, 357
Symmetric growth retardation, 427
Symphyseal separation, 362; *see also* Pubis
Symphysis pubis, 500-501, 570
 separation of, 265, 362, 606
 urethra and, 562
Synclitism, 410, 504
Syncytial knob, 147-148
Syncytiotrophoblast, 150, 151, 155
Syncytium, 147
Syndrome
 Albright's, 49
 amenorrhea-galactorrhea, 106, 606
 Asherman's, 101
 Cushing's, 311
  amenorrhea and, 109
  placenta and, 161
 Down's, 148, 459
 Eisenmenger's, 319
 empty-sella, 107
 Guillain-Barré, 357
 Halban's, 89
 Kallmann's, 108, 178
 Klinefelter's, 45
  chromosomal aberration and, 148
  fertilization and, 144
  infertility and, 178
 Marfan's, 319
 Mayer-Rokitansky-Kuster-Hauser, 99
 Meigs', 675
 premenstrual, 86, 118-120
 Reye's, 330
 Sheehan's, 454, 606
  amenorrhea and, 107-108
 Swyer's, 102, 113
 testicular feminizing, 101, 103-104

Syndrome—cont'd
 toxic shock, 86, 196
 Turner's; *see* Turner's syndrome
Synechiae, 42
Syphilis
 breast lesions and, 136
 fetus and, 459
 placental infection and, 168
 pregnancy and, 344-345
 rape and, 74
  preadolescent, 40
 spontaneous abortion and, 211
 testing for, 275, 612
 treatment for, 344-345
 vulva and, 612
 young primigravidas and, 428
Systemic lupus erythematosus, 361
Systolic murmurs, 260, 315

T

T_3; *see* Triiodothyronine
T_4; *see* Thyroxine
Tachycardia
 hyperthyroidism and, 309
 paroxysmal, 316
Tamoxifen, 140
Tampon, 86
Tay-Sachs disease, 149
TBG; *see* Thyroxine-binding globulin
Teenagers; *see* Adolescence
Teeth care in pregnancy, 326
Telangiectasia, 256
Telecobalt therapy, 663
Temperature
 basal body, 25-27
  natural family planning and, 195, 196
  ovulation and, 186
  pregnancy testing and, 29
  progesterone and, 23
 eclampsia and, 373
 infected abortion and, 581
 puerperium and, 601
Tensilon; *see* Edrophonium chloride
Teratogenesis
 diabetes mellitus and, 300-301
 medical abortion and, 206
Teratoma
 benign cystic, 669-670, 677
 solid, 671
Term placenta, 162-166
Test
 androgen, 23
 cancer, 29-32

Test—cont'd
  diagnostic, 16-18
  estrogen, 18-20
  gonadotropin, 23
  nonstress; *see* Nonstress test
  ovulation, 23-28
  phentolamine, 311
  pregnancy, 28-29, 280
  progesterone, 23
  renal function, 302, 336
  Rubin, 184
  Schiller's, 29, 640
  Sims-Huhner, 187
  stress incontinence, 563
  syphillis, 275, 612
  thyroid function, 308-309
  tolbutamide, 299
  tuberculin skin, 275, 313
  urine concentration, 263
Test tube assay, 28, 29
Testicular feminizing syndrome
  amenorrhea and, 101, 103-104
  male pseudohermaphroditism and, 48
Testis
  diethylstilbestrol and, 42
  undescended, 178
Testosterone, 23
  aging and, 682
  fetus and, 61-62
  lichen sclerosus and, 615
  oral contraception and, 199
  placenta and, 159
  plasma, 23
  pseudocyesis and, 280
  sexual desire and, 61
Tetany, 309, 310
Tetracaine, 440
Tetracyclines, 588, 589
  breast-feeding and, 603
  fetus and, 339, 457
  gonorrheal vulvovaginitis and, 38
  granuloma inguinale and, 612
  newborn eye ointment and, 473
  pancreatitis and, 331
  postpartum infection and, 594
  pregnancy and, 339
  rape and, 74
  salpingo-oophoritis and, 587
  ureaplasma and, 221
Tetralogy of Fallot, 319
Thalassemia, 149, 323
Thalidomide, 457
Thayer-Martin culture medium, 17
Theca granulosa cell, 76
Theca interna, 104

Theca-lutein cyst, 666
  hydatidiform mole and, 241
Thecomas, 675
Theophylline, 314
Therapeutic insemination, 188-189
Thermal cautery; *see* Cautery
Thermography, 135
Thermometer, 25, 27
Thiazides
  hypertension and, 377
  pancreatitis and, 331
Thiouracil, 603
Third-degree laceration, 549
Third-degree uterine prolapse, 568
Thorax development, 279
Threatened abortion, 213-216
  ectopic pregnancy and, 235
  treatment of, 215-216
Thrombocytopenia
  abnormal uterine bleeding and, 91
  cytomegalovirus and, 295
  eclampsia and, 369
  purpura and, 324
Thromboembolism; *see also* Thrombosis
  oral contraception and, 201
  valve disease and, 318
Thrombophlebitis, 583, 594-595; *see also* Thrombosis
  estrogens and, 691
  infected abortion and, 585
  pelvic, 595
    septic, 578
  prenatal, 594
  puerperal, 594-595
Thrombosis; *see also* Thromboembolism
  coronary, 319
  renal vein, 301
Thrombotic thrombocytopenic purpura, 324
Thromboxane B_2, 127
Thrush, 623
Thymectomy, 357
Thymoma, 357
Thyroid gland
  amenorrhea and, 108-109, 112
  diseases of, 307-309
  infertility and, 188
  pregnancy and, 266
  puerperium and, 602
Thyroid hormone, 309
  pregnancy and, 263
Thyroidectomy, 308-309
Thyroid-stimulating hormone
  aging and, 682
  pregnancy and, 266
  serum, 93

Thyrotoxicosis, 670
Thyrotropin-releasing hormone, 266
Thyroxine, 266, 307, 308, 309
 amenorrhea diagnosis and, 109
 carbohydrate metabolism and, 269
Thyroxine-binding globulin, 266, 308
Tincture of belladonna, 326
Tobacco; *see also* Smoking
 fetus and, 458
 pregnancy and, 289
 premenstrual syndrome and, 120
Tobramycin, 588
Tocodynamometer, 468-469
Tocolysis, 522
Tolbutamide tests, 299
Toluidine blue, 616
Tonus, uterine, 406
TORCH syndrome, 459
Total parenteral nutrition, 287
Tourniquet test, 359
Toxemia, 364, 369-370; *see also* Eclampsia
Toxic shock syndrome, 196
 tampon and, 86
Toxoplasmosis
 fetus and, 459
 pregnancy and, 296
Traction, scalp, 386
Traction force, 537
Tranquilizers
 fetus and, 458
 hot flushes and, 692
Transcortin, 267
Transferrin, 179
Transfusions
 multifetal pregnancy and, 510, 514
 placental separation and, 390
 sickle cell trait and, 323
 whole blood, 390
Transitional metaplasia, 669
Translocation of chromosomes, 148
Transmigration, 226
Transplantation, renal, 310
Transverse arrest, 504
Transverse diameter, 494, 500
Transverse incision, 543
Transverse lie, 393, 399
 diagnosis of, 484
 dystocia and, 483-486
 malposition of uterus and, 353
 placenta previa and, 382
Transvestism, 63
Trauma; *see also* Injury
 placental separation and, 386
 preadolescent and, 40

Trauma—cont'd
 rape and, 71
 spontaneous abortion and, 212
Traumatic neuritis, 359
Travel during pregnancy, 288
TRH; *see* Thyrotropin-releasing hormone
Trial forceps application, 539
Trial labor, 505-506, 544
Trichloroacetic acid, 611
Trichomoniasis, 622-623, 629
 preadolescent and, 38
 pregnancy and, 347
 rape and, 74
 suspensions and, 17-18
 vaginal, 630
 vulva and, 609, 610
Triiodothyronine, 308
 amenorrhea and, 109
 hyperthyroidism and, 309
Triiodothyronine resin uptake, 308
Trimethoprim/sulfamethoxazol, 611
Trisomies, 34, 149
Trophoblast
 death of embryo and, 212
 fertilization and, 147
 gestational neoplasm of, 239-250; *see also* Gestational trophoblastic neoplasm
 glucose synthesis and, 150
 placenta and, 150
 pregnancy and, 211-212
True conjugate, 494, 500
True hermaphroditism, 48
True pelvis, 494
True precocity, 48
TSH; *see* Thyroid-stimulating hormone
Tubal cautery, 204
Tubal ligation
 cesarean section and, 545
 sickle cell-hemoglobin C disease and, 323
 sterilization and, 204
Tubal patency, 184-186
Tubal peristalsis, 144-145
Tubal pregnancy; *see also* Ectopic pregnancy
 blood count and, 17
 intrauterine device and, 199
 retrograde, 127
 ruptured, 230-231
 surgical sterilization and, 226
 treatment of, 235-237
Tubal reversal, 189
Tubal rupture, 230
Tubal spasm, 226
Tubal sterilization, 317, 319
Tubercle, Montgomery's, 256
Tuberculin skin testing, 275, 313

Tuberculosis
  breast lesions and, 136
  endometrial, 596
  pelvic, 596
  placental infection and, 154, 168
  pulmonary, 313-314
  renal, 339
  spontaneous abortion and, 211
Tuboovarian abscess, 588
Tuboplasty, 189
Tubular necrosis, 391
Tumor, 649, 650
  adrenal, 47
  Brenner, 669, 672
  feminizing, 44, 48-49
  granulosa-thecal cell, 103
  Krukenberg, 675, 676
  liver, 483
  masculinizing hilus cell, 106
  mixed mesodermal, 43-44, 661
  ovarian estrogen-producing, 96
  pedunculated, 349
  placental, 168
  Sertoli, 675
  solid, 617
  vaginal, 626
  vulvar, 616-617
Turner's syndrome
  amenorrhea and, 101-102
  chromosomal aberrations and, 148
  fertilization and, 143-144
  infertility and, 189
Twins; Multifetal pregnancy
  abdominal palpation of, 511, 512
  conjoined, 507
  delivery of, 513-514
  dizygotic, 507, 508
  locking of, 514, 515
  monoamniotic, 507
  monozygotic, 507, 508
    arteriovenous shunt and, 169
  mortality and, 514
  placenta and membranes and, 507
Twisted ovarian neoplasm, 675-676
Typhoid fever, 295
Tyramine test, 311

U

Ulcer
  cervical cancer and, 640
  peptic, 330
  vulva and, 613

Ulcerative colitis, 331
Ulcus molle, 611
Ultrasonography; *see* Sonography
Ultraviolet lamp, 72
Umbilical artery, single, 473
Umbilical cord, 163
  advancement of, 446
  compression of, 466, 467
  disorders of, 168-169
  entanglement of, 471
  formation of, 150
  ligation of, 472-473
  long, 168
  loops of, around neck, 487
  placental separation and, 386
  prolapsed, 469-471
    cesarean section and, 542
    multifetal pregnancy and, 514
    neonatal death and, 11
  short, 168
    cesarean section and, 542
Umbilical cord blood, thyroid tests on, 309
Umbilical hernia, 333
Underweight women, pregnancy and, 284-285
Unification operation for double uterus, 354
UN/TN; *see* Urea nitrogen/total nitrogen ratio
Upper respiratory disease, 314
Upper zone, 461
Urea, 259, 263
Urea nitrogen, 336
Urea nitrogen/total nitrogen ratio, 268
Ureaplasma urealyticum, 211, 219, 221
Ureter
  calculi in, 332
  cervical cancer and, 638
  dilatation of, 262, 335
  ectopic, 40-41
  muscle tone of, 335
Ureterocele, 40
Ureteroneocystostomy, 570
Ureteropelvic dilatation, 340
Ureterovaginal fistula, 570
Urethra
  prolapsed, 39
  pubis and, 562
Urethral axis, 562
Urethral closure pressure profile, 563
Urethral meatus, 14
Urethrocele, 559, 560
Urethrocystitis, 337-339
Urethrocystometry, 564
Urethroscopy, 563
Urethrovesical angle, posterior, 562
Urge incontinence, 561, 565

Uric acid, 263
  preeclampsia-eclampsia and, 368, 371
Urinalysis, 74
Urinary estriol, 303
Urinary incontinence, 560-564, 565
  menopause and, 683, 690-691
Urinary protein excretion, 371
Urinary retention, infant, 483
Urinary system, 262-264
  abnormality of, 561
  calculi in, 339-340
  disorders of, 335-342
  endometriosis and, 124
  fistula of, 570
  infections of
    appendicitis and, 332
    postoperative, 589, 590
    postpartum, 594
    single kidney and, 341
  lesions of, 128
  puerperium and, 600
  x-ray study of, 336
Urinary-free catecholamines, 267
Urine, 335, 337
  concentration of, 263
  eclampsia treatment and, 373
  estriol in, 303
  examination of, 16, 275
  labor and, 419
  preeclampsia and, 367, 371
  protein excretion in, 371
  reducing substances in, 298
Urogenital sinus, 46
Urography
  pregnancy and, 336
  stress incontinence and, 563
Uterine atony, 450
Uterine bleeding; *see also* Bleeding
  abnormal, 88-96
  aging and, 691
  dysfunctional, 89-90
    adolescent, 50
  psychogenic, 90-91
Uterine blood flow, preeclampsia-eclampsia and, 367
Uterine cavity, 147
Uterine contractions, 402-406
  inhalation anesthesia and, 438
  after orgasm, pregnancy and, 288
  postpartum hemorrhage and, 451
  pregnancy and, 253-255
Uterine displacement
  anterior, 350
  posterior, 548, 572-575
    postpartum, 606

Uterine dressing forceps, 22
Uterine dysfunction
  dystocia and, 474-479
  multifetal pregnancy and, 510
  normal active phase and, 475
Uterine enlargement, ultrasound and, 33
Uterine fibromyoma, 348-349
  diagnosis of pregnancy and, 280
  infertility and, 190
  spontaneous abortion and, 211
Uterine fusion defect, 219
Uterine growth, cessation of, 281
Uterine inertia, 353
Uterine isthmus, pregnancy and, 277
Uterine leiomyoma, 649-655
  abnormal uterine bleeding and, 89
  abortion and, 211, 220, 221
  diagnosis of pregnancy and, 280
Uterine muscle fiber, 402
Uterine retrodisplacement, 548, 572-575
  postpartum, 606
Uterine segment, 402
Uterine support, childbirth and injury to, 567-570
Uterine suspension, endometriosis and, 130
Uterine weight, 401, 402
Uterine work, 407
Uteroplacental apoplexy
  abruptio placentae and, 387
  complete placental separation and, 391
Uteroplacental insufficiency, late deceleration and, 466, 467
Uterosacral block, 437
Uterosacral ligament, uterine retrodisplacement and, 572
Uterotonic drug, 447
Uterus, 401; *see also* Uterine entries
  abnormality of
    abortion and, 211, 220
    amenorrhea and, 99, 101
    pregnancy and, 352-354
  absence of, 99, 101
  adhesions of, 101
  atony of, 450
  bimanual palpation of, 15
  bleeding from; *see* Uterine bleeding
  blood flow in, preeclampsia-eclampsia and, 367, 369
  changes in
    ectopic pregnancy and, 227
    menstruation and, 81-84
    pregnancy and, 277
  childbirth and injury to, 565-567
  contractility of; *see* Uterine contractions
  diethylstilbestrol exposure and, 42
  diseases of, 649-665
    benign, 649-656
    malignant, 656-664

Uterus—cont'd
  displacement of
    anterior, 350
    posterior, 548, 572-575, 606
  double, 352, 353
    absence of kidney and, 351, 352
    amenorrhea and, 100
    unification operation and, 354
  enlarged, 315
    pregnancy and, 251
  expected delivery date and, 282
  height of, during pregnancy, 283
  incarceration of gravid, 351
  infertility and, 180
  inversion of, 453-454
  irregular shedding of, 90
  lower segment of, labor and, 253, 254
  malposition of, during pregnancy, 350-351
  operation on
    cesarean section and, 542; *see also* Cesarean section
    incomplete abortion and, 216-218
    induction of labor and, 432
  overdistention of
    postpartum hemorrhage and, 450
    uterine dysfunction and, 476
  pelvic examination and, 15
  pelvic tuberculosis and, 596
  pendulous, 487
  perforated or ruptured
    childbirth injury and, 566-567
    infected abortion and, 582, 585
    intrauterine device and, 198
  prolapse of, 568, 683
    puerperium and, 598
  retrocession of, 572
  retrodisplacement of, 351, 548, 572-575
  retroversion of, 64, 572
  sarcoma of, 659, 660
  scar of
    induction of labor and, 432
    previous cesarean section and, 544
    separation of, 566, 567
  septate, habitual abortion and, 220
  surgical evacuation of, abortion and, 216-218
  ventrofixation of, 350-351
  weight of, 401, 402
  work of, 407
Uterus arcuatus, 352, 353
Uterus bicornis unicollis, 352, 353
  amenorrhea and, 100
Uterus didelphys
  amenorrhea and, 100
  pregnancy in rudimentary horn of, 354
Uterus didelphys bicollis with septate vagina, 352, 353

Uterus duplex bicornis bicollis, 352, 353
Uterus septus, 352, 353
  amenorrhea and, 100
Uterus subseptus, 352, 353
Uterus unicornis, 352, 353

V

Vabra aspiration, 23
Vaccine, Salk, 357
Vacuolization, subnuclear, 82, 83
Vacuum extraction, 540
Vagina; *see also* Vaginal entries
  absence of, 99, 101
    preadolescent and, 40
  aging and, 683
  atresia of, 99, 100
    preadolescent, 39
  benign tumor of, 626
  changes of
    pregnancy and, 277
    puerperium and, 600
  cyst of, 626
    infants and, 41
  disease of, 621-626
  epithelium of, 18-19
    age and, 622
    menstruation and, 85
  estrogens and abnormal bleeding from, 691
  examination of, 290
    threatened abortion and, 215
  laceration of
    childbirth injury and, 554
    postpartum hemorrhage and, 451
  metastasis of, 663
  pH of, 683
  posterior hernia of, 557, 558
  pregnancy and, 255
  septate, 353
Vaginal adenosis, 41-43, 626
  diethylstilbestrol and, 42
Vaginal bulge, cystocele and, 559
Vaginal candidiasis
  bacterial culture and, 17, 18
  fecal culture and, 624
Vaginal delivery
  diabetes mellitus and, 304
  incomplete placenta previa and, 384
Vaginal discharge
  cancer and, 625
  decrease in, 683
  diagnosis of, 13-14
    cultures, smears and suspensions in, 17-18

Vaginal discharge—cont'd
  labor and, 416
  pH of, 621, 622
Vaginal ectopic anus, 41
Vaginal hood, 42
Vaginal inclusion cyst, 626
Vaginal smear, 17, 18-20
Vaginal terminus of ectopic ureter, 40-41
Vaginal vault, pediatric gynecology and, 36-37
Vaginal wall injury in childbirth, 558-565
Vaginismus, 64, 65
  infertility and, 179
Vaginitis, 624-625
  atrophic, 687, 690
  monilial, 38
  rape and, 74
Vaginosis; *see* Vaginitis
Valium; *see* Diazepam
Valproic acid, 459
Valve lesions, 316
Valvulotomy, 317-318
Vancomycin, 318
Vanillylmandelic acid, 311
Variable deceleration, 466, 467
Varicocele, 179
Varicose veins, 320, 510
Vasa previa, 169
Vasectomy, 205
Vasomotor symptoms of menopause, 686-687, 689, 692
Vasopressin, 266, 307
Vegetarian diet, 284-285
Veillonella, 578
Veins
  ovarian, thrombosis of, 595
  thrombophlebitis of; *see* Thrombophlebitis
  varicose, 320, 510
Velamentous insertion of placental cord, 168-169
Vena cava syndrome, 260-261
Vena caval compression, 316
Venereal disease; *see* Sexually transmitted disease
Venous oxygen saturation, 173
Venous pressure, 260
Ventrofixation of uterus, 350-351
Vernix caseosa, 430
Version
  cephalic, 522, 523
  second twin delivery and, 514
Vertex of fetal skull, 396
Vertex position, 536
Vesicovaginal fistula, 570
Vestibular gland infection, 613
Viable infant, 400
Villus, 147
  testing of, 35, 149

Vincristine, 324
Vinegar douche, 630
Virilization, 46, 47-48, 49
Virus, placenta and, 154
Vital respiration capacity, 261
Vitamins
  B_6, deficiency of, 119
  B_{12}
    megaloblastic anemia and, 322
    deficiency of, 270
  B complex, 328
  C
    deficiency of, 322
    dehydration and, 328
  D
    aging and, 688
    deficiency of, 119
  K, 356
Vitiligo, 613
VMA; *see* Vanillylmandelic acid
Voided specimen, 16
Volvulus, 333
Vomiting; *see also* Nausea
  diabetes mellitus and, 298
  inhalation anesthesia and, 438
  intestinal obstruction and, 333
  multifetal pregnancy and, 510
  physiologic, 331
  pregnancy and, 276, 326-328
Voyeurism, 63
Vulva
  diseases of, 32, 608-620
    benign conditions in, 608-617
    malignant lesions in, 618-619
  irritation of, 609
  pigment defect of, 613
  varicosities of, 320
Vulvectomy, 618
Vulvitis, 343, 609
Vulvovaginal disorders, 343-347
Vulvovaginitis, 38
  mycotic, 347

W

Wandering fibroid, 650
Warfarin
  breast-feeding and, 603
  prenatal thrombophlebitis and, 594
  valve disease and, 318
Water, body, 268
Water balance, 299
Water intoxication, 448

Watery discharge, cervical, 639
Weight
  amenorrhea and, 108, 111
  birth
    dystocia and, 480
    maternal weight gain and, 284
  cervical cancer and, 639
  gain in, during pregnancy, 283-287
    dystocia and, 480
  preeclampsia treatment and, 371
  puerperium and, 601
  uterine, 251
Wet compress, vulvar dermatitis and, 614
Wharton's jelly, 163
White blood cells
  abortion and, 581
  pregnancy and, 321
  pyelonephritis and, 338
White infarct, placental, 167, 168
White lesion, 613
Whole blood transfusion, 390; *see also* Transfusions
Whooping cough, 295
Wide conization, 642
Withdrawal as contraception, 193-194
Wolffian duct, 44-45
Wood's ultraviolet lamp, 72
Work during pregnancy, 287
Wound drape, 589

X

Xeroradiography, 134
X-linked disorders, 149
X-linked inheritance, 149
X-ray examination, 32-33, 313
  breast and, 134
  breech delivery and, 520
  ectopic pregnancy and, 235
  fetus and, 458
  infected abortion and, 582
  multifetal pregnancy and, 511
45 XO; *see* Turner's syndrome
47 XXY; *see* Klinefelter's syndrome
Xylocaine; *see* Lidocaine

Y

Y chromatin, 144
Y chromosome, 44
Yeast infection, 623
Yolk sac, 147

Z

Zatuchni and Andros breech score, 524
Zovirax; *see* Acyclovir
Zygote, 143, 144
  spontaneous abortion and, 210-211